THIRD EDITION

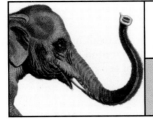

APPLETON & LANGE

REVIEW FOR THE

ULTRASONOGRAPHY EXAMINATION

Carol A. Krebs, RT, RDMS, RVT
Ultrasound Consultant
Shreveport, Louisiana

Charles S. Odwin, BS, RDMS, PA-C
Physician Assistant in OB/GYN
Department of Obstetrics and Gynecology
North Central Bronx Hospital
Clinical Instructor, Emergency Medicine Residency Training Program
Jacobi Medical Center and Montefiore Medical Center
Bronx, New York
Clinical Instructor, Ultrasound
University of Medicine and Dentistry of New Jersey
School of Allied Health Professions
Newark, New Jersey
Sonographer, Department of Radiology
Bronx-Lebanon Hospital Center
Bronx, New York

Arthur C. Fleischer, MD
Professor of Radiology and Radiological Sciences
Professor of Obstetrics and Gynecology
Chief of Diagnostic Sonography
Vanderbilt University Medical Center
Nashville, Tennessee

Appleton & Lange Reviews/McGraw-Hill
Medical Publishing Division

New York   Chicago   San Francisco   Lisbon   London   Madrid
Mexico City   Milan   New Delhi   San Juan   Seoul   Singapore   Sydney   Toronto

Appleton & Lange Review for the Ultrasonography Examination, Third Edition

7 8 9 IMA / IMA 9

ISBN 0-07-136516-8

Notice

Medicine is an ever-changing science. As new research and clinical experience broaden our knowledge, changes in treatment and drug therapy are required. The authors and the publisher of this work have checked with sources believed to be reliable in their efforts to provide information that is complete and generally in accord with the standards accepted at the time of publication. However, in view of the possibility of human error or changes in medical sciences, neither the authors nor the publisher nor any other party who has been involved in the preparation or publication of this work warrants that the information contained herein is in every respect accurate or complete, and they disclaim all responsibility for any errors or omissions or for the results obtained from use of the information contained in this work. Readers are encouraged to confirm the information contained herein with other sources. For example and in particular, readers are advised to check the product information sheet included in the package of each drug they plan to administer to be certain that the information contained in this work is accurate and that changes have not been made in the recommended dose or in the contraindications for administration. This recommendation is of particular importance in connection with new or infrequently used drugs.

This book was set in New Century Schoolbook by Circle Graphics.
The editors were Michael Brown and Christie Naglieri.
The production supervisor was Sherri Souffrance.
Project management was provided by Columbia Publishing Services.
The printer and binder was Imago (U.S.A.), Inc., Singapore.

This book is printed on acid-free paper.

Library of Congress Cataloging-in-Publication Data

Appleton & Lange's review for the ultrasonography examination / [edited by] Carol A.
  Krebs, Charles S. Odwin, Arthur C. Fleischer.—3rd ed.
      p. ; cm.
  Includes bibliographical references.
  ISBN 0-07-136516-8 (alk. paper)
   1. Diagnosis, Ultrasonic—Examinations, questions, etc. I. Title: Appleton and Lange's
review for the ultrasonography examination. II. Title: Review for the ultrasonography
examination. III. Title: Ultrasonography examination. IV. Krebs, Carol V. Odwin,
Charles S. VI. Fleischer, Arthur C.
  [DNLM: 1. Ultrasonography—Examination Questions. WN 18.2 A649 2003]
  RC78.7.U4O38 2003
  616.07´543´076—dc21
                                                        2003054186

Please tell the authors and publisher what you think of this book by sending your comments to sonography@mcgraw-hill.com. Please put the author and title of the book on the subject line.

We dedicate this edition of
Appleton & Lange Review for the Ultrasonography Examination
to those individuals who strive to teach others,
to those who share their knowledge and expertise to further the education of others,
and to those who help students achieve their goals and grow
within the field of sonography.

And to the memory of Trudy Dubinsky MA, RDMS,
the founder and Program Director of the
New York University Medical Center School of Diagnostic Medical Sonography.

Contributors

Dunstan Abraham, MPH, RDMS, PA-C
Physician Assistant
Department of Surgery, Division of Urology
Lincoln Hospital Medical Center
Bronx, New York
Sonographer, Department of Radiology
Bronx-Lebanon Hospital Center
Bronx, New York
Endorectal Prostate Sonography

Mark N. Allen, MBA, RDMS, RDSC, RVT
Senior Clinical Sales Specialist
Siemens Medical
Mountain View, California
Adult Echocardiography

Teresa M. Bieker, BS, RT, RDMS, RVT
Lead Sonographer
Division of Ultrasound, Department of Radiology
University of Colorado Health Sciences Center
Denver, Colorado
Fetal Echocardiography

Julia A. Drose, BA, RDMS, RDCS, RVT
Associate Professor
Division of Ultrasound, Department of Radiology
University of Colorado Health Sciences Center
Denver, Colorado
Fetal Echocardiography

Arthur C. Fleischer, MD
Professor of Radiology and Radiological Sciences
Professor of Obstetrics and Gynecology
Chief of Diagnostic Sonography
Vanderbilt University Medical Center
Nashville, Tennessee
Transvaginal Sonography

Thomas G. Hoffman, BS, RT, RDMS, RVT
Clinical and Adjunct Instructor
New York University Diagnostic Medical
    Sonography Program
New York, New York
Clinical and Adjunct Instructor, Diagnostic
    Medical Imaging Program
College of Health Related Professions
SUNY/Health Sciences Center
Brooklyn, New York
Supervisor, Department of Ultrasound
Weiler Hospital of the Albert Einstein College
    of Medicine
Montefiore Medical Center
Bronx, New York
Abdominal Vascular Sonography;
    Vascular Sonography-Cerebrovascular;
    Vascular Sonography-Peripheral Veins;
    Vascular Sonography-Peripheral Arterial

Sandra L. Hughes, RT, RDMS, RVT
Ultrasound Department Head
Division of Radiology, Department of Ultrasound
Willis-Knighton Health Systems
Shreveport, Louisiana
Abdominal Vascular Sonography;
    Vascular Sonography-Cerebrovascular;
    Vascular Sonography-Peripheral Veins;
    Vascular Sonography-Peripheral Arterial

Carol A. Krebs, RT, RDMS, RVT
Ultrasound Consultant
Shreveport, Louisiana
Adult Echocardiography;
    Abdominal Vascular Sonography;
    Vascular Sonography-Cerebrovascular;
    Vascular Sonography-Peripheral Veins;
    Vascular Sonography-Peripheral Arterial;
    Neurosonology

Jayne C. Moser, BS, RDMS
Lead Perinatal Sonographer
Mount Carmel-St. Ann's OB/GYN Clinic
Columbus, Ohio
OB/GYN Sonography

Christine Nicoleau, MD
Associate Professor of Radiology
Weiler Hospital of Albert Einsten College
    of Medicine
Bronx, NY
Transvaginal Sonography

Charles S. Odwin, BS, RDMS, PA-C
Physician Assistant in OB/GYN
Department of Obstetrics and Gynecology
North Central Bronx Hospital
Clinical Instructor, Emergency Medicine Residency
    Training Program
Jacobi Medical Center and Montefiore Medical
    Center
Bronx, New York
Clinical Instructor, Ultrasound
University of Medicine and Dentistry of New Jersey
School of Allied Health Professions
Newark, New Jersey
Sonographer, Department of Radiology
Bronx-Lebanon Hospital Center
Bronx, New York
Transvaginal Sonography; Neurosonology

Chandrowti Devi Persaud, RT, RDMS, PA
Clinical Sonography Instructor
New York University Medical Center
Diagnostic Ultrasound Technology Program
    Sonographer
Bronx-Lebanon Hospital Center
Bronx, New York
Neurosonology

Raymond L. Powis, PhD
Ultrasound Consultant
Greeley, Colorado
Doppler Color Flow Imaging Instrumentation

Ronald R. Price, PhD
Professor of Radiology and Radiological Sciences
Vanderbilt University School of Medicine
Nashville, Tennessee
Ultrasonic Physics and Instrumentation

Karen K. Rawls, RT(R), RDMS, RVT, APS
Medical Sonographer Manager
Louisiana State University Health Science Center
Shreveport, Louisiana
Abdominal Vascular Sonography;
    Vascular Sonography-Cerebrovascular;
    Vascular Sonography-Peripheral Veins;
    Vascular Sonography-Peripheral Arterial;
    Neurosonology

Kerry E. Weinberg, MPA, RT, RDMS, RDCS
Director, Diagnostic Medical Sonography Program
New York University
New York, New York
General Abdominal Sonography

Michael W. Yates, BS, MBA
Director
Department of Echocardiography
Louisiana State University Health Science Center
Instructor
School of Allied Health, Department of
    Cardiopulmonary Science
Louisiana State University Health Science Center
Shreveport, Louisiana
Pediatric Echocardiography

Contents

Preface

The clinical application of diagnostic medical ultrasound has expanded considerably since the first and second editions of this book were published. Accordingly, we have developed a comprehensive up-to-date self-examination and study guide which incorporates these new applications.

This new edition is comprised of thirteen examination specialties with each specialty containing a study guide followed by numerous questions and explanations. Of primary interest are the new sections in vascular sonography, which include cerebrovascular and abdominal vascular. The chapters on peripheral venous and arterial sonography have also been updated and expanded to further the students' knowledge in vascular technology.

Candidates seeking RDMS, RDCS, and RVT certifications will find this edition informative and invaluable. In addition, this review guide was carefully revised for sonography students as a supplement to classroom lectures. Hopefully, you will find this new edition not only a means to study for the Registry but a useful tool to enhance your professional growth and clinical effectiveness.

We applaud you in your search for knowledge and we thank you for the opportunity of sharing our experience with you.

Acknowledgments

The preparation of this edition has been hard work and without the support of many sonographers and students, it would not have been achieved. We wish to extend our thanks to all the contributing authors who gave of their valuable time and expertise to make this edition a reality. We also want to thank all of our colleagues and students for their support and encouragement.

We wish to thank Paul Bobby, MD and George Mussalli, MD of the North Central Bronx Hospital, Department of OB-GYN, who were kind enough to allow flexible work schedules which allowed time for working on this edition and also Robert Chin, MD, Medical Director and Rajesh Verma, MD, Associate Medical Director of the Emergency Medicine Department at North Central Bronx Hospital, for their support.

How to Use This Book

This book has been written as a study guide for review and self-examination and serves as a useful tool for preparation for the American Registry of Diagnostic Medical Sonography Examination and the ultrasound portion of the American Board of Radiology Examination.

To get the most from this book, first read the Study Guide then go through the questions answering them all regardless of difficulty, just as you would take the actual test. The questions are either multiple choice or matching, and many are accompanied by a sonogram or illustration.

At the end of each set of questions, there is a section of answers and explanations. In this section the answer is explained and a reference is given for each answer. The first number of the reference indicates a book or journal, as numbered in the reference section. The second number or numbers indicate the page or pages on which the relevant material can be found. If only one number is given, the reference is to the entire book.

Do not be discouraged if you are unable to answer all of the questions on the first try. We encourage you to try again.

Best wishes for success in your study of ultrasonography.

CHAPTER 1

ULTRASONIC PHYSICS AND INSTRUMENTATION

Ronald R. Price

Study Guide

WHAT IS ULTRASOUND?

Ultrasound is a mechanical, longitudinal wave that carries variations of quantities referred to as *acoustic variables*. Ultrasound is above the range of human hearing (20,000 hertz [or cycles per second] or greater).

Ultrasound waves are produced by oscillatory motion of the particles in a medium, creating regions of compression and rarefaction. The continued movement of particles propagating through a medium is the result of collision between particles that make up the medium.

Ultrasound can be continuous or pulsed. In the *continuous* mode, the vibratory motions are produced by the source in an uninterrupted stream, whereas in the *pulsed* mode, the sound is delivered in a series of packets, or pulses. In almost all diagnostic applications of ultrasound, *pulsed ultrasound* is used.

The following terms are commonly used in diagnostic medical sonography.

Mechanical wave is a wave that requires a medium in which to travel and, therefore, cannot propagate in a vacuum.

Longitudinal wave is a wave in which the particle motion travels parallel to the energy source (as opposed to shear or transverse waves, which travel perpendicularly).

Acoustic variable. Each of the following is considered an acoustic variable: *pressure, temperature, density, particle motion*. Note that all of these variables change as an acoustic wave passes through the medium.

Parameters of a wave (Fig. 1–1A). The following terms are common to all waves:

Cycle. A cycle is composed of one compression and one rarefaction, or a complete positive and negative change in an acoustic variable.

Frequency (*f*) is the number of cycles per second. Frequency describes how many times the acoustic variable (whether it be pressure, density, particle motion, or temperature) changes in one second. *Units:* hertz (Hz), megahertz (MHz).

$$\text{frequency } (f) = \frac{\text{propagation speed}}{\text{wavelength}}, \quad f = \frac{c}{\lambda}$$

Period is the time it takes for 1 cycle to occur; the inverse of frequency. *Units:* seconds (s), microseconds (μs).

$$\text{period} = \frac{1}{\text{frequency}}, \quad p = \frac{1}{f}$$

As the frequency increases, the period decreases. Conversely, as the frequency decreases, the period increases.

Wavelength (λ) is the distance the wave must travel in 1 cycle. Wavelength is determined by both the source of the wave and the medium in which it is propagating (Fig. 1–1B). *Units:* meters (m), millimeters (mm).

$$\text{wavelength } (\lambda) = \frac{\text{propagation speed } (c)}{\text{frequency } (f)}, \quad \lambda = \frac{c}{f}$$

With a velocity or propagation speed (*c*) of 1540 m/s, the wavelength of 1 MHz is 1.54 mm, of 2 MHz is 0.77 mm, and of 3 MHz is 0.51 mm.

Propagation speed is the maximum speed with which an acoustic wave can move through a medium, determined by the density and stiffness of the medium. Propagation speed increases proportionally with the stiffness (i.e., the stiffer the medium, the faster the variable will travel). Density is the concentration of mass per unit volume, and propagation speed is

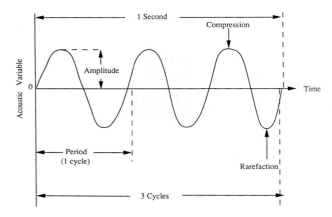

Figure 1–1A. The parameters of a wave. The frequency of this wave variable is 3 Hz (or cycles per second). A period is one complete cycle; therefore, this wave consists of three periods. *Note:* The vertical direction is compression and downward direction is rarefaction and both represent pressure and density. Otherwise, it represents a positive (upward) or negative (downward) change in the acoustic variable.

inversely proportional to density. *Units:* meters/second (m/s), millimeters/microsecond (mm/μs).

$$\text{propagation speed} = \sqrt{\frac{\text{elasticity (stiffness)}}{\text{density}}}, \quad c = \frac{e}{\rho}$$

It should be emphasized that *compressibility* is the opposite of stiffness. If compressibility increases, then the propagation speed decreases.

Propagation speed is greater in solids > liquids > gases. Propagation speed (c) is equal to frequency (f) times wavelength (λ) $\{c = f \times \lambda\}$. Because the propagation speed is constant for a given medium, if the frequency increases, the wavelength will decrease. Conversely, if the frequency decreases, the wavelength will increase.

Example

If the frequency of an ultrasound wave traveling through soft tissue is increased from 5 to 10 MHz, what happens to the wavelength?

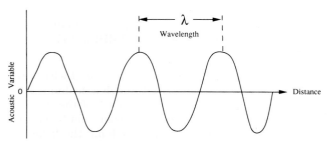

Figure 1–1B. A wavelength represents the distance between two adjacent wave peaks.

Steps to Solution:

propagation speed = 1540 m/s or 1.54 mm/μs

frequency = 5 MHz

$$\frac{\text{propagation speed}}{\text{frequency}} = \text{wavelength}$$

1.54 mm/μs/5 MHz = 0.31 (mm)

frequency = 10 MHz

1.54 mm/μs/10 MHz = 0.154 (mm)

Doubling the frequency halves the wavelength in a given medium. Note how the wavelength gets smaller.

PARAMETERS USED TO DESCRIBE PULSED WAVES

Pulse repetition frequency (PRF) is the number of pulses per second. *Units:* hertz (Hz), kilohertz (kHz).

The PRF used depends on imaging depth. As the imaging depth increases, the PRF must decrease. This phenomenon is characteristic of the pulse-listening period-receiving cycle of the transducer. The longer it takes the returning signals (echoes) to come back to the transducer, the greater the interval between pulses. Therefore, the farther away a target, the longer the return trip, and the greater the interval between transmissions of the pulses wave.

Pulse repetition period (PRP) is the time from the beginning of one pulse to the beginning of the next (Fig. 1–2A). *Units:* seconds (s), milliseconds (ms).

$$PRP = \frac{1}{PRF}$$

The PRP increases as imaging depth increases. When depth decreases, the PRP decreases.

Pulse duration (PD) is the time it takes for a pulse to occur: the period of the ultrasound in the pulse multiplied by the number of cycles in the pulse (see Fig. 1–2A). *Units:* seconds (s), milliseconds (ms), pulse duration = number of cycles (n) × period (p)

Duty factor is the fraction of time that the transducer is generating a pulse.

Maximum value: 1.0. In continuous wave, the transducer is always generating a pulse. A second transducer acts as the listening device.

Minimum value: 0.0. The transducer is *not* being excited (therefore, no pulse will be generated). In clinical imaging, using pulse echo system the duty factor ranges from 0.001 to 0.01. *Units:* unitless.

$$\text{duty factor} = \frac{PD \ (\mu s)}{PRP \ (ms) \times 1000}$$

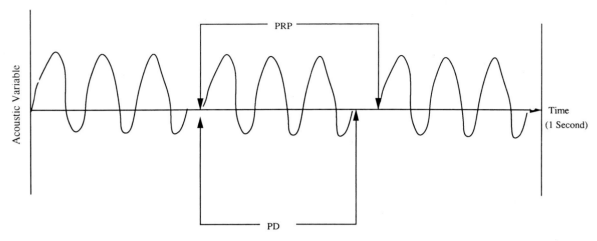

Figure 1–2A. Pulse repetition period (PRP).

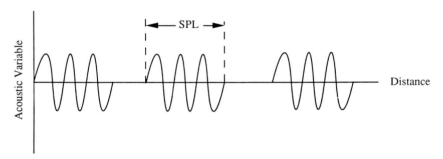

Figure 1–2B. Spatial pulse length (SPL).

Note: Because the duty factor is unitless, and PD is usually in microseconds, it is necessary to divide by 1000 to cancel out the units in the formula. In using this formula, the units must match (PD and PRP both must be in seconds, milliseconds, or microseconds). If not, a correction factor, such as the 1000 in the denominator, must be used.

The duty factor can also be computed by the following formula:

$$\text{duty factor} = \frac{\text{PD} \times \text{PRF}}{1000}$$

Spatial pulse length (SPL) is the distance over which a pulse occurs (Fig. 1–2B). *Unit:* millimeters (mm). Spatial pulse length (SPL) = wavelength (λ) × number of cycles in a pulse *(n)*.

Amplitude is the maximum variation that occurs in an acoustic variable. It indicates the strength of the sound wave. To arrive at this variation, the undisturbed value is subtracted from the maximum value, and the unit for the acoustic variable is applied (Fig. 1–3). Peak-to-peak amplitude (P–P) is the maximum to minimum value.

Power is the rate of energy transferred. The power is proportional to the wave amplitude squared. *Unit:* watts (W).

$$\text{power} \sim \text{amplitude}^2$$

Intensity is the power in a wave divided by the area of the beam. *Unit:* Watts per centimeter squared (W/cm²).

$$\text{intensity} = \frac{\text{power (W)}}{\text{area (cm}^2)}$$

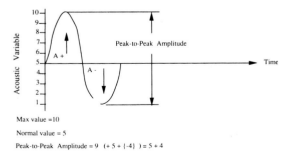

Max value =10

Normal value = 5

Peak-to-Peak Amplitude = 9 (+ 5 + (-4)) = 5 + 4

Figure 1–3. A wave amplitude. Amplitude is equal to the maximum value minus the normal value. Peak-to-peak amplitude (P–P) is equal to the maximum plus absolute value of the minimum.

Note: The intensity is proportional to the amplitude squared. If the amplitude doubles, then the intensity quadruples.

POWER AND INTENSITY

The ultrasound power and the intensity of the ultrasound beam are not identical, although the two terms are sometimes used interchangeably. The *ultrasound power* is the rate at which work is done; it is equal to the work done divided by the time required to do the work. The intensity is the power per unit area and represents the strength of the ultrasound beam. The intensities used in diagnostic medical sonography applications range from 1 to 50 mW/cm². Understanding of the ultrasound intensity is important when studying the biologic effects of ultrasound in tissue (discussed later in this chapter).

Intensities have both a peak value and an average value. The intensity of the sound beam as it travels through a medium varies across the beam (*spatial intensity*) and with time (*temporal intensity*).

Spatial peak (SP) is intensity at the center of the beam.

Spatial average (SA) is intensity averaged throughout the beam.

Temporal peak (TP) is maximum intensity in the pulse (measured when the pulse is on).

Temporal average (TA) is intensity averaged over one on-off beam cycle (takes into account the intensity from the beginning of one pulse to the beginning of next).

Pulse average (PA) is intensity averaged over the duration of the single pulse.

Six intensities result when spatial and temporal considerations are combined:

spatial peak–temporal peak	SPTP (highest)
spatial average–temporal peak	SATP
spatial peak–temporal average	SPTA
spatial average–temporal average	SATA (lowest)
spatial average–pulse average	SAPA
spatial peak–pulse average	SPPA

In pulsed ultrasound, the TP is greater than the PA, which is greater than the TA. When using continuous wave ultrasound, however, TP and TA intensities are the same.

Spatial peak intensity is related to SA by the beam uniformity ratio (BUR).

BUR is a unitless coefficient that describes the distribution of ultrasound beam intensity in space. The higher the SP, the more concentrated and the higher the SA, the less concentrated the intensity. *Units:* unitless.

$$\text{spatial average} = \frac{\text{spatial peak intensity (W/cm}^2)}{\text{beam uniformity ratio}},$$

$$SA = \frac{SP}{BUR}$$

$$\text{spatial peak} = \text{beam uniformity ratio} \times \text{spatial average}$$

$$(SP) = BUR \times SA$$

Temporal average intensity is related to TP by the duty factor (DF). *Units:* unitless.

$$\text{duty factor} = \frac{\text{temporal average}}{\text{temporal peak}}, \quad DF = \frac{TA}{TP}$$

Attenuation

Attenuation is the reduction of the sound beam's amplitude and intensity as it travels through a medium. This is why the echoes from deep structures are weaker than those from more superficial structures. The factors that contribute to attenuation are the following

Absorption is the conversion of sound energy into heat. Absorption is the major source of attenuation in soft tissues.

Scattering. *Diffuse scattering* is the redirection of the sound beam after it strikes rough or small boundaries, when the wavelength is larger than the reflecting surface. Liver parenchyma and red blood cells represent diffuse scattering.

Reflection is the return of a portion of the ultrasound beam back toward the transducer (an echo). Of interest in diagnostic sonography is *specular reflection,* which occurs when the wavelength of the pulse is much smaller than the boundary it is striking, and the surface is smooth. The best examples of specular reflectors are the diaphragm, liver capsule, and gallbladder walls. Reflection of the ultrasound beam depends on the *acoustic impedance mismatch* at the boundary between two media (discussed in detail later in this chapter).

The unit in which attenuation is given is the decibel (dB). *The decibel is the unit of intensity ratio, or power; it is the quantity obtained by taking 10 times the log of the ratio of two intensities.*

$$\text{decibels (dB)} = 10 \log \frac{\text{final intensity}}{\text{initial intensity}}$$

Attenuation coefficient is the attenuation per unit length of sound wave travel. For soft tissue, it is approximately half of the operating frequency of the transducer; that is, for every centimeter per MHz there is approximately 0.5 dB of attenuation. For example, if the operation frequency of a transducer is 5 MHz, then the attenuation coefficient is approximately 2.5 dB/cm.

$$\text{attenuation (dB)} = \text{attenuation coefficient (dB/cm)}$$
$$\times \text{pathlength (cm)}$$

Note: Pathlength is the distance the sound beam travels in a medium. The actual calculation of decibel values is complex and need not be part of the sonographer's bank of common knowledge, but the sonographer should understand that because decibels are exponents, a small change in decibels can mean a large change in resulting values. The most useful way to handle these values is to memorize the commonly encountered ones (Table 1–1).

Example 1

The ultrasound beam produced by a 4-MHz transducer has an initial intensity of 20 mW/cm² after traveling through 3 cm of tissue. What is the intensity of the beam at the end of this path?

> *Given:* Frequency is 4 MHz; original intensity is 20 mW/cm²; pathlength is 3 cm; attenuation coefficient is ½ frequency, i.e., ½ (4 MHz) = 2 dB/cm.
>
> *Then:* If attenuation is attenuation coefficient × pathlength, then attenuation is 2 dB/cm × 3 cm = 6 dB.
> If attenuation is 0.25, then the decibel value is –6 dB.
> (See Table 1–1.)

To obtain the final intensity, multiply the intensity ratio by the original intensity:

$$20 \text{ mW/cm}^2 \times 0.25 = 5 \text{ mW/cm}^2$$

The intensity was, therefore, reduced to 25% of its original value. Another way to do this example is to note that a 3-dB reduction means halving a value. Because 6 dB = 3 dB + 3 dB, an attenuation of 6 dB reduces the power by one-half (20 W → 10 W), then by one-half again (10 W → 5 W).

Example 2

After passing through soft tissue media, an ultrasound beam with an initial intensity of 100 mW/cm². Calculate the amount of attenuation.

> *Given:* Initial intensity is 100 mW/cm²; final intensity is 0.01 mW/cm².

TABLE 1–1. DECIBEL VALUES OF ATTENUATION

Decibels (dB)	Value
–3 dB	(1/2) 0.5
–6 dB	(1/4) 0.25
–9 dB	(1/8) 0.13
–10 dB	(1/10) 0.10
–20 dB	(1/100) 0.01
–30 dB	(1/1000) 0.001

> *Then:* If decibels = $10 \log \dfrac{0.01}{100} = 10 \log \dfrac{1}{10,000}$
>
> $= 10 \, (-4) = 40$ dB

Note: In strict mathematical terms, the 40 dB should be negative, but for our purpose, it can be simply stated as 40 dB of attenuation. The attenuation, therefore, was 40 dB (–40 dB).

The *half-intensity depth* is the distance at which the intensity will be half that of the original; the distance the sound beam will travel through a medium before its intensity is reduced by 50%. It is calculated by the formula:

$$\text{half-intensity depth} = \frac{3}{\text{attenuation coefficient (dB/cm)}}$$

The half-intensity depth can also be calculated from the frequency:

$$\text{half-intensity depth} = \frac{6}{\text{frequency (MHz)}}$$

The half-intensity depth is a good indicator of the frequency that should be selected to view different structures in the body. For example, if 50% of the intensity is gone before one reaches a certain depth, then it is obvious that deeper structures will receive less of the sound beam and, thus, generate weaker echoes. Therefore, to visualize deep structures it is necessary to use a lower frequency.

Time gain compensation (TGC) is an electronic compensation for tissue attenuation.

Echoes

Echoes are the reflections of the sound beam as it travels through the media. An echo is generated each time the beam encounters an acoustic impedance mismatch, but its strength depends on a number of factors. One very important factor, the *angle of incidence,* is the angle at which the incident beam strikes a boundary. The angle of incidence is equal to the angle of reflection (Fig. 1–4A).

Perpendicular Incidence is a beam traveling through a medium perpendicular to a boundary and encountering the boundary at a 90° angle (Fig. 1–4B). Perpendicular incidence is also known as *normal incidence.*[1] The portion of the beam that is not reflected continues in a straight line; this is called *transmission.*

Perpendicular incidence will produce a reflection when the acoustic impedance changes at the boundary. *Acoustic impedance is the product of the density of a medium and the velocity of sound in that medium.*

Acoustic impedance (rayls) = density (kg/m) × propagation speed (m/s)

$$Z = \rho \times c$$

At an acoustic impedance mismatch, the sound beam will proceed (transmission), be reflected, or both. The relationship between *perpendicular incidence* and the

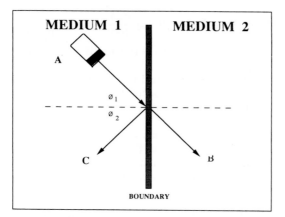

Figure 1–4A. (A) An oblique incidence striking a boundary; **(B)** refraction of the sound beam; **(C)** reflection of the sound beam. *Note:* An oblique incidence is *not* a normal incidence. A normal incidence is 90° (perpendicular). An incidence beam can be

1. Perpendicular (normal)
2. Oblique incidence (an incidence beam at an oblique angle) not perpendicular. The angle of incidence is the angle of any of the incidence beams.

intensity of the echoes can be characterized by the following formulas:

$$\text{intensity reflection coefficient (IRC)} = \left(\frac{z_2 - z_1}{z_2 + z_1}\right)^2$$

$$\text{intensity reflection coefficient (IRC)} = \frac{\text{reflected intensity}}{\text{incident intensity}}$$

$$\text{intensity transmission coefficient (ITC)} = \frac{\text{transmitted intensity}}{\text{incident intensity}}$$

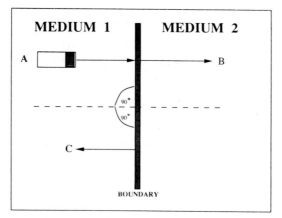

Figure 1–4B. The transmission of the perpendicular incidence sound beam, also called *normal incidence*. **(A)** Normal incidence striking a boundary perpendicularly; **(B)** the intensity transmitted; **(C)** reflection of energy at the boundary of medium 1 and medium 2. *Note:* Beam **(C)** actually travels back along the beam coming from **(A)**, but it is depicted separately.

The ITC can also be calculated by the formula:

$$\text{ITC} = 1 - \text{IRC}$$

$$\text{Incident intensity} = \text{IRC} \times \text{incident intensity} + \text{ITC}$$
$$\times \text{incident intensity}$$

Example

Given two media, one with an acoustic impedance of 20 rayls and the other with an acoustic impedance of 40 rayls, calculate the intensity reflection coefficient (IRC), the intensity transmission coefficient (ITC), the reflected intensity, and the transmitted intensity. (Assume that the incident intensity is 10 mW/cm².)

$$Z_1 = 20 \text{ rayls}; \ Z_2 = 40 \text{ rayls}$$

$$\text{IRC} = \left(\frac{40 - 20}{40 + 20}\right)^2 = \left(\frac{20}{60}\right)^2 = \left(\frac{1}{3}\right)^2 = \frac{1}{9} = 0.11$$

Given: The IRC is 0.11

Then: ITC = 1 – IRC
ITC = 1 – 0.11 = 0.89

If the reflected intensity is equal to the IRC times the original intensity, then reflected intensity = 0.11 × 10 mW/cm² = 1.1 mW/cm².

If the transmitted intensity is equal to the ITC times the original intensity, then transmitted intensity = 0.89 × 10 mW/cm² = 8.9 mW/cm².

Oblique incidence is an angle of incidence that is not 90° perpendicular to a boundary. The angle of transmission will be equal to the angle of incidence as long as the propagation speeds of the media on each side of the boundary are equal. If the propagation speeds are different, however, then the angle of incidence will not be equal to the angle of transmission. The change in direction, the difference in the angle of incidence and the angle of transmission (Fig. 1–5A, B, and C), is called *refraction* (Snell's law).

The angle of incidence is equal to the angle of reflection, but the angle of transmission is variable and can be calculated as follows:

angle of transmission = angle of incidence

$$\times \frac{\text{propagation speed (medium 2)}}{\text{propagation speed (medium 1)}}$$

$$\phi_2 = \text{angle of transmission}$$

$$\phi_1 = \text{angle of incidence}$$

$$\phi_2 = \phi_1 \times \frac{C_2}{C_1}$$

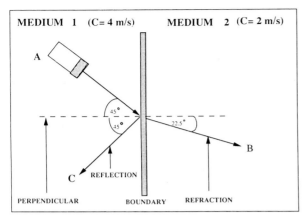

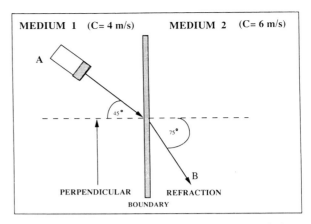

Figure 1–5A. In medium 1, the propagation speed is 4 m/s; in medium 2, the propagation speed is 2 m/s; therefore, the beam bends toward the normal plane. **(A)** Incidence striking a boundary; **(B)** refraction of the sound beam; **(C)** reflected beam.

Figure 1–5C. In medium 1, the propagation speed is 4 m/s; in medium 2, the propagation speed is 6 m/s; therefore, the beam bends away from the normal angle. **(A)** Incidence striking a boundary; **(B)** refraction of the sound beam; **(C)** reflected beam.

Note: The above equation is only an approximation; at larger angles, it is subject to larger error. To obtain true accuracy, use the full form of Snell's law.

$$\sin \phi_2 = \sin \phi_1 \times \frac{C_2}{C_1}$$

The *range equation* is the relationship between the round-trip travel time of the pulse and the distance to a reflector. This equation determines the position a reflector will have in depth on the display monitor.

$$\text{distance to the reflector (mm)} = \frac{1}{2} \times \text{propagation speed (mm/µs)} \times \text{pulse round-trip time (µs)}$$

If we assume the propagation speed to be constant at 1540 m/s or 1.54 mm/µs, then one-half the propagation speed is equal to 0.77 mm/µs, and the formula can be simplified:

$$\text{distance to the reflector } (d) = 0.77 \times \text{pulse round-trip time } (t)$$

If we assume that for every 13 µs the pulse travels 1 cm, then $d = t/13$. the value of (t) must be given in microseconds if the propagation speed is in millimeters per microseconds. The range equation defines the position a reflector will have in depth on the display monitor.

Contrast Agents and Tissue Harmonic Imaging

Contrast agents for ultrasound have included colloidal suspensions, emulsions, liquids, solid particles, and gas-filled bubbles. At the present time, contrast agents based on gas-filled bubbles dominate those that are FDA-approved and in common clinical use. The first gas-filled bubbles used air; however, more recent agents are microspheres containing trapped perfluorocarbon gas. The choice of a gas-filled structure to enhance reflectivity is obvious if we refer back to the intensity reflection coefficient (IRC). In the IRC, it is the difference between the acoustic impedance (Z) of the contrast agent and its surroundings that is important. By making the Z of the agent very small relative to the surrounding tissue (achieved by using a gas), the reflectivity of the agent becomes much greater than the surrounding tissue reflectivity.

Harmonic imaging is a result of the nonlinear propagation of the sound beam as it passes through tissue. Harmonic images were first recognized when imaging gas-filled contrast agents in which a portion of the energy being transmitted at a fundamental frequency (f) was being reflected (backscattered) at higher harmonic frequencies ($2f$, $3f$, etc.).

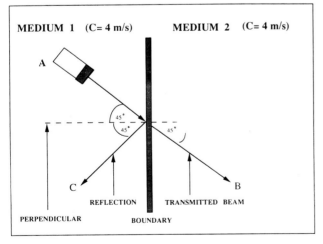

Figure 1–5B. In medium 1, the propagation speed is 4 m/s; in medium 2, the propagation speed is 4 m/s; therefore, the angle incidence will be equal to the angle of transmission with *no* refraction. **(A)** Incidence striking a boundary; **(B)** transmitted beam; **(C)** reflected beam.

Later, it was recognized that harmonic frequencies were also being produced in tissues. The advantage of the harmonic beam is that it has less dispersion (narrower) than the fundamental frequency and also has smaller side lobes. The narrower beam results in increased lateral resolution, and the reduced side-lobes reduces image clutter. Harmonic images are created by eliminating the fundamental frequency and selectively recording the higher-frequency echo components.

TRANSDUCERS

A *transducer* is a device that converts one form of energy to another. In diagnostic sonography, the transducer converts electrical energy to pressure energy (acoustic energy) and vice versa.

1. *Active element*
   A. *Piezoelectric principle* is the conversion of electrical energy to pressure energy and vice versa. Ultrasound (pressure energy) is generated by electric stimulation of the piezoelectric element causing expansions and contractions of the element, which, in turn, generate the ultrasound pulse. The resultant ultrasound pulse produces a similar distortion of the element and then converts back to an electric signal (Fig. 1–6).
   B. *Material.* The active element can be *natural* (e.g., quartz, tourmaline, Rochelle salt) or *synthetic* (e.g., lead zirconate titanate [PZT], barium titanate, lithium sulfate). Synthetic elements are most commonly used in today's diagnostic equipment because of their availability and low cost. To turn one of these manufactured substances into a piezoelectric element, it is heated to its Curie point, or the temperature at which a ferroelectric material, such as many piezoelectric materials, loses its magnetic properties. The dipoles within the material are then polarized with an electric current. When the element cools, the dipoles are fixed (Fig. 1–7). The material is cut and shaped, then housed in the transducer.
   C. *Properties of elements (crystals).* The frequency of the acoustic wave produced by a standard

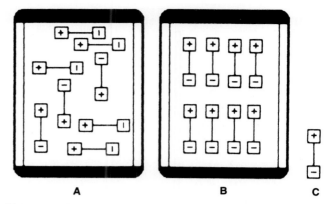

Figure 1–7. Synthetic material with dipoles. **(A)** nonpolarized; **(B)** polarized; **(C)** dipole.

pulsed-wave imaging system is determined by the *thickness* of the piezoelectric element and the *propagation speed* of the crystal. The propagation speed of the crystal is approximately three to five times greater than the speed of ultrasound in soft tissue, namely, 4 to 8 mm/μs. The thinner the crystal, the greater the frequency.

$$\text{frequency (MHz)} = \frac{\text{propagation speed of the crystal (mm/μs)}}{2 \times \text{thickness (mm)}}$$

The diameter of the crystal does not affect the pulse frequency; it does, however, determine the *lateral resolution.* Neither the impedance of the matching layer nor the thickness of the backing material is a primary determinant of ultrasound frequency.

In contrast to pulse wave, *the frequency of continuous wave ultrasound is equal to the frequency of the electric voltage that drives the piezoelectric crystal.* In simpler terms, when the pulser of a continuous wave system produces an electric signal with a frequency of 6 MHz, the frequency of the emitted acoustic signal will also be 6 MHz.

2. *Damping material (backing material)* is an epoxy resin attached to the back of the element that absorbs the vibrations and reduces the number of cycles in a pulse (Fig. 1–8). By reducing the number of cycles, the following are accomplished:
   A. Pulse duration (PD) and spatial pulse length (SPL) are reduced. PD = number of cycles (n) × time (t), where t = period of ultrasound in pulse. Spatial pulse length (SPL) = number of cycles (n) × wavelength (λ).

   By reducing these two factors the axial resolution will be improved.

$$\text{axial resolution } (R_A) = \frac{\text{SPL}}{2}$$

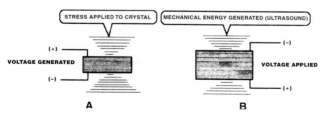

Figure 1–6. Applied electrical voltage. **(A)** Physical compression on the crystal will generate a potential difference across the faces of the crystal. The effect is called *piezoelectric effect.* **(B)** Voltage applied on the crystal will generate mechanical energy (ultrasound). The effect is called *reverse piezoelectric effect.*

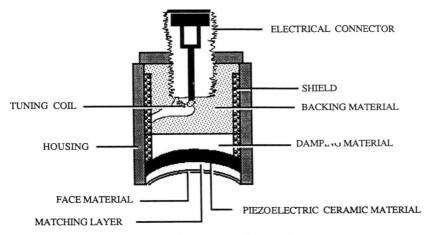

Figure 1–8. Components of a transducer.

B. *Bandwidth* (the width of the frequency spectrum) is increased by increasing the damping. When the bandwidth increases, the quality factor (*Q* factor) of the transducer decreases.

C. The duty factor is decreased.

3. *Matching layer* is a substance placed in front of the transducer element's face material to decrease the reflection at the transducer–tissue interface. The matching layer is necessary because the impedance difference between the transducer crystal and the soft tissue is so large that most of the energy will be reflected back at the skin surface. The matching layer provides an intermediate impedance, allowing transmission of the ultrasound beam into the body.

The thickness of the matching layer is usually equal to one-quarter of the wavelength.[1] Multiple layers are often used to avoid reflections caused by the variety of frequencies and wavelengths present in short pulses. In addition to the matching layer of the transducer, a *coupling gel* is used to form a transducer surface–skin contact that will eliminate air and prevent reflection at this boundary.

Bandwidth and Quality Factor

The transducer produces more than one frequency. For example, the operating frequency may be 3.5 MHz, but a spectrum of other frequencies are also generated, known as the *bandwidth*. The shorter the pulse, the more of these other frequencies are generated. Therefore, the bandwidth and the pulse length are inversely proportional; as the pulse length decreases, the bandwidth increases (Fig. 1–9). Continuous-wave ultrasound has a very narrow bandwidth.

If the bandwidth increases, the Q factor decreases. If, however, the operating frequency increases, the Q factor increases. A low Q factor indicates:

1. broad bandwidth
2. low operating frequency
3. shortened pulse length

4. uniform near field (Many frequencies in a pulse result in a more uniform intensity distribution.)

Types of Transducers

There are several ways to classify transducers; one is the way the sound beam is swept (or steered). This process can be either mechanical or electrical.

A *mechanical transducer* (Fig. 1–10) has a scan head that contains a single disk-shaped active element. One type of mechanical transducer is the *oscillatory* or *rotary type,* which has an element physically attached to a mechanical device to move it through a pathway (see Fig. 1–10A). A second type has an *oscillatory mirror* that mechanically moves while the element remains stationary (see Fig. 1–10B).

Focusing the beam produced by a mechanical transducer is achieved by curvature of the crystal, a curved lens on the crystal, or the reflecting mirror. Focusing occurs at a *specific depth* on both the horizontal and vertical planes. To change the focal depth, the operator must select another transducer with the desired focal zone. The mechanical transducer produces a sector-shaped image (see Fig. 1–10C). *Mechanical transducers are mechanically steered (MS) and mechanically focused (MF).*

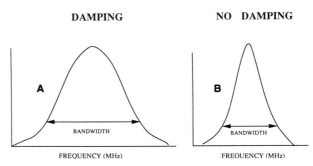

Figure 1–9. Bandwidth **(A)** with damping, **(B)** with damping. *Note:* Damping increases bandwidth.

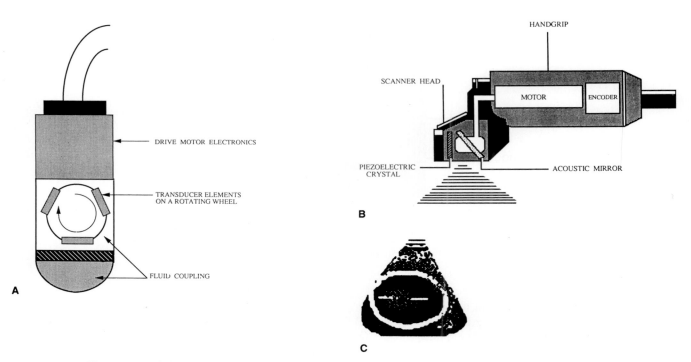

Figure 1–10. (A) mechanical sector real-time transducer that is mechanically steered and mechanically focused. **(B)** A mechanical sector real-time transducer that moves a mirror instead of the transducer. **(C)** Image presentation from a mechanical sector.

The *annular array* is a mechanical transducer. The transducer element consists of 5–11 rings of transducer elements mounted on a mechanically moved (steered) arm (Fig. 1–11). The advantage of the annular array over the single element transducer is the presence of many elements, allowing for electronic focusing. By focusing transmission and reception of the ultrasound energy, greater depth resolution is achieved. The image produced by an annular array is also a sector. *Annular arrays are mechanically steered (MS) and electronically focused (EF).*

An *electronic transducer* is an assembly of multiple elements called an *array*. There are many types of arrays, each with a particular set of characteristics:

Linear sequential array (linear array). Shown in Fig. 1–12. This type of transducer produces a rectangular image (Fig. 1–13B).

Curved array (radial array, convex array). The array of transducer elements are arranged with specific curvature (Fig. 1–14). Focusing the beam is achieved by internal and electronic focusing; there is no beam steering. The curved design of the transducer head creates a *sector* or *trapezoid image*.

Sector phased array (phased array). The voltage pulses are applied to the entire groups of elements with varying time delays. The beam can be electronically focused (EF) and steered (ES). The image format is sector (Fig. 1–15).

Focusing Techniques

Transducers can be either mechanically or electronically focused. *Mechanical focusing* is accomplished by using a curved crystal or an acoustic lens for each element. This type of focusing is usually applied to mechanical transducers and will improve lateral resolution by limiting the beam width.

There are two types of electronic focusing: transmit focusing and receive focusing.

Transmit focusing. Electronic focusing during transmission it is accomplished by firing a group of elements with a small time delay (nanoseconds) between various elements in the group. The wavefront generated by each element in the group will arrive at a specific point in space, resulting in a focused beam. Using transmit focus will improve lateral resolutions and create several possible focal zones. Multizone transmit focusing will result in a slower frame rate. If, for example, there are three focal zones, then the frame rate will be reduced as compared to a single focus zone. If the rate is very slow, then the image will flicker causing a "perceived" distortion of the image.

Received focusing. Electronic focusing of the received echoes, by electronically delaying the return of the signals to the processing system within the diagnostic unit, the optimum range of the focal zone can be extended. This process will enhance image clarity.

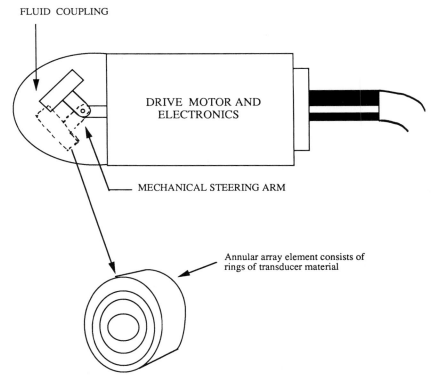

FLUID COUPLING

DRIVE MOTOR AND
ELECTRONICS

MECHANICAL STEERING ARM

Annular array element consists of
rings of transducer material

Figure 1–11. Annular array real-time transducer probe that contains four transducer rings (multielement) on a mechanically steered shaft.

Sound Beam

A *sound beam* is the acoustic energy emitted by the transducer. The beam can be pulsed or continuous wave. *Ultrasound waves follow Huygen's principle, which states that the resultant beam is a combination of all sound arising from different sources (wavelets) on the transducer crystal face. Focusing is the superimposition (algebraic summation) of all sound waves in the beam.*[1-3] As the various wavelets within a beam collide, interference (constructive and destructive) results in the formation of a sound beam (Fig. 1–16).

Constructive interference. The waves are not in phase, producing a decrease in amplitude or even zero amplitude. Zero amplitude occurs if the out-of-phase waves completely cancel each other.

The beam is composed of a near zone, focal point, and a far zone.

1. *Near zone (near field, fresnel zone)* is the portion of the sound beam in which the beam diameter narrows as the distance from the transducer increases until it reaches its narrowest diameter. This distance is the *near zone length* (NZL). At the far end of the NZL, the diameter of the beam is equal to one-half the diameter of the transducer. The NZL is also related to the frequency: increasing the frequency increases the NZL, and vice versa. Compo-

nents of the beam of a focused transducer are shown in Fig. 1–17.

2. *Focal point* is the point at which the beam reaches its narrowest diameter. As the diameter narrows, the beam width resolution improves, becoming the best at the focal point. The *focal zone* is the distance between equal beam diameters that are some multiple of the diameter of the focal point (often two times the diameter of the focal point). The focal zone extends toward the transducer from the focal point, and toward the far zone. The *focal length* is the region of the beam from the transducer to the focal point.

3. *Far field (far zone, Fraunhofer zone)* is the portion of the sound beam (after the NZL) in which the diameter of the beam increases as the distance from the transducer increases. At a distance of two times the NZL, the beam diameter once again equals the diameter of the transducer. The divergence of the beam in the far field is inversely proportional to the crystal diameter and frequency. The larger the transducer element and the higher the frequency, the smaller the angle of divergence in the far field (Fig. 1–18A, B).

Resolution

There are two types of resolution, lateral and axial (Figs. 1–19A, B).

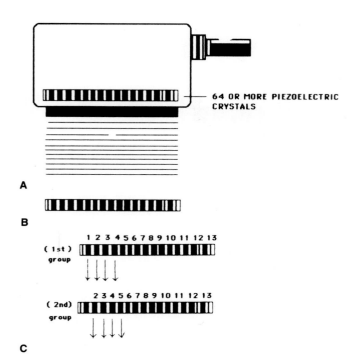

64 OR MORE PIEZOELECTRIC CRYSTALS

A

B

Figure 1–12. Linear sequential array. **(A)** A real-time linear-array transducer. **(B)** Design of a linear segmental phased-array transducer. These transducers consist of a long strip of piezoelectric crystals divided into elements, which are arranged next to each other; **(C)** operation of a linear segmental phased-array transducer. The crystal elements are pulsed in groups of four in this example, with each group sending and receiving in succession.

Lateral resolution (azimuthal, transverse, or angular resolution) is equal to the beam diameter (see Fig. 1–19A). The distance between two interfaces has to be greater than the beam diameter (width) for the two interfaces to be resolved as separate entities. Lateral resolution applies to interfaces perpendicular to the direction of the sound beam. With an unfocused transducer, lateral resolution is best in the near field; with a focused transducer, the lateral resolution is best

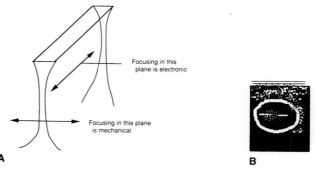

Figure 1–13. Linear sequential array. **(A)** Focusing in the plane of the long axis of the transducer is electronic; focusing in the plane perpendicular to the long axis is mechanical. **(B)** Image presentation from a linear phased array transducer. Note the rectangular image.

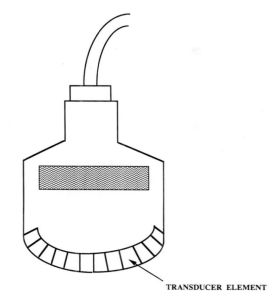

TRANSDUCER ELEMENT

Figure 1–14. Curved linear array. The array of transducer elements are arranged with a specific curvature. There is no beam steering; focusing of the beam is achieved internally by mechanical and electronic means.

at the focal point. A transducer with a smaller diameter will improve lateral resolution as the beam diverges in the far zone.

Axial resolution (linear, range longitudinal, or depth resolution) is related to the spatial pulse length (SPL). Two interfaces at different depths will be dis-

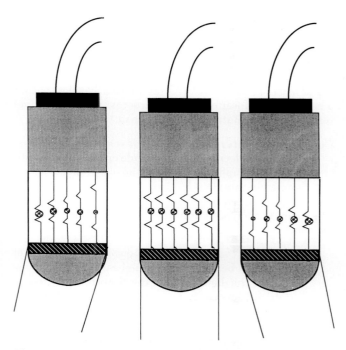

Figure 1–15. Sector phased array real-time transducer. This diagram illustrates how electronic pulses are used to steer the ultrasound beam.

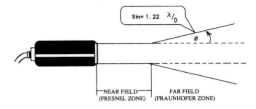

Figure 1–16. The ultrasound beam from an unfocused transducer.

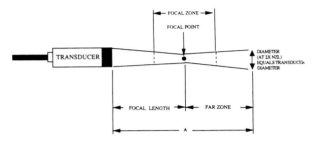

Figure 1–17. The components of the ultrasound beam in a focused transducer. **(A)** Note that the diameter of the beam is equal to the diameter of the transducer face.

tinguished from each other only if the distance between them is equal to or greater than one-half the SPL (see Fig. 1–19B).

$$\text{axial resolution} = \frac{\text{spatial pulse length (SPL)}}{2}$$

To obtain maximum image quality, axial resolution (R_A) should be as small as possible. Axial resolution improves when wavelength or the number of cycles per second decreases (both of these factors are related to SPL). Frequency also affects the axial resolution. As the frequency increases, the wavelength decreases, thus the axial resolution improves. However, as the fre-

quency increases, the depth of penetration decreases, creating a need to compromise resolution for adequate penetration into the tissues. This compromise is why the frequency range for diagnostic procedures is usually between 2 and 10 MHz.

IMAGING PROCESS

The components of a pulsed-echo diagnostic ultrasound system are the pulser, receiver, scan converter, and display (Fig. 1–20).

Pulser

The *pulser* produces an electric voltage that activates the piezoelectric element, causing it to contract and expand to produce the longitudinal compression wave (sound beam). A second function of the pulser is to signal the receiver and scan converter that the transducer has been activated. Each electric pulse generates an ultrasonic pulse. The number of ultrasonic pulses per second is defined as the *pulse repetition frequency* (PRF). With array transducers, the pulser is responsible for the delay and variations in pulse amplitude needed for electronic control of beam scanning, steering, and shaping. In improving the dynamic range of multi-element transducers, the pulser suppresses grating lobes, a process termed *dynamic apodization*.[1]

Increasing the power output control of a system will raise the intensity by signaling the pulser to put out more voltage. To reduce the potential for harmful bioeffects, it is desirable to keep the power low. Therefore, to increase the number of echoes displayed, it is recommended that the operator increase the gain control, not the power.

Receiver

The receiver processes electric signals returned from the transducer (i.e., ultrasonic reflections converted into electric signals by the transducer). Processing involves

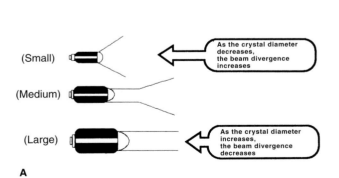

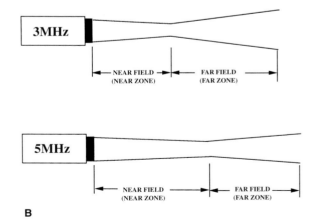

A

B

Figure 1–18A. (A) Beam diversion with increasing crystal diameter. **(B)** Transducer crystal size shown in relationship to frequency. *Note:* The higher the frequency of the transducer, the smaller the beam diameter, and the longer the near-zone. The angle of beam divergences in the far field is smaller with a higher frequency transducer.

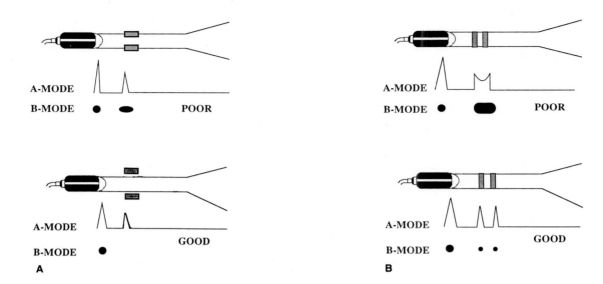

Figure 1–19. (A) *Lateral Resolution:* the ability of the ultrasound beam to separate two structures lying at a right angle (perpendicular) to the beam direction. Lateral resolution is also referred to as azimuthal, transverse, angular, or horizontal. **(B)** *Axial Resolution:* The ability of the ultrasound beam to separate two structures lying along the path of (parallel to) the beam direction. Axial resolution is also referred to as linear, longitudinal, depth, or range.

amplification, compensation, compression, demodulation, and rejection (Fig. 1–21).

Amplification is the process that increases small electric voltages received from the transducer to a level suitable for further processing. This process is sometimes referred to as "over-all-gain" enhancement or increase. Gain is the ratio of output electric power to input electric power and is measured in decibels (dB). *Dynamic range* is the range of values between the minimum and maximum echo amplitudes. It is the ratio of the largest power to the smallest power in the working range of the diagnostic unit. Dynamic range is also expressed in decibels.

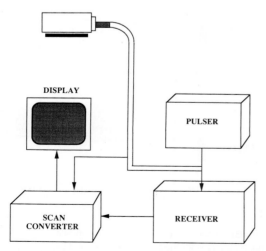

Figure 1–20. Components of a pulsed-echo ultrasound system.

Compensation is also referred to as gain compensation, swept gain, or time gain compensation. It is the mechanism that compensates for the loss of echo strength caused by the depth of the reflector. It allows reflectors with equal reflection coefficients to appear on the screen with equal brightness and to compensate, to a certain extent, for the effects of attenuation caused by greater depth. For the average soft tissues, the attenuation coefficient is equal to one-half the frequency (expressed in decibels per centimeter).

Compression is the internal process in which larger echoes are equalized with smaller echoes. Compression decreases dynamic range.

Demodulation is the process of converting voltages delivered to the receiver to a more useful form. Demodulation is done by rectification (removal of negative components, replacement with positive values) and smoothing (averaging of the new wave form).

Rejection is also termed suppression or threshold. Rejection is the elimination of smaller amplitude voltage pulses produced by weaker reflections. This mechanism helps to reduce noise by removing low-level signals that do not contribute to meaningful information in the image.

Scan Converter (Memory)

The *scan converter,* or *memory,* transforms the incoming echo data into a suitable format for the display, storing all of the necessary information for the two-dimensional image. As the tissue is scanned, several images (frames) are acquired per second. Memory allows for a single scan consisting of one or more frames to be displayed. Most

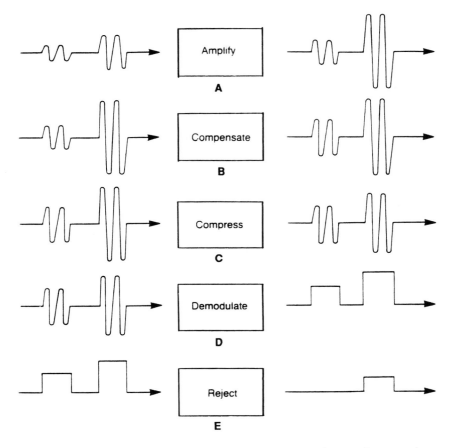

Input to each process

Output from each process

Figure 1–21. The five functions of the receiver. **(A)** Amplification of both pulses. **(B)** Amplification of the weaker pulses. **(C)** The difference between the pulse amplitudes is reduced. **(D)** The pulses are converted to another form. **(E)** The weaker pulse is rejected. (Kremkaw FW. *Diagnostic Ultrasound: Principles, Instruments, and Exercises.* 3rd ed. Philadelphia: WB Saunders; 1989.)

instruments have enough memory to store the last several frames scanned (cine loop). There are two types of scan converters (memories): analog and digital.

Analog scan converters are found in older machines, these consist of semiconductors arranged in square matrices. As the ultrasound pulse transverses the tissues, an electronic beam scans the square matrix. It is swept in the same direction as the beam in the body. The current within the electronic beam corresponds to the intensity of the returning echoes. If the echoes are weak, the current in the electronic beam is decreased and vice versa. The strengths of the electrical charges are precisely what are stored in the individual insulators of the matrix. These electronic charges have values that correspond to brightness levels. To read the stored images, the electronic beam is scanned across the stored matrix. The stored charge in each element affects the current in the electronic beam, and together these charges are used to vary the brightness of display.

Digital scan converters store image brightness values as numbers instead as of electrical charges. A digital scan converter consists of three components: an analog-to-digital (A–D) converter, which changes the voltages of received signals into numeric values; a digital memory, which stores these image echo values; and a circuit, which translates these stored numbers back into analog (voltage) values when needed (a digital-to-analog, or D–A, converter).

The digital memory component is the same as computer memory. Modern computers use circuits that have only two states: off and on. Within the computer these states may be represented; for example, by the absence or presence of electrical current, the open or closed condition of switches, or the direction of magnetization on a magnetic disk or tape. Each of these examples has two states, which the computer considers zero (0) or one (1). At first, it seems that this system, called the *binary number system,* or binary,[4] is not very useful for computing, but it can represent any number that the more common decimal system can. Instead of using increasing powers of 10, as the decimal system does, the binary system uses increasing powers of 2. In the decimal system, the right-most digit represents units, the next to the left tens, the next hundreds, etc. In the binary system, the right-most binary digit or bit is ones, the next left twos, the next fours, the next eights, etc.[1] (Fig. 1–22).

Display

How is this system used to represent ultrasound images? Imagine that the image is divided into many small squares similar to a checkerboard. Each square is assigned a number that represents the ultrasound echo amplitude. For example, for white-on-black displays, the highest echo value is white, and the lowest is black (the reverse is true for black-on-white displays).[2] A square located in a part of the image that has the highest echo values (e.g., echoes in a gallstone) would be assigned a high number value, whereas, a square in the surrounding bile would receive a small number value. In color flow imaging, each square would be assigned a number that represents the Doppler shift value. If the squares are made small enough, then the eye will not be able to see them as separate. Typically, ultrasound images are divided into 512 by 512 of these small squares.[1]

The squares are called picture elements, or *pixels*. The number 512 is a power of two (two to the ninth power) and also happens to fit well in a standard television frame. This number yields an image containing 262,144 pixels.

If each of these pixels could store only one binary value, then the results would be very much like an old bistable image, having only black and white values. Each pixel could be either black or white, with no gray values. To store gray scale images, each pixel must have more than one binary digit (or bit). For example, with three bits per pixel each pixel could represent eight different shades of gray. To calculate how many different shades of gray can be represented by a pixel containing a set number (n) of databits, the following formula can be applied:

$$\text{number of shades} = 2^n$$

The largest value that can be represented by a given number of bits is calculated by the formula:

$$\text{largest value of } n \text{ bits} = 2^n - 1$$

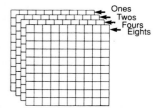

Figure 1–22. A 10×10 pixel, 4-bit-deep digital memory. (Kremkaw FW. *Diagnostic Ultrasound: Principles, Instruments, and Exercises.* 3rd ed. Philadelphia: WB Saunders; 1989.)

If, for example, we are considering three bits, we could represent eight different shades of gray with the largest gray value equal to seven.

Most ultrasound machines generate images with four to eight bits of gray scale (16 to 256 shades of gray). Color-flow Doppler machines need more bits to represent the various colors. Because the machine makes no distinction of color (to the machine, the image is merely an array of numbers), the color values are stored as a number value for each of three primary colors. Combinations of these three primaries (usually red, green, and blue) can yield almost any color.

Fig. 1–22 is an example of a 10×10 pixel matrix with four bits/pixel. To calculate how many bits an ultrasound image contains, the following formula can be applied:

$$\frac{\text{number of}}{\text{bits/image}} = \frac{\text{number of image rows} \times \text{number of}}{\text{image columns} \times \text{number of bits/pixel}}$$

or

$$\text{number of bits/image} = \text{total number of pixels}$$
$$\times \text{number of bits/pixels}$$

In computer terminology, eight binary digits or eight bits equals 1 *byte*. To determine the number of bytes of memory an image requires, divide the number of bits per image by eight:

$$\text{number of bytes/image} = \frac{\text{number of bits per image}}{8}$$

Examples

If an image has 10 pixel columns and rows with 2 bits/pixel, then:

$$\text{number of bits/image} = 10 \times 10 \times 2 = 200 \text{ bits}$$

$$\text{number of bytes/image} = \frac{200 \text{ bits/image}}{8} = 25 \text{ bytes}$$

If a 512×512 pixel image has eight bits/pixel, then:

$$\text{number of bits/image} = 512 \times 512 \times 8$$
$$= 2,097,152 \text{ bits}$$

$$\text{number of bytes/image} = \frac{2,097,152}{8} = 262,144 \text{ bytes}$$

Thus, a single image can contain over 2 million bits or more than $\frac{1}{4}$ million bytes. To reduce the number of digits used to describe these values, multipliers are applied, such as kilo-, mega-, giga- (Table 1–2). These multipliers are not identical to their counterparts in the metric system, however. For example, 1 kilobit is not 1000 bits, but 1024 bits or 2 to the 10th power. For convenience, large numbers may be rounded (e.g., 262,144 bytes may be rounded to 260 kilobytes).

TABLE 1–2. UNIT OF MEASUREMENT IN COMPUTER TERMINOLOGY

Unit	Prefix	Symbol	Quantity
byte[a]	kilo-	K	1000[a]
byte	mega-	M	1,000,000
byte	giga-	G	1,000,000,000

[a] 1 kilobyte equals 1024 characters, but can be rounded off to 1000.

The image can be stored in the digital memory as numbers, but it cannot be viewed unless the numbers are converted back to an image. Otherwise, a large list of numbers is all that would be displayed. The third part of the digital scan converter does the following conversion. It takes the number values stored in the memory and changes them back into an analog voltage. The voltage varies the brightness of a spot on the cathode ray tube, generating an image that the human eye can interpret. The hardware that performs this function is the digital-to-analog (D–A) converter.

DYNAMIC IMAGING

Dynamic imaging is simply the process of viewing an image in motion. The dynamic image is displayed on a *cathode-ray tube* (CRT), the unit of visual display that receives electrical impulses and translates them into the picture on the screen by varying the brightness of the trace or lines displayed. The CRT in Fig. 1–23 is an electrostatic deflection CRT; another type, the magnetic deflection CRT, substitutes a magnetic coil to serve the same function as the deflection plates (i.e., to move the electron beam). The front face of the CRT, the screen, is phosphor coated and displays

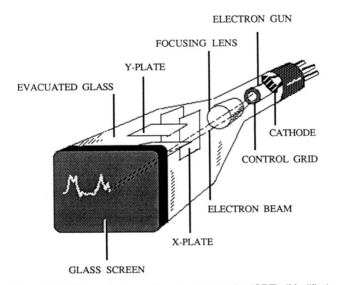

Figure 1–23. Basic structure of a cathode ray tube (CRT). (Modified from McDicken W: *Diagnostic Ultrasonics: Principles and use of Instruments.* 2nd ed. New York: Wiley; 1981; p. 15.)

the product of the aforementioned process in the form of a recognizable image.

A *frame* is a single image composed of multiple scan lines. To produce a dynamic or moving image, numerous frames are required. To freeze a frame, or stop the image to record or view it, the memory of the system is activated. The *frame rate* (FR) is the number of frames displayed or scanned per second. In most diagnostic medical sonography or echocardiography systems, the frame rate is usually 10 to 60 frames/s. If the display frame rate is below 20/s, then the real-time image appears to flicker, preventing the eye from integrating the images.

The pulse repetition frequency (PRF) is the number of pulses produced by the transducer in a given time period. It is related to the number of lines per frame and the frame rate by the formula:

$$\frac{\text{pulse repetition}}{\text{frequency (PRF)}} = \frac{\text{lines per frame (LPF)}}{\times \text{ frame rate (FR)}}$$

The PRF, LPF, and FR are directly related to the propagation speed. The maximum effective velocity is 77,000 cm/s, or one-half the propagation speed of ultrasound in soft tissues (1540 m/s or 154,000 cm/s). The one-half value results from the pulse having to make a round-trip to be received.

$$\text{depth} \times \text{LPF} \times \text{FR} = 77,000$$

Note: LPF × FR = PRF. Hence the equation can also be stated

$$\text{depth} \times \text{PRF} = 77,000$$

Improving image quality by increasing the lines per frame will reduce the frame rate if the depth remains constant. Increasing the depth of penetration while maintaining a constant number of lines per frame also reduces the frame rate. The frame rate can be increased if the depth of penetration is decreased, assuming the LPF is constant.

The *display format* refers to how the image appears on the screen, as either a rectangular display or a sector display. A *rectangular display* image appears in the form of a rectangle. The width of the display is given in centimeters; the *line density* is expressed as the number of lines per centimeter. To determine the line density for a rectangular display the lines per frame are divided by the display width in centimeters.

$$\text{line density (lines/cm)} = \frac{\text{lines per frame (LPF)}}{\text{display width (cm)}}$$

A *sector display* yields a pie-shaped image. The scans form an angle so that the line density is expressed as lines per degree.

$$\text{line density (lines/degree)} = \frac{\text{lines per frame (LPF)}}{\text{sector angle (degrees)}}$$

The *scan converter,* electronic circuitry in the machine's display, transforms a rectangular or arc-shaped image into a rectangular video frame, and adds the text and graphics (such as depth markers).

Modes of Display

The *A-mode,* or amplitude mode, is a one-dimensional graphic display with vertical deflections of the baseline. The height of the deflection represents the amplitude, or strength, of the echo; the distance in time is a function of where on the baseline the deflection occurs.

The *B-mode,* or brightness mode, displays the echoes as variations in the brightness of a line of spots on the CRT. The position of the spot on the baseline is related to the depth of the reflecting structure; the brightness is proportional to the strength of the echo. Each row of spots represents information obtained from a single position of the transducer or scanning beam. When successive rows of these spots are integrated into an image, a B-scan is produced.

The *M-mode,* or motion mode, is a two-dimensional recording of the reflector's change in position, or motion, against time. Most M-modes display the brightness of the signal in proportion to the strength of the echo. This mode is most commonly used for the study of dynamic structures such as the heart.

ARTIFACTS

Unlike a Grecian urn, which is an *artifact* from a past culture, the term in diagnostic medical sonography has a very different implication. If refers to something seen on an image that does not, in reality, exist in the anatomy studied. An artifact can be beneficial to the interpretation of the image, or it can detract from this process. For example, certain artifacts are known to occur in cystic structures and are notably absent from a solid mass, and this information can, therefore, be used in a beneficial way when determining the nature of a mass. Conversely, there are artifacts that can appear similar to the placenta, making delineation of the limits of the placenta more difficult. Artifacts can be subdivided by the physical principals that produce them; namely, resolution artifacts, propagation artifacts, attenuation artifacts, or miscellaneous artifacts.

Resolution Artifacts

Axial resolution is the failure to resolve two separate reflectors parallel to the beam.

Lateral resolution is the failure to resolve two separate reflectors perpendicular to the beam.

Speckle is scatter in tissues, causing interference effects referred to as *noise.*

Section thickness is the finite width of the beam producing extraneous echoes, or debris, in normal anechoic, or echo-free structures.

Propagation Artifacts

Reverberation is repetitive reflections between two highly reflective layers. The bouncing back and forth increases travel time, causing the signals to be displayed at different depths. The reverberations are seen on the image as equally spaced bands of diminishing amplitude.

Refraction is the change in direction of the sound beam as it passes from one medium to another. This phenomenon will cause a reflection to appear improperly positioned on the image.

Multipath. Because the returning signal does not necessarily follow the same path as the incident beam, the time required for some parts of the signal to return to the transducer will vary, causing reflections to appear at incorrect depths.

Mirror image is generated when objects present on one side of a strong reflector are also shown on the other side of the reflector. Such artifacts are commonly seen around the diaphragm.

Attenuation Artifacts

Shadowing is the reduction in echo strength of signals arising from behind a strong reflector or attenuating structure. Structures such as gallstones, renal calculi, and bone will produce shadowing.

Enhancement is an increase in the amplitude of echoes located behind a weakly attenuating structure. The increase pertains to the relative strength of the signals as compared with neighboring signals passing through more highly attenuating media. For example, stronger reflections may be seen behind a fluid-filled structure than behind a solid structure (e.g., the urine-filled bladder versus a sold tumor of the uterus).

Refraction or edge shadowing. The beam may bend at a curved surface and lose intensity, producing a shadow. If the beam is traveling from a higher velocity medium (less dense) to a low-velocity medium, a narrower shadow will be generated. Conversely, a sound beam traveling from a low-velocity medium to a higher one will project a wider shadow.

Miscellaneous Artifacts

Comet tail is produced by a strong reflector; similar in appearance to reverberation. The comet tail, however, is composed of thin lines of closely spaced discrete echoes.

Ring down is thought to be caused by a resonance phenomenon and is associated with gas bubble. It also appears very similar to reverberation, producing numerous parallel echoes. Sometimes discrete echoes cannot be differentiated, giving the appearance of a continuous emission of sound.

Propagation speed error. Most diagnostic ultrasound equipment operates on the assumption that the speed of sound in the body is 1540 m/s. This is not always true because different tissues have different propagation speeds. If the beam passes from a medium of one speed into a medium of a greater speed, then the calculated distance will be less than the actual distance, causing the echo to be erroneously displayed too close to the transducer. If the propagation speed decreases, then the echo will appear farther from the transducer than it actually is.

Side lobes are the result of the transducer element being finite in size. The difference in vibration at the center and edge results in acoustic energy emitted by the transducer flowing along the main axis of the sound beam. The energy that diverts from the main path is the cause of the side lobes, which will generate reflections at improper, off-axis locations in the image.

Grating lobes are seen with linear array transducers, which also produce off-axis acoustic waves as a result of the regular spacing of the active elements. All grating lobes will cause reflections to appear at improper, off-axis locations in the image.

Range ambiguity. As noted earlier, the range equation relates the depth of a reflector to the propagation speed and the pulse round-trip time. The maximum depth (d_{max}) of a reflector that can be unambiguously recorded is:

$$d_{max} = \tfrac{1}{2} \times \text{propagation speed} \times \text{PRP}$$

Thus, the pulse repetition period (PRP) that controls the field-of-view (FOV) also determines the maximum depth of a reflector that can be unambiguously recorded. Echoes from a transmitted pulse that return after a time equal to the PRP will be erroneously recorded at a depth closer to the transducer.

QUALITY OF PERFORMANCE

To guarantee efficiency of performance, all ultrasound diagnostic equipment is tested under a quality assurance (QA) program. To ensure that the instrument is operating correctly and consistently, it is checked for

1. imaging performance
2. equipment performance and safety
3. beam measurements
4. acoustic output
5. preventative maintenance

AIUM Test Object

The American Institute of Ultrasound in Medicine (AIUM) has designed a test object specifically to measure imaging performance of an ultrasound system (Fig. 1–24). The AIUM test object is a "tank" consisting of a series of stainless steel rods, 0.75 mm in diameter, arranged in a specific pattern between two transparent plastic sides, with the other boundaries formed by thin, acrylic plastic sheets.[1,4] The tank is filled with a mixture of alcohol, an algae inhibitor, and water, which allows the propagation speed to approximate the speed of sound in soft tissues (1540 m/s). The

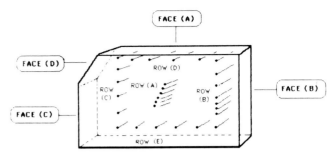

Figure 1–24. AIUM 100-mm test object.

results obtained are not affected by normal fluctuations in room temperature; the speed varies less than 1% for a temperature variation of 5°Celsius (5°C).

The following factors are measured by the AIUM test object (Table 1–3):

System sensitivity is measured by determining the weakest signal that the system will display.

Axial resolution is determined by placing the transducer on face A and scanning rod group (a). The six rods are separated by 4, 3, 2, and 1 mm, respectively. The system's axial resolution in millimeters is equal to the distance between the two closest yet distinguishable echoes.

Lateral resolution is measured by placing the transducer on face B and scanning rod group (b). The lateral resolution is equal to the distance between the two closest rods in this group.

Dead zone is the region of the sound beam in which imaging cannot be performed; the area closest to the transducer. To determine the extent of the dead zone, the transducer is placed on face A and rod group (d) is scanned. The distance from the transducer to the first rod imaged is equal to the length of the dead zone.

Range accuracy (depth accuracy) is measured by placing the transducer on face A and scanning rod group (e). For the system to be operating properly, the echoes should appear at their actual depths and spacings within 1 mm (The rods in this group are 2 cm apart). Checking the range accuracy ensures the accuracy of the internal calipers of the system.

In addition to the AIUM test object, other devices have been designed to measure different parameters of imaging performance. The *beam profiler* is designed to record three-dimensional reflection amplitude information. It consists of a pulser, receiver, transducer, and tank equipped with rods placed at different distances from the transducer.[1]

The transducer is pulsed and scanned across the rods. The fluctuation in amplitude of each reflection returning to the transducer is recorded in an A-mode pattern. The *hydrophone* is one of several devices that measure acoustic output; it consists of a small transducer element mounted on a narrow tube.[1] When used with an oscilloscope, the

TABLE 1–3. PERFORMANCE MEASUREMENTS FOR THE AIUM TEST OBJECT

Measurement	Row	Test Object Face	Parameter Tested
Dead zone	D	Face (A)	The distance measured between the transducer face and the first rod depicted
Lateral resolution	B	Face (B)	Linear measurement of the echoes produced by row D
Depth calibration	C or E	Face (A) or (B)	The distance measured between the first and the last line in Row E
Registration	E	Face (A), (B), (C), and (D)	Good Poor
Axial resolution	A	Face (A)	5-mm to 1-mm pins spaced at decreasing intervals of 1-mm in Row A
Digital calipers	E	Face (C)	A distance of 10 cm or 100 mm measured on the horizontal pins in Row E, indicating the digital calipers are functioning correctly
Liquid velocity	E	Face (C)	The cursors are positioned at the leading edge echo to the other end leading edge echo, on the horizontal pins in Row E. A 100-mm measurement indicates the liquid medium velocity is correct.

voltage produced in response to variations in pressure can be displaced and evaluated. The output produced by the hydrophone permits calculation of the period, pulse repetition period, and pulse duration. The hydrophone can also be used as a beam profiler.

Tissue/Cyst Phantom

This test device contains a medium that simulates soft tissue (Fig. 1–25). Enclosed in the phantom are structures that mimic cysts and solid masses and a series of 0.375-mm targets, in two groups. Each group measures depth and angular resolution. The phantom is used to evaluate the ultrasound system and transducer performance. Sonographic equipment can be evaluated for depth and angular resolution, vertical and horizontal distance calibration, and ring down.[5]

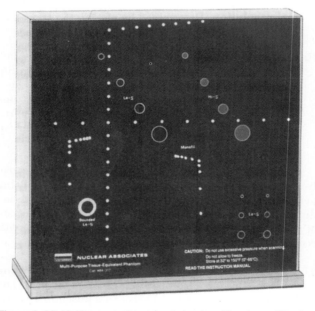

Figure 1–25. Multipurpose tissue/cyst phantom (Courtesy of Nuclear Associates, Carle Place, NY. Reprinted with permission.)

Bioeffects

To date, there is no concrete evidence to support any truly detrimental bioeffects from the application of diagnostic ultrasound to human tissues.[1] The study of possible effects is ongoing, however, and the definitive answer has not been found. It is generally agreed that the potential value of the information obtained from the procedure far outweighs the possibility of deleterious effects. Greater study of the microscopic effects of sound on tissue will have to take place before additional conclusions can be reached. To clarify what is known to date, the potential bioeffects are categorized in three groups: mechanical effects, thermal effects, and cavitation.

Mechanical effects include all types of damage not categorized as thermal or cavitational. There is very little information on this type of effect.

Thermal effects are produced primarily by the mechanisms of attenuation. As a major component of attenuation, absorption by the tissue leads to a rise in tissue temperature. Increased temperatures can cause irreversible damage, depending on the extent of the exposure. It is generally agreed that *exposure producing a maximum temperature of 1°C can be used without any effects. A rise in temperature of the tissues to 41°C or above is considered dangerous to a fetus. The longer that this temperature is maintained, the greater the potential risk for damage.*[1]

Cavitation is the result of pressure changes in the medium causing gas bubbles to form; it can produce severe tissue damage. The two types of cavitation are stable cavitation and transient cavitation. *Stable cavitation* involves microbubbles already present in tissue that respond by expanding and contracting when pressure is applied. These bubbles can intercept and absorb a large amount of the acoustic energy. Stable cavitation can result in shear stresses and microstreaming in the surrounding tissues.

Transient cavitation is dependent on the pressure of the ultrasound pulses. The tissue bubbles expand and collapse violently. This type of cavitation can cause highly localized, violent effects involving enormous pressures, markedly elevated temperatures, shock waves, and mechanical stress.

Cavitation may occur with short pulses. It has been shown that pulses with peak intensities of greater than 3300 W/cm² can induce cavitation in mammals.[1] Precise determination of when cavitation will occur is not currently within our capabilities. For specific conditions of homogeneous media, it is possible to estimate an index for the cavitation threshold.

The following guidelines are adapted from an official statement by the American Institute of Ultrasound in Medicine (AIUM). *Bioeffects Considerations for the Safety of Diagnostic Ultrasound.* Bethesda, MD, American Institutes of Ultrasound Medicine, 1988. The reader is urged to read the full AIUM text.

Intensity. There are no independently confirmed significant biological effects in mammalian tissues exposed in vivo with unfocused transducers with intensities below 100 mW/cm² and below 1 W/cm² for focused transducers.

Exposure. Exposure times can be > 1 s and < 500 s for an unfocused transducer; and < 50 s/pulse for a focused transducer. No significant bioeffects have been observed even at higher intensities than noted above (as long as the intensity × time product is < 50 J/cm²).

Thermal. A maximum temperature rise of 1°C is acceptable, but an increase in the in situ temperature to 41°C or greater is hazardous to fetuses.

Cavitation. Can result if pressure peaks are greater than 3300 W/cm². However, it is not possible to specify a threshold at which cavitation will occur.

Randomized studies are the best method for assessing potential effects. *There are no independent confirmed biologic effects on patients or operators.*[1]

COMPUTERS AND ULTRASOUND

Most modern ultrasound equipment is computerized or has some computer capabilities. Today's ultrasound equipment can calculate gestational age, store nomograms, store patient data, and transfer sonographic images from one hospital to another via a modem (modulator/ demodulator).

What is a Computer?

A computer is a device that contains a microprocessor and can perform high-speed mathematical calculations, assemble and store data, and perform logic operations. The graphics in this book, for example, were processed and stored by a computer.

The Computer Brain. The "brain" of the computer (Fig. 1–26) comprises three general parts:

1. the central processing unit (CPU)
2. the memory unit
3. the input–output unit

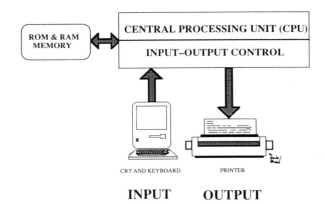

Figure 1–26. Computer organization.

The *main computer storage* (MCS) is the memory of the computer. There are two kinds of computer memory.[6]

ROM (Read-only memory). ROM is permanent and unchangeable. It is installed by the computer manufacturer and contains instructions needed by the CPU when the computer is turned on.

RAM (Random-access memory, or read and write). RAM is temporary and changeable. It is usable memory for the operator to change depending on needs. This is temporary memory because when the computer is turned off, the RAM is lost. However, data can be extracted from the RAM before the computer is turned off to be stored permanently on a floppy disk or hard disk for use at a later time.

When the sonographer looks at the contents of the memory, he or she is *reading*. When the sonographer is entering or changing information, he or she is *writing* (read and write memory).

REFERENCES

1. Kremkau FW. *Diagnostic Ultrasound: Principles, Instruments and Exercises.* 3rd ed. Philadelphia: WB Saunders; 1989.
2. Edelman SK. *Understanding Ultrasound Physics: Fundamentals and Exam Review.* Houston: EPS Publishers; 1990.
3. Pinkney N. *A Review of the Concepts of Ultrasound Physics and Instrumentation.* 4th ed. Philadelphia: Sonior; 1983.
4. Bushong SC, Archer RB. *Diagnostic Ultrasound: Physics, Biology, and Instrumentation.* St. Louis: Mosby-Year Book; 1991.
5. *Diagnostic Ultrasound: Test Equipment and Accessories.* New York: Nuclear Associates, Catalog U-2; 1991; 2–3.
6. Shelly G, Cashman T. *Computer Fundamentals for an Information Age.* Brea, CA: Anaheim Publishing; 1984; 1984.

Questions

GENERAL INSTRUCTIONS: For each question, select the best answer. Select only one answer for each question unless otherwise specified.

1. An example of a nonspecular reflector is

   (A) the liver surface
   (B) the diaphragm
   (C) red blood cells
   (D) any structure that does *not* produce a strong echo

2. The spatial pulse length

   (A) determines penetration depth
   (B) usually decreases with frequency
   (C) is improved with rectification
   (D) determines lateral resolution

3. Axial resolution

   (A) is improved in the focal zone
   (B) depends on the TGC slope
   (C) is improved by digital scan converters
   (D) depends on the wavelength

4. Lateral resolution

   (A) and ring-down are the same
   (B) depends on the beam diameter
   (C) improves with frequency
   (D) cannot be measured in the far zone

5. The beam of an unfocused transducer diverges

   (A) because of inadequate damping
   (B) in the Fresnel zone
   (C) in the Fraunhofer zone
   (D) when the pulse length is long

6. Reverberation artifacts are a result of

   (A) electronic noise
   (B) improper TGC settings
   (C) the presence of two or more strong reflecting surfaces
   (D) an angle of incidence that is too small

7. Grating lobes are essential for the proper operation of a linear phased array.

   (A) true
   (B) false

8. Electronically steered scanners always produce higher resolution images than do mechanically steered scanners.

   (A) true
   (B) false

9. An annular array scanner uses mechanical beam steering.

   (A) true
   (B) false

10. A linear sequenced array cannot be dynamically focused.

    (A) true
    (B) false

Questions 11 through 15: Match the following group of wires with its function for the AIUM test object (Fig. 1–27).

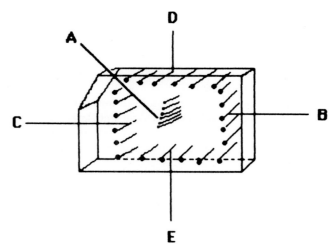

Figure 1–27. AIUM 100-mm test object.

11. registration or B-mode alignment _____

12. axial resolution _____

13. lateral resolution _____

14. dead zone _____

15. depth calibration _____

16. Decreasing the spatial pulse length

    (A) reduces the field of view
    (B) reduces lateral resolution
    (C) improves axial resolution
    (D) improves lateral resolution

17. How much will a 3.5 MHz pulse be attenuated after passing through 2 cm of soft tissue?

    (A) 7 dB
    (B) 3.5 dB
    (C) 17 dB
    (D) 1.75 dB

18. Propagation speed errors result in

    (A) reverberation
    (B) improper axial position
    (C) shadowing
    (D) a Doppler shift

19. Enhancement is caused by

    (A) strongly reflected structures
    (B) propagation speed errors
    (C) Snell's law
    (D) weakly attenuating structures

20. The Doppler shift frequency is

    (A) directly proportional to the velocity of the reflector
    (B) greater in pulsed Doppler systems
    (C) greater at high intensity levels
    (D) dependent on the number of transducer elements being used

21. The number of frames per second necessary for a real-time image to be flicker free is

    (A) more than 15
    (B) less than 10
    (C) between 6 and 10
    (D) between 3 and 6

22. The SPTA intensity will always be larger than the SATA intensity.

    (A) true
    (B) false

23. The intensity of the ultrasound beam is usually greater at the focal zone because of

    (A) decreased attenuation
    (B) the smaller beam diameter
    (C) diffraction effects
    (D) a shorter duty factor

24. If the amplitude is doubled, the intensity is

    (A) doubled
    (B) cut in half
    (C) increased by four times
    (D) unchanged

25. The attenuation for soft tissue is

    (A) increased with tissue thickness
    (B) determined by the scope of he TGC curve
    (C) increased with decreasing wavelength
    (D) unimportant when using digital scan converters

26. The acoustic impedance of the matching layer

    (A) can be chosen to improve transmission into the body
    (B) must be much larger than the transducer material to reduce attenuation
    (C) is not necessary with real-time scanners
    (D) must be made with the same material as the damping material

27. In a pulse–echo system, the quality factor should be made as large as possible.

    (A) true
    (B) false

28. The beam diameter is constant in the near zone.

    (A) true
    (B) false

29. The operating frequency

    (A) depends on the transducer's ring-down time
    (B) depends on the thickness of the crystal
    (C) is increased as the crystal diameter is decreased
    (D) depends on the strength of the pulser

30. The period of an ultrasound wave is

    (A) the time at which it is no longer detectable
    (B) determined by the duty factor
    (C) the time of one wavelength
    (D) independent of the frequency

31. The dynamic range of a system

    (A) is increased when specular reflectors are scanned
    (B) is decreased when shadowing is present
    (C) can be increased through the use of coupling gel
    (D) is the ratio of smallest to largest power level that the system can handle

32. The intensity of an ultrasonic beam can be measured with radiation force balance

    (A) true
    (B) false

33. Increasing the pulse repetition period

    (A) improves resolution
    (B) increases the maximum depth that can be imaged
    (C) decreases the maximum depth that can be imaged
    (D) increases refraction

34. Ultrasound bioeffects

    (A) do not occur
    (B) do not occur with diagnostic instruments
    (C) are not confirmed below 100 mW/cm² SPTA
    (D) are not confirmed below 1 W/cm² SPTA

35. No refraction can occur at an interface if the media impedances are equal.

    (A) true
    (B) false

36. Smaller transducers always produce smaller beam diameters.

    (A) true
    (B) false

37. The ultrasound beam profile can be measured with a hydrophone.

    (A) true
    (B) false

38. The pulsed-Doppler system yields better depth resolution than the continuous wave (CW) system.

    (A) true
    (B) false

39. The gray-scale display was made possible when digital scan converters replaced analog scan converters.

    (A) true
    (B) false

40. Videotape recorders operating at 30 frames per second cannot be used with mechanical real-time units because the frame rate is too slow.

    (A) true
    (B) false

41. Linear phased array scanners need no form of mechanical focusing because focusing is performed electronically.

    (A) true
    (B) false

42. The frame rate of real-time scanners depends on the number of lines used to form the image.

    (A) true
    (B) false

43. It is *not* possible to steer an annular phased array electronically.

    (A) true
    (B) false

44. The near zone length should be kept as short as possible.

    (A) true
    (B) false

45. What percentage of intensity of an ultrasound pulse incident on an interface of 0.25 and 0.75 rayls is reflected?

    (A) 50%
    (B) 100%
    (C) 25%
    (D) 75%

46. Axial resolution can be improved by using

    (A) higher frequency transducers
    (B) lower frequency transducers
    (C) larger transducers
    (D) poorly damped transducers

47. When particle motion of a medium is parallel to the direction of a wave propagation, the wave being transmitted is called a

    (A) longitudinal wave
    (B) shear wave
    (C) surface wave
    (D) lamb wave

48. The wavelength in a material having a wave velocity of 1500 m/s employing a transducer frequency of 5 MHz is

    (A) 0.3 mm
    (B) 0.3 cm
    (C) 0.6 mm
    (D) 0.6 cm

49. The factor that determines the amount of reflection at the interface of two dissimilar materials is

    (A) the index of refraction
    (B) the frequency of the ultrasonic wave
    (C) Young's modulus
    (D) difference in specific acoustic impedances

50. The equation that describes the relationship among propagation, wavelength, and frequency is

    (A) $V = f\lambda$
    (B) wavelength = 2(frequency × velocity)

(C) $Z = pV$
(D) wavelength = frequency + velocity

51. Which of the following can occur when an ultrasonic beam reaches the interface of two dissimilar materials?

(A) reflection
(B) refraction
(C) mode conversion
(D) all of the above

52. The acoustic impedance of a material is

(A) directly proportional to density and inversely proportional to velocity
(B) directly proportional to velocity and inversely proportional to density
(C) inversely proportional to density and velocity
(D) equal to the product of density and velocity

53. The average velocity of ultrasonic waves in soft tissue is

(A) 1540 ft/s
(B) 3300 m/s
(C) 1540 m/s
(D) 300×10^6 m/s

54. Receiver-angle values in CW Doppler analysis do *not* influence the final Doppler shift.

(A) true
(B) false

55. Refraction occurs because of difference in _____ across an interface between two materials.

(A) acoustic impedance
(B) wave velocity
(C) density
(D) none of the above

56. Reflection factor at an interface between two materials depends primarily on the change in _____ across the interface.

(A) acoustic impedance
(B) wave velocity
(C) density
(D) none of the above

57. The velocity of sound waves is primarily dependent on

(A) angulation
(B) reflection
(C) the material through which the sound is being transmitted and the mode of vibration
(D) none of the above

58. Increasing the frequency of an ultrasonic longitudinal wave will result in _____ in the velocity of that wave.

(A) an increase
(B) a decrease
(C) no change
(D) a reversal

59. The change in direction of an ultrasonic beam, when it passes from one medium to another, in which elasticity and density differ from those of the first medium is called

(A) refraction
(B) rarefaction
(C) angulation
(D) reflection

60. A long near zone can be obtained by

(A) using a higher frequency transducer
(B) adding a convex lens to the transducer
(C) decreasing the diameter of the transducer
(D) increasing the damping

61. If a 2-MHz frequency is used in human soft tissue, the wavelength is approximately

(A) 0.75 mm
(B) 0.15 mm
(C) 0.21 mm
(D) 0.44 mm

62. The ratio of particle pressure to particle velocity at a given point within the ultrasonic field is

(A) interference
(B) impedance
(C) incidence
(D) noise

63. What is the following formula used to determine?

$$\frac{2 \times \text{velocity of reflector} \times \text{original frequency}}{\text{velocity of sound}}$$

(A) shift in frequency caused by the Doppler effect
(B) degree of attenuation
(C) distance a wave front travels
(D) amount of amplification necessary to produce diagnostic ultrasound

64. The principle that states that all points on a wavefront can be considered as point sources for the production of spherical secondary wavelets was postulated by

(A) Doppler
(B) Young
(C) Huygens
(D) Langevin

65. A 10-dB difference in signal intensity is equivalent to a _____ difference.

(A) twofold
(B) tenfold
(C) hundredfold
(D) thousandfold

66. The level below which signals are *not* transmitted through an ultrasound receiver system is the

   (A) intensity level
   (B) threshold, negative, or reject level
   (C) impedance level
   (D) dynamic range level

67. Gray-scale systems typically use _____ as a means of signal dynamic range reduction.

   (A) rejection
   (B) compression
   (C) relaxation
   (D) elimination

68. The strength of the echo is related to the height of the deflection on the oscilloscope for the _____ display.

   (A) A-mode
   (B) B-mode
   (C) B-scan
   (D) M-mode

69. Which of the following is *not* a method for restricting the dynamic range of the signal?

   (A) suppression
   (B) rejection
   (C) compression
   (D) relaxation

70. Most of the scan converters currently in use are of the _____ type.

   (A) analog
   (B) digital
   (C) bistable
   (D) static

71. The fraction of time that pulsed ultrasound is actually on is the

   (A) duty factor
   (B) frame rate
   (C) cavitation
   (D) intensity transmission coefficient

72. The ability of an imaging system to detect weak reflections is called

   (A) compression
   (B) demodulation
   (C) gain
   (D) sensitivity

73. Which of the following image shapes is produced by a linear sequenced array real-time transducer?

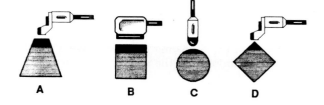

A   B   C   D

74. The major factor in determining the acoustic power output of the transducer is the

   (A) size of the transducer
   (B) magnitude of the voltage spike
   (C) amount of amplification at the receiver
   (D) amount of gain

75. Two primary mechanisms that produce tissue biological effects are

   (A) oscillations and radiation
   (B) absorption and reflection
   (C) direct and indirect
   (D) thermal and cavitational

76. The _____ relates bandwidth to operating frequency.

   (A) near zone
   (B) piezoelectric crystal
   (C) quality factor
   (D) far zone

77. The extraneous beams of ultrasound generated from the edges of individual transducer elements and not in the direction of the main ultrasonic beam are called

   (A) a phased array
   (B) impedance artifacts
   (C) side lobes
   (D) acoustic errors

78. The product of the period and the number of cycles in the pulse is the

   (A) pulse repetition frequency
   (B) continuous wave
   (C) pulse repetition period
   (D) pulse duration

79. The substance typically used as a matrix on the imaging surface of an analog scan converter tube is

   (A) mercurous chloride
   (B) silicon oxide
   (C) manganese sulfide
   (D) lithium fluoride

80. Specular reflection occurs when

   (A) the frequency is small compared with the wavelength

(B) the object that causes the reflection is small
(C) the reflector surface is smooth as compared with the wavelength
(D) The angle of incidence and the angle of reflection differ by at least 45°

81. The refractive index of water is slightly altered when a sound beam passes through it, thus causing compression and rarefaction of the water molecules. The phenomenon is the basis for the _____ technique of beam measurement.

(A) isoamplitude
(B) Schlieren
(C) relative echo
(D) attenuator calibration

82. Artifacts appearing as parallel, equally spaced lines are characteristic of

(A) acoustic shadowing
(B) off-normal incidence
(C) specular reflection
(D) reverberation

83. An increase in reflection amplitude from reflectors that lie behind a weakly attenuating structure is called

(A) the incidence angle
(B) enhancement
(C) the intensity reflection coefficient
(D) the effective reflecting area

84. The amount of dispersion in the far field of an ultrasound beam can be decreased by

(A) using a transducer with a convex face
(B) using a larger diameter transducer
(C) decreasing the intensity of the beam in the near field
(D) using a lower frequency transducer

85. Longitudinal or axial resolution is directly dependent on

(A) depth of penetration
(B) spatial pulse length
(C) damping
(D) the angle of incidence

86. The transducer ____ is equal to the ratio of the operating frequency to the frequency bandwidth.

(A) frequency
(B) Q factor
(C) resolution
(D) polarity

87. The technique that uses an optical system to produce a visible image of an ultrasonic beam is the ____ technique.

(A) M-mode
(B) B-scan
(C) Schlieren
(D) kinetic scanning

88. Which of the following is the least obstacle to the transmission of ultrasound?

(A) muscle
(B) fat
(C) bone
(D) blood

89. The ratio of the largest power to the smallest power that the ultrasound system can handle is the

(A) dynamic range
(B) gain
(C) rejection
(D) amplification factor

90. Ultrasound waves in tissues are called ____ waves

(A) shear
(B) lateral displacement
(C) rotational vibration
(D) longitudinal

Questions 91 through 99 refer to Fig. 1–28.

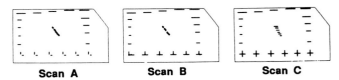

Scan A   **Scan B**   **Scan C**

Figure 1–28. Diagram of the AIUM 100-mm test object.

91. The row of wires in the middle are used to check

(A) lateral resolution
(B) axial resolution
(C) dead zone
(D) horizontal distance calibration
(E) all of the above

92. Which of the diagrams shows correct arm registration?

(A) scan A
(B) scan B
(C) scan C
(D) all of the above
(E) none of the above

93. The row of wires on top is used to check

(A) dead zone
(B) vertical distance calibration
(C) horizontal distance calibration
(D) axial resolution
(E) none of the above

94. While using the AIUM test object to test an articulated-arm scanner you obtain an image similar to scan A. You should

    (A) call for service
    (B) increase the contrast setting
    (C) switch to another type of transducer
    (D) try another test object

95. The row of wires on the bottom is used to check for

    (A) axial resolution
    (B) lateral resolution
    (C) horizontal caliper check
    (D) vertical distance calibration
    (E) dead zone

96. All except the following can be checked when the test object is scanned from the top only.

    (A) axial resolution
    (B) lateral resolution
    (C) vertical distance calibration
    (D) horizontal distance calibration

97. Which of the following parameters cannot be evaluated by the AIUM test object?

    (A) gray scale
    (B) dynamic range
    (C) azimuthal resolution
    (D) depth resolution
    (E) both A and B
    (F) all of the above

98. Scanning a test object from three sides without erasing would be used to check

    (A) gray scale
    (B) depth resolution
    (C) horizontal distance calibration
    (D) registration
    (E) all of the above

99. When using the AIUM test object, which of the following should be kept constant for comparisons?

    (A) output power
    (B) TGC
    (C) reject
    (D) transducer, MHz, and focus
    (E) all of the above

100. Which type of ultrasound machine can be used with AIUM test object?

    (A) linear array
    (B) static scanner
    (C) phased array
    (D) annular array
    (E) sector scanner
    (F) all of the above
    (G) A and C only

101. There are many types of natural and synthetic crystals that possess and exhibit piezoelectric properties. Which of the following are not natural?

    (A) tourmaline
    (B) quartz
    (C) lead zirconate titanate (PZT-4 or PZT-5)
    (D) barium titanate
    (E) Rochelle salt
    (F) lithium sulfate
    (G) lead metaniobate
    (H) ammonium dihydrogen phosphate

102. Which of the following materials would not be suitable as acoustic insulators for transducer backing?

    (A) cork
    (B) rubber
    (C) oil
    (D) araldite loaded with tungsten powder
    (E) epoxy resin
    (F) B and E only
    (G) all of the above

103. Ultrasound can be described as a(n)

    (A) mechanical vibration that can be transmitted through matter
    (B) mechanical vibration that can be transmitted through a vacuum
    (C) electromagnetic wave that can be transmitted through tissues
    (D) x-ray that can be transmitted through soft tissues

104. If the frequency of sound is below 16 Hz it is called

    (A) infrasound (subsonic)
    (B) audible sound
    (C) ultrasound
    (D) x-rays

105. If the frequency of sound is above 20 kHz it is called

    (A) infrasound (subsonic)
    (B) ultrasound
    (C) audible sound
    (D) x-rays

106. If the frequency of sound is between 16 Hz and 20 kHz it is called

    (A) x-rays
    (B) audible sound
    (C) ultrasound
    (D) infrasound (subsonic)

107. Which of the following is not among the spectrum of electromagnetic waves?

    (A) x-rays
    (B) ultrasound
    (C) ultraviolet

(D) infrared

(E) visible light

108. The term Hertz denotes

(A) density

(B) milliwatts per centimeter square (mW/cm²)

(C) kilogram

(D) cycle per second

109. An ultrasound transducer converts

(A) electrical energy into light and heat

(B) electrical energy into mechanical energy and vice versa

(C) mechanical energy into radiation

(D) sound into ultrasound

110. Which of the following is (are) an example(s) of a transducer?

(A) battery

(B) loudspeaker

(C) light bulb

(D) human being

(E) all of the above

(F) none of the above

(G) A and B only

111. When electric voltage is applied on both faces of a piezoelectric crystal, the crystal will

(A) increase in size

(B) decrease in size

(C) lose its polarization

(D) increase or decrease in size depending on the voltage polarity

112. The abbreviation 5 MHz denotes

(A) five hundred thousand cycles per second

(B) five hundred million cycles per second

(C) 5,000 cycles per second

(D) five million cycles per second

113. The function of the damping material in the transducer housing is to

(A) reduce pulse duration

(B) improve axial resolution

(C) reduce spatial pulse length

(D) improve lateral resolution

(E) A and B only

(F) A and D only

(G) A, B, and C only

114. What is the velocity of ultrasound in human soft tissue at 37°C?

(A) 1,540 meters per second

(B) 1,540 miles per second

(C) 741 miles per hour

(D) 1,087 meters per second

115. In physical science, the word period denotes

(A) the pressure or height of a wave

(B) the speed of a wave

(C) the time it takes to complete a single cycle

(D) propagation

116. Longitudinal waves are characterized by

(A) motion of particles parallel to the axis of wave propagation

(B) motion of particles perpendicular to the axis of wave propagation

(C) twisting action of the particles in motion

(D) surface vibrating particles

117. Transverse waves are characterized by

(A) motion of particles parallel to the axis of wave propagation

(B) surface vibrating particles

(C) motion of particles perpendicular to the axis of wave propagation

(D) twisting action of the particles in motion

118. Ultrasound wave propagation causes displacement of particles in a medium. The regions of greatest particle concentration are called

(A) acoustic impedance

(B) compression

(C) rarefactions

(D) attenuation

119. Ultrasound wave propagation causes displacement of particles in a medium. The regions of lowest particle concentration are called

(A) acoustic impedance

(B) condensations

(C) rarefactions

(D) attenuation

120. The prefix piezo is derived from a Greek word that denotes

(A) electric

(B) transducer

(C) crystal

(D) pressure

121. Axial resolution is

(A) the ability to distinguish two objects parallel to the ultrasound beam

(B) the ability to distinguish two objects perpendicular to the ultrasound beam

(C) the same as depth, longitudinal, and range resolution

(D) the same as azimuthal, angular, and transverse resolution

(E) both A and D

(F) both A and C

122. Lateral resolution is

(A) the same as depth, longitudinal, and range resolution
(B) the ability to distinguish two objects perpendicular to the ultrasound beam
(C) the ability to distinguish two objects parallel to the ultrasound beam
(D) the same as azimuthal, angular, and transverse resolution
(E) both A and B
(F) both B and D

Questions 123 through 131: Match the structures in Fig. 1–29 with the list of parts given.

123. _____
124. _____
125. _____
126. _____
127. _____
128. _____
129. _____
130. _____
131. _____

(A) tuning coil
(B) damping material
(C) electrical connector
(D) piezoelectric ceramic material
(E) housing
(F) shield
(G) matching layer
(H) backing material
(I) face material

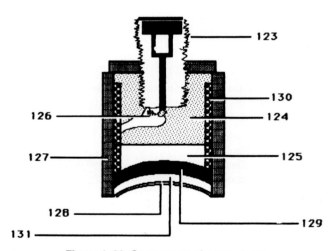

Figure 1–29. Components of a transducer.

Questions 132 through 140: Match the structures in Fig. 1–30 with the list of parts given.

132. _____
133. _____
134. _____
135. _____
136. _____
137. _____
138. _____
139. _____
140. _____

(A) cathode
(B) Y-plate
(C) glass screen
(D) electron gun
(E) evacuated glass
(F) X-plate
(G) control grid
(H) electron beam
(I) focusing lens

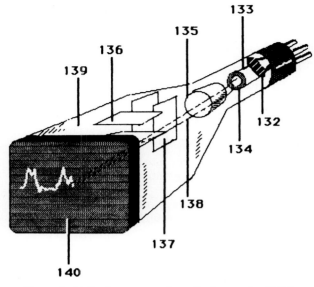

Figure 1–30. Basic structure of a cathode ray tube (CRT).

141. If frequency increases, the wavelength will

(A) decrease
(B) increase
(C) increase 10 times
(D) remain the same

142. If frequency decreases, the wavelength will

(A) decrease
(B) increase
(C) increase 10 times
(D) remain the same

143. As frequency increases, the resolution will

(A) decrease
(B) increase
(C) increase 10 times
(D) remain the same

144. As frequency increases, the resolution will

(A) decrease
(B) increase
(C) increase 10 times
(D) remain the same

145. As frequency increases, the beam width will

(A) decrease
(B) increase
(C) increase 10 times
(D) remain the same

146. Ultrasound has difficulty in propagating through

(A) air
(B) bone
(C) $BaSO_4$
(D) IVP contrast
(E) all of the above
(F) A, B, and C only
(G) A and B only

147. Which of the following *cannot* be used a coupling medium?

(A) water
(B) saline
(C) barium sulfate
(D) aqueous gels

148. Attenuation denotes

(A) progressive weakening of the sound beam as it travels
(B) density of tissue and the speed of sound in the tissues
(C) the redirection of the ultrasound back to the transducer
(D) bending of the transmitted wave after crossing an interface

149. The piezoelectric effect can be best described as

(A) density of tissue and the speed of sound in the tissues
(B) mechanical deformation that results from high voltage applied on faces of the crystal, and in turn generate ultrasound
(C) Piezoelectric crystals subject to pressure resulting in an electrical charge appearing on their surfaces.
(D) having a damaging effect on crystal because of high voltage

150. The reverse piezoelectric effect can be best described as

(A) density of tissue and the speed of sound in the tissues
(B) mechanical deformation that results from high voltage applied on faces of the crystal, and, as a result, generate ultrasound
(C) piezoelectric crystals subjected to pressures resulting in electrical charges appearing on their surfaces
(D) having a damaging effect on crystal because of high voltage

151. The parameter used to express attenuation is

(A) $\left(\dfrac{z_2 - z_1}{z_2 + z_1} \right)^2 \times 100$

(B) $dB = 10 \log_{10} \dfrac{l_2}{l_1}$

(C) $Z = pV$

(D) $\dfrac{\sin i}{\sin r} = \dfrac{V_1}{V_2}$

152. A waveform transfers ____ from one point in space to another point in space.

(A) particles
(B) matter
(C) energy
(D) mass

153. In a mechanical wave, there are material particles that

(A) oscillate around an equilibrium point
(B) move forward at a set rate
(C) move away from an equilibrium point
(D) move backward at a set rate

154. Wavelength is a measure of

(A) time
(B) voltage
(C) distance
(D) pulse duration

155. Ultrasonic waves are

(A) mechanical
(B) x-ray
(C) electromagnetic
(D) solar

156. Acoustic impedance is

(A) the amount of tissue × the speed of sound in tissue
(B) the density of tissue × the speed of sound in tissue
(C) the transducer frequency × the speed of sound in tissue
(D) the distance from one interface to the next

157. Amplitude is measured in

(A) W/cm^2
(B) $A = pV$
(C) $\dfrac{\sin i}{\sin r} = \dfrac{V_1}{V_2}$
(D) dB

158. The spectrum of ultrasonic frequency is

(A) less than 20 Hz
(B) above 20,000 Hz
(C) 20–20,000 Hz
(D) 1–3 million Hz

159. Period is inversely proportional to

(A) velocity
(B) watts
(C) hertz
(D) frequency

160. In a pulse–echo system, as the ultrasound beam becomes more perpendicular to the organ interface

(A) scattering becomes greater
(B) there are more refracted echoes
(C) there are fewer specular echoes
(D) the received echoes will be larger

161. A decibel (dB) describes the

(A) ratio of two sound intensities
(B) sum of two sound intensities
(C) amount of scattering
(D) velocity of the sound wave

162. Axial resolution is also known as all of the following except

(A) depth
(B) range
(C) azimuthal
(D) longitudinal

163. Which of the following has the highest sound velocity?

(A) soft tissue
(B) bone
(C) air
(D) water

164. According to the AIUM, no significant biologic effects have been proved in mammals exposed to

(A) SPTA intensities above 100 mW/cm^2
(B) SPTA intensities below 100 mW/cm^2
(C) SPTP intensities below 10 mW/cm^2
(D) SATP intensities below 2 mW/cm^2

165. Temporal peak intensity is measured at

(A) the time the pulse is present
(B) the center of the beam
(C) the time cavitation occurs
(D) none of the above

166. Which of the following has the lowest intensity?

(A) SPTP
(B) SATP
(C) SPTA
(D) SATA

167. What is the definition of the beam uniformity ratio?

(A) the spatial average intensity divided by the spatial intensity

(B) the spatial peak intensity divided by the spatial average intensity
(C) the temporal average intensity divided by the spatial average intensity
(D) the temporal peak intensity divided by the spatial peak intensity

168. The duty factor of a pulsed echo system is normally less than

(A) 10%
(B) 100%
(C) 1%
(D) 25%

169. A shortened spatial pulse length results in

(A) better lateral resolution
(B) low frequency
(C) poor resolution
(D) better axial resolution

170. The equation for measuring the relationship among velocity, frequency, and wavelength is

(A) $\left(\dfrac{z_2 - z_1}{z_2 + z_1} \right)^2 \times 100$

(B) $V = f \lambda$

(C) $Z = pV$

(D) $\dfrac{\sin i}{\sin r} = \dfrac{V_1}{V_2}$

171. Attenuation of an ultrasound beam can occur by

(A) divergence of a beam
(B) scattering
(C) reflection
(D) all of the above

172. Attenuation coefficient of sound can be defined by which of the following?

(A) dB/cm/MHz
(B) dB/cm^2/Hz
(C) cm/Hz/dB
(D) m/dB/cm^3

173. If the transducer Q factor is low, the bandwidth will be

(A) narrow
(B) high
(C) wide
(D) low

174. Axial resolution can be improved by

(A) reducing the spatial pulse length
(B) increasing the spatial pulse length
(C) lowering the transducer frequency
(D) all of the above

175. Axial resolution is primarily affected by

    (A) beam width
    (B) spatial pulse length
    (C) strength of the echo
    (D) velocity of the medium

176. Which of the following will improve both axial and lateral resolution?

    (A) short pulse length
    (B) narrow beam width
    (C) increase beam diameter
    (D) increase transducer frequency

177. All of the following are also known as lateral resolution except

    (A) azimuthal
    (B) transverse
    (C) range
    (D) angular

178. Continuous wave Doppler has a duty factor of

    (A) less than 1%
    (B) 100%
    (C) greater than 100%
    (D) 50%

179. Acoustic impedance is defined as

    (A) density × propagation speed
    (B) frequency × propagation
    (C) elasticity + propagation
    (D) density × elasticity

180. Acoustic impedance is defined by which of the following?

    (A) rayons
    (B) meters/dB
    (C) mW/cm^2
    (D) rayls

181. Acoustic impedance is not dependent on which of the following?

    (A) frequency
    (B) density
    (C) stiffness
    (D) none of the above

182. The height of the vertical spike on the A-mode display corresponds to

    (A) the strength of the echo
    (B) the distance to the reflector
    (C) round-trip time of the echo
    (D) the pulse repetition frequency

183. B-mode ultrasound includes all of the following except

    (A) static scans
    (B) M-mode scans
    (C) real-time scans
    (D) all of the above are B-mode

184. The correct equation for calculating the percentage of reflection is

    (A) $R = \left(\dfrac{Z_2 - Z_1}{Z_2 + Z_1} \right)^2 \times 100$

    (B) $R = \dfrac{Z_1 \times Z_2}{2}$

    (C) $R = \sqrt{Z_1 + Z_2 \times \pi}$

    (D) $R = \dfrac{Z_1 \times Z_2}{Z_1 + Z_2}$

185. The reflection coefficient between water and air is

    (A) 1%
    (B) 50%
    (C) 75%
    (D) nearly 100%

186. What happens to the ultrasound beam beyond the critical angle?

    (A) 100% is transmitted
    (B) 100% is reflected
    (C) 75% is transmitted, 25% is reflected
    (D) 75% is reflected, 25% is transmitted

187. Rayleigh scattering occurs if the particle dimensions are

    (A) less than the wavelength
    (B) greater than 3 mm
    (C) greater than the wavelength
    (D) none of the above

188. One of the acoustic parameters that determines the intensity of an ultrasound wave is

    (A) waveform
    (B) particle displacement
    (C) period
    (D) power

189. Power is defined as energy per unit

    (A) mass
    (B) distance
    (C) time
    (D) force

190. The ability to resolve structures lying perpendicular to the axis of the ultrasound beam is called

    (A) lateral resolution
    (B) axial resolution
    (C) depth resolution
    (D) longitudinal resolution

191. In most soft tissue, the attenuation coefficient varies approximately

    (A) inversely with frequency
    (B) with the square of the frequency
    (C) logarithmically with frequency
    (D) directly with frequency

192. Ultrasound absorption in a medium results in

    (A) conversion of ultrasound into heat
    (B) dissipation of ultrasound into x-rays
    (C) conversion of ultrasound into visible light
    (D) dissipation of ultrasound into gamma rays

193. The typical value of attenuation in soft tissue is

    (A) 2 dB/cm²/Hz
    (B) 1 dB/cm/Hz
    (C) 2 dB/cm²/MHz
    (D) 0.5 dB/cm/MHz

194. False echoes are produced by

    (A) reflection
    (B) rarefaction
    (C) reverberation
    (D) diffraction

195. Approximately what percentage of the ultrasound beam will be transmitted between fat and muscle?

    (A) 1%
    (B) 10%
    (C) 50%
    (D) 99%

196. Huygens' principle describes

    (A) multiple point sources
    (B) refraction
    (C) velocity
    (D) cathode ray tubes

197. Enhancement occurs posterior to

    (A) strong attenuations
    (B) weak attenuations
    (C) strong diffractors
    (D) weak diffractors

198. The role of sound attenuation in tissue is expressed in terms of

    (A) half-value layer
    (B) Huygens's principle
    (C) duty cycle
    (D) spatial peak

199. Improper location of an echo may be attributable to

    (A) shadowing
    (B) Huygens's principle
    (C) density error
    (D) propagation speed error

200. The range equation explains

    (A) side lobes
    (B) distance to reflector
    (C) attenuation
    (D) calibration

201. For a specular reflector

    (A) the angle of incidence is equal to the angle of reflection
    (B) the angle of incidence is greater than the angle of reflection
    (C) there is no dependence on beam angle
    (D) the angle of incidence is less than the angle of reflection

202. Which of the following is determined by the medium?

    (A) intensity
    (B) period
    (C) propagation speed
    (D) amplitude

203. Which of the following is not an acoustic variable?

    (A) density
    (B) pressure
    (C) temperature
    (D) force

204. TGC denotes

    (A) tissue gain characteristic
    (B) time gain compensation
    (C) transducer generator control
    (D) temperature generator control

205. The propagation speed for fat is

    (A) higher than 1540 m/s
    (B) lower than 1540 m/s
    (C) equal to 1540 m/s
    (D) cannot be measured

206. Which of the following has a propagation speed closest to the average soft tissue?

    (A) bone
    (B) air
    (C) fat
    (D) muscle

207. Arrange the following media in terms of propagation velocity, from lowest to highest.

    (A) air, fat, muscle, bone
    (B) bone, fat, air, muscle
    (C) bone, muscle, fat, air
    (D) muscle, air, fat, bone

208. As frequency increases, backscatter

    (A) decreases
    (B) is not affected
    (C) increases
    (D) is reflected

209. The angle at which total reflection occurs is called

    (A) critical angle
    (B) warp angle
    (C) reflectivity angle
    (D) diffraction angle

210. The pulse repetition frequency is the number of pulses occurring per

    (A) wave
    (B) returning echo
    (C) microsecond
    (D) second

211. The unit(s) used for the duty factor is (are)

    (A) rayls
    (B) m/s/Hz
    (C) m/μs/MHz
    (D) unitless

212. The typical value for attenuation coefficient for 6 MHz ultrasound in soft tissue is

    (A) 3 dB/cm
    (B) 1 dB/cm/Hz
    (C) 3 dB/cm^2
    (D) 2 dB

213. Normal incidence occurs when the ultrasound beam travels ____ to the boundary between the two media

    (A) parallel
    (B) perpendicular
    (C) obliquely
    (D) at 1540 m/s

214. The amount of energy transmitted and/or reflected at the boundary between two media depends on

    (A) acoustic impedance mismatch
    (B) the frequency of the beam
    (C) the propagation speed of the first medium
    (D) the propagation speed of the second medium

215. Which of the following has a higher acoustic impedance coefficient?

    (A) solid
    (B) liquid
    (C) gas
    (D) all the above have an equal acoustic impedance coefficient

216. According to Snell's law, the transmission angle is greater than the incidence angle if the propagation speed

    (A) of medium 2 is greater than that of medium 1
    (B) of medium 1 is greater than that of medium 2
    (C) of the two media are equal
    (D) is calculated at 3 dB down

217. According to the range equation, which of the following are necessary to calculate the distance to the reflector?

    (A) attenuation coefficient and type of reflector
    (B) density and type of reflector
    (C) propagation speed and pulse round-trip time
    (D) density and pulse round-trip time

218. The mirror image artifact is commonly seen around which of the following structures?

    (A) kidney
    (B) pancreas
    (C) spleen
    (D) diaphragm

219. The comet tail artifact can be seen posterior to an object that has

    (A) a much lower acoustic impedance than its surroundings
    (B) a much higher acoustic impedance than it surroundings
    (C) either a much lower or a much higher acoustic impedance than its surroundings
    (D) the same acoustic impedance as its surroundings

220. Which of the following may produce the comet tail artifact?

    (A) liver–kidney interface
    (B) spleen–kidney interface
    (C) tissue–gas interface
    (D) gas–fluid interface

221. If the ultrasound beam passes through a mass in the liver that contains fat, how might the diaphragmatic echo posterior to it appear?

    (A) closer than it really is
    (B) farther than it really is
    (C) will not be affected
    (D) will not be visualized

222. Bandwidth can be increased by

    (A) increasing the quality factor
    (B) increased frequency
    (C) increasing pulse length
    (D) increasing damping

223. Which of the following will not affect the echo intensity in the image?

    (A) output power
    (B) overall gain
    (C) time gain curve
    (D) all of the above

224. On some sonographic equipment, adjusting the compression will affect which of the following processes?

(A) slope position
(B) dynamic range
(C) output
(D) balance

225. Generally, ultrasound transducers have

(A) better axial resolution than lateral resolution
(B) better lateral resolution than axial resolution
(C) better azimuthal resolution than radial resolution
(D) equal axial resolution and lateral resolution

226. The pulse repetition frequency of an ultrasound unit is typically

(A) 1 Hz
(B) 10 Hz
(C) 100 Hz
(D) 1,000 Hz

227. B-mode display denotes

(A) basic modulator
(B) beam motion
(C) beam modulator
(D) brightness modulation

228. What percentage of the time is a typical pulsed ultrasound system capable of receiving echoes?

(A) 100%
(B) 99.9%
(C) 75%
(D) 50%

229. If the frequency doubles, what happens to the wavelength?

(A) increases fourfold
(B) increases twofold
(C) decreases by one-half
(D) no relationship to wavelength

230. Which of the following does not display a sector format?

(A) linear-sequenced array
(B) electronic-phased array
(C) mechanical rotating wheel
(D) mechanical wobbler

231. The equation for measuring acoustic impedance is

(A) $\left(\dfrac{z_2 - z_1}{z_2 + z_1}\right)^2 \times 100$

(B) $V = f\lambda$

(C) $Z = \rho V$

(D) $\dfrac{\sin i}{\sin r} = \dfrac{V_1}{V_2}$

232. Which of the following are most commonly used ultrasound transducers?

(A) lead zirconate titanate (PZT)
(B) barium sulfate
(C) metaniobate
(D) quartz

233. Transmit-delay focusing in a linear array transducer will

(A) improve axial resolution
(B) improve lateral resolution
(C) improve the frequency
(D) decrease the depth of penetration

234. For real-time systems, which of the following is not related to the other?

(A) frame rate
(B) lines per frame
(C) pulse repetition frequency
(D) frequency

235. The pulse repetition frequency is

(A) pulses emitted per second
(B) time from the beginning of one pulse to the beginning of the next
(C) the time during which the purse actually occurs
(D) cannot be defined

236. Which of the following is not a role of the pulser?

(A) driving the transducer
(B) telling the receiver when the ultrasound pulses are produced
(C) telling the memory when ultrasound pulses are produced
(D) beam steering

237. Demodulation is a process of

(A) converting the voltage delivered to the receiver from one form to another
(B) decreasing the differences between the smallest and largest amplitudes
(C) eliminating the smaller amplitude voltage produced by electronic noise
(D) rejecting weak echoes to reduce noise

238. Which of the following are not operator adjustable?

(A) compensation and rejection
(B) amplification and compensation
(C) demodulation and compression
(D) rejection and amplification

239. Which of the following varies with distance from the transducer?

(A) lateral resolution
(B) frequency

(C) axial resolution
(D) spatial pulse length

240. A period can be described by which number on the following diagram?

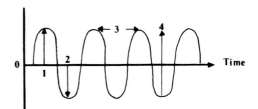

(A) #2
(B) #1
(C) #3
(D) #4

241. Increasing axial resolution by increasing frequency also results in

(A) increasing penetration
(B) decreasing half-intensity depth
(C) decreasing the pulse repetition frequency
(D) none of the above

242. Reflection refers to

(A) the bending of the ultrasound beam as it crosses a boundary
(B) conversion of ultrasound to heat
(C) redirection of a portion of the ultrasound beam from a boundary
(D) the scattering of the ultrasound beam in many directions

243. Digital computers use a special number system called

(A) digital number system
(B) alphanumeric system
(C) chronologic system
(D) binary number system

244. The term *bit* in computer science denotes

(A) binary digit
(B) buffer
(C) baud rate
(D) BASIC programming

245. An 8-bit binary number is referred to as

(A) byte
(B) baud rate
(C) buffer register
(D) BUS

246. Which of the following is not an example of computer hardware?

(A) monitor
(B) program
(C) disk drive
(D) printer

247. The acronym RAM denotes

(A) reset-auxiliary memory
(B) random-access memory
(C) retailing American microcomputers
(D) retailing American machines

248. The acronym ROM denotes

(A) read-only memory
(B) read-only modem
(C) retailing only microcomputers
(D) run-output machine

249. Which of the following is not an input device?

(A) keyboard
(B) printer
(C) disk drive
(D) magnetic disk

250. The type of permanent memory that is produced at the time of manufacture and cannot be changed by the computer user is called

(A) RAM
(B) ROM
(C) PROM
(D) EPROM

251. The type of programmable memory that allows the user to write, store, or erase data is called

(A) PLA
(B) ROM
(C) PROM
(D) EPROM

252. CPU denotes

(A) computer program update
(B) central processing unit
(C) capacitor power unit
(D) computer portable unit

253. The most common binary word length in microprocessors is

(A) 8, 16, or 32 bits
(B) 12 or 24 bits
(C) 128K bytes
(D) 64K bytes

254. An 8-bit word microcomputer with 128K words of memory can store how many bits of data?

(A) 1000
(B) 128,000

(C) 1,048,576
(D) 128

255. The contents of EPROM can be completely erased by which of the following applications?

(A) light waves
(B) infrared
(C) ultrasound
(D) ultraviolet light

256. A sonographic image can be transferred from one computer to another by way of

(A) fixed disk drive
(B) modem
(C) printer
(D) keyboard

257. The most commonly used programming language for personal computer is

(A) COBOL
(B) FORTRAN
(C) BASIC
(D) LOGO

258. The unit for measuring the speed of data communication is called

(A) buffer
(B) booting
(C) output unit
(D) baud rate

259. Which of the following disks has the highest storage capacity and fastest access time?

(A) $3\frac{1}{2}$-in microfloppy double density
(B) hard disk
(C) $5\frac{1}{4}$-in minifloppy
(D) $3\frac{1}{2}$-in microfloppy high density

260. The acronym BASIC denotes

(A) basic American scientific instructional code
(B) basic American scientific information center
(C) beginner's all-purpose symbolic instruction code
(D) business application software information center

261. A modem is an electronic device that

(A) simulates human voice
(B) prints data
(C) translates signals from digital into analog and analog into digital
(D) senses data from a card inserted into it

262. Each binary digit in a binary number is represented in memory by a memory element, which at any time is in one of ____ states.

(A) many
(B) 2
(C) 10
(D) none of the above

263. In binary numbers, how many values are used for each digit?

(A) 10
(B) multiples of 10
(C) 2
(D) 5

264. The number 30 in binary is

(A) 0110
(B) 1110
(C) 1001
(D) 1111
(E) none of the above

265. How many gray levels (echo amplitude levels) can a 4-bit deep digital scan converter store?

(A) 2
(B) 4
(C) 8
(D) 16
(E) 32

266. An ultrasound instrument that could represent 64 shades of gray would required a(n) ____ bit memory

(A) 8
(B) 6
(C) 4
(D) 16

267. Which of the following are effects seen in tissue at high ultrasound intensities?

(A) fusion, ionization
(B) heating, cavitation
(C) expansion, encrustation
(D) reabsorption, dehydration

268. Which of the following is the correct list of functions performed by the receiver system in the ultrasound machine (B-scanner)?

(A) inspection, detection, correction, rejection, depression
(B) randomization, amplification, modulation, rectification, limitation
(C) amplification, compensation, compression, rejection
(D) expansion, contraction, band limitation, sonification

269. A large amplitude pulse from the pulser results in

(A) a long duration pulse from the transducer
(B) a short duration pulse from the transducer

(C) shutdown of the receiver
(D) a large amplitude pulse from the transducer
(E) a large amplitude pulse from the display

270. Voltage pulses from the pulser go to the

(A) transducer and display
(B) transducer and receiver
(C) transducer and TGC control
(D) display and image memory
(E) amplifier and receiver

271. The five major components of a pulse–echo ultrasound system are

(A) flux capacitor, image memory, transducer, scan arm, amplifier
(B) interrossitor, pulser, receiver, display, power supply
(C) image memory, display, scan arm, TGC control, foot switch
(D) transducer, receiver, image memory, pulser, display

272. Transducers are focused by two major methods: internal focusing and external focusing. These methods can be accomplished by

(A) thickening the crystal and adding a water path
(B) cutting a curved transducer element and/or using an acoustic lens
(C) "doping" the crystal with metal ions and damping
(D) using a crystal pulse and a bandwidth limiter
(E) all of the above will focus a transducer element

273. The unit applied to the Q factor (quality factor) that describes the ratio of operating frequency to bandwidth is called

(A) megahertz (MHz)
(B) percentage
(C) millimeter per microsecond
(D) Fresnel
(E) none of the above; Q factor is unitless

Questions 274 through 282: Match the terms in Column A with the correct definition in Column B.

COLUMN A

274. acoustic shadow _____

275. acoustic enhancement _____

276. anechoic _____
277. artifact _____
278. echogenic _____
279. hyperechoic _____
280. hypoechoic _____
281. interface _____
282. sonolucent _____

COLUMN B

(A) without echoes
(B) echoes of lower amplitude than the normal surrounding tissues
(C) the surface forming the boundary between two media having different acoustic impedance
(D) an echo that does not correspond to the real target
(E) reduction in echoes from a region distal to an attenuating structure
(F) a tissue or structure that does not have internal echoes (echo-free)
(G) an increase in echoes from a region distal to a weakly attenuating structure or tissue
(H) echoes of higher amplitude than the normal surrounding tissues
(I) a structure that possesses echoes

283. The backing material that is usually constructed in a continuous-wave Doppler transducer is

(A) epoxy resin
(B) cork
(C) air
(D) tungsten powder

284. Transducers with continuous-wave operation are commonly used in which of the following applications?

(A) diagnostic, surgical, therapeutic, and Doppler
(B) diagnostic and surgical
(C) diagnostic and Doppler
(D) surgical, therapeutic, and Doppler

285. Which of the following waves are visible under normal conditions?

(A) water waves
(B) x-ray waves
(C) radio waves
(D) sound waves

286. Ultrasound can travel in all of the following *except*

(A) IVP contrast
(B) solid tissue
(C) vacuum
(D) blood

287. Lambda (λ) represents

(A) period
(B) wavelength
(C) frequency
(D) velocity

288. The time it takes to complete a single cycle is called

(A) period
(B) wavelength
(C) frequency
(D) velocity

289. A wave vibration at 20 cycles per second has frequency of

(A) 20 MHz
(B) 20 Hz
(C) 20 kHz
(D) 120 kHz

290. A wave vibrating at 1 million cycles per second has a frequency of

(A) 1 GHz
(B) 1 kHz
(C) 1 MHz
(D) 100 MHz

291. The device that produces the ultrasound beam is commonly called a

(A) cathode-ray tube (CRT)
(B) scan converter
(C) transducer
(D) mechanical arm

Questions 292 through 294: Match the question in Column A with the correct answer in Column B.

COLUMN A

292. Which statement best describes A-mode? _____

293. Which statement best describes B-mode? _____

294. Which statement best describes M-mode? _____

COLUMN B

(A) a graphic presentation with vertical spikes arising from a horizontal baseline; the height of the vertical spikes represents the amplitude of the deflected echo

(B) a two-dimensional image of internal body structures displayed as dots; the brightness of the dots is proportional to the amplitude of the echo; the image is applicable to both real-time and static scanners

(C) a graphic presentation of moving structures in a waveform; the display is presented as a group of lines representing the motion of moving interfaces versus time

(D) unidimensional presentation of moving structures displayed in a pie-shaped or rectangular image; the image is applicable only to real-time scanners

295. Which of the following is *not* an essential part of the cathode-ray tube (CRT)?

(A) electron gun
(B) fluorescent screen
(C) silicon
(D) deflection system (horizontal and vertical plates)

296. The CRT used in ultrasound usually encloses

(A) air
(B) vacuum
(C) oil
(D) gas

297. The positively (+) charged CRT terminal is called the

(A) anode
(B) cathode
(C) both anode and cathode
(D) diode

298. The negatively (–) charged CRT terminal is called the

(A) anode
(B) cathode
(C) both anode and cathode
(D) diode

299. The intensity of the ultrasound beam

(A) is measured in watts
(B) is always constant
(C) depends on the beam diameter
(D) is measured with the AIUM phantom

300. Whose principal states, "All points on an ultrasound waveform can be considered as point sources for the production of secondary spherical wavelets"?

(A) Doppler's
(B) Curie's
(C) Huygens's
(D) Young's

301. The fraction of time that a pulsed ultrasound system is actually producing ultrasound is called the

(A) duty factor
(B) Curie factor
(C) frame rate
(D) transmission factor

302. Real-time ultrasound instrumentation can be classified as

(A) annular, sector, linear, and static scanners
(B) sector scanners only
(C) sector, linear, and annular scanners
(D) static scanners only

303. The speed at which ultrasound propagates within a medium depends primarily on

(A) its frequency
(B) the compressibility of the medium
(C) its intensity
(D) the thickness of the medium

304. An artifact that results from a pulse that has traveled two or more round-trip distances between the transducer and the interface is called

(A) a multipath
(B) a side lobe
(C) reverberation
(D) scattering

305. The ratio of output of electric power to input electric power is termed

(A) power
(B) intensity
(C) gain
(D) voltage

306. Multipath artifacts result from

(A) echoes that return directly to the transducer
(B) shotgun pellets
(C) echoes that take an indirect path back to the transducer
(D) none of the above

307. A scan converter will accept echo signals from the receiver and store them in the "memory" of the instrument. Identify the types of memory used in scan converters.

(A) gray scale and bistable
(B) analog and digital
(C) static and real-time
(D) none of the above

308. To achieve the best possible digital representation of an analog system, the echo signals should undergo

(A) postprocessing
(B) preprocessing
(C) rectification
(D) amplification

309. Near zone length may be increased by increasing

(A) wavelength
(B) wavelength and bandwidth
(C) transducer diameter
(D) frequency and transducer diameter

Questions 310 through 319: Match the terms in Column A with the correct definition in Column B.

COLUMN A

310. density _____

COLUMN B

(A) rate at which work is done

311. propagation _____
312. frequency _____
313. power _____
314. duty factor _____
315. bandwidth _____
316. acoustic impedance _____
317. absorption _____
318. quality factor _____
319. intensity _____

(B) mass divided by volume
(C) conversion of sound to heat
(D) number of cycles per unit time
(E) density multiplied by sound propagation speed
(F) range of frequencies contained in the ultrasound pulse
(G) the product of pulse duration and pulse repetition rate
(H) progression or travel
(I) operating frequency divided by bandwidth
(J) power divided by area

320. Which of the following is a true definition for a highly damped transducer?

(A) increased efficiency, sensitivity, and spatial pulse length
(B) decreased efficiency, sensitivity, and spatial pulse length
(C) increased efficiency and sensitivity, but decreased spatial pulse length
(D) decreased efficiency, but increased sensitivity and spatial pulse length

321. Gain compensation is necessary due to

(A) reflector motion
(B) gray scale
(C) attenuation
(D) resolution

322. The frequency bandwidth may be determined by which of the following?

(A) spectral analysis
(B) Schlieren system
(C) hydrophone analysis
(D) cathode analysis

323. Analog scan converters

(A) function perfectly as peak deflectors
(B) have greater image sharpness than digital
(C) store any increment of signal amplitude
(D) have better image uniformity than digital scan converters

324. The gray-scale resolution for a 5-bit digital instrument that has a dynamic range of 42 dB is

(A) 1.9 dB
(B) 3 dB
(C) 1.3 dB
(D) 0.07 dB

325. If it takes 0.01 second for a pulse emitted by the transducer to reach an echo source of soft tissue, what distance must the pulse travel to be recorded?

(A) 1,540 cm
(B) 30.8 m
(C) 15.4 m
(D) both A and C

326. An artifact that is produced from interaction of the incident beam with a curved surface and results in an acoustic shadow is referred to as

(A) a ghost artifact
(B) an edge artifact
(C) a comet tail artifact
(D) a ring down artifact

327. An artifact that results from refraction of the ultrasound beam at a muscle–fat interface and give rise to double images is called

(A) a split image artifact
(B) an edge artifact
(C) a comet tail artifact
(D) a ring down artifact

328. An artifact that would *least* likely produce a pseudo-mass is

(A) a comet tail artifact
(B) a multipath artifact
(C) a mirror image artifact
(D) a slide lobe artifact

329. Split image artifact is more noticeable in

(A) athletic patients and mesomorphic habitus patients
(B) patients with underdeveloped rectus muscle
(C) mesomorphic habitus patients and patients with underdeveloped rectus muscle
(D) all of the above

330. Select the least likely cause or causes for a split image artifact.

(A) abdominal scar
(B) lateral margins of the rectus muscles
(C) gas bubble
(D) refraction of the sound beam at a muscle–fat interface

331. The most likely cause for a beam thickness artifact is

(A) metallic surgical clips
(B) gas bubble
(C) partial volume effect
(D) shotgun pellets

332. Beam thickness artifact is primarily dependent on

(A) position of the patient
(B) gas bubble
(C) beam angulation
(D) gravity

333. Which of the following is not true for side lobe artifact?

(A) caused by multiple side lobes of the transducer
(B) apparent in real-time image
(C) may be diffuse or specular in appearance
(D) not visible on real-time image

334. Which of the following is least likely to produce an acoustic shadow?

(A) bone interface
(B) metallic surgical clips
(C) gallstones
(D) gas interface

335. The most common type of artifact encountered in patients with shotgun wounds is

(A) comet tail artifact
(B) multipath artifact
(C) mirror image artifact
(D) side lobe artifact

336. The type of reverberation echo that usually results from a small gas bubble and appears as a high-amplitude echo occurring at regular intervals is called a

(A) multipath artifact
(B) mirror image artifact
(C) side lobe artifact
(D) ring-down artifact

337. The amount of splitting that occurs in a split image artifact for a given structure

(A) can be calculated using Snell's law
(B) cannot be calculated because it is an artifact
(C) can be calculated using the equation $Z = pV$
(D) can be calculated using a 5-MHz transducer with the equation: split (m/s) $= D\pi/T$

338. The first vertical deflection on the A-mode that corresponds to the transducer face is called

(A) bistable
(B) side lobe
(C) main bang
(D) gain

339. The type of real-time system that employs a combination of electronic and mechanical means is called

(A) wobbler sector real-time
(B) rotating wheel real-time
(C) annular-array real-time
(D) linear-sequenced array

340. If the amount of acoustic coupling medium is insufficient, what changes could result?

(A) decrease in amplitude of the returning echo
(B) increase in amplitude of the returning echo
(C) the transducer will slide on the skin easier
(D) no effect on the image

341. Which of the following is not a hard copy?

(A) x-ray film
(B) Polaroid film
(C) dye sublimation color print
(D) videotape recorder

Questions 342 through 344: Each diagram represents modes of operation used in diagnostic ultrasound.

342. Identify the type of mode displayed in the following diagram.

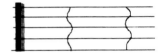

(A) B-mode
(B) A-mode
(C) M-mode
(D) R-mode

343. Identify the type of mode displayed in the following diagram.

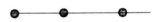

(A) B-mode
(B) A-mode
(C) M-mode
(D) R-mode

344. Identify the type of mode displayed in the following diagram.

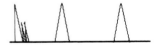

(A) B-mode
(B) A-mode
(C) M-mode
(D) R-mode

345. The effects of diagnostic ultrasound on human soft tissue are called

(A) sensitivity effects
(B) biologic effects
(C) neurologic effects
(D) pressure effect

346. The average propagation speed of ultrasound in soft tissue is

(A) 1.54 mm/µs
(B) 741 mph
(C) 1560 m/s
(D) 331 mm/s

Questions 347 through 350: Identify the regions on the diagram below by filling in the blanks.

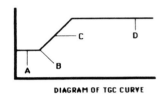

DIAGRAM OF TGC CURVE

347. slope _____
348. delay _____
349. far gain _____
350. near gain _____

Questions 351 through 360: Match the terms in Column A with the correct definition in Column B.

COLUMN A

351. attenuation _____
352. bistable _____
353. bit _____
354. cavitation _____
355. coupling medium _____
356. damping _____
357. gray scale _____
358. matching layer _____
359. pixel _____
360. static imaging _____

COLUMN B

(A) picture element
(B) the production and behavior of bubbles in sound
(C) progressive weakening of the sound beam as it travels through a medium
(D) a liquid placed between the transducer and the skin
(E) the number of intensity levels between black and white
(F) having two stages
(G) binary digit
(H) a method of reducing pulse duration by electrical or mechanical means
(I) single-frame imaging
(J) plastic material placed in front of the transducer face to reduce the reflection at the transducer surface

361. The intensity of ultrasound is measured in

(A) kg/m³
(B) N/m²
(C) Hz
(D) W/cm²

362. There is no known adverse biologic effect in tissue at intensities below

(A) 100 mW/cm² SPTA
(B) 1000 mW/cm² SAPA
(C) 10 W/cm² SPTP
(D) 500 m/Wcm² SATA

363. The acronym SPTA denotes

(A) static probe transmission amplitude
(B) static probe transmission absorption
(C) spatial peak temporal average
(D) sound propagation temperature artifact

Questions 364 through 370: Match the quantity in Column A with the correct unit in Column B.

COLUMN A   COLUMN B

364. density _____   (A) W/cm²
365. speed _____   (B) kg/m³
366. frequency _____   (C) m
367. work _____   (D) m/s
368. intensity _____   (E) J
369. wavelength _____   (F) Hz
370. attenuation _____   (G) dB

371. The general range of intensities in diagnostic ultrasound is

(A) 0.5 W/cm²–2.0 W/cm² SPTA
(B) 0.002 W/cm²–0.5 W/cm² SPTA
(C) 50 W/cm²–100 W/cm² SPTA
(D) the general range of intensities in diagnostic ultrasound is unknown

372. The general range of intensities in therapeutic ultrasound is

(A) 0.5 W/cm²–2.0 W/cm² SPTA
(B) 0.002 W/cm²–0.5 W/cm² SPTA
(C) 50 W/cm²–100 W/cm² SPTA
(D) the general range of intensities in therapeutic ultrasound is unknown

373. Which of the following characteristics does *not* apply to diagnostic ultrasound at normal diagnostic intensity levels?

(A) noninvasive
(B) atraumatic
(C) ionizing
(D) nontoxic

374. The most common result of high intensity ultrasound is

(A) cavitation
(B) brain damage
(C) fetal developmental anomalies
(D) heat

375. In the study of bioeffects, cavitation denotes

(A) production and behavior of gas bubbles
(B) necrosis
(C) cell membrane rupture
(D) chromosome breakage

376. The two types of cavitation are

(A) silent and noisy
(B) micro and macro
(C) membrane and nonmembrane
(D) stable and transient

377. An instrument used to detect frequency shift is called

(A) Doppler
(B) real-time
(C) A-mode
(D) static scanner

378. Specular reflections

(A) occur when the interface is larger than the wavelength
(B) occur when the interface is smaller than the wavelength
(C) arise from interfaces smaller than 3 mm
(D) are not dependent on the angle of incidence

379. Nonspecular reflections

(A) occur when the interface is larger than the wavelength
(B) occur when the interface is smaller than the wavelength
(C) arise from mirror-like surfaces
(D) are beam-angle dependent

380. The acronym SATA denotes

(A) static amplitude transmission average
(B) spatial average temporal average
(C) spatial average tissue absorption
(D) sound attenuation transmission average

381. SPPA denotes

(A) static probe power average
(B) static probe transmission absorption
(C) spatial peak pulse average
(D) sound propagation performance average

382. The mode not applicable to a Doppler instrument is

    (A) static
    (B) pulsed
    (C) continuous
    (D) audible

383. Which of the following transducers would be most useful for imaging superficial structures?

    (A) 5-MHz, short-focus
    (B) 3-MHz, long-focus
    (C) 5-MHz, long-focus
    (D) 2.5 MHz, short-focus

384. Which of the following transducers would be most useful for good penetration on an obese patient?

    (A) 5-MHz, short-focus
    (B) 3-MHz, long-focus
    (C) 5-MHz, long-focus
    (D) 2.5 MHz, short-focus

385. The digital memory represents a picture element called a

    (A) pixel
    (B) bistable
    (C) real-time
    (D) matrix

386. How many shades of gray can the human eye distinguish?

    (A) about 16 shades
    (B) between 16 and 32 shades
    (C) more than 64 shades
    (D) more than 124 shades

387. The most recent digital storage employs what size memory?

    (A) $512 \times 512 \times 6$-bit deep
    (B) $64 \times 64 \times 2$-bit deep
    (C) $128 \times 128 \times 4$-bit deep
    (D) $16 \times 16 \times 2$-bit deep

388. A disadvantage of pulsed-wave Doppler (PW) relative to continuous-wave Doppler (CW) is that

    (A) It is unidirectional.
    (B) The Doppler shift depends on frequency.
    (C) It is subject to "aliasing."
    (D) It does not provide in-depth information.

389. Which of the following utilize a TGC?

    (A) static system
    (B) real-time system
    (C) bistable system
    (D) all of the above

390. What is the effect of ultrasound absorption on tissues at normal intensity levels?

    (A) dissipation of heat by conduction
    (B) significant temperature elevations
    (C) significantly lowered temperature
    (D) necrosis

391. Video monitors normally have how many horizontal lines?

    (A) 16
    (B) 64
    (C) 100
    (D) 525

392. How many frames per second are displayed by a video monitor?

    (A) 525
    (B) 30
    (C) 16
    (D) 60

393. How many times each second does the electron beam scan each field on a standard video monitor to produce a flicker-free display?

    (A) 30
    (B) 60
    (C) 40
    (D) 10

394. The dynamic range of the dots on the average oscilloscope or CRT monitor is

    (A) 50–60 dB
    (B) 20–25 dB
    (C) 125 dB
    (D) 525 dB

395. The term matrix, when referring to digital memory, denotes

    (A) number of rows and columns
    (B) analog
    (C) pixel
    (D) buffer

396. Digital memory can be visualized as

    (A) squares on a checkerboard
    (B) a transducer
    (C) an electron beam
    (D) a hydrophone

397. A region that is anechoic is displayed as

    (A) echo-free
    (B) echogenic
    (C) hyperechoic
    (D) hypoechoic

398. A region that is hyperechoic is

(A) anechoic
(B) echogenic
(C) echo-free
(D) transonic

399. Which of the following cannot be measured by a hydrophone?

(A) pressure amplitude
(B) spatial pulse length
(C) impedance
(D) intensity

400. The hydrophone is made up of

(A) x-rays
(B) transducer elements
(C) ultraviolet lights
(D) all of the above

401. Bioeffects at medium intensity levels on laboratory animals have resulted in

(A) cancer
(B) death
(C) growth retardation
(D) no effects

402. Which of the following is the least likely cause for attenuation?

(A) absorption
(B) reflection
(C) refraction
(D) scattering

403. Absorption refers to

(A) bending of the sound beam crossing a boundary
(B) conversion of sound to heat
(C) redirection of a portion of the sound from a boundary beam
(D) redirection of the sound beam in several directions

404. Diffraction refers to

(A) spreading-out of the ultrasound beam
(B) conversion of sound to heat
(C) redirection of a portion of the sound from a boundary beam
(D) bending of the sound beam crossing a boundary

405. Scattering refers to

(A) bending the sound beam crossing a boundary
(B) conversion of sound to heat
(C) redirection of a portion of the sound from a boundary beam
(D) redirection of the sound beam in several directions

406. The method for sterilizing transducers is

(A) heat sterilization
(B) steam
(C) recommended by the transducer manufacturer
(D) autoclave

407. An example of an acoustic window is

(A) liver interface
(B) rib interface
(C) tissue/air interface
(D) tissue/bone interface

408. The binary number 1010 equals the decimal number

(A) 10
(B) 11
(C) 110
(D) 200

409. Real-time imaging is similar to

(A) static scanning
(B) fluoroscopy
(C) MRI
(D) all of the above

410. When attempting to identify fetal heart motion, the frame rate of the real-time system should be

(A) turned off to avoid confusion
(B) set at a slow rate
(C) set at a fast rate
(D) set at five frames per second

411. Select the recommended orientation for a transverse scan.

(A) all transverse scans should be viewed from the patient's feet
(B) all transverse scans should be viewed from the patient's head
(C) all transverse scans should be viewed lateral from the patient's right side
(D) all transverse scans should be viewed lateral from the patient's left side

412. The recommended orientation for longitudinal scans is

(A) the patient's head to the right of the image and feet to the left of the image
(B) the patient's head to the left of the image and feet to the right of the image
(C) the patient's head to the top (anterior) of the image and feet to the bottom (posterior) of the image
(D) none of the above

413. Demodulation is a function performed by the

(A) pulser
(B) amplifier

(C) receiver

(D) transmitter

414. Which of the following statements about ultrasound waves is not true?

(A) Ultrasound waves are mechanical vibrating energy.

(B) Ultrasound waves can be polarized.

(C) Ultrasound waves are not part of the electromagnetic spectrum.

(D) Ultrasound waves cannot travel in a vacuum.

415. The transducer crystal *most* likely to be employed in high-frequency work, above 18 MHz, is

(A) lithium sulfate

(B) PZT-5

(C) Rochelle salt

(D) quartz

416. The advantage that PZT-5 has over other ceramic materials is that it is

(A) easy to shape

(B) effective at low voltage

(C) inexpensive

(D) all of the above

417. The trade name for lead zirconate titanate is

(A) $BaSO_4$

(B) quartz

(C) PZT-5

(D) synthetic-P

418. How many shades of gray can be displayed using a scan converter with 8 bits per memory element?

(A) 8

(B) 16

(C) 128

(D) 256

419. The transducer that would be best suited for intercostal scanning is

(A) linear-sequenced array real-time

(B) mechanical sector real-time transducer

(C) static with large diameter

(D) no type of transducer can scan between the intercostal space

420. The difference between real-time and fluoroscopy is

(A) Ultrasound does not need contrast media.

(B) Fluoroscopy has potential biologic effects; whereas, ultrasound has no known biologic effects at normal intensity level.

(C) Ultrasound is nonionizing.

(D) A movie-like image is displayed; whereas, real-time displays a single frame image.

(E) all of the above

(F) A and D

(G) A, B, and C

421. Which of the following contract media used in x-ray do *not* obscure the propagation of ultrasound?

(A) barium sulfate ($BaSO_4$) for upper GI examination

(B) hypaque for IVP examination

(C) air for lower GI examination

(D) telepaque for oral cholecystogram

(E) C and D

(F) B and D

(G) none of the above

(H) all of the above

Questions 422 through 430: Match each term in Column A with the correct definition in Column B.

COLUMN A	COLUMN B
422. acoustic lens _____	(A) unit of impedance
423. pixel _____	(B) the portion of the sound beam outside of the main beam
424. sector _____	
425. acousto-optical converter _____	(C) picture element
426. side lobe _____	(D) pie shaped
427. wavefront _____	(E) a change in frequency as a result of reflector motion between the transducer and the reflector
428. rayl _____	
429. Snell's law _____	
430. Doppler effect _____	(F) a device that changes sound waves into visible light patterns
	(G) the ratio between the angle of incidence and the refraction
	(H) imaginary surface passing through particles of the same vibration as an ultrasound wave
	(I) a device used to focus sound beams

431. Lateral resolution is equal to

(A) the wavelength

(B) the beam diameter

(C) the near-zone length

(D) the wave number

432. Which of the following materials are used to make acoustic lenses?

(A) aluminum

(B) Perspex (acrylic plastic)

(C) polystyrene

(D) ethylene oxide

(E) all of the above
(F) A, B, and C
(G) B and D

433. Ultrasound beams can be focused and defocused with the use of

(A) a concave or convex mirror
(B) acoustic lenses
(C) both A and B
(D) ultrasound beam cannot be focused, only light can

434. The normal range of wavelength in medical application is

(A) 0.1–1.5 mm
(B) 1.5–2 mm
(C) 2–5 mm
(D) 5.5–15 mm

435. Which of the following cannot be distinguished on diagnostic ultrasound?

(A) tissue
(B) solid mass
(C) individual cells
(D) male and female genitalia

436. Density is defined as

(A) unit of impedance
(B) force divided by area
(C) force multiplied by displacement
(D) mass per unit volume

437. Ultrasound absorption is directly proportional to

(A) viscosity
(B) frequency
(C) distance
(D) all of the above

438. The confirmed bioeffect(s) on pregnant women with the use of real-time diagnostic instruments is (are)

(A) brain damage
(B) fetal developmental anomalies
(C) growth retardation
(D) no known effect

439. The confirmed bioeffects on pregnant mice exposed to continuous wave ultrasound in a laboratory setting have resulted in

(A) cancer
(B) death
(C) neurocranial damage
(D) no known effect

440. Which of the following combinations of frequency and intensity would *most* likely result in cavitation?

(A) high frequency and low intensity
(B) low frequency and high intensity
(C) high frequency and high intensity
(D) intensity has no effect on cavitation

Questions 441 through 448: Match each term in Column A with the correct definition in Column B.

COLUMN A

441. in vivo _____
442. in vitro _____
443. spectral analysis _____
444. viscoelasticity _____
445. rejection _____
446. relaxation _____
447. real cell stasis _____
448. acoustic power _____

COLUMN B

(A) an in vivo phenomenon characterized by erythrocytes within small vessels stopping the flow and collecting in the low pressure regions of the standing wavefield
(B) elimination of small amplitude echo
(C) a process of acoustic energy absorption
(D) energy transported per unit time
(E) tissue cultures in a test tube
(F) a method of analyzing a waveform
(G) the property of a medium characterized by energy distortion in the medium and irreversibly converted to heat
(H) living human tissue

449. Which of the following statements about bioeffects is (are) unconfirmed?

(A) Ultrasound exposure in humans is accumulative.
(B) Most harmful bioeffects that occurred in experimental conditions have been confirmed in humans in a clinical setting.
(C) Intensity, frequency, and exposure time used on experimental animals were compatible to those used in a clinical setting.
(D) Continuous wave used in experimental studies gives the same tissue exposure as pulsed ultrasound used in a clinical setting.
(E) The exposure of pregnant women to high intensity levels resulted in growth retardation of their offspring.
(F) *A* and E
(G) All of the above are false or unconfirmed.
(H) All of the above are true.

450. The number of known human injuries resulting from diagnostic medical ultrasound exposure is

(A) 2500 in England
(B) 115 in the United States
(C) 1500 in Japan
(D) no exposure injuries in humans have been reported

451. What is the distinction between real-time scans and B-scans?

(A) No distinction; real-time scans are B-scans.
(B) Real-time scans display gray-scale images; whereas, B-scans display bistable images.
(C) Real-time scans exhibit motion images; whereas, B-scans exhibit static images.
(D) B-scans are specific for static scanners; real-time scans are not.

452. Transonic regions are always

(A) echo-free
(B) anechoic
(C) echogenic
(D) uninhibited to propagation

453. Which of the following is not related to real-time?

(A) A-mode
(B) static imaging
(C) dynamic imaging
(D) M-mode

454. Which of the following is *not* a component of the time-gain compensation (TGC) curve?

(A) gray scale
(B) far gain
(C) knee
(D) delay

455. The range of pulse repetition frequencies used in diagnostic ultrasound is

(A) 0.5–4 kHz
(B) 1–10 MHz
(C) 1–7 kHz
(D) 10–15 MHz

456. The spatial pulse length is defined as the product of the ____ multiplied by the number of ____ in a pulse.

(A) cycles, frequency
(B) frequency, velocity
(C) wavelength, cycles
(D) frequency, wavelength

457. Which of the following is (are) one-dimensional?

(A) B-mode and A-mode
(B) A-mode and M-mode
(C) B-mode
(D) static imaging

458. Continuous wave ultrasound is

(A) applicable to real-time instruments only
(B) used in all Doppler instruments
(C) used in some Doppler instruments
(D) applicable only to static scanners

459. Which imaging modality is audible?

(A) x-ray
(B) ultrasound
(C) Doppler
(D) computed tomography (CT)

460. Which mode requires two crystals: one for transmitting and one for receiving?

(A) A-mode
(B) M-mode
(C) continuous wave mode
(D) pulse-echo mode

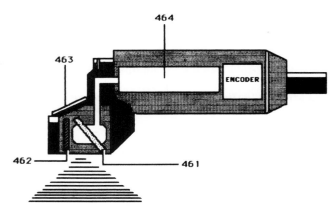

Figure 1–31. Diagram of a mechanical sector real-time transducer.

Questions 461 through 464: Identify the components in Fig. 1–31 by correlating them with the list of terms given.

461. _____   (A) motor
462. _____   (B) acoustic mirror
463. _____   (C) scanner head
464. _____   (D) piezoelectric crystal

465. The normal range of intensities used in Doppler instruments is

(A) 0.2–400 W/cm^2
(B) 0.2–400 mW/cm^2
(C) 400–800 mW/cm^2
(D) 800–900 mW/cm^2

466. If the media boundary is moving toward the source, the reflected sound wave will have

(A) a higher frequency than the incident frequency
(B) a lower frequency than the incident frequency

(C) no change in frequency

(D) be delayed

467. If the media boundary is moving away from the source, the result will be

(A) a higher frequency than the incident frequency

(B) a lower frequency than the incident frequency

(C) no change in frequency

(D) be delayed

468. A Doppler instrument that can distinguish between positive and negative shifts is called

(A) bistable

(B) a modulator–demodulator

(C) bidirectional

(D) a polarized shifter

469. Which statement about Doppler application is not true?

(A) Color Doppler is not beneficial.

(B) Doppler can produce audible sound.

(C) Doppler instruments use both pulsed and continuous wave.

(D) Doppler can display an image.

Questions 470 through 474: Match the time gain compensation (TGC) controls in Column A with the control functions in Column B.

COLUMN A

470. near gain _____
471. far gain _____
472. slope _____
473. delay _____
474. knee _____

COLUMN B

(A) control used to suppress or increase echoes in the far field

(B) control used to suppress or increase echoes in the near field

(C) control used to delay the start of the slope

(D) control the upward incline of the TGC, used to display an even texture

(E) controls the point where the slope ends

475. The range of frequencies contained in an ultrasound pulse is called

(A) propagation

(B) bandwidth

(C) refraction

(D) rejection

476. Which quantity is unitless?

(A) Q-factor

(B) volume

(C) intensity

(D) force

477. Which of the following would be *most* likely to cause acoustic enhancement?

(A) a solid mass

(B) a fluid-filled mass

(C) a calcified mass

(D) a gallstone

478. Which of the following would be *most* likely to cause acoustic shadowing?

(A) gallbladder

(B) a fluid-filled mass

(C) a calcified mass

(D) urinary bladder

479. Continuous-wave Doppler uses how many piezo-electric element(s)?

(A) 1

(B) 2

(C) 64

(D) none

480. The greatest Doppler angle is achieved

(A) when the beam strikes a vessel at a sharp angle

(B) when the beam strikes a vessel perpendicular

(C) when the beam strikes a vessel at a 30° angle

(D) when the beam strikes a vessel at a 70° angle

481. If the power output of an amplifier is 100 times the power at the input, the gain is

(A) 10 dB

(B) 20 dB

(C) 30 dB

(D) 40 dB

482. Which control is used to minimize the effects of attenuation?

(A) reject

(B) field-of-view

(C) frame rate

(D) depth-gain compensation

483. When an ultrasound beam passes obliquely across the boundary between two materials, ____ will occur if there is a difference in ____ in the two materials.

(A) reflection, impedance

(B) reflection, density

(C) refraction, impedance

(D) refraction, propagation speed

484. A decreased pulse duration leads to

(A) better axial resolution

(B) decreased spatial resolution

(C) decreased longitudinal resolution

(D) better lateral resolution

485. What is the reflected intensity from a boundary between two materials if the incident intensity is 1 mW/cm^2 and the impedances are 25 and 75?

(A) 0.25 mW/cm^2
(B) 0.33 mW/cm^2
(C) 0.50 mW/cm^2
(D) 1.00 mW/cm^2

486. The near zone length of an unfocused transducer depends on

(A) frequency and thickness
(B) frequency and diameter
(C) resolution and field of view
(D) diameter and field of view

487. The frequency of a transducer depends primarily on

(A) overall gain
(B) the speed of ultrasound
(C) the element diameter
(D) the element thickness

488. An ultrasound beam that is normally incident on an interface will experience no

(A) attenuation
(B) refraction
(C) reflection
(D) absorption

489. The average speed of propagation of ultrasound in soft tissue is

(A) 1540 ft/s
(B) 1.54 dB/cm
(C) 1.54 mm/μs
(D) 1540 mW/cm^2

490. The duty factor for a system with a pulse duration (PD) of 5 μs and a pulse repetition period (PRP) of 500 μs is

(A) 0.1%
(B) 0.5%
(C) 1.0%
(D) 10.0%

491. Ultrasound is defined as sound with frequencies above

(A) 20 Hz
(B) 20 kHz
(C) 20 MHz
(D) 20 GHz

492. Frequency is a significant factor in

(A) propagation speed
(B) tissue compressibility
(C) tissue attenuation
(D) transducer diameter

493. In a pulse–echo system, a 3.5 MHz beam of 2 cm of tissue will be attenuated by

(A) 3.5 dB/cm
(B) 7.0 dB/cm
(C) 3.5 dB
(D) 7.0 dB

494. The characteristic acoustic impedance of a material is equal to the product of the material density and

(A) path length
(B) wavelength
(C) frequency
(D) propagation speed

495. For a focused transducer, the beam intensity will remain constant through the scan field.

(A) true
(B) false

496. For normal incidence, if the intensity reflection coefficient is 30%, the intensity transmission coefficient will be

(A) 30%
(B) 60%
(C) 70%
(D) 100%

497. A Fourier transform of a returning echo will result in a presentation of the ____ contained within the echo.

(A) frequencies
(B) wavelength
(C) intensity
(D) power

498. The range equation relates

(A) frequency, velocity, and wavelength
(B) frequency, velocity, and time
(C) distance, velocity, and time
(D) distance, frequency, and time

499. The axial resolution of a system is determined by

(A) spatial pulse length
(B) beam intensity
(C) beam diameter
(D) spatial resolution

500. The Doppler shift frequency is zero when the angle between the receiving transducer and the flow direction is

(A) 0°
(B) 45°
(C) 90°
(D) 180°

501. The frame rate of real-time scanner that uses an electronic array will be limited only by the speed of the scan converter memory.

(A) true
(B) false

502. The dynamic range of a pulse–echo ultrasound system is defined as

(A) the ratio of the maximum to the minimum intensity that can be processed
(B) the range of propagation speeds
(C) the range of gain settings allowed
(D) none of the above

503. The digital scan converter will generally have a dynamic range that is ____ than other components of the system.

(A) larger
(B) smaller

504. The time-gain or depth-gain compensation control

(A) compensates for attenuation effects
(B) compensates for increased patient scan time
(C) compensates for machine malfunctions
(D) compensates for video-image drifts

505. A digital scan converter is essentially a

(A) radio receiver
(B) video monitor
(C) television set
(D) computer memory

506. A mechanical real-time scanner will always produce images at a slower frame rate than does an electronic real-time scanner.

(A) true
(B) false

507. Acoustic enhancement can be observed when scanning

(A) highly attenuating structures
(B) weakly attenuating structures
(C) highly reflective structures
(D) structures with large speed differences

508. Changes in the preprocessing controls will not affect the numbers stored in the scan converter.

(A) true
(B) false

509. The lateral resolution of a system

(A) is equal to the beam diameter
(B) is better at higher frequencies

(C) is constant throughout the image
(D) changes with gain settings

510. If the lines per degree in a mechanical sector scanner remain constant, a decreased sector angle can result in

(A) decreased resolution
(B) increased frame rate
(C) decreased frame rate
(D) increased resolution

511. The threshold control is equivalent to the

(A) TGC control
(B) DGC control
(C) modulation control
(D) reject control

512. If the actual propagation speed in soft tissue is 1,700 m/s, current diagnostic scanners will display a reflector at a location ____ the transducer.

(A) too close to
(B) too far from
(C) displaced to the left of
(D) displaced to the right of

513. Continuous-wave (CW) ultrasound is used in

(A) static B-scanners
(B) bistable systems
(C) most modern B-scan systems
(D) some Doppler systems

514. If the gain of an amplifier is 18 dB, what will the new gain setting be if the gain setting is reduced by one-half?

(A) 9 dB
(B) 36 dB
(C) 15 dB
(D) 0.5 dB

515. Decreasing the pulse repetition period

(A) decreases spatial resolution
(B) decreases axial resolution
(C) decreases the maximum depth imaged
(D) increases the maximum depth imaged

516. The AIUM 100-mm test object

(A) measures power output
(B) measures beam intensity
(C) measures frequency
(D) measures spatial resolution

517. Real-time imaging is impossible without electronic arrays.

(A) true
(B) false

518. Grating lobes in electronic array systems

(A) increase with increased steering angle
(B) decrease with increased steering angle
(C) are eliminated at high frame rates
(D) are not likely to produce artifacts

519. The attenuation coefficient is expressed in units of

(A) mW/cm^2
(B) dB
(C) dB/cm
(D) mW

520. The wave equation relates

(A) time, mass, and distance
(B) time, velocity, and frequency
(C) wavelength, velocity, and frequency
(D) wavelength, distance, and frequency

521. The ability of a system to detect low-amplitude echoes accurately is referred to as

(A) resolution
(B) sensitivity
(C) accuracy
(D) dynamic range

522. The primary mechanisms whereby ultrasound can produce biologic effects are

(A) thermal and cavitation
(B) absorption and reflection
(C) reflection and transmission
(D) heat and cold

523. The near-zone length of a transducer depends on

(A) propagation speed and frequency
(B) frequency and transducer diameter
(C) field of view and transducer diameter
(D) path length

524. The AIUM Committee on Biological Effects (1982) stated that ____ biologic effects have been observed for ultrasound intensities below 100 mW/cm^2.

(A) no
(B) no confirmed
(C) few
(D) many

525. The intensity of a focused beam is generally

(A) constant
(B) highest at the transducer surface
(C) highest at the focal zone
(D) lowest at the transducer surface

526. The wavelength of a 5 MHz wave passing through soft tissue is approximately

(A) 0.1 mm
(B) 0.3 mm
(C) 0.5 mm
(D) 1.0 mm

527. An echo that has undergone an attenuation of 3 dB will have an intensity that is ____ than its initial intensity.

(A) three times smaller
(B) three times larger
(C) two times smaller
(D) two times larger

528. A pulse–echo system should have a high Q factor (quality-factor).

(A) true
(B) false

529. A 5 MHz transducer used in a pulse–echo system will generally produce

(A) a wide band of frequencies centered at 5 MHz
(B) frequencies only at 5 MHz
(C) frequencies only at 5 MHz or multiples of 5 MHz
(D) a wide band of frequencies above 5 MHz

530. The transducer ____ determines its ____.

(A) diameter, intensity
(B) damping, lateral resolution
(C) thickness, sensitivity
(D) thickness, resonance frequency

531. The axial resolution of a transducer can be improved with ____ but at the expense of ____.

(A) increased damping, sensitivity
(B) frequency, lateral resolution
(C) focusing, sensitivity
(D) focusing, lateral resolution

532. A material that changes its dimensions when an electric field is applied is called ____ material.

(A) piezoelectric
(B) elastic
(C) inelastic
(D) compressible

533. The process of making the impedance values on either side of a boundary as close as possible to reduce reflections is called

(A) damping
(B) refracting
(C) matching
(D) compensating

534. When the pressure peaks of two waves coincide at a point to produce a new pressure that is larger than either of the two initial waves, the effect is called

(A) phase cancellation
(B) destructive interference
(C) enhancement
(D) constructive interference

535. Shadowing occurs with

(A) highly attenuating structures
(B) large changes in propagation speed
(C) low frequencies more often than with high frequencies
(D) weak reflectors

536. Reverberation artifacts

(A) occur most often at high frequencies
(B) occur with multiple strong reflecting structures
(C) occur only with real-time arrays
(D) cannot occur in color Doppler systems

537. A transducer with a large bandwidth is likely to have

(A) good axial resolution
(B) a large ring-down time
(C) poor resolution
(D) a high Q factor

538. The near zone is also referred to as the

(A) Fraunhofer zone
(B) Fresnel zone
(C) focal zone
(D) divergence zone

539. Refraction will not occur at an interface

(A) when high frequencies are used
(B) if the acoustic impedances are equal
(C) if the propagation speeds are significantly different
(D) with normal incidence of the ultrasound beam

540. Acoustic power output is determined primarily by

(A) the diameter of the transducer
(B) the thickness of the transducer
(C) the pulser voltage spike
(D) focusing

541. Specular reflections occur when

(A) the reflecting object is small with respect to the wavelength
(B) the reflecting surface is large and smooth with respect to the wavelength
(C) the reflecting objects are moving
(D) the angle of incidence and angle of reflection are unequal

542. The angle at which an ultrasound beam is bent as it passes through a boundary between two different materials is described mathematically by

(A) Huygen's principle
(B) Curie's principle

(C) Snell's law
(D) Doppler's law

543. An annular array real-time scanner

(A) is steered electronically
(B) is steered mechanically
(C) is not capable of electronic focusing
(D) is not used with digital-scan converters

544. The percentage of an ultrasound beam reflected at an interface between gas and soft tissue is approximately

(A) 90–100%
(B) 40–50%
(C) 1–10%
(D) < 1%

545. The percentage of an ultrasound beam reflected at an interface between fat and muscle is approximately

(A) 90–100%
(B) 40–50%
(C) 1–10%
(D) 0%

546. By using a waterpath offset

(A) Tissue attenuation can be reduced.
(B) The focal zone can be moved to the skin surface.
(C) Lower frequencies can be used.
(D) No reflections will occur at the skin surface.

547. Ultrasound waves in tissue are referred to as

(A) shear waves
(B) transverse waves
(C) vibrational waves
(D) longitudinal compression waves

548. High-frequency transducers have

(A) shorter wavelengths and less penetration
(B) longer wavelengths and greater penetration
(C) shorter wavelengths and greater penetration
(D) longer wavelengths and less penetration

549. When the piezoelectric crystal continues to vibrate after the initial voltage pulse, this is referred to as

(A) ring-down time
(B) pulse delay
(C) pulse retardation
(D) overdamping

550. Annular phased arrays unlike linear phased arrays

(A) can be dynamically focused
(B) electronically focus in two dimensions rather than one
(C) can be used in Doppler systems
(D) can achieve high frame rates

551. Which group is arranged in the correct order of increasing propagation speed?

   (A) gas, bone, muscle
   (B) bone, muscle, gas
   (C) gas, muscle, bone
   (D) muscle, bone, gas

552. The lower useful range of diagnostic ultrasound is determined primarily by ____; whereas, the upper useful range is determined by ____.

   (A) resolution, penetration
   (B) scattering, propagation speed
   (C) cost, resolution
   (D) scattering, resolution

553. Color Doppler systems are not subject to aliasing.

   (A) true
   (B) false

554. Which of the following is true?

   (A) SPTA is always equal to or greater than SPTP.
   (B) SPTP is always equal to or greater than SPTA.
   (C) SATA is always equal to or greater than SATP.
   (D) SPTA is always equal to or greater than SATP.

555. A beam-intensity profile is often mapped with

   (A) a radiation force balance
   (B) a SUAR phantom
   (C) a hydrophone
   (D) AIUM phantom

556. Real-time scanners are generally classified as either

   (A) electronic or mechanical
   (B) dynamic or fixed
   (C) programmable or fixed
   (D) static or electronic

557. The technique of passing an ultrasound beam through water so that compression and rarefaction of the water molecules allow the beam pattern to be measured is referred to as the

   (A) Doppler method
   (B) Schlieren method
   (C) hydrostatic method
   (D) water-density method

558. Pulse duration is the ____ for a pulse to occur.

   (A) space
   (B) range
   (C) intensity
   (D) time

559. The frame rate of a real-time scanner will not depend on

   (A) the depth of view
   (B) the line density
   (C) the frequency
   (D) the propagation speed

560. The unit of measure of SPTA is

   (A) dB
   (B) W/cm^2
   (C) W
   (D) Hz

561. The piezoelectric properties of a transducer will be lost if the crystal is heated above the

   (A) dew point
   (B) dynamic range
   (C) Curie point
   (D) linear range

562. If the amplitude of a wave is increased threefold, the intensity will

   (A) decrease threefold
   (B) increase threefold
   (C) increase ninefold
   (D) increase sixfold

563. A videotape recorder records at a rate of 30 frames/s and therefore cannot be used to record images from a mechanical scanner operating a lower frame rates.

   (A) true
   (B) false

564. If the frequency is increased, the ____ will be ____.

   (A) velocity, increased
   (B) attenuation, decreased
   (C) velocity, decreased
   (D) velocity, unchanged

565. Beam steering is achieved in a linear phased array by

   (A) mechanical motion
   (B) electronic time-delay pulsing
   (C) an acoustic lens
   (D) dynamic focusing

566. Dynamic focusing

   (A) is made possible by array-based systems
   (B) is made possible by acoustic lens
   (C) is not possible in a linear-switched array
   (D) is often used in single-element systems

567. Quality assurance measurements are not required with electronic scanners with digital scan converters.

   (A) true
   (B) false

568. Sound will travel ____ in 1 μs in soft tissue.

   (A) 1540 m
   (B) 1.54 cm
   (C) 1.54 mm
   (D) 0.75 mm

569. The arrow in Fig. 1–32 points to a

(A) ring-down artifact
(B) mirror image artifact
(C) side lobe artifact
(D) ghost artifact

570. In the image in Fig. 1–33, which represents a tissue-equivalent phantom, the small open arrows point to

(A) rods for measuring "ring-down"
(B) parallel rods used for horizontal calibration
(C) rods used for axial resolution
(D) rods used for measure registration

571. In the image in Fig. 1–33, which represents a tissue-equivalent phantom, the curved open arrow points to

(A) a dead zone
(B) a simulated solid lesion
(C) a ghost artifact
(D) a side lobe artifact

572. In the image in Fig. 1–33, which represents a tissue-equivalent phantom, the solid black arrow points to

(A) a ghost artifact
(B) a dead zone
(C) a simulated cyst
(D) a side lobe artifact

573. When the FOV is reduced by decreasing the PRP, the following is more likely to occur

(A) greater beam attenuation
(B) higher lateral resolution
(C) greater range ambiguity artifacts
(D) higher reflection amplitudes

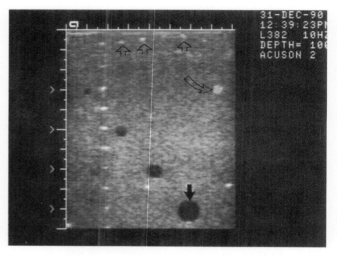

Figure 1–33. Image from a tissue-equivalent phantom.

574. At the present time, most ultrasound contrast agents are based upon

(A) suspended particles
(B) higher viscosity liquids
(C) MRI contrast agents
(D) gas-filled bubbles

575. Microspheres filled with this material is currently used as an ultrasound contrast agent

(A) xenon
(B) perfluorocarbon
(C) iodine
(D) gadolinium

576. In harmonic imaging, received echoes used for the image have ____ than in ordinary pulse-echo imaging.

(A) higher frequencies
(B) higher echo amplitudes
(C) lower resolution
(D) lower attenuation

577. Harmonic imaging relative to conventional pulse-echo imaging has

(A) better lateral resolution
(B) more image clutter
(C) higher intensity echoes
(D) less image contrast

578. Compounding, in the context of real-time ultrasound scanners, refers to

(A) addition of color Doppler capability
(B) using two or more transducers at once
(C) steering the beam to achieve larger echoes at a specific image location
(D) adding images following the injection of a contrast agent

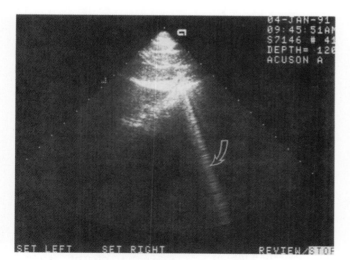

Figure 1–32. Sonogram of an artifact.

Answers and Explanations

At the end of each explained answer there is a number combination in parentheses. The first number identifies the reference source; the second number or set of numbers indicates the page or pages on which the relevant information can be found.

1. **(C)** Red blood cells. Structures smaller than a wavelength will scatter sound in all directions and are sometimes called diffuse reflectors. *(2:42)*

2. **(B)** Spatial pulse length is defined as the product of the number of cycles in the pulse and its wavelength. This is generally shorter for higher frequencies since the wavelength is shorter. *(2:64)*

3. **(D)** Axial resolution, also called longitudinal, range, or depth resolution, is determined by the wavelength, damping, and frequency. Axial resolution improves with increased frequency. *(2:64)*

4. **(B)** Lateral resolution is defined as being equal to the beam diameter. *(2:65)*

5. **(C)** The beam of an unfocused transducer diverges in the Fraunhofer (far) zone. *(1:360)*

6. **(C)** Reverberation artifacts are present when two or more strong reflectors are located within the beam. One of these may be the transducer itself. *(2:142)*

7. **(B)** False. Grating lobes are an undesirable property of multi-element array transducers. *(4:31)*

8. **(B)** False. Resolution is a function of the focusing characteristics of any scanner and cannot be assumed to be better for any particular scanner configuration. *(1:390–399)*

9. **(A)** True. Annular arrays may be used for creating variable focusing in two dimensions but are not capable of electronic steering of the beam. *(5:233)*

10. **(B)** False. The focusing of a linear array is controlled by timing and is thus capable of dynamic focusing. *(4:29)*

11. **(A, B, C, D, E)** All rods must be used to check registration accuracy. *(2:158)*

12. **(A)** See Fig. 1–24 and Table 1–3, Study Guide. *(2:156)*

13. **(B)** See Fig. 1–24 and Table 1–3, Study Guide. *(2:156)*

14. **(D)** See Fig. 1–24 and Table 1–3, Study Guide. *(2:156)*

15. **(C or E)** See Fig. 1–24 and Table 1–3, Study Guide. *(2:156)*

16. **(C)** Decreasing the spatial pulse length improves axial resolution. Axial resolution is equal to one-half of the spatial pulse length. *(2:64)*

17. **(B)** A rule of thumb approximating the attenuation coefficient of a reflected echo in soft tissue is 0.5 dB/cm/MHz. Thus, the attenuation coefficient will be one-half the operating frequency.

    attenuation (dB) = attenuation coefficient (dB/cm) × path length (cm)

    dB = 1.75 dB/cm × 2 cm = 3.5 dB *(2:23)*

18. **(B)** Improper axial (along-the-beam) position *(2:139)*

19. **(D)** Weakly attenuating structures *(2:139)*

20. **(A)** Directly proportional to the velocity of the reflector *(1:386)*

21. **(A)** More than 15 frames per second *Note:* The scan converter in most modern systems turns the scanning frame rate (which is the subject of this question) into a display frame rate (or video frame rate), which is usually faster (30 video frames/s). This is done by displaying the same scan frame more than once if the scan frame is less than video rate. *(4:34)*

22. **(A)** True. Spatial peak (SP) values will always be greater than spatial average (SA) intensity values. *(2:21)*

23. **(B)** Smaller beam diameter. Intensity is defined as power per unit beam area; as the beam area decreases the intensity increases. *(2:18)*

24. **(C)** Increased by four times. Intensity equals the square of the amplitude. *(2:18)*

25. **(A)** Increased with tissue thickness. Attenuation is the product of the attenuation coefficient and path length. *(2:23)*

26. **(A)** Should be chosen to be at a value approximately equal to the mean of impedances of the material on either side of it *(1:370)*

27. **(B)** False. The Q factor, or quality factor, of a transducer refers to the length of time that the sound persists. High-Q transducers tend to ring for a long time, whereas low-Q transducers ring for a shorter time. A low Q produces a short pulse length, which is necessary to provide good images. *(1:359)*

28. **(B)** False. The beam diameter reduces to one-half of the transducer diameter from the face of the transducer to the focal point. *(2:58)*

29. **(B)** Depends on crystal thickness. Thickness equals one-half the wavelength. *(2:50)*

30. **(C)** The time of one wavelength *(2:6)*

31. **(D)** Ratio of smallest to largest power level *(2:84)*

32. **(A)** True. Radiation pressure can be measured with a sensitive balance and converted to intensity. *(5:89)*

33. **(B)** Increases the maximum depth that can be imaged *(4:36)*

34. **(C)** Are not confirmed below 100 mW/cm^2 SPTA *(3:9)*

35. **(B)** False. Refraction comes as a result of changes in sound velocity across a boundary, not impedance. *(4:7)*

36. **(B)** False. Beam diameter depends on whether or not the transducer is focused, the distance from the transducer, and whether one is in the near field or far field. Small transducers produce greatly diverging beams in the far field. *(1:364)*

37. **(A)** True. A hydrophone is usually a very small piezoelectric crystal that can be moved in front of the transmitting crystal to map its beam characteristics. *(5:85)*

38. **(A)** True. Pulse Doppler utilizes range gating to localize the signals to specific depths. *(5:385)*

39. **(B)** False. Gray-scale ultrasound images were also possible with analog storage devices. *(5:198)*

40. **(B)** False. If the imaging rate is slower than the video framing rate, frames are duplicated to fill in. *(4:44)*

41. **(B)** False. Linear arrays must also be focused in the direction perpendicular to the array axis to reduce the slice thickness. This is usually accomplished by mechanical focusing. *(1:394)*

42. **(A)** True. Real-time scanners display 15 to 60 images per second, called the frame rate. This rate must be greater than 15 frames per second to produce flicker-free image. Each frame is made of scan lines, the number of lines per frame, and the number of frames per second are related to one another. *(4:35; 2:105)*

43. **(A)** True. Annular phased arrays must be steered mechanically, most frequently through the use of an oscillating acoustic mirror. *(3:4)*

44. **(B)** False. Images produced in the near zone have the best lateral resolution; therefore, the near zone length should be long enough to include all time regions-of-interest. *(1:362)*

45. **(C)** Twenty-five percent. The reflection coefficient *(R)* is equal to:

$$R = \left(\frac{Z_2 - Z_1}{Z_2 + Z_1}\right)^2 = \left(\frac{0.75 - 0.25}{0.75 + 0.25}\right)^2 = 0.25$$

where Z_1 and Z_2 are the acoustic impedance of each material. *(1:366)*

46. **(A)** Higher frequency transducers usually produce shorter spatial pulse lengths and thus improve axial resolution. *(2:64)*

47. **(A)** Longitudinal wave *(4:2)*

48. **(A)** 0.3 mm *(4:2)*

$$\text{wavelength (mm)} = \frac{\text{velocity (mm/µs)}}{\text{frequency (MHz)}} = \frac{1.5}{5} = 0.3 \text{ mm}$$

49. **(D)** The difference in specific acoustic impedances. The fraction of sound reflected at an interface *(r)* is given by:

$$R = \left(\frac{Z_2 - Z_1}{Z_2 + Z_1}\right)^2,$$

where Z_1 and Z_2 are the acoustic impedance of the boundary material. *(1:366)*

50. **(A)** V or C = propagation velocity (cm/s)

f = frequency (cycles/s)
λ = wavelength (cm)
$V = f\lambda$ *(31:9; 12:2)*

51. **(D)** All of the above. Reflection refers to echoes; refraction refers to the bending of the beam; and mode conversion refers to a change in the propagation mode transverse, shear, surface, or longitudinal waves.   *(5:15–19)*

52. **(D)** Equal to the product of density and velocity for longitudinal waves   *(1:365)*

53. **(C)** 1540 meters per second   *(1:353)*

54. **(B)** False. The magnitude of the Doppler shift frequency is directly related to the cosine of the angle between the direction of the blood flow and the receiver angle. The maximum shift frequency is, therefore, observed when the flow is along the receiver line-of-sight.   *(1:386)*

55. **(B)** Wave velocity. Refraction is described by Snell's law, which relates the incident angle (θ_i) to the transmitted angle (θ_t) to the relative velocities of the two media making up the interface:

$$\frac{\sin \theta_i}{\sin \theta_t} = \frac{C_1}{C_2}$$ *(1:367)*

56. **(A)** Acoustic impedance   *(1:366)*

57. **(C)** The material through which the sound is being transmitted and the mode of vibration   *(1:353)*

58. **(C)** No change. The velocity of sound propagation depends on the material through which it is being transmitted and is independent of frequency.   *(1:353)*

59. **(A)** Refraction   *(1:367)*

60. **(A)** Using a higher frequency transducer. The near zone length (x) is given by:

$$x = \frac{r^2}{\lambda},$$

where r is the radius of the transducer, and λ is the wavelength. Thus, a longer near zone length is achieved by increasing the transducer diameter or increasing the frequency.   *(1:367)*

61. **(A)** 0.75 mm. The wavelength can be determined by using the following equation:

$$\lambda = \frac{v}{f}$$

v = propagation velocity (m/s)
f = frequency (Hz)
λ = wavelength (m)

For example $\lambda = \dfrac{1500 \text{ meters per second}}{2 \text{ MHz}}$

$\lambda = \dfrac{1.5 \times 10^3 \text{ meters per second}}{2 \times 10^6 \text{ cycles per second}}$

$\lambda = 0.75 \times 10^{-3}$ meters

$\lambda = 0.75$ mm   *(2:8; 12:2)*

62. **(B)** Impedance

$\begin{array}{l} Z \text{ (impedance) for} \\ \text{longitudinal waves} \end{array} = \dfrac{\text{particle pressure}}{\text{particle velocity}}$ *(5:13)*

63. **(A)** Doppler-shift formula   *(2:125)*

64. **(C)** Huygens   *(1:362; 5:26)*

65. **(B)** Tenfold difference in intensity or power   *(2:255)*

66. **(B)** Threshold, negative, or reject level   *(1:376)*

67. **(B)** Compression   *(2:84)*

68. **(A)** A-mode   *(1:370)*

69. **(D)** Relaxation processes are modes by which ultrasound may be attenuated in passing through a material. Suppression is another name for rejection.   *(2:79–85)*

70. **(B)** Digital scan converter   *(3:31)*

71. **(A)** Duty factor   *(2:55)*

72. **(D)** Sensitivity   *(2:155)*

73. **(B)** Linear array transducers produce a rectangular image. (Sector scanners produce a pie-shaped image.)   *(3:18–26)*

74. **(B)** Magnitude of the voltage spike applied to the transducer by the pulser   *(2:77)*

75. **(D)** Thermal and cavitational   *(2:171)*

76. **(C)** Quality factor, or Q factor, is equal to the operating frequency divided by the bandwidth.   *(1:36)*

77. **(C)** Side lobes *(5:29)*

78. **(D)** Pulse duration *(2:15)*

79. **(B)** The silicon oxide matrix is charged by a scanning electron beam, producing an image pattern that can be displayed on a video monitor. *(5:198)*

80. **(C)** Reflectors whose boundaries are smooth relative to a wavelength behave as mirrors and are called specular reflectors. *(2:42)*

81. **(B)** Schlieren technique of measurement *(1:362)*

82. **(D)** Reverberation *(2:140)*

83. **(B)** Enhancement *(2:146)*

84. **(B)** Using a larger diameter transducer. The dispersion angle in the far field (θ) is given as: $\sin \theta = 1.22\ \lambda/d$, where λ is the wavelength, and d is the diameter of the transducer. The angle can be reduced by using either a larger transducer or a higher frequency (smaller wavelength). *(1:364)*

85. **(B)** Spatial pulse length

$$\text{axial resolution (mm)} = \frac{\text{spatial pulse length (mm)}}{2}$$

(2:64)

86. **(B)** Quality factor (Q factor)

$$Q = \frac{f_0}{f_2 - f_1}$$

where f_0 is the central resonance frequency and $(f_2 - f_1)$ is the frequency bandwidth. *(2:53; 1:360)*

87. **(C)** Schlieren technique *(1:362)*

88. **(D)** Blood *(1:369)*

89. **(A)** Dynamic range *(2:84)*

90. **(D)** Longitudinal waves *(1:352)*

91. **(B)** Axial resolution *(2:156)*

92. **(C)** Scan C *(2:158)*

93. **(A)** Dead zone *(2:156)*

94. **(A)** Call for service *(6:23–24)*

95. **(C)** Horizontal caliper check *(6:15)*

96. **(B)** Lateral resolution *(6:19–26)*

97. **(E)** Gray scale and dynamic range *(2:158; 6:19–24)*

98. **(D)** Registration *(6:18)*

99. **(E)** All of the answers given are correct. *(6:10–24)*

100. **(F)** All of the answers given are correct. *(6:10–24)*

101. **(C, D, F, G, H)** Lead zirconate titanate, barium titanate, lithium sulfate, lead metaniobate, and ammonium dihydrogen phosphate are not natural. *(7:85–87; 8:28)*

102. **(A, B, D, E)** Cork, rubber, epoxy resin, and tungsten powder in araldite are good acoustic insulators. Water and oil are not. *(8:38–39)*

103. **(A)** Sound and ultrasound are mechanical vibrations that can propagate in matter, such as liquid and solid. However, sound or ultrasound cannot travel in a vacuum. *(10:1)*

104. **(A)** Infrasound (subsonic) *(10:1)*

105. **(B)** Ultrasound *(10:1)*

106. **(B)** Audible sound *(10:1)*

107. **(B)** The electromagnetic spectrum is a large family of electromagnetic waves. Light, x-rays, and infrared, and ultraviolet rays are among its spectrum; ultrasound is not. *(1:1–3)*

108. **(D)** Cycle per second (cps) *(10:1)*

109. **(B)** Electrical energy into mechanical energy and vice versa *(2:48)*

110. **(E)** All of the answers given are correct. *(2:48)*

111. **(D)** Increase or decrease depending on the polarity applied *(2:49)*

112. **(D)** 1 mega = 1 million. Therefore, 5 MHz = 5 million cycles per second or 5 million Hz. *(10:1)*

113. **(G)** The damping material reduces pulse duration and spatial pulse length, and as a result is improves axial resolution. *(2:51)*

114. **(A)** Velocity of ultrasound transmitted through a medium depends on the properties of the medium: (1) temperature, (2) elasticity, and (3) density. The speed of ultrasound varies with temperature. However, temperature/velocity in human soft tissue can usually be ignored because body temperature is usually constant within a narrow range, for example, 94°F (low) to 106°F (high). The velocity of ultrasound in soft tissue at 37°C or 98.6°F (body temperature) is 1,540 meters per second (1540 m/s).   *(11:3; 9:55; 10:5)*

115. **(C)** A single cycle   *(11:2)*

116. **(A)** Particle motion parallel to (or in the same direction of) the axis of wave propagation   *(7:4)*

117. **(C)** Particle motion perpendicular to the axis of wave propagation   *(7:4)*

118. **(B)** Compression   *(7:4)*

119. **(C)** Rarefactions   *(7:4)*

120. **(D)** Pressure   *(2:64)*

121. **(F)**   *(2:64)*

122. **(F)**   *(2:64)*

123–131. See Fig. 1–8 in the Study Guide.   *(1:367; 2:98)*

132–140. See Fig. 1–23 in the Study Guide.   *(12:2; 1:373)*

141. **(A)** If frequency increases, the wavelength decreases.   *(2:140–141)*

142. **(B)** If frequency decreases, the wavelength increases.   *(2:140–141)*

143. **(A)** As frequency increases, the penetration decreases.   *(2:140–141)*

144. **(B)** As frequency increases, the resolution increases.   *(2:140–141)*

145. **(A)** Higher frequency transmits shorter pulse and narrower beam width.   *(9:31)*

146. **(F)** Air, bone, and barium sulfate ($BaSO_4$). The contrast material used for intravenous pyelogram (IVP) does not prevent the propagation of ultrasound.   *(12:2; 13:413)*

147. **(C)** Barium sulfate ($BaSO_4$). A coupling medium is a liquid medium placed between the transducer and the skin to eliminate air gap. Air has a reflection coefficient approaching 100%, which results in almost zero transmission. Water or saline can also be used, but they dry out faster than gel.   *(13:10–11; 11:52)*

148. **(A)** The progressive weakening of the sound beam as it travels. Attenuation occurs because of (1) absorption, (2) reflection, and (3) scatter. Barium sulfate and air impair ultrasound transmissions.   *(11:4)*

149. **(C)** When crystals are subjected to pressure resulting in an electrical charge on their surfaces, it is called a piezoelectric effect.   *(10:12)*

150. **(B)** When crystals are subjected to electrical impulse and generate ultrasound as a result, it is called reverse piezoelectric effect.   *(10:12)*

151. **(B)** Attenuation is the amount of energy lost per unit of depth into the tissue. The parameter used to express the energy loss is the decibel (dB).

$$dB = 10 \log_{10} \frac{I_2}{I_1}$$ *(12:5)*

152. **(C)** Waves carry energy from one place to another through a medium.   *(14:1)*

153. **(A)** A mechanical wave causes particles to oscillate around its equilibrium point.   *(14:2)*

154. **(C)** Wavelength is the distance between two identical points on the waveform.   *(14:4)*

155. **(A)** Ultrasonic waves are mechanical. A medium is required for propagation of sounds.   *(14:1)*

156. **(B)** Acoustic impedance is defined as the density of tissue × the speed of sound in tissue ($Z = pc$).   *(15:30)*

157. **(D)** Amplitude is defined as the height of the wave. For amplitude, dB = 20 log (amplitude ratio).   *(15:3)*

158. **(B)** Ultrasound is above 20,000 cycles per second (Hz) and is above the audible range of sound.   *(15:2)*

159. **(D)** The equation for period is:

$$period = \frac{1}{frequency}$$ *(14:2)*

160. **(D)** The direction of the returning echo is related to the beam angle. The more perpendicular the beam gets to an organ interface, the greater the portion of the reflected echo that will be received by the transducer.   *(15:5)*

161. **(A)** A decibel is the ratio of two sound intensities, highest to lowest (or vice versa).   *(14:1)*

162. **(C)** Azimuthal is another name for *lateral* resolution.   *(14:6)*

163. **(B)** Bone has the highest sound velocity because of its stiffness.   *(14:8)*

164. (B) No significant biologic effects have been proved in mammals exposed below 100 mW/cm² spatial peak, temporal average (SPTA). *(2:175)*

165. (A) Temporal peak intensity is measured at the time the pulse is present. *(14:5)*

166. (D) SATA has the lowest intensity because the intensity is averaged over the whole beam profile (SA), and over the whole duration of exposure (TA). *(2:21)*

167. (B) The beam uniformity ratio is defined as the spatial peak intensity (measured at the beam center) divided by the spatial average intensity (the average intensity across the beam). *(2:19)*

168. (C) The duty factor is the fraction of time the transducer is emitting sound. In a pulsed echo system, it is normally less than 1%. *(14:5)*

169. (D) Axial resolution is defined as one-half the spatial pulse length. Therefore, the shorter the spatial pulse length, the better the axial resolution. *(14:6)*

170. (B) V = velocity of sound (cm/s); f = frequency (cycle/s); and λ = wavelength (cm). *(1:364)*

171. (D) Attenuation of an ultrasound beam can occur by divergence of a beam, scattering and reflection. It can also occur by absorption. *(14:8)*

172. (A) Attenuation coefficient of sound is determined by knowing dB/cm/MHz and then multiplying that quantity by the frequency expressed in MHz. *(14:12)*

173. (C) Transducer Q factor (quality factor) is equal to the operating frequency divided by the bandwidth. Therefore, if the transducer Q factor is low, the bandwidth is wide. *(14:6)*

174. (A) Axial resolution can be improved by shortening pulse length, increasing damping, and a higher-frequency transducer. *(14:6)*

175. (B) Axial resolution is primarily affected by spatial pulse length. Because the spatial pulse length is the product of wavelength, reducing the wavelength or increasing the frequency will affect axial resolution. *(2:64)*

176. (D) Increasing transducer frequency will improve both lateral and axial resolution but decrease depth of penetration. *(2:69)*

177. (C) Range resolution is another name for *axial* resolution. *(2:65)*

178. (B) The duty factor is the fraction of time that sound is being emitted from the transducer. In continuous wave the sound is being emitted 100% of the time. *(2:20)*

179. (A) Acoustic impedance (Z) is defined as density (p) × propagation speed (c). Z = pc. *(2:10)*

180. (D) Acoustic impedance is defined by the unit rayl. Density is defined by kg/m³, and propagation speed by meters per second. *(2:10)*

181. (A) Acoustic impedance is dependent on density and stiffness. It does not depend on frequency. *(2:10)*

182. (A) The height of the vertical spike corresponds to the strength of the echo received by the transducer. *(6:60)*

183. (B) B-mode is a short form for brightness modulation. Both real-time and static scanning are B-mode display. *(6:60)*

184. (A) The correct equation for calculating reflection percentage is:

$$R = \left(\frac{Z_2 - Z_1}{Z_2 + Z_1}\right)^2 \times 100$$

(31:14–15)

185. (D) The reflection coefficient between water and air interface is nearly 100%. Air prevents the sound from entering the body. It is for this reason that a coupling gel is necessary. *(13:8)*

186. (B) Beyond the critical angle, 100% of the sound beam is reflected and 0% is transmitted. *(13:9)*

187. (A) Rayleigh scattering occurs when the particle size is smaller than a wavelength (for ultrasound typically in the 1-mm range). *(13:9)*

188. (B) Particle displacement is an acoustic parameter related to the intensity of an ultrasound wave. Other intensity-related factors include sound velocity, pressure, amplitude, and density of the medium. *(13:4)*

189. (C) Power is defined as the rate at which work is done or energy is transferred (energy per unit time). *(2:269)*

190. (A) Lateral resolution is the minimum separation between two reflectors perpendicular to the sound path. *(2:65)*

191. (D) In most soft tissues, the attenuation coefficient increases directly with frequency. As frequency is increased the attenuation coefficient increases, thereby limiting depth of perception. *(13:9)*

192. (A) Absorption is the conversion of sound into heat. Absorption, scattering, and reflection are all factors of attenuation. *(2:23)*

193. (D) The rule of thumb for attenuation in soft tissue is 0.5 dB per centimeter per megahertz. Therefore, an ultrasound beam of 1 MHz frequency will lose 0.5 dB of amplitude for every centimeter traveled. *(11:4)*

194. (C) Reverberations produce false echoes. *(2:142)*

195. (D) The acoustic mismatch between fat and muscle is small; therefore, approximately 99% of the sound beam is transmitted. *(14:10)*

196. (A) Huygens's principle states that all points on a wavefront can be considered as a source for secondary spherical wavelets. *(14:3)*

197. (B) Enhancement is the "burst of sound" visualized posterior to weak attenuations. *(2:151)*

198. (A) Half-value layer (HVL—sometimes called half-intensity depth) is defined as the thickness of tissue that reduces the beam intensity by half. *(13:10)*

199. (D) Propagation speed error. The ultrasound machine assumes a speed of 1540 meters per second (1540 m/s). If the sound passes through a medium of a different velocity, the result is an error in the range equation. *(2:146)*

200. (B) Range equation explains the distance to the reflector, which is equal to one-half of the propagation speed × the pulse round-trip time. *(2:44)*

201. (A) For a specular reflector, the angle of incidence is equal to the angle of reflection. *(14:9)*

202. (C) Propagation speed is determined by the medium. Amplitude, period, and intensity are determined by the transducer. *(2:5)*

203. (D) Acoustic variables include density, pressure, temperature, and particle motion. *(2:5)*

204. (B) Time gain compensation *(15:19)*

205. (B) The propagation speed for fat is 1440 meters per second (1440 m/s), which is lower than that of average soft tissue. *(2:10)*

206. (D) Muscle has a propagation speed of 1585 meters per second (1585 m/s), which is very close to average soft tissue at 1540 m/s. *(14:8)*

207. (A) A is correct, with the propagation velocity in this order respectively: 331 m/s, 1450 m/s, 1585 m/s, and 4080 m/s. *(2:9, 180)*

208. (C) Backscatter is increased by increasing frequency and increasing heterogeneous media. *(2:32)*

209. (A) Critical angle is the angle at which sound is totally reflected and none is transmitted. *(13:9)*

210. (D) The pulse repetition frequency (PRF) is the number of pulses occurring per second. The PRF is inversely proportional to the pulse repetition period. *(2:16)*

211. (D) The duty factor is the fraction of time that the transducer is emitting a pulse. It is unitless. *(2:15)*

212. (A) The attenuation coefficient is the attenuation per unit length of sound travel. Its typical value is 3 dB/cm, for 6 MHz sound in soft tissue (0.5 dB/cm/MHz × 6 MHz = 3 dB/cm). *(2:28)*

213. (B) Normal incidence is also known as perpendicular incidence. At normal incidence, sound may be reflected or transmitted in various degrees. *(2:32)*

214. (A) The difference (mismatch) of acoustic impedance between two media is what determines how much energy will be transmitted and/or reflected. *(14:10)*

215. (A) Acoustic impedance is equal to the product of the density of a substance and the velocity of sound. The propagation speed in solids is higher than in liquids, and the propagation speed in gas is low. The increase in propagation speed is caused by increasing stiffness of the media, not by the density. *(2:180)*

216. (A) According to Snell's law,

$$\frac{\sin i}{\sin r} = \frac{V_1}{V_2}$$

the transmission angle is proportional to the incidence angle times the medium 2 propagation speed divided by the medium 1 propagation speed. *(2:30)*

217. (C) The propagation speed of the medium must be known in order to calculate the distance to the reflector. In addition, the round-trip must be measured. The distance to the reflector is equal to the product of the propagation speed and the pulse round-trip divided by 2. *(2:45)*

218. (D) The mirror image artifact occurs around strong reflectors, for example, the diaphragm. *(2:144–146)*

219. (C) The comet tail is a type of reverberation artifact. The greater the acoustic impedance mismatch, the greater the possibility of this artifact to occur. *(16:7)*

220. **(C)** The acoustic impedance mismatch between tissue and gas is very great; therefore, it may produce the comet tail artifact. *(16:7)*

221. **(B)** Fat has a slower velocity than the liver. Therefore, the returning time of the echo to the transducer is delayed. Because the ultrasound machine assumes that everything in its path has a velocity of 1540 meters per second (1540 m/s), the diaphragm posterior to the fat is registered as farther than it actually is. *(19:58)*

222. **(D)** By increasing damping one also increases the bandwidth. Bandwidth is the range of frequency involved in a pulse. *(2:54)*

223. **(D)** All of the above. *(14:12)*

224. **(B)** The compression controls on some sonographic equipment, when adjusted, will reduce the dynamic range. Compression is the process of decreasing the difference between small and large amplitude echoes. *(14:13)*

225. **(A)** Ultrasound transducers generally can resolve reflectors along the sound path better than it can those perpendicular to it. *(2:69)*

226. **(D)** The number of electrical pulses produced per second is typically 1000 Hz. *(2:77)*

227. **(D)** Brightness modulation. This display is used in two-dimensional ultrasound images, real-time, and static. *(6:60)*

228. **(B)** With a typical PRF of 1000 Hz, each pulse–receive interval is 1 millisecond (1000 microseconds) long. Because an average pulse is 1 microsecond long, this leaves 999 microseconds for receiving. 999/1000 is 99.9%. *(20:190)*

229. **(C)** Frequency equals velocity divided by wavelength. Because velocity is standard at 1540 m/s, doubling the frequency will result in decreasing the wavelength by one-half. *(2:8)*

230. **(A)** Real-time transducers display two formats: sector and rectangular. The linear-sequenced array transducer displays a rectangular format. *(2:120)*

231. **(C)** Z is the acoustic impedance; P is the material density; and V is the propagation velocity. *(12:2)*

232. **(A)** Lead zirconate titanate (PZT) is a ceramic material with piezoelectric properties. It is most commonly used in transducers because of its greater efficiency and sensitivity. *(6:50)*

233. **(B)** Transmit-delay focusing creates a narrow beam, which improves lateral resolution. *(14:19)*

234. **(D)** Pulse repetition frequency is equal to lines per frame and is related to time frame rate. Frequency has no relationship to this equation. *(2:77)*

235. **(A)** Pulse repetition frequency is the number of pulses emitted per second or pulse rate. *(2:140)*

236. **(D)** The pulser produces the electric voltage pulses; this, in turn, drives the transducer to emit ultrasound pulses. It also tells both the memory and receiver when the ultrasound pulses were produced. *(2:77)*

237. **(A)** Demodulation converts the voltage delivered to the receiver from one form to another by rectification and smoothing. *(2:82)*

238. **(C)** Demodulation and compression are not operator adjustable. Amplification, compensation, and rejection functions are operator adjustable. *(2:85)*

239. **(A)** Lateral resolution is dependent on beam diameter, which varies with distance from the transducer. *(2:65)*

240. **(C)** A period is the time it takes for one full cycle to occur. *(2:7)*

241. **(B)** Half-intensity depth decreases with increasing frequency. *(2:64)*

242. **(C)** Redirection of a portion of the sound beam from a boundary *(11:5)*

243. **(D)** Computers use a special number system called binary numbers. The system uses two digits, 0 and 1. *(18:8.2)*

244. **(A)** Bit is an acronym for binary digit and represents the basic unit for storing data in the main computer memory. *(18:8.1)*

245. **(A)** Eight bits equal 1 byte. A bit is a unit of data in binary notation and assumes one of two states: "on" representing the number 1, or "off" representing the number 0. *(17:136)*

246. **(B)** A computer and its peripherals are categorized into hardware and software. Hardware is the term used to describe any of the physical embodiments of the computer, for example, the keyboard, disk drive, CRT, and printer. Computer programs are software. The software, in turn, runs the hardware. *(17:139)*

247. **(B)** Random-access memory. This type of memory is called random because it provides access to any storage location in the memory. *(18:8.13)*

248. **(A)** Read-only memory. This type of program memory provides access to read out only. *(18:8.13)*

249. **(B)** Any set of computer devices that transfers information or data from an external medium into the internal storage of the computer is called an input device. A printer is an output device. *(18:3.2)*

250. **(B)** ROM (read-only memory) is programmed into the computer at the time of manufacture. PROM (programmable read-only memory) can be written to by the programmer. *(18:8.13)*

251. **(D)** Erasable programmable read-only memory (EPROM) can be programmed or erased. *(18:8.13)*

252. **(B)** Central processing unit (CPU). *(18:8.1)*

253. **(B)** Most microprocessors use 8-, 16-, or 32-bit word length. The most common is a 16-bit. *(18:8.1–8.17)*

254. **(C)** While the symbol K represents kilo or 1000 in metric, in computer terminology K = 1024. Then, the amount that can be stored in memory is $128 \times 1024 \times 8$ bits = 1,048,576 bits, referred to as 1 megabit. *(18:8.1–8.17)*

255. **(D)** Contents of EPROM are erased by exposing them to ultraviolet light. *(18:8.13)*

256. **(B)** Modem *(18:11.5)*

257. **(C)** BASIC *(18:13.8)*

258. **(D)** Baud rate. The measured speed is expressed in the number of bits per second (bps). *(18:11.9)*

259. **(B)** Hard disks have a larger storage capacity and faster access than do floppy disks. *(18:9.9)*

260. **(C)** Beginner's all purpose symbolic instruction code (BASIC). *(18:13.8)*

261. **(C)** A modem is an acronym for modular/demodulator. It is a device that translates digital data to analog signals and vice versa over standard telephone lines. *(18:11.5)*

262. **(B)** Two: off or on. "Off" represents the number 0. "On" represents the number 1. *(19:33; 17:137)*

263. **(C)** Two (0 or 1) *(19:31)*

264. **(E)** The number 30 is represented by 011110. To convert from decimal to binary, repeatedly divide by two and note the remainder.

$30 \div 2 = 15$ remainder 0 $3 \div 2 = 1$ remainder 1
$15 \div 2 = 7$ remainder 1 $1 \div 2 = 0$ remainder 1
$7 \div 2 = 3$ remainder 1 $0 \div 2 = 0$ remainder 0
(2:259)

265. **(D)** The binary system, which is used in digital scan converter memory, is based on the powers of two. For four bits, 2^4 ($2 \times 2 \times 2 \times 2$) or 16 different gray levels can be represented. Another way of looking at this is to list all possible states:

0000	0100	1000	1100
0001	0101	1001	1101
0010	0110	1010	1110
0011	0111	1011	1111

There are 16 possible unique states. *(19:32)*

266. **(B)** Digital memory, where the electronic components are either on (1) or off (0), is based on the binary number system. We can say that the number of discrete levels possible, *N,* is equal to 2 raised to the power of that number of bits. $N = 2^n$. Therefore, to make 64 shades of gray would require 2^6 bit memory.

$$(2 \times 2 \quad 4 \times 2 \quad 8 \times 2 \quad 16 \times 2 \quad 32 \times 2 = 64)$$
$$1 \quad 2 \quad 3 \quad 4 \quad 5 \quad 6 \qquad (19:32)$$

267. **(B)** At high ultrasound intensities, tissue damage has been observed to be caused by heat and cavitation. *(7:185)*

268. **(C)** The receiver processes echoes detected by the transducer. These echoes may be amplified (gain), compensated for depth (TGC), compressed (to fit into the dynamic range of the system), and rejected (eliminating low-level signals). *(19:27)*

269. **(D)** The greater the pulse amplitude (electronic voltage applied to the transducer), the greater the amplitude of the ultrasound pulse provided by the transducer. *(2:77)*

270. **(B)** The pulser produces electric voltage pulses that drive the transducer and at the same time tell the receiver that the transducer has been driven. *(2:77)*

271. **(D)** Components of a pulse–echo system include the *pulser* that produces the electrical pulse, which drives the *transducer.* For each reflection received from the tissue by the transducer, an electrical voltage is produced that goes to the *receiver,* where it is processed for display. Information on transducer position and orientation is delivered to the *image memory.* Electric information from the memory drives the *display* (oscilloscope). *(2:75)*

272. **(B)** Transducers may be focused by using a curved piezoelectric transducer element (internal focusing) or by using an acoustic lens. *(19:20)*

273. **(E)** Quality factor (Q factor) is equal to the operating frequency divided by the bandwidth and is unitless.
(2:54)

274. **(E)** Reduction in echoes from a region distal to an attenuating structure *(2:216)*

275. **(G)** An increase in echoes from a region distal to a weakly attenuating structure or tissue *(2:212)*

276. **(A or F)** A structure that is echo-free; not necessarily cystic unless there is good through transmission. A solid mass can be anechoic but will not have good through transmission. *(15:27)*

277. **(D)** An echo that does not correspond to the real target *(21)*

278. **(I)** A structure that possesses echoes *(15:27)*

279. **(H)** Echoes of higher amplitude than the normal surrounding tissues *(21)*

280. **(B)** Echoes of lower amplitude than the normal surrounding tissues *(21)*

281. **(C)** The surface forming the boundary between two media having different acoustic impedances *(15:28)*

282. **(A or F)** A structure without echoes and with low absorption; not necessarily cystic unless there is good through transmission. *Sonolucent* is a misnomer for *anechoic*. *(15:29; 21)*

283. **(C)** Air. There are numerable backing materials used for damping. Pulse-echo transducer backing materials are: (1) epoxy resin, (2) tungsten, (3) cork, and (4) rubber. Continuous-wave Doppler transducers have little or no backing materials. They are usually air backed. *(9:263; 22:33)*

284. **(D)** Surgical, therapeutic, and Doppler. Diagnostic application uses a pulse–echo transducer. *(9:311; 19:23; 22:33)*

285. **(A)** Not all waves are visible. Waves that appear on the surface of water (water waves) are visible. X-rays, radio waves, and sound waves are invisible waves. *(17:3)*

286. **(C)** For ultrasound to propagate a medium, that medium must be composed of particles of matter. A vacuum is a space empty of matter; therefore, ultrasound cannot travel in a vacuum. *(10:1; 25:19)*

287. **(B)** Wavelength *(17:5)*

288. **(A)** Period *(17:5)*

289. **(B)** Hertz (Hz) represents cycle per second (cps). Therefore, 20 cps = 20 Hz. *(17:5)*

290. **(C)** One MHz *(17:5)*

291. **(C)** Ultrasound is produced by piezoelectric crystal. The crystal, damping material, and matching layer are enclosed in a device called a transducer. *(17:31)*

292. **(A)** A-mode is a shortened form of amplitude mode. This mode is presented graphically with vertical spikes arising from a horizontal baseline. The height of the vertical spikes represents the amplitude of the deflected echo. *(22:2)*

293. **(B)** B-mode is a shortened form of brightness modulation. This mode presents a two-dimensional image of internal body structures displayed as dots. The brightness of the dots is proportional to the amplitude of the echo. B-mode display is employed in all two-dimensional images, static or real-time.
(6:60; 22:2)

294. **(C)** M-mode is a shortened form of time-motion modulation. This mode is a graphic display of movement of reflecting structures related to time. M-mode is used almost exclusively in echocardiography.
(6:60; 22:2)

295. **(C)** The cathode-ray tube (CRT) is formed by three essential elements: (1) the electron gun, (2) the fluorescent screen, and (3) the deflection system (vertical and horizontal plates). Silicon is a nonmetallic element found in the earth and used in computer semiconductors. *(24:234)*

296. **(B)** The cathode-ray tube (CRT) is enclosed by a glass tube containing a high vacuum. The manufacturer normally "degases" the tube (removes trapped air or gas) to provide a free passage for electrons.
(17:88; 9:13–15)

297. **(A)** The anode is the counterpart of the cathode and is positively (+) charged. *(17:88)*

298. **(B)** The cathode consists of the electron gun and filament and is negatively (–) charged. *(17:88)*

299. **(C)** The intensity of the ultrasound beam depends on the beam diameter. Intensity is defined as the beam power divided by the beam cross-sectional area.
(2:18)

300. **(C)** Huygens's principle *(1:362)*

301. **(A)** The fraction of time that a pulsed ultrasound is actually producing ultrasound is called the duty factor.

$$\text{duty factor (DF)} = \frac{\text{pulse duration (PD)}}{\text{pulse repetition period (PRP)}}$$

(2:55)

302. **(C)** Real-time ultrasound instrumentation is classified as

1. Sector
   - Linear phased array (pie shaped)
   - Wobbler or rotating wheel (pie shaped)
2. Linear-sequenced array _____ rectangular image
3. Annular _____ employs both mechanical and electronic (combination systems)

(3:15–30; 22:6–9)

303. **(B)** The speed at which ultrasound propagates within a medium depends primarily on the compressibility of the medium.   *(34:1)*

304. **(C)** The reverberation artifact occurs when two or more reflections are present along the path of the beam. This gives rise to multiple reflections, which will appear behind one another at intervals equal to the separation of the real reflectors.   *(11:40; 19:50)*

305. **(C)** Gain is the ratio of electric power. Gain governs the electric compensation for tissue attenuation and is expressed in decibels (dB).   *(2:80; 9:89)*

306. **(C)** Multipath reverberation artifacts result from sound reflected from a highly curved specular surface when the echo takes an indirect path back to the transducer.   *(6:28–29)*

307. **(B)** Both analog and digital scan converters are memory devices. An analog converter stores image information gathered during the scanning process and then retrieves and reads out the information to a vacuum tube similar to a CRT oscilloscope without the phosphor screen. A digital scan converter takes the incoming analog signals from the detector and converts them to binary numbers that are used to represent signal levels. These numbers are then stored in memory.   *(19:31–32)*

308. **(B)** Echo signals that are in analog format as they emerge from the receiver are transferred to a digital format by an analog-to-digital (A–D) converter. Pre-processing then produces the best possible digital representation of the analog signal.   *(19:32)*

309. **(D)** By increasing frequency (MHz) *(f)* and/or transducer diameter (mm), the near zone length (mm) is increased, as shown in the equation:

$$\text{near zone length} = \frac{(\text{transducer diameter})^2 f}{6}$$

(2:59)

310. **(B)** Mass divided by volume   *(2:209–217)*

311. **(H)** Progression or travel   *(2:209–217)*

312. **(D)** Number of cycles per unit time   *(2:209–217)*

313. **(A)** Rate at which work is done   *(2:209–217)*

314. **(G)** The product of pulse duration and pulse repetition rate   *(2:209–217)*

315. **(F)** Range of frequencies contained in the ultrasound pulse   *(2:209–217)*

316. **(E)** Density multiplied by sound propagation speed   *(2:209–217)*

317. **(C)** Conversion of sound to heat   *(2:209–217)*

318. **(I)** Operating frequency divided by bandwidth   *(2:209–217)*

319. **(J)** Power divided by area   *(2:209–217)*

320. **(B)** The damping material reduces spatial pulse length, efficiency, and sensitivity.   *(2:15)*

321. **(C)** Gain is electric compensation for tissue attenuation.   *(15:19)*

322. **(A)** Spectral analysis allows the determination of the frequency spectrum of a signal.   *(17:16)*

323. **(C)** Analog scan converters store any increment of signal amplitude, whereas digital scan converters store the signal amplitude in discrete steps.   *(17:30)*

324. **(C)** Gray-scale resolution is the ability of a gray-scale display to distinguish between echoes of slightly different amplitudes or intensities. The first step in this problem is to figure out how many shades of gray are contained in a 5-bit digital system. The total number of shades of gray is 32 ($2^5 = 32$). The next step is to divide the dynamic range (42 dB) by the number of levels. This will give the number of dB per level. 42 dB ÷ 32 gray levels = 1.3 dB/gray level.   *(2:93)*

325. **(B)**

$$\begin{aligned}\text{Distance} &= \text{velocity} \times \text{time} \\ &= 1540 \text{ m/s} \times 0.01 \text{ s} \\ &= 15.4 \text{ m}\end{aligned}$$

However, 0.1 seconds is only the time to reach the echo source. The time of the round trip must be calculated by multiplying by 2. Round-trip distance = 15.4 m × 2 = 30.8 m.   *(14:2)*

326. **(B)** An edge artifact. Edge shadowing results from refraction and reflection of the ultrasound beam on a rounded surface, for example, the fetal skull.

(28:42)

327. **(A)** A split image artifact (ghost artifact) may produce duplication or triplication of an image, resulting in ultrasound beam refraction at a muscle-fat interface. *(26:29–34; 27:49–52)*

328. **(A)** Multipath, mirror image and side lobe artifacts are most likely to produce a pseudomass. A comet tail artifact is least likely. *(28:27–43)*

329. **(A)** Split image artifact is more noticeable in athletic and mesomorphic habitus patients. *(27:49–52)*

330. **(C)** Split image artifact (ghost artifact) is *not* caused by a gas bubble. The most likely cause is refraction of the sound beam at a muscle–fat interface. The artifact is more evident at an interface between subcutaneous fat and abdominal muscle or between rectus muscle and fat in the pelvis. The artifact can also be produced by an abdominal scar.

(26:29–34; 27:49–52)

331. **(C)** The most likely cause of beam thickness artifact is partial volume effect. This type of artifact occurs most often when the ultrasound beam interacts with a cyst or other fluid-filled structures. *(28:27–45)*

332. **(C)** Beam thickness artifacts depend on beam angulation, not gravity. Therefore, if an image of the gallbladder has what appears to be sludge, a change in the patient's position relative to the beam could differentiate pseudosludge caused by artifact from layering of biliary sludge. *(28:27–45)*

333. **(D)** Side lobe artifact is apparent in both static and real-time images. *(28:27–45)*

334. **(B)** Shotgun pellets and metallic surgical clips produce a trail of dense continuous echoes. Bone, gas, and gallstones produce distal acoustic shadow.

(28:27–45)

335. **(A)** The most common type of artifact observed in patients with shotgun pellets or metallic surgical clips is the comet tail artifact. This type of reverberation artifact is characterized by a trail of dense continuous echoes distal to a strongly reflecting structure.

(16:1–17; 29:225–230)

336. **(D)** A ring-down artifact is characterized sonographically as high-amplitude parallel lines occurring at regular intervals distal to a reflecting interface. This type of artifact is commonly associated with bowel gas. *(30:21–28)*

337. **(A)** It is possible to calculate the displacement in split images by using Snell's law. *(26:29–34)*

338. **(C)** The first vertical deflection at the start of the A-mode is called "main bang," or transducer artifact.

(11:26–27)

339. **(C)** Annular-array real-time uses a combination of mechanical and electronic devices. The annular-array is used for dynamic focusing; the mechanical part for beam steering. *(22:9)*

340. **(A)** A decrease in the amplitude of the returning echo results in a fade-away picture. *(11:52; 22:21)*

341. **(D)** Hard copy is a term applied to forms of picture storage that can be directly viewed. A videotape recorder is hardware. *(11:35; 22:23)*

342. **(C)** M-mode stands for time-motion modulation. This mode displays a graphic representation of motion of reflecting surfaces. It is used primarily in echocardiography. *(10:44)*

343. **(A)** B-mode stands for brightness modulation. This mode displays a two-dimensional view of internal body structures in cross section or sagittal section. The images, displayed as dots on the monitor, result from interaction between ultrasound and tissues. The brightness of the dots is proportional to the amplitude of the echo. Both static and real-time equipment use B-mode. *(10:44; 22:2)*

344. **(B)** A-mode stands for amplitude modulation. This mode displays a graphic representation of vertically deflected echoes arising from a horizontal baseline. The height of the vertical deflection is proportional to the amplitude of the echo, and the distance from one vertical deflection to the next represents the distance from one interface to another. A-mode is one-dimensional. *(10:44; 11:26; 22:2)*

345. **(B)** The effects of ultrasound on human soft tissue are called bioeffects or biologic effects. *(2:2)*

346. **(A)** 1.54 millimeters per microsecond (1.54 mm/μs) or 1540 meters per second (1540 m/s).

347. **(C)** Slope

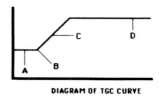

DIAGRAM OF TGC CURVE

348. **(B)** Delay

349. **(D)** Far gain

350. **(A)** Near gain   *(17:299–318; 19:26–27)*

351. **(C)** Progressive weakening of the sound beam as it travels through a medium   *(2:209–217)*

352. **(F)** Having two stages (on or off), black-and-white image, no range of gray   *(2:209–217)*

353. **(G)** Binary digit   *(2:209–217)*

354. **(B)** The production and behavior of bubbles in sound at high intensities   *(2:209–217)*

355. **(D)** A liquid placed between the transducer and the skin   *(2:209–217)*

356. **(H)** A method of reducing pulse duration by mechanical or electrical means   *(2:209–217)*

357. **(E)** The number of intensity levels between black and white   *(2:209–217)*

358. **(J)** Plastic material used in front of the transducer face to reduce the reflection at the transducer surface   *(2:209–217)*

359. **(A)** Picture element   *(2:209–217)*

360. **(I)** Single-frame imaging   *(2:209–217)*

361. **(D)** W/cm^2 *(17:242)*

362. **(A)** 100 mW/cm^2 SPTA   *(2:168)*

363. **(C)** Spatial peak temporal average   *(17:242)*

364. **(B)** kg/m^3 *(2:261)*

365. **(D)** m/s   *(2:261)*

366. **(F)** Hz   *(2:261)*

367. **(E)** J   *(2:261)*

368. **(A)** W/cm^2 *(2:261)*

369. **(C)** m   *(2:261)*

370. **(G)** dB   *(2:261)*

371. **(B)** 0.002 W/cm^2–0.5 W/cm^2 SPTA   *(17:250)*

372. **(A)** 0.5 W/cm^2–2.0 W/cm^2 SPTA   *(17:250)*

373. **(C)** Under normal intensity ranges, diagnostic ultrasound is atraumatic, nontoxic, noninvasive, and nonionizing. It is nonionizing because the intensity in diagnostic ultrasound range is not sufficient to eject an electron from an atom.   *(10:26)*

374. **(D)** Heat. However, at the diagnostic intensity range, the heat produced has no known effect.   *(10:26)*

375. **(A)** The production and behavior of gas bubbles (microbubbles) is called cavitation. Cavitation occurs when dissolved gases grow into microbubbles during the negative pressure phase of ultrasound wave propagation. There are two types of cavitation, stable and transient. Stable cavitation is a phenomenon in which microbubbles are formed and persist in a diameter with the passing pressure variations of the ultrasound wave. In transient cavitation, the microbubbles continue to grow in size until they collapse, producing shock waves.   *(10:26–27; 35:156)*

376. **(D)** There are two types of cavitation, stable and transient. Stable cavitation is a phenomenon in which bubbles are formed and persist. In transient cavitation, the bubbles continue to grow in size until they collapse.   *(10:26–27)*

377. **(A)** Doppler   *(10:61)*

378. **(A)** When an interface is smooth, or "mirror-like," or larger than the wavelength, it is called a specular reflector. When the ultrasound beam strikes a specular reflector, the angle of reflection can be a critical factor when performing sonograms. The maximum amount of reflected echo occurs when the transducer is perpendicular to the interface.   *(11:6, 12)*

379. **(B)** When an interface is smaller than the wavelength, usually less than 3 mm, it is called a nonspecular reflector. Nonspecular reflectors are not beam-angle dependent.   *(11:6; 12)*

380. **(B)** Spatial average temporal average   *(17:242)*

381. **(C)** Spatial peak pulse average   *(17:242)*

382. **(A)** Because Doppler instruments are used for moving structures, static imaging does not apply. The Doppler instrument employs pulsed or continuous waves. The signal is amplified by a loudspeaker, thus the resulting sound is audible.   *(22:10)*

383. **(A)** 5-MHz, short-focus. The choice of focal zone depends on what structure is to be imaged. The choice of transducer frequency depends on the amount of penetration and/or resolution needed. High-frequency transducers display good axial resolution but reduced tissue penetration. For superficial structures, a high-frequency transducer is most useful; for deep structures, low frequency is most useful.   *(4:26–29)*

384. **(B)** 3-MHz, long-focus. See explanation for Question 383. *(4:26–29)*

385. **(A)** Pixel is short for picture element. *(11:32)*

386. **(A)** Under normal circumstances, the human eye can distinguish as many as 16 shades of gray. *(4:38)*

387. **(A)** $512 \times 512 \times 6$-bit deep *(11:32)*

388. **(C)** "Aliasing" results when the velocity exceeds the pulse repetition frequency (PRF). Aliasing is an artifact seen in Doppler ultrasound. *(34:1)*

389. **(D)** All of the above *(4:43)*

390. **(A)** As ultrasound propagates through body tissue it undergoes attenuation, which is the progressive weakening of the sound wave as it travels. The causes of attenuation are:

1. absorption
2. reflection
3. scattering

When the sound wave is absorbed, it is then converted to heat. The heat generated from absorption is mostly removed by conduction. *(10:28; 11:5, 19:74)*

391. **(D)** Most commercial video monitors produced in the United States use 525 horizontal lines. *(11:34)*

392. **(B)** Video monitors in the United States display 30 frames per second. *(11:34)*

393. **(B)** Every one-sixtieth of a second reduces the flicker. *(11:34)*

394. **(B)** 20–25 dB *(11:34)*

395. **(A)** Digital memory stores information in an array of memory locations. The number of rows and columns of the array is called a matrix. *(11:32)*

396. **(A)** Digital memory can be visualized as squares on a checkerboard in which echoes are stored in a square corresponding to the location of the scanning plane. *(11:32)*

397. **(A)** Echo-free *(21)*

398. **(B)** Echogenic *(21)*

399. **(C)** Impedance cannot be measured by a hydrophone. *(2:163)*

400. **(B)** The hydrophone is made up of transducer elements. *(2:163)*

401. **(C)** When a beam is applied for 2–3 minutes on laboratory animals, the results are growth retardation and hemorrhage. These effects were observed in laboratory animals, not humans, and with continuous wave ultrasound. *(17:251)*

402. **(C)** Refraction and diffraction are least likely associated with attenuation. Refraction is the bending of the sound beam as it crosses an acoustic impedance mismatch. The spreading-out of an ultrasound beam is referred to as diffraction. *(9:48; 11:5)*

403. **(B)** Conversion of sound to heat *(11:5)*

404. **(A)** The spreading-out of an ultrasound beam is referred to as diffraction. *(9:48; 11:5)*

405. **(D)** Redirection of the sound beam in several directions *(2:215; 11:5; 9:60)*

406. **(C)** The transducer's piezoelectric ceramic is heat sensitive and should not be subjected to excessive heat sterilization because the crystal in the transducer housing could become depolarized and lose it piezoelectric properties. Transducers are made up of a variety of materials, including plastic, crystals, bounding seals, steel or metal casing, but they are not all constructed alike. A disinfectant that is safe for some transducers may be destructive to others. The recommended method for sterilizing transducers is available from the manufacturer's user manual or from the manufacturer's technical support department. Any product used on transducers against the manufacturer instructions or precautionary measures could result in damage to the transducer and loss of the transducer warranty. *(33:130–131)*

407. **(A)** An acoustic window is a pathway through which the sound beam travels without interference. Examples are the liver and urinary bladder. *(31:77)*

408. **(A)** The decimal number 10 may also be represented by the binary number 1010. *(2:96)*

409. **(B)** Real-time imaging is similar to x-ray fluoroscopy in that each displays motion of internal body parts. *(31:167)*

410. **(C)** The frame rate for real-time systems vary from 15 frames per second to 60 frames per second. A slow frame rate causes flickering. A frame rate higher than 15 frames per second is required to produce a flicker-free image. For fast-moving structures, a high frame rate is needed. *(4:34; 31:167)*

411. **(A)** All images of transverse scans should be viewed from the patient's feet, supine, or prone. *(31:86)*

412. (B) In longitudinal (sagittal) scans the images are presented with the patient's head to the left of the image and feet to the right of the image in both supine and prone positions. *(31:86)*

413. (C) Within the receiver, a number of signal-processing functions take place: amplification, compensation, demodulation, compression, and rejection. *(2:84)*

414. (B) Because the particles in ultrasound waves oscillate in the same direction of wave propagation, no plane is defined. Therefore, ultrasound waves cannot be polarized. *(9:359; 10:1)*

415. (D) Quartz is the transducer crystal most likely to be employed. *(9:310)*

416. (D) All of the above *(9:310)*

417. (C) PZT-5 *(9:310)*

418. (D) Two hundred fifty-six (256), or the number 2 raised to the power of 8 (the number of bits per memory element): $256 = 2^8$. *(34:32)*

419. (B) A real-time mechanical sector transducer allows greater maneuverability for small intercostal space scanning. *(3:173–174)*

420. (G) Both ultrasound and fluoroscopy evaluate moving structures in movie-like appearance. However, ultrasound is nonionizing because its intensity is insufficient to eject an electron from the atom. Fluoroscopy is ionizing and results in potential biologic effects. *(10:26)*

421. (F) The contrast media used for roentgenographic oral cholecystogram (x-ray of the GB) and intravenous pyelogram (x-rays of the kidneys) do not obscure the propagation of ultrasound. *(10:329)*

422. (I) A device used to focus sound beams *(2:209–217)*

423. (C) Picture element *(2:209–217)*

424. (D) Pie shaped *(2:209–217)*

425. (F) A device that changes sound waves into visible light patterns *(2:209–217)*

426. (B) The portion of the sound beam outside of the main beam *(2:209–217)*

427. (H) Imaginary surface passing through particles of the same vibration as an ultrasound wave *(2:209–217)*

428. (A) Unit of impedance *(2:209–217)*

429. (G) The ratio between the angle of incidence and the refraction *(2:209–217)*

430. (E) A change in frequency as a result of reflector motion between the transducer and the reflector *(22:233–238)*

431. (B) The lateral resolution is defined as being equal to the beam diameter. *(32:32)*

432. (F) Perspex, aluminum, and polystyrene. Ethylene oxide is a gas, not a material used for lenses. *(9:317)*

433. (C) Both ultrasound and light can be focused and defocused by mirrors and lenses. *(9:317)*

434. (A) 0.1–1.5 mm *(10:7)*

435. (C) Individual cells cannot be identified because they are smaller than the wavelength used in the medium. *(10:10)*

436. (D) Mass per unit volume *(10:5)*

437. (D) The longer the distance traveled, the greater the absorption. Absorption increases with increased frequency, and the amount of frictional force encountered by the propagating sound wave (viscosity) determines the amount of absorption. *(10:18)*

438. (D) There are no confirmed biologic effects on human tissue exposed to intensities used in the diagnostic range below 100 m/Wcm². However, laboratory experiments on pregnant mice with intensities far greater than that used in the diagnostic range resulted in growth retardation in the offspring of the mice. *(17:251; 2:168)*

439. (C) Pregnant mice exposed to continuous wave ultrasound, applied for 2–3 minutes, experienced neurocranial damage, hemorrhage, and growth retardation. *(2:168)*

440. (B) A combination of low frequency and high intensity is most likely to cause cavitation resulting in tissue damage. *(17:250)*

441. (H) Living human tissue *(2:1–12; 32:1–3)*

442. (E) Tissue cultures in a test tube *(2:1–12; 32:1–3)*

443. (F) A method of analyzing a waveform *(2:1–12; 32:1–3)*

444. (G) The property of a medium characterized by energy distortion in the medium and irreversibly converted to heat *(2:1–12; 32:1–3)*

445. (B) Elimination of small amplitude echo *(2:1–12; 32:1–3)*

446. **(C)** A process of acoustic energy absorption
(2:1–12; 32:1–3)

447. **(A)** An in vivo phenomenon, characterized by erythrocytes within small vessels stopping the flow and collecting in the low pressure regions of the standing wavefield
(2:1–12; 32:1–3)

448. **(D)** Energy transported per unit time
(2:1–12; 32:1–3)

449. **(G)** All of the statements are false or unconfirmed at the present time. Experimental studies were conducted on pregnant mice, not pregnant women. The intensity, frequency, and exposure time were far greater than those used in a diagnostic setting. Continuous ultrasound was used in many of the experiments.
(17:251; 2:173–174)

450. **(D)** At present, there are no known exposure injuries in humans in the clinical setting. Injuries have been reported only in laboratory animals.
(17:251; 2:173–174)

451. **(A)** No distinction. All real-time scans are B-scans, and both static and real-time instruments employ B-mode.
(28:44–45)

452. **(D)** The word transonic implies a region uninhibited to the propagation of ultrasound. An echo-free (anechoic) region does not guarantee the region to be transonic. For example, a homogenous solid mass can be echo-free but not transonic. Conversely, a region can exhibit echoes and be transonic.
(2:179)

453. **(B)** Real-time is also referred to as dynamic imaging. A-mode and M-mode are also real-time modes.
(2:179)

454. **(A)** The TGC is comprised of near gain, delay, slope, knee, and far gain.
(31:58–61)

455. **(A)** The range of pulse repetition frequencies used in diagnostic ultrasound is 0.5 to 4 kHz.
(2:192)

456. **(C)** Cycles, wavelength. The spatial pulse length (SPL) is defined as the product of the wavelength multiplied by the number of cycles in a pulse.
(35:61)

457. **(B)** A-mode and M-mode
(2:105–107)

458. **(C)** Used in some Doppler instruments. Doppler instruments use both continuous or pulse waves.
(2:128)

459. **(C)** Doppler. Doppler instruments employ an audio mode.
(10:62)

460. **(C)** Continuous wave mode. Continuous wave mode requires two crystals, one for transmitting and the other for receiving.
(10:14)

461. **(B)** Acoustic mirror. See Fig. 1–10B, p. 10, in the Study Guide.

462. **(D)** Piezoelectric crystal

463. **(C)** Scanner head

464. **(A)** Motor

465. **(B)** $0.2–400 \text{ mW/cm}^2$
(2:123)

466. **(A)** Higher frequency than the incident frequency
(2:123)

467. **(B)** Lower frequency than the incident frequency
(2:123)

468. **(C)** Bidirectional
(2:128)

469. **(A)** Color Doppler is not beneficial. Color Doppler is very helpful in improving the ability to depict abnormal blood flow.
(2:129)

470. **(B)** Control used to suppress or increase echoes in the near field
(15:19–22)

471. **(A)** Control used to suppress or increase echoes in the far field
(15:19–22)

472. **(D)** Control the upward incline of the TGC. Used to display an even texture throughout an organ
(15:19–22)

473. **(C)** Control used to delay the start of the slope
(15:19–22)

474. **(E)** Controls the point where the slope ends
(15:19–22)

475. **(B)** Bandwidth. Bandwidth is the range of frequencies contained in an ultrasound pulse.
(2:210)

476. **(A)** Q factor. The Q factor is unitless.
(2:54)

477. **(B)** A fluid-filled mass. Fluid-filled masses are characterized by sharp posterior walls and distal acoustic enhancement. The enhancement is associated with low attenuation. Solid and calcified masses demonstrate a different phenomenon, distal attenuation, the degree of which is determined by the attenuating properties of the mass.
(13:32)

478. **(C)** A calcified mass. Calcified masses, gallstones, or any high reflective or attenuating structure can produce an acoustic shadow. This results from failure of the sound beam to pass through the object. The urinary bladder, gallbladder, and any fluid-filled structure will demonstrate acoustic enhancement. In some circumstances, both acoustic enhancement and acoustic shadowing can be seen, for example, a gallbladder with stones.   *(2:216; 15:29)*

479. **(B)** 2. Continuous-wave Doppler uses two piezo-electric crystals, one for transmitting and the other for receiving the returning echoes.   *(1:391)*

480. **(C)** When the beam strikes a vessel at a 30° angle. Doppler angle is the angle between the direction of propagation of the ultrasound beam and the direction of flow. Unlike real-time imaging of the abdominal organs in which the best images are obtained when the ultrasound beam has a perpendicular incidence, Doppler has minimum shift at 90° (perpendicular) incidence, and a maximum shift when the transducer is oriented parallel to the direction of flow, even though parallel transducer orientation is not possible in most cases. Doppler application employs a Doppler angle of 30°–60° with respect to the vessel.   *(1:391)*

481. **(B)** 20 dB

$$dB = 10 \log\left(\frac{\text{power out}}{\text{power in}}\right)$$

$$= 10 \log(100) = 20 \text{ dB} \qquad (34:3)$$

482. **(D)** Depth-gain compensation   *(1:376)*

483. **(D)** Refraction, propagation speed. Refraction occurs only if there is a change in propagation speed. *(1:367)*

484. **(A)** Better axial resolution. Axial resolution is related to the length of the pulse. The shorter the pulse, the better the axial resolution.   *(1:378)*

485. **(A)** 0.25 mW/cm². The reflection fraction R:

$$R = \left(\frac{Z_2 - Z_1}{Z_2 + Z_1}\right)^2 = \left(\frac{75 - 25}{75 + 25}\right)^2 = 0.25 \qquad (1:366)$$

486. **(B)** Frequency and diameter. Near zone length (NZL) is the same as the Fresnel zone:

$$\text{NZL} = \frac{D^2}{4\lambda}$$

where D is diameter transducer (cm), and λ is wavelength (cm).   *(1:362)*

487. **(D)** The element thickness

$$\text{thickness} = \tfrac{1}{2} \text{ wavelength} \qquad (2:50)$$

488. **(B)** Refraction. Refraction is described by Snell's Law, which relates the incident angle (ϕ_i) and the transmitted angle (ϕ_t) to the relative velocities of the two media.

$$\frac{\sin \phi_i}{\sin \phi_t} = \frac{V_1}{V_2}$$

When there is normal incidence, $\phi_i = 0$, and the sound will only change velocity and will not be bent.   *(1:367)*

489. **(C)** 1.54 mm/µs or 1540 m/s   *(1:353)*

490. **(C)** 1.0%

$$\text{DF} = \frac{\text{PD}}{\text{PRP}} = \frac{5}{500} = \frac{1}{100} = 1\% \qquad (2:155)$$

491. **(B)** 20 kHz (or 20,000 Hz). This is the upper limit of the audible range for human beings.   *(34:1)*

492. **(C)** Tissue attenuation. Tissue attenuation increases with increased frequency.   *(1:369)*

493. **(C)** 3.5 dB

total attenuation = attenuation coefficient × path length

$$dB = 1.75 \text{ dB/cm} \times 2 \text{ cm}$$

$$= 3.5 \text{ dB}$$

The attenuation coefficient in dB/cm is by a rule-of-thumb equal to one-half the frequency in MHz; that is, at 3.5 MHz, the attenuation coefficient is 1.75 dB/cm.   *(2:23)*

494. **(D)** Propagation speed.

$$Z = \rho C,$$

where ρ is density, and C is propagation speed. *(34:7)*

495. **(B)** False. Intensity depends upon beam diameter, which is not constant.

$$\text{intensity} = \frac{\text{power}}{\text{beam area}} \qquad (34:2)$$

496. (C) 70%

$$100\% = \text{percentage reflected}$$
$$+ \text{percentage transmitted} \qquad (1{:}366)$$

497. (A) Frequencies   *(1:360)*

498. (C) Distance, velocity, and time

$$\text{distance} = \text{velocity} \times \text{time} \qquad (34{:}1)$$

499. (A) Spatial pulse length. (See answer for question 456.)   *(2:64)*

500. (C) 90°

$$\text{Doppler shift frequency} = \frac{2fV}{C}\cos\theta,$$

where V = velocity of blood flow; f, transducer frequency; c, velocity of sound. Because cos 90° is 0, then the Doppler shift frequency is 0.   *(1:386)*

501. (B) False. Frame rate depends upon the velocity of sound, the image depth, and the number of lines in an image.   *(34:14)*

502. (A) The ratio of the maximum to the minimum intensity that can be processed.   *(2:6)*

503. (B) Smaller. The scan converter dynamic range is determined by its bit depth.   *(34:30)*

504. (A) Compensates for attenuation effects   *(1:376)*

505. (D) Computer memory   *(34:32)*

506. (B) False. Frame rate is determined by the velocity of sound, the depth of the image, and the lines per frame and does not necessarily get reduced by the mechanical scanner.   *(34:14)*

507. (B) Weakly attenuating structures   *(2:146)*

508. (B) False. Preprocessing alters the echo amplitudes before storage; thus, changes will cause the memory content to change.   *(34:32)*

509. (A) Is equal to the beam diameter   *(2:65)*

510. (B) Increased frame rate. If the line density is kept constant, then the number of lines per image will decrease, making the time required per image smaller.   *(34:14)*

511. (D) Reject control   *(1:376)*

512. (A) Too close to. The arrival time will be sooner than expected, causing the system to position the echoes too close.   *(1:353)*

513. (D) Some Doppler systems   *(34:34)*

514. (C) 15 dB. For every change of 3 dB, the intensity will change by a factor of 2.   *(2:255)*

515. (C) Decreases the maximum depth imaged. The pulse repetition period is the length of time allowed to collect echoes for each image line; a short PRP means less image depth.   *(34:14)*

516. (D) Measures spatial resolution. Using different rod-sets in the phantom, estimates of both axial and lateral resolution may be made.   *(2:155)*

517. (B) False. Real-time scanning is achieved using a number of different designs of mechanically steered single-element transducers.   *(34:26)*

518. (A) Increase with increased steering angle. In electronic array systems, minimum grating lobe artifacts are generated when the beam is projected normal to the plane of the array. Beams steered away from the normal will experience greater grating lobe artifacts.   *(34:29)*

519. (C) dB/cm. Total attenuation is expressed in terms of dB, intensity in units of mW/cm^2 and power in units of mW.   *(34:6)*

520. (C) Wavelength, velocity, and frequency

$$C = \lambda f,$$

where C = velocity; λ, wavelength, f, frequency.   *(34:1)*

521. (B) Sensitivity   *(2:155)*

522. (A) Thermal and cavitation. Thermal or heating effects are normally unmeasurable with diagnostic instruments. Further cavitation is also unlikely at current diagnostic levels. Cavitation refers to the growth and behavior of gas bubbles produced in tissue by ultrasound.   *(34:17)*

523. (B) Frequency and transducer diameter. High frequencies and/or large diameter transducers produce long near-zones (Fresnel) lengths.   *(1:362)*

524. (B) No confirmed   *(2:168)*

525. (C) Highest at the focal zone. This is true because the intensity is equal to the power/beam area, and the beam area is smallest at the focal zone.   *(2:18)*

526. **(B)** 0.3 mm

$$\lambda = \frac{V}{f} = \frac{1.54 \text{ mm/}\mu\text{s}}{5 \text{ MHz}}$$

$$\lambda = 0.3 \text{ mm} \qquad (2:8)$$

527. **(C)** Two times smaller. A 3-dB attenuation change would correspond to a factor-of-two reduction; that is, one-half. For each decrease in intensity of 3 dB, the intensity is decreased by one-half. Thus, for 6 dB attenuation, the intensity is decreased by one-fourth. *(1:356)*

528. **(B)** False. A low Q factor implies a short spatial pulse length, which means higher spatial resolution. *(1:359)*

529. **(A)** A wide band of frequencies centered at 5 MHz *(1:360)*

530. **(D)** Thickness, resonance frequency. Specifically, thickness equals one-half wavelength, where wavelength is velocity divided by frequency. *(1:358)*

531. **(A)** Increased damping, sensitivity. Increased damping does improve axial resolution by making the spatial pulse length shorter; however, the result is to make the transducer less sensitive to small echoes. *(1:360)*

532. **(A)** Piezoelectric *(34:4)*

533. **(C)** Matching. Usually a matching layer is added to the front surface of the transducer acoustic impedance intermediate between the impedance of the transducer and that of soft tissue. *(1:370)*

534. **(D)** Constructive interference *(1:361)*

535. **(A)** Highly attenuating structures *(2:139)*

536. **(B)** Occur with multiple strong reflectors. Reverberation artifacts are present when two or more strong reflectors are located in the beam. One of these may be the transducer itself. The sound, in essence, gets trapped between these reflectors. *(2:142)*

537. **(A)** Good axial resolution. A large bandwidth is equivalent to a short spatial pulse length. *(1:360)*

538. **(B)** Fresnel zone. The far zone is also known as the Fraunhofer zone. *(1:363)*

539. **(D)** With normal incidence of the ultrasound beam. At oblique incidence, a sound beam will be bent if there is a change in propagation speed across the boundary. With normal incidence, however, the beam will either slow down or speed up, but will not bend. *(34:7)*

540. **(C)** The pulser voltage spike. The larger the applied voltage, the greater the deformation of the crystal and, consequently, the amplitude of the pressure wave produced. However, a larger crystal (same thickness) experiencing the same voltage will produce more acoustic energy. *(34:8)*

541. **(B)** The reflecting surface is large and smooth with respect to the wavelength. Reflectors whose boundaries are smooth relative to the wavelength behave as mirrors and reflect all frequencies equally. Small reflectors (diffuse or nonspecular) scatter the sound in all directions and show a frequency dependence. *(2:42)*

542. **(C)** Snell's law *(34:6)*

543. **(B)** Is steered mechanically. An annular array is capable of focusing the beam electronically in both x and y directions, but is unable to steer electronically. It must be steered, therefore, by physically moving the transducer or, alternatively, an acoustic mirror. *(34:31)*

544. **(A)** 90–100%. Because the acoustic impedance of gas is so much smaller than that of soft tissue, there is almost 100% of the energy reflected. *(1:366)*

545. **(C)** 1–10%

$$Z_{\text{fat}} = 1.38$$

$$Z_{\text{muscle}} = 1.70$$

$$R = \left(\frac{1.70 - 1.38}{1.70 + 1.38}\right)^2 = 0.011 \ (1.1\%),$$

where R is the percentage of beam reflected. *(1:366)*

546. **(B)** Focal zone can be moved to the skin surface. Often a detachable water path is used to allow the focal zone of a fixed focus transducer to be placed at a superficial location. *(34:28)*

547. **(D)** Longitudinal compression waves. Longitudinal implies that the variation in the pressure occurs in the direction of propagation. This is opposed to a transverse wave, where variations occur perpendicular to the propagation. Transverse waves can occur in bone. *(34:1)*

548. **(A)** Short wavelength and less penetration. The wavelength is inversely related to the frequency, and the attenuation is directly related to frequency.

$$\text{half-intensity depth (cm)} = \frac{3 \text{ dB}}{f},$$

where f is the frequency in MHz. *(34:6)*

549. **(A)** Ring-down time. A long ring-down time is undesirable. It increases the spatial pulse length and, thus, decreases axial resolution.   *(1:360)*

550. **(B)** Electronically focus in two dimensions rather than one. An annular phased array can be focused dynamically in two dimensions. A linear array can be focused dynamically only in the plane of the array. In the slice-thickness direction, perpendicular to the array plane, focusing is achieved by shaping the transducer elements or by acoustic lens. This is often referred to as double focusing.   *(34:30)*

551. **(C)** Gas, muscle, bone. This ordering proceeds along increasing stiffness or lack of compressibility.   *(34:2)*

552. **(A)** Resolution, penetration. At low frequencies, the axial resolution becomes unacceptable (< 1 MHz), whereas at high frequencies, the depth of penetration in the body becomes prohibitively small (10 MHz).   *(34:6)*

553. **(B)** False. Color Doppler is basically a pulsed Doppler system with color encoding. As such, it suffers from aliasing at high flow velocities; that is, shift frequencies greater than one-half the pulse repetition frequency.   *(34:37)*

554. **(B)** SPTP is always equal to or greater than SPTA. SPTP refers to spatial peak–temporal peak, and SPTA refers to spatial peak–temporal average. In all cases, peak values will be at least as great as the average values by definition. For continuous wave ultrasound, there is no variation of the intensity in time, and peak values will be equal.   *(2:21)*

555. **(C)** A hydrophone. A hydrophone is a small piezoelectric crystal that is moved in front of a transducer in a manner so that the beam pattern is mapped. A radiation force balance is used to quantify the total beam power. Other phantoms can be used to give qualitative estimates of beam profiles.   *(2:163)*

556. **(A)** Electronic or mechanical. Electronic generally also refers to a transducer array, either linear or annular. Mechanical generally refers to a single element or physically moved annular arrays.   *(34:26)*

557. **(B)** Schlieren method. Schlieren photography gives a two-dimensional photograph of the beam pressure profile.   *(1:362)*

558. **(D)** Time. Pulse duration is equal to the period of a wave times the number of waves in a pulse, usually microseconds in length.   *(2:14)*

559. **(C)** The frequency. The propagation speed does not significantly depend upon frequency, and, thus, the frame rate is not dependent.   *(34:14)*

560. **(B)** W/cm^2. SPTA refers to intensity, which is power (Watts) per unit beam area (cm^2).   *(2:21)*

561. **(C)** Curie point. Crystals heated above the Curie point lose their piezoelectric property. The Curie point for quartz is 573°C and for PET-4 is 328°C.   *(1:358)*

562. **(C)** Increase ninefold. $I = A^2 = (3)^2 = 9$, where I is intensity, and A is amplitude.   *(1:388)*

563. **(B)** False. In many cases, electronic and mechanical scanners demonstrate a frame rate lower than 30 frames/s.   *(34:32)*

564. **(D)** Velocity, unchanged. The velocity is essentially independent of frequency and is rather dependent upon the physical properties of the medium.   *(34:1)*

565. **(B)** Electronic time-delay pulsing. The delay pulsing of the array elements can be used to form a wavefront directed at different angles. Pulsing can also be used to focus the beam at different depths.   *(34:30)*

566. **(A)** Is made possible by array-based systems. Dynamic focusing is possible only with array-based systems because it is necessary to monitor individually echoes received from each location.   *(34:30)*

567. **(B)** False. Quality assurance is essential for all systems to operate in a reproducible manner.   *(34:37)*

568. **(C)** 1.54 mm. The velocity of ultrasound in tissues is 1.54 mm/µs.   *(34:2)*

569. **(A)** Ring-down artifact. The arrow points to a ring-down artifact produced most probably by gas bubbles resulting in a tail of reverberation echoes.   *(30:21–28)*

570. **(A)** Rods for measuring ring-down. The small open arrows point to a rod group used in measurement of the transducer dead-zone or ring-down distance.   *(17:261–276)*

571. **(B)** A simulated solid lesion   *(17:261–276)*

572. **(C)** A simulated cyst   *(17:261–276)*

573. **(C)** Greater range ambiguity artifacts. Echoes arriving at times greater than the PRP will be placed in the wrong image line and at the wrong depth.

574. **(D)** Gas-filled bubbles. The earliest agents used air-filled bubbles. More recently perfluorocarbon gas is used.

575. **(B)** Perfluorocarbon

576. **(A)** Higher frequencies

577. **(A)** Better lateral resolution. The higher frequency beam has less divergence leading to better lateral resolution and has smaller side-lobes leading to less image clutter.

578. **(C)** Steering the beam to achieve larger echoes at a specific image location. By steering the beam between image lines, it is possible to achieve a more perpendicular angle of incidence and, thus, larger echoes. In the compounding process, the largest echo from an image location is recorded.

REFERENCES

1. Christensen EE, Curry T, Dowdey J. *Introduction to the Physics of Diagnostic Radiology.* 3rd ed. Philadelphia: Lea & Febiger; 1984.
2. Kremkau FW. *Diagnostic Ultrasound: Principles, Instrumentation, and Exercises.* 2nd ed. New York: Grune & Stratton; 1984.
3. Fleischer AC, James E. *Real-Time Sonography.* Norwalk, CT: Appleton-Century-Crofts; 1984.
4. Sanders R, James E. *The Principles and Practice of Ultrasonography in Obstetrics and Gynecology.* 3rd ed. Norwalk, CT: Appleton-Century-Crofts; 1984.
5. Wells PNT. *Biomedical Ultrasonics.* London: Academic Press; 1977.
6. Raymond H, Zwiebel W, et al. *Seminars in Ultrasound: Physics 4(1).* New York: Grune & Stratton; 1983.
7. Rose J, Goldberg B. *Basic Physics in Diagnostic Ultrasound.* New York: Wiley; 1979.
8. Wells PNT. *Physical Principles of Ultrasonic Diagnosis.* New York: Academic Press; 1969.
9. McDicken W. *Diagnostic Ultrasonics: Principles and Use of Instruments.* 2nd ed. New York: Wiley; 1981.
10. Goldberg B, Kotler M, Ziskin M, et al. *Diagnostic Uses of Ultrasound.* New York: Grune & Stratton; 1975.
11. Bartrum R, Crow H. *Real-time Ultrasound: A Manual for Physicians and Technical Personnel.* Philadelphia: WB Sanders; 1983.
12. Powis R. *Ultrasound Physics: For the Fun of It.* Denver: Unirad; 1978.
13. Sarti D, Sample W. *Diagnostic Ultrasound Text and Cases.* Boston: GK Hall; 1980.
14. Pinkney N. *A Review of the Concept of Ultrasound Physics and Instrumentation.* Philadelphia: Sonior; 1983.
15. Saunders R. *Clinical Sonography: A Practical Guide.* Boston: Little, Brown; 1984.
16. Ziskin MC, Thickman DI, Goldberg NJ. The comet tail artifact. *J Ultrasound Med.* 1982; 1:1–7.
17. Powis R, Powis W. *A Thinker's Guide to Ultrasonic Imaging.* Baltimore: Urban & Schwarzenberg; 1984.
18. Shelly G, Cashman T. *Computer Fundamentals for an Information Age.* Brea, CA: Anaheim Publishing; 1984.
19. Hagen-Ansert S. *Textbook of Diagnostic Ultrasonography.* 2nd ed. St. Louis: CV Mosby; 1983.
20. Skelly A: Beyond 100 mW/cm². In: *A Bioeffects Primer: Part 1—Fundamentals.* Vol 1. No 5. Philadelphia: JB Lippincott; 1985.
21. Eggleton R. *American Institute of Ultrasound in Medicine: Recommended Nomenclature: Physics and Engineering.* Oklahoma City: AIUM; 1979.
22. Wells P, Ziskin M. New Techniques and Instrumentation in Ultrasonography. In: *Clinics in Diagnostic Ultrasound.* Vol 5. New York: Churchill Livingstone; 1980.
23. Beiser A. *Modern Technical Physics.* 2nd ed. Menlo Park, CA: Cummings; 1973.
24. Rose J, Goldberg B. *Basic Physics in Diagnostic Ultrasound.* New York: Wiley; 1979.
25. Hussey M. *Diagnostic Ultrasound: An Introduction to the Interactions Between Ultrasound and Biological Tissues.* Glasgow: Blackie & Son; 1975.
26. Sauerbrei E. The split image artifact in pelvic ultrasonography: The anatomy and physics. *J Ultrasound Med.* 1985; 29–34.
27. Buttery B, Davison G. The ghost artifact. *J Ultrasound Med.* 1984; 49–52.
28. Laing F. Commonly encountered artifacts in clinical ultrasound. In: Raymond H, Zwiebel W, eds. *Seminars in Ultrasound: Physics 4(1).* New York: Grune & Stratton; 1983.
29. Thickman D, Ziskin M, Goldenberg J, et al. Clinical manifestations of the comet tail artifact. *J Ultrasound Med.* 1983; 225–230.
30. Avruch L, Cooperberg P. The ring-down artifact. *J Ultrasound Med.* 1985; 21–28.
31. Wicks J, Howe K. *Fundamentals of Ultrasonographic Technique.* Chicago: Yearbook; 1983.
32. Edmonds P. *American Institute of Ultrasound in Medicine: Appendix Relating to Ultrasound Tissue Signatures.* Oklahoma City: AIUM-11375; 1976.
33. Odwin C, Fleischer AC, Kepple DM, et al. Probe covers and disinfectants for transducers. *J Diag Med Sonogr.* 1990; 6:130–135.
34. Fleischer AC, Romero R, Manning FA, et al. *The Principles and Practice of Ultrasonography in Obstetrics and Gynecology.* 4th ed. Norwalk, CT: Appleton & Lange; 1991.
35. Bushong SC, Archer BR. *Diagnostic Ultrasound: Physics, Biology, and Instrumentation.* St. Louis: Mosby-Year Book; 1991.

CHAPTER 2

DOPPLER COLOR FLOW IMAGING INSTRUMENTATION

Raymond L. Powis

Study Guide

Color flow imaging arrived on the medical scene in answer to a basic medical need: an ability to look at cardiovascular blood flow noninvasively. The technology emerged from the development of multigate Doppler systems, which first appeared in 1975.[1] Although these systems used color Doppler only inside an M-mode display, they established both the multigate approach and the use of color to encode motion. In 1983, the first real-time echocardiography color flow system became commercially available.[2] The first commercial color flow vascular imaging device followed in 1986. Since then, nearly all ultrasound manufacturers have added color flow imaging capabilities to their product lines.

Because the ultrasound community had no terminology standards for displaying color-coded information, color flow imaging (CFI) has acquired several alternate names including color Doppler imaging (CDI), color flow Doppler, and angiodynography. In fact, CFI includes both Doppler and non-Doppler depictions of flow in color such as color velocity imaging (CVI).[3] Based on the number of instruments in use, however, Doppler-based CFI (DCFI) is the most common technology sonographers will see. In addition, CVI is not currently being produced or marketed. As a consequence, this chapter focuses only on DCFI instrumentation and how it fits into the major applications of imaging.

The current applications of DCFI are extensive and increasing vigorously. Basic and clinical research is extending the usefulness of this imaging modality. And within the research departments of many ultrasound companies, new technologies are shaping the speed and capabilities of DCFI. As in other parts of ultrasound, understanding the instrumentation can go a long way toward understanding how to conduct clinical examinations and read the images.

THE ESSENTIAL DOPPLER COLOR FLOW IMAGE

The primary feature of the color flow image is its simultaneous depiction of stationary soft tissues in gray scale and moving soft tissues in color. For the most part, the moving soft tissue we are interested in is blood within the cardiovascular system. The technology, however, can be configured to provide a color depiction of myocardial motion as well as flowing blood.[4] Despite this special application, the gray scale and color relationship opens the use of DCFI for two major applications: echocardiography and vascular imaging. But, as you will discover, any moving echo source within and sometimes outside the scanning field can produce color in the image. Setting up the system correctly, however, can limit the color flow information to moving blood.[2]

DCFI is the son of duplex imaging and Doppler multigate analysis. Duplex imaging is older than multigate analysis and has several different forms. It includes the combination of either a continuous wave or a single-point (pulsed-Doppler) spectrum with an image.[5] The image can be an M-mode trace, a real-time B-mode image, or, almost paradoxically, a color flow image. (The paradox is not real, however. DCFI and a single-point spectrum look at the same events, but they do so from different points of view. As a result, they can be profitably combined into a common presentation.)

Multigate analysis is a method of collecting Doppler data from several adjacent spatial locations. A multigate system analyzes each of several sampling sites for flow events using Doppler signal processing. The limitation on this form of signal processing is time. Multigate systems look at each of several sites serially; thus, as the number of sites increases, the time required to make a composite image also increases.[3] As a result, as the time needed to form a composite image frame *increases,* the corresponding image frame rate *decreases.*

Current machines use a number of modern signal handling techniques to keep the image frame rates as high as possible. The essential color flow presentation provides the following pieces of information directly from the image: (1) the existence of flow, (2) its location in the image,

(3) its location in the anatomy, (4) its direction relative to the transducer, (5) its direction relative to the anatomy, and (6) its pattern over space and time.

Because the color image shows flow over space and time, we can use the image to locate specific characteristics within the flow pattern. For example, the higher-velocity flow segments (major streamlines and poststenotic jets) are visible within the heart and larger vessels. In addition, the image clearly shows the difference between a complex flow pattern resulting from anatomy and the poststenotic flow pattern (turbulence) associated with disease.[6]

The ability to clearly show the patterns of flow depends on advanced technologies focused on asking the right technological questions. Everything comes together at the image, where we begin the discussion.

DOPPLER COLOR FLOW IMAGING TECHNOLOGY

Producing an Image

DCFI begins by making a multigate image for both the gray-scale and the Doppler segments of the image. By design, the system divides each beam location in the scanning field into a series of small sampling sites, each of which translates into a specific location in the digital scan converter image.[7] Fig. 2–1 is an example of this division using a linear array. The digital scan converter design in the ultrasound machine determines the size and spacing of these sampling sites.[8]

The sampling intervals used to make the gray scale and color segments of the DCFI depend on the image. For example, a gray-scale image requires sampling intervals no greater than one wavelength.[7] The gray-scale image rests on detection of the echo signal amplitudes, which the signal processing converts into gray-scale intensities. Sampling intervals that are greater than one wavelength simply do not display tissue texturing well enough to support good gray-scale imaging. To show the differences among tissues, a gray-scale image must be able to show the differences among the various tissue textures.

Sampling for Doppler information has a different set of requirements. At the outset, Doppler signal processing requires more time than does amplitude detection. For example, a single pulse–listen cycle can provide the information for a single gray-scale image line-of-sight (LOS). Doppler, however, requires anywhere from 4 to 100 pulse–listen cycles to build a single Doppler image LOS.[3] The increased time is needed to detect the phase shifts in the echo signals that encode the reflector motion. This extended sitting on a single LOS to detect motion is called *dwell time* or *ensemble time*. Practicalities will limit the dwell time on each line of sight to a range of 4 to 32 cycles. As a result, the sampling intervals are usually larger and fewer than in conventional gray-scale imaging. The smallest Doppler sampling sites are at one-wavelength intervals. Often, to shorten the time to form one frame of the combined gray scale and color real-time image, the Doppler sampling sites may be several wavelengths long. There is a limit here, too. Sampling sites larger than 1 mm provide a poor depiction of vascular flow patterns. Fig. 2–2 shows how the sampling intervals can affect the depiction of flow patterns in a vessel.

The heart poses a different set of requirements. Because we do not need to see the same detailed flow patterns required in vascular imaging, color flow echocardiography can use larger sampling intervals.[2] By reducing the time required to make the colored portion of an image, the combined frame rates can be speeded up enough to depict events in both adult and pediatric hearts. Even these techniques, however, may be inadequate. In these cases, the system can still obtain higher frame rates by limiting the flow interrogation to a smaller number of Doppler lines of sight in the image. Limiting Doppler signal processing to a specific region of interest (ROI) or window can help restore the frame rates to usable levels. Despite a limited ROI, the interrogation window can be moved to permit a look at flow over the entire field of view. At each Doppler sampling site, the DCFI system looks at the returning echo signals for changes in phase and the presence of Doppler shift frequencies.

Changes in Phase. Changes in the phase or timing of an echo signal show that an echo source is moving and reveal its direction of motion.[9] The ultimate reference for this motion is the transducer. As in duplex Doppler

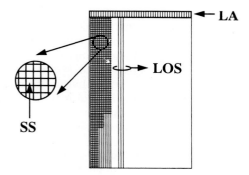

Figure 2–1. Sampling the scanning beams. LA is the linear array, SS is a sample site, and LOS represents the scanning lines-of-sight. Each sampling site represents a position in the digital scan converter.

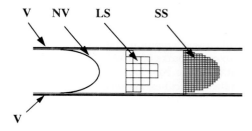

Figure 2–2. Flow image resolution and sampling intervals. W is the vessel wall, NV is the normal velocity profile, LS is the profile with large-interval sampling, and SS is the profile with small-interval sampling. The smaller the sampling, the better the depiction of flow.

imaging, movement toward the transducer is called *forward* motion; movement away from the transducer is called *reverse* motion. The color-flow system encodes this directional information into color, typically red and blue. Fig. 2–3 shows this color assignment geometry for a linear array. These same rules apply to every ultrasound beam in either a sector or linear scanning field. Because no universally accepted standard exists for assigning color to direction, most systems have a flow reverse button that switches the color assignment. This often permits setting arterial flow in red and venous flow in blue. Obviously, in complex vascular patterns, this rule may not hold throughout the image. In this case, a pulsatile flow pattern usually identifies an artery from a vein with lower velocities and a respiratory dependence.

Doppler Shift Frequencies. Each Doppler image sampling site is a range gate that represents the position of the Doppler sample volume. If the sample volume is within a blood flow pattern, a spectrum of Doppler shift frequencies compose the resulting signal. The system, however, cannot display a frequency spectrum within each colored pixel that combines to form a color flow image. Instead, most color flow systems determine a representative frequency and encode this frequency into a color quality.[10]

All current color-flow systems use some form of average frequency to represent the Doppler shift frequency within a sample site. The average frequency is a good choice because it is less sensitive to noise than are most alternatives. In some systems, the average frequency comes from an on-line spectral analysis.[10] In others, autocorrelation and signal-averaging techniques produce the average value. Regardless of the type of system, the signal processing encodes the average frequency into one of several color qualities.

Color has three inherent qualities we can use to encode information: hue, brightness, and saturation. The hue of a color represents its basic frequency or wavelength. For example, red and blue are different hues; so are yellow and green. Some systems encode the Doppler shift frequency information into hue, presenting a variety of different col-

ors, each color representing a different average Doppler shift frequency.[2]

The brightness of a color represents its energy content. For example, increasing or decreasing the illumination on a color patch changes the brightness of the perceived color without changing its hue. Most DCFI designs use changes in hue rather than color brightness to encode the average frequency. At the same time, the brightness of the color may be modulated to smooth the color edges.

Saturation expresses the purity of a color. A color with 100% saturation is considered completely pure. For example, a pure or 100%-saturated red would appear on the display screen as a deep red. Changing the saturation means adding some white light to the color, thus, a less saturated red appears whiter. Many systems allow the user to choose color assignment rules including the use of color saturation to encode the average frequency information.[11] These color assignments make jets and major streamlines appear whiter than the surrounding color.

Beam Contributions to Sampling

Forming the ultrasound beam and the beam's subsequent motion have a strong role to play in making a color flow image. Most DCFI systems use a phased array, linear array, or curved linear array transducer. Only a few systems use a mechanical scan. This preference for electronic scanning is not merely a matter of chance.

The Doppler effect cannot distinguish between a moving ultrasound beam and stationary echo source or a stable ultrasound beam with moving echo source. Without special techniques to control the pattern of beam motion, a mechanical scanner has a steadily moving beam (Fig. 2–4). This continuous motion means that the Doppler signal processing always sees some movement between the tissue echo sources and the ultrasound beam. This movement produces a set of low Doppler shift frequencies that can hide low blood flow velocities.

One clear advantage of the electronic systems is the formation of a stationary ultrasound beam (Fig. 2–4) in

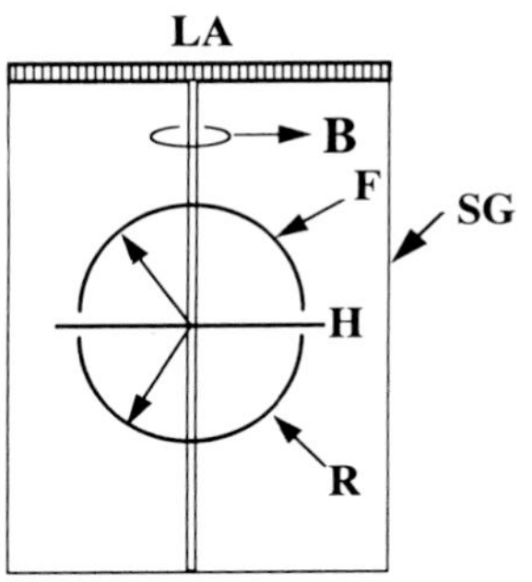

Figure 2–3. Color assignment to the direction of flow. LA is the linear array, B is the ultrasound beam, SG is the scanning field geometry, F is forward motion, R is a reverse motion, and H is a horizontal line. Flow vectors pointing on the F arc are all one color. Flow vectors pointing on the R arc are the opposite color. Anatomy further restricts blood flow to the geometry of the vessel.

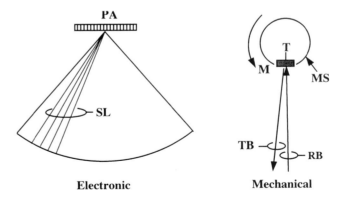

Electronic   **Mechanical**

Figure 2–4. Electronic and mechanically steered beams. PA is a phased array, SL represents the scanning lines, MS is the mechanical scanning head, T is a transducer, M is the direction of motion, TB is the position of the transmit beam, and RB is the position of the receive beam. Electronic steering permits fixed positions for each scan line.

each LOS position. In this scanning pattern, a stationary beam appears at each LOS in the scanning plane.[12] Electronic beam forming and steering have a price as well, however. Every transducer, regardless of size, acts as if it were a hole or aperture in space. In this model (Fig. 2–5), the ultrasound comes from a point source behind the aperture. As the waves travel through the aperture, the waves and aperture interact to produce a diffraction pattern. Most of the energy comes through the aperture and forms a large central lobe of energy. The remaining energy diffracts into a set of *side lobes* that can broaden and smear the beam.

An array of transducer elements (whether linear or curved) produces a similar set of side lobes. Because these lobes come from the summation of side lobes from each transducer element as if from a diffraction grating, and they are called *grating lobes*. When the electronic control positions the beam perpendicular to the array, the grating lobes can be relatively small. By using several different cancellation techniques, however, engineers can suppress the grating lobes as much as –60 dB (1/1000th) or more below the main lobe of energy. When the steered beam points off to the side, however, the number and size of the grating lobes increase (Fig. 2–6).[2] Again, the result can be a smearing of the ultrasound beam and a loss of lateral resolution, a loss that can affect the accurate placement of color within an image.

Signal Processing

Once the echo signals are inside the machine, they face a diverse set of analyses. When and how these analyses occur will determine the character of the final color flow image.

Within the Doppler-based machines, signal processing can take on two different forms. First, a system can use the same signal to make both the gray-scale and Doppler images. This is *synchronous* signal processing.[3] Alternatively, the system can use different signals to form the gray-scale and Doppler images. This is *asynchronous* signal processing.[3] Nearly all DCFI machines designed for vascular applications are now asynchronous, dividing the data collection between gray-scale imaging and color mapping to form each composite image frame.

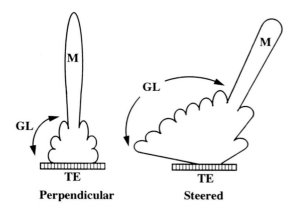

Figure 2–6. Grating lobe formation with beam steering. TE represents transducer elements, GL represents grating lobes, and M is the main lobe. Steering increases the formation of side lobes, smearing the ultrasound beam.

Synchronous Signal Processing. Fig. 2–7 shows the basic organization of a synchronous signal-processing system. Replacing the linear array with a single transducer and replacing the B-mode image with an M-mode trace produced the earliest synchronous system: the M/Q system.[13,14] This system used the same signals to produce both an M-mode display and a point spectrum. All synchronous systems use the same transducer, coherent transmitter, and receiver because they extract different information from a common signal. After reception, the signals divide into two pathways: one for the gray-scale image, the other for the Doppler image. The system uses a priority function to place color properly within the gray-scale image.

To form image frames at speeds useful to echocardiography, most echocardiography color flow systems use synchronous signal processing.[2] These systems use a phased array to form and steer the ultrasound beams (Fig. 2–8). Although beam steering spreads the beam because of grating lobes and side lobes, the effects of these beam distortions do not detract seriously from echocardiography images.

In synchronous vascular imaging, the system shapes and focuses an ultrasound beam along an LOS perpendic-

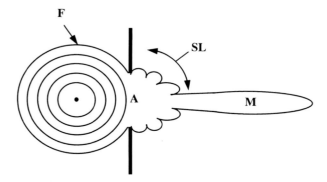

Figure 2–5. The transducer is a diffracting apertures. F is the virtual ultrasound field behind the aperture, A is the aperture, SL represents the diffraction side lobes, and M is the main beam. Each transducer including individual array elements acts as a diffracting hole in space.

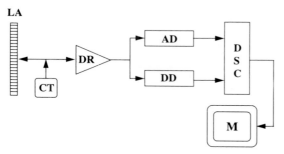

Figure 2–7. Synchronous signal processing. LA is the linear array, CT is a coherent transmitter, R is a receiver, AD represents amplitude detection, DD represents Doppler detection, DSC is the digital scan converter, and M is the color monitor. Synchronous signal processing uses the same signal to make the gray-scale and Doppler images.

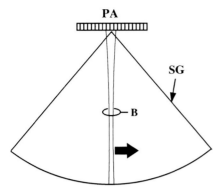

Figure 2–8. Formation of a phased array beam and steering. PA represents the phased array elements, B is the beam, SG is the scanning field geometry, and the arrow shows beam movement. The phased array has a limited aperture size that limits the focal point size and focal range. Thus, focusing is poorest at the edges of the sector.

ular to the linear array. Fig. 2–9 shows the organization of such a system. The beam scans down the array to form a rectangular scanning field. Zone focusing on "transmit" and dynamic focusing on "receive" provide a narrow beam over the field of view.[15]

The system tests each sample site along each beam for flow. If flow exists, the corresponding image pixel becomes colored; if not, the pixel becomes gray scale. In this manner, the processing builds the image on a sample-site by sample-site basis.

Synchronous DCFI for the vascular system faces a Doppler angle requirement. Most of the vessels in the neck, arms, and legs are parallel, or nearly so, to the skin surface, which places an unsteered beam from a linear array 90° to the flow pattern. In this situation, the system can either beam steer or use a wedge stand-off to provide the necessary Doppler angle. A wedge standoff is a water-filled plastic device that slips on and off a linear array as needed. Despite the apparent simplicity of a wedge, most synchronous vascular imaging systems use electronic beam steering to provide the Doppler angle.

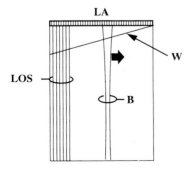

Figure 2–9. Scanning field organization in synchronous signal processing. LA is the linear array, LOS represents the scanning lines-of-sight, W is a wedge, B is the beam, and the arrow shows beam motion. The wedge provides a Doppler angle between the moving blood and the ultrasound beam.

The physical simplicity of the wedge can be deceiving. For example, design engineers must not only consider beam formation, but also how the wedge may change the beam because of refraction, scattering from air bubbles, bacterial growth inside the wedge, and antiseptic treatments of the wedge that do not destroy the plastics that compose the wedge.

Asynchronous Signal Processing. Asynchronous signal-processing systems use different ultrasound beams and signals to create the composite gray-scale and Doppler images.

Asynchronous systems use separate transmitters for the gray-scale and Doppler portions of the image. Only the transducer array and a central coordinating timer are common to the separate signal pathways to the scan converter. Fig. 2–10 shows the organization of an asynchronous imaging system.

Most asynchronous systems use beam steering to obtain the Doppler image while keeping the gray-scale image beams perpendicular to the transducer. Fig. 2–11 shows how the two scanning fields overlay. Because the system uses two different transmitters, the Doppler carrier frequency can be different from the imaging frequency. For example, gray-scale imaging might be at 5.0 MHz and Doppler imaging at 3.0 MHz.

The operating cycle interweaves the Doppler and gray-scale beams to produce two separate images. This interweaving reduces the potential frame rates for the system. Because the sample sites for the two fields of view do not coincide, they cannot accumulate into a common memory in a simple manner. Instead, they pass to separate memories and finally overlay one over the other in the digital scan converter.

Because the two scanning fields have different orientations, the color and gray-scale imaging do not have a one-to-one correspondence over the composite image field (Fig. 2–11). Portions of the steered Doppler image are out-

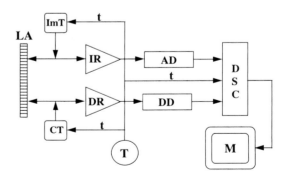

Figure 2–10. Asynchronous signal processing. LA is the linear array, ImT is the image transmitter, CT is the coherent transmitter, R is a receiver, AD represents amplitude detection, DD represents Doppler detection, DSC is the digital scan converter, M is the color monitor, T is a common timer with control signals (t), IR is the gray-scale imaging receiver, and DR is the Doppler receiver. Asynchronous signal processing uses different signals for the gray-scale and color portions of the image.

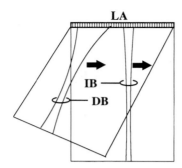

Figure 2–11. Scanning organization for asynchronous signal processing. LA is the linear array, DB is the Doppler beam, IB is the gray-scale beam, and the arrows show beam motion. Beam steering provides a Doppler angle for making the Doppler image. The operating Doppler and gray-scale frequencies can differ.

side the gray-scale field, just as portions of the gray-scale scanning field are outside the Doppler scanning field. One way of keeping the overall image frame rate high is to confine the color signal processing to a small mobile window or region of interest (ROI). This technology arrangement is a common practice for all color flow systems, both vascular and cardiac.

Amplitude Signal Processing (Power Doppler Imaging). Doppler signal processing is generally one of deriving the Doppler frequency components within a returning echo signal. Fast Fourier Transform (FFT) analysis operates on the composite wave form and produces a range of discrete frequency components. Thus, an FFT provides two properties of these component signals for analysis and portrayal in color: (1) Doppler signal frequencies and (2) Doppler signal amplitudes. DCFI encodes the Doppler shift frequencies into color to show both the direction and speed of blood flow. An alternative to frequency analysis is to determine the *power spectrum* of the Doppler signal amplitudes using the system directional (in-phase and quadrature) channels. Although this technique may have different trade names, the technology is most often called *amplitude* or *power Doppler* imaging.[16] Importantly, although the name of the technique includes the word *power, it does not increase the acoustic power* delivered to the patient. Rather, it is a different method of signal processing using normal signal amplitudes and output power values.

Signal processing for Doppler frequency information offers advantages and disadvantages. At the outset, frequency information shows both the direction and relative velocity of the blood flow in the image. At the same time, it is very sensitive to noise, the Doppler angle, and is subject to high-frequency aliasing.

Power Doppler on the other hand, is not as sensitive to system noise as frequency-based Doppler, but it is more sensitive at displaying flow boundaries. In addition, power Doppler is relatively angle independent, and is nonaliasing. Because of these last three advantages, power Doppler can better show overall vascularity and better supports

three-dimensional depictions of perfusion into organs and masses.[16]

Power Doppler, however, forfeits detailed flow information within the vessels. In addition, it is very sensitive to soft tissue motion and the so called "flash artifact" produced by this motion. To date, much effort has gone into developing techniques that can suppress the flash artifact and improve power Doppler imaging.

PRACTICAL ISSUES

Cardiac Imaging Requirements

In general, viewing the heart with ultrasound requires intercostal and subcostal imaging with low-frequency ultrasound.[2] Parasternal DCFI naturally places the ultrasound beam approximately 90° to the flow pattern. As a result, apical and subcostal views of the heart are needed to place flow patterns parallel to the ultrasound beams. The phased array and the short-radius, curved linear arrays are the transducers of choice for viewing through these thoracic and abdominal windows. The sector angles range from 30° to 180°.

Because blood is a low attenuator (0.15 dB/cm per MHz), viewing the heart with ultrasound does not require the same sort of front-end design (delay lines and receivers) that vascular imaging requires. In addition, the high frame rates, combined with large fields of view, impose large sampling intervals on the cardiac image, and the scanning uses a sector format. All of these factors combine to make the cardiac color flow device right for the heart and wrong for the vascular system.

Because the Doppler sampling intervals can be relatively large in echocardiography, detecting a regional turbulence is not always easy. To help locate flow disorganization (spectral broadening) for any sampling location, most cardiac systems determine not only the mean frequency at a sample site, but the signal variance as well.[2] In many cardiac devices, color coding for an increasing variance introduces a green tint to the primary color.

Vascular Imaging Requirements

Vascular DCFI involves all available peripheral vessels, the large, upper thoracic vessels, and the deeper vessels in the abdomen. A linear array typically is used to view the peripheral vessels. This linear scanning field sets the stage for using changes in color to show changes in the direction of flow. In contrast, a sector scan of a linear vessel produces a continuously changing Doppler angle (Fig. 2–12) and, thus, continuously changing color. Instead, sector scanning transducers, such as the phased array and the curved linear array, are used to view abdominal vasculature. These transducers permit both subcostal and intercostal scanning to visualize the deeper abdominal vessels that may be within the rib cage.

The sector fields, however, make reading the images more difficult. Identifying arteries and veins requires knowing both the direction and the pulsatility of the flow. Large fields of view and longer processing times for the

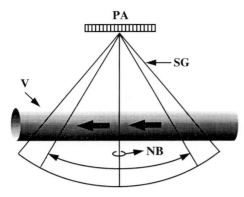

Figure 2–12. Vascular imaging with a sector scanning field. PA is a phased array, SG is the scanning field geometry, V is the vessel, and NB is the beam perpendicular to flow in the vessel (arrows). Because each beam position has a different Doppler angle, the colors in the image change rapidly.

color flow image often make the effective frame rates too low to permit an easy determination of pulsatility. Using a single-point spectrum and a color flow image together as well as decreasing the ROI can yield information about vascular pulsatility.

Displays of Frequency and Velocity

All current color flow images using Doppler are two-dimensional maps of the Doppler shift frequencies. After all, color flow uses Doppler, too.

Many systems show the color values in velocity (cm/s) rather than frequency (Hertz). This sort of display suggests a direct measurement of velocity in color. As in all color-flow Doppler determinations of velocity, the values represent a solution to the Doppler equation (Fig. 2–13). In this display, however, the velocity is not the absolute velocity of the red cells. Instead, the image values represent the *closing velocity* along the ultrasound beam. Absolute velocities would require a continuous correction of for all angles to the flow patterns throughout the image. Fig. 2–14 shows this closing velocity relationship.

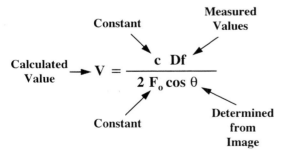

Figure 2–13. Calculation of velocity with the Doppler equation. V is the velocity, c is the ultrasound propagation velocity, Df is the Doppler shift frequency, F_o is the carrier frequency, and θ is the Doppler angle. Doppler machines measure frequency and calculate "true" velocity, V, based on an estimated Doppler angle entered by the sonographer.

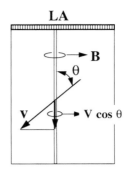

Figure 2–14. The closing velocity geometry. LA is the linear array, B is the ultrasound beam, SG is the scanning field geometry, V is the target velocity, and V cos θ is the closing velocity. Closing velocity is the component of motion along the ultrasound beam.

Color Flow Imaging Artifacts

Because DCFI incorporates both B-mode imaging and Doppler signal processing, it is subject to the same artifacts that affect ultrasound in general. Three primary sources of confusion in DCFI are: (1) range ambiguity artifacts, (2) Doppler high-frequency aliasing, and (3) soft-tissue vibrations.

Fig. 2–15 shows the organization of events required to obtain a range ambiguity artifact. The high power and faster frame rates typical of DCFI offer ample opportunities for this artifact.[17] In DCFI, the artifact appears as diffuse, nonpulsatile colors, suggesting flow that may not actually exist where it appears in the image.

In a pulsed Doppler system, the Doppler shift frequencies are being sampled at the pulse repetition frequency (PRF) of the system. High-frequency *aliasing* occurs when the Doppler shift frequency exceeds the system PRF sampling frequency. This aliasing limit is known as the *Nyquist*

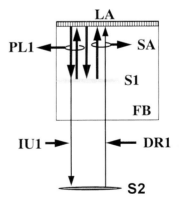

Figure 2–15. The range ambiguity artifact. LA is the linear array, PL1 is the initial pulse–listen cycle, IU1 is the incident ultrasound from PL1, S1 is a phantom echo source inside the field boundary (FB), S2 is a real echo source outside the scanning field, DR1 is the deeper returning echo, and SA represents the simultaneous arrival of the two echo signals. Range ambiguity occurs when echo sources outside the scanning field appear in the image.

limit, which is PRF/2. When aliasing occurs in CFI, both the colors and the single point Doppler spectra "wrap around" the display format (that is, the high frequencies in one direction appear as lower frequencies in the opposite direction) and confuse the appearance of flow. To remove aliasing, a sonographer must either increase the PRF (shorten the field of view) or decrease the Doppler shift frequency associated with the highest velocity.[13] You can decrease the Doppler shift frequency by either decreasing the Doppler carrier frequency or moving the transducer to place the Doppler angle closer to 90°. Because of the increasingly pronounced error production with Doppler angles above 70°, however, it is better to choose a lower carrier frequency than to increase the Doppler angle above 70° (e.g., at 75°, the velocity calculation has an inherent error rate of 6.5%/degree; thus, an error of +/– 3° in estimating the true Doppler angle creates a velocity calculation error of +/– 19.5%).[9]

A not uncommon source of DCFI confusion is the mechanical vibration of soft tissues. For example, tissue vibrations can occur if a patient talks or if the blood flow happens to be producing a *bruit* or noise.[18] These tissue vibrations can fill an image of an artery or vein with lots of color outside the vessel walls. The low-frequency pulse from the heart also can fill an abdominal image with a burst of color known as a *flash artifact,* which can cause problems for power Doppler as noted earlier.[16]

Applying the Technology to Real Images

Using these ideas of how the various color flow systems work, we are now in a position to examine some examples of DCFI. They range from the depiction of flow within an M-mode recording to high-resolution imaging of the vascular system.

Fig. 2–16 shows the combination of an M-mode recording with DCFI. All motion in this image is referenced to the transducer as a closing velocity; that is, only as motion directly toward or away from the transducer. In this example, the Doppler frequencies have been calculated into closing velocities, which *do not* necessarily represent the true velocities of the cardiac blood flow. This system encodes the presence of spectral broadening by adding green to the primary directional colors. The green color flow in diastole demonstrates: (1) the presence of aortic regurgitation and (2) the ensuing turbulence as the left ventricle fills through an open mitral valve.

Determining the true flow pattern is easier with a two-dimensional image of the heart. Fig. 2–17 provides a clear view of the heart in long axis, with the color flow confined to the heart's chambers. Again, the Doppler frequency map is calculated into closing velocity values. This image shows a nonaxial regurgitating jet extending from the aortic root into the left ventricle. In this case, the color flow images show not only the existence of the jet but also its nonaxial geometry.

Fig. 2–18 (normal carotid artery flow) depicts a normal carotid artery with an early synchronous DCFI system. The Doppler angle comes from a wedge standoff at the top of the image. The sampling rate in this image is at one-

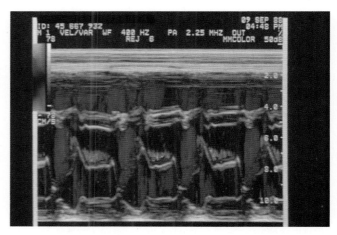

Figure 2–16. Color flow imaging of a mitral valve. The M-mode tracing views the mitral valve from the upper portion of the cardiac window, aimed down toward the mitral valve. Red is flow toward the transducer; blue is flow away. Closing velocity values (aliasing limits) appear on the color bar. The red flow between the interventricular septum and closed mitral valve is ejection through the left ventricular outflow tract. During ventricular filling, the blue–green flow along the anterior mitral valve leaflet is reversed, turbulent flow produced by an aortic regurgitation. Depth markers are at the right of the image, and an EKG trace provides timing at the bottom of the image. *(Reproduced with permission from Advanced Technology Labs, Bothell, WA.)*

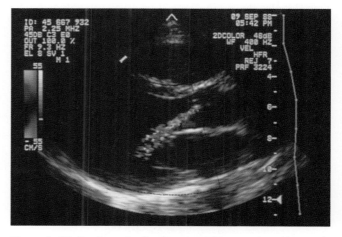

Figure 2–17. Cardiac color flow imaging. This parasternal long-axis view of the heart shows (from the top down) the right ventricle, the interventricular septum, and the left ventricle containing the mitral valve leaflets. Red is flow toward the transducer; blue is away. Closing velocity values (aliasing limits) appear on the color bar. The color-imaging window (blue boundary) shows a nonaxial blue–green turbulent jet (regurgitation) originating at the aortic root. Without color, the nonaxial quality of the jet could not be easily determined. *(Reproduced with permission from Advanced Technology Labs, Bothell, WA.)*

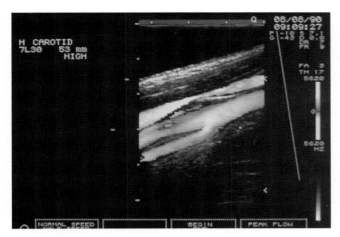

Figure 2–18. Color flow imaging of a carotid artery. The long-axis view of a normal carotid artery bifurcation shows the common carotid artery branching into internal (upper branch) and external (lower branch) carotid arteries. Flow is right to left, away from the transducer (red bar at the top of the image). The vessel above the carotid (blue) is the jugular vein. Within the carotid bulb is a normal flow separation and reversal (blue). Because higher Doppler shift frequencies are whiter, the major streamlines appear whiter in the image. The required Doppler angle comes from the wedge standoff (black triangular space at the top of the image). The peripheral dots are 1-cm markers, and the aliasing frequencies appear at the top and bottom of the color bar. *(Reproduced with permission from Siemens Ultrasound Group, Issaquah, WA.)*

Figure 2–19. Color flow imaging of a carotid artery. The image shows the internal carotid artery and bulb. Flow in the artery (red) is from right to left, with a flow separation and reversal in blue. The major, nonaxial streamline (yellow) in the bulb is along the anterior wall. A small segment of aliasing (green) appears in the streamline. The more anterior blue vessel is the jugular vein. The Doppler angle is this image comes from beam steering. The white parallelogram shows the steering angle and the boundary for color signal processing in the image. The aliasing frequency limits appear on the color bar, with depth markers and a transmit focal point position on the right side of the image. *(Reproduced with permission from Advanced Technology Labs, Bothell, WA.)*

wavelength intervals (0.2 mm at 7.5 MHz) for both the gray-scale image and the color portion of the image. The internal flow pattern of the vessel shows a normal flow separation and reversal in the carotid bulb. The flow direction is from image right to left, away from the transducer, causing the vessel to appear red. The higher Doppler shift frequencies appear whiter, depicting the higher-velocity portions of the flow.

The beam steering that is typical of asynchronous signal processing changes the organization of a similar image of a normal carotid artery. This system depicts different average Doppler shift frequencies in different color hues. As in Fig. 2–19, however, the image clearly shows the flow separation and reversal (blue portion in the red vessel) that is typical of a normal carotid bulb. The beam steering in this image limits simultaneously showing flow and soft tissue anatomy throughout the image. Moving the color flow processing window and changing the scanning position, however, permits a full interrogation of most vessels.

Any highly vascular tissue or structure is a good candidate for DCFI when trying to separate out ambiguous anatomy. Flow within major fetal vessels appears in Fig. 2–20. This image is formed with a convex linear array, producing a sector image pattern. Because of the complexity of the vascular anatomy and the changing angle between the vessels and the beams, the immediate color encoding does not always indicate arteries and veins. Instead, the vessel pulsatility and its position relative to internal ana-

tomical landmarks tell the story. If the system frame rate is too slow, however, a single point, pulsed Doppler spectrum will be the most reliable means of determining the

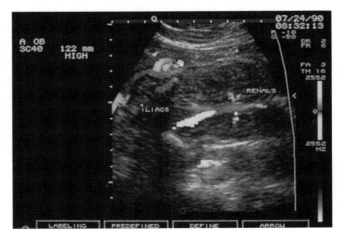

Figure 2–20. Color flow imaging of a fetal abdomen. This image shows the fetal aorta with renal and iliac branches. Flow away from the transducer is blue; flow toward the transducer is red. The peripheral dots are 1-cm markers, and the aliasing frequencies appear at the top and bottom of the color bar. A convex curved array forms a sector scanning field. *(Reproduced with permission from Siemens Ultrasound Group, Issaquah, WA.)*

pulsatile flow patterns of arteries and the steadier flow patterns of veins.

When wall disease in a vessel or simply vascular anatomy disturbs the flow pattern, a single point spectrum cannot show the source or character of the disturbance. High-resolution DCFI, however, as shown in Fig. 2–21 clearly depicts not only curving vessel walls, but also a major streamline moving across the vessel in response to flow inertia.

In the presence of stenosis, the flow within the narrowing increases velocity. The narrowing also often appears in the image as a physical narrowing of the color distribution as the spatial signal processing maps a reduced lumen. Fig. 2–22 shows these two results, the narrowing of the color distribution and the acceleration (central green portion of the color in the lumen poststenosis) due to a carotid artery stenosis.

When frame rates are high enough and the Doppler sampling is fine enough, we begin to see some of the subtler flow physiology. For example, each pulse in the vascular system is a mechanical wave that travels down the vessels to be reflected at changes in hydraulic impedance. Fig. 2–23 shows the intersection of two traveling pulse waves: The red portion is the incident wave, and the blue portion is the reflected wave. The color flow image and the Doppler spectrum show the connection between the triphasic flow pattern of this high-resistance vessel and the passing of forward and reversed pulse waves within the artery.

Although power Doppler can fill an image with color as in Fig. 2–24, the processing looses the information about flow direction. As a consequence, the carotid arteries and the jugular vein have the same color. As the sampling ap-

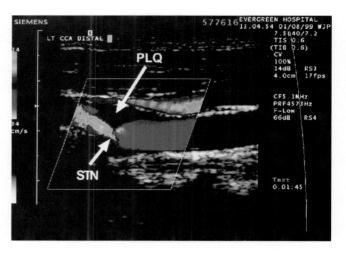

Figure 2–22. Color flow imaging of a carotid artery stenosis. This artery has a significant stenosis that is narrowing the flow channel (narrow color distribution), causing a poststenotic turbulence (mixed colors). Prestenotic flow is right to left, away from the transducer and colored red. The poststenotic flow is toward the transducer and colored blue. The markers on the image left are 0.5-cm intervals. The aliasing closing velocities appear at the top and bottom of the color bar. PLQ is a soft, anechoic plaque. STN is the narrowest region of the stenosis. (*Reproduced with permission from Siemens Ultrasound Group, Issaquah, WA.*)

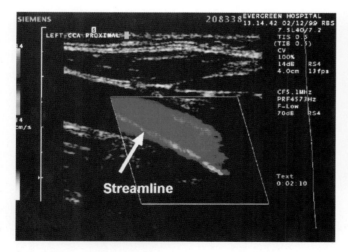

Figure 2–21. Color flow imaging of a common carotid artery. This artery has a curve that sends a major streamline (arrow) across the vessel lumen. Flow is from right to left toward the transducer. The upper red color bar represents motion toward the transducer. The flow deviation is about 15° steeper than the vessel wall. The vertical markers on image left indicate 0.5-cm intervals. The aliasing closing velocities appear at the top and bottom of the color bar. (*Reproduced with permission from Siemens Ultrasound Group, Issaquah, WA.*)

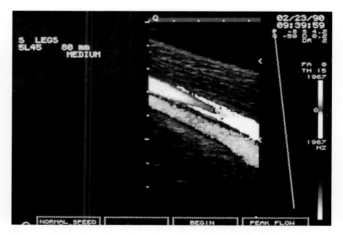

Figure 2–23. Color flow imaging of a superficial femoral artery and vein. These normal vessels show typical flow patters during the cardiac and respiratory cycle. Arterial flow from left to right, and a distally reflected pulse wave (blue) arriving to cross the incident pulse wave (red). The superficial femoral vein (blue posterior vessel) is flowing right to left as flow and color fill the vein's residual lumen. This color flow image clearly shows the reversal of flow in a triphasic or biphasic flow pattern comes from a traveling pulse wave. The peripheral dots are 1-cm markers, and the aliasing frequencies appear at the top and bottom of the color bar. The black space at the top of the image is a wedge standoff. (*Reproduced with permission from Siemens Ultrasound Group, Issaquah, WA.*)

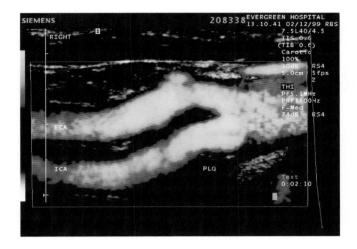

Figure 2–24. Power Doppler depiction of flow in a carotid artery. ECA is the external carotid; ICA is the internal carotid, PLQ is an anechoic plaque narrowing the carotid bulb. The depth marker on the image left shows 0.5-cm intervals. The upper right corner of the ROI includes a portion of the jugular vein flowing in opposite direction to the carotid arteries with the same color as the arteries.

proaches the vessel walls, the signals are coded for a decrease in signal brightness.

SUMMARY

DCFI is a combination of gray-scale anatomical information and a colored depiction of flow events. It is an integrated image of form and function, anatomy, and physiology. The color portion of the image is not an image of blood, however; it is an image of motion. Using power Doppler, the color can depict the presence of flow with great sensitivity, but without some flow details.

Within each Doppler color flow system, the amplitudes of echo signals become gray-scale intensities, while the frequency content of the signals becomes color. The echo signals for both may be the same or be different, even in carrier frequency. This imaging modality depends on the sophistication and speed of contemporary digital signal processing. It also is an imaging modality that is changing and will continue to change the fields of ultrasound and medicine.

Questions

GENERAL INSTRUCTIONS: For each question, select the best answer. Select only one answer for each question unless otherwise specified.

1. Duplex imaging combines gray scale with Doppler and can appear as

   (A) M-mode and spectrum
   (B) B-mode and spectrum
   (C) color flow imaging and spectrum
   (D) all of the above

2. Doppler color flow imaging produces an image composed of

   (A) tissue echoes in gray scale and blood echoes in color
   (B) moving soft-tissue echoes in gray scale and blood motion in color
   (C) stationary tissues in gray scale and moving tissues in color
   (D) stationary tissues in gray scale and stationary blood in color

3. Color Doppler imaging is a term used to describe

   (A) a form of color flow imaging
   (B) a form of magnetic resonance imaging
   (C) a new form of imaging relying on high-speed propagation velocities in soft tissues
   (D) a form of detecting flow with lasers

4. The Doppler effect occurs

   (A) only to waves traveling more than 1,000 m/s
   (B) only to ultrasound waves with intensities greater than 500 mW/cm², SPTA
   (C) to all waves coming from a moving wave source
   (D) in ultrasound, but only when the targets are moving faster than 1.0 m/s

5. The Doppler effect depends on

   (A) the carrier frequency, the angle between echo source velocity and beam axis, and the reflectivity of blood
   (B) the closing velocity between transducer and tissue, carrier frequency, and ultrasound propagation velocity
   (C) the lowest Doppler-shift frequency detectable and the highest frequency without aliasing
   (D) the largest change in acoustical impedance within the moving blood

6. To calculate blood velocity using color flow imaging, a sonographer must

   (A) place a sample volume in the major streamline or jet within the vessel and set an angle correction parallel to the vessel wall
   (B) assume that all flow is parallel to the vessel wall
   (C) locate the major streamline and place the sampling angle at 60° to the vessel wall
   (D) place a sample volume in the major streamline or jet and set the angle correction parallel to the streamline

7. To preserve gray-scale texture, digital sampling for gray-scale images must be at intervals of

   (A) 0.6 mm
   (B) one wavelength or less
   (C) 1.0 mm
   (D) 3 dB

8. To preserve flow detail, digital Doppler sampling intervals for a vascular color flow image must be at intervals of

   (A) 1–2 mm
   (B) 1–2 cm
   (C) one wavelength or more but less than 1 mm
   (D) −6 dB

9. Gray-scale tissue texture in a color flow imaging system depends on

   (A) transmit focusing only
   (B) receive focusing only
   (C) the product of transmit and receive focusing
   (D) the speed at which the ultrasound beam is moved by the scanhead

10. The shape of the sample volume in pulsed Doppler has a major effect on the content of the Doppler signal.

    (A) true
    (B) false

11. To form the color patterns in a Doppler color flow image, a color flow system samples down each Doppler image line of sight for

    (A) the amplitude of the Doppler signal
    (B) the velocities of red blood cells
    (C) the average Doppler shift frequency
    (D) the velocity spread within the sample site

12. The Doppler portion of a color flow image is a map of red-cell velocities.

    (A) true
    (B) false

13. Separating moving soft tissue from moving blood in a color flow image tests for

    (A) Doppler signal amplitudes only
    (B) tissue signal amplitudes only
    (C) Doppler signal frequencies only
    (D) the relationship between the amplitudes and frequencies of the Doppler signals

14. A curving vessel within a color flow image shows color in the vessel when the beam and vessel are parallel but shows no color as the vessel turns perpendicular to the beam. The loss of color means that

    (A) the vessel is occluded
    (B) the vessel is open, but the blood velocity is too low to complete the image
    (C) the dark region is diseased
    (D) The Doppler effect works only when the vessel is parallel to the ultrasound beam.

15. The smallest vessels that appear in a color flow image are about 1 mm in diameter. The smaller vessels are absent because

    (A) arterial blood velocities are too low in vessels that are less than 1 mm in diameter
    (B) the smaller vessels are shadowed by the surrounding soft tissue
    (C) soft tissue does not have many vessels that are less than 1 mm in diameter
    (D) the smaller vessels do not reflect ultrasound as well as the larger vessels do

16. The color flow image provides information on (1) the existence of flow, (2) the location of flow in the image, (3) flow direction relative to transducer, (4) the maximum flow velocity.

    (A) all of the above
    (B) 1, 3, and 4
    (C) 3 and 4
    (D) 1, 2, and 3

17. Detecting flow in a color flow imaging system depends on the detection of

    (A) changes in Doppler signal amplitude
    (B) changes in Doppler signal frequency content
    (C) changes in echo signal phase and frequency content
    (D) changes in echo signal phase

18. One begins reading a color flow image by

    (A) determining the maximum systolic frequency
    (B) knowing the position of the scan plane on the patient's body
    (C) knowing the direction of flow relative to the transducer
    (D) determining the Doppler carrier frequency

19. Changes in the Doppler shift frequencies within a color flow image sample site appear in the image as

    (A) nothing; the image only shows changes in phase
    (B) different colors (hues)
    (C) different levels of color saturation (purity)
    (D) different colors (hues) or different levels of saturation (purity)

20. A Doppler color flow image can show changes in the frequency content at a Doppler sample site by

    (A) changes in gray scale
    (B) changes in saturation
    (C) changes in color hue
    (D) the introduction of green markers

21. Cardiac color flow imaging shows changes in the frequency content of the Doppler sample site by

    (A) changes in color
    (B) changes in saturation
    (C) changes in color texture
    (D) the introduction of red markers

22. Color flow imaging systems determine the maximum Doppler shift frequency at each sample site.

    (A) true
    (B) false

23. A measurement of the peak systolic frequency in a carotid artery with a single-point spectrum will be lower than a measurement of the color-encoded frequency at the same point.

    (A) true
    (B) false

24. The synchronous signal processing uses a Doppler carrier frequency that is the same as the imaging center operating frequency.

    (A) true
    (B) false

25. Asynchronous signal processing in color flow imaging requires the same frequency for both Doppler and gray-scale imaging.

   (A) true
   (B) false

26. Beam steering in asynchronous color flow imaging is used to provide

   (A) a Doppler angle significantly less than 90° to typical blood flow
   (B) a way of looking at the same soft-tissue targets at an angle different from the perpendicular beams
   (C) an enlarged Doppler beam to improve Doppler sensitivity
   (D) improved Doppler sensitivity to smaller vessels

27. The mechanical wedge in synchronous color flow imaging is used to provide

   (A) improved penetration through impedance matching
   (B) improved beam focusing for the gray-scale image
   (C) an attenuation system to remove side lobes
   (D) a Doppler angle between the typical flow patterns in vessels

28. The ability to see flow in deep vessels is limited by the fact that

   (A) blood has scattering units that are about the same size as soft tissue
   (B) blood is moving faster than the surrounding tissues
   (C) blood has an extremely low attenuation rate
   (D) blood reflectivity is about 40–60 dB below that of soft tissue

29. Levels of output power and intensity for color flow imaging are generally higher than those for conventional gray-scale imaging.

   (A) true
   (B) false

30. Because Doppler signal processing requires more energy, synchronous signal processing always produces Doppler power levels that are higher than those for gray-scale imaging.

   (A) true
   (B) false

31. In general, tissue ultrasonic intensity levels are higher for single-point spectra than for color flow imaging with the same system.

   (A) true
   (B) false

32. Moving from gray-scale only to full-screen color flow imaging in a system means that the image frame rate will probably do which of the following?

   (A) decrease
   (B) increase
   (C) stay the same
   (D) color signal processing has no effect on frame rate

33. Color flow imaging in the heart uses larger Doppler sampling intervals to increase the image frame rate than does vascular imaging.

   (A) true
   (B) false

34. Cardiac color flow imaging also works well in the vascular system because the design can handle the high attenuation rates in cardiac imaging.

   (A) true
   (B) false

35. Sampling intervals for cardiac color flow imaging and vascular color flow imaging are similar.

   (A) true
   (B) false

36. Cardiac color flow imaging is limited with a mechanical sector scanner because

   (A) the cardiac attenuation rate is too high
   (B) the ultrasound beams are always moving
   (C) the beam has a fixed focal point
   (D) the beam has too many side lobes

37. The phased array sector scanner and the linear array share common beam forming properties of (1) a stationary beam at each line of sight, (2) increased grating lobes with beam steering, (3) three-dimensional dynamic focusing on receive, (4) the same aperture sizes for dynamic focusing.

   (A) 1 and 2
   (B) 1, 2, and 4
   (C) 2, 3, and 4
   (D) all of the above

38. Color flow imaging in the peripheral vascular system typically uses

   (A) the phased sector scan
   (B) the linear array scan
   (C) the curved linear scan
   (D) a combination of A and B

39. Color flow imaging in the heart typically uses

   (A) the phased sector scan
   (B) the linear array scan
   (C) the curved linear scan
   (D) a combination of A and C

40. You are imaging a small vessel using 7.5 MHz DCFI with the lowest displayable velocity of 6.0 cm/s. Changing only the carrier frequency to 5.0 MHz will change the *lowest* displayable velocity to

(A) 1.5 cm/s
(B) 9 cm/s
(C) 6.0 cm/s; the vessel does not change
(D) 15 cm/s

41. Doppler color flow imaging is unique because it does not have a major problem with high-frequency aliasing.

(A) true
(B) false

42. Both the color and a point spectrum in a stenosis show high-frequency aliasing. One strategy for removing the aliasing involves

(A) doing nothing. Aliasing cannot be removed from the system.
(B) decreasing the system PRF
(C) decreasing the carrier frequency
(D) decreasing the Doppler angle toward zero

43. Increasing a sonograph's output power levels and PRF to increase penetration and frame rates opens the system to the following artifact:

(A) high-frequency aliasing
(B) loss of low velocities
(C) tissue mirroring
(D) range ambiguity

44. The color coding of red arteries and blue veins and the slow high-resolution frame rates make the identity of arteries and veins in the abdomen direct and easy.

(A) true
(B) false

45. Turbulence in a vascular color flow image appears as

(A) a mottled pattern of colors
(B) a mottled pattern of red and blue with changing saturations
(C) a mottled green region
(D) A or B

46. Turbulence in a cardiac color flow image appears as

(A) a mottled pattern of colors
(B) a mottled pattern of red and blue with changing saturations
(C) a bright red region
(D) a mottled green region

47. Power Doppler Imaging is so named because

(A) it increases output power for image improvement
(B) it encodes the power spectrum of the Doppler signal into color
(C) it uses the phase of the amplitude to detect flow
(D) none of the above

48. Power Doppler Imaging is limited because

(A) it has a serious aliasing problem
(B) it does not work with low carrier frequencies
(C) it does not show the directionality of vessel flow
(D) A and B

49. Power Doppler imaging is a good choice when you

(A) want to show tissue perfusion
(B) want to show tissue velocity
(C) want to easily separate blood flow form simple tissue motion
(D) A and B

Answers and Explanations

At the end of each explained answer there is a number combination in parentheses. The first number identifies the reference source; the second number or set of numbers indicates the page or pages on which the relevant information can be found.

1. **(D)** All of the above. Color flow images can be used to position a single point, pulsed-Doppler, sample volume, as is the case with more conventional duplex imaging. *(5:1241)*

2. **(C)** Stationary tissue in gray-scale and moving tissues in color. All moving tissues in a color flow imaging can produce color. Thus, stationary tissues are in gray scale, whereas moving tissues, including blood, are in color. *(3:236)*

3. **(A)** A form of color flow imaging. Color flow imaging includes both Doppler and non-Doppler forms of imaging. *(3:236, 5:1241, 9:27)*

4. **(C)** To all waves coming from a moving wave source. The Doppler effect happens to all waves coming from a moving source, regardless of propagating velocity or power levels. *(12:172)*

5. **(B)** The closing velocity between transducer and tissue, carrier frequency, and ultrasound propagation velocity. The Doppler equation looks like the following,

$$Df = 2(f_o/c) \, V \cos \theta,$$

where F_o is the carrier frequency, c is the propagation velocity, and θ is the Doppler angle. $V \cos \theta$ is the closing velocity between the transducer and moving tissue. *(12:173)*

6. **(D)** Place a sample volume in the major streamline or jet and set the angle correction parallel to the streamline. Because the color pattern shows the location of the major streamline or jet, calculating velocity requires correction relative to the flow geometry, not the vessel. *(12:195)*

7. **(B)** One wavelength or less. This is necessary for textural information to reach the display in a digital scan converter. *(7:654)*

8. **(C)** One wavelength or more but less 1 mm. Digital sampling for vascular flow information requires such an interval because larger intervals cannot show the flow patterns within the vessel. *(3:236)*

9. **(C)** The product of transmit and receive focusing. The effective beam width results from the mathematical product of both functions. *(13:155, 11:620)*

10. **(A)** True. The sample volume and flow interact in a manner that depends on the geometry of the sample volume. *(8:9)*

11. **(C)** The average Doppler shift frequency. At each sample site, the color flow system determines the average Doppler shift frequency. *(3:236)*

12. **(B)** False. At each sample site, the system determines the average Doppler shift frequency. The display is then either these average frequencies or, in some cases, the calculated closing velocity. This velocity is the rate at which the flow is approaching or moving away from the transducer along the line of sight. *(3:236)*

13. **(D)** The relationship between the amplitudes and frequencies of the Doppler signals. The system will then avoid coloring strong slow-moving echo sources (tissue) but still color moderately fast weak echo sources (blood). *(15:647)*

14. **(B)** The vessel is open, but the blood velocity is too low to complete the image. As the vessel curves away from the beam, the Doppler frequencies become too low to be portrayed. The completeness of a color flow image depends on the velocity of the blood flow and the Doppler angle. *(2:19, 44)*

15. **(D)** The smaller vessels do not reflect ultrasound as well as the larger vessels do. Every living cell in the body is no more than two cell layers away from a red

94

blood cell. The smaller vessels, however, are not suf-
ficiently echogenic and vanish from the color display
first because of their small echo signals.   *(8:7)*

16. **(D)** 1, 2, and 3. Color provides information about
the existence of flow, its location in the image, its
location in the anatomy, the direction of the flow relative to the transducer, the direction of flow within
the vessel, the flow pattern within the vessel, and
the pulsatility of the flow. It does not indicate the
velocity of the flow.   *(5:1245)*

17. **(D)** Changes in echo signal phase. As with all directional Doppler systems, color flow systems detect
the existence of motion with a change in echo signal
phase. By measuring the direction of the phase
change, the system shows whether the direction of
motion is toward or away from the transducer. *(8:34)*

18. **(B)** Knowing the position of the scan plane on the
patient's body. The expected flow pattern in any vessel comes from knowing how the scan plane is positioned on the patient. For example, the patient's
head is always placed on the image left in long axis
scans, and the patient's right side is on the image
left in cross-sectional scans.   *(12:407)*

19. **(D)** Different colors (hues) or different levels of saturation (purity). The average frequency within each
Doppler sample site is portrayed as a change in either
color saturation (purity or whiteness) or hue (color).
The object is to use the color to show flow patterns
within the vessel lumen or heart chambers.   *(2:44)*

20. **(C)** Changes in color hue. The variance in Doppler
frequencies can be shown with a change in hue, such
as green tones with increasing variance. *(3:236, 9:27)*

21. **(A)** Changes in color. Cardiac systems change color
hues (frequencies) along red and blue lines to show
changes in Doppler shift frequencies. Broadening frequencies in a sample site become shades of green.
(2:44)

22. **(B)** False. Because only one frequency can come to
the screen for each Doppler image pixel, all current
systems use some estimate of the mean frequency.
(3:236)

23. **(B)** False. Because color uses the average frequency
at each location, the maximum systolic frequency
will always be greater than the mean value.
(3:236, 9:27, 10:591)

24. **(A)** True. Because synchronous signal processing
uses the same echo signal for both Doppler and gray-
scale signal processing, the frequency must be the
same.   *(3:236)*

25. **(B)** False. Asynchronous signal processing can, and
often does, use different frequencies for the gray-
scale image and the Doppler image. For example, it
could image at 5.0 MHz and have a Doppler carrier
of 3.0 MHz.   *(3:236)*

26. **(A)** A Doppler angle significantly less than 90° to
typical blood flow. All Doppler imaging requires a
Doppler angle. In asynchronous systems that do not
use a wedge, the angle comes from beam steering.
(12:173)

27. **(D)** A Doppler angle between the typical flow patterns in vessels. Synchronous systems that keep the
beams perpendicular to the transducer array (angiodynography) use a mechanical wedge to obtain the
Doppler angle to the flow pattern of the vessel.
(9:27, 3:236)

28. **(D)** Blood reflectivity is about 40–60 dB below that
of soft tissue. The fact that blood reflectivity is about
1/100th to 1/1,000th that of soft tissues translates
into reflectivities that are much lower than those of
soft tissues.   *(8:18)*

29. **(A)** True. Because the reflectivity of blood is low,
many color flow systems improve color penetration
by greatly increasing the power of the transmitted
Doppler output.   *(3:236)*

30. **(B)** False. Synchronous signal processing systems
are limited by the power levels of the common transmitter used for both gray-scale imaging and Doppler
imaging. As a result, imaging with and without
Doppler produces similar power levels. *(3:236, 9:27)*

31. **(A)** True. The single-point spectrum requires the
ultrasound beam to linger over its position longer
than is the case in either real-time gray-scale imaging or color flow imaging.   *(3:236, 9:27)*

32. **(A)** Decrease. Color flow imaging requires dwelling
on each line of sight for as few as four pulse–listen
cycles to as many as 32 pulse–listen cycles. Various
systems have different dwell times. The typical end
result is a reduction in image frame rate for color
flow imaging.   *(3:236)*

33. **(A)** True. Real-time color flow imaging of the heart
requires relatively high frame rates. In general,
Doppler requires dwelling on each line of sight for
some period of time. In addition, each Doppler sample
site requires processing time to extract the average
Doppler shift frequency. Restoring suitable cardiac
frame rates requires decreasing the number of color
flow lines of sight and the number of samples along
each line.   *(12:17, 9:27)*

34. **(B)** False. Cardiac color flow imaging does not work well for vascular imaging because the Doppler sampling intervals are too large. Imaging the heart also involves a problem with reflectivities, not with tissue attenuation. *(3:236)*

35. **(B)** False. Doppler sampling for vascular imaging may be well below intervals of 1 mm. In contrast, sampling for echocardiography may be at intervals or several millimeters or more. *(2:17)*

36. **(B)** The ultrasound beams are always moving. This is the case because mechanical systems lack a special motor that could move the beam in small steps. Because Doppler signal processing is keyed to relative movement, and the beam is always moving, color does not work well in mechanical systems. *(2:17)*

37. **(A)** 1 and 2. The linear phased array and the phased linear array have stationary ultrasound beams at each line of sight in the scanning plane. Both arrays also have increased grating lobes with beam steering. They do not have three-dimensional dynamic focusing or apertures necessarily of the same size. *(9:27, 2:21)*

38. **(B)** The linear array scan. The linear array with a rectangular scanning field is the geometry used for vascular imaging. The sector-scanning geometry makes reading color ambiguous in the straighter segments of a vessel. *(2:44)*

39. **(D)** A combination of A and C. Color flow imaging of the heart uses the phased array sector scan and the curved-linear array sector scan. These scanheads permit cardiac imaging from intercostal and subcostal windows. *(2:41)*

40. **(B)** Nine cm/s. Lowering the Doppler carrier frequency means that the same Doppler shift frequency requires a higher velocity to be just visible. *(13:280)*

41. **(B)** False. Like all pulsed Doppler systems, color systems will alias when the Doppler frequencies exceed the PRF sampling limit. *(8:37)*

42. **(C)** Decreasing the carrier frequency. This moves all Doppler frequencies downward and may bring the high aliasing frequencies below the aliasing limit. *(12:192)*

43. **(D)** Range ambiguity. High frame rates (high PRF) and high output power permit structures from outside the field of view to enter the image as a range ambiguity artifact. *(14:83)*

44. **(B)** False. The large fields of view for abdominal imaging slow the frame rate. In addition, vessel anatomy goes in all directions. Sorting out arteries and veins requires the spectrum to determine pulsatility. *(10:591)*

45. **(D)** A or B. In vascular color flow imaging, turbulence appears as broken streamlines. The image then takes on a mottled appearance either in color or in color saturation. *(10:591)*

46. **(D)** A mottled green region. In color flow echocardiography, the sampling intervals are too large to show turbulence. As a result, the system determines the spectral variance at each sampling site and expresses increased turbulence (increased variance) with increasing tones of green. *(2:12)*

47. **(B)** It encodes the power spectrum of the Doppler signal into color. Power Doppler looks at only the amplitudes of the Doppler signals in the I and Q channels. *(16:13)*

48. **(C)** It does not show the directionality of vessel flow. Power Doppler uses only the amplitudes of the signals in the I and Q channels. Without phase information, power Doppler cannot show the direction of flow. *(16:14)*

49. **(A)** Want to show tissue perfusion. Power Doppler will show wherever the system detects Doppler signal amplitudes. Thus, the color will distribute according to this signal map for both arteries and veins. *(16:16)*

REFERENCES

1. Fish PJ. Multichannel, direction resolving Doppler angiography. *Abstracts of 2nd European Congress of Ultrasonics in Medicine.* 72, 1975.
2. Omoto R, ed. *Color Atlas of Real-Time Two-Dimensional Doppler Echocardiography.* Tokyo: Shindan-ToChiryo; 1984.
3. Powis RL. Color flow imaging: understanding its science and technology. *JDMS.* 1988; 4:236–245.
4. Gorcsan J. Tissue Doppler echocardiography. *Curr Opin Cardiol.* 2000; Sept 15: 323–329.
5. Burns PN. Instrumentation and clinical interpretation of the Doppler spectrum: carotid and deep Doppler. In: *Conventional & Color-Flow Duplex Ultrasound Course.* Proc AIUM Spring Education Meeting. 1989; 29–38.
6. Persson AV, Powis RL. Recent advances in imaging and evaluation of blood flow using ultrasound. *Med Clin North Am.* 1986; 70:1241–1252.
7. Ophir J, Maklad NF. Digital scan converters in diagnostic ultrasound imaging. *Proc IEEE.* 1979; 67:654–664.
8. Atkinson P, Woodcock JP. *Doppler Ultrasound and Its Use in Clinical Measurement.* New York: Academic Press; 1982.

9. Goldstein A, Powis RL. Medical ultrasonic diagnostics in ultrasonic instruments and devices: reference for modern instrumentation, techniques and technology. In: Mason WP, Thurston RN, eds. *Physical Acoustics Series*. Vol. 23A. New York: Academic Press; 1999.

10. Powis RL. Color flow imaging technology. In: *Basic Science of Flow Measurement*. Proc Syllabus AIUM 1989 Spring Education Meeting. 1989; 27–33.

11. Merritt RBC. Doppler color flow imaging. *J Color Ultrasonog*. 1987; 15:591–597.

12. Havlice JF, Taenzer JC. Medical ultrasonic imaging: an overview of principles and instrumentation. *Proc IEEE*. 1979; 67:620–641.

13. Powis RL, Powis WJ. *A Thinker's Guide to Ultrasonic Imaging*. Baltimore: Urban & Schwarzenberg; 1984.

14. Baker DW, Daigle RE. Noninvasive ultrasonic flowmetry. In Hwang, NHC, Normann NA, eds. *Cardiovascular Flow Dynamics and Measurements*. Baltimore: University Park Press; 1977.

15. McDicken WN. *Diagnostic Ultrasonics: Principles and Use of Instruments*. 2nd ed. New York: John Wiley & Sons, 1981.

16. Murphy KJ, Rubin JM. Power Doppler: It's a good thing. *Semin Ultrasound CT MRI*. 1997; Feb. 18:13–21.

17. Goldstein A. Range ambiguities in real-time. *Ultrasound*. 1981; 9:83–90.

18. Middleton WD, Erickson S, Melson GL. Perivascular color artifact: pathologic significance and appearance on color Doppler US images. *Radiology*. 1989; 171:647–652.

CHAPTER 3

ADULT ECHOCARDIOGRAPHY

Mark N. Allen and Carol A. Krebs

Study Guide

INTRODUCTION

Echocardiography has evolved into a highly specialized field of ultrasound. It originally began with M-mode techniques and developed into two-, three-, and even four-dimensional imaging combined with Doppler and color flow capabilities. Innovative technical advances, such as transesophageal examinations and contrast agents, added yet further diagnostic capabilities. Echocardiology serves as an ideal non-invasive method to examine cardiac anatomy in the normal as well as abnormal states. The combination of anatomical and functional information provided by echocardiography make it the diagnostic method of choice in a variety of clinical situations.[1]

The heart is an extremely complex organ, and echocardiography provides a variety of techniques that can be applied to obtain comprehensive information about a very dynamic organ. When performing an echocardiographic examination, it is important to consider not only the two-dimensional imaging information but also the Doppler and color flow findings.[1] These techniques are performed as an integral part of an echocardiographic examination and should be used to complement one another.

TECHNIQUES AND INSTRUMENTATION

Transthoracic Exam

Real-time imaging combined with M-mode and Doppler are the foundation of the basic echocardiographic examination. EKG provides timing for electrical events, which are used in making measurements and calculations. There are specific protocols established by each laboratory that govern the performance and interpretation of the examination. These protocols usually include the guidelines recommended by the American Society of Echocardiography. The positions are specifically designed for viewing of specific heart structures. The structures viewed form the various positions and windows are listed below:

LEFT PARASTERNAL LONG-AXIS VIEW

- Anterior right ventricular free wall
- Right ventricular cavity
- Interventricular septum, including membranous portion
- Left ventricle
- Left ventricular posterior wall
- Mitral valve and apparatus
- Left ventricular outflow tract
- Aortic valve-left and noncoronary cusps
- Aortic root
- Left atrium
- Descending thoracic aorta
- Coronary sinus
- Pericardium

RIGHT VENTRICULAR INFLOW VIEW

- Obtained by starting in a left parasternal long axis view and angling anteriorly
- Right atrium
- Right ventricle
- Tricuspid valve and apparatus (chordea tendinea and papillary muscles)

PARASTERNAL SHORT-AXIS VIEW

- Left ventricle-all wall segments
- Aortic valve—all three cusps
- Pulmonic valve
- Tricuspid valve
- Right atrium
- Right ventricle
- Main pulmonary artery (left and right branches)
- Interatrial septum
- Pericardium
- Left atrium

APICAL FOUR-CHAMBER VIEW

- Left ventricle (septal wall, apex, lateral wall)
- Right ventricle
- Left atrium
- Right atrium
- Mitral valve-anterior and posterior leaflets
- Tricuspid valve
- Interatrial and interventricular septae
- Pulmonary veins

APICAL TWO CHAMBER VIEW

- Left ventricle (anterior wall, inferior wall, apex)
- Left atrium and left atrial appendage
- Coronary sinus
- Mitral valve

APICAL LONG-AXIS VIEW

- Left ventricle (septum, posterior wall, apex)
- Left atrium
- Aortic valve
- Ascending aorta
- Mitral valve (both leaflets) and apparatus
- Right ventricle (small portion)

APICAL FOUR-CHAMBER VIEW WITH AORTA

- Left ventricle (septal wall, apex, lateral wall)
- Right ventricle
- Left atrium
- Right atrium
- Atrioventricular valves
- Aortic valve
- Ascending aorta/left ventricular outflow tract

SUBCOSTAL FOUR-CHAMBER VIEW

- Left ventricle (septal wall, lateral wall)
- Right ventricle
- Left atrium
- Right atrium
- Atrioventricular valves
- Interatrial septum
- Interventricular septum

SUBCOSTAL SHORT-AXIS VIEW

- Left ventricle-short axis
- Right ventricle

- Tricuspid valve
- Pulmonic valve
- Right ventricular outflow tract
- Main pulmonary artery

SUBCOSTAL INFERIOR VENA CAVA VIEW

- Inferior vena cava
- Hepatic veins
- Right atrium

SUPRASTERNAL VIEW

- Ascending aorta
- Aortic arch
- Descending aorta
- Left common carotid artery
- Left subclavian artery
- Innominate artery
- Right pulmonary artery

Stress and Pharmacologic Examination

Stress echocardiography can be performed using a treadmill, supine or upright bike, pacing techniques or by using such pharmacologic agents as dobutamine, adenosine, or dipyridamole. The combination of echocardiography, ECG and stress has been used since the 1980s. The use of exercise ECG only is unreliable in such subgroups of patients as women or patients who have a history of myocardial infarction or coronary bypass surgery, as well as in patients on certain medications such as antiarrhythmic agents, diuretics, and antidepressive agents. In addition, exercise ECG is unreliable in patients with certain arrhythmias, such as left bundle branch block or other repolarization abnormalities, and valvular heart disease.

The ischemic cascade is a series of events that take place with an ischemic episode (see Table 3–1).

The fact that systolic changes occur before ECG changes and patient symptoms, the addition of imaging

TABLE 3–1. ISCHEMIC CASCADE

Imbalance in supply and demand	Myocardial perfusion is decreased by obstructed coronary vessel
Decreases in LV compliance	Changes in diastolic function occur such as slowed relaxation, increased L stiffness and increased end-diastolic pressure (LVEDP)
Decreased or changes in systolic function	Segmental or regional wall motion abnormalities develop
ECG changes develop	Significant changes in ST segment (elevation or depression)
Patient symptoms	Chest pain

techniques to the exercise ECG improves the diagnostic accuracy of the test.

Myocardial ischemia occurs when the regional oxygen supply is insufficient to meet the body's demand. When the myocardial blood flow reserve becomes inadequate, such as during exercise or inotropic stimulation, it results in ischemia and impaired myocardial function. Coronary artery stenoses may have little or no effect in the resting state but becomes manifested during stress or exercise. Therefore, evaluation of patients with exercise has become a standard part of the echocardiographic examination.

Exercise echocardiography has evolved as a test ideally suited for the evaluation of patients with coronary artery disease (CAD) or valvular heart disease. It is a cost-effective, reliable tool for detecting the presence, extent, and distribution of coronary stenosis. Echocardiography rapidly detects regional wall motion at rest and after exercise, which allows highly accurate predictions of the extent and distribution of CAD.[1] Other capabilities of stress echocardiography include:

- Assessment of left ventricular size and ejection fraction
- Identification of thrombus or aneurysm that may of resulted from previous myocardial infarction
- Identification of other causes of chest pain unrelated to vascular obstruction, such as hypertrophic cardiomyopathy, aortic dissection or pericardial disease
- The evaluation of valvular heart lesions, especially if used in conjunction with Doppler echocardiography

Indications for stress echocardiography include: (1) screening of new patients for CAD, (2) assessing states before and after intervention, (3) determining prognosis after myocardial infarction and, (4) evaluate hemodymanic significance of valvular heart disease.[1]

Contraindications include: (1) recent myocardial infarction, (2) unstable angina, (3) potentially life threatening dysrhythmias, (4) acute pericarditis, (5) severe hypertension, (6) acute pulmonary embolism, and (7) critical aortic valve stenosis. Interpretation of the test includes the evaluation of the patient's blood pressure, ECG, symptoms and the echocardiographic response to exercise. The LV myocardial segments are divided into three perfusion zones, each dictated by coronary artery anatomy. The left anterior descending artery or LAD supplies the anterior, septal, and apex. The left circumflex coronary artery supplies the posterolateral segments, but may also supply the inferior segments depending on dominance. The right coronary artery or posterior descending (PDA) supplies the inferior segments.

An exercise echocardiogram is considered positive if any of these three findings are present: (1) there is an exercise-induced wall-motion abnormality, (2) there is an increase in LV volume, and/or (3) there is a decrease in global LV ejection fraction. The greater the wall motion abnormality the more severe the disease. There are many factors that affect wall motion abnormalities. Perhaps the most important of these include the duration of exercise, the less exercise the patient does, the less likely the patient achieved an adequate

TABLE 3–2. FALSE POSITIVES AND NEGATIVES

False-Negative Exams	False-Positive Exams
Mild coronary artery disease	Cardiomyopathies
Inability to reach maximal heart rate	Inadequate exercise
Presence of extensive collateral vessels (improves flow to diseased area)	Preexisting myocardial dysfunction
	Left ventricular hypertrophy
	Left ventricular fibrosis
	Aging of the heart
	High blood pressure (220/110 mmHg)
	Severe hypertension

heart rate. A list of false positives and false negatives follows in Table 3–2.

Contrast Echocardiography

The use of contrast agents has gained wide spread use in the field of echocardiography. Their uses range from the evaluation of left and right heart structures and function, enhancements of regurgitant and stenotic lesions, enhanced assessment of pulmonary artery pressures, presence of various shunts such as patent foramen, ASD and VSDs and other shunts, and patency coronary artery perfusion.[1]

Contrast agents come in many forms from the simplest, such as agitated saline solution, to complex agents composed of perfluorocarbon shells (or other substances) filled with gases. These later forms of contrast agents hold special promise not only in aiding in the identification of cardiac structures and function, but more recently in the evaluation of myocardial perfusion imaging. Currently (at the time of this writing), contrast agents are only approved by the FDA in the evaluation of left ventricular opacification or "LVO" and not for the evaluation of myocardial perfusion imaging. Still, research continues in the use of microbubbles to help identify coronary distribution.

Internal contrast or spontaneous contrast (SEC) is the discrete reflections in the blood within the cardiac chambers or vessels without the injection of contrast media. SEC is observed when blood becomes echogenic in a region of decreased flow. It is not seen with shear rates greater than 40 seconds. SEC may be seen in normal states as well as abnormal conditions. SEC has the potential to induce embolic events caused by thrombus formation.[1] As technology and equipment improve, visualization of SEC may become more prevalent, even in totally normal patients.

Contrast agents in the form of microbubbles range in size from 0.1 to 8 μm. These tiny spheres are strong reflectors of ultrasound but small enough to pass through the capillary bed. The microbubbles must be small to avoid harmful effects, must remain tiny after injection, and must stay in the circulation long enough to be detected by ultrasound. The reflective property of the microbubbles comes from the material within the bubbles or spheres, which is usually gas or air bodies. Because of the acoustic impedance

TABLE 3–3. MICROBUBBLE AGENTS

Available Agents	Manufacturer	Uses (FDA approved)
Optison	Amersham	• Left Ventricular Function (LVO)
Definity	Bristol-Myer Squibb	• LVO

of the air or gas versus blood there is a strong signal. Other factors that affect reflective properties are:

- Transmitted frequency
- Microbubble diameter
- Microbubble concentration
- Microbubble survival rate

The microbubble eventually disappears through natural processes of the body. Table 3–3 lists the currently available agents in the US and their potential uses.

Transesophageal Examination

Transesophageal (TEE) echocardiography is another echocardiographic technique routinely used to evaluate cardiac structure and function. It is performed by a physician with specialized training on TEE performance and interpretation.[1] Transesophageal echocardiography examinations provide complete evaluation of all regions of the heart, including the great vessels. Although it is considered more invasive than a transthoracic or surface echocardiogram, it is a relatively simple procedure tolerated by most patients.

Atrial paced TEE is performed by attaching a flexible silicone-coated pacing catheter to the TEE probe. Pacing is increased incrementally to 85% of patient age predicted maximum heart scale. Left ventricular function is monitored by TEE examination at baseline, during and immediately after maximal pacing. This technique has a high sensitivity and specificity for detection or coronary artery disease and a high success rate of 90–100% of patients.[1]

TEE plus pharmacologic agents is used to assess coronary artery disease and has proved to be feasible and accurate. At each stage of dobutamine infusion, it is important to use longitudinal and transverse planes to optimize visualization of all wall segments.

There are several advantages of using TEE, which include the following:

- TEE provides higher resolution than the transthoracic echocardiographic (TTE) exam because of the use of the transesophageal window, which allows the use of higher frequencies. The transducer is mounted on a flexible gastroscope that is sufficient in length to be advanced down the esophagus. It is positioned behind the posterior wall of the left ventricle.
- TEE provides additional viewing of structures that are often not seen well on the TTE exam in technically difficult studies. These structures include the posterior cardiac structures such as the aorta, atria, left atrial appendage, and cardiac valves.

TABLE 3–4. INDICATIONS FOR TEE

Left ventricular function	• Regional wall motion abnormalities
	• Global LV function
Endocarditis	• Valvular vegetations
	• Valvular strands
Valvular disorders/pathology	• Mitral valve prolapse
	• Mitral, aortic, pulmonic, tricuspid stenosis.
	• Mitral, aortic, pulmonic, tricuspid regurgitation
	• Flail leaflets
	• Torn chordal structures
Pericardial disease	• Pericarditis
	• Pericardial fluid
	• Tamponade
Aortic abnormalities	• Presence and extent of arteriosclerotic disease
	• Traumatic aortic rupture
	• Aortic dissection
	• Nondissecting aneurysms
Shunts (atrial, ventricular, other)	• Atrial septal defects
	• Ventricular septal defects
	• Patent foramen ovale
	• Atrial septal aneurysms
Source of embolus	• Can help identify patients at risk for stroke
	• Used to screen patients for cardioversion
	• Allows interrogation of left atrial appendage
Right heart function	• Monitoring during and after open heart surgery

- TEE provides "off-axis planes" in addition to the standard planes, which often provides a clearer view of the anatomy or anomalies.

There are contraindications to performing the TEE examination. These include: esophageal tumors or tumors of the mouth, esophageal stenosis or strictures, diverticulum, esophageal varices, perforated viscus, gastric volvulus or perforation, active gastrointestinal bleeding, and patient refusal or unwillingness to cooperate.[1] Occasionally, the TEE probe cannot easily be passed and should never be forced.

Table 3–4 lists the indications for TEE.

ANATOMY

To become proficient in the techniques of echocardiography a thorough understanding of cardiac anatomy is essential. One must know the normal structures and be able to recognize normal variants from pathologic states. One must also understand the anatomic orientation of the heart within the chest cavity.

The heart is cone-shaped, hollow, fibromuscular organ located in the middle mediastinum between the lungs and the pleurae. It has a base, apex, and multiple surfaces and borders. It is enclosed in pericardium. The pericardium is made of fibrous and serosal components. The fibrous pericardium is the tough outer sac that completely surrounds the heart but does not adhere to it. The serosal component is the inner layer which has two components. The visceral or epicardial layer, which adheres to the surface of the heart and makes up the epicardium and the serosal pericardium, which is the outer or parietal layer. The serosal pericardium lines the inside surface of the fibrous pericardium. Within the serosal layers is a thin film of pericardial fluid. The purpose of the pericardium is to (1) reduce friction with cardiac movement; (2) allow the heart to move freely with each beat, facilitating ejection and volume changes; (3) contain the heart within the mediastinum, especially during trauma; and (4) serve as a barrier to infection.[1]

The average adult heart measures approximately 12 cm from the apex to the base, 8–9 cm transversely in the broadest diameter, and 6 cm anterior–posterior. The weight varies in males ranging from 280–340 g and in females 230–280 g. Cardiac weight is approximately 0.45% of total body weight in men and 0.40% of total body weight in women.[1,2]

The heart is divided into four chambers two atria and two ventricles. The external surface contain numerous grooves and sulci. The coronary or atrioventricular groove separates the atria from the ventricles and contains the main trunk of the coronary arteries and coronary sinus. The interventricular groove separates the right and left ventricles. The anterior interventricular groove runs on the anterior surface and contains the descending branch of the left coronary artery. The posterior interventricular groove lies on the diaphragmatic surface of the heart and contains the posterior interventricular descending coronary artery and the middle cardiac vein. The interatrial grooves separate the atria. The interatrial grooves are shallow and less prominent than the other grooves. The interatrial, atrioventricular, and posterior interventricular grooves meet and form the crux of the heart. The terminal groove or sulcus terminalis demarcates the true atrium and the venous component of the right atrium. These external grooves are filled with fatty tissue that varies with overall body fat and increases with age.[1]

There are basically two important types of heart valves: the semilunar and the atrioventricular. Semilunar valves are the aortic and pulmonary. Atrioventricular valves are the tricuspid and the mitral.

There are numerous pathologies that affect the heart in the adult. These disease states can cause a variety of primary as well as secondary anatomical changes in the heart. Knowing what these changes are greatly enhances the echocardiographic examination. Once the student has an understanding of heart anatomy, the echocardiographic images are better understood. The basic two-dimensional echocardiographic views are illustrated in Figs. 3–1 to 3–8. These figures are from the American Society of Echocardiography and are the accepted nomenclature for two-dimensional imaging.

Left Ventricle

Anatomy. The left ventricle is the largest cardiac chamber, accounting for 75% of the heart mass. It consists of two papillary muscles, has trabeculations in the apex, and a smooth-walled basal area. Its end-diastolic diameter is

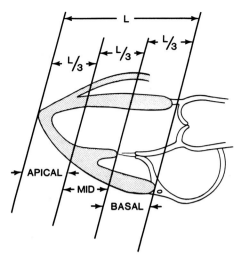

Figure 3–1. Parasternal long-axis view of the heart demonstrating the method of subdividing the myocardial walls along the long axis (L) into three regions of equal length using the left ventricular papillary muscles as landmarks. (*Reprinted with permission from the American Society of Echocardiography. Report of the ASE Committee on Nomenclature and Standards: Identification of Myocardial Wall Segments, November 1982.*)

3.6–5.6 cm, and its end-systolic diameter is 2.3–4.0 cm. Normal fractional shortening (difference between diastolic and systolic diameters is:

$$FS = \frac{LV\ Dd\text{-}LVLVIDS}{LVIDd}$$

Normal LV wall thickness in diastole ranges from 0.6–1.1 cm.

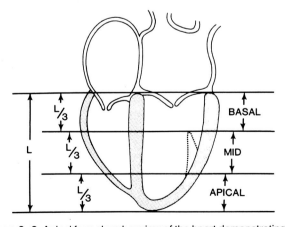

Figure 3–2. Apical four-chamber view of the heart demonstrating the method of subdividing the myocardial walls into three regions using the left ventricular papillary muscles as landmarks. (*Reprinted with permission from the American Society of Echocardiography. Report of the ASE Committee on Nomenclature and Standards: Identification of Myocardial Wall Segments, November 1982.*)

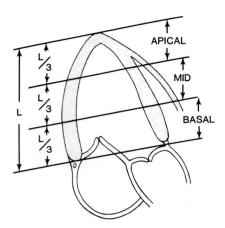

Figure 3–3. Apical long-axis view of the heart demonstrating the method of subdividing the myocardial walls into three regions of equal length. (*Reprinted with permission from the American Society of Echocardiography. Report of the ASE Committee on Nomenclature and Standards: Identification of Myocardial Wall Segments, November 1982.*)

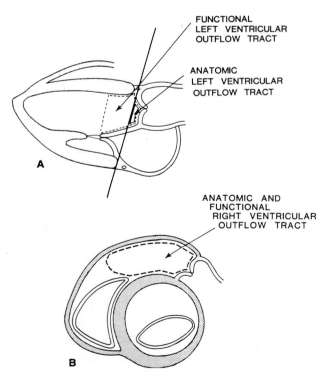

Figure 3–4. The functional and anatomic left ventricular outflow tracts of the heart are diagrammed in the upper panel (**A**), whereas the functional and anatomic right ventricular outflow tract is illustrated in the bottom panel (**B**). (*Reprinted with permission from the American Society of Echocardiography. Report of the ASE Committee on Nomenclature and Standards: Identification of Myocardial Wall Segments, November 1982.*)

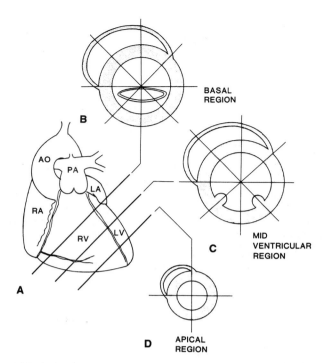

Figure 3–5. Diagram of the heart (**A**) and the short-axis views of the basal region (**B**), midventricular region (**C**), and apical region (**D**). (*Reprinted with permission from the American Society of Echocardiography. Report of the ASE Committee on Nomenclature and Standards: Identification of Myocardial Wall Segments, November 1982.*)

Hemodynamics. The ventricle receives oxygenated blood from the left atrium and pumps it through the aortic valve to the body by way of arteries, arterioles, and capillaries. Its systolic pressure is 100–120 mm Hg.

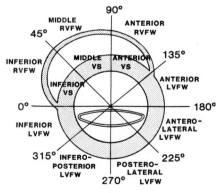

Figure 3–6. Short-axis view of the basal region of the heart demonstrating the method of subdividing the myocardial walls into segments using a coordinate system consisting of eight lines that are 45° apart. With this system, the left ventricular free wall (LVFW) is divided into five segments, whereas the ventricular septum (VS) and right ventricular free walls (RVFW) are subdivided into three segments each. (*Reprinted with permission from the American Society of Echocardiography. Report of the ASE Committee on Nomenclature and Standards: Identification of Myocardial Wall Segments, November 1982.*)

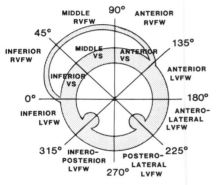

Figure 3–7. Short-axis view of the midventricular region of the heart demonstrating the method of subdividing the myocardial walls into segments using a coordinate system consisting of eight lines that are 45° apart. With this system, the left ventricular free wall (LVFW) is divided into five segments, whereas the ventricular septum (VS) and right ventricular free walls (RVFW) are subdivided into three segments each. (*Reprinted with permission from the American Society of Echocardiography. Report of the ASE Committee on Nomenclature and Standards: Identification of Myocardial Wall Segments, November 1982.*)

Echocardiographic Views. Almost all the standard views allow visualization of at least part of the left ventricle. The apical views allow examination of the apex, which can be difficult to see in other views. The maximum internal dimensions are seen at end systole and should be taken at the peak posterior motion of the interventricular septum (see Table 3–5).

Left Atrium

Anatomy. The left atrium is a smooth-walled sac, the walls of which are thicker than those of the right atrium. The chamber receives four pulmonary veins: two (sometimes three) on the right and two (sometimes one) on the left. The interatrial septum divides the left and right atria.

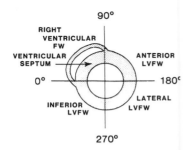

Figure 3–8. Short-axis view of the apical region of the heart demonstrating the method of subdividing the myocardial walls into segments using a coordinate system consisting of four lines that are 90° apart. With this system, the left ventricular free wall (LVFW) is subdivided into three segments, whereas the ventricular septum and right ventricular free wall (FW) are subdivided into one segment each. (*Reprinted with permission from the American Society of Echocardiography. Report of the ASE Committee on Nomenclature and Standards: Identification of Myocardial Wall Segments, November 1982.*)

TABLE 3–5. TEE LEFT VENTRICLE EXAMINATION

Views	Structures/Walls
Long axis (LAX)	• Septum • Posterior wall • Papillary muscles • Trabeculations
Short axis (SAX)	• Septum (inferior, mid, anterior) • Lateral wall • Posterior wall • Inferior wall
Apical 4 chamber	• Apex • Lateral wall • Septum • Papillary muscles
Apical 2 chamber	• Apex • Posterior wall • Anterior wall
Apical long axis	• Apex • Septum • Posterior wall
Subcostal four chamber	• Apex • Septum • Lateral wall
Subcostal short axis	• Septum • Lateral wall • Posterior wall • Inferior wall

It is thinnest in its central portion, the fossa, and varies in thickness elsewhere due to fat deposits. These normally increase with age. The left auricle, or left atrial appendage, arises from the upper anterior part of the left atrium and contains small pectinate muscles. The average dimension of the chamber in the adult is 29–38 mm.

Hemodynamics. The mean pressure in the left atrium ranges from 1 mm Hg to 10 mm Hg. Oxygenated blood flows from the lungs and enters the atrium through the pulmonary veins. As left atrial pressure increases over that of the left ventricle, the mitral valve opens, and blood then passes through the mitral valve and enters the left ventricle.

Echocardiographic Views. Maximal dimensions should be measured at end-systole. Measurements may be made from the leading edge of the posterior wall of the aorta to the leading edge of the posterior wall of the left atrium. This chamber is best seen from the parasternal long and short-axis views; however, it also can be seen from the apical and subcostal views. In the left parasternal long-axis view, the descending aorta can be seen from running posteriorly to the left atrium. Care must be given when measuring the diameter of the left atrium so that descending aorta is not included in the measurement because this will give an erroneous left atrial diameter. The left atrial appendage can be seen from the transthoracic two chamber and parasternal short axis views.

Transesophageal echocardiography can also be used to evaluate this area and is typically carefully evaluated in patients where source of embolus is a consideration or when patients may be scheduled for cardioversion.

Right Atrium

Anatomy. The right atrium has two parts: an anterior portion and a posterior portion. The two portions are separated by a ridge of muscle called the crista terminalis. This area is typically not seen well from the transthoracic approach.

The smooth-walled posterior portion of the atrium is derived from the embryonic sinus venosus and receives the inferior and superior vena cavae. Guarding the opening (ostium) of the inferior vena cava is a thin fold of tissue called the eustachian valve, which is sometimes large and complex and forms a network of tissues known as the network of Chiari. The coronary sinus also enters the right atrium anterior to the inferior vena cava. The coronary sinus also can be guarded by a thin fold of tissue called the thebesian valve.

The anterior portion, which represents the embryonic right atrium, is extremely thin and is trabeculated. The right atrial appendage, or right auricle, arises from the superior portion of the right atrium and contains pectinate muscle. The dimensions of the right atrium in adults range from 26 to 34 mm.

Hemodynamics. Deoxygenated blood from the body, head, and heart flows into the right atrium through the inferior vena cava, the superior vena cava, and the coronary sinus, respectively. When pressures in the right atrium increase above the pressures in the right ventricle, the tricuspid valve opens, allowing the blood to flow forward into the right ventricle. Mean pressures in this chamber range from 0 to 8 mm Hg.

Echocardiographic Views. Apical views are best for assessing the right atrium. Others include the subcostal and, to a lesser extent, the parasternal short-axis views.

Right Ventricle

Anatomy. The right ventricle is divided into a posterior inferior inflow portion and an anterior superior outflow portion. The inflow portion contains the tricuspid valve and is heavily trabeculated. The outflow portion, also called the infundibulum, gives rise to the pulmonary trunk. The subpulmonic area is smooth walled.

The right ventricle contains numerous papillary muscles that anchor the tricuspid valve. The ventricle contains numerous bands of muscle. One band, the moderator band, is readily seen in the apex of the ventricle by two-dimensional imaging. Internal diameters range from 7 to 26 mm.

Hemodynamics. Systolic pressures range from 15 to 30 mm Hg, and diastolic pressures range from 0 to 8 mm Hg.

Echocardiographic Views. The right ventricle is seen best from the apical and subcostal views. It also can be seen from the left parasternal long and short axis views and right ventricular inflow view.

Aorta

Anatomy. The aorta arises from the base of the heart and enters the superior mediastinum, where it almost reaches the sternum, then courses obliquely backward and to the left over the left bronchus. It then becomes the descending aorta and courses downward anterior to and slightly left of the vertebral column. The aorta is highly elastic and has three layers: (1) a thin inner layer called the tunica intima, (2) a thick middle layer called the tunica media, and (3) a thin out layer called the tunica adventia. The diameter of the aortic root measures 2.5–3.3 cm.

Hemodynamics. Maximal velocities of blood flow in adults are 1.0–0.7 m/s.

Echocardiographic Views. The aortic root is seen from the parasternal views. A good portion of the ascending aortic arch can be seen by beginning with the transducer in a standard left parasternal long axis view and sliding the probe up an intercostal space. The ascending aorta, aortic arch, and descending aorta can be seen from the suprasternal view. As was mentioned earlier, part of the descending aorta also can be seen behind the left atrium in the long-axis view. The subcostal views allow visualization of the aortic root and valve.

Main Pulmonary Artery

Anatomy. The main pulmonary artery is located superior to and originates from the right ventricle. Immediately after leaving the pericardium, it bifurcates into a right pulmonary artery and a left pulmonary artery that enter the right and left lung, respectively.

Hemodynamics. This artery delivers deoxygenated blood from the right ventricle to the lungs. Flow velocities range from 0.6 to 0.9 m/s.

Echocardiographic Views. The artery is seen best from the parasternal short-axis view.

Mitral Valve

Anatomy. The mitral valve is an atrioventricular valve. It is located between the left atrium and the left ventricle, is a thick yellowish-white membrane that originates at the annulus fibrous, a fibrous ring that surrounds the orifice of the valve. The valve has an anterior leaflet and a posterior leaflet, both of which have sawtoothlike edges. Both leaflets are attached to papillary muscles by cordae tendinae. The surface on the atrial side of the valve is smooth; whereas, the surface on the ventricular side is irregular. Normal mitral valve area is 4–6 cm².

Hemodynamics. Flow velocities across the valve range from 9.6 to 1.3 m/s. The valve's function is to prevent backflow of blood from the left ventricle into the left atrium.

Echocardiographic Views. The mitral valve is seen best from the long and short-axis parasternal views and the apical view. Doppler measurements are obtained best from the apical four and two-chamber views.

Aortic Valve

Anatomy. The aortic valve consists of three pocket-shaped thin smooth cusps named according to their location in relation to the coronary arteries. The cusp near the left coronary artery is the left coronary cusp, the cusp near the right coronary artery is the right coronary cusp, and the cusp that is not near a coronary artery is the noncoronary cusp. Because of its lunar or half-moon shape, the aortic valve is referred to as semilunar. Normal aortic valve area is 3–4 cm^2.

Hemodynamics. The function of the aortic valve is to prevent backflow of blood from the aorta into the left ventricle. The velocity of flow ranges from 1.0 to 1.7 m/s.

Echocardiographic Views. The valve is seen best from the parasternal views. It also can be seen from the apical four-chamber view with anterior angulation. The best Doppler measurements are obtained from the apical four-chamber view with anterior angulation, from the right parasternal window, and from the suprasternal view.

Tricuspid Valve

Anatomy. The tricuspid valve is an atrioventricular valve. It is located between the right atrium and ventricle. The atrial side is smooth; the ventricular side is irregular. As in the mitral valve, it is a thick yellowish-white membrane that originates at the annulus fibrous, a fibrous ring that surrounds the orifice of the valve. The valve has three leaflets—anterior, posterior, and medial—all of which are sawtoothlike in appearance. Each leaflet is attached to papillary muscles by cordae tendinae.

Hemodynamics. The function of this valve is to prevent backflow of blood from the right ventricle to the right atrium. The velocity of flow ranges from 0.3 to 0.7 m/s.

Echocardiographic Views. The valve is seen best from the parasternal short-axis, parasternal 4-chamber, apical 4 chamber, and subcostal views. Measurements are best obtained in the parasternal 4-chamber view. The best Doppler measurements are taken from the parasternal short-axis and apical four-chamber views.

Pulmonic Valve

Anatomy. The pulmonic valve consists of three thin smooth pocket s-shaped cusps. Because of its shape, this valve, like the aortic valve, is called semilunar.

Hemodynamics. The function of this valve is to prevent backflow of blood from the main pulmonary artery to the right ventricle. The velocity of flow ranges from 9.6–0.9m/s.

Echocardiographic Views. The pulmonic valve is seen best from the parasternal short-axis view. The best Doppler recordings are taken from the left parasternal short axis.

PHYSIOLOGY

The hearts functions as a pump to distribute blood to the body. To be adequately distributed, the blood pressure must be maintained. Pressure and flow are controlled by a complex control mechanism that responds to the metabolic requirements of the body.

There are two fluid pumps within the heart, one on the right and one on the left, lying side by side. The right side supplies the pulmonary circulation. From the lungs, blood returns to the left side and ultimately supplies the body via the systemic circulation. The volume pumped by both sides is equal to ensure normal circulation of flow. The blood is pumped from the ventricles during systole and received during diastole, the relaxation phase. The cardiac cycle includes all of the electrical and mechanical events that occur during the cycle of one heartbeat (see Fig. 3–9). Each side of the heart has specific characteristics and functions, which are listed below.

RIGHT HEART CHARACTERISTICS AND FUNCTION

- Blood returns to right atrium from superior and inferior vena cava
- Supplies the pulmonary circulation
- Normal pressure in the right ventricle is approximately 22 mm Hg
- Blood returning to the right heart has a lower oxygen saturation (75%)
- Contains the tricuspid valve which closes during right ventricular systole and contained blood in right ventricle is propelled out of right ventricle outflow tract through the open semilunar pulmonic valve to the pulmonic circulation

LEFT HEART CHARACTERISTICS AND FUNCTION

- Left ventricular pressure is approximately 120 mm Hg
- Blood pumped from the left ventricle has a high oxygen saturation (95–100%)
- Left atrium receives blood from the lungs through the pulmonary veins in the back of the left atrium
- During left atrial systole the mitral valve opens and allowed blood in the left atrium to be propelled into the left ventricle. When ventricular systole occurs the mitral valve closes and blood is propelled out of the left ventricle through the outflow tract

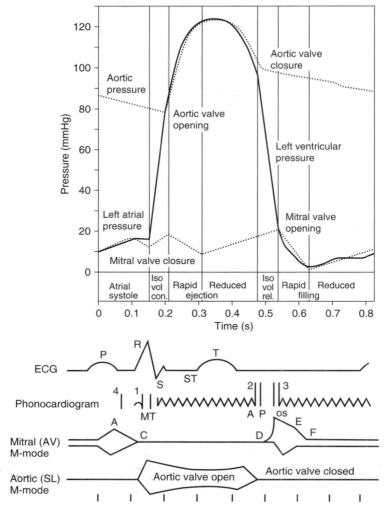

Figure 3–9. Events of the cardiac cycle.

The blood supply to the heart is derived from the right and left coronary arteries and their respective tributaries (see Fig. 3–10).

CONDUCTION SYSTEM OF THE HEART/ INTRINSIC INNERVATION OF THE HEART

The conduction system of the heart is responsible for the initiation, propagation, and coordination of the heartbeat. Fig. 3–11 demonstrates this system.

The SA node is also called the pacemaker of the heart. It provides the bursts of electrical impulses that are conducted throughout the walls of the heart. The activation conduction is from the SA node to the AV node, where it is slows and delays. The impulse is conducted to the ventricles by way of the AV bundle and the right and left bundle branches. It becomes continuous with the fibers of the purkinje network. The ventricles contract and blood is ejected to the pulmonic and systemic circulation. The heart contains its own intrinsic conduction system; however, its rate is modified by the autonomic nervous system. Fibers from both the sympathetic and parasympathetic nervous system are received by the heart. Sympathetic nervous system fibers are received by the atria via the right and left vagus nerves, which contribute to the control of the SA and AV nodes. The parasympathetic nerves are derived from the vagus and come off in the neck as vagal cardiac nerves. They connect to the SA node. Stimulation of the parasympathetic nervous system fibers to the heart cause the following:

- Decrease in the heart rate
- Retardation of transmission between the atria and ventricles
- Decrease in the force of contraction
- Decrease in conduction rate of the nodes and atria

The sympathetic and parasympathetic nervous system have opposite effects on the heart. The reflex center for both are in the medulla oblongata.

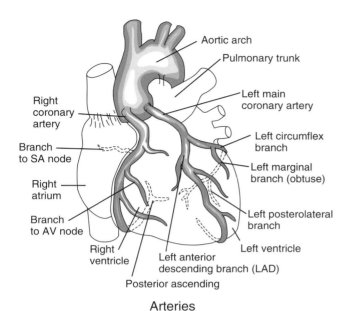

Figure 3–10. Anatomic drawing of the heart and vessels.

DISEASE AND PATHOLOGY

Diseases Affecting the Valves

Anomalies or diseases of the valves can be divided into two main categories. Valve anomalies that occur in fetal development are known as congenital anomalies. Valve anomalies that develop after fetal development or in the adult stages are referred to as acquired valve disease. This later category can further be divided into rheumatic and nonrheumatic heart disease.

Mitral Valve Disease

Stenosis. Mitral valve stenosis results primarily from rheumatic disease. The valves may not become involved for many decades following rheumatic fever. Congenital mitral stenosis can occur but is extremely rare.

M-mode findings include (1) a flattened E–D slope (reduced diastolic filling), (2) anterior motion of the posterior leaflet, (3) thickened leaflets, and (4) an absent A wave in the absence of atrial fibrillation. Two-dimensional imaging also indicates thickening and shows doming of the leaflets in diastole.

Doppler measurements reveal a reduced rate of decrease in diastolic flow (reduced diastolic slope), a higher than normal peak velocity of flow, and spectral broadening on Doppler display. Secondary findings and complications include left atrial dilatation, pulmonary hypertension, a left atrial clot, and an exaggerated diastolic dip of the interventricular septum.[22] Color Doppler shows turbulent left ventricular inflow.

Stenosis–Severity of Mitral Stenosis (Valve Area)

Normal	4–6 cm^2
Mild	1.6–2.0 cm^2
Moderate	1.1–1.5 cm^2
Severe	1.0 cm^2 or less

Regurgitation. Mitral regurgitation (shunting back and forth of blood) can occur as a result of mitral annular calcification, rheumatic mitral disease, flail mitral valve leaflet, conditions that may stretch the mitral annulus, such as cardiomyopathies, myocardial infarction, mitral valve vegetations or other masses on the mitral valve or within the left atrium, papillary dysfunction, and mitral valve prolapse.

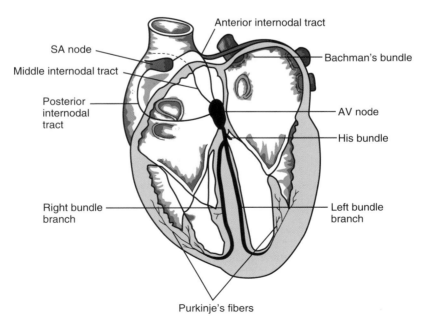

Figure 3–11. Intrinsic conduction system of the heart.

The hallmark sign of regurgitation is a systolic murmur most often maximal over the left ventricular apex.

M-mode findings include (1) increased size of the left atrium, (2) exaggerated motion of the interventricular septum, (3) pulsations of the left atrial wall, and (4) preclosure of the aortic valve during systole. The first three findings are the result of volume overload.

Two-dimensional imaging reveals an increase in the size of the left atrium and exaggerated motion of the interventricular septum-all of which are the result of volume overload. In addition, pulsations of the left atrial wall and preclosure of the aortic valve during systole are observed.

Doppler may be used to evaluate the regurgitant fraction. Color Doppler displays the turbulent jet in the left atrium, and is useful for estimating the severity of regurgitation.

Prolapse. (Protrusion or buckling of the mitral leaflets into the left atrium in systole) The classic clinical findings in mitral valve prolapse are a systolic click (a sound that corresponds with the posterior displacement of the mitral valve leaflet into the left atrium) and a late systolic murmur (a sound that corresponds with the resulting mitral regurgitation that often occurs because of the prolapsing leaflets).

M-mode findings include late systolic posterior displacement of the anterior and posterior leaflets and anterior motion of the mitral valve in early systole. To achieve the best views for making the diagnosis, the ultrasound beam should be perpendicular to the valve from the parasternal windows. The two-dimensional findings reveal that the valve is bowing into the left atrium and, in many cases, thickened.

Flail Leaflet. The most common cause of flail leaflet is rupture of the chordae tendineae, which often occurs secondary to myocardial infarction. Rupture of papillary muscle is a less common etiology.

M-mode findings indicate coarse diastolic fluttering and systolic fluttering of the leaflet and visualization of part of the leaflet in the left atrium. Two-dimensional imaging indicates protrusion of the flail leaflet into the left atrium, noncoaptation of the two leaflets, a systolic and coarse diastolic motion of the flail leaflet. Doppler measurements indicate harsh, turbulent mitral regurgitation.

Annular Calcification. Mitral annular calcification results from the deposition of calcium in the annulus of the mitral valve. This is normally associated with aging. This condition can be caused by mitral regurgitation, conduction abnormalities, aging, or obstruction of the left ventricular outflow tract (LVOF).

M-mode findings reveal high-density echoes between the valve and the posterior wall of the left ventricle. Two-dimensional imaging reveals high-density bright echoes between the valve and the posterior wall of the left ventricle.

Aortic Valve Disease

Stenosis (versus Sclerosis). The cause of stenosis of the aortic valve can be congenital, the result of rheumatic heart disease, or degeneration. Degenerative disease is the most common cause of aortic valve stenosis. Clinical symptoms include chest pain, shortness of breath, and syncope. These symptoms do not present until the aortic valve stenosis becomes moderate to severe. Patients with aortic valve stenosis often present with a harsh systolic murmur heard at the right sternal border, which often radiates to the carotids.

The normal aortic vale has three leaflets. In congenital or rheumatic stenosis, the body of the cusps may appear to be thin and pliable, but the cusp tips are tethered resulting in a systolic doming effect, best seen in the early systole from a left parasternal or apical long axis view. In degenerative stenosis, the cusps frequently appear to be bright reflectors with little or no discernable cusp separation. Because of the increased pressure from the valve stenosis the walls of the left ventricle become thickened or hypertrophied.

M-mode findings indicate thickened cusps and restricted excursion of the cusps to less than 1.5 cm. Continuous wave Doppler is used in the apical long axis or apical "five" chamber views to evaluate the velocity across the valve. The peak instantaneous and mean aortic gradients are recorded. The continuity equation is commonly used to evaluate the severity of the aortic valve stenosis by calculating the valve area. This equation is based upon the principle of "conservation of mass." All blood flow going across the left ventricular outflow tract must be equal to the blood flow across the aortic valve. By determining the flow in the LVOT the flow in the aortic valve can also be determined. This is measured by calculating the velocity time integral of flow in the left ventricular outflow tract and at the aortic valve leaflet tips. The diameter of the LVOT is also measured to obtain a cross-sectional area. The continuity equation is as follows: Flow 1 = Flow 2, where Flow 1 = LVOT VTI × LVOT CSA and Flow 2 = AV VTI × AV CSA. The aortic valve area or AVA is calculated by dividing LVOT VTI × LVOT CSA by AV VTI. It is important to note that the LVOT VTI is obtained using pulsed wave Doppler; whereas, the AV VTI is obtained using continuous wave Doppler. The LVOT diameter is a two-dimensional measurement. Current equipment normally performed this calculation for the user, but an understanding of these principles is important. The normal aortic valve area is 2.5–4.5 cm². The normal diameter of the LVOT ranges from 1.8 to 2.4 cm with an LVOT VTI of 18–22 cm (see Table 3–6). Color Doppler can also be used to help identify aortic valve stenosis by demonstrating turbulent flow in the ascending aorta.

Parasternal Long and Short Axis Views. These views can be used to help evaluate the aortic valve cusps, making measurements of the left ventricular walls in M-mode or two dimensional planes. The diameter of the LVOT is usually taken from a left parasternal long axis view although the apical long axis view may also be used.

Apical Views. The apical views are used to obtain Doppler measures across the valve because the blood flow is parallel to the sound beam and, therefore, well suited to obtain maximal and accurate blood velocities.

TABLE 3–6. CRITERIA RANGE FOR AORTIC VALVE STENOSIS

	Mild Aortic Stenosis	Moderate Aortic Stenosis	Severe/Critical Aortic Stenosis
Peak gradient	16–36 mm Hg	37–79 mm Hg	>80 mm Hg
Mean gradient	<20 mm Hg	21–49 mm Hg	>50 mm Hg
Valve area	1.1–1.9 cm^2	0.75–1.0 cm^2	<0.74 cm^2

Regurgitation. The effects of regurgitation on atria, ventricles, and cardiac vessels result in dilation of the left ventricle. The condition can be caused by any one of the following: congenital (bicuspid cusp), rheumatic heart disease (the most common cause in adults), degeneration of the leaflet caused by infection or aortic dilatation (Marfan syndrome).

M-mode finding reveal fluttering of the interventricular septum and diastolic fluttering of the mitral valve. Two-dimensional imaging indicates fine diastolic fluttering of the aortic valve, diastolic fluttering of the mitral valve, and fluttering of the interventricular septum. Spectral Doppler studies reveal diastolic flow, which appears above the baseline when in an apical position.

Tricuspid Valve Diseases

Stenosis. Stenosis of the tricuspid valve is most often caused by rheumatic heart disease. It can be caused by other conditions, which include: systemic lupus erythematosus, carcinoid heart disease, Löffler's endocarditis, metastatic melanoma, and congenital heart disease.[1] In stenotic disease of the tricuspid valve, the effects on atria, ventricles, and vessels cause dilatation of the right atrium.

M-Mode findings indicate a reduced diastolic slope and thickening and decreased separation of the leaflets. Two-dimensional imaging reveals the most specific finding, systolic doming, as well as thickening of the leaflets. In Doppler measurements, the sample is placed in the right ventricle, the results indicate turbulent diastolic flow and slowed reduction in the velocity of flow during diastole.

Doppler is used to qualify and quantitate the severity of stenosis.

Regurgitation. Regurgitation is a common abnormality associated with the tricuspid valve in adults.[1] The primary cause of regurgitation is secondary to pulmonary hypertension. In rare cases, the condition can be caused by rheumatic heart disease, prolapse of the valve, or carcinoid heart disease. A secondary effect is dilatation of the right atrium and ventricle. CW Doppler is used to measure the velocity of the regurgitant jet. Pulmonary artery pressure may be calculated by adding the pressure gradient across the tricuspid valve to right atrial pressure (normally 5–10 mm Hg) Generally a TR velocity at 3 m/s or greater indicates pulmonary hypertension.

M-mode findings indicate a dilated right ventricle and anterior motion of the interventricular septum during isovolumetric contraction. Two-dimensional imaging reveals incomplete closure and diastolic fluttering of the leaflets, ruptured chordae, dilation of the right ventricle, and flattening of the interventricular septum. With Doppler measurements, turbulent flow can be detected on the right atrium during systole.

Pulmonic Valve Disease

Stenosis. The causes of pulmonic valve disease are atherosclerosis, infections, endocarditis, and papillary fibroma. This disease is extremely rare in adults. CW Doppler reveals velocities greater than 2 m/s in the main pulmonary artery. Color Doppler reveals turbulent flow distal to the pulmonic valve.

Regurgitation. M-Mode findings reveal fluttering of the tricuspid leaflets, and Doppler measurements reveal early diastolic high-velocity, turbulent flow. The cause can be pulmonary hypertension or bacterial endocarditis or secondary to pulmonary valvotomy.

Endocarditis

Endocarditis is an inflammation of the endocardium characterized by vegetations on the surface and in the endocardium.[1]

Types. Endocarditis can be caused by either bacteria or vegetation (fungus-like growth) and, depending on the infecting organism, is classified as acute or subacute. Although the disease can occur in the endocardium of the heart, the infection usually affects the endocardium in specific valves and is more likely to affect the left heart than the right. Infection of the tricuspid and pulmonic valves is usually the result of intravenous (IV) drug abuse.

Bacterial Endocarditis. Predisposing factors for bacterial endocarditis include dental procedures, tonsilloadenoidectomy, cirrhosis, drug addiction, surgery, and burns. Infectious endocarditis is mainly caused by two bacteria groups; staphylococci and streptococci.[1]

Nonbacterial Endocarditis. Among the nonbacterial forms of the disease are systemic lupus erythematosus (SLE) and fungal (mycotic), nonbacterial thrombotic, Löffler's, marantic, and Libman–Sacks endocarditis. The most common manifestation of SLE is vegetation. Although this nonbacterial form of endocarditis primarily involves the mitral valve, it also can affect the mural endocardium. The mycotic form of the disease is usually subacute and can be caused by a variety of fungi—most commonly, Candida, Aspergillus, and histoplama. In the thrombotic form of nonbacterial endocarditis, the vegetation consists of fibrin and other blood elements.

Löffler's endocarditis is characterized by a marked increase of eosinophils. It primarily affects men in their 40s who live in temperate climates. The disease affects both ventricles equally. Thickening of the inflow portions of the ventricles and the apices can be observed, as can formation of mural thrombi. Hemodynamically, diastolic filling is impaired because of increased stiffness of the heart. Atrio-ventricular valve regurgitation is a typical finding.

In the marantic form of the disease, the vegetation is nondestructive and sterile. It occurs in patients with malignant tumors and primarily affects the valves on the left side of the heart. Embolus is the most serious complication.

Libman–Sacks endocarditis is characterized by vegetation or verrucae on the echocardium.

Hemodynamic Mechanisms. One common cause of subacute infectious endocarditis occurs when a high velocity jet consistently hits a surface. Damage results when blood from a high-pressure area flows to a low-pressure area; this is called the Venturi effect. The site where vegetation has formed will usually be in the low pressure area. When the mitral valve is involved and mitral regurgitation is present, the atrial side of the leaflets is the susceptible area. In this case, the high-pressure area is the ventricle and, because the mitral leaflets fail to coapt, the low-pressure area is the atrial side of the leaflets. The atrial wall that bears the brunt of the regurgitation also may become infected.

When the aortic valve is involved and aortic insufficiency is present, the aorta is the high-pressure area, and the ventricle is the low-pressure area. Vegetations tend to form on the ventricular side of the aortic cusps because the cusps do not close completely in aortic regurgitation. The section of the ventricular wall hit by the regurgitant jet also may be damaged.

In ventricular septal defects (VSDs), the high pressure area is the left ventricle in left-to-right shunting and the low-pressure area is the right ventricular side of the defect. The right ventricular wall directly across from the defect also can suffer damage and become prone to vegetation.

The presence of a mass on any valve leads to a diagnosis of infection caused by vegetation. However, echocardiography cannot differentiate between a new and and old infection. M-mode patterns indicate shaggy echoes on the infected valve and detect 52% of vegetations. Transesophageal echo (TEE) is the imaging modality of choice.

Aortic Valve. Vegetation is seen best in diastole and is attached to the ventricular side of the cusps. This condition can cause reduced cardiac output and acute aortic regurgitation. The best views for two-dimensional imaging are the left parasternal long and short axes.

Mitral Valve. Predisposing factors to vegetational infection of the mitral valve include mitral valve prolapse, rheumatic valvulitis, and dysfunction of the papillary muscles with secondary mitral regurgitation and mitral annular calcification. Infection occurs most commonly on the atrial side of the leaflet.

The best views include the left parasternal short and long axes; the apical two and four chamber views also can be used. Vegetations as small as 2 mm in diameter are

detectable or can be as large as 40 mm in diameter. Whereas M-mode imaging detects 14–65% of the vegetation, two-dimensional imaging detects 43–100%. Differential diagnoses include myomas, lipomas, and fibromas.

Tricuspid or Pulmonic Valve. Infections of the tricuspid or pulmonic valves are usually caused by IV drug abuse. Such infections are less common than left-sided infections; however, when they occur on the tricuspid valve, the infections can become larger than is typical of left-sided infections. They rarely occur on the pulmonic valve.

Prosthetic Valves

Types. The two types of prosthetic valves are available: mechanical and bioprosthetic. The mechanical types are ball-in-cage, disc-in-cage, and tilting-disc valves. The Starr–Edwards valve is the most common ball-in-cage type. The best view for observing excursion of the ball is the apical view when in the mitral and aortic positions. The disc-in-cage valve has less excursion than does the ball-in-cage type. The most common type of tilting-disc valve is the Bjork–Shiley, which consists of one disc that tilts. The less common St. Jude valve contains two tilting discs.

All bioprosthetic valves are made from biological tissue which include; heterografts or xenograft (porcine tissue or bovine pericardial tissue), homografts (human cryopreserved from autopsy), and allografts (patients own tissue).[1] The most common bioprosthetic valve is the xenograft. A porcine heterograft is the most commonly used tissue; porcine pericardial tissue also can be used. Human homografts and facia lata tissue are sometimes used as valves.

Malfunctions. The following factors cause both types of prosthetic valves to malfunction: thrombi, regurgitation, stenosis, dehiscence, and vegetation.

Thrombi. Blood clots, the most common cause of valve malfunction, reduce the effective orifice and impair motion of the ball, disc, or leaflet tissue. Their major complication is the potential for an embolus. Two-dimensional imaging is the echocardiographic technique of choice for detecting the presence of a clot. The limitation of the technique is the masking effect produced by the highly reflective nature of the prosthetic valves. In the Bjork–Shiley mitral prosthesis, there is a rounding to the E point on M-mode.

Regurgitation. Regurgitation can occur through the valve or around the sewing ring. Doppler echocardiography is the procedure of choice for detecting the problem. When masking is a problem from apical views, color Doppler is especially useful. Color flow Doppler not only allows spatial orientation but also demonstrates the direction of blood jets. Secondary echocardiographic findings for aortic prosthetic regurgitation include: (1) fluttering of the mitral valve, (2) fluttering of the interventricular septum, and (3) evidence of volume overload in the left ventricle. Doppler echocardiography also is a procedure of choice for detecting paravalvular leaks with a high degree of sensitivity and specificity. In the Bjork–Shiley mitral valve, an early diastolic bump is noted by M-Mode and two dimensional imaging.

Stenosis. All prosthetic valves have some degree of obstruction. Doppler echocardiography can detect a valve with moderate to severe stenosis.

Dehiscence. In dehiscence, the valve becomes detached from its sewing bed. Disruption of suture lines securing the prosthesis to the sewing ring is usually the cause. The result is severe regurgitation, heart failure, or both, which can be detected by a Doppler examination. Two-dimensional imaging demonstrates an unusually rocking motion away from its normal excursion. Cinefluoroscopy can be helpful in assessing abnormal rocking motion.

Vegetation. As was mentioned earlier, vegetation is difficult to assess with echocardiographic techniques because it is often masked by the highly reflective properties of the prosthesis. These infections area usually found on bioprosthetic valves, are extremely mobile, and are more common in the aortic than the mitral position.

Degeneration. Degeneration is most common in the bioprosthetic valves and usually occurs as a result of calcification of the area where the valve is joined to the surrounding tissue.

DISEASES AFFECTING THE PERICARDIUM

The pericardium is composed of two layers. The inner layer is a serous membrane called the visceral pericardium, which is attached to the surface of the heart. This layer folds back upon itself to form an outer fibrous layer called the parietal pericardium. Between the two layers is the pericardial space, which is filled with a thin layer of fluid throughout. The functions of the pericardium are to (1) fix the heart anatomically,[1] (2) prevent excessive motion during changes in body position, (3) reduce friction between the heart and other organs, (4) provide a barrier against infection, and (5) help maintain hydrostatic forces on the heart. Pericardial disease can be caused by any one of the following: malignant disease that spreads to the pericardium, pericarditis, acute infarction, cardiac perforation during diagnostic procedures, radiation therapy, SLE, or postcardiac surgery.

Effusion
In the normal pericardium, the pressure within the pericardial space is similar to the intrapleural pressure and lower than the right and left ventricular diastolic pressures. Increased intrapericardial pressure depends on three factors: the volume of the effusion, the rate at which fluid accumulates, and the characteristics of the pericardium. The normal intrapericardial space contains 15–50 mL of fluid, and it can tolerate the slow addition of as much as 1–2 L of fluid without increasing the intrapericardial pressure. However, if the fluid is added rapidly, the intrapericardial pressure increases dramatically.

Pericardial effusion can be diagnosed using M-mode and two-dimensional techniques. Three diagnostic criteria

can be used: (1) posterior echo-free space, (2) obliteration of echo-free space at the left atrioventricular groove, and (3) decreased motion of the posterior pericardial motion.

Cardiac tamponade results when intrapericardial pressures increase. This problem is characterized by increased intracardiac pressures, impaired diastolic filling of the ventricles, and reduced stroke volume. The following echocardiographic findings are associated with cardiac tamponade:

- Increased dimensions of the right ventricle during inspiration
- Decreased mitral diastolic slope (E–F)
- Decreased end diastolic dimension of the right atrium or ventricle
- Posterior motion of the anterior wall of the right ventricle
- Collapse of the right ventricular free wall
- Diastolic collapse of the right atrial wall
- Increased flow velocities across the tricuspid pulmonic valve during inspiration

Several findings can create a false-positive diagnosis of pericardial effusion:

- Epicardial fat located on the anterior wall
- Misinterpretation of normal cardiac structures such as the descending aorta or coronary sinus
- Other abnormal cardiac or noncardiac structures
- Confusion of pleural effusions with pericardial effusions

Pericardial effusion can be differentiated from pleural effusion in several ways. First, in pericardial effusion, a large amount of fluid can collect posterior to the heart without any anterior collection. Second, a pericardial effusion tapers as it approaches the left atrium; a pleural effusion does not. Third, if both types of effusion occur simultaneously, a thin echogenic line should be noted between the two collections of fluid. And fourth, the descending aorta lies posterior to a pericardial effusion; whereas, it lies anterior to a pleural effusion.

Pericarditis
Pericarditis comes in two forms: acute and constrictive. In acute pericarditis, the pericardium is inflamed. This form of the disease has a variety of etiologies: idiopathic causes, viruses, uremia, bacterial infections, acute myocardial infarction, tuberculosis, malignancies, and trauma. Echocardiography reveals thickening of the pericardium, with or without pericardial effusion.

In constrictive disease, the pericardium thickens and restricts diastolic filling of the heart chambers. As in the acute form, it has a variety of causes: tuberculosis, hemodialysis used to treat chronic renal failure, connective tissue disorders (e.g., SLE, rheumatoid arthritis), metastatic infiltration, radiation therapy to the mediastinum, fungal or parasitic infections, and complications of surgery. Echocardiographic findings may include:

- Thickened pericardium
- Flattening of the left ventricular wall in mid and late systole
- A rapid mitral valve E–F slope

- Exaggerated anterior motion of the interventricular septum
- Mid-diastolic premature opening of the pulmonic valve
- Inspiratory dilatation of hepatic veins and the inferior vena cava
- Inspiratory leftward motion of the interatrial and interventricular septa

DISEASES AFFECTING THE MYOCARDIUM

The term cardiomyopathy is used to describe a variety of cardiac diseases that affect the myocardium. Cardiomyopathies have been classified into three categories: (1) hypertrophic, which may or may not obstruct the left ventricular outflow tract, (2) dilated, and (3) restrictive. The classification depends on the anatomical characteristics of the left ventricular cavity as well as systolic ejection and diastolic-filling properties of the left ventricle.

Hypertrophic Cardiomyopathy

Hypertrophic cardiomyopathy is characterized by concentric or asymmetric left ventricular hypertrophy, which results in an increase in left ventricular mass, with normal or reduced dimensions of the left ventricular cavity. Normal systolic function usually is preserved. Although asymmetric hypertrophy can occur anywhere within the left ventricle, the most common site is the proximal portion of the ventricular septum near the outflow tract. Asymmetric septal hypertrophy can be diagnosed when the ratio of septal thickness to posterior wall thickness is 1.3:1. When asymmetric hypertrophy is present obstruction most frequently occurs. Concentric hypertrophy may or may not lead to obstruction. A number of names are used to describe the obstructive forms of cardiomyopathy, including idiopathic hypertrophic subaortic stenosis, muscular subaortic stenosis, asymmetric septal hypertrophy, and hypertrophic obstructive cardiomyopathy.

Several echocardiographic findings, when found in conjunction, are highly specific for the diagnosis of obstructive cardiomyopathy. M-mode and two-dimensional findings include systolic anterior motion of the mitral valve, asymmetric septal hypertrophy, premature midsystolic closure of the aortic valve, septal hypokinesis, and anterior displacement of the mitral valve. The size of the anterior displacement of the mitral valve. The size of the left ventricle is small to normal. Doppler examination reveals a decreased E wave to mitral flow with an exaggerated A wave. These findings suggest a decrease in diastolic compliance and an increase in left ventricular end diastolic pressures. In aortic flow, there is a midsystolic reduction of velocity. Fifty percent of patients demonstrate regurgitation in the mitral valve. Pulsed-wave Doppler is used to determine the obstructed area. At rest, systolic anterior motion of the mitral valve may not be demonstrated. Because this motion is a diagnostic indication for this disease, provocative maneuvers are used to bring it out. Such techniques include the Valsalva maneuver, amyl nitrate, and IV isoproterenol.

Dilated Cardiomyopathy

Dilated cardiomyopathy is characterized by globally reduced systolic function, with an ejection fraction of less than 40%, increased end-systolic and end-diastolic volumes, and, eventually, congestive heart failure. M-mode findings include increased end-diastolic and end-systolic dimensions of the left ventricle, reduced septal and posterior wall excursion, increased E point-to-septal separation, decreased aortic root movement, and a structurally normal aortic valve that opens slowly and drifts closed during systole because of reduced cardiac output. The principal two-dimensional echocardiographic findings include left ventricular dilatation and dysfunction, abnormal closure of the mitral valve, and dilatation of the left atrium. The abnormal closure of the aortic valve also is noted. Mitral regurgitation is a frequent Doppler finding in dilated cardiomyopathy. Hemodynamically, the left ventricle demonstrates signs of increased diastolic pressure in the left ventricle and decreased compliance. The walls of the left ventricle are normal in size. The right heart also may become enlarged as a result of the increased diastolic pressures in the left heart. The most common complication of dilated cardiomyopathy is the formation of thrombi and a potential cardiac source of emboli.

Dilated cardiomyopathies can be the result of a familiar or x-linked cardiomyopathy, pregnancy, systemic hypertension, ingestion of toxic agents such as alcohol or other drugs, and a variety of viral infections. They also can be of an unknown cause or idiopathic. This form of cardiomyopathy also can be found in severe coronary artery disease.

Restrictive Cardiomyopathy

Restrictive cardiomyopathy falls into two categories: endomyocardial fibrosis and infiltrative myocardial disease, which includes amyloidosis, sarcoidosis, hematochromatosis, Pompe's disease, and Fabry's disease. The characteristic feature of restrictive cardiomyopathy is increased resistance to left ventricular filling. The associated cardiac findings include elevated diastolic pressure in the left ventricle, hypertension and enlargement of the left atrium, and secondary pulmonary hypertension. The echocardiographic features include an increase in the thickness and mass of the left ventricular wall, a small-to-normal sized left ventricular cavity, normal systolic function, and pericardial effusion. Restrictive cardiomyopathies are most common in East Africa; they account for only 5% of noncoronary cardiomyopathies in the western world.

Endomyocardial fibrosis involves formation of fibrotic sheets of tissue in the subendocardium. These sheets vary in thickness and result in increased stiffness of the ventricles. The bright reflective characteristic of this tissue is easily seen with two-dimensional echocardiography. Other characteristic echocardiographic findings include a normal-sized left ventricle, increased thickness of the left ventricular wall, thrombus, and left atrial enlargement, which usually occurs because of elevated diastolic pressure of the left ventricle. The right heart is normal in size, with mildly reduced systolic function and increased wall dimensions. Tricuspid regurgitation is present because of the pulmonary hypertension that occurs because of elevated pressures in the left heart.

There are two basic varieties of endomyocardial fibrosis. One form, found primarily in temperate regions, results from hypereosinophilia and is, therefore, termed hypereosinophilic syndrome. This syndrome, also referred to as Löffler's endocarditis parietalis fibroblastic or Löffler's endocarditis, mainly affects men in their 40s and is characterized by increased eosinophils of more than 1500/mm.[3] The second form, obliterative endomyocardial fibrosis,[3] occurs primarily in subtropical climates and is especially common in Uganda and Nigeria. It accounts for 10–20% of all cardiac deaths in those countries. Large pericardial effusions are typical in this cardiomyopathy.

Diastolic Dysfunction

The importance of diastolic function has become apparent over recent years. Many patients with symptoms of congestive heart failure (shortness of breath, edema) have normal systolic function. The inability of the left ventricle to relax properly can result in diastolic heart failure. This is often seen in patients with hypertrophic cardiomyopathies and similar conditions. Doppler echocardiography is the diagnostic tool of choice for evaluation of diastolic function.

CARDIAC MASSES

Benign Tumors

Myxomas. Myxomas are neoplasms that arise from the endocardial tissue and typically arise from the left atrium.[1] They are the most common type of benign tumor, accounting for 30–50% of all benign tumors. Three times as many females as males are affected, and 90% of the tumors are found in the atria: 75–86% are found in the left atrium; 9–20% in the right atrium; and 5–11%, in the right atrium or left ventricle but rarely in both atria. Ninety percent of myxomas are pedunculated; the most common site of attachment is the interatrial septum near the fossa avalis. This tumor may be hereditary (autosomal dominant).

M-Mode findings reveal echoes behind the anterior leaflet of the mitral valve. Two-dimensional imaging reveals an echogenic mass in the affected chamber. The echo may be brightly echogenic to sonolucent because of hemorrhage or necrosis.

The clinical findings include the following: symptoms similar to those of mitral valve disease, embolic phenomena, no symptoms, symptoms similar to those of tricuspid valve disease, sudden death, pericarditis, myocardial infarction, symptoms similar to pulmonic valve disease, and a fever or unknown origin.

Rhabdomyomas. Rhabdomyoma, is a benign tumor derived from striated muscle most commonly associated with tuberous sclerosis. It is also called myocardial hamartoma, and the most common cardiac tumor found in infants and children. In 90% of the cases, multiple rhabdomyomas are involved. The tumor is yellow gray in appearance, ranges from 1-mm to several centimeters in diameter, and most commonly involves the ventricles. Large tumors may lead to intracavitary obstruction resulting in death.

Lipomas. Lipoma is a benign tumor usually containing mature fat cells. It is the second most common benign tumor of the heart. It affects people of all ages and is found equally often in males and females. Most of these tumors are sessile. Fifty percent are located in the subendocardium, 25% are intramuscular. The most common sites are the left ventricle, right atrium, and interatrial septum.

Fibromas. Fibromas occur in the connective tissue and contain fibrous connective tissue. They are usually well circumscribed and the second most common benign tumors found predominantly in children (most of whom are younger than 10 years) almost all of these tumors occur in the ventricular myocardium. On the echocardiogram, they typically, present as a large mass within the interventricular system.

Angiomas. Angiomas are extremely rare. They may occur in any part of the heart.[5]

Teratomas. Teratomas are extremely rare and occur more often in children. They contain all three germ cell layers. They are found most frequently in the right heart, but also can occur in the interatrial or interventricular septum.[5]

Malignant Tumors

Primary Cardiac Tumors. Angiosarcomas usually occur in adults and are twice as common in men as in women. They are the fourth most common primary tumor but the most common malignant cardiac tumor. They are soft tissue tumors of the blood vessels and usually found in the right atrium; the most common site is the interatrial septum. Other primary cardiac tumors area rhabdomyosarcomas, fibrosarcomas, lymphosarcomas, and sarcomas of the pulmonary artery.

Secondary Metastatic Tumors. Metastatic and secondary tumors usually invade the right heart and are far more common than primary tumors. Usually they are clinically silent. However, they can cause superior vena cava syndrome because of obstruction, supraventricular arrhythmias, myocardial infarction, cardiomegaly, congestive heart failure, or nonbacterial endocarditis, bronchogenic carcinomas, breast carcinomas, malignant melanomas, and leukemias. Spread of these tumors varies. Bronchogenic carcinomas spread via the lymphatic channels, and metastases of malignant melanomas spread through the blood. Usually metastases involve the pericardium or the myocardium.[5]

Cardiac Thrombi

Left Ventricular Thrombi. Thrombi of the left ventricle occur in myocardial infarctions, left ventricular aneurysms, and cardiomyopathies. They usually form in the apex of the ventricle. Two-dimensional imaging can diagnose the clot with a 90% sensitivity and specificity. Echocardiography reveals that the clot has distinct margins, is usually located near an akinetic or dyskinetic area, and may protrude within the ventricle or move with the adjacent wall. Protruding thrombi tend to be more echodense than mural thrombi;

whereas, mural thrombi have a layered appearance and are often echolucent along the endocardial border.

Thrombi form within the first 4 days after an infarction and occur in 30% of all anterior wall infarctions; they rarely occur in inferior wall infarctions. If they do not dissolve spontaneously, they may disappear with the use of anticoagulants.

Left Atrial Thrombi. Thrombi usually form in the left atrium in the presence of mitral valve disease (stenosis), an enlarged left atrium, and atrial fibrillation—conditions that predispose to blood stasis. The most common site is the atrial appendage. The echocardiographic appearance of these thrombi varies. In many cases, they are attached to the atrial wall and can be round or ovoid in shape. Their borders are often well defined, they demonstrate mobility, and their texture is uniform. Occasionally, they appear as a flat immobile mass or as a free-floating ball.

Thrombi of the Right Heart. Most thrombi form in the right heart in the presence of right ventricular infarction, cardiomyopathies, or cor pulmonale. They usually are immobile, heterogeneous sessile masses. In addition, secondary thrombi may occur. Their source is embolization from deep-vein thrombosis. Echocardiography typically reveals a long, serpentine, apparently free-floating mass with no obvious site of attachment. Patients are at a much higher risk for an embolus when the thrombus in any area of the heart is protruding or free floating.

Other Cardiac Masses. Because a number of foreign objects can mimic a thrombus, one must be aware of their presence and location. For example, right-heart catheters are often seen in both the right atrium and the right ventricle. These appear as highly reflective linear echoes.

Normal cardiac structures also can mimic intracardiac masses. The moderator band seen in the apex of the right ventricle appears as a thick muscular band extending from the free wall of the right ventricle to the interventricular septum. Occasionally, a prominent eustachian valve can be seen in the right atrium at the junction of the inferior vena cava. It appears as a thin, long, mobile structure in the right atrium, which also may contain thin filamentous structures known as the Chiari network that is a remnant of embryonic structures. The left ventricle also may contain long thin fibers known as false tendons or ectopic chordae tendineae. These filamentous structures traverse the left ventricle and typically are brightly reflective structures of no clinical significance.

DISEASES OF THE AORTA

Aortic Dilatation

The aorta is considered dilated when its diameter is greater than 37 mm. The average diameter of the adult aorta is 33–37 mm. M-mode measurements of the aorta should be taken at the level of the aortic annulus and the sinus of Valsalva. Aortic dilatation is seen most frequently in patients with annuloaortic ectasia or Marfan syndrome. In these patients, the medial layer of the aorta weakens, and the aorta dilates. The dilatation occurs not only in the wall of the aorta, but in the aortic annulus as well. This often leads to aortic insufficiency because the cusps of the aorta are unable to coapt during closure. Two-dimensional echocardiography can easily detect a dilated aorta.

Aortic Aneurysm

An aortic aneurysm can occur anywhere along the thoracic aorta. The most common sites are the arch and descending aorta, with most occurring just beyond the left subclavian artery. Aneurysms of the thoracic aorta often extend into the abdominal aorta. There are several types of aneurysms, which include; saccular (sack-like dilatation), fusiform (spindle-shaped aneurysm), and dissecting (separation of the arterial wall creating a false and true lumen).

A dissecting aortic aneurysm results from intimal tears of the aortic wall. The driving force of the blood destroys the media further and strips the intimal layer from the adventitial layer. Aortic dissections are classified according to the area and extent of the intimal tear. Type I tears extend from the ascending aorta and continue beyond the arch. Type II tears also begin a few centimeters from the aortic valve but are confined to the ascending aorta. Type III tears begin in the descending aorta, usually just distal to the origin of the left subclavian artery. More than 90% of patients with dissecting aneurysms experience severe pain. Dissections occur twice as often in men as in women and usually in the sixth and seventh decade of life. M-mode findings reveal extra linear echoes within the aorta. Two-dimensional imaging is the echocardiographic tool of choice. Two-dimensional imaging is the echocardiographic tool of choice. Two-dimensional imaging allows visualization of the intimal flap, which divides the true lumen of the aorta from the false lumen. Color flow Doppler can be invaluable in localizing the site of intraluminal communication. Other echocardiographic evidence for dissection includes aortic regurgitation—the most commonly noted complication. Doppler is useful for detecting disturbed flow patterns in the left ventricular outflow tract. The left ventricle may become enlarged because of volume overload from the aortic regurgitation; pericardial effusion can be noted, and left pleural effusion also may be noted. The diagnosis of dissection should be made when an intima flap is seen in more than one view.

Aneurysms that occur in the sinus of Valsalva are seen best using two-dimensional imaging. They are observed most easily in the short-axis view during diastole. Rupture usually occurs into the right side of the heart, but it also can occur in the left heart and interventricular septum. Sinus of Valsalva aneurysms can be acquired or congenital in nature.

CONGENITAL HEART DISEASE

Aortic Stenosis

Abnormalities of the left ventricular outflow tract are the most common congenital heart disease found in the adult population. Obstruction can occur at the subvalvular, supravalvular, or valvular level. Congenital abnormalities of the aortic valve occur in 1% of the population, with a higher prevalence among males. The most common malformation of the aortic valve is a bicuspid valve. Aortic coarctation, VSD, and isolated pulmonic stenosis are associated with the condition. As the valve ages, it becomes fibrotic and may calcify. By the fourth decade, 50% of all bicuspid aortic valves become stenotic.

Subvalvular stenosis also can occur. There are two types of subvalvular stenosis: discrete and subaortic. In discrete stenosis, a thin membrane obstructs the outflow tract or a more fibromuscular ridge obstructs the flow of blood. Subaortic stenosis, too, is more common in males. Aortic regurgitation is a frequent finding in subaortic stenosis. Discrete subvalvular stenosis is primarily an acquired rather than a congenital problem when it is present in adults.

Supravalvular stenosis also can be classified into two categories. The most frequent supravalvular narrowing is found in the ascending aorta just above the valve. Less frequently, the obstruction involves the ascending aorta, the aortic arch, and the descending aorta. Supravalvular obstruction can be a familial finding, but it also can be sporadic or as a result of rubella infection. When found in association with mental retardation, a diagnosis of Williams syndrome can be made.

Patients with congenital outflow obstruction usually present with left ventricular systolic hypertension and develop concentric left ventricular hypertrophy. The physical examination reveals a harsh systolic ejection murmur over the right parasternal border. Echocardiography has become the diagnostic tool of choice in making this diagnosis. M-mode echocardiography reveals a thickened valve with an eccentric closure line. Normally, the closure line of the aortic valve is centrally located. In a bicuspid aortic valve, however, the closure line is displaced toward either the anterior or the posterior wall of the aorta. Two-dimensional echocardiography reveals systolic doming of the cusps, which is seen in the left parasternal long-axis view. The left parasternal short-axis view reveals the presence of only two cusps. Pulsed-wave Doppler echocardiography can localize the area of obstruction and determine what type of obstruction is present. Continuous wave Doppler examination allows quantification of peak and mean pressure gradients across the obstruction. Color flow Doppler examination allows assessment of blood flow direction.

Atrial Septal Defects

Atrial septal defects (ASD) is the second most common congenital abnormality found in adults. There are three classifications of ASDs, depending on their location: ostium secundum defects, ostium primum defects, and sinus venosus defects. Ostium secundum defects make up 70% of all ASDs found in adults. These are located near the fossa ovalis. Women are three times more likely than men to have this defect. Twenty percent of patients with this type of ASD have mitral valve prolapse. Other associated findings include mitral or pulmonic stenosis and atrial septal aneurysm. When an ASD and mitral stenosis exist simultaneously, the condition is called Lutembacher's syndrome. In isolated mitral stenosis, the left atrium is dilated because the valve area is reduced. With ASD, the blood can escape across the atrial defect, thereby preserving the size of the left atrium.

Fifteen percent of all ASDs are the ostium primum type. These defects occur in the region of the ostium primum or the lower portion of the atrial septum. A commonly associated finding is a clefted anterior mitral valve leaflet.

Sinus venosus ASDs account for the other 15%. The defects occur in the upper portion of the atrial septum near the orifice of the interior vena cava. The most common finding associated with this defect is partial anomalous pulmonary venous drainage.

Two-dimensional and M-mode echocardiography reveal a volume overload in the right heart. Findings indicative of right-sided volume overload include a dilated right ventricle and a flattening of the septum in diastole. Two-dimensional imaging of the atrial septum allows direct visualization and localization of the defect. The view most commonly used to assess the atrial septum includes: the parasternal short-axis, the apical four-chamber, and the subcostal views. The latter view is the best one for visualizing the atrial septum. In addition to the secondary findings already described, two-dimensional imaging allows direct visualization of the defect. In septal defects, a dropout of echoes is noted in the area of the defect. On echocardiography, the dropout of echoes is characterized by a bright echo perpendicular to the atrial septum. This finding has been described as the "T" sign.

Doppler echocardiography also can help detect ASDs. In the absence of elevated pressures in the right heart, blood flows from the higher-pressure left ventricle to the lower-pressure right heart. In the subcostal view, a pulsed Doppler sample gate can be placed in the right heart near the atrial septum. The spectral display will reveal turbulent flow toward the transducer in late systole and throughout diastole. Color flow Doppler allows visualization of the interatrial shunt by superimposing a color coding on a two-dimensional image.

Contrast echocardiography can be used when imaging and when Doppler are unable to identify the atrial defect clearly. When used in conjunction with two-dimensional imaging, 92–100% of ASDs can be detected. Contrast agents injected into a vein enter the right heart, which is often highly opacified. In the presence of an ASD, small amounts of contrast material can be seen crossing the atrial septum into the left atrium and to the left ventricle. When the shunt is left to right, which is normally the case, a negative contrast effect can be noted. Contrast enhancement can be increased by having the patient perform the Valsalva maneuver or cough.

Patent Foramen Ovale

Patent (open) foramen ovale can be found in 27% of older patients. Left-to-right shunting does not normally occur when pressures are normal. A potential complication of the condition is paradoxical embolus.

Ventricular Septal Defects

VSDs are the most common defects found in infants and children. In the adult, ASDs are much more common.

VSDs fall into two major classifications: muscular septal defects and membranous defects. Like ASDs VSDs are classified according to the region involved.

Muscular Septal Defects. Muscular septal defects are entirely surrounded by muscle. Outlet defects occur in the most superior portion of the septum and make up part of the outflow region of the left ventricle. They are also referred to as outflow defects, subpulmonic or infundibular defects, or bulbar defects. These defects are bordered by the trabecula septomarginalis (right ventricular septal band) and the pulmonary valve annulus. Thus, they are the most difficult VSDs to image and are seen best from the subcostal and high parasternal positions.

A special form of outlet defect occurs above the crista supraventricularis. This defect is known as supracristal ventricular defect; it also is referred to as the doubly committed subarterial defect because of its proximity to both semilunar valves. This defect also is seen best from the subcostal and high parasternal positions. Associated findings in this defect include (1) aortic valve prolapse because of lack of support, usually involving the right coronary cusp, (2) dilatation of the right coronary sinus of Valsalva, and (3) aortic insufficiency. The defect is usually small.

Inlet ventricular defects are bordered superiorly by the tricuspid valve annulus, apically by the tips of the papillary muscles, and anteriorly by the trabecula septomarginalis. They are also referred to as endocardial cushion defects, retrocristal defects, sinus defects, and inflow defects, which can be seen in several planes, including the parasternal, apical, and subcostal views. Because these defects are usually large, they can be confused with a double-inlet ventricle.

Trabecular defects are bordered by the chordal attachments of the papillary muscle to the apex. They extend from the smooth outlet septum to the inlet septum, are heavily trabeculated, and are usually large. They also can be multiple. These defects typically lead to hypertension of the right ventricle and may produce a right-to-left shunt if the pressures in the right heart exceed those in the left. A special type of muscular septal defect that occurs in the muscular septum is characterized by numerous small defects resembling Swiss cheese. This "Swiss cheese" defect occurs primarily in the apex.

Membranous Defects. Membranous septal defects occur in the region bordered by the inlet and outlet septums and the junctions between the right and noncoronary cusps of the aortic valve. This part of the septum is located at the base of the heart. Defects in this area are often referred to as perimembranous because they usually involve part of a surrounding muscular septum. Almost all planes can be used to image these defects, which occur more frequently than the muscular varieties.

Using two-dimensional imaging allows visualization of the septum. When the defect is large, a dropout of echoes is appreciated. In addition a "T" artifact is observed. When imaging does not allow localization of the defect, color-flow Doppler can be used. High-velocity turbulent flow usually can be seen as a mosaic color pattern in the area of the jet.

Contrast echocardiography also can be used to localize the defect. Agitated solution can be injected into the right heart through a peripheral vein. Even a few bubbles seen entering the left ventricle are indicative of a right-to-left shunt when right-sided pressures are slightly elevated.

Tetralogy of Fallot

In adults, tetralogy of Fallot is the primary congenital disease producing cyanosis. In this condition, four specific findings are noted. The aorta overrides the perimembranous VSD. Infundibular or valvular pulmonic stenosis is present, resulting in right ventricular hypertrophy. M-mode criteria for diagnosing tetralogy of Fallot includes a break in the continuity of the anterior wall of the aorta from that of the interventricular septum as well as a narrowing of the right ventricular outflow tract. Two-dimensional imaging, however, allows direct visualization of the cardiac anatomy and is, therefore, the echocardiographic procedure of choice. Imaging often allows visualization of the VSD and gives valuable information about the amount of aortic override. Doppler echocardiography allows quantification of gradients across the obstruction of right ventricular outflow.

Pulmonic Stenosis

Eighty percent of all congenital obstructions of right ventricular outflow occur at the level of the pulmonic valve. The valve is often thickened with fusion of the cusps and can be seen doming in systole. Right ventricular hypertrophy occurs as a result of the increased resistance to flow. Two-dimensional imaging allows visualization of the valve, which usually appears thickened and with reduced excursion.

Persistent Ductus Arteriosus

Persistent ductus arteriosus (PDA) occurs when the ductus fails to close after birth. In utero, communication exists between the pulmonary circulation and the systemic circulation, the purpose of which in fetal circulation is to direct the flow of desaturated blood away from the coronary and cerebral circulation and toward the placenta. The ductus is located near the isthmus of the aorta near the origin of the left subclavian artery; it extends to the left pulmonary artery just beyond the bifurcation. In the absence of elevated pulmonary pressures, blood flows from the aorta to the pulmonary artery. In adults, the most common symptom of a PDA is dyspnea on exertion. In persistent ductus, the increased blood flow to the lungs results in dilatation of the pulmonary arteries, the left atrium and ventricle, and the aorta. If pulmonary pressure increases, the blood flow may reverse and travel from the pulmonary circulation toward the aorta. This condition is known as Eisenmenger's complex and is characterized by right-to-left shunting.

Coarctation of the Aorta

Coarctation is a stricture or contraction of the aorta. Twice as many men as women are likely to have coarctation of the aorta. Most patients with this condition are asymptomatic. The coarctation is manifested as left ventricular hypertension. On physical examination, a systolic murmur can be heard. The most common site of narrowing occurs in the thoracic aorta just distal to the left subclavian artery. This condition is often found in association with other congenital abnormalities such as; VSD, PDA, a bicuspid aortic valve, and mitral valve abnormalities. It is the most common cardiac malformation found in Turner's syndrome.

The suprasternal notch offers the best view of the ascending aorta, the arch, and the descending aorta. Direct visualization of the coarctation is possible using two-dimensional imaging. Doppler echocardiography typically reveals increased velocities across the site of coarctation.

Ebstein's Anomaly

Ebstein's anomaly is characterized by downward displacement of the anterior or septal leaflet of the tricuspid valve into the right ventricle. As a result, the ventricle becomes "atrialized" and loses some of its pumping capacity. Associated findings include secundum-type ASDs, pulmonic stenosis or atresia, VSD, and mitral valve prolapse. Symptoms may not be evident until the patient is between 30 and 40 years old. The most common complication of this abnormality is failure of the right ventricle.

The M-mode criterion for this anomaly includes visualization of a large tricuspid valve leaflet, simultaneously seen with the anterior leaflet of the mitral leaflet. A delay time in closure of the tricuspid valve of 80 m/s or more to that of closure of the mitral valve is the second M-mode finding. Two-dimensional imaging allows direct visualization of the anatomy. Specific findings in imaging include an apically located tricuspid leaflet and a functionally small right ventricle. Ebstein's anomaly can be diagnosed if the leaflet is displaced 20 mm or more.

HYPERTENSIVE DISEASE

Systemic Hypertension

There are two basic types of systemic hypertension: essential or idiopathic and secondary hypertension. Both affect the diastolic and systolic pressure. The classification of blood pressure is shown in Table 3–7.

TABLE 3–7. CLASSIFICATION OF BLOOD PRESSURE

Range (mm Hg)	Category
Diastolic	
<85	Normal blood pressure
85–89	High normal blood pressure
90–104	Mild hypertension
105–114	Moderate hypertension
≥115	Severe hypertension
Systolic, when diastolic blood pressure is <90 mm Hg	
<140	Normal blood pressure
140–159	Borderline isolated systolic hypertension
≥160	Isolated systolic hypertension

Reprinted with permission from The 1984 Report of the Joint National Committee on Detection, Evaluation, and Treatment of High Blood Pressure. Arch Intern Med. 144, May, 1984.

The cause of essential hypertension is unknown. Although several mechanisms may come into play, no specific cause has been well described. Secondary hypertension results in high blood pressure associated with any of the following: renal disease, endocrine disease, coarctation of the aorta, pregnancy, neurological disorders, acute stress, increased intravascular volume, alcohol and other drug abuse, increased cardiac output, and rigidity of the aorta.

The hemodynamic properties of systemic hypertension, whatever the cause, are similar. Initially cardio output increases, as does fluid volume. This increased fluid volume is transferred to the various organs and tissues. Once tissues receive more blood than they need, the blood vessels that deliver the blood constrict. This is known as vasoconstriction, which is an intrinsic property of such systemic vessels as arterioles and the bicep increases in size when one does curls, so the arteries. If this state continues, the vessels continue to exert resistance on the incoming blood (peripheral resistance). As a result, the heart beats gain greater resistance and the vessel themselves become thicker.

As is the case with any muscle, hypertrophy occurs when stress is exerted. Just as the bicep increases in size when one does curls, so does the heart increase in size as it is forced to pump blood against increased peripheral resistance. Therefore, the main echocardiographic findings are increased muscle mass of the heart, especially the left ventricle. By M-mode criteria, the walls of the left ventricle are thick. The principal Doppler findings include (1) decreased transmitral E wave, (2) increased A wave, and (3) increased A-to E-wave ratios.

Pulmonary Hypertension

In normal physiology, the pulmonary blood flow allows passage of blood to the lungs for three basic functions: oxygenation, filtration, and pH balance by excreting carbon dioxide. Blood coming in from the various tissues and organs of the body is directed to the right heart through the superior and inferior vena cavae. Once this deoxygenated blood enters the right atrium, it passes through the tricuspid valve into the right ventricle across the pulmonic valve and into the main pulmonary artery, which bifurcates into a left and right branch and directs blood to the left and right lobes of the lungs. Normally the pulmonary circulation offers little resistance to blood flow. The normal peak systolic pressure ranges from 18–25 mm Hg, and the normal diastolic pressure ranges from 6–10 mm Hg. Pulmonary artery pressure in excess of 30 mm Hg systolic pressure and 20 mm Hg diastolic pressure represents elevated pulmonary pressures, or pulmonary hypertension.

As with systemic hypertension, pulmonary hypertension has two basic forms: primary and secondary. Primary pulmonary hypertension—also known as idiopathic, essential, or unexplained pulmonary hypertension—has no known discernible cause. Secondary pulmonary hypertension can be the result of any one of the following factors:

- Increased resistance to pulmonary venous drainage
- Elevated left ventricular diastolic pressure
- Left atrial hypertension (mitral stenosis)

- Pulmonary parenchyma disease
- Pulmonary venous obstruction (cor triatriatum or pulmonary veno-occlusive disease

Cor triatriatum is a congenital abnormality in which the common embryonic pulmonary vein is not incorporated into the left atrium. Instead, the pulmonary veins empty into an accessory chamber and communicate with the left atrium through a small opening. The result is obstruction of pulmonary venous flow that simulates mitral stenosis. In pulmonary veno-occlusive disease, the veins and venules of the lung become fibrotic. M-mode findings reveal an absent or decreased A wave in the absence of right ventricular failure: a lack of respiratory variation in the A wave; an extended pre-ejection period; midsystolic closure of the pulmonic valve, also known as midsystolic notch; and reduced ejection time of the right ventricle. Two-dimensional imaging indicates a dilated pulmonary artery and abnormalities in interventricular septal motion.

Doppler measurements reveal the following: a decreased acceleration time, a longer pre-ejection period, a shorter ejection time, and tricuspid regurgitation. The acceleration time is the time interval between the onset of flow and the peak systolic flow. In pulmonary hypertension, the velocity of blood flow increases rapidly and peaks early in systole. This measurement is made by identifying the beginning of the Doppler signal and the peak velocity of the same signal. The time between the two is the acceleration time.

The pre-ejection period is the time interval between the onset of the ORS complex to onset of flow in the pulmonary artery. In pulmonary hypertension, this time period increases.

Ejection time is the time from the onset of flow to the cessation of flow. In pulmonary hypertension, this time period becomes shorter. This measurement is made by taking the time between the beginning and end of the Doppler signal.

Tricuspid regurgitation occurs in the majority of patients with elevated pressures in the pulmonary artery. Continuous-wave Doppler can be used to localize the regurgitant jet and obtain the peak transtricuspid gradient using the modified Bernoulli equation. The peak gradient is the difference in systolic pressure between the right atrium and right ventricle. Estimation of the pulmonary pressures is accomplished by adding the right atrial pressures, which are determined by visual inspection of the jugular venous pulse. A more common way is to add the constant "10" to the peak systolic transtricuspid gradient. When stenosis of the pulmonic valve is present, however, one cannot determine pulmonary artery pressures using the peak transtricuspid regurgitant gradient.

CORONARY ARTERY DISEASE

The normal right and left coronary arteries supply the heart muscle with oxygenated blood (see Table 3–8). The left coronary artery originates from the left coronary sinus of Valsalva, which bifurcates into two branches: the ante-

TABLE 3–8. NORMAL BRANCHES OF THE CORONARY ARTERIES

Coronary Artery	Major Branches	Area Supplied
Left coronary	Left anterior descending	Anterior left ventricular wall
		Anterior two-thirds of apical septum
		Anteroapical portions of left ventricle
		Anterior-lateral papillary muscle
		Midseptum
		Bundle of His
		Anterior right ventricular papillary muscle
	Circumflex*	Lateral left ventricular wall
		Left atrium
Right coronary	Numerous branches	Anterior right ventricular wall
		Posterior third (or more) of the interventricular septum
		Diaphragmatic wall of right ventricle
		Atrioventricular node

*If the circumflex terminates at the crux of the heart, it supplies the entire left ventricle and interventricular septum.

rior interventricular or descending branch, also known as the left anterior descending branch, and the circumflex branch. The right coronary artery originates from the right coronary sinus of Valsalva.

The coronary anatomy can vary considerably in humans. In 67% of cases, the right coronary artery is the dominant artery. In these cases, this artery supplies the parts of the left ventricle and septum. In 15% of cases, the left coronary artery is the dominant one and supplies blood to all of the left ventricle and septum. In 18% of cases, the two arteries are equal; this situation is called the balanced coronary arterial pattern.

Abnormal Wall Motion

When the blood supply to the heart muscle is interrupted, the muscle is damaged, and immediate changes in motion can be observed. The affected area can be identified using the various echocardiographic views. The wall segment should be identified using the American Society of Echocardiography's recommendation (see the section of wall segment in the "Normal Anatomy" section.[4]

Complications of Ischemic Heart Disease

Ventricular Aneurysm. One complication of ischemic heart disease is ventricular aneurysm. Although aneurysm can form in any part of the left ventricle, more than 80% form in the apex and are the result of an anterior infarction. Of the 5–10% that form in the posterior wall, nearly half are false aneurysms.

The echocardiographic appearance of aneurysms includes thin walls that do not thicken in systole, a bulging wall, and dyskinetic motion to the affected area.

There are three types of ventricular aneurysms: anatomically true, functionally true, and anatomically false aneurysms. An anatomically true aneurysm is composed of fibrous tissue, may or may not contain a clot, and protrudes during both diastole and systole. Its mouth is wider or as wide as its maximum diameter, and its wall is the former left ventricular wall. An anatomically true aneurysm almost never ruptures once healed. A functionally true aneurysm also consists of fibrous tissue but protrudes only during ventricular systole.

An anatomically false aneurysm always contains a clot. Its mouth is considerably smaller than its maximum diameter, and it protrudes during both systole and diastole and may even expand. Its wall is composed of parietal pericardium. Because a false aneurysm often ruptures, immediate surgery is usually required.

Ventricular Septal Defect. A VSD occurs when a rupture occurs in the septum. Several echocardiographic techniques can be used to make the diagnosis. Two-dimensional imaging allows direct visualization of the defect. With contrast echocardiography with imaging, contrasting material can be seen filling the right ventricle and entering the left ventricle as blood moves back and forth through the defect. Negative contrast effect also can be noted. Doppler measurements can detect turbulent high-velocity signals on the right side of the ventricular septum. The best views include the left parasternal long and short-axis views and the apical four-chamber view. Color Doppler can demonstrate communication between the left and right ventricles. The color jet appears as a mosiac pattern of high-velocity flow.

Thrombus. Thrombus, the most common complication of infarction, usually occurs in the apex in areas of dyskinesis. It can be laminar, lay close to the wall of the ventricle, or protrude into the cavity and be highly mobile. The diagnosis should be made when the thrombus is seen in several views.

Valve Dysfunction. An infarction is most likely to affect the mitral valve. Mitral regurgitation results if the papillary muscle is ruptured; if it becomes fibrosed; or if the mitral annulus is affected, resulting in incomplete closure of the leaflets.

Right Ventricular Involvement. Involvement of the right ventricle occurs primarily when the infarction is in the inferior wall or when the proximal right coronary artery is obstructed. Echocardiography reveals that the ventricle is dilated and its free wall moves abnormally.

REFERENCES

1. Allen MN, *Echocardiography.* 2nd ed. New York: Lippincott; 1999.
2. *Grays Anatomy.* Williams PL, Warwick R, Dyson M, eds. 37th ed. New York: Churchill Livingston; 1989.
3. *Report of the American Society of Echocardiography Committee on Nomenclature and Standards Identification of Myocardial Wall Segments.* 1982.
4. Feigenbaum H. *Endocardiopathy.* 4th ed. Philadelphia: Lea & Febiger; 1986.
5. Braunwald E. *Heart Disease: A Textbook of Cardiac Medicine.* 3rd ed. Philadelphia: WB Saunders; 1988.

Questions

GENERAL INSTRUCTIONS: For each question, select the best answer. Select only one answer for each question unless otherwise specified.

1. Which heart groove or sulci separates the atria from the ventricles?

   (A) interventricular
   (B) interatrial
   (C) anterior interventricular
   (D) coronary or atrioventricular

2–10. Identify the coronary arteries in Fig. 3–12

2. _____   left posterolateral branch

3. _____   left circumflex branch

4. _____   pulmonary trunk

5. _____   left marginal branch

6. _____   AV node branch

7. _____   left main coronary artery

8. _____   right coronary artery

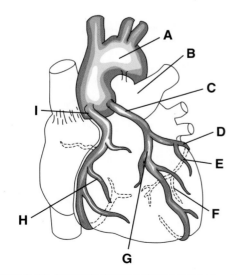

Figure 3–12. Anatomic drawing of the heart and vessels.

9. _____   aortic arch

10. _____   left anterior descending branch

11. Indications for stress echocardiography does not include

    (A) screening of new patients for CAD
    (B) assessing states before and after intervention
    (C) determining prognosis after myocardial infarction
    (D) unstable angina

12. Which of the following cardiology examination requires a physician to perform?

    (A) echocardiography
    (B) stress echocardiography
    (C) transesophageal echocardiography
    (D) Color flow Doppler

13. The purpose of the pericardium is

    (A) allow the heart to move freely with each beat
    (B) facilitating ejection and volume changes
    (C) contain the heart within the mediastinum
    (D) serve as a barrier to infection
    (E) all of the above

14. What is the largest cardiac chamber?

    (A) right atrium
    (B) right ventricle
    (C) left atrium
    (D) left ventricle

15. The left atrium receives how many pulmonary veins?

    (A) one
    (B) two
    (C) three
    (D) four

16. Crista terminalis is

    (A) anterior portion of the right atrium
    (B) posterior portion of the right atrium
    (C) a ridge of muscle separating the right atrium
    (D) a heart groove or sulci

17. Which valve is located between the left atrium and the left ventricle?

    (A) tricuspid
    (B) mitral
    (C) aortic
    (D) foramen ovale

18. Which of the following is not a right heart characteristic and/or function?

    (A) supplies blood to the pulmonary circulation
    (B) normal pressure in the ventricle is approximately 140 mm Hg
    (C) blood returning to the right heart has a lower oxygen saturation
    (D) contains the tricuspid valve

19. Mitral valve stenosis results primarily from

    (A) atherosclerosis
    (B) endocarditis
    (C) hypertension
    (D) rheumatic disease

20. Vegetations are more commonly associated with

    (A) pulmonary hypertension
    (B) aneurysms
    (C) endocarditis
    (D) mitral valve disease

21. Which of the following is not a type of bioprosthetic heart valve?

    (A) xenograft
    (B) heterograft
    (C) homograft
    (D) Bjork–Shiley valve

22. Which of the following would indicate pericardial effusion?

    (A) 5–10 mL of fluid
    (B) 10–15 mL of fluid
    (C) 15–50 mL of fluid
    (D) 75–100 mL of fluid

23. The term cardiomyopathy is used to describe

    (A) pericardial effusion
    (B) variety of cardiac diseases that affect the pericardium
    (C) variety of cardiac diseases that affect the myocardium
    (D) variety of cardiac diseases that affect the endocardium

24. The most common type of benign tumor of the heart is

    (A) myxoma
    (B) rhabdomyoma
    (C) lipoma
    (D) fibroma

25. The most common malignant cardiac tumor is

    (A) teratoma
    (B) rhabdomyoma
    (C) carcinoma
    (D) angiosarcoma

26. Which type of aneurysm results from intimal tears of the aortic wall?

    (A) saccular
    (B) fusiform
    (C) pseudo
    (D) dissecting

27. What is the most common congenital heart disease?

    (A) atrial septal defects
    (B) ventricular septal defects
    (C) muscular septal defects
    (D) abnormalities of the left ventricular outflow tract

28. What is the primary congenital disease in adults that produces cyanosis?

    (A) pulmonic stenosis
    (B) coarctation of the aorta
    (C) persistent ductus arteriosus
    (D) tetralogy of Fallot

29. Which of the following is not a characteristic of cardiomyopathy?

    (A) dilatation
    (B) pericarditis
    (C) restrictive
    (D) hypertrophic

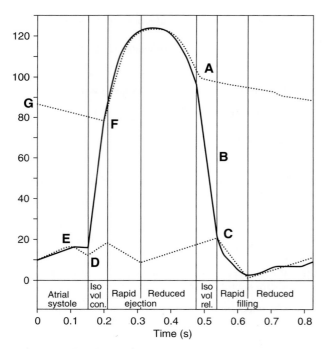

Figure 3–13. Events of the cardiac cycle.

30–36. Identify the structures in Fig. 3–13.

30. _____   aortic valve closure

31. _____   aortic valve opening

32. _____   aortic pressure

33. _____   left ventricular pressure

34. _____   mitral valve closure

35. _____   left atrial pressure

36. _____   mitral valve opening

37. In stenotic diseases of the tricuspid there is dilatation of

(A) left atrium
(B) left ventricle
(C) right atrium
(D) right ventricle

38. In tricuspid valve disease, the primary cause of regurgitation is

(A) carcinoid heart disease
(B) prolapse of the valve
(C) rheumatic heart disease
(D) secondary to pulmonary hypertension

39. Which of the following is not a type of endocarditis?

(A) Ebstein's anomaly

(B) bacterial
(C) mycotic
(D) Löffler's

40. Clinical symptoms associated with aortic valve stenosis does not include

(A) chest pain
(B) dyspnea on exertion
(C) shortness of breath
(D) syncope

41. Which of the following is the bicuspid valve with two major leaflets?

(A) tricuspid valve
(B) aortic valve
(C) pulmonic valve
(D) mitral valve

42. The classic finding in mitral valve prolapse is

(A) systolic doming
(B) fluttering of the mitral valve
(C) pulmonary edema
(D) a systolic click

43. The most common cause of a flail leaflet is

(A) rupture of the chordal tendineae
(B) rupture of the papillary muscle
(C) annular calcification
(D) congenital defect

44. Which cardiac examination provides the highest resolution?

(A) transthoracic echocardiography
(B) contrast transthoracic echocardiography
(C) stress echocardiography
(D) transesophageal echocardiography

45. In which cardiac sinus is a thin fold of tissue guards called the thebesius valve?

(A) sinus of Morgagni
(B) aortic sinus
(C) coronary sinus
(D) sinus of Valsalva

46. The average length of an adult heart is

(A) 12 cm
(B) 8–9 cm
(C) 6 cm
(D) 16 cm

47. The atrioventricular node (AV) is located in which triangle region of the right atrium?

(A) posterior region
(B) anterior region
(C) triangular region
(D) triangle of Koch

48. Which vessel drains the head and parts of the upper extremities?

(A) aorta
(B) superior vena cava
(C) inferior vena cava
(D) portal venous system

49. Which of the following views would best demonstrate all four cardiac chambers simultaneously?

(A) left parasternal
(B) right parasternal
(C) subcostal
(D) suprasternal

50. The three orthogonal planes for two-dimensional echocardiographic imaging are termed

(A) long axis, short axis, and four chamber
(B) apical, subcostal, and parasternal
(C) suprasternal, right sternal border, and left sternal border
(D) anterior, posterior, and coronal

51. Which of the following abnormalities are usually best demonstrated with the subcostal four-chamber view?

(A) atrial septal defects and ventricular septal defects
(B) mitral regurgitation and tricuspid regurgitation
(C) mitral stenosis and tricuspid stenosis
(D) aortic insufficiency and pulmonic insufficiency

52. The control that suppresses near-field echoes and enhances the intensity of the far-field echoes is called

(A) attenuation
(B) time-gain compensation
(C) reject
(D) compression

53. The tricuspid valve opens when

(A) the right ventricular pressure drops below the right atrial pressure
(B) the papillary muscle contracts
(C) the velocity of blood flow in the right ventricle exceeds the velocity of flow in the right atrium
(D) the pulmonic valve opens

54. Which of the following is *not* a remnant of the fetal circulation?

(A) the eustachian valve
(B) the coronary ligament
(C) the foramen ovale
(D) the ligamentum arteriosus

55. Blood normally flows from the right ventricle to the

(A) pulmonary artery
(B) aorta
(C) right atrium
(D) pulmonary vein

56. A pulmonary vein is normally attached to the

(A) right ventricle
(B) left ventricle
(C) left atrium
(D) right atrium

57. Which of the following statements regarding cardiac anatomy is false?

(A) the heart tends to assume a more vertical position in tall thin people and a more horizontal position in short heavy people
(B) the ligamentum arteriosum runs from the left pulmonary artery to the descending aorta
(C) the coronary arteries arise from the sinuses within the pockets of the left and right coronary cusps of the aortic valve
(D) the left ventricle constitutes most of the ventral surface of the heart

58. Left ventricular ejection time can be assessed from an M-mode echocardiogram by measuring the distance between the

(A) aortic valve opening and closing points
(B) mitral D and C points
(C) R wave and T wave
(D) mitral valve closure and aortic valve opening

59. Often, the best two-dimensional view for examining patients with chronic obstructive pulmonary disease is

(A) parasternal
(B) apical
(C) suprasternal
(D) subcostal

60. The two best transducer positions for Doppler investigation of systolic blood flow across the aortic valve are

(A) parasternal and suprasternal
(B) apical and right sternal border
(C) suprasternal and subcostal
(D) subcostal and apical

61. The size of the left atrium is measured on the M-mode

(A) at end-systole
(B) at the peak of the R wave
(C) with the onset of aortic valve opening
(D) at the beginning of the P wave

62. Doming of any cardiac valve on two-dimensional echocardiography is consistent with

(A) regurgitation
(B) decreased cardiac output
(C) stenosis
(D) congenital malformation

63. Two-dimensional images are best obtained when the ultrasound beam is directed _____ to the structure of interest. Doppler signals are best obtained when the ultrasound beam is directed _____ to the flow of blood.

(A) oblique, perpendicular
(B) parallel, perpendicular
(C) perpendicular, parallel
(D) perpendicular, oblique

64. Right ventricular systolic pressure overload can be caused by

(A) pulmonary insufficiency
(B) an atrial septal defect
(C) aortic stenosis
(D) pulmonary hypertension

65. Left ventricular measurements should be obtained from the parasternal long-axis view at the level of the

(A) mitral valve annulus
(B) tips of the mitral leaflets
(C) chordae tendineae
(D) papillary muscle

66. All of the following can cause paradoxical interventricular septal motion except

(A) left bundle branch block
(B) postpericardiotomy
(C) left ventricular volume overload
(D) severe tricuspid regurgitation

67. In a patient with volume overload of the right ventricle, the onset of ventricular systole is likely to show the interventricular septum moving

(A) toward the right ventricular free wall
(B) toward the left ventricular wall
(C) laterally
(D) not at all

68. A murmur that is associated with a thrill is likely to be

(A) organic in origin
(B) insignificant
(C) functional
(D) the result of an atrial septal defect

69. The Valsalva maneuver and the inhalation of amyl nitrite are techniques that are sometimes used during an echocardiographic examination when checking for

(A) mitral valve prolapse or systolic anterior motion of the mitral valve
(B) aortic stenosis or mitral stenosis
(C) aortic stenosis or aortic regurgitation
(D) a ventricular septal defect or pulmonic stenosis

70. Clubbing of the fingers and nail beds is a sign of

(A) cyanotic heart disease
(B) Marfan syndrome
(C) Barlow syndrome
(D) increased cardiac output

71. Even though two-dimensional echocardiography has largely replaced M-mode echocardiography for cardiac diagnosis, M-mode still has the advantage of

(A) defining spatial relationships of cardiac structures
(B) providing enhanced temporal resolution
(C) providing dynamic assessment of the velocity of blood flow
(D) providing superior lateral resolution

72. When attempting a parasternal short-axis view, if the left ventricle appears oval rather than circular, the echocardiographer should move the transducer

(A) medially
(B) laterally
(C) to a higher intercostal space
(D) to a lower intercostal space

73. A Doppler tracing of the mitral valve in which the A point is higher than the E point indicates

(A) high cardiac output
(B) low cardiac output
(C) decreased left ventricular compliance
(D) high left ventricular end-diastolic pressures

74. Which of the following is usually not a secondary finding in patients with mitral stenosis?

(A) a dilated left atrium
(B) a dilated right atrium
(C) a left ventricular thrombus
(D) a left atrial thrombus

75. The Doppler signal obtained from the apex in a patient with mitral stenosis is most likely to demonstrate all of the following except

(A) an increased diastolic peak velocity
(B) spectral broadening
(C) a decreased E-F slope
(D) a peak gradient occurring in late diastole

76. Torn chordae tendineae will cause

    (A) aortic insufficiency
    (B) myocardial infarction
    (C) mitral insufficiency
    (D) mitral stenosis

77. All of the following can produce false positive signs of mitral valve prolapse on an M-mode except

    (A) pericardial effusion
    (B) premature ventricular contractions
    (C) improper placement of the transducer
    (D) hypertrophic obstructive cardiomyopathy

78. Which of the following is a secondary echocardiographic finding in mitral regurgitation?

    (A) a dilated left atrium
    (B) left ventricular hypertrophy
    (C) a hypokinetic left ventricle
    (D) a dilated aortic root

79. The degree of mitral regurgitation is best estimated by measuring the

    (A) width and length of the systolic jet by color Doppler
    (B) peak velocity of the continuous-wave Doppler systolic mitral signal
    (C) pressure half-time of the continuous-wave Doppler diastolic signal
    (D) integral of the continuous-wave systolic curve

80. Which of the following is least likely to occur as a sequela of rheumatic fever?

    (A) mitral stenosis
    (B) mitral insufficiency
    (C) aortic stenosis
    (D) pulmonic stenosis

81. the two-dimensional echocardiogram of a patient with combined mitral and aortic stenosis is most likely to demonstrate

    (A) a dilated left atrium and left ventricular hypertrophy
    (B) a dilated left atrium and a dilated left ventricle
    (C) a small left atrium and a small left ventricle
    (D) systolic anterior motion of the mitral valve and left ventricular hypertrophy

82. The M-mode of the mitral valve in mitral stenosis is often missing an A wave. The reason is

    (A) high initial diastolic pressures in the left ventricle
    (B) concurrent atrial fibrillation
    (C) decreased compliance of the left ventricle
    (D) a dilated left atrium

83. A Doppler tracing that demonstrates a late diastolic mitral inflow velocity (A point) that is higher than the initial diastolic velocity (E point) can be seen with which of the following pathologies?

    (A) aortic insufficiency
    (B) hypertrophic cardiomyopathy
    (C) mitral regurgitation
    (D) a ventricular septal defect

84. If the two-dimensional examination demonstrates a markedly dilated and hyperkinetic left ventricle and a left atrium of normal size, one should suspect the presence of

    (A) mitral regurgitation
    (B) aortic regurgitation
    (C) a ventricular septal defect
    (D) aortic stenosis

85. Which group of echocardiographic findings would give a definitive diagnosis of mitral stenosis?

    (A) a decreased E–F slope, a dilated left atrium, and a small left ventricle
    (B) a thickened mitral valve, a dilated left atrium, and a small left ventricle
    (C) a decreased E–F slope, a thickened mitral valve, and diastolic doming of the mitral valve
    (D) a thickened mitral valve and a mitral diastolic velocity >1.5 m/s

86. A patient with mitral stenosis will usually have all of the following except

    (A) a diastolic rumble on auscultation
    (B) an increased E–F slope on M-mode
    (C) a history of rheumatic fever
    (D) a dilated left atrium

87. To obtain the true circumference of the mitral valve, one should obtain a short-axis view at the level of the

    (A) papillary muscle
    (B) chordae tendineae
    (C) tips of the mitral leaflets
    (D) mitral annulus

88. Secondary echocardiographic findings of mitral stenosis include all of the following except

    (A) a dilated left atrium
    (B) a dilated right atrium
    (C) a dilated left ventricle
    (D) a left atrial thrombus

89. A successful mitral valve commissurotomy would be *least* likely to demonstrate

    (A) doming of the mitral valve
    (B) mitral valve thickening
    (C) an increase in pressure half-time
    (D) a dilated left atrium

90. Left ventricular dilatation in a patient with mitral stenosis suggests

(A) severe mitral stenosis
(B) concomitant mitral regurgitation
(C) aortic stenosis
(D) hypertrophic cardiomyopathy

91. Early diastolic closure of the mitral valve is usually a sign of

(A) severe acute aortic regurgitation
(B) a left bundle branch block
(C) poor function of the left ventricle
(D) first-degree A–V block

92. Degenerative calcification of the mitral annulus can be accelerated by all of the following conditions except

(A) systemic hypertension
(B) aortic stenosis
(C) hypertrophic obstructive cardiomyopathy
(D) a ventricular septal defect

93. A mitral valve pressure half-time of 220 ms is consistent with a mitral valve area of

(A) 0.6 cm²
(B) 1 cm²
(C) 2.2 cm²
(D) 5 cm²

94. Echocardiographic findings of significant aortic stenosis include all of the following except

(A) reduced separation of the aortic valve cusp
(B) diastolic fluttering of the anterior mitral leaflet
(C) Doppler systolic velocities greater than 4 m/s
(D) thickened left ventricular walls

95. Which of the following causes the left ventricular walls to appear thick on an echocardiogram?

(A) mitral stenosis
(B) aortic insufficiency
(C) mitral regurgitation
(D) systemic hypertension

96. The presence of a systolic ejection murmur should alert one to look for

(A) a ventricular septal defect
(B) mitral regurgitation
(C) aortic stenosis
(D) patent ductus arteriosus

97. All of the following statements regarding a bicuspid aortic valve are true except

(A) the problem is a congenital one
(B) it may be associated with aortic stenosis
(C) it is often seen in conjunction with mitral stenosis

(D) it may be associated with coarctation of the aorta

98. The continuity equation is used to calculate the _____. It is most helpful in patients with _____.

(A) mitral valve area, mitral stenosis
(B) aortic valve area, poor left ventricular function
(C) aortic valve velocity, systemic hypertension
(D) degree of shunting, a ventricular septal defect

99. In patients with combined aortic stenosis and aortic insufficiency, which of the following parameters is best for assessing the severity of aortic stenosis?

(A) the maximum pressure gradient
(B) the mean pressure gradient
(C) the high pulse-repetition frequency
(D) the analog waveform

100. Which of the following two-dimensional views will best illustrate a color Doppler jet of aortic insufficiency?

(A) the apical long-axis view
(B) the suprasternal view
(C) the subcostal fine-chamber view
(D) the short axis view of the base

101. Which of the following is a secondary echocardiographic sign of aortic stenosis?

(A) a thickened aortic valve
(B) left ventricular hypertrophy
(C) a hyperdynamic left ventricle
(D) a dilated left ventricle

102. An M-mode finding of fine diastolic fluttering of the anterior mitral leaflet is consistent with

(A) aortic insufficiency
(B) mitral stenosis
(C) atrial fibrillation
(D) a prolonged heart rate

103. Diastolic velocity signals were detected in a patient's left ventricular outflow tract using pulsed Doppler. They could be detected between the tip of the anterior mitral leaflet and the aortic valve from the parasternal position. This is

(A) normal
(B) consistent with severe mitral regurgitation
(C) consistent with severe aortic regurgitation
(D) consistent with moderate aortic regurgitation
(E) consistent with moderate mitral regurgitation

104. The referring physician hears an Austin–Flint murmur. The M-mode echocardiogram of this patient is most likely to demonstrate

(A) a thickened mitral valve with a decreased E–F slope
(B) fine diastolic fluttering and possible flattening of the anterior mitral leaflet
(C) a thickened aortic valve with a decreased opening
(D) systolic posterior motion of the tricuspid valve

105. The best approach for obtaining the maximum aortic velocity in patients with aortic stenosis is from the

(A) left sternal border
(B) left supraclavicular region
(C) subcostal region
(D) right sternal border view

106. The best way to rule out an aortic dissection is with

(A) M-mode echocardiography
(B) transthoracic two-dimensional imaging
(C) color Doppler
(D) transesophageal echocardiography

107. Which echocardiographic finding is not associated with tricuspid insufficiency?

(A) a dilated right atrium
(B) tricuspid prolapse
(C) a dilated right ventricle
(D) a thickened anterior right ventricle wall

108. A tricuspid regurgitant velocity of 4 m/s indicates the presence of

(A) tricuspid stenosis
(B) severe tricuspid regurgitation
(C) a flail tricuspid leaflet
(D) pulmonary hypertension

109. Which of the following regarding tricuspid stenosis is *not* true?

(A) it occurs as a sequela to rheumatic fever
(B) Doppler echocardiography demonstrates a decreased pressure half-time
(C) two-dimensional echocardiography shows diastolic doming, and M-mode reveals a decreased E–F slope
(D) it is usually seen as part of the aging process

110. A peripheral contrast injection into the arm of a patient with severe tricuspid regurgitation is likely to demonstrate

(A) contrast in the pulmonary veins during diastole
(B) right-to-left shunting
(C) contrast in the inferior vena cava during ventricular systole
(D) left-to-right shunting

111. If the physician suspects carcinoid heart disease, the echocardiographer should pay special attention to the

(A) mitral valve
(B) tricuspid valve
(C) inferior vena cava
(D) interatrial septum

112. The velocity of a tricuspid regurgitant jet can be used to calculate

(A) the severity of tricuspid regurgitation
(B) right ventricular systolic pressure
(C) the severity of pulmonic regurgitation
(D) left atrial pressure

113. Coarse systolic fluttering of the pulmonic valve with an extremely high systolic velocity in the right ventricular outflow tract is most likely to be found in a patient with

(A) pulmonic regurgitation
(B) paradoxical interventricular septal motion
(C) infundibular pulmonic stenosis
(D) pulmonary hypertension

114. The most common window used to record peak pulmonic systolic velocity is

(A) suprasternal
(B) apical
(C) right parasternal
(D) left parasternal

115. The pulmonic valve is located where in relation to the aortic valve?

(A) cranial and lateral
(B) caudal and lateral
(C) cranial and medial
(D) caudal and medial

116. All of the following echocardiographic findings are associated with pulmonic stenosis except

(A) right ventricular hypertrophy
(B) M-mode demonstration of a steep pulmonic A wave
(C) midsystolic notching noted on M-mode
(D) systolic pulmonic Doppler velocities greater than 3 m/s

117. Valvular vegetations are best detected with

(A) M-mode echocardiography
(B) two-dimensional echocardiography
(C) Doppler echocardiography
(D) contrast injection

118. A 30-year-old intravenous drug abuser presents with an embolus to the right leg. The most likely cause of the embolic event is the presence of

(A) a left atrial myxoma
(B) mitral valve vegetation
(C) a right ventricular thrombus
(D) a myocardial abscess

119. Color Doppler assessment of prosthetic heart valves is especially helpful when checking for the

(A) presence of valve stenosis
(B) presence of paravalvular regurgitation
(C) presence of a clot
(D) valve area

120. A normally functioning Starr–Edwards valve

(A) may exhibit high Doppler velocities
(B) will echocardiographically resemble a bioprosthetic valve
(C) has a major and a minor orifice
(D) may exhibit mild-to-moderate regurgitation

121. A Bjork–Shiley is

(A) an example of a mechanical heart valve
(B) an example of a bioprosthetic heart valve
(C) not noticeable on the two-dimensional image
(D) a surgical procedure used to correct for transposition of the great vessels

122. Which of the following echocardiographic examinations is best used for evaluating the function of a prosthetic valve?

(A) M-mode echocardiography
(B) high-pulse repetition-frequency Doppler echocardiography
(C) transesophageal echocardiography
(D) contrast echocardiography

123. All of the following are examples of mechanical prosthetic valves *except*

(A) St. Jude
(B) Bjork–Shiley
(C) Starr–Edwards
(D) Hancock

124. To check for prosthetic valve dehiscence, the echocardiographer should look for

(A) decreased valve excursion
(B) an abnormal mass of echoes on the valve
(C) abnormal rocking motion of the valve
(D) Doppler evidence of stenosis

125. A 26-year-old woman with significant mitral insufficiency is about to receive a mitral valve replacement. The surgeons are most likely to use a porcine valve because

(A) it tends to last longer
(B) it preserves myocardium better
(C) it often makes anticoagulation unnecessary
(D) it obstructs flow less

126. Prophylactic antibiotics are often recommended for individuals with mitral valve prolapse who are undergoing dental or surgical procedures

(A) because these patients are at a higher risk for endocarditis
(B) to prevent possible mitral regurgitation
(C) to prevent pneumonia
(D) because incisions on patients with mitral valve prolapse usually take longer to heal

127. One can be reasonably certain that a large amount of pericardial effusion is present by noting

(A) echocardiographic signs of cardiac tamponade
(B) a crescent-shaped pattern on the short-axis view
(C) a "swinging heart" on the two-dimensional examination
(D) a posterior echo-free space

128. Constrictive pericarditis

(A) impairs diastolic filling
(B) is sometimes referred to as "Dressler's syndrome"
(C) is detected by noting increased echogenicity of the pericardium
(D) is usually associated with a large pericardial effusion

129. Cardiac tamponade is most likely to occur when

(A) pressure in the pericardial cavity rises to equal or exceed the diastolic pressure in the heart
(B) there is a small pericardial effusion
(C) there is a large chronic pericardial effusion
(D) the pericardium becomes a sheath of fibrous tissue that interferes with diastolic filling

130. Which one of the following statements about pericardial effusion is false?

(A) pericardial effusion may be confused with epicardial fat
(B) an effusion may accumulate anteriorly without accumulating posteriorly
(C) a pericardial effusion can consist of blood or clear fluid
(D) in Dressler's syndrome, a pericardial effusion develops as a result of renal disease

131. A 38-year-old woman with a history of breast cancer is referred for an echocardiogram because she is experiencing shortness of breath. The echocardiogram is most likely to reveal

(A) metastasis to the left atrium
(B) metastasis to the right atrium

(C) a left atrial myxoma

(D) a pericardial effusion

132. All of the following can lead to a false-positive diagnosis of pericardial effusion on M-mode except

(A) the descending aorta
(B) a calcified mitral annulus
(C) ascites
(D) mitral valve prolapse

133. A false-negative sign of tamponade may occur in patients with

(A) pulmonic stenosis
(B) a pleural effusion
(C) mitral regurgitation
(D) loculated effusions

134. The pericardium appears as an extremely bright linear structure on the echocardiogram because

(A) it is a thick structure
(B) it is a fibrous band
(C) there is a large acoustic mismatch between lung tissue and pericardial tissue
(D) it contains calcium

135. Two echocardiographic techniques that are useful when evaluating for the presence of pericardial effusion are

(A) increasing reject and decreasing frame-rate
(B) decreasing time-gain control and increasing overall gain
(C) decreasing overall gain and increasing depth setting
(D) increasing reject and decreasing depth setting

136. The structure that often aids in differentiating a pericardial effusion from a pleural effusion on two-dimensional examination is the

(A) liver
(B) inferior vena cava
(C) pleural sac
(D) descending aorta

137. Flat mid-diastolic motion of the posterior wall on an M-mode echocardiogram suggests

(A) constrictive pericarditis
(B) left ventricular volume overload
(C) myocardial infarction
(D) dilated cardiomyopathy

138. The most striking echocardiographic feature of patients with an absent pericardium is

(A) excessive cardiac motion
(B) absence of bright linear pericardial echoes
(C) hypokinesis of the heart
(D) dyskinetic motion of the heart

139. The effect of systemic hypertension on the heart is

(A) thickening of the right ventricular free wall
(B) decreased systolic function of the left ventricle
(C) reduced compliance of the left ventricle
(D) right ventricular dilatation

140. Echocardiographic signs of outflow tract obstruction in hypertrophic cardiomyopathy include all of the following except

(A) midsystolic notching of the aortic valve
(B) left ventricular hypertrophy
(C) systolic anterior motion of the mitral valve
(D) high systolic velocity in the left ventricular outflow tract

141. A definitive diagnosis of amyloid heart disease is best made with

(A) M-mode echocardiography
(B) transthoracic echocardiography
(C) transesophageal echocardiography
(D) endomyocardial biopsy

142. All of the following can cause dilated (congestive) cardiomyopathy except

(A) coronary artery disease
(B) sarcoidosis
(C) viral myocarditis
(D) long-term alcohol abuse

143. All of the following are echocardiographic findings seen in dilated cardiomyopathy except

(A) increased systolic velocity in the left ventricular outflow tract
(B) dilated chambers
(C) global hypokinesis
(D) an increased E point-to-septal separation

144. Cardiac contusion

(A) is more likely to affect the right ventricle than the left ventricle
(B) is the same as a myocardial infarction
(C) occurs when there is underlying coronary artery disease
(D) leads to hypercontractility of the left ventricle

145. A 64-year-old man presents with an acute myocardial infarction of the anterior wall and an embolus to the right leg. Before beginning the examination, the echocardiographer should suspect the possibility of (choose the most likely diagnosis)

(A) an apical aneurysm with a mural thrombus
(B) mitral stenosis and a left atrial clot
(C) a right ventricular infarct with a clot
(D) vegetation on the mitral or aortic valve

146. All of the following echocardiographic findings are consistent with diastolic dysfunction of the left ventricle except

(A) M-mode demonstration of a mitral valve B notch
(B) M-mode demonstration of a high mitral A wave
(C) two-dimensional demonstration of an ejection fraction lower than 50%
(D) Doppler demonstration of a mitral valve E-to-A ratio >1.0

147. Akinesis of the anterior left ventricular wall is most likely to indicate obstruction of the

(A) right coronary artery
(B) left circumflex artery
(C) left anterior descending artery
(D) posterior descending artery

148. Pseudoaneurysms

(A) are usually hyperkinetic
(B) have a low risk of rupture
(C) have walls comprised of endocardium, myocardium, epicardium, and pericardium
(D) have a narrow neck

149. An increased E point-to-septal separation is usually a good indicator of

(A) high end-diastolic pressures in the left ventricle
(B) a reduced ejection fraction
(C) high initial diastolic pressures
(D) poor compliance of the left ventricle

150. A segment of the left ventricle that lacks systolic wall thickening and motion is best described as

(A) hypokinetic
(B) akinetic
(C) dyskinetic
(D) aneurysmal

151. Aneurysms in the inferior wall of the left ventricle may be associated with all of the following except

(A) an increased E point-to-septal separation
(B) thrombus formation
(C) mitral regurgitation
(D) occlusion of the left anterior descending coronary artery

152. The echocardiogram of a patient with a ruptured papillary muscle will exhibit

(A) mitral valve prolapse
(B) severe mitral regurgitation
(C) some degree of aortic insufficiency
(D) dyskinesis of the posterior left ventricular wall

153. Stress echocardiography

(A) is used instead of standard stress testing
(B) studies the acoustic properties of the myocardium
(C) allows for visualization of myocardial perfusion
(D) is used in diagnosing ischemic heart disease

154. Which of the following statements regarding left atrial myxomas is not true?

(A) they usually attach to the interatrial septum
(B) they may be pedunculated
(C) they do not recur once they are surgically removed
(D) clinically, they can mimic mitral stenosis

155. The QP/QS ratio is used to evaluate the severity of

(A) pulmonic stenosis
(B) ventricular septal defects
(C) aortic stenosis
(D) systemic hypertension

156. Which of the following would best describe the pulsed Doppler pattern of a patent ductus arteriosus if the sample volume were placed in the pulmonary artery from a short-axis view of the base of the heart?

(A) systolic flow below baseline
(B) continuous flow (systolic and diastolic) above baseline
(C) diastolic flow above baseline
(D) a biphasic systolic flow pattern below baseline

157. The best way to detect a small atrial septal defect is with

(A) two-dimensional echocardiography
(B) contrast injection echocardiography
(C) M-mode echocardiography
(D) pulsed-wave Doppler echocardiography

158. The most common type of atrial septal defect is

(A) primum
(B) secundum
(C) fenestrated
(D) sinus venosus

159. A ventricular septal defect with right-to-left shunting is consistent with

(A) Ebstein's anomaly
(B) tetralogy of Fallot
(C) Eisenmenger's syndrome
(D) a double-outlet right ventricle

160. Which of the following is not associated with Ebstein's anomaly?

(A) an abnormally large tricuspid valve
(B) infundibular pulmonic stenosis

(C) "atrialization" of the right ventricle

(D) an atrial septal defect

161. The echocardiogram of a patient with an endocardial cushion defect might exhibit

(A) a muscular ventricular septal defect and tricuspid valve vegetation

(B) a hypokinetic left ventricle and mitral valve vegetation

(C) overriding of the aorta and subpulmonic stenosis

(D) ostium primum atrial septal defect and an inlet ventricular septal defect

162. An echocardiographic diagnosis of coarctation of the aorta can be made by detecting a high-velocity Doppler jet in the

(A) left branch of the pulmonary artery

(B) aortic arch, proximal to the subclavian artery

(C) descending thoracic aorta

(D) abdominal aorta

163. The four principal components of tetralogy of Fallot include all of the following except

(A) a ventricular septal defect

(B) an override of the aorta

(C) an obstruction of pulmonary blood flow

(D) an atrial septal defect

164. Cor triatriatum

(A) is a fairly common congenital abnormality

(B) is a congenital malformation in which a fibrous membrane divides the left atrium into an upper and lower chamber

(C) results in mitral stenosis

(D) is a condition in which the pulmonary veins drain into the right atrium

165. The echocardiographic finding most commonly associated with left bundle branch block is

(A) left ventricular hypertrophy

(B) a hypercontractile interventricular septum

(C) paradoxical septal motion

(D) a dilated left ventricle

166. The echocardiographic pattern of the mitral valve in Fig. 3–14 is consistent with

(A) mitral stenosis

(B) mitral valve vegetation

(C) a mechanical prosthetic valve

(D) a calcified mitral valve annulus

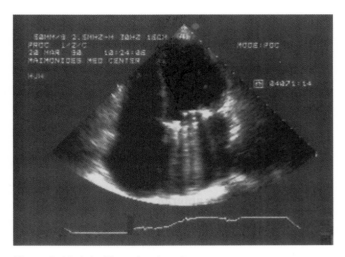

Figure 3–14. Apical four-chamber view.

167. The M-mode pattern in Fig. 3–15 suggests that the ejection fraction of the left ventricle is

(A) normal

(B) mildly increased

(C) significantly increased

(D) significantly decreased

168. What other hemodynamic information could be derived from the M-mode (Fig. 3–15)?

(A) cardiac output is increased

(B) left ventricular end-diastolic pressure is increased

(C) the systolic ejection period is prolonged

(D) atrial flutter is present

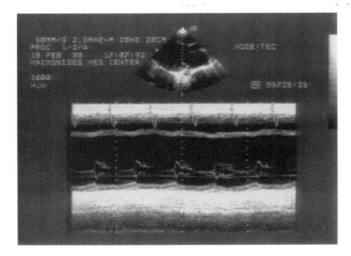

Figure 3–15. M-mode echocardiogram at the level of the mitral valve.

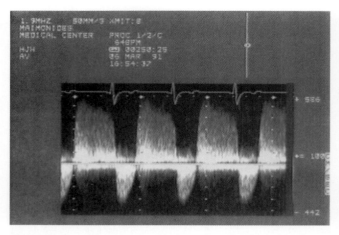

Figure 3–16. Continuous-wave Doppler tracing obtained from the apical position.

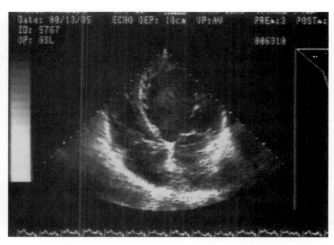

Figure 3–18. Apical four-chamber view showing a dilated left ventricle.

169. The Doppler tracing in Fig. 3–16 demonstrates

(A) aortic stenosis and aortic insufficiency
(B) mitral stenosis and mitral regurgitation
(C) tricuspid stenosis and tricuspid regurgitation
(D) mitral stenosis and aortic stenosis

170. The echocardiographic findings in Fig. 3–17 indicate that the patient probably has a history of

(A) hypertension
(B) diabetes mellitus
(C) rheumatic fever
(D) coronary artery disease

171. The arrow in Fig. 3–17 is pointing to

(A) a side-lobe artifact
(B) papillary muscle
(C) chordae tendineae
(D) the anterior mitral leaflet

172. Fig. 3–18 demonstrates echoes within the left ventricular cavity. These echoes are

(A) artifactual
(B) caused by a mural thrombus
(C) caused by stagnant blood
(D) caused by a high near-gain setting

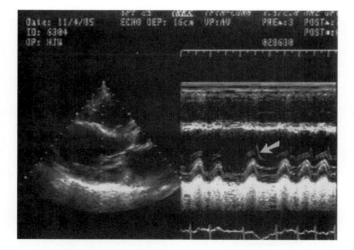

Figure 3–17. Split-screen display of a two-dimensional long-axis (left) and a correlating M-mode pattern (right). Note M-mode scan plane indicated by cursor (arrow).

Questions 173 through 179: Match the numbered structures in Fig. 3–19 with the correct term given in Column B.

COLUMN A	COLUMN B
173. _____	left ventricle
174. _____	coronary sinus
175. _____	left atrium
176. _____	right ventricle
177. _____	pericardial effusion
178. _____	descending aorta
179. _____	pleural effusion
	aortic root
	right atrium

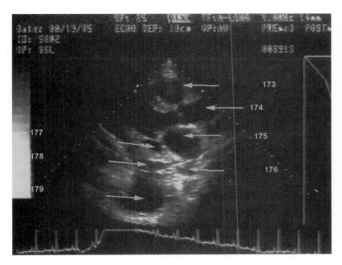

Figure 3–19. Parasternal long-axis view with an increased depth setting.

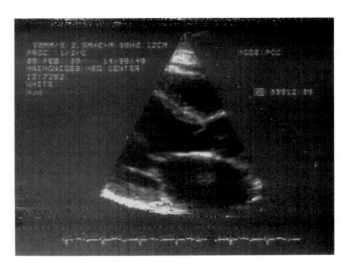

Figure 3–21. Narrow sector parasternal long-axis view.

180. Fig. 3–20 demonstrates

    (A) a large pleural effusion
    (B) pneumomediastinum
    (C) ascites
    (D) a large pericardial effusion

181. The echocardiographic examination of this patient should include analysis of the motion of the

    (A) interventricular septum
    (B) right ventricular wall
    (C) left ventricular wall
    (D) tricuspid valve

182. Color Doppler interrogation of the aortic valve shown in Fig. 3–21 is most likely to demonstrate

    (A) a narrow diastolic jet directed at the anterior mitral leaflet

    (B) a diastolic jet filling the left ventricular outflow tract and extending deep into the left ventricle
    (C) a normal pattern of blood flow
    (D) a narrow systolic jet directed at the anterior mitral leaflet

183. The arrow in Fig. 3–22 is pointing to

    (A) a fistula between the aorta and right ventricle
    (B) the coronary sinus
    (C) the left main coronary artery
    (D) the origin of the right coronary artery

184. The right ventricular outflow tract is located medial to the arrow in Fig. 3–22.

    (A) true
    (B) false

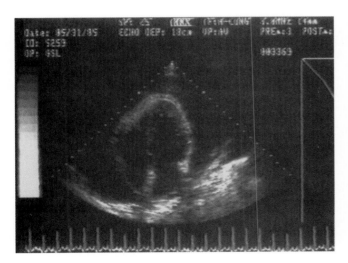

Figure 3–20. Apical four-chamber view.

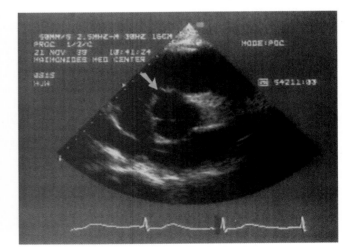

Figure 3–22. Short-axis view of the base of the heart.

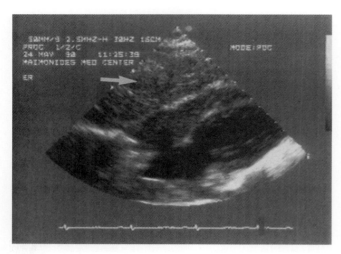

Figure 3–23. Subcostal four-chamber view with contrast injection.

185. The contrast study in Fig. 3–23 shows

(A) left-to-right shunting at the atrial level
(B) no shunting of blood
(C) right-to-left shunting at the atrial level
(D) right-to-left shunting at the ventricular level

186. A secondary finding noted on Fig. 3–23 is a moderate-sized pericardial effusion.

(A) true
(B) false

187. The arrow in Fig. 3–23 is pointing to

(A) lung tissue
(B) liver parenchyma
(C) a mediastinal tumor
(D) the spleen

188. The absence of an A wave and midsystolic notching of the pulmonic valve on the M-Mode in Fig. 3–24 is consistent with

(A) pulmonic stenosis
(B) tricuspid stenosis
(C) mitral stenosis
(D) pulmonary hypertension

189. What other abnormality should be ruled out in the presence of the abnormality noted on the M-mode of the tricuspid valve in Fig. 3–25?

(A) tricuspid stenosis
(B) pulmonary hypertension
(C) mitral valve prolapse
(D) atrial septal defect

190. An 85-year-old woman with a long history of chest pain is sent for an echocardiogram. The M-mode of the mitral valve is shown in Fig. 3–26. The M-mode of the aortic valve would be likely to demonstrate

(A) diastolic fluttering
(B) delayed opening
(C) midsystolic notching
(D) systolic fluttering

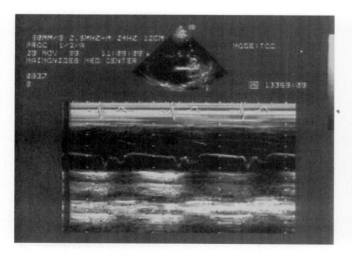

Figure 3–24. M-mode of the pulmonic valve.

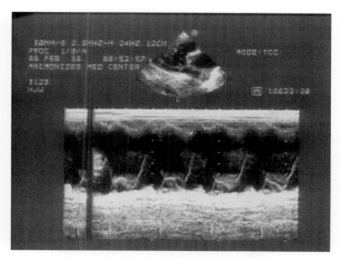

Figure 3–25. M-mode of the tricuspid valve.

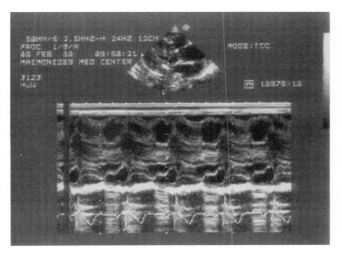

Figure 3–26. M-mode echocardiogram at the level of the mitral valve.

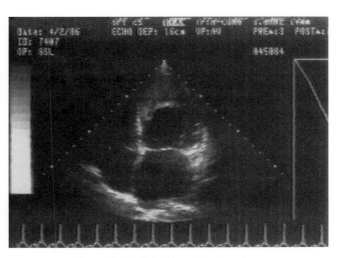

Figure 3–28. Apical four-chamber view.

191. An extremely tall slender young man was referred for an echocardiogram because he has a murmur. Echocardiographic findings in Fig. 3–27 include

   (A) a biscupid aortic valve
   (B) a cleft mitral valve
   (C) a dilated aortic root
   (D) left ventricular hypertrophy

192. Which echocardiographic view would be best for further evaluation of this abnormality?

   (A) the long-axis suprasternal view
   (B) the short-axis view of the base of the heart
   (C) the apical four-chamber view
   (D) the subcostal four-chamber view

193. The left ventricle in Fig. 3–28 demonstrates

   (A) hypertrophic cardiomyopathy
   (B) an infiltrative tumor
   (C) a large apical thrombus
   (D) a myxoma

194. The mitral valve in Fig. 3–29 is

   (A) normal
   (B) flail
   (C) stenotic
   (D) prolapsing

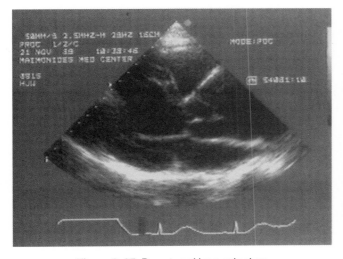

Figure 3–27. Parasternal long-axis view.

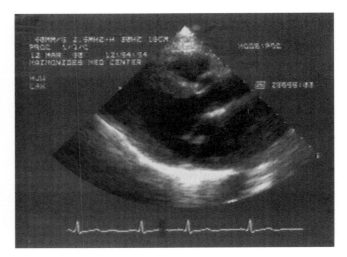

Figure 3–29. Parasternal long-axis view.

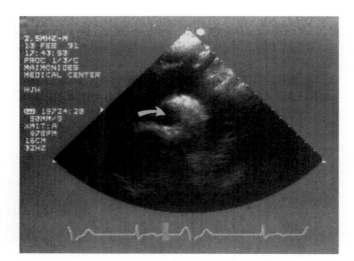

Figure 3–30. Suprasternal notch long-axis view of the aorta and transverse arch.

195. The arrow in Fig. 3–30 is pointing to the

(A) left subclavian artery
(B) right pulmonary artery
(C) superior vena cava
(D) left pulmonary vein

196. Posterior to this structure is an echo-free space. This represents

(A) the left atrium
(B) a pleural effusion
(C) pericardial effusion
(D) the superior vena cava

197. The curved arrow in Fig. 3–31 is directed at

(A) a pacemaker wire
(B) the Chiari network

(C) false chordae tendineae
(D) the moderator band

198. The arrow in Fig. 3–31 is pointing to a structure that most likely represents

(A) a right atrial myxoma
(B) a left atrial thrombus
(C) the left pulmonary vein
(D) the eustachian valve

199. The echocardiographic findings in the long-axis view presented in Fig. 3–32 include

(A) a dilated left atrium, mitral stenosis, and a pericardial effusion
(B) aortic stenosis, a calcified mitral annulus, and basal septal hypertrophy
(C) a dilated coronary sinus, left ventricular hypertrophy, and mitral valve vegetation
(D) a dilated aortic root, a dilated left ventricle, and a thickened mitral valve

200. These findings are most consistent with

(A) rheumatic heart disease
(B) congenital heart disease
(C) subacute bacterial endocarditis
(D) an aged heart

201. The mitral valve diastolic waveforms in Fig. 3–33C are not uniform. This is caused by

(A) high end-diastolic pressure of the left ventricle
(B) faulty technique
(C) inspiration
(D) atrial fibrillation

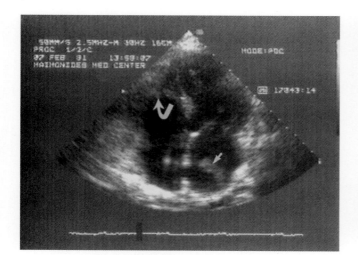

Figure 3–31. Apical four-chamber view.

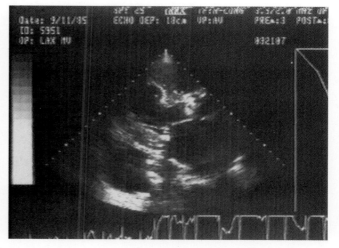

Figure 3–32. Parasternal long-axis view with slightly increased depth setting.

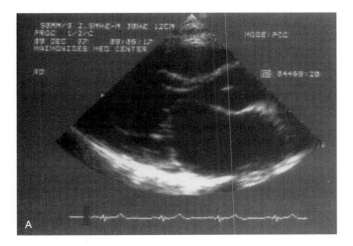

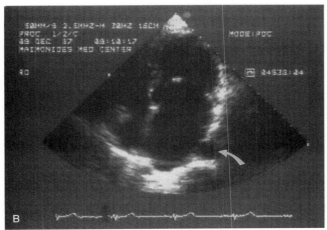

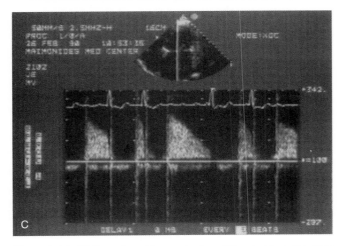

The following study is of a 58-year-old woman who vaguely remembers a childhood illness that included pain in her joints. She was presented with a trans-ischemic attack and atrial fibrillation. For questions 202 through 204, refer to Fig. 3–33A, B, and C.

202. The mitral valve demonstrates

(A) systolic prolapse
(B) diastolic doming
(C) myxomatous degeneration
(D) hyperkinesis

203. Which chamber is significantly dilated?

(A) the left atrium
(B) the left ventricle
(C) the right atrium
(D) the right ventricle

204. Auscultation of this patient is most likely to reveal

(A) a midsystolic click
(B) a systolic ejection murmur
(C) a systolic rumble
(D) an opening snap

205. The arrow in Fig. 3–33B is pointing to the

(A) coronary sinus
(B) inferior vena cava
(C) descending aorta
(D) left pulmonary vein

206. The pressure half-time derived from the Doppler tracing of the mitral valve in Fig. 3–33C can be used to estimate

(A) the mitral valve area
(B) the mitral valve gradient
(C) the severity of aortic insufficiency
(D) the ejection fraction

Figure 3–33. (**A**) Parasternal long-axis view; (**B**) apical four-chamber view; (**C**) continuous-wave Doppler tracing of mitral inflow from the apical position.

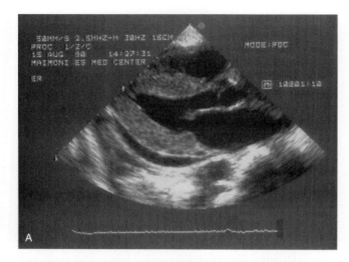

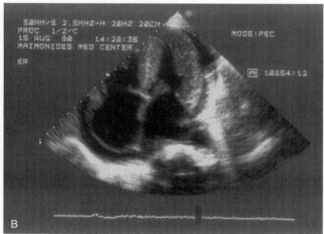

Figure 3–34. (A) Parasternal long-axis view; **(B)** apical four-chamber view.

A 52-year-old woman presents with chronic dyspnea. Chest x-ray reveals cardiomegaly. For questions 207 through 210, refer to Fig. 3–34A and B.

207. The most striking feature of this echocardiogram is

    (A) left atrial compression
    (B) mitral valve doming
    (C) left ventricular hypertrophy
    (D) right ventricular dilatation

208. Additional findings on this echocardiogram include

    (A) a dilated aortic root, mitral valve prolapse, and a dilated coronary sinus
    (B) a thickened mitral valve, a prominent inter-atrial septum, a small left ventricle, and a pericardial effusion

    (C) a calcified mitral annulus, an extracardiac mass, and pleural effusion
    (D) left atrial dilatation, systolic anterior motion of the mitral valve, and a thickened aortic valve

209. Given all the above information, the most likely diagnosis is

    (A) hypertrophic obstructive cardiomyopathy
    (B) Marfan syndrome
    (C) endomyocardial fibrosis
    (D) amyloid cardiomyopathy

210. The best way to substantiate this diagnosis is by obtaining

    (A) a CT scan
    (B) an endomyocardial biopsy
    (C) a cardiac catheterization
    (D) an electrocardiogram

A 64-year-old male sustained a myocardial infarction 1 week before this echocardiogram. He developed congestive heart failure and became hypotensive. A new murmur was detected on auscultation. For questions 211 through 215, refer to Fig. 3–35A and B.

211. The echocardiogram reveals a

    (A) dilated cardiomyopathy
    (B) ventricular septal defect
    (C) cleft mitral valve
    (D) pseudoaneurysm

212. Which of the following would be the most helpful in confirming the diagnosis?

    (A) color-flow Doppler imaging
    (B) M-mode echocardiography
    (C) continuous-wave Doppler imaging
    (D) pulsed-wave Doppler imaging

213. The arrow in Fig. 3–35B is pointing to a linear structure called the

    (A) coronary sinus
    (B) left anterior descending coronary artery
    (C) left pulmonary vein
    (D) left circumflex coronary artery

214. This linear structure contains

    (A) serous fluid
    (B) deoxygenated blood
    (C) oxygenated blood
    (D) air

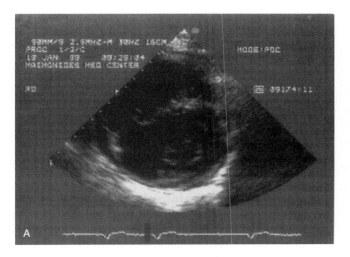

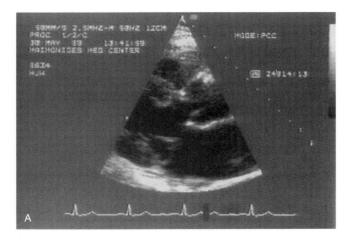

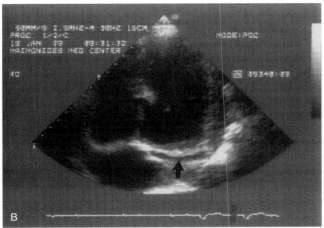

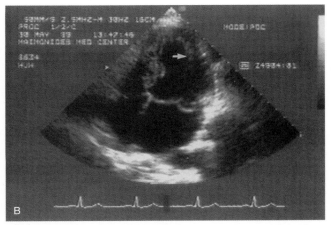

Figure 3–35. (**A**) Parasternal short-axis view at the level of the papillary muscles; (**B**) modified apical four-chamber view: The transducer is angled posteriorly and the depth setting is decreased.

Figure 3–36. (**A**) Narrow sector parasternal long-axis view; (**B**) apical four-chamber view.

215. In Fig. 3–35B, in what direction would the transducer need to be directed to visualize the left ventricular outflow tract?

   (A) anteriorly
   (B) medially
   (C) laterally
   (D) inferiorly

A 34-year-old woman is extremely nervous at the time of the examination. She states that she often experiences chest pain and palpitations. Auscultation reveals a systolic murmur. For questions 216 through 219 refer to Fig. 3–36A and B.

216. The mitral valve demonstrates

   (A) diastolic doming
   (B) prolapse of the anterior leaflet
   (C) prolapse of the posterior leaflet
   (D) systolic anterior motion

217. Continuous-wave Doppler evaluation of the mitral valve from the apical position would most likely demonstrate a

   (A) systolic curve below baseline greater than 3 m/s
   (B) diastolic signal above baseline with a decreased pressure half-time
   (C) systolic curve above baseline less than 3 m/s
   (D) diastolic curve below baseline greater than 3 m/s

218. The arrow in Fig. 3–36B is pointing to the posterior wall of the left ventricle.

   (A) true
   (B) false

219. The dropout of echoes in the interatrial septum in Fig. 3–36B is most likely

   (A) a primum atrial septal defect
   (B) a secundum atrial septal defect
   (C) artifactual
   (D) the result of interatrial septal prolapse

A 23-year-old male was referred for an echocardiogram because a systolic ejection murmur was heard on auscultation. For questions 220 through 223, refer to Fig. 3–37A and B.

220. The M-mode of the aortic valve in Fig. 3–37A demonstrates

(A) slight thickening of the valve with a normal opening
(B) the absence of aortic valve echoes
(C) systolic fluttering of the aortic valve
(D) a thickened aortic valve with a markedly decreased opening

221. According to the Doppler tracing in Fig. 3–37B, the peak aortic gradient using the simplified Bernoulli formula is approximately

(A) 4 mm Hg
(B) 16 mm Hg

(C) 36 mm Hg
(D) 100 mm Hg

222. The most likely diagnosis for this patient is

(A) aortic valve vegetation
(B) congenital aortic stenosis
(C) moderate aortic insufficiency
(D) rheumatic heart disease

223. Two-dimensional examination of the aortic valve is most likely to demonstrate

(A) systolic doming
(B) a mass of echoes in the left ventricular outflow tract
(C) diastolic doming
(D) four aortic cusps

A 38-year-old woman, who recently had extensive dental work performed, presented with fever, chills, and a transischemic attack. Auscultation revealed a grade 2/6 systolic murmur. For questions 224 through 229, refer to Fig. 3–38A, B, and C.

224. The mitral valve is

(A) normal
(B) doming
(C) exhibiting shaggy irregular echoes
(D) flail

225. The most likely diagnosis for this patient is

(A) rheumatic heart disease
(B) subacute bacterial endocarditis
(C) ruptured papillary muscle
(D) mitral valve prolapse

226. The mitral valve excursion is most likely

(A) reduced
(B) increased
(C) normal
(D) absent

227. Apical continuous-wave Doppler examination of the mitral valve is most likely to demonstrate a

(A) systolic waveform below baseline
(B) diastolic waveform below baseline
(C) diastolic waveform above baseline greater than 3 m/s
(D) systolic waveform above baseline

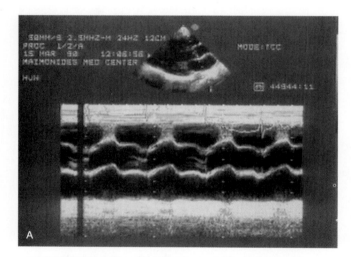

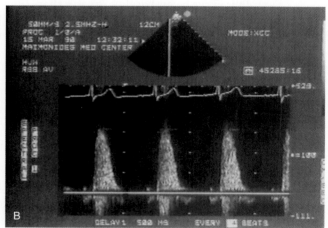

Figure 3–37. (**A**) M-mode tracing at the aortic valve level; (**B**) Continuous-wave Doppler tracing of aortic flow from the right sternal border (calibration marks are 1 m/s).

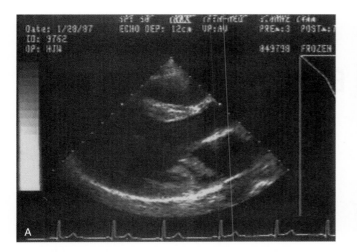

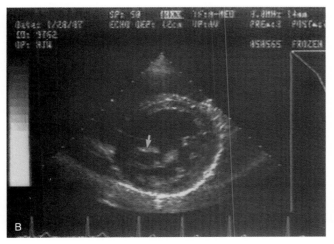

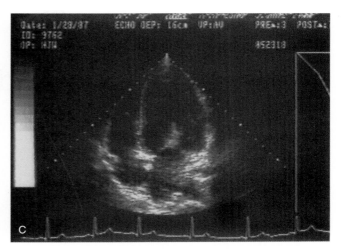

Figure 3–38. (A) Parasternal long-axis view; **(B)** parasternal short-axis view at the papillary muscle level; **(C)** apical four-chamber view.

228. By referring to all three echocardiographic views presented in this case, one could suggest that the mass of echoes on the mitral valve

(A) is stationary
(B) prolapses into the left atrium
(C) prolapses into the left ventricle
(D) prolapses into the left atrium and left ventricle

229. The arrow in Fig. 3–38B points to

(A) a mural thrombus
(B) the posteromedial papillary muscle
(C) vegetation
(D) a cleft mitral valve

Answers and Explanations

At the end of each explained answer there is a number combination in parentheses. The first number identifies the reference source; the second number or set of numbers indicates the page or pages on which the relevant information can be found.

1. **(D)** The coronary or atrioventricular groove separates the atria from the ventricles. Within this groove lies the main trunk of the coronary arteries and the coronary sinus. *(31:13)*

2. **(F)** *(31:378)*

3. **(D)** *(31:378)*

4. **(B)** *(31:378)*

5. **(E)** *(31:378)*

6. **(H)** *(31:378)*

7. **(C)** *(31:378)*

8. **(I)** *(31:378)*

9. **(A)** *(31:378)*

10. **(G)** *(31:378)*

11. **(D)** Indications for stress echocardiography does not include unstable angina. In fact, this is a contraindication for stress echocardiography. *(31:138)*

12. **(C)** Transesophageal echocardiography is performed by a physician with specialized training on TEE performance and interpretation. TEE is routinely used to evaluate cardiac structure and function although it is considered more invasive than a transthoracic or surface echocardiogram. *(31:209)*

13. **(E)** The purposes of the pericardium is to (1) reduce friction with the cardiac movement, (2) allow the heart to move freely with each beat, facilitating ejection and volume changes, (3) contain the heart within the mediastinum, especially during trauma, and (4) serve as a barrier to infection; whereas, the grooves or sulci separate the heart chambers and contain the vessels. *(31:12,13)*

14. **(D)** Left ventricle. In the adult, the left ventricle is larger and has an outer wall which is 8–12 mm thick. *(31:16)*

15. **(D)** There are four pulmonary veins, two from each lung. They carry oxygenated blood from the lungs to the left atrium of the heart. *(31:14)*

16. **(C)** The right atrium has two parts; an anterior portion and a posterior portion. These two portions are separated by a ridge of muscle called the crista terminalis. *(Study Guide: 106)*

17. **(B)** The mitral valve is an atrioventricular valve that is located between the left atrium and the left ventricle. *(31:14,15)*

18. **(B)** The normal pressure in the right ventricle is approximately 15–30 mm Hg. *(Study Guide: 106)*

19. **(D)** Mitral valve stenosis results primarily from rheumatic disease. The valves may not become involved for many decades following rheumatic fever. Other rare causes include; congenital mitral stenosis, calcification of the mitral annulus that involves the mitral leaflets, thrombus, vegetations, atrial myxomas, and parachute mitral valve deformity. *(31:241)*

20. **(C)** Endocarditis. Endocarditis is caused by bacterial, yeast, or fungal infections that seed and grow on the valves of the heart, papillary muscles, and in some cases, the endocardial surface of the ventricles. Vegetations, commonly associated, form as a result of complex interactions between the immune system, the coagulation system, hemodynamic forces, and the invading microorganisms. *(31:477)*

21. **(D)** Bjork–Shiley is a tilting disc valve that is a mechanical prosthetic valve. The xenograft, heterograft, homograft, and allograft are all bioprosthetic heart valves. *(31:310–311)*

22. **(D)** The normal intrapericardial space contains 15–50 mL of fluid. In cases of pericardial effusion as the fluid is added rapidly, the intrapericardial pressure increases dramatically. Initially, pericardial effusion is recognized in the posterior basal region, and as it increases, it occurs medially and laterally and involves the apex. *(31:489)*

23. **(C)** The term cardiomyopathy is used to describe a variety of cardiac diseases that affect the myocardium. Cardiomyopathies affect an otherwise structurally normal heart and are classified into three categories; hypertrophic, dilated, and restrictive. *(31:586)*

24. **(A)** Myxoma is the most common benign tumor of the heart. Almost 75% of all primary tumors are benign, with myxomas accounting for almost half of this group. They can occur in all age groups. *(31:463)*

25. **(D)** Angiosarcomas are the most common malignant cardiac tumors of the heart. Usually occurring in adults and more frequent in men. They are soft tissue tumors of the blood vessels and lymphatic endothelium. *(31:467)*

26. **(D)** A dissecting aneurysm results from intimal tears of the aortic wall. The driving force of the blood destroys the media and strips the intimal layer from the adventitial layer. They are classified as a Type I, II, or III, according to the area and extent of the intimal tear. *(31:606–607)*

27. **(D)** Abnormalities of the left ventricular outflow tact are the most common congenital heart disease in the adult population, with obstruction occurring at the subvalvular, supravalvular or valvular level. *(Study Guide)*

28. **(D)** In adults tetralogy of Fallot is the primary congenital disease producing cyanosis. It comprises four defects; aorta overriding IVS, VSD, infundibular stenosis, and right ventricular hypertrophy. *(31:549)*

29. **(B)** Pericarditis is not a characteristic of cardiomyopathy. Cardiomyopathy is a term describing a variety of cardiac diseases affecting the myocardium. They are classified into three categories according to the characteristics. The categories are hypertrophic, dilated, and restrictive. *(31:586–588)*

30. **(A)** *(31:28)*

31. **(F)** *(31:28)*

32. **(G)** *(31:28)*

33. **(B)** *(31:28)*

34. **(D)** *(31:28)*

35. **(E)** *(31:28)*

36. **(C)** *(31:28)*

37. **(C)** Right atrium. In stenotic disease of the tricuspid valve, the effects on atria, ventricles, and vessels cause dilatation of the right atrium. Tricuspid stenosis is most often caused by rheumatic heart disease but can also be caused by such other conditions as: systemic lupus erythematosus, carcinoid heart disease, Löffler's endocarditis, metastatic melanoma, and congenital heart disease. *(31:295–296.)*

38. **(D)** In tricuspid valve disease the primary cause of regurgitation is secondary to pulmonary hypertension. In rare cases, regurgitation can be caused by rheumatic heart disease. *(31:297)*

39. **(A)** Ebstein's anomaly of the tricuspid valve is a condition where the tricuspid valve leaflets are displaced toward the apex of the right ventricle. *(31:571)*

40. **(B)** Clinical symptoms of aortic valve stenosis include; chest pain, shortness of breath, and syncope. Most patients do not develop these classic symptoms until the degree of aortic stenosis is moderate to severe. *(31:277)*

41. **(D)** The mitral valve has two major leaflets and is the only cardiac valve with this characteristic and, therefore, it is occasionally called the bicuspid valve. *(31:15)*

42. **(D)** The classic clinical finding in mitral valve prolapse is a systolic click, which corresponds with the posterior displacement of the mitral valve leaflet into the left atrium, and a late systolic murmur, which corresponds with the resulting mitral regurgitation that often occurs because of the prolapsing leaflets. *(31:263)*

43. **(A)** The most common cause of flail leaflet is rupture of the chordae tendineae, which often occurs secondary to myocardial infarction. Rupture of the papillary muscle is a less common etiology. The chordae tendineae support the leaflets and prevent them from prolapsing during systole. *(31:19)*

44. **(D)** Transesophageal echocardiography provides complete evaluation of all regions of the heart, including the great vessels. It provides higher resolution because of the transesophageal window, allowing the use of higher-frequency transducers. *(31:92)*

45. **(C)** The coronary sinus is guarded by the thebesius valve. This valve is often continuous with the eustachian valve. *(31:18)*

46. (A) The average length of an adult heart is 12 cm, width 8–9 cm in the broadest diameter, and 6 cm at its narrowest portion. The weight is roughly 280–340 g in males and 230–280 g in females. Cardiac weight is approximately 0.45% of total body weight in men and 0.40% of total body weight in women.

(31:12,13)

47. (D) The AV node and its atrial branches are located in a triangular zone lying between the attachment of the septal leaflet of the tricuspid valve, the antero-medial orifice of the coronary sinus, and the tendon of Todaro. It is referred to as the triangle of Koch.

(31:17)

48. (B) The blood circulates through the body and returns to the heart to be transported to the lungs for reoxygenation. The IVC drains the trunk and lower extremities and the superior vena cava drains the head and parts of the upper extremities. *(31:17)*

49. (C) Subcostal. Standard parasternal and suprasternal views do not demonstrate all four cardiac chambers. Only the apical and subcostal windows allow visualization of all cardiac chambers. *(1:80)*

50. (A) Long axis, short axis, and four chamber. The American Society of Echocardiography has standardized two-dimensional views of the heart into three basic orthogonal planes for which all views can basically be categorized. *(2:212)*

51. (A) Atrial septal defect and ventricular septal defect. If the ultrasound beam is not oriented perpendicular to the interatrial and interventricular septum, there may be false dropout of echoes. The subcostal approach allows the ultrasound beam to be perpendicular to the cardiac chambers, thereby allowing a better demonstration of atrial or ventricular septal defects. In addition, any gap noted in the interatrial or interventricular septum when the subcostal four-chamber view is used should be considered real.

(1:92)

52. (B) Time-gain compensation. The time-gain compensation control allows the echocardiographer to selectively increase or decrease the gain at different depths of tissue. The objective is to achieve a uniform echocardiographic image without artifactually adding or eliminating information. *(3:52)*

53. (A) The right ventricular pressure drops below the right atrial pressure. The atrioventricular valves open when ventricular pressure drops below atrial pressure. *(3:38)*

54. (B) The coronary ligament. This ligament defines the bare area of the liver and is the only choice that does not represent a remnant of fetal circulation.

(4:30)

55. (A) Pulmonary artery. The right side of the heart pumps deoxygenated blood through the pulmonary artery to the lungs for reoxygenation. (The pulmonary artery is the only artery in the body that carries deoxygenated blood.) *(3:9)*

56. (C) Left atrium. Four pulmonary veins transport oxygenated blood from the lungs to the left atrium. (The pulmonary veins are the only veins in the body that carry oxygenated blood.) *(3:9)*

57. (D) The left ventricle constitutes most of the ventral surface of the heart. The right ventricle, although less muscular than the left ventricle, dominates the ventral surface of the heart. *(3:25)*

58. (A) Aortic valve opening and closing points. Left ventricular ejection time—the time it takes for blood to be ejected from the left ventricle—can be obtained from an M-mode tracing of the aortic valve by measuring the time interval between opening and closing of the valve. *(3:156)*

59. (D) Subcostal. Lung expansion in patients with chronic obstructive pulmonary disease often obliterates the apical and parasternal position. This lung expansion also tends to shift the heart inferiorly, making the subcostal view the best approach for scanning the heart. *(5:79)*

60. (B) Apical and right sternal border. The most common windows used to record systolic blood flow across the aortic valve are the apical, right parasternal, and suprasternal. *(6:128)*

61. (A) At end-systole. M-mode measurements of the left atrium, left ventricle, and right ventricle are done at a point when the chambers are at their largest. The left atrium is largest at end-systole. *(3:82)*

62. (C) Stenosis. Doming is a main two-dimensional feature of any stenotic valve. The valve domes when it opens because the commissures are fused, causing the body of the valve to separate more widely than the tips. *(1:251)*

63. (C) Perpendicular, parallel. Because of the differences in transducer orientation for optimum two-dimensional and Doppler studies, one rarely obtains excellent quality images and waveforms simultaneously and may have to relinquish quality in one to obtain excellent-quality images in the others. *(1:104)*

64. (D) Pulmonary hypertension. The constant pressure overload of pulmonary hypertension causes right ventricular hypertrophy until the ventricle fails, at which point the right ventricle wall dilates. *(3:217)*

65. (C) Chordae tendineae. Left ventricular dimensions have been standardized to be obtained at the level of the chordae tendineae. *(7:1072)*

66. (C) Left ventricular volume overload. Right ventricular volume overload may cause paradoxical interventricular septal motion (anterior motion of the interventricular septum at the onset of systole).
(1:164)

67. (A) Toward the right ventricular free wall. Right ventricular volume overload causes paradoxical septal motion, whereby the septum moves toward the right side of the heart in systole rather than toward the left side of the heart.   *(1:164)*

68. (A) Organic in origin. A thrill is a murmur that produces a vibratory sensation when palpated. It is almost always organic in origin.   *(8:51)*

69. (A) Mitral valve prolapse or systolic anterior motion of the mitral valve. The Valsalva maneuver and the inhalation of amyl nitrite decrease left ventricular volume and reduce the diameter of the left ventricular outflow tract, thereby stimulating mitral valve prolapse or systolic anterior motion of the mitral valve.   *(3:222)*

70. (A) Cyanotic heart disease. Clubbing occurs when there is widening and cyanosis of the distal ends of the fingers and toes.   *(9:18)*

71. (B) Providing enhanced temporal resolution. M-mode is still used in many laboratories to take measurements and to evaluate events that occur too rapidly for the eye to perceive, such as diastolic fluttering of the anterior mitral leaflet. This is the case because M-mode provides far better temporal (time) resolution than does two-dimensional echocardiography and allows for better analysis of intracardiac events.
(3:78)

72. (C) To a higher intercostal space. If the transducer is placed too low relative to the position of the heart, the sector plane passes obliquely through the left ventricle, producing an ovoid image.   *(3:110)*

73. (C) Decreased left ventricular compliance. This situation, referred to as reversed E-to-A ratio, indicates decreased left ventricular diastolic compliance. Conditions that cause this include left systemic hypertension, hypertrophic cardiomyopathy, and coronary artery disease.   *(3:240)*

74. (C) A left ventricular thrombus. Left ventricular function is not impaired in mitral stenosis. Because thrombi tend to form in areas of poor blood flow, the likelihood of finding a left ventricular thrombus is low.   *(1:489)*

75. (D) A peak gradient occurring in late diastole. The peak gradient in mitral stenosis usually occurs in early diastole.   *(10:132)*

76. (C) Mitral insufficiency. Ruptured chordae tendineae always result in mitral regurgitation, the onset of which is often abrupt and acute.   *(3:189)*

77. (D) Hypertrophic obstructive cardiomyopathy. This causes anterior motion of the mitral valve. It is not a source of confusion for mitral valve prolapse, in which the mitral valve moves posteriorly in systole.
(11:211)

78. (A) A dilated left atrium. This is a secondary sign of mitral regurgitation. The left ventricle usually dilates as well and becomes hyperkinetic in response to the volume overload.   *(1:266)*

79. (A) Width and length of the systolic jet by color Doppler. Color Doppler provides a spatial display of regurgitant flow. Quantification of the severity of mitral regurgitation is based roughly on the size and configuration of the regurgitant jet.   *(12:87)*

80. (D) Pulmonic stenosis. The pulmonic valve is the valve that is least likely to be deformed by rheumatic fever. When pulmonic stenosis is noted on an echocardiogram, it is usually a congenital abnormality rather than a sequela of rheumatic fever.   *(9:1711)*

81. (A) A dilated left atrium and left ventricular hypertrophy. Mitral stenosis causes the left atrium to dilate, and aortic stenosis leads to left ventricular hypertrophy.   *(3:186,206)*

82. (B) Concurrent atrial fibrillation. Mitral stenosis often leads to atrial fibrillation. The A wave of the mitral valve corresponds to the P wave on the electrocardiogram. Because the P wave is absent in atrial fibrillation, the A wave will be absent as well.   *(11:333)*

83. (B) Hypertrophic cardiomyopathy. Under normal circumstances, the mitral E point, which represents rapid ventricular filling, is higher than the mitral A point, which corresponds to atrial contraction. This relationship between the two points is altered when there is decreased left ventricular compliance (as is the case with hypertrophic cardiomyopathy).
(6:155)

84. (B) Aortic regurgitation. Aortic regurgitation causes a left ventricular volume overload pattern on the echocardiogram (a dilated and hypercontractile left ventricle). Mitral regurgitation usually causes dilatation of both the left atrium and the left ventricle.
(5:231)

85. (C) A decreased E–F slope, a thickened mitral valve, and a mitral distal velocity >1.5 m/s. Both thickening of the mitral valve and a reduced E–F slope must be noted to be sure the pathology is mitral stenosis. Diastolic doming of the mitral valve also is a specific sign of mitral stenosis.   *(1:251)*

86. **(B)** An increased E–F slope on M–mode. One M-mode criterion for mitral stenosis is a decreased E–F slope. *(1:249)*

87. **(C)** Tips of the mitral leaflets. The mitral valve is funnel shaped, with the true orifice at the narrow end. Measurement of the size of the orifice should therefore be done at the tips of the leaflets at the point where the chordae tendineae merge with the body of the valve. *(3:161)*

88. **(C)** A dilated left ventricle. Unless there is concomitant mitral regurgitation, the size of the left ventricle will be normal or smaller than normal. *(13:64)*

89. **(C)** An increase in pressure half-time. A successful mitral valve commissurotomy should lead to a decrease in the pressure half-time. The other findings will usually remain, although the left atrium may decrease slightly in size. *(13:65)*

90. **(B)** Concomitant mitral regurgitation. Pure mitral stenosis leads to a dilated left atrium and a normal or smaller-than-normal left ventricle. Aortic stenosis and hypertrophic cardiomyopathy cause the left ventricular walls to appear thickened. Only concomitant mitral regurgitation will cause left ventricular dilatation as well. *(1:139)*

91. **(A)** Severe acute aortic regurgitation. Severe acute aortic insufficiency can cause an elevated left ventricular diastolic pressure, which, in turn, causes the mitral valve to close early. *(1:295)*

92. **(D)** A ventricular septal defect. Such conditions as systemic hypertension that stress the area of the mitral annulus can lead to premature calcification of the mitral annulus. *(9:1035)*

93. **(B)** 1 cm². Studies by Hatle and co-workers found that a mitral valve with an area of 1 cm² exhibits a Doppler pressure half-time of 220 m/s. *(14:1096)*

94. **(B)** Diastolic fluttering of the anterior mitral leaflet. This is a finding of aortic insufficiency. *(3:210)*

95. **(D)** Systemic hypertension. This produces pressure overload of the left ventricle that, in turn, leads to left ventricular hypertrophy. Choices B and C cause a left ventricular volume overload pattern on the echocardiogram (dilated and hyperkinetic left ventricle). *(15:104)*

96. **(C)** Aortic stenosis. A systolic ejection murmur can be heard with this disorder. *(3:204)*

97. **(C)** It is often seen in conjunction with mitral stenosis. A bicuspid aortic valve is a congenital abnormality in which one of the aortic commissures is fused, leading to the formation of two aortic cusps instead of the usual three. Bicuspid valves tend to become

stenotic in adulthood. Although they are sometimes seen in conjunction with coarctation of the aorta, a bicuspid valve and mitral stenosis have no direct association. *(3:202)*

98. **(B)** Aortic valve area, poor left ventricular function. When aortic stenosis is found in conjunction with a poorly moving left ventricle, standard estimations of the degree of aortic stenosis will be inaccurate. The continuity equation compensates for ventricular hypocontractility, allowing for a more accurate estimate of the aortic valve area. *(3:207, 16:105)*

99. **(B)** The mean pressure gradient. Aortic insufficiency may cause a high initial instantaneous gradient. When there is combined aortic stenosis and insufficiency, the mean pressure gradient is more specific for estimating the severity of aortic stenosis. *(6:137)*

100. **(A)** The apical long-axis view. All Doppler procedures are best performed with the ultrasound beam directed parallel to the flow of blood. Of the choices presented, the apical long-axis view provides the optimum angle to image acquisition. *(1:104)*

101. **(B)** Left ventricular hypertrophy. Aortic stenosis causes pressure overload of the left ventricle. This overload leads to left ventricular hypertrophy. *(11:203)*

102. **(A)** Aortic insufficiency. The anterior mitral leaflet flutters rapidly when hit by an aortic insufficiency jet. These oscillations are best detected by M-mode. Atrial fibrillation causes coarse diastolic fluttering of the anterior mitral leaflet. *(1:294)*

103. **(D)** Consistent with moderate aortic regurgitation. The grading of aortic insufficiency with Doppler echocardiography is similar to the grading method used in cardiac catheterization laboratories. An aortic insufficiency jet that extends from the aortic valve to the tips of the anterior mitral leaflet is consistent with moderate aortic regurgitation. *(17:339)*

104. **(B)** Fine diastolic fluttering and possible flattening of the anterior mitral leaflet. An Austin–Flint murmur represents functional mitral stenosis caused by inhibition of anterior leaflet motion resulting from compression by a strong aortic insufficiency jet. This would appear on M-mode as fine diastolic fluttering of the anterior mitral leaflet with inhibition of opening. *(9:77)*

105. **(D)** The right sternal border view. When obtainable, the right sternal border approach is usually best for acquiring maximum aortic valve velocities. The patient is turned onto his or her right side, and the Doppler probe is directed into the aortic root. *(18:89)*

106. (D) Transesophageal echocardiography. Because of the high-resolution images it provides of the thoracic aorta, transesophageal echocardiography has been highly successful in evaluating patients with suspected aortic dissection. *(19:216)*

107. (D) A thickened anterior right ventricle wall. Thickening of the right ventricular walls is usually caused by right ventricular pressure overload. Tricuspid insufficiency causes right ventricular volume overload. *(1:162)*

108. (D) Pulmonary hypertension. The right ventricular systolic pressure in this ventricle is approximately 74 mm Hg (using the formula $4 V^2 + 10$). Because right ventricular pressures are basically equal to pulmonary artery pressures, the pulmonary artery pressure in this instance is roughly 74 mm Hg, thus indicating the presence of pulmonary hypertension. *(3:161)*

109. (D) It is usually seen as part of the aging process. Tricuspid stenosis is a rare condition that usually occurs as a sequela to rheumatic fever. Its echocardiographic findings are similar to those of mitral stenosis. *(3:198)*

110. (C) Contrast in the inferior vena cava during ventricular systole. With severe tricuspid regurgitation, the regurgitant volume extends all the way back into the right atrium and sometimes into the inferior vena cava as well. By injecting contrast, this regurgitant volume can be "seen" with M-mode or two-dimensional echocardiography. *(1:305)*

111. (B) Tricuspid valve. The echocardiographer should pay special attention to this valve because carcinoid heart disease presents as thickening and rigidity of the tricuspid valve leaflets. Severe tricuspid regurgitation is usually detected with Doppler. *(1:305)*

112. (B) Right ventricular systolic pressure. By using the modified Bernoulli equation and an estimate of jugular venous pressure, systolic pressure in the right ventricle can be determined. *(3:112)*

113. (C) Infundibular pulmonic stenosis. This is caused by hypertrophied muscle bands in the right ventricular outflow tract. Echocardiographically, it can be distinguished from valvular pulmonic stenosis by noting a step-up in Doppler velocities proximal to the pulmonic valve. In addition, the muscular ridge produces turbulence of blood, which hits the pulmonic valve and causes it to flutter. *(1:393)*

114. (D) Left parasternal. Pulmonary artery flow velocities are usually obtained from the left parasternal short-axis view at the level of the aortic root. *(10:80)*

115. (A) Cranial and lateral. This relationship is best appreciated from the short-axis view of the base of the heart. *(3:27)*

116. (C) Midsystolic notching noted on M-mode. Midsystolic notching is a sign of pulmonary hypertension. *(3:388)*

117. (B) Two-dimensional echocardiography. The spatial orientation of two-dimensional echocardiography provides for a better assessment of the size, location, and motion of valvular vegetations. *(3:277)*

118. (B) Mitral valve vegetation. Intravenous drug abusers have an increased incidence of endocarditis because of microorganisms that enter the bloodstream via unsterile needles. Vegetations usually form on the valves of the right side of the heart, but they may settle on left-sided valves as well. One complication of valvular vegetation is an embolic event. *(3:276)*

119. (B) Presence of paravalvular regurgitation. The spatial orientation of color Doppler allows for a quick assessment of blood flow in the region surrounding the prosthetic valve. *(12:141)*

120. (A) May exhibit high Doppler velocities. The normal Doppler velocities across any prosthetic valve will be slightly higher than those of a native valve. A Starr–Edwards, or ball-in-cage valve, tends to exhibit the highest velocities. *(3:349)*

121. (A) An example of a mechanical heart valve. The Bjork–Shiley is a tilting-disc mechanical heart valve. *(3:314)*

122. (C) Transesophageal echocardiography. This is a major application in the evaluation of prosthetic heart valves, particularly in the mitral position. *(3:358)*

123. (D) Hancock. This valve is an example of a heterograft (bioprosthetic) valve. *(3:334)*

124. (C) Abnormal rocking motion of the valve. Valve dehiscence refers to a condition in which the prosthetic valve loosens or separates from the sewing ring and causes an abnormal rocking motion and a paravalvular leak. *(3:346)*

125. (C) It often makes anticoagulation unnecessary. Mechanical valves require constant anticoagulation. Women during childbearing years would, therefore, be more likely to receive a bioprosthetic valve, which would not require anticoagulation. *(20:1392)*

126. (A) Because these patients are at a higher risk for endocarditis. Because bacteremias occur during dental or surgical procedures, prophylactic antibiotics are often administered to susceptible patients (such as mitral valve prolapse patients) in an attempt to prevent bacterial endocarditis. *(20:1151)*

127. (C) A "swinging heart" on the two-dimensional examination. Excessive motion of the heart can sometimes be noted with massive pericardial effusion. *(1:558)*

128. (A) Impairs diastolic filling. The rigid and fibrotic pericardial sac impairs diastolic filling of the cardiac chambers. *(3:268)*

129. (A) Pressure in the pericardial cavity rises to equal or exceed the diastolic pressure in the heart. Tamponade occurs when intrapericardial pressures rise and impair cardiac filling. Although cardiac tamponade is usually seen in association with a large pericardial effusion, a small effusion may cause tamponade if the rate of accumulation of pericardial fluid exceeds the ability of the pericardium to accommodate the increased volume. *(15:213)*

130. (D) In Dressler's syndrome, a pericardial effusion develops as a result of renal disease. Dressler's syndrome, also known as postmyocardial infarction syndrome, is the development of pericardial effusion 2 to 10 weeks after infarction. *(9:1287)*

131. (D) A pericardial effusion. Neoplasms from the thoracic region often lead to pericardial effusion. *(20:1254)*

132. (D) Mitral valve prolapse. The descending aorta, a calcified mitral annulus, and ascites can cause echo-free spaces that may be misleading on an echocardiogram. Although a large effusion in which the heart exhibits excessive motion may lead to false mitral valve prolapse, prolapse will not lead to a false-positive diagnosis of pericardial effusion. *(1:552)*

133. (A) Pulmonic stenosis. Diastolic collapse of the right ventricular walls is a good indicator of tamponade. Pulmonic stenosis, or any other form of right ventricular pressure overload, leads to thickening of the right ventricular walls. A thickened wall is unlikely to collapse in diastole. *(1:565)*

134. (C) There is a large acoustic mismatch between lung tissue and pericardial tissue. A greater mismatch between two structures results in brighter reflected echoes from the interface between them. Because there is an extremely large acoustic mismatch between lung (air) and pericardium (tissue), the interface created by the two will cause a bright echo to appear on the echocardiogram. *(1:2)*

135. (C) Decreasing overall gain and increasing depth setting. Decreasing the gain allows for differentiation between the pericardium and epicardium, and increasing the depth setting helps define the borders of the effusion. *(11:249)*

136. (D) Descending aorta. Because the descending aorta lies posterior to the pericardial effusion and anterior to the pleural effusion, it often aids in differentiating between the two. *(1:554)*

137. (A) Constrictive pericarditis. The pericardium limits cardiac motion. When the pericardium is surgically removed (e.g., in constrictive pericarditis), the heart expands and exhibits excessive motion. *(1:575)*

138. (A) Excessive cardiac motion. Again, because the pericardium limits cardiac motion, the heart exhibits excessive motion when the pericardium is surgically removed. *(1:575)*

139. (C) Reduced compliance of the left ventricle. Systemic hypertension causes pressure overload of the left ventricle. As in all pressure-overload situations (e.g., aortic stenosis), the left ventricle hypertrophies and may become noncompliant, leading to diastolic dysfunction. *(11:273)*

140. (B) Left ventricular hypertrophy. This condition can be present in the absence of an obstruction. *(1:522)*

141. (D) Endomyocardial biopsy. Several echocardiographic signs are suggestive of amyloid heart disease, but a definitive diagnosis can be made only with an endomyocardial biopsy performed in the catheterization laboratory. *(20:1215)*

142. (B) Sarcoidosis. This is an infiltrative process that can lead to restrictive cardiomyopathy. *(11:317)*

143. (A) Increased systolic velocity of the left ventricular outflow tract. Velocities are low because of decreased cardiac output. *(3:230)*

144. (A) Is more likely to affect the right ventricle than the left ventricle. Cardiac contusion may be seen following a blunt trauma to the chest (such as a steering-wheel injury). Because the right ventricle is the most anterior structure of the heart, it is the one most susceptible to injury. *(3:301)*

145. (A) An apical aneurysm with a mural thrombus. Apical aneurysms sometimes develop following an anterior wall myocardial infarction. Because aneurysms are a likely site for thrombus, choice A is the most likely answer. *(1:489)*

146. (C) Two-dimensional demonstration of an ejection fraction lower than 50%. The ejection fraction is a measure of systolic left ventricular function. *(20:51)*

147. (C) Left anterior descending artery. This artery supplies the anterior wall of the left ventricle and the anterior portion of the interventricular septum.

(3:237)

148. **(D)** Have a narrow neck. The best way to differentiate a true aneurysm from a pseudoaneurysm is to look at the width of its neck. Pseudoaneurysms tend to have a narrow neck because they result from a tear in the myocardium. *(1:486)*

149. **(B)** A reduced ejection fraction. An E point-to-septal separation of more than 10 mm correlates with a reduced ejection fraction. *(11:205)*

150. **(B)** Akinetic. Lack of systolic thickening and motion is referred to as akinesis. *(11:287)*

151. **(D)** Occlusion of the left anterior descending coronary artery. Blood to the inferior wall of the left ventricle is usually supplied by the right coronary artery. *(1:467, 21:93)*

152. **(B)** Severe mitral regurgitation. Doppler interrogation of a patient with ruptured papillary muscle will usually demonstrate this condition. *(3:249)*

153. **(D)** Is used in diagnosing ischemic heart disease. Stress echocardiography is used as an adjunct to standard stress testing in diagnosing patients with suspected coronary artery disease. Resting wall motion is compared to wall motion during and after stress. *(3:250)*

154. **(C)** They do not recur once they are surgically removed. Although characterized as a benign tumor, a myxoma may recur if some cells remain after excision of the tumor. *(20:1285)*

155. **(B)** Ventricular septal defects. The QP/QS ratio refers to the ratio of pulmonary-to-systemic blood flow. It can be calculated echocardiographically to determine the magnitude of left-to-right shunting of blood. *(6:161)*

156. **(B)** Continuous flow (systolic and diastolic) above baseline. Shunting of blood from the aorta to the pulmonary artery occurs in both systole and diastole. *(18:220)*

157. **(B)** Contrast injection echocardiography. Even a small atrial septal defect can be detected by noting the presence or absence of microbubbles. *(1:406)*

158. **(B)** Secundum. Atrial septal defects occur most commonly in the area of the foramen ovale, where they are termed ostium secundum defects. *(3:381)*

159. **(C)** Eisenmenger's syndrome. In this syndrome, the pulmonary vascular resistance is equal to or greater than the systemic vascular resistance, leading to right-to-left shunting. *(20:589)*

160. **(B)** Infundibular pulmonic stenosis. In Ebstein's anomaly, the tricuspid valve is large and partially adherent to the walls of the right ventricle so that the valve orifice is displaced apically. Therefore, most of the right ventricle functions as part of the right atrium. It is frequently associated with an atrial septal defect. Infundibular pulmonic stenosis is not part of the spectrum of this disorder. *(3:406)*

161. **(D)** Ostium primum atrial septal defect and an inlet ventricular septal defect. Endocardial cushion defects occur when the atrial and ventricular components of the cardiac septum fail to develop properly. *(3:381)*

162. **(C)** Descending thoracic aorta. Coarctation of the aorta is a constrictive malformation of the aortic arch, usually located just distal to the origin of the left subclavian artery. The obstruction increases the velocity of blood flow beyond the point of constriction. *(3:396)*

163. **(D)** An atrial septal defect. The fourth component is right ventricular hypertrophy. *(3:421)*

164. **(B)** Is a congenital malformation in which a fibrous membrane divides the left atrium into an upper and lower chamber. Cor triatriatum is a rare abnormality in which an embryonic membrane in the left atrium fails to regress. It can be detected echocardiographically by noting a linear echo traversing the left atrium. Doppler echocardiography will detect high-velocity flow across a hole in the membrane. *(3:402)*

165. **(C)** Paradoxical septal motion. Left bundle branch block often causes this motion. *(1:231)*

166. **(C)** A mechanical prosthetic valve. This high echogenicity of the mitral valve is characteristic of a mechanical prosthetic valve. *(3:347)*

167. **(D)** Significantly decreased. The M-mode demonstrates a dilated and hypokinetic left ventricle. The markedly increased E point-to-septal separation is consistent with a decreased left ventricular ejection fraction. *(23:140)*

168. **(B)** Left ventricular end-diastolic pressure is increased. There is a mitral valve B notch, which is consistent with high end-diastolic pressure in the left ventricle. *(24:69)*

169. **(A)** Aortic stenosis and aortic insufficiency. The systolic waveform below baseline is consistent with moderate aortic stenosis. A mitral regurgitation waveform would be wider and is usually of higher velocity. The diastolic waveform above baseline is too high a velocity to be caused by mitral or tricuspid stenosis and is consistent with aortic insufficiency.   *(6:78)*

170. **(D)** Coronary artery disease. The interventricular septum is hypokinetic and more echogenic than the posterior left ventricular wall. These findings are consistent with an old myocardial infarction. *(1:478)*

171. **(C)** Chordae tendineae. The M-mode cursor in this long-axis view is directed beyond the tips of the mitral leaflets at the level of the chordae tendineae—the level at which left ventricular measurements are obtained.   *(11:12)*

172. **(C)** Caused by stagnant blood. The cloud of fuzzy smokelike echoes in the left ventricle is the result of blood stasis. It is usually seen when there is a severe decrease in left ventricular contractibility.   *(1:492)*

173–179. If you are having a difficult time orienting yourself to an echocardiographic image, find a structure that is easy for you to recognize and work your way from there. For example, if you can identify the aortic root, you can then follow the anterior wall of the root as it continues into the interventricular septum. The posterior wall of the root will follow into the anterior mitral leaflet, and so on. **173.** Right ventricle. **174.** Aortic root. **175.** Left atrium. **176.** Descending aorta. **177.** Left ventricle. **178.** Pericardial effusion. **179.** Pleural effusion.   *(1:558)*

180. **(D)** A large pericardial effusion. A massive circumferential pericardial effusion is demonstrated in this four-chamber view.   *(11:253)*

181. **(B)** Right ventricular wall. The presence of tamponade should be ruled out in patients with pericardial effusion, especially a massive one. A fairly specific echocardiographic sign of tamponade is diastolic collapse of the right ventricle, the right atrium, or both.   *(25:561)*

182. **(B)** A diastolic jet filling the left ventricular outflow tract and extending deep into the left ventricle. This long-axis view demonstrates a flail right coronary cusp of the aortic valve. The cusp is seen extending into the left ventricular outflow tract in diastole. Color Doppler would be likely to demonstrate severe aortic insufficiency, which choice B describes.   *(12:100)*

183. **(D)** The origin of the right coronary artery. With slight superior angulation from a standard short-axis view of the aortic valve, the ostia and proximal segments of the right coronary artery can be visualized.   *(11:23)*

184. **(B)** False. The right ventricular outflow tract is located lateral to the origin of the right coronary artery.   *(1:102)*

185. **(A)** Left-to-right shunting at the atrial level. There is a washout effect in the right atrium as blood from the left side of the heart enters the contrast-filled right atrium.   *(11:355)*

186. **(B)** False. A pericardial effusion would appear on a subcostal four-chamber view as an echo-free space anterior to the right ventricle.   *(11:251)*

187. **(B)** Liver parenchyma. To obtain a subcostal four-chamber view, the transducer is placed on the abdomen and angled in a cephalic direction. Therefore, liver parenchyma will occupy the near field of the image.   *(3:129)*

188. **(D)** Pulmonary hypertension. An absent A wave and midsystolic notching (flying W sign) are consistent with this condition.   *(3:388)*

189. **(C)** Mitral valve prolapse. The M-mode in Fig. 3–25 demonstrates late-systolic tricuspid valve prolapse. Tricuspid valve prolapse almost always occurs in patients with concomitant mitral valve prolapse.   *(1:305)*

190. **(C)** Midsystolic notching. Fig. 3–26 is an example of systolic anterior motion of the mitral valve. This is one classic echocardiographic sign of hypertrophic obstructive cardiomyopathy. The midsystolic obstruction of the left ventricular outflow tract will often be demonstrated on the M-mode of the aortic valve as well as by midsystolic notching.   *(26:6)*

191. **(C)** A dilated aortic root. This patient exhibits characteristic findings of Marfan syndrome, a connective tissue disorder. There is a linear echo near the aortic valve suggesting aortic root dissection, another complication of Marfan syndrome. This syndrome often causes ascending aortic dilatation as well as myxomatous degeneration of the aortic and mitral valves.   *(11:242)*

192. **(A)** The long-axis suprasternal view. Because the aortic root is dilated, echocardiographic evaluation should follow the length of the aorta to determine the extent of the aneurysm. The suprasternal long-axis view allows for visualization of the aortic arch and the proximal portion of the descending aorta. Further investigation should include a modified apical two-chamber view for evaluating the thoracic aorta and a subcostal approach for interrogating the abdominal aorta.   *(3:121, 137)*

193. **(C)** A large apical thrombus. This thrombus is seen filling the apex, with a piece of the medial segment protruding into the left ventricle. Most thrombi are associated with anterior infarctions and are located in the apex in the majority of cases. *(1:489)*

194. (B) Flail. The tip of the posterior leaflet can be seen protruding into the left atrium, which is consistent with a flail mitral valve. *(27:1383)*

195. (B) Right pulmonary artery. The artery is seen in its short axis. *(11:36)*

196. (A) The left atrium. This atrium can sometimes be visualized posterior to the right pulmonary artery on the suprasternal long-axis view. *(11:36)*

197. (D) The moderator band. This is a muscular strip located in the apical third of the right ventricle. It is sometimes misdiagnosed as a right ventricular apical thrombus. *(3:117, 294)*

198. (B) A left atrial thrombus. This is seen protruding into the left atrium. (The bright linear echo in the right atrium originates from a pacemaker wire.) *(1:592)*

199. (B) Aortic stenosis, a calcified mitral annulus, and a pericardial effusion. The aortic valve is markedly calcified; there is a bright echo posterior to the mitral valve, representing a calcified mitral annulus; and the base of the interventricular septum is hypertrophied. The posterior echo-free space represents pleural effusion, as opposed to a pericardial effusion, because it does not taper at the descending aorta. *(1:345, 283)*

200. (D) An aged heart. When seen together, these findings usually indicate signs of aging. *(9:1658)*

201. (D) Atrial fibrillation. The electrocardiogram at the top of the Doppler tracing indicates this fibrillation. The variations from beat to beat reflect the altering lengths in diastolic filling periods that occur with atrial fibrillation. *(11:333)*

202. (B) Diastolic doming. The mitral valve is bulging into the left ventricle in diastole because the valve is stenotic and cannot accommodate all the blood available for delivery into the left ventricle. *(1:251)*

203. (A) The left atrium. Even without using the centimeter markers as a gauge, one can determine that the left atrium is dilated. On the long axis-view, the aortic root and left aorta should be approximately the same size. The apical four-chamber view is extremely useful for assessing relative chamber size. The right and left atria should be roughly the same size (although the left atrium is usually slightly larger), and they should be smaller than the ventricles. *(11:368)*

204. (D) An opening snap. The opening snap often affords the first clue to the diagnosis of mitral stenosis. *(20:185)*

205. (C) Descending aorta. A portion of the aorta can be seen lying behind the left atrium on the apical four-chamber view. *(1:98)*

206. (A) The mitral valve area. The pressure half-time, or the time it takes for the initial pressure drop of the mitral valve to be halved, can be used to measure mitral valve area. A pressure half-time of 220 ms has been shown to correlate with a valve area of 1.0 cm². *(18:117)*

207. (C) Left ventricular hypertrophy. The left ventricular walls are thickened and exhibit increased echogenicity. *(28:188)*

208. (B) A thickened mitral valve, a prominent interatrial septum, a small left ventricle, and pericardial effusion. The mitral valve and interatrial septum are slightly thickened, there is a small-to-moderate-sized pericardial effusion, and the left ventricle is small. *(1:535)*

209. (D) Amyloid cardiomyopathy. This patient exhibits classic features of this disease. The infiltrative process of the disease causes thickening of the ventricles, interatrial septum and valves. Pericardial effusion is another finding sometimes associated with this disease. *(3:232)*

210. (B) An endomyocardial biopsy. This has been shown to be helpful in identifying amyloid cardiomyopathy. *(3:232)*

211. (B) Ventricular septal defect. The short-axis and modified four-chamber views demonstrate a gap in the posterior aspect of the midsection of the interventricular septum. Given the patient's history and the irregular borders on the echocardiogram, one can assume that this defect is acquired rather than congenital. *(29:506)*

212. (A) Color-flow Doppler imaging. This is particularly useful for quickly determining the location and quantifying the extent of abnormal blood flow in patients with ventricular septal defects. *(3:243)*

213. (A) Coronary sinus. When imaged from the apical two-chamber view, the coronary sinus appears as a circular structure in the atrioventricular groove. By rotating to a four-chamber view and angling posteriorly, one can follow the coronary sinus as it courses along the length of the posterior atrioventricular groove. *(20:29)*

214. (B) Deoxygenated blood. The coronary sinus carries venous blood to the right atrium.   *(30:211)*

215. (A) Anteriorly. By tilting the scan plane anteriorly from this posteriorly directed apical four-chamber view, the aorta and left ventricular outflow tract can be imaged.   *(3:131)*

216. (C) Prolapse of the posterior leaflet. The posterior mitral leaflet bulges beyond the plane of the mitral annulus, which is consistent with prolapse. *(3:189)*

217. (A) A systolic curve below baseline greater than 3 m/s. Mitral valve prolapse, especially to the degree shown in this study, is most likely to be accompanied by some degree of mitral regurgitation, which is detected from the apical window with Doppler echocardiography by noting a systolic curve below baseline usually greater than 3 m/s.   *(6:74)*

218. (B) False. The arrow is pointing to the lateral wall of the left ventricle.   *(11:25)*

219. (C) Artifactual. A dropout of echoes in the interatrial septum is not an uncommon finding when visualized from the apical four-chamber view. If this were a true atrial septal defect, a "T sign" would likely be noted.   *(1:404)*

220. (A) Slight thickening of the valve with a normal opening. This thickening is noted best in diastole. The leaflets appear to open widely in systole. (They open in close proximity to the walls of the aortic root.)   *(1:279)*

221. (C) 36 mm Hg. Using the simplified Bernoulli equation, the peak aortic gradient can be obtained by squaring the peak velocity (in this case 3 m/s) and then multiplying by 4.   *(18:23)*

222. (B) Congenital aortic stenosis. In this disorder, the valve may be thin or minimally thickened, and M-mode may demonstrate a normal opening if the cursor was directed at the body of the leaflets rather than at the restricted tips. The best way to determine if congenital aortic stenosis is present is by noting Doppler evidence of increased velocities across the valve.   *(1:384)*

223. (A) Systolic doming. This occurs in congenital aortic stenosis because the body of the leaflets expands to accommodate systolic flow while the tips of the leaflets restrict blood flow. (Normally, the tips of the aortic valve open wide and lie parallel to the aortic root in systole.)   *(1:383)*

224. (C) Exhibiting shaggy irregular echoes. The mitral valve has a mass of shaggy echoes with irregular borders attached to it.   *(3:277)*

225. (B) Subacute bacterial endocarditis. Because of the patient's history and the echocardiographic demonstration of an irregular mass attached to the mitral valve, this is the most likely diagnosis.   *(20:1141)*

226. (B) Increased. Unlike calcium, which tends to inhibit valve opening, vegetations are likely to increase valve excursion. Because calcium and vegetations can look similar echocardiographically this difference can aid in the diagnosis.   *(3:277)*

227. (A) Systolic waveform below baseline. A mitral valve vegetation will usually cause the mitral valve to be regurgitant. Mitral regurgitation can be detected by continuous-wave Doppler from the apical four-chamber view by noting systolic flow below baseline.   *(6:74)*

228. (D) Prolapses into the left atrium and left ventricle. In Fig. 3–38A, the mass is in the left atrium. In Fig. 3–38B and C, the mass appears in the left ventricle. Therefore, one could deduce that the mass is prolapsing into the left atrium in systole and into the left ventricle in diastole.   *(1:312)*

229. (B) The posteromedial papillary muscle. On the opposite wall of the left ventricle, one can see the anterolateral papillary muscle. Between the two papillary muscles, the tip of the mitral valve vegetation can be seen protruding into the left ventricle.   *(3:113)*

REFERENCES

1. Feigenbaum H. *Echocardiography.* 4th ed. Philadelphia: Lea & Febiger; 1986.
2. Henry WL, DeMaria A, Gramik R. *Nomenclature and Standardization in Two-Dimensional Echocardiography.* Raleigh, NC: American Society of Echocardiography; 1980.
3. Craig M. *Diagnostic Medical Sonography: A Guide to Clinical Practice. Vol. 2. Echocardiography.* Philadelphia: JB Lippincott; 1991.
4. Cosgrove DO, McCready VR. *Ultrasound Imaging: Liver, Spleen, Pancreas.* New York: John Wiley & Sons; 1982.
5. Weyman AE. *Cross-Sectional Echocardiography.* Philadelphia: Lea & Febiger; 1982.
6. Kisslo J, Adams D, Mark DB. *Basic Doppler Echocardiography.* New York: Churchill Livingstone; 1986.
7. Sahn DJ, DeMaria A, Kisso J, Weyman A. Recommendations regarding quantitation in M-mode echocardiography: results of a survey of echocardiographic measurements. *Circulation.* 1978; 58:1072–1083.
8. Sokolow M, McIlroy MB, Cheitlin MD. *Clinical Cardiology.* 5th ed. Norwalk, CT: Appleton & Lange; 1990.
9. Braunwald E. *Heart Disease: A Textbook of Cardiovascular Medicine.* 3rd ed. Philadelphia: WB Saunders; 1988.

10. Goldberg SJ, Allen HD, Marx GR, Flinn CJ. *Doppler Echocardiography.* Philadelphia: Lea & Febiger; 1985.

11. Harrigan P, Lee R. *Principles of Interpretation in Echocardiography.* New York: John Wiley & Sons; 1985.

12. Kisso J, Adams DB, Belkin RN. *Doppler Color-Flow Imaging.* New York: Churchill Livingstone; 1988.

13. Salcedo E. *Atlas of Echocardiography,* 2nd ed. Philadelphia: WB Saunders; 1985.

14. Hatle L, Angelsen B, Tromsdal A. Noninvasive assessment of atrioventricular pressure half-time by Doppler ultrasound. *Circulation.* 1979; 60:1096–1104.

15. Gravanis MB. *Cardiovascular Pathophysiology.* New York: McGraw-Hill; 1987.

16. Popp RL. Echocardiography. *N Engl J Med.* 1990; 323:101–109.

17. Aobanu J, et al. Pulsed Doppler echocardiography in the diagnosis and estimation of severity of aortic insufficiency. *Am J Cardiol.* 1982; 49:339–343.

18. Hatle L, Angelsen B. *Doppler Ultrasound in Cardiology: Physical Principles and Clinical Applications.* Philadelphia: Lea & Febiger; 1985.

19. Currie PJ. Transesophageal echocardiography: new window to the heart. *Circulation.* 1989; 80:215–218.

20. Hurst JW. *The Heart,* 6th ed. New York: McGraw-Hill; 1986.

21. Wasser HJ, Greengart A, et al. Echocardiographic assessment of posterior left ventricular aneurysms. *J Diagn Med Sonography.* 1986; 2:93–95.

22. Driscoll DJ, Fuster V, McGoon DC. Congenital heart disease in adolescents and adults: atrioventricular canal defect. In: Brandenburg RO, Fuster V, Giulani ER, et al., eds. *Cardiology: Fundamentals and Practice.* Chicago: Year Book Medical Publishers; 1987.

23. D'Cruz IA, Lalmalani GG, et al. The superiority of mitral E point-ventricular septum separation to other echocardiographic indicators of left ventricular performance. *Clin Cardiol.* 1979; 2:140.

24. D'Cruz IA, Kleinman D, Aboulatta H, et al. A reappraisal of the mitral B-bump (B-inflection): its relationship to left ventricular dysfunction. *Echocardiography.* 1990; 7:69–75.

25. Williams GJ, Partidge JB, Right ventricular diastolic collapse: an echocardiographic sign of tamponade. *Br Heart J.* 1983; 49:292.

26. Doi YL, McKenna WJ, et al. M-mode echocardiography in hypertrophic cardiomyopathy: diagnostic criteria and prediction of obstruction. *Am J Cardiol.* 1980; 45:6–14.

27. Child JS, Skorton DJ, Taylor RD, et al. M-mode and cross-sectional echocardiographic features of flail posterior mitral leaflets. *Am J Cardiol.* 1979; 44:1383–1390.

28. Sigueira-Filho AG, Cunha CL, Tajik AJ, et al. M-mode and two-dimensional echocardiographic features in cardiac amyloidosis. *Circulation.* 1981; 63:188–196.

29. Chandraratna PAN, Balachandran PK, Shah PM, Hodges M. Echocardiographic observations on ventricular septal rupture complicating myocardial infarction. *Circulation.* 1975; 51:506–510.

30. Berne RM, Levy MN. *Cardiovascular Physiology.* 4th ed. St. Louis: CV Mosby; 1981.

31. Allen MN. *Diagnostic Medical Sonography: A Guide to Clinical Practice Echocardiography.* 2nd ed. Philadelphia: Lippincott; 1999.

CHAPTER 4

PEDIATRIC ECHOCARDIOGRAPHY

Michael W. Yates

Study Guide

INTRODUCTION

Effective echocardiographic evaluation of congenital heart disease requires an appreciation of malformation severity and cardiovascular hemodynamics. A complete echocardiographic study involves the use of every modality available. Anatomy should be carefully delineated by two-dimensional (2-D) imaging because malformations frequently occur in combination rather than as isolated lesions. Doppler techniques provide information on shunt patterns, flow volumes, gradients through obstructions, and severity of regurgitation. Color flow Doppler facilitates rapid detection of flow abnormalities and qualitative assessment of such flow characteristics as direction, timing, and degree of turbulence. Pulsed-wave (PW) Doppler provides range (spatial) resolution of flow patterns. Quantification of high-velocity flows require the use of continuous-wave (CW) Doppler. M-mode is used primarily to evaluate subtle movements and to measure chamber, vessel, and wall size. Contrast echocardiography is useful in the demonstration of intracardiac and extracardiac shunts, particularly in cases in which 2-D and color flow imaging is suboptimal.

The study outline is intended as a guide for the entry-level pediatric echocardiographer and, as such, includes malformations that occur with relative frequency as well as those that occur rarely but are relatively straightforward. The outline includes a definition of the anatomic malformation, a list of variants, the hemodynamic effect of the lesion, characteristic clinical findings, key echocardiographic concepts, the natural history of the disease, commonly associated cardiac malformations, interventional catheterization techniques, and palliative as well as corrective surgical procedures. Complex malformations, such as single ventricle, double-inlet ventricle, and double-outlet ventricle are beyond the scope of this chapter. For information regarding these malformations, the reader is referred to more extensive texts.

Sample examination questions are provided following the text to give the reader an appreciation of the scope of knowledge required to perform routine diagnostic pediatric echocardiograms. The questions are *not* intended to be a comprehensive review but to assist the reader in determining what needs to be studied in greater detail.

For discussions of normal anatomy, general scanning technique, echocardiographic physics and instrumentation, and acquired heart disease that is not specific to the pediatric population, the reader is referred to other chapters within this book. Acquired pathologies that occur in the pediatric as well as adult population include mitral valve prolapse, rheumatic heart disease, cardiac masses, cardiomyopathies, pericardial effusions, and bacterial endocarditis. Evaluation of ventricular function in the pediatric population is identical to that of the adult population and, therefore, will not be repeated within this chapter.

SEGMENTAL ANATOMY

When evaluating congenital heart disease, the echocardiographer begins by determining whether the heart is located in the left chest (levocardia), right chest (dextrocardia), or directly posterior to the sternum (mesocardia). The direction in which the apex is pointing is also noted. The echocardiographer should demonstrate segmental anatomy by delineating situs, ventricular looping, and great vessel relationship. This may be done by documenting anatomic landmarks for each chamber and vessel, as follows:

1. Situs[1,2]
    A. Types
        (1) Solitus—normal
            • Descending aorta and left atrium to the left
            • Inferior vena cava to the right
        (2) Inversus—mirror image visceral placement
            • Very rare

(3) Left atrial isomerism—double left-sidedness
  • Both atria have left atrial morphology
  • 70% have interrupted inferior vena cava with dilated azygos vein located posterior to the aorta on the same side of the spine or direct hepatic vein drainage into atria bilaterally (2-D transverse subcostal views; confirm venous versus arterial structures by Doppler from sagittal views)
  • Usually have polysplenia
  • Frequently have complex cardiac anomalies
(4) Right atrial isomerism—double right-sidedness
  • Inferior vena cava located anterior to the aorta on the same side of the spine
  • Usually have asplenia
  • Frequently have other cardiac lesions
B. Determined by
  (1) Positions of descending aorta and inferior venae cavae in the abdomen
  (2) Positions of the atria as proven by anatomic landmarks
    a. Right atrium
      • Entrance of superior and inferior venae cavae (contrast echo)[3]
      • Presence of Eustachian valve
      • Right atrial appendage (broad connection to atrium)
        — parasternal or subcostal sagittal views
    b. Left atrium
      • Entrance of pulmonary veins (posterior subcostal coronal plane)
      • Left atrial appendage (tubular, with narrow connection)
        — parasternal long or short axis, subcostal, apical four-chamber views
2. Ventricular connection (looping)[4–6]
  A. Types
    (1) Dextro—right ventricle to the right
    (2) Levo—right ventricle to the left
  B. Determined by positions of the ventricles as proven by anatomic landmarks
    (1) Right ventricle
      • Trabeculated endocardial surface
      • Tricuspid valve (three leaflets)
        — annulus inserts more apically than the mitral valve
        — chordal insertion into ventricular septum or free wall
      • Moderator band
    (2) Left ventricle
      • Smooth endocardial surface
      • Mitral valve (two leaflets)
      • Two prominent papillary muscles
3. Great vessel relationship[1]
  A. Types
    (1) Dextro—aortic valve to the right of the pulmonic valve

(2) Levo—aortic valve to the left of the pulmonic valve
B. Determined by positions of the great arteries as proven by anatomical landmarks
  (1) Pulmonary artery
    • Bifurcates soon after exiting the heart
    • Posterior course from base of the heart
  (2) Aorta
    • Superior course from base of the heart, to form aortic arch
    • Coronary arteries

NORMAL HEMODYNAMICS[7]

Chamber/ vessel	Mean	Diastolic	Systolic
Right atrium		<9 mm Hg	<9 mm Hg
Right ventricle		<7mm Hg	<30 mm Hg
Pulmonary artery	<20mm Hg		<30 mm Hg
Left atrium	<12 mm Hg		<17mm Hg
Left ventricle		<12mm Hg	<140 mm Hg (within 5 mm Hg of arm pressure)
Aorta	determined by blood pressure cuff on arm		

IMPORTANT DOPPLER CALCULATIONS

1. Conversion of frequency shift into velocity by use of the Doppler equation[8]
2. Estimation of pressure gradient by application of the modified Bernoulli equation[8]
3. Determination of flow volume[9]
4. Determination of pulmonary to systemic flow ratio, referred to as Q_p; Q_s[10–12]
5. Estimation of valve area by use of the continuity equation[13]

ESTIMATION OF PULMONARY ARTERY PRESSURE

The development and progression of elevated pulmonary artery pressure is of concern in any patient with congenital heart disease. Pulmonary artery pressures rise in response to increased flow volume and/or pressure as pulmonary vascular resistance becomes elevated. Increased flow volume and/or high pressure cause the intimal and medial layers of the pulmonary arterioles to hypertrophy, thereby increasing pulmonary vascular resistance. With prolonged exposure to high-flow volume and/or pressure, the patient develops pulmonary hypertension and eventually pulmonary vascular obstructive disease, which is irreversible. When pulmonary artery pressures exceed systemic pressures, blood flow through intra- and extracardiac shunts reverses, so that they become pulmonary-to-systemic or right-to-left shunts. Mixing of deoxygenated blood with oxygenated blood leads to cyanosis. The right ventricle eventually fails because of the increased resistance against which it must work to eject blood. Pulmonary vascular disease that results from prolonged increased volume and pressure to the pulmonary vascular bed from a systemic to pulmonary (left to right) shunt is referred to as Eisenmenger's syndrome.[14]

Echocardiographic Signs of Elevated Pulmonary Artery Pressure (Pulmonary Hypertension)
- Dilated right ventricle with thickened right ventricular free wall
- Disappearance of the "a" wave on the pulmonic valve M-mode[15,16]
- Midsystolic closure of the pulmonic valve on M-mode, also known as the "flying W"[17]
- Tricuspid and/or pulmonic regurgitation in the absence of structural abnormalities of the valves[18]

Estimation of Systolic Pulmonary Artery Pressure
- Peak tricuspid regurgitation gradient plus 7 mm Hg (assumed central venous pressure)[18,19]
- Enhancement of tricuspid regurgitation Doppler tracing by use of echocardiographic contrast[20]

Estimation of Diastolic Pulmonary Artery Pressure
- End-diastolic pulmonary regurgitation gradient plus 7 mm Hg (assumed central venous pressure)[21]

Estimation of Mean Pulmonary Artery Pressure
- Acceleration time (AcT) divided by ejection time (ET) flow through the right ventricular outflow tract as recorded by PW Doppler[22]

SIMPLE SHUNT LESIONS

Persistent Patent Ductus Arteriosus (PDA)
Anatomy. The ductus arteriosus is a vessel connecting the left pulmonary artery to the descending aorta (immediately distal to the level of the left subclavian artery) that allows blood to bypass the pulmonary circulation during fetal life. Shortly after birth, this vessel should close so blood can enter the pulmonary circulation to be oxygenated. When the vessel remains patent, it is referred to as a persistent patent ductus arteriosus.

Hemodynamics. During fetal life, pulmonary vascular resistance is higher than systemic vascular resistance; therefore, pulmonary pressure is higher than systemic pressure, so blood flows from the pulmonary artery to the descending aorta. After birth, pulmonary vascular resistance decreases and becomes much lower than systemic vascular resistance. The reversal in pressure differences between the pulmonary and systemic circulations causes a reversal of flow through a persistently patent ductus arteriosus, so that the blood from the descending aorta enters the pulmonary circulation. The resulting increase in pulmonary flow continues into the left atrium as a volume overload, causing the left atrium and ventricle to dilate. The magnitude of the systemic to pulmonary shunt is determined by the difference between the pulmonary and systemic vascular resistances, the difference in pulmonary artery and descending aortic pressures, and by the luminal diameter of the ductus arteriosus.[7]

Clinical Presentation.[7,23] Patients are usually asymptomatic; in cardiac failure if the shunt is large.

- Physical exam: bounding pulses
- Auscultation: systolic murmur in infants, continuous murmur at older age
- ECG (electrocardiogram): variable
- Chest x-ray: enlarged pulmonary artery and aorta, increased vascular markings, ductus "bump" off the descending aorta

Key Echocardiographic Concepts
- 2-D visualization of the ductus entering the pulmonary artery (parasternal short axis or high parasternal view)[24,25]
- 2-D visualization of the ductus entering the descending aorta (suprasternal notch or high parasternal view)[26,27]
- Continuous flow in the pulmonary artery by PW or color flow Doppler[28,29]
- Diastolic flow reversal in the descending aorta distal to the left subclavian artery by PW or color flow Doppler[13,30]
- Demonstration of shunt by contrast echocardiography[24,31]
- Left atrial to aortic root ratio (LA/Ao ratio) greater than 1.2 in the absence of left ventricular failure[31]
- Estimation of pulmonary artery pressure by determining the pressure gradient through the duct by CW Doppler and subtracting this value from the systolic blood pressure[13]

Populations at Increased Risk[7]
- Preterm infant
- Infant born at altitudes greater than 4500 m above sea level
- Rubella syndrome
- Family history
- Complex congenital heart disease[14]

Natural History.[7] A large shunt may cause congestive heart failure, failure to thrive, and recurrent respiratory infections. Pulmonary vascular obstructive disease will develop if left untreated.

Treatment[7]

- Indomethacin: to close ductus medically
- Prostaglandin E_1: to keep ductus patent in the presence of a "duct-dependent" lesion, in which the ductus is necessary to provide pulmonary circulation
- Umbrella closure (interventional catheterization)[32]
- Foam plastic plug closure (interventional catheterization)
- Surgical ligation

Postoperative Echocardiographic Evaluation. Left atrial and ventricular size should regress to normal. Color flow or PW Doppler should be used to check for residual shunting.

Other Systemic to Pulmonary Shunts

Echocardiographic Concepts

- PW Doppler documentation of diastolic descending aortic flow reversal to evaluate patency of the shunt
- Localization of shunt by PW Doppler (determine the level at which the diastolic reversal begins)
- Visualization of shunt on 2-D and color flow Doppler

Types

A. Aorticopulmonary Window: a defect in the walls of the ascending aorta and main pulmonary artery resulting in blood shunting between these structures; Doppler findings are similar to persistent patent ductus arteriosus, except reversal of flow may be detected in the ascending as well as descending aorta.[13]

B. Surgically Created Systemic to Pulmonary Shunts[7,33]

1. Blalock–Taussig: subclavian artery to pulmonary artery on side opposite the aortic arch; modified versions may be placed on either side; current shunt of choice
2. Central: anastomosis or conduit between the pulmonary artery and aorta
3. Glenn: superior vena cava to right main pulmonary artery; persistent left superior vena cava with innominate vein communication results in a steal phenomenon; occlusion may lead to various complications; including superior vena cava syndrome
4. Potts: descending aorta to pulmonary artery; difficult to control size; older technique
5. Waterston: ascending aorta to right pulmonary artery; difficult to control size; older technique

Atrial Septal Defects (ASDs)

Anatomy. ASD is incomplete septation of the atrial septum that results in a "hole" or communication through which blood can flow directly from one atrium to the other. Types of atrial septal defects, as determined by physical location, are listed below.[25,34]

- Secundum: area of the foramen ovale; most common
- Primum: posterior, near the atrioventricular valves; associated with cleft mitral valve and mitral regurgitation

- Sinus venosus: posterior and superior, near the entrance of the superior vena cava; associated with anomalous right pulmonary venous return into the right atrium
- Coronary sinus: area of the entrance of the coronary sinus; rare; associated with persistent left superior vena cava, absent coronary sinus, and complex congenital heart disease.[35]

Hemodynamics. Blood is "shunted" from the higher pressure left atrium to the lower pressure right atrium causing a volume overload and, therefore, dilation of the right atrium, right ventricle, and pulmonary arteries. Doppler interrogation reveals blood flow through the interatrial septum and increased flow velocities through the tricuspid and pulmonic valves.

Clinical Presentation.[7,23] Patients are usually asymptomatic.

- Physical exam: systolic impulse may be felt at the lower left sternal border
- Auscultation: fixed splitting of the second heart sound, systolic crescendo–decrescendo (ejection) murmur that is heard best at upper left sternal border
- ECG: right ventricular hypertrophy
- Chest x-ray: enlarged heart and increased pulmonary vascular markings

Key Echocardiographic Concepts

- Visualization of defect on 2-D and with color flow Doppler (subcostal long and short, parasternal short axis, and apical four-chamber views)[25,29]
- PW Doppler tracing characteristic of left to right shunt through an atrial septal defect[36]
- Degree of right atrial and ventricular dilatation to estimate severity
- PW Doppler technique to calculate Q_p:Q_s (i.e., magnitude of the shunt)
- Use of echocardiographic contrast to confirm the presence of a shunt[37,38]

Associated Disease[23,31]

- Mitral valve prolapse
- Left ventricular inflow obstruction (Lutenbacher's syndrome)
- Subaortic stenosis
- Atrial septal aneurysm

Natural History[7,23]

- May close spontaneously
- Pulmonary vascular obstructive disease may develop, usually in adulthood

Treatment

- Elective surgical suture closure
- Elective surgical patch closure with pericardial or Teflon patch

Postoperative Echocardiographic Evaluation
- Right atrial and ventricular size should regress to normal
- Color flow, PW Doppler, or contrast echo[3] should be used to check for residual shunting around the patch

Ventricular Septal Defects (VSDs)

Anatomy. A communication exits between the ventricles as a result of incomplete septation. Type is determined by location, as listed below.[25,39]

- Perimembranous: including the membranous septum and frequently portions of the muscular septum directly under the aortic valve
- Malalignment: the aorta or pulmonary artery overrides the interventricular septum
- Inflow (atrioventricular canal, endocardial cushion): posterior, at the level of the atrioventricular valves
- Doubly committed subarterial (subpulmonic, supracristal): immediately proximal to the pulmonic valve, in the right ventricular outflow tract
- Muscular: in the body of the ventricular septum
- Apical: in the apical septum
- Left ventricular to right atrial shunt: rare; mimics tricuspid regurgitation[40]

Hemodynamics. Blood from the higher-pressure left ventricle courses through the communication into the lower-pressure right ventricle. The greatest volume of blood is shunted during systole, when the pressure difference between the ventricles is most pronounced. Because the pulmonic valve is open during systole, the high-velocity jet from the left ventricle proceeds through the right ventricle directly into the pulmonary artery. The pulmonary vasculature, therefore, is affected more by the increased volume and pressure than the right ventricle. The increased blood volume proceeds into the left atrium and ventricle causing dilatation of these chambers.

Clinical Presentation.[23] Patients usually are asymptomatic; may present in cardiac failure if shunt is large.

- Physical exam: palpable thrill over the chest
- Auscultation: harsh holosystolic murmur; variably split second heart sound
- ECG: dilated pulmonary artery, pulmonary vessels, left atrium, left ventricle
- Chest x-ray: left ventricular hypertrophy with or without right ventricular hypertrophy

Key Echocardiographic Concepts
- Visualization of defect on 2-D or of the shunt (jet) by color flow Doppler[25,29,41]
- Systolic flow into the right ventricle through the interventricular septum by PW or CW Doppler[11,42]
- Evidence of shunt by contrast echocardiography[39]
- Estimation of right ventricular pressure by determining the pressure gradient through the VSD by CW Doppler and subtracting this value from the systolic blood pressure[43]

- Restrictive versus nonrestrictive VSD[14]
- Estimation of the magnitude of the shunt by calculation of the $Q_p:Q_s$ by Doppler technique

Associated Disease
- Multiple ventricular septal defects may occur
- Aortic insufficiency (particularly with doubly committed subarterial and perimembranous types)[25,44]
- Membranous subaortic stenosis[45]

Natural History[7,14]
- Small defects may close spontaneously
- Risk of developing endocarditis
- Aneurysms of tricuspid valve tissue may partially or completely occlude perimembranous VSDs[39]
- Doubly committed subarterial VSDs may develop aortic valve herniation (prolapse) and subsequent aortic insufficiency of increasing severity[44]
- Development of pulmonary vascular obstructive disease if a significant defect remains open
- Increased risk of progression of pulmonary vascular obstructive disease if closure is delayed beyond 2 years of life.

Treatment
- Elective surgical stitch or patch closure
- Repair of aortic valve herniation

Postoperative Echocardiographic Evaluation
- Left atrial and ventricular size should regress to normal[31]
- Assess for peripatch residual shunts by PW Doppler, color flow, or contrast echo[3,14,28]
- Assess for patch dehiscence[31]

Atrioventricular Septal Defects (AVSDs)

Anatomy. A spectrum of malformations that occur at the crux of the heart where the atrioventricular valves, interatrial septum, and interventricular septum intersect. These malformations may also be referred to as endocardial cushion defects or atrioventricular canals. Any combination of the following malformations may exist. When there are atrial, ventricular, and atrioventricular valve involvement, the patient is said to have a complete atrioventricular septal defect[46]:

- Ostium primum atrial septal defect
- Inlet ventricular septal defect
- Atrioventricular valve malformation: including cleft mitral valve, single atrioventricular valve, overriding atrioventricular valve, straddling atrioventricular valve
- Common atrium: interatrial septum is completely absent (associated with atrial isomerism)

Hemodynamics. The defects are generally large; therefore, equalization of pressures may occur between chambers, resulting in bidirectional shunting through septal defects. The right heart is dilated because of volume and/or pressure increase. Atrioventricular valve regurgitation may cause atrial dilatation.

Clinical Presentation[7,23] Patients are usually symptomatic during infancy.

- Physical exam: failure to thrive, fatigue, dyspnea, heart failure, recurrent respiratory infections
- Auscultation: variety of murmurs
- ECG: left axis deviation, biventricular hypertrophy
- Chest x-ray: gross cardiomegaly with increased vascular markings

Key Echocardiographic Concepts
- 2-D evaluation of size and positions of ventricular and atrial septal defects
- Relative right ventricular and left ventricular size by 2-D[46]
- Atrioventricular valve competency by PW or color flow Doppler[11]
- Structure of the atrioventricular valves, particularly chordal attachments[39]
- Assessment of pulmonary artery pressure by Doppler methods

Associated Disease[7,31,46]
- Left heart and aortic obstructive lesions
- Muscular ventricular septal defects
- Atrial isomerisms

Natural History
- Pulmonary vascular obstructive disease develops at an early age[23]

Treatment.[7] Surgery is usually done during the first year of life

- Elective surgical repair of atrioventricular valves and patch closure of septal defects
- Pulmonary artery band: surgical palliation in which supravalvular pulmonary stenosis is created to limit blood flow to the pulmonary vascular bed to retard progression of pulmonary vascular disease

Postoperative Echocardiographic Evaluation
- After definitive repair, evaluate ventricular function, check for residual shunts and assess competency of atrioventricular valves.
- After pulmonary artery banding, determine the anatomic position of the band and the pressure gradient across it by CW Doppler.

OBSTRUCTIVE LESIONS

Left Ventricular Outflow Obstructions
Anatomy. Various types of obstruction are listed below.[7,14,25,31]

- Bicuspid aortic valve: one of the commissures remains fused; the most common type of congenital heart dis-

ease; frequently hemodynamically insignificant until adulthood
- Unicuspid aortic valve: in place of a valve, there is a membrane with an orifice
- Discrete subaortic stenosis: membrane or ridge in the left ventricular outflow tract; may also affect the anterior leaflet of the mitral valve
- Dynamic subaortic stenosis (idiopathic hypertrophic subaortic stenosis, hypertrophic obstructive cardiomyopathy): thickened interventricular septum; genetically transmitted
- Tunnel aortic stenosis: diffuse narrowing of the left ventricular outflow tract; rare
- Supravalvular aortic stenosis: localized or diffuse narrowing of the ascending aorta, generally just distal to the sinuses of Valsalva; usually associated with the William syndrome

Hemodynamics. Obstruction increases resistance to flow out of the left ventricle. The left ventricle must, therefore, generate higher systolic pressures to force the blood past the obstruction. This pressure overload results in thickening of the left ventricular walls.

Clinical Presentation.[7,23] Patients are usually asymptomatic unless obstruction is severe.

- Physical exam: anacrotic notch and prolonged upstroke in peripheral arterial pulse; left ventricular lift and precordial systolic thrill may be palpable
- Auscultation: ejection click and systolic ejection murmur, narrowed splitting of the second heart sound; reversed splitting of the second heart sound if obstruction is severe
- ECG: left ventricular hypertrophy
- Chest x-ray: enlarged left ventricle, dilated ascending aorta

Key Echocardiographic Concepts
General Concepts
- High-velocity turbulent jet distal to obstruction by PW or color flow Doppler[8,28]
- Increased thickness of left ventricular walls[31]
- Prolonged time to peak velocity (acceleration time to left ventricular ejection time ratio greater than 0.30 suggests pressure greater than 50 mm Hg, greater than 0.55 requires surgery)[8]
- Estimation of pressure gradient through the obstruction by CW Doppler-peak systolic pressure gradient greater than 75 mm Hg with a normal cardiac output is critical aortic stenosis and a surgical emergency[2,7,8]
- Estimation of valve area by continuity equation—area less than 0.5 cm^2/m^2 of body surface area is critical aortic stenosis and a surgical emergency[7]
- Calculation of left ventricular wall stress[31]
- Estimation of left ventricular pressure as posterior left ventricular wall thickness at end systole divided by end-systolic diameter multiplied by 225[47]

Bicuspid Aortic Valve
- Delineation of configuration of cusps by 2-D
- Doming of cusps on 2-D
- Aortic eccentricity index greater than 1.5 determined by M-mode[31]

Discrete Subaortic Stenosis[25,31]
- 2-D visualization of the membrane from the parasternal long axis or apical five-chamber view
- Premature closure or midsystolic notch on the aortic valve M-mode or PW Doppler tracing
- Coarse systolic fluttering of the aortic cusps on M-mode
- Increased velocity of flow proximal to the aortic valve by PW and color flow Doppler

Dynamic Subaortic Stenosis[48]
- 2-D demonstration of distribution of myocardial thickening
- Late systolic peak on CW Doppler tracing

Tunnel Aortic Stenosis
- 2-D visualization of diffusely narrow left ventricular outflow tract, hypoplastic aortic valve with thick cusps, and hypoplastic ascending aorta[25]

Associated Disease[7]
- Bicuspid aortic valve: aortic insufficiency, coarctation of the aorta
- Unicuspid aortic valve: aortic insufficiency
- Discrete subaortic stenosis: aortic insufficiency

Natural History[7]
- Obstruction usually progresses
- Development of aortic regurgitation

Treatment.[7,14] Patients are generally prophylaxed and restricted from participating in competitive sports.

- Valvular aortic stenosis: intervention when peak systolic pressure gradient exceeds 75 mm Hg or orifice size decreases to 0.5 cm^2/m^2 of body surface area
  — Percutaneous balloon valvuloplasty[49]
  — Commissurotomy
  — Aortic valve replacement
- Discrete subaortic stenosis: surgical resection of the membrane
- Supravalvular aortic stenosis: surgical resection of obstruction when pressure gradient exceeds 50 mm Hg
- Tunnel aortic stenosis: left ventricular to descending aorta valved conduit,[50] Konno procedure (widening of aortic root and left ventricular outflow tract)

Postoperative Echocardiography Evaluation. Evaluate for residual or restenosis and aortic insufficiency.

Coarctation of the Aorta
Anatomy. There is a discrete or diffuse narrowing of the aorta, most commonly located immediately distal to the left subclavian artery in the area of the ductus arteriosus. Infrequently, the coarctation will occur proximal to the ductus arteriosus or a portion of the aortic arch may be hypoplastic. In either of these cases, patency of the ductus arteriosus may be necessary to perfuse the descending aorta and maintain life.[7]

Hemodynamics. Obstruction to flow at the level of the coarctation results in a build-up of pressure proximal to the obstruction and decreased flow distal to it.[14] Left ventricular walls thicken in response to increased resistance. A high-velocity jet through the obstruction may weaken the aortic wall immediately distal to the obstruction causing post-stenotic dilatation.

Clinical Presentation.[7,23] Patients are usually asymptomatic; if severe during infancy, will present in heart failure.

- Physical exam: systemic hypertension, with systolic blood pressure much higher in the upper extremities than in the lower extremities;[14] weak femoral pulses; upper body may be more well developed than the lower body
- Auscultation: systolic murmur along the left sternal border transmitting to back and neck; bruits from collateral vessels in older children
- ECG: right ventricular hypertrophy in symptomatic infants; left ventricular hypertrophy in older children
- Chest x-ray: inverted "3" sign at level of coarctation; prominent descending aorta; rib notching in children older than 8 years

Key Echocardiography Concepts
- 2-D visualization of obstruction within the aortic lumen[51,52]
- Determination of gradient by CW Doppler tracing through the coarctation[53]
  — Velocity of flow proximal to the obstruction should be taken into consideration[11]
- Decreased pulsatility on the PW Doppler tracing of the descending aorta (blunted acceleration and slow deceleration of flow that does not return to baseline during diastole)[11]

Associated Disease[7,52]
- Bicuspid aortic valve (found in as many as 50% of patients with coarctation of the aorta)
- Additional levels of left heart obstruction
- Ventricular septal defects
- Transposition of the great arteries
- Double-outlet right ventricle

Natural History. If unrelieved, as many as 80% of patients die before reaching the age of 50 years.[7]

Treatment.[7,14] Early repair seems to decrease probability of residual systemic hypertension

- Surgical resection of constricted area and primary anastomosis or graft placement
- Subclavian artery to widen aortic lumen

Postoperative Echocardiographic Evaluation
- Assessment of the lumen size and pressure gradient in the area of the reanastomosis
- PW Doppler spectral tracing of the descending aortic flow may continue to appear somewhat blunted

Hypoplastic Left Heart Syndrome
A spectrum of left-sided hypoplasia in which the left atrium, mitral valve, left ventricle, aortic valve, and aorta may be hypoplastic, stenotic, or atretic. Frequently associated with an atrial septal defect through which pulmonary venous return flows into the right atrium and a patent ductus arteriosus, which in turn supplies the descending aorta.[25]

Treatment[54]
- Cardiac transplantation
- Norwood procedure

Pulmonary Stenosis
Anatomy. Obstruction may occur at various levels along the right ventricular outflow tract and the pulmonary arterial system. Types are listed below.[7,23]

- Valvular stenosis: fusion or dysplasia of cusps
- Infundibular stenosis: hypertrophy of muscle bands in the right ventricular outflow tract; usually associated with a ventricular septal defect or Valvular pulmonary stenosis[25]
- Double chamber right ventricle: hypertrophied anomalous muscle bundles in the right ventricle, effectively dividing the right ventricle into two chambers with a communication between them; associated with valvular pulmonary stenosis, perimembranous ventricular septal defects, and subaortic stenosis[39,45]
- Peripheral pulmonary stenosis: may occur as a distinct shelf in the pulmonary artery, discrete narrowing of the pulmonary artery branches, or as diffuse tapered narrowing of the pulmonary artery branches[55]

Hemodynamics. Increased resistance to right ventricular outflow results in a pressure overload to this chamber. The right ventricular walls thicken and the chamber dilates. Blood flow into the pulmonary arterial system is at high velocity and turbulent. Eddy currents produced distal to the obstruction may cause poststenotic dilatation of the pulmonary artery.[25]

Clinical Presentation.[7] Patients are usually asymptomatic.

- Auscultation: systolic ejection murmur
- ECG: right ventricular hypertrophy
- Chest x-ray: prominent pulmonary artery trunk; large right atrium

Key Echocardiographic Concepts
- Thickened right ventricular free wall
- 2-D visualization and measurement of pulmonary valve annulus in candidate for balloon angioplasty of valvular stenosis[56]
- 2-D visualization of anomalous muscle bundle and orifice from parasternal and subcostal views[56]
- Accentuation of the "a wave" on M-mode[7]
- Doppler estimation of pressure gradient from all available positions[57]

Natural History[7]
- Increased risk of endocarditis
- Mild valvular and peripheral stenosis (right ventricular pressure less than 50 mm Hg and a pressure gradient of less than 40 mm Hg) is considered benign and may or may not progress
- Severe stenosis (right ventricular pressure greater than 100 mm Hg and a pressure gradient greater than 80 mm Hg) requires relief
- Infundibular stenosis and anomalous muscle bundles tend to become progressively more obstructive

Treatment. When patient becomes symptomatic or pressure gradient exceeds 50 mm Hg[14]

- Balloon valvuloplasty: to relieve valvular and peripheral stenosis[49]
- Surgical valvotomy[7]
- Surgical resection of infundibular muscle or anomalous muscle bundles

Postoperative Echocardiographic Evaluation
- Assess patency of area of former obstruction
- Assess presence and severity of pulmonary insufficiency

Pulmonary Atresia
Anatomy. There is an imperforate membrane or thick fibrous band in place of a pulmonary valve or complete absence of the main pulmonary artery.[55]

Hemodynamics. Life is dependent upon a persistent patent ductus arteriosus or collateral vessels. A ventricular septal defect usually coexists and acts as an outlet to systemic venous return.[14]

Clinical Presentation.[7] Severe cyanosis and hypoxemia are seen in the neonate.

- Auscultation: possibly the murmur of a persistent ductus arteriosus
- ECG: right ventricular hypertrophy; right axis deviation
- Chest x-ray: boot-shaped heart; reticular or decreased pulmonary vascular markings

Key Echocardiographic Concepts[7,56]
- 2-D delineation of anatomy
  — right ventricular outflow tract, location, and size of main pulmonary artery and branches (subcostal coronal and parasternal short axis)
  — associated malformations
- Contrast echocardiography to delineate anatomy
- Doppler and color flow delineation of flow patterns

Associated Disease[56]
- Persistent ductus arteriosus
- Atrial septal defect or patent foramen ovale
- Malformations of the tricuspid valve
- Coronary arterial sinusoids

Natural History
- Death when the persistent ductus arteriosus closes or systemic to pulmonary collateral flow becomes insufficient to sustain minimal blood oxygenation requirements[7]

Treatment[7,14]
- Prostaglandin E_2: to keep the ductus arteriosus patent
- Palliation with a surgically created systemic to pulmonary shunt
- Surgical reconstruction and/or placement of prosthetic valve

Postoperative Echocardiographic Evaluation
- Evaluate patency of systemic to pulmonary shunt
- Evaluate patency of reconstructed area

Left Ventricular Inflow Obstruction
Anatomy. Left ventricular inflow is obstructed by a membrane in the left atrium or a decrease in the mitral orifice size. Various forms exist, as listed below.[25,39]

- Valvular mitral stenosis: rare; dysplastic valve leaflets, chordae and papillary muscles
- Parachute mitral valve: all chordae insert onto a single papillary muscle
- Arcade mitral valve: chordae insert onto multiple papillary muscles; may be regurgitant
- Double orifice mitral valve: rare; tissue bridge divides mitral valve into two halves and chordae from each half inserting onto a particular papillary muscle; may be regurgitant; associated with atrioventricular malformation[58]
- Cortriatriatum: rare; left atrial membrane immediately superior to the fossa ovalis and left atrial appendage
- Supravalvular ring: more common than cortriatriatum; left atrial membrane immediately superior to the mitral valve annulus; usually associated with other mitral valve anomalies[35,59]
- Mitral valve hypoplasia: small mitral valve annulus and leaflets
- Mitral Atresia: imperforate mitral valve may be associated with a large ventricular septal defect, straddling tricuspid valve, or double-outlet right ventricle

Hemodynamics. Obstruction to left ventricular inflow results in a build-up of pressure in the left atrium causing it to dilate. Pulmonary veins become congested because they cannot empty easily into the left atrium.

Clinical Presentation[7]
- Physical exam: history of recurrent respiratory infections
- Auscultation: diastolic murmur heard best at the apex
- ECG: left atrial enlargement
- Chest x-ray: left atrial enlargement; increased pulmonary vascular markings; right heart enlargement

Key Echocardiographic Concepts
- Delineation of anatomy by 2-D
- Doppler estimation of pressure gradient
- Estimation of orifice size by application of the continuity equation

Associated Disease[7]
- Other levels of left heart obstruction
- Secundum and primum atrial septal defects
- Transposition of the great arteries
- Double-outlet right ventricle

Natural History. Left ventricle inflow obstruction eventually develops into pulmonary vascular obstructive disease.[7]

Treatment[7]
- Valvular: commissurotomy or valve replacement
- Cortriatriatum and supramitral ring: surgical excision of membrane[56]

Postoperative Echocardiographic Evaluation
- Evaluate residual stenosis and regurgitation

Tricuspid Atresia
Anatomy. A dense band of tissue replaces the tricuspid valve preventing direct communication between the right atrium and ventricle. A large atrial septal defect or patent foramen ovale must coexist to provide an outlet to the right atrium (obligatory shunt).[39] The right ventricle is usually small.[14]

Hemodynamics. Deoxygenated systemic venous blood returns to the right atrium and is shunted into the left atrium, where it mixes with oxygenated pulmonary venous return. This mixing of deoxygenated blood with the pulmonary venous return results in a desaturation of the oxygenated blood and, therefore, cyanosis. The right atrium and left heart are generally dilated because of increased flow volume. Because the right ventricle receives blood only indirectly through a ventricular septal defect, it is generally small.[23]

Clinical Presentation.[7,23] Patients are cyanotic with a history of hypoxic spells.

- Physical exam: clubbing of the fingers; delayed growth; hyperactive cardiac impulse at the apex
- Auscultation: single first heart sound; no murmur
- ECG: left ventricular hypertrophy; left axis deviation
- Chest x-ray: decreased vascular markings

Key Echocardiographic Concepts
- 2-D visualization of dense fibrous band across tricuspid annulus and absence of tricuspid valve leaflets
- Dilated right atrium[39]
- Atrial septal defect or single atrium
- Small right ventricle or right ventricular outflow tract

Associated Disease[7,23]
- Atrial septal defect or patent foramen ovale
- Ventricular septal defect and pulmonary stenosis
- Pulmonary atresia
- Transposition of the great vessels

Natural History
- Early death without intervention[7]

Treatment[1]
- Pulmonary artery band (surgical palliation to restrict flow to the pulmonary bed)
- Systemic to pulmonary shunt (surgical palliation to increase flow to the pulmonary bed)
- Balloon atrial septostomy (interventional catheterization to increase interatrial shunting)
- Park blade septostomy (interventional catheterization to increase interatrial shunting)
- Fontan procedure: definitive physiologic correction; the right atrium is connected to the pulmonary artery by placement of a patch or conduit in the hope of increasing pulmonary flow[34]

Postoperative Echocardiographic Evaluation
- Assess for right atrial contractility and adequacy of flow through the pulmonary artery

Tricuspid Hypoplasia/Stenosis
Anatomy. There is a small tricuspid valve annulus, usually associated with critical pulmonary stenosis, pulmonary atresia with intact interventricular septum, or Ebstein anomaly.[39]

Imperforate Tricuspid Valve
Anatomy. Membrane exists in place of a tricuspid valve, which may be surgically opened.[39]

MALFORMATION OF THE TRICUSPID VALVE

Ebstein Anomaly of the Tricuspid Valve
Anatomy. The septal leaflet is tethered to the interventricular septum and attaches at least 8 mm distal to the tricuspid valve annulus.[31] Other tricuspid leaflets may also adhere to the ventricular wall and be dysplastic.[60] This malformation results in a large "functional" right atrium and small "functional" right ventricle. The dysplastic nature of the leaflets and chordae prevents effective coaptation resulting in varying degrees of tricuspid insufficiency and

stenosis.[39] Contractility of the right ventricle is affected by its size.

Hemodynamics. The right atrium is dilated because of the volume overload that results from the tricuspid regurgitation. The size of the right ventricle varies with the severity of tricuspid valve leaflet displacement.

Clinical Presentation.[7,23,60] Cyanosis, dyspnea, or exertion, and profound weakness or fatigue may be present.

- Physical exam: prominent left chest
- Auscultation: systolic and diastolic murmurs; loud, widely split first heart sound—"sail sound"; triple or quadruple rhythm
- ECG: right atrial hypertrophy; right bundle branch block; Wolff–Parkinson–White syndrome; paroxysmal supraventricular tachycardia
- Chest x-ray: enlarged heart; decreased pulmonary vascular markings; right atrial enlargement

Key Echocardiographic Concepts
- 2-D delineation of the anatomy of the tricuspid valve and degree of displacement and tethering of each leaflet from parasternal short axis, apical four-chamber and subcostal long- and short-axis views[61]
- Determination of the size of the functional right ventricle—if less than 35% of the size of the anatomic right ventricle, prognosis is poor[31]
- Severity of tricuspid regurgitation
- Tricuspid valve closure delayed greater than 90 m/s after mitral valve closure on M-mode[31]

Associated Disease[7,60,61]
- Persistent patent ductus arteriosus
- Atrial septal defect or patent foramen ovale with right to left shunting
- MVP
- Pulmonary stenosis
- Pulmonary atresia with intact ventricular septum
- Congenitally corrected transposition of the great vessels
- Ventricular septal defect

Natural History[7,60,61]
- Increased risk of endocarditis
- Prognosis is better with a larger functional right ventricle
- Prognosis is good if the child survives infancy but generally poor if there are associated lesions

Treatment[7,60,61]
- Annuloplasty: repair of the valve annulus to make it smaller
- Valve replacement
- Valve repair
- Plication of some of the atrialized portion of the right ventricle

Postoperative Echocardiographic Evaluation
- Assess right ventricular function and residual tricuspid insufficiency and/or stenosis

COMPLEX CONGENITAL HEART DISEASE

Tetralogy of Fallot
Anatomy. In this malformation, a large perimembranous ventricular septal defect is associated with a malalignment of the aorta, so that the aortic root overrides the septal defect. The malalignment of the aortic root contributes to the infundibular pulmonary stenosis that occurs as part of this malformation.[56]

Hemodynamics. The large size of the ventricular septal defect allows equalization of left and right ventricular pressures, so that the shunting through the defect is bidirectional. The overriding aorta receives blood from both ventricles, thereby mixing deoxygenated with oxygenated blood.

Clinical Presentation.[7,23] Cyanosis and a history of "tet spells" (transient cerebral ischemia resulting in limpness, paleness, and unconsciousness); history of squatting may present.

- Physical exam: prominent left chest, "clubbing" of fingers, right ventricular heave
- Auscultation: single second heart sound; systolic ejection murmur
- ECG: right ventricular hypertrophy; right axis deviation
- Chest x-ray: boot-shaped heart with decreased vascular markings

Key Echocardiographic Concepts[56]
- 2-D visualization of large perimembranous VSD and assessment of degree of aortic override
- 2-D assessment of degree and levels of right ventricular outflow obstruction
- Size of pulmonary artery and branches from high parasternal short axis and suprasternal notch views (aneurysmally dilated in cases of absent pulmonic valve)[62]
- Thickened RV free wall
- 2-D delineation of coronary artery and aortic arch anatomy to determine surgical approach[63]

Associated Disease[7,31,56,62]
- Valvular pulmonary stenosis or pulmonary atresia
- Congenitally absent pulmonic valve
- Right-sided aortic arch
- Atrioventricular malformation
- Mitral stenosis
- Coronary artery anomalies
- Persistent left superior vena cava

Natural History.[7] Severe infundibular stenosis may result in a fatal "tet spell," in which the infundibulum becomes totally occluded. Pulmonary vascular obstructive disease develops.

Treatment[7]
- Palliation by surgical creation of a systemic to pulmonary shunt
- Patch closure of ventricular septal defect and possible myomectomy of the right ventricular outflow tract, or pulmonary valvotomy

Postoperative Echocardiographic Evaluation
- Evaluation of patency of surgically created systemic to pulmonary shunt
- Evaluation of residual right ventricular outflow obstruction and residual shunting around ventricular septal defect

Transposition of the Great Arteries (TGA)
Anatomy. The aorta arises from the embryologic right ventricle, and the pulmonary artery arises from the embryologic left ventricle. Terminology is listed below.

- C-transposition of the great arteries (congenitally corrected, L-transposition): ventricular inversion with the great vessels originating from the incorrect ventricle; blood flow sequence is normal; however, there is a high incidence of associated congenital heart disease
- D-transposition of the great arteries (frequently referred to simply as transposition of the great arteries or complete transposition): the ventricles are concordant with the atria; however the aorta originates from the right ventricle and the pulmonary artery originates from the embryologic left ventricle

Hemodynamics
- C-TGA: Blood flows in the normal sequence—from the systemic veins into the right atrium, through the mitral valve into the left ventricle, and out the pulmonary artery, returns to the left atrium via the pulmonary valves, courses through the tricuspid valve, into the right ventricle and out the aorta.
- D-TGA: Blood flows in two parallel circuits. It flows from the systemic veins into the right atrium, through the tricuspid valve, into the right ventricle and out the aorta, to return again through the systemic veins. Pulmonary venous return flows into the left atrium, through the mitral valve into the left ventricle, and out the pulmonary artery, to return again through the pulmonary veins. In short, deoxygenated blood flows in a continuous loop, and oxygenated blood flows in a separate continuous loop. Unless a communication exists between the systemic and pulmonary circulations (i.e., an obligatory shunt), this situation is incompatible with life. In the newborn period, a left-to-right shunt occurs at the level of the foramen ovale

and through a persistent ductus arteriosus, allowing mixing of oxygenated with deoxygenated blood.

Clinical Presentation for D-TGA.[7,23] Newborns become cyanotic, as the ductus arteriosus closes.

- Physical exam: normal weight, healthy-looking infant
- Auscultation: no murmurs; single second heart sound
- ECG: right ventricular hypertrophy
- Chest x-ray: cardiomegaly; narrow mediastinum; increased vascular markings

Key Echocardiographic Concepts[64]
- Identify situs by delineating anatomic atrial landmarks on 2-D.
- Identify ventricular morphology (embryologic origins) by delineating anatomic landmarks on 2-D.
- Identify great vessel morphology and relationship (will course in parallel fashion).
- Identify and evaluate magnitude of shunt through the obligatory shunt defect(s).
- Delineate coronary artery anatomy for consideration of surgical approach.[63]
- Identify and evaluate associated congenital heart disease.

Associated Disease for D-TGA[31,64]
- Patent ductus arteriosus: obligatory shunt; most commonly associated heart disease
- Aortic arch anomalies: coarctation, hypoplastic segment, interrupted aortic arch
- Atrial septal defect or patent foramen ovale: obligatory shunt
- Ventricular septal defect: obligatory shunt; with or without juxtaposed atrial appendages
- Outflow tract obstruction: fixed or dynamic
- Straddling atrioventricular valve: chordae from one atrioventricular valve attach into both ventricles
- Atrioventricular malformation: rare
- Pulmonary origin of coronary artery

Natural History. Patients with congenitally corrected transposition may never know they have congenital heart disease unless there is associated congenital heart disease, in which case, the natural history is determined by the associated disease.

Patients with D-transposition of the great vessels must be palliated or repaired on an emergent basis because occlusion of the obligatory shunt would result in immediate death. The mortality rate in the absence of intervention is 95% at the end of 2 years of life.[16]

Treatment[7,31,33]
Prostaglandin E₁ Treatment. Palliation; to keep ductus arteriosus patent until an atrial shunt or definitive surgical procedure can be performed

Balloon Atrial Septostomy (Rashkind Procedure). Palliative interventional catheterization technique in which a distended balloon catheter is torn across a patent foramen

ovale or small atrial septal defect creating a large atrial septal defect

Surgical Atrial Septectomy (Blalock–Hanlon Operation). Palliation

Mustard Procedure (Atrial Switch). Surgical excision of the interatrial septum and placement of a baffle made of pericardium or synthetic material to redirect right atrial flow through the mitral valve into the left ventricle and allow pulmonary venous return to flow around the baffle into the tricuspid valve

Senning Procedure (Atrial Switch). Surgical reconstruction of the atrial wall and interatrial septum to create an intraatrial baffle redirecting venous flow through the atria

Rastelli Procedure (Intraventricular Repair and Extracardiac Conduit). Surgical procedure in which a tunnel is constructed through a large ventricular septal defect, so that the left ventricular outflow is directed to the aortic valve and a valved conduit is placed between the right ventricle and pulmonary artery

Jatene Procedure (Arterial Switch). Surgical procedure in which the great arteries are taken off their trunks and moved so that each is reanastomosed to the trunk that will restore a normal blood flow sequence; coronary arteries also are removed and reimplanted into the neoaorta.

Postoperative Echocardiographic Evaluation. Evaluation of left ventricular function

- Balloon atrial septostomy: 2-D visualization of definitive tear in the interatrial septum and calculation of atrial septal defect size to interatrial septal length ratio[16]
- Mustard and Senning procedures: rule out superior vena cava or pulmonary venous obstruction and baffle leaks[7,13] by PW Doppler, color flow Doppler, or contrast echocardiography[3]
- Jatene procedure: evaluate anastomotic sites of great arteries for possible constriction[7]

Truncus Arteriosus
Anatomy.[7,23] A rare malformation in which a single large great artery (common trunk) arises from the heart and receives outflow from both ventricles. In most cases, the common trunk overrides the large ventricular septal defect, which must be present. The valve of the common trunk frequently has more than three cusps. Pulmonary circulation occurs in one of the following ways:

- Type I: main pulmonary trunk arises from the common trunk (usually from the posterior aspect) and bifurcates into right and left branches
- Type II: right and left pulmonary arteries arise separately from the left posterolateral aspect of the common trunk
- Type III: right and left pulmonary arteries arise separately from lateral aspects of the common trunk

- Type IV: no pulmonary arteries exist; pulmonary circulation is through bronchiole arteries arising from the descending aorta

Hemodynamics.[7] The large ventricular septal defect causes equalization of pressures between the ventricles. Flow into the pulmonary circulation is at systemic pressures because the pulmonary arteries arise from the aorta, and there is no pulmonary valve. There may be decreased flow to the pulmonary circulation if there is stenosis of the pulmonary branches or in Type IV.

Clinical Presentation.[7,23] Patients are cyanotic.
- Physical exam: early congestive heart failure or hypoxic spells
- Auscultation: single second heart sound; systolic ejection click and murmur
- ECG: biventricular hypertrophy
- Chest x-ray: cardiomegaly; biventricular enlargement; wide mediastinum

Key Echocardiographic Concepts
- 2-D delineation of anatomy
- Color flow and PW Doppler evaluation of truncal valve (rule out stenosis or insufficiency)
- 2-D and color flow localization of pulmonary arteries (suprasternal notch views may be most helpful)
- Evaluation of size of pulmonary arteries

Associated Disease.[7] Usually, truncus arteriosus is an isolated lesion.

- Right aortic arch
- Truncal valve stenosis and/or insufficiency
- Aortic arch anomalies
- Persistent patent ductus arteriosus
- Coronary ostial anomalies
- Absence of a branch pulmonary artery on the side of the arch
- Atrial septal defect

Natural History.[7] If left untreated, death in infancy from heart failure or later from pulmonary vascular obstructive disease will result. Without intervention, survival beyond 1 year is unusual.

Treatment[7]
- Removal of the pulmonary arteries from the aorta and placement of a valved conduit between the right ventricle and pulmonary arteries
- Pulmonary artery banding palliation; may make definitive repair difficult or impossible

Postoperative Echocardiographic Evaluation
- Evaluate competency of the conduit valve and evaluate anastomatic areas for stenosis
- Evaluate placement of pulmonary artery band and gradient across it

ANOMALIES OF THE CORONARY ARTERIES

Kawasaki Syndrome (Mucocutaneous Lymph Node Syndrome)

Anatomy. Acquired coronary artery disease may occur as a sequela to a childhood disease known as Kawasaki disease. Around 15% of patients develop cardiovascular involvement in the form of coronary artery aneurysm formation. The proximal branches seem to be most frequently involved. Distal aneurysms may occur in addition, although rarely without proximal involvement.[66]

Clinical Presentation.[67] Usually seen January to April, patients have fever over a 5 day duration, lethargy, and irritability.

- Physical exam: bilateral conjunctivitis; dry, fissured lips, strawberry tongue; polymorphous truncal rash; erythema of palms and soles; desquamation of fingertips and toes; cervical lymphadenopathy
- Lab tests: elevated white count, platelet count, erythrocyte sedimentation rate, α_2-globulin, immunoglobulin E, transaminase, and lactic acid dehydrogenase
- ECG: infrequent, minimal changes

Key Echocardiographic Concepts
Acute Phase[63,65]
- Left ventricular dysfunction
- Valvular regurgitation
- Pericardial effusion

Convalescent Phase
- 2-D demonstration of saccular or fusiform coronary aneurysms (Table 4–1)
- Segmental wall motion abnormalities

TABLE 4–1. ECHOCARDIOGRAPHIC VIEWS USED TO EVALUATE CORONARY ARTERY ANATOMY

Coronary Artery	Echocardiographic View
Proximal right, left main, proximal left anterior descending, proximal left circumflex	Parasternal short axis
	High parasternal short axis (caudal angle)
	Subcostal 4 coronal
Distal right coronary	Subcostal coronal (acute margin of heart)
	Subcostal short axis (sagittal)
	Posterior apical 4 chamber (posterior atrioventricular groove)
Posterior descending	Parasternal short axis
	Subcostal coronal
	Apical 4 chamber
Left circumflex	Parasternal short
	Parasternal long
	Subcostal sagittal
Distal left anterior descending	Parasternal long
	Parasternal short
	Subcostal coronal

(Data from references 6 and 41.)

Natural History. The majority of aneurysms resolve; however, those with diameters larger than 8 mm are at increased risk for thrombosis, which may result in myocardial infarction.[65]

Treatment. Patients with aneurysms are usually treated with one aspirin per day to decrease risk of thrombosis. Serial echocardiographic exams are generally performed, with coronary angiography at intervals to determine whether coronary artery bypass surgery is indicated.[7]

Anomalous Origin of the Left Coronary Artery

Anatomy. A rare malformation in which the left coronary artery originates from the main pulmonary artery rather than from the aortic root.[63]

Hemodynamics. The myocardium of the left ventricle is inadequately perfused with oxygen because the blood flowing into the left coronary artery is deoxygenated blood from the pulmonary artery.

Clinical Presentation.[63] It is symptomatic in infancy.
- Physical exam: irritable, dyspneic, tachypneic
- Auscultation: mitral insufficiency murmur
- ECG: left ventricular hypertrophy with anterolateral myocardial infarction
- Chest x-ray: enlarged heart

Key Echocardiographic Concepts[63]
- 2-D visualization of left coronary artery originating from the pulmonary artery
- 2-D visualization of a dilated right coronary artery originating from the right sinus of Valsalva
- PW Doppler or color flow demonstration of diastolic flow entering the main pulmonary artery just distal to the pulmonary valve
- Decreased left ventricular contractility
- Mitral insufficiency

Natural History. In the absence of intervention, permanent myocardial damage occurs.

Treatment. Surgery to reimplant the left coronary artery into the aortic root is recommended.[63]

Coronary Arteriovenous Fistula

Anatomy. A variably tortuous coronary artery courses along the surface of the heart or within the myocardium to empty into a cardiac chamber or great vessel. Generally, it is the right coronary artery that is involved, and the site of drainage is usually a right heart structure.[63]

Hemodynamics. Rather than perfusing the myocardium, blood from the coronary artery flows into the cardiac chamber or vessel into which it empties.

Clinical Presentation. Generally, patients remain asymptomatic until the fourth decade of life.[67]
- Auscultation: atypical continuous murmur

Key Echocardiographic Concepts[68]
- 2-D demonstration of a dilated coronary artery
  — normal ratios of coronary artery diameter to aortic root diameter
    — left coronary artery = 0.17 ± 0.03
    — right coronary artery = 0.14 ± 0.03
- 2-D demonstration of origin, course, and site of drainage of the fistula
- Color flow Doppler visualization and PW Doppler confirmation of a continuous, turbulent jet entering a cardiac chamber or great vessel in a location in which shunt lesions do not enter
- PW Doppler demonstration of turbulent late systolic, early diastolic flow in a dilated coronary artery supplying the fistula

Natural History[68]
- Spontaneous closure may occur
- Bacterial endocarditis
- Congestive heart failure due to volume overload and myocardial ischemia

Treatment. Elective surgical ligation of the fistula.[68]

Postoperative Echocardiographic Evaluation. Check for residual flow through the fistula.

VENOUS MALFORMATIONS

Persistent Left Superior Vena Cava

Anatomy. In this relatively common malformation (0.5% of the general population and 3–5% of patients with congenital heart disease), a superior vena cava persists in the left chest. The left superior vena cava may empty into coronary sinus (62%), pulmonary venous atrium (21%), common atrium (17%), or rarely into a left-sided pulmonary vein. In most cases, there is also a right superior vena cava, and in 45–60% of cases, a communication exists between the two superior venae cavae.[69]

Hemodynamics. Systemic venous blood returns to the cardiac chamber to which the left superior vena cava connects. Deoxygenated blood mixes with oxygenated blood (right to left shunt) if the left superior vena cava drains into a left heart structure.

Key Echocardiographic Concepts[34]
- Dilated coronary sinus
- Contrast echocardiography[70]
- 2-D and color flow visualization of the left superior vena cava
- Absent or small innominate vein

Associated Disease[69]
- Atrial septal defect
- Complex congenital heart disease

Total Anomalous Pulmonary Venous Return

Anatomy. All of the pulmonary veins drain into something other than the left atrium. The types of anomalous drainage are listed below.[34,71]

- Supracardiac: pulmonary veins drain directly into the superior vena cava or form a vertical vein that empties into the innominate vein, superior vena cava, or persistent left superior vena cava
- Cardiac: pulmonary veins drain into the right atrium or coronary sinus
- Infracardiac: pulmonary veins form a common vein that descends below the diaphragm and empties into the portal vein

Hemodynamics. There is increased flow into a systemic vein, right atrium, or coronary sinus[71] and ultimately, the right heart. There is an obligatory right-to-left shunt at the atrial level.[23]

Clinical Presentation Without Obstruction.[23] There is mild cyanosis; asymptomatic.

- Physical exam: poor growth; prominent left chest; right ventricular heave
- Auscultation: fixed, widely split second sound
- ECG: right ventricular hypertrophy
- Chest x-ray: enlarged right heart; increased pulmonary vascular markings; snowman- or figure 8-shaped mediastinum

Clinical Presentation in the Presence of Obstruction.[23] There is cyanosis; symptomatic during the newborn period.

- Physical exam: tachypnea; dyspnea; right ventricular failure
- Auscultation: no murmurs
- ECG: right ventricular hypertrophy
- Chest x-ray: normal size heart; increased pulmonary vascular markings

Key Echocardiographic Concepts[35,71]
- Absence of normal pulmonary venous return into the left atrium by 2-D and color flow Doppler
- Dilated coronary sinus
- Turbulent flow noted in systemic vein or right atrium by color flow Doppler
- Localization of anomalous venous structures by use of 2-D and color flow Doppler from the subcostal and suprasternal positions
- Color flow Doppler interrogation of anomalous venous structures to rule out obstruction
- Contrast echocardiography

Associated Disease
- Atrial septal defect

Natural History.[23] Obstruction of the common vein or entry into a systemic venous structure will result in pulmonary edema and right heart failure, complete obstruction will cause death. Eventually, pulmonary vascular obstructive disease will develop.

Treatment. Surgical anastomosis of the common vein with the left atrium and closure of the atrial communication is the indicated treatment.

Postoperative Echocardiographic Evaluation
- Assessment of ventricular function
- Evaluate area of anastomosis to rule out obstruction

TRANSESOPHAGEAL ECHOCARDIOGRAPHY

Transesophageal echocardiography (TEE) is a more invasive echo technique that requires sedation of the patient. A biplane or multiplane echo probe, similar to an endoscope, allows visualization of the heart from the esophagus and stomach. Most of the ultrasound's limiting factors are removed in this technique, allowing for much better imaging and resolution.

TEE is becoming a standard of care in the operating room during pediatric cardiovascular procedures. It enables the surgeon to delineate anatomy before surgery and evaluate repair effectiveness after surgery. TEE allows the probe to be left in the patient for the entire procedure with continuous monitoring. Comparison of the preoperative and postoperative left ventricular systolic function has proved helpful in perioperative medical management. Intraoperative TEE is most commonly performed by the anesthesiologist. An echocardiographer is not normally required. Routine TEE is performed in cases where acceptable images are not obtained by Transthoracic echography (TTE). TEE is superior to TTE in most cases, allowing better visualization of valve apparatus, interatrial septum, and most other cardiac structures. Color flow Doppler is also superior in TEE. Flow measurements by pulsed, and continuous-wave Doppler are often better obtained by TTE because of imaging angles alone. TEE requires the presence of a physician who performs the procedure, and a nurse who administers conscious sedation and monitors vital signs. The echocardiographer is normally responsible for optimizing the images, directing Doppler flow sampling, and recording the study. At some institutions, the echocardiographer manipulates the TEE probe under the direction of a cardiologist, but this is rare.

TEE is a valuable alternative to transthoracic echo. Its use in the OR has proved invaluable. Outside the OR, TEE in pediatrics is less common than in adults because pediatric patients usually offer adequate imaging because patient habitus and respiratory interference are not often factors.

HYPERTENSION

Long recognized as a contributor to heart disease in adults, hypertension is being diagnosed much more frequently in pediatric patients than in the recent past. Echocardiography is required to assess the effect on the heart.

Clinical Presentation
- Normally asymptomatic and usually noted during routine examinations

Hemodynamics
- In adults, systolic and diastolic pressures may be elevated.

Key Echocardiographic Findings
- Long-standing hypertension can result in left ventricular hypertrophy and increased left ventricular mass, resulting in impaired left ventricular filling.

Natural History
- Untreated hypertension will result in myriad cardiac abnormalities, including left ventricular outflow obstruction, coronary artery disease, stroke, and kidney failure.

CHEST PAIN AND FATIGUE

Chest pain and fatigue are fairly common complaints among older children and adolescents. The cause is seldom cardiac. However, if cardiac causes are present, they are generally serious.

Causes of Chest Pain in Children
1. Congenital coronary abnormalities
   a. Anomalous coronary origin
   b. Coronary fistula
2. Acquired Coronary Disease
   a. Kawasaki's disease
   b. Emboli
3. Aortic Stenosis
4. Hypertrophic cardiomyopathy
5. Dilated cardiomyopathy
6. Pericarditis
7. Sinus of Valsalva aneurysm

As previously stated, these are rare, but their seriousness requires that the echo exam for chest pain in children must be accurate and comprehensive. Particular attention should be paid to the coronary arteries.

Fatigue in children is also rarely cardiac related, but some cardiac findings may be:

Dilated cardiomyopathy
Hypertrophic cardiomyopathy
Shunts
Aortic stenosis
Pulmonic stenosis

As in cases of chest pain, a complete echo exam is required to rule out any cardiac source.

REFERENCES

1. Anderson R, Ho SY. Echocardiographic diagnosis and description of congenital heart disease: anatomic principles and philosophy. In: St. John Sutton M, Oldershaw PJ, eds. *Textbook of Adult and Pediatric Echocardiography and Doppler.* Boston: Blackwell Scientific; 1989: 573–606.
2. Silverman NS, Araujo LML. An echocardiographic method for the diagnosis of cardiac situs and malpositions. *Echocardiography.* 1987; 4:35–57.
3. Van Hare GF, Silverman NH. Contrast two-dimensional echocardiography in congenital heart disease: techniques, indications and clinical utility. *J Am Coll Cardiol.* 1989; 13:673–686.
4. Foale R, Stefanini L, Rickards A, et al. Left and right ventricular morphology in complex congenital heart disease defined by two-dimensional echocardiography. *Am J Cardiol.* 1982; 49:93.
5. Sutherland GR, Smallhorn JF, Anderson RH, et al. Atrioventricular discordance: cross-sectional echocardiographic morphological correlative study. *Br Heart J.* 1983; 50:8.
6. Tani L, Ludomirsky A, Murphy DJ, et al. Ventricular morphology: echocardiographic evaluation of isolated ventricular inversion. *Echocardiography.* 1988; 5:39–42.
7. Adams FH, Emmanouilides GC, Riemenschneider TA, eds. *Moss' Heart Disease in Infants, Children, & Adolescents.* 4th ed. Baltimore: Williams & Wilkins; 1989.
8. Hatle L, Angelsen B. *Doppler Ultrasound in Cardiology: Physical Principles and Clinical Applications.* 2nd ed. Philadelphia: Lea & Febiger; 1985.
9. Sahn DJ, Valdes-Cruz LM. Ultrasound Doppler methods for calculating cardiac volume flows, cardiac output and cardiac shunts. In: Kotler MN, Steiner RM, eds. *Cardiac Imaging: New Technologies and Clinical Applications.* Philadelphia: FA Davis; 1986: 19–31.
10. Cloez JL, Schmidt KG, Birk E, Silverman NS. Determination of pulmonary to systemic blood flow ratio in children by a simplified Doppler echocardiographic method. *J Am Coll Cardiol.* 1987; 11:825–830.
11. Stevenson JG. Doppler evaluation of atrial septal defect, ventricular septal defect, and complex malformations. *Acta Paediatr Scand.* 1986; 329 (suppl):21–43.
12. Stevenson JG. The use of Doppler echocardiography for detection and estimation of severity of patent ductus arteriosus, ventricular septal defect and atrial septal defect. *Echocardiography.* 1987; 4:321–346.
13. Silverman NH, Schmidt KG. The current role of Doppler echocardiography in the diagnosis of heart disease in children. *Cardiol Clin.* 1989; 7:265–297.
14. Fuster V, Driscoll DJ, McGoon DC. Congenital heart disease in adolescents and adults. In: Brandenburg RO, Fuster V, Giulani ER, McGoon DC, eds. *Cardiology: Fundamentals and Practice.* Chicago: Year Book Medical; 1987: 1386–1458.
15. Kosturakis D, Goldberg SJ, Allen HD, et al. Doppler echocardiographic prediction of pulmonary arterial hypertension in congenital heart disease. *Am J Cardiol.* 1984; 53:1110–1114.

16. Marantz P, Capelli H, Ludomirsky A, et al. Echocardiographic assessment of balloon atrial septostomy in patients with transposition of the great arteries: prediction of the need for early surgery. *Echocardiography.* 1988; 5:99–104.

17. Weyman AE, Dillon JC, Feigenbaum H, et al. Echocardiographic patterns of pulmonic valve motion with pulmonary hypertension. *Circulation.* 1974; 50:905–910.

18. Stevenson JG. Comparison of several noninvasive methods for estimation of pulmonary artery pressure. *J Am Soc Echo.* 1989; 2:157–171.

19. Yock PG, Popp RL. Noninvasive estimation of right ventricular systolic pressure by Doppler ultrasound in patients with tricuspid regurgitation. *Circulation.* 1984; 70:657–662.

20. Beard JT, Byrd BF. Saline contrast enhancement of trivial Doppler tricuspid regurgitation signals for estimating pulmonary artery pressure. *Am J Cardiol.* 1988; 62:486–488.

21. Masuyama T, Kodama D, Kitabatake A, et al. Continuous wave Doppler echocardiographic detection of pulmonary regurgitation and its application to noninvasive estimation of pulmonary artery pressure. *Circulation.* 1986; 74:484–492.

22. Kitabatake A, Inoue M, Asao M, et al. Noninvasive evaluation of pulmonary hypertension by a pulse Doppler technique. *Circulation.* 1983; 68:302–309.

23. Fink, BW. *Congenital Heart Disease: A Deductive Approach to Its Diagnosis.* 2nd ed. Chicago: Year Book Medical; 1985.

24. Sahn DJ, Allen HD. Real-time cross-sectional echocardiographic imaging and measurement of the patent ductus arteriosus in infants and children. *Circulation.* 1978; 58:343–354.

25. Seward JB, Tajik AJ, Edwards WD, Hagler DJ. *Two-Dimensional Echocardiographic Atlas.* vol I: *Congenital Heart Disease.* New York: Springer, 1987.

26. Smallhorn JF. Patent ductus arteriosus—evaluation by echocardiography. *Echocardiography.* 1987; 4:101–118.

27. Smallhorn JF, Huhta JC, Anderson RH, et al. Suprasternal cross-sectional echocardiography in assessment of patent ductus arteriosus. *Br Heart J.* 1982; 48:321–330.

28. Kyo S. Congenital heart disease. In: Omoto R., ed. *Color Atlas of Real-Time Two-Dimensional Doppler Echocardiography.* 2nd ed. Philadelphia: Lea & Febiger; 1987: 149–209.

29. Ritter SB. Application of Doppler color flow mapping in the assessment and the evaluation of congenital heart disease. *Echocardiography.* 1987; 4:543–556.

30. Snider AR. Doppler echocardiography in congenital heart disease. In: Berger M, ed. *Doppler Echocardiography in Heart Disease.* New York: Marcel Dekker; 1987.

31. Armstrong, WF. Congenital heart disease. In: Feigenbaum H, ed. *Echocardiography.* 4th ed. Philadelphia: Lea & Febiger; 1986: 365–461.

32. Perry SB, Keane JF, Lock JE. Interventional catheterization in pediatric congenital and acquired heart disease. *Am J Cardiol.* 1988; 61:109G–117G.

33. NeSmith J, Philips J. The sonographer's beginning guide to surgery for congenital heart disease. *J Am Soc Echo.* 1988; 1:384–387.

34. Sanders SP. Echocardiography and related techniques in the diagnosis of congenital heart defects Part I: Veins, atria and interatrial septum. *Echocardiography.* 1984; 1:185–217.

35. Schmidt KG, Silverman NH. Cross-sectional and contrast echocardiography in the diagnosis of interatrial communications through the coronary sinus. *Int J Cardiol.* 1987; 16:193–199.

36. Lin F, Fu M, Yeh, S, et al. Doppler atrial shunt flow patterns in patients with secundum atrial septal defect: determinants, limitations and pitfalls. *J Am Soc Echo.* 1988; 1:141–149.

37. Fraker TD, Harris PJ, Behar VS, et al. Detection and exclusion of interatrial shunts by two-dimensional echocardiography and peripheral venous injection. *Circulation.* 1979; 59:379–384.

38. Valdez-Cruz LM, Sahn DJ. Ultrasonic contrast studies for the detection of cardiac shunts. *J Am Coll Cardiol.* 1984; 3:978–985.

39. Sanders SP. Echocardiography and related techniques in the diagnosis of congenital heart defects Part II: Atrioventricular valves and ventricles. *Echocardiography.* 1984; 1:333–391.

40. Goldfarb BL, Wanderman KL, Rovner M, et al. Ventricular septal defect with left ventricular to right atrial shunt: documentation by color flow Doppler and avoidance of the pitfall of the diagnosis of tricuspid regurgitation and pulmonary hypertension. *Echocardiography.* 1989; 6:521–525.

41. Ritter S, Rothe W, Kawai D, et al. Identification of ventricular septal defects by Doppler color flow mapping. *Clin Res.* 1988; 36:311A.

42. Stevenson JG, Kawabori I, Dooley T, et al. Diagnosis of ventricular septal defects by pulsed Doppler echocardiography. *Circulation.* 1978; 58:322–326.

43. Murphy DJ, Ludomirsky A, Huhta JC. Continuous-wave Doppler in children with ventricular septal defect: noninvasive estimation of interventricular pressure gradient. *Am J Cardiol.* 1986; 57:428–432.

44. Schmidt KG, Cassidy SC, Silverman, NH. Doubly committed subarterial ventricular septal defects: echocardiographic features and surgical implications. *Am Coll Cardiol.* 1988; 12:1538–1546.

45. Cassidy SC, Van Hare GF, Silverman NH. The probability of detecting a subaortic ridge in children with ventricular septal defect or coarctation of the aorta. *Am J Cardiol.* 1990; 66:505–508.

46. Silverman NH, Zuberbuhler JR, Anderson RH. Atrioventricular septal defects: Cross-sectional echocardiographic and morphologic comparisons. *Int J Cardiol.* 1986; 13:309–331.

47. Brenner JI, Baker KR, Berman MA. Prediction of left ventricular pressure in infants with aortic stenosis. *Br Heart J.* 1980; 44:406–410.

48. Rakowski H, Sasson Z, Wigle ED. Echocardiographic and Doppler assessment of hypertrophic cardiomyopathy. *J Am Soc Echo.* 1988, 1:31–47.

49. McKay RG. Balloon valvuloplasty for treating pulmonic, mitral, and aortic valve stenosis. *Am J Cardiol.* 1988; 61:102G–108G.

50. Sweeney MS, Walker WE, Cooley DA, et al. Apicoaortic conduits for complex left ventricular outflow obstruction: 10-year experience. *Ann Thorac Surg.* 1986; 42: 609–611.

51. Huhta JC, Gutgesell HP, Latson LA, et al. Two-dimensional echocardiographic assessment of the aorta in infants and children with congenital heart disease. *Circulation.* 1984; 70:417–424.

52. Nihoyannopoulos P, Karas S, Sapsford RN, et al. Accuracy of two-dimensional echocardiography in the diagnosis of aortic arch obstruction. *J Am Coll Cardiol.* 1987; 10:1072–1077.

53. George B, DiSessa TG, Williams R, et al. Coarctation repair without cardiac catheterization in infants. *Am Heart J.* 1987; 114:1421–1425.

54. Bash SE, Huhta JC, Vick GW, et al. Hypoplastic left heart syndrome: Is echocardiography accurate enough to guide surgical palliation? *J Am Coll Cardiol.* 1986; 7: 610–616.

55. Burrows PE, Freedom RM, Rabinovitch M, et al. The investigation of abnormal pulmonary arteries in congenital heart disease. *Radiol Clin North Am.* 1985; 23: 689–717.

56. Smallhorn J. Right ventricular outflow tract obstruction. In: St. John Sutton M, Oldershaw P, eds. *Textbook of Adult and Pediatric Echocardiography and Doppler.* Boston: Blackwell Scientific; 1989: 761–790.

57. Frantz, EG, Silverman, NH. Doppler ultrasound evaluation of valvar pulmonary stenosis from multiple transducer positions in children requiring pulmonary valvuloplasty. *Am J Cardiol.* 1988; 61:844–849.

58. Lipshultz SE, Sanders SP, Mayer JE, et al. Are routine preoperative cardiac catheterization and angiography necessary before repair of ostiuum primum atrial septal defect? *J Am Coll Cardiol.* 1988; 11:373–378.

59. Sullivan ID, Robinson PJ, DeLeval M, et al. Membranous supravalvular mitral stenosis: a treatable form of congenital heart disease. *J Am Coll Cardiol.* 1986; 8: 159–164.

60. Zuberbuhler JR, Anderson RH. Ebstein's malformation of the tricuspid valve: morphology and natural history. In Anderson RH, Neches WH, Park SC, Zuberbuhler JR, eds. *Perspectives in Pediatric Cardiology.* Mt. Kisco, NY: Futura Publishing; 1988: 99–112.

61. Silverman NS, Birk E. Ebstein's malformation of the tricuspid valve: cross-sectional echocardiography and Doppler. In: Anderson RH, Neches WH, Park SC, Zuberbuhler JR, eds. *Perspectives in Pediatric Cardiology.* Mount Kisco, NY: Futura Publishing; 1988: 113–125.

62. McIrvin DM, Murphy DJ, Ludomirsky A. Tetralogy of Fallot with absent pulmonary valve. *Echocardiography.* 1989; 6:363–367.

63. Caldwell RL, Ensing GJ. Coronary artery abnormalities in children. *J Am Soc Echo.* 1989; 2:259–268.

64. Smallhorn J. Complete transposition. In: St. John Sutton M, Oldershaw P, eds. *Textbook of Adult and Pediatric Echocardiography and Doppler.* Boston: Blackwell Scientific; 1989: 791–808.

65. Meyer RA. Echocardiography in Kawasaki disease. *J Am Soc Echo.* 1989; 2:269–275.

66. Neches WH. Kawasaki syndrome. In: Anderson RH, Neches WH, Park SC, Zuberbuhler JR, eds: *Perspectives in Pediatric Cardiology.* Mount Kisco, NY: Futura Publishing; 1988: 411–424.

67. Lloyd TR, Mahoney LT, Marvin WJ, et al. Identification of coronary artery to right ventricular fistulae by color flow mapping. *Echocardiography.* 1988; 5:115–120.

68. Velvis H, Schmidt KG, Silverman NH, et al. Diagnosis of coronary artery fistula by two-dimensional echocardiography pulsed Doppler ultrasound and color flow imaging. *J Am Coll Cardiol.* 1989; 14:968–976.

69. Zellers TM, Hagler DJ, Julsrud PR. Accuracy of two-dimensional echocardiography in diagnosing left superior vena cava. *J Am Soc Echo.* 1989; 2:132–138.

70. Huhta, JC, Smallhorn JF, Macartney FJ, et al. Cross-sectional echocardiographic diagnosis of systemic venous return. *Br Heart J.* 1980; 44:718–723.

71. Van Hare GF, Schmidt KG, Cassidy SC, et al. Color Doppler flow mapping in the ultrasound diagnosis of total anomalous pulmonary venous connection. *J Am Soc Echo.* 1988; 1:341–347.

Questions

GENERAL INSTRUCTIONS: For each question, select the best answer. Select only one answer for each question unless otherwise specified.

1. The most common type of atrial septal defect is

   (A) primum
   (B) secundum
   (C) sinus venosus
   (D) single atrium

2. Which transducer position is most helpful in the 2-D visualization of atrial septal defects?

   (A) left parasternal
   (B) apical
   (C) subxiphoid
   (D) right parasternal

3. Partial anomalous pulmonary venous return is most commonly associated with which type of atrial septal defect?

   (A) secundum
   (B) primum
   (C) sinus venosus
   (D) coronary sinus

4. What is the most common congenital heart lesion in the pediatric population?

   (A) mitral stenosis
   (B) atrial septal defect
   (C) ventricular septal defect
   (D) pulmonary stenosis

5. A "T-sign" artifact demonstrated by _____ is useful in the detection of ventricular septal defects.

   (A) M-mode
   (B) 2-D
   (C) pulsed-wave Doppler
   (D) continuous-wave Doppler
   (E) color flow Doppler

6. A small muscular ventricular septal defect may be most easily localized by

   (A) M-mode
   (B) 2-D
   (C) pulsed-wave Doppler
   (D) continuous-wave Doppler
   (E) color flow Doppler

7. Which of the following will *not* cause a reversal of flow in the descending aorta during diastole?

   (A) large patent ductus arteriosus with severe pulmonary hypertension (suprasystemic pulmonary pressures)
   (B) severe aortic insufficient
   (C) surgically created systemic to pulmonary shunt with normal pulmonary artery pressures
   (D) large patent ductus arteriosus with normal pulmonary artery pressures

8. Which of the following may be associated with valvar aortic stenosis?

   (A) patent ductus arteriosus
   (B) coarctation of the aorta
   (C) ventricular septal defect
   (D) pulmonary stenosis
   (E) all of the above

9. The most commonly associated lesion in patients with coarctation of the aorta is

   (A) ventricular septal defect
   (B) bicuspid aortic valve
   (C) patent ductus arteriosus
   (D) aortic stenosis
   (E) mitral stenosis

10. In the normally related heart, the aortic valve lies

    (A) anterior and to the left of the pulmonary valve
    (B) anterior and to the right of the pulmonary valve
    (C) posterior and to the right of the pulmonary valve
    (D) posterior and to the left of the pulmonary valve

11. Which of the following surgical procedures is *not* frequently used to treat transposition of the great arteries?

(A) Senning procedure
(B) Mustard procedure
(C) Jatene procedure
(D) Fontan procedure

12. Which of the following is also known as the arterial switch procedure?

(A) Rashkind procedure
(B) Mustard procedure
(C) Jatene procedure
(D) Senning procedure

13. When the aorta and pulmonary artery are transposed, they course _____ as they exit the heart.

(A) parallel to each other
(B) perpendicular to each other
(C) wound around each other
(D) in no particular relationship to each other

14. Balloon atrial septostomy is most commonly performed in infants who have

(A) Ebstein anomaly of the tricuspid valve
(B) transposition of the great arteries
(C) truncus arteriosus
(D) tetralogy of Fallot

15. Of all children who suffer from Kawasaki disease, _____ will develop coronary artery aneurysms.

(A) 2%
(B) 15%
(C) 50%
(D) 75%
(E) 100%

16. Which of the following groups is most likely to develop coronary artery aneurysms as a complication of Kawasaki disease?

(A) toddlers
(B) infants
(C) adolescents
(D) adults

17. Which of the following is *not* useful in the assessment of pulmonary artery pressure?

(A) peak Doppler gradient through a patent ductus arteriosus
(B) peak Doppler gradient of tricuspid regurgitation
(C) end-diastolic Doppler gradient of pulmonary insufficiency
(D) acceleration time to ejection time ratio calculated from a right ventricular outflow tract velocity curve
(E) all of the above are useful in estimating pulmonary artery pressure

18. A child with tetralogy of Fallot is upset and crying during the echocardiogram. The Doppler gradient through the right ventricular outflow tract will be _____ than if the child were sleeping peacefully.

(A) greater
(B) less
(C) outflow obstruction in tetralogy of Fallot is not affected by the patient's activity

19. A 3-year old child with Kawasaki disease is referred to echocardiology. Which of the following views is not really necessary in the 2-D evaluation of the coronary arterial system?

(A) subcostal transverse
(B) parasternal short axis
(C) apical five chamber
(D) subcostal coronal
(E) all views are helpful

20. Which of the following Doppler findings is *not* characteristic of coarctation of the aorta?

(A) forward flow through the descending aorta extending throughout diastole
(B) normal or slightly increased velocity of flow in the aorta proximal to the left subclavian artery
(C) rapid acceleration and deceleration of the Doppler signal taken from the descending aorta
(D) Doppler signal from the descending aorta does not return to baseline during diastole
(E) high-velocity flow detected in the descending aorta distal to the left subclavian artery

21. Careful echocardiographic evaluation of a child with complex congenital heart disease reveals absence of the inferior vena cava above the level of the renal arteries. The aorta is to the left of the spine. What is this child's situs mostly likely to be?

(A) solitus
(B) inversus
(C) left atrial isomerism
(D) right atrial isomerism

22. The characteristic aortic valve M-mode tracing from a patient with discrete membranous subaortic stenosis demonstrates

(A) an asymmetric closure line
(B) early closure and partial reopening
(C) gradual closure (drifting closed)
(D) prolonged ejection time

23. Which of the following should *not* be included in the differential diagnosis when a Doppler tracing such as that in Fig. 4–1 is obtained from the descending aorta?

(A) patent ductus arteriosus
(B) severe aortic regurgitation
(C) arteriovenous malformation
(D) aortic to pulmonary window
(E) coarctation of the aorta

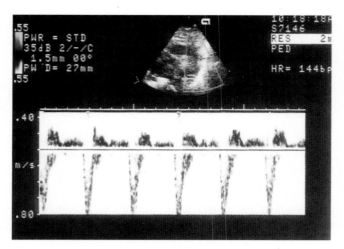

Figure 4–1. Pulsed Doppler spectral tracing of flow in the descending aorta as obtained from the suprasternal notch view.

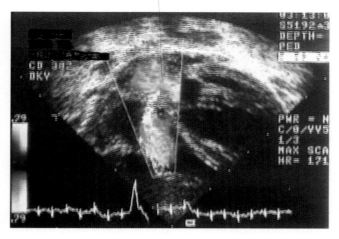

Figure 4–3. Color flow Doppler image of a subcostal four-chamber view presented with the apex down (anatomically correct) presentation. The patient is an 8-month-old female with trisomy 21.

24. An echocardiogram was requested for a premature infant in the neonatal intensive care unit who appeared clinically to be in congestive failure and in whom a murmur was heard. The color flow Doppler image in Fig. 4–2 was taken from the ductus view, which is a parasternal sagittal view. The closed aortic valve may be appreciated in the center of the image. This image demonstrates

   (A) a small patent ductus arteriosus
   (B) a moderate patent ductus arteriosus
   (C) a large patent ductus arteriosus
   (D) no ductus arteriosus

25. The image in Fig. 4–3 was taken from an 8-month-old female with trisomy 21. The color flow Doppler image was taken from the subcostal four-chamber view. The image demonstrates

   (A) a left-to-right shunt through a primum atrial septal defect
   (B) a right-to-left shunt through a primum atrial septal defect
   (C) a left-to-right shunt through a secundum atrial septal defect
   (D) a right-to-left shunt through a secundum atrial septal defect
   (E) a normal heart

26. The images presented in Fig. 4–4 were taken from the cardiac apex of a cyanotic infant. These images demonstrate

   (A) a normal heart
   (B) an isolated inflow ventricular septal defect
   (C) single atrium
   (D) tricuspid atresia with ventricular septal defect
   (E) tricuspid atresia with intact ventricular septum

27. The color flow Doppler image presented in Fig. 4–5 was taken from an 8-year-old male with a systolic murmur. The image is of the parasternal short axis view during early systole and demonstrates a left to right shunt through a(n)

   (A) inflow ventricular septal defect
   (B) membranous ventricular septal defect
   (C) muscular ventricular septal defect
   (D) doubly committed subarterial ventricular septal defect

28. The 2-D image in Fig. 4–6 was taken from the cardiac apex and demonstrates

   (A) a normal apical four-chamber view
   (B) tricuspid atresia
   (C) Ebstein anomaly of the tricuspid valve
   (D) ventricular inversion

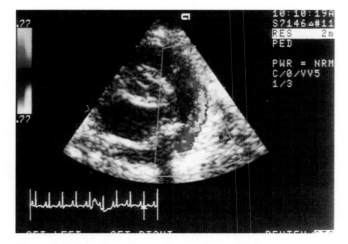

Figure 4–2. Color flow Doppler image of a modified short-axis parasternal view, known as the "ductus view." The patient is a premature infant in congestive heart failure in whom a murmur is heard.

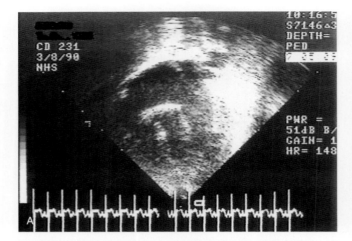

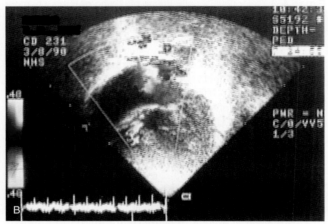

Figure 4–4. Apical four-chamber view presented with the apex down. (A) 2-D image. (B) Color flow Doppler image. The patient is a cyanotic infant.

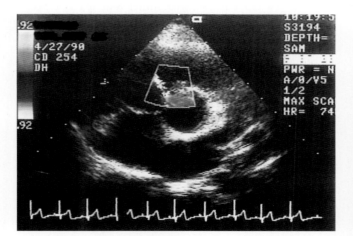

Figure 4–5. Color flow Doppler image of the parasternal short-axis view at the level of the semilunar valves taken in early systole. The patient is an 8-year-old male in whom a systolic murmur may be heard.

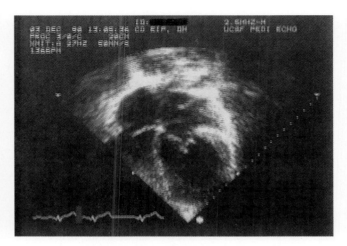

Figure 4–6. 2-D image of the apical four-chamber view presented with the apex down.

29. The 2-D image of the parasternal long-axis view presented in Fig. 4–7 was taken during diastole and demonstrates

    (A) a normal heart
    (B) valvular aortic stenosis
    (C) discrete membranous subaortic stenosis
    (D) idiopathic hypertrophic subaortic stenosis

30. If the left ventricular outflow tract of the patient presented in Fig. 4–7 was interrogated by PW Doppler, what is the most proximal location at which an increase in velocity would be detected?

    (A) just proximal to the aortic valve
    (B) at the aortic valve
    (C) just distal to the aortic valve
    (D) in the aortic root
    (E) distal to the left subclavian artery

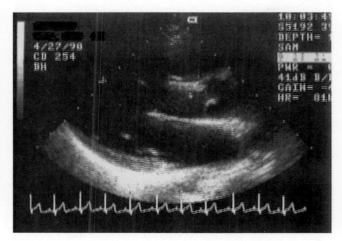

Figure 4–7. 2-D image of a parasternal long-axis view taken in diastole.

31. The 2-D parasternal short-axis view image pre-sented in Fig. 4–8 was taken from a young child who had recently had Kawasaki disease. This view demonstrates

    (A) left coronary artery involvement
    (B) right coronary artery involvement
    (C) both left and right coronary arteries are involved
    (D) normal coronary arteries

32. The 2-D parasternal short-axis view image pre-sented in Fig. 4–9 was taken from an infant who was diagnosed as having tetralogy of Fallot. This image demonstrates

    (A) a normal right ventricular outflow tract
    (B) infundibular pulmonary stenosis only
    (C) infundibular and valvular pulmonary stenosis
    (D) infundibular pulmonary stenosis with hypo-plasia of the pulmonary valve and main pulmonary artery

33. Which of the following views would *not* be helpful in delineating the size of left and right pulmonary arter-ies in the patient imaged for Fig. 4–9?

    (A) suprasternal coronal view
    (B) apical outflow view
    (C) subcostal short axis (sagittal) view
    (D) high left parasternal view
    (E) all of the above views would be useful

34. Which of the following methods is most reliable for estimating pulmonary artery pressures?

    (A) thickness of the right ventricular free wall
    (B) determination of the peak regurgitant gradient through the tricuspid valve

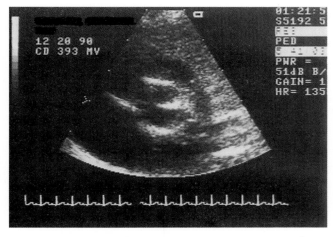

Figure 4–9. 2-D image of a parasternal short-axis view at the level of the semilunar valves. This infant has been diagnosed as having tetral-ogy of Fallot.

    (C) determination of the peak regurgitant gradient through the pulmonic view
    (D) dividing the acceleration time by the ejection time of flow as obtained from the main pul-monary artery

35. In which of the following surgically created shunts is the subclavian artery used?

    (A) Central
    (B) Glenn
    (C) Waterston
    (D) Blalock-Taussig
    (E) Potts

36. What is needed to estimate Q_p:Q_s in a patient with a ventricular septal defect?

    (A) diameters and peak flow velocities through the pulmonary and aortic valves
    (B) peak pressure gradient through a tricuspid regurgitation jet
    (C) diameters and peak flow velocities through the tricuspid and aortic valves
    (D) diameters and peak flow velocities through the pulmonary and mitral valves

37. The shunt through the atrial septal defect of a patient with tricuspid atresia is

    (A) always left to right
    (B) always right to left
    (C) may be bidirectional
    (D) nonexistent

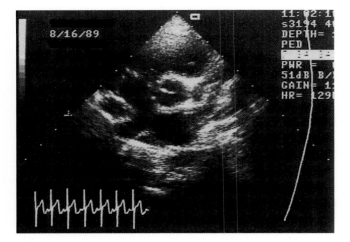

Figure 4–8. 2-D image of a parasternal short-axis view at the level of the semilunar valves. The patient is a young child who is in the con-valescent phase of Kawasaki's disease.

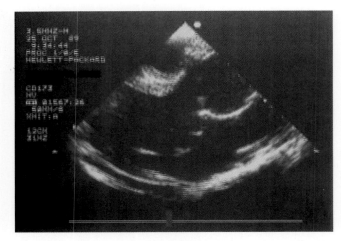

Figure 4–10. 2-D image of a parasternal long-axis view. The patient is an adolescent girl thought to have Marfan syndrome.

38. The 2-D image parasternal view presented in Fig. 4–10 was taken from an adolescent girl with Marfan syndrome. What abnormalities may be seen which are frequently associated with Marfan syndrome?

    (A) dilated aortic root and mitral valve prolapse
    (B) aortic aneurysm dissection
    (C) idiopathic hypertrophic subaortic stenosis
    (D) herniation of the sinus of Valsalva

39. The 2-D image presented in Fig. 4–11 was taken from the apex in a child who has had corrective surgery for transposition of the great arteries. The echogenic line in the left atrium represents

    (A) cortriatriatum
    (B) supramitral ring
    (C) total anomalous pulmonary venous return
    (D) an interatrial baffle

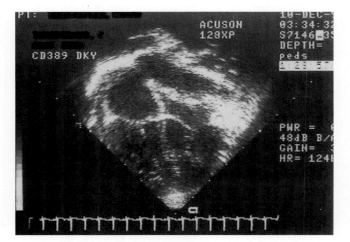

Figure 4–11. 2-D image of an apical four-chamber view presented with the apex down. This young child has had a previous repair for transposition of the great vessels.

40. If a patient has total anomalous pulmonary venous return, the right atrium should be

    (A) atretic
    (B) small
    (C) normal in size
    (D) dilated

41. The most useful modality in the delineation of anatomy in total anomalous pulmonary venous return is

    (A) 2-D
    (B) M-mode
    (C) PW Doppler
    (D) CW Doppler
    (E) color flow Doppler

TRUE OR FALSE: Indicate whether each of the following statements is true or false.

42. Patent ductus arteriosus is more commonly seen in low birth weight premature infants than in term infants.

43. Patency of the ductus arteriosus may be desirable in some cases.

44. In cortriatriatum, the left atrial appendage is continuous with the anatomic left atrium and not with the proximal chamber that receives flow directly from the pulmonary veins.

45. Children with trisomy 21 frequently have partial atrioventricular septal defects.

46. Patients with truncus arteriosus are usually quite cyanotic in infancy.

47. Individuals with Ebstein anomaly of the tricuspid valve are always symptomatic.

48. Distal coronary artery aneurysms are common in the absence of proximal aneurysm formation in patients who have had Kawasaki disease.

49. In patients with coarctation of the aorta, the gradient through the obstruction should approximate the difference in systolic blood pressures taken from the arm and leg of the patient.

50. Persistent left superior vena cava may exist in the absence of a dilated coronary sinus.

For each of the following transducer positions, indicate (true or false) whether the position could yield the highest pressure gradient estimate in a patient with valvular pulmonary stenosis.

51. parasternal

52. apical

53. subcostal

54. suprasternal

The 2-D image in Fig. 4–12 was obtained by placing the transducer at the cardiac apex of an infant. The infant was referred to echocardiology because of an enlarged heart on chest x-ray and cardiac failure. A systolic murmur may be heard at the apex. Indicate whether statements 55–60 are true or false for this image.

55. There is a secundum atrial septal defect.

56. There is a primum atrial septal defect.

57. The tricuspid valve appears normal.

58. The left ventricle is significantly smaller in size than the right ventricle.

59. The diagnosis for this patient is Ebstein anomaly of the tricuspid valve.

60. The systolic murmur is probably caused by aortic stenosis.

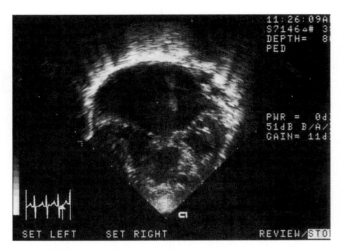

Figure 4–12. 2-D image of an apical four-chamber view presented with the apex down. This infant was in cardiac failure and reportedly had an enlarged heart on chest-x-ray. A systolic murmur may be heard at the apex.

Answers and Explanations

At the end of each explained answer there is a number combination in parentheses. The first number identifies the reference source; the second number or set of numbers indicates the page or pages on which the relevant information can be found.

1. **(B)** Sinus venosus is the rarest form, and the single atrium is not considered to be an atrial septal defect because there is complete absence of the atrial septum. *(14:1391)*

2. **(C)** In the subxiphoid position, the sound beam is perpendicular to the interatrial septum, thereby utilizing the axial resolution of the transducer. The atrial septum may also be visualized from the parasternal short axis view but it is more parallel to the sound beam and, therefore, may not be resolved optimally. In the apical position, the sound beam is parallel to the atrial septum, and the atrial septum is a great distance from the transducer, so echo-cardiographic dropout may be mistaken for an atrial communication. *(25:144–147)*

3. **(C)** Sinus venosus atrial septal defects are bordered posteriorly by the posterior atrial wall and superiorly by the entrance of the superior vena cava. Because of this, the upper right pulmonary vein may empty into the right atrium or superior vena cava. *(7:175)*

4. **(C)** Atrial septal defect and pulmonary stenosis are also common. Mitral stenosis is relatively uncommon in the pediatric population. *(7:190)*

5. **(B)** The "T" artifact is visualized on 2-D echocardiography as a prominence of echoes at the edges of the septal tissue. *(31:415)*

6. **(E)** Muscular VSDs may occur anywhere and be very small. Color flow Doppler allows relatively repaid evaluation of the entire interventricular septum. Visualization of a jet of turbulent flow identifies a VSD, PW, or CW Doppler interrogation can be tedious and may miss a small muscular defect in an unusual position. *(29:544–548)*

7. **(A)** When pulmonary pressures exceed systemic pressures, the flow through the patient ductus arteriosus will be right to left; therefore, there would be no reversal in the descending aorta. All of the other choices should cause a reversal of flow in the descending aorta. *(13:285–287)*

8. **(E)** Although patent ductus arteriosus and coarctation of the aorta are more commonly associated with valvar aortic stenosis, ventricular septal defect and pulmonary stenosis may also be associated. *(7:224)*

9. **(B)** Although all of the listed malformations may be associated findings, bicuspid aortic valve has been reported to be an associated finding in as much as 85% of cases. *(7:244)*

10. **(C)** The aortic view is posterior and to the right of the pulmonic valve in the normally related heart. The aortic valve is located centrally in the base of the heart, whereas the pulmonic valve is anterior and left. *(1:578–581)*

11. **(D)** The Fontan procedure was originally developed to treat patients with tricuspid atresia. Although it is now used in a modified form to treat other forms of complex congenital heart disease, it is not commonly used to treat patients with transposition of the great arteries. *(7:357–359, 402–417)*

12. **(C)** The Rashkind procedure is an interventional catheterization technique that also is known as a balloon atrial septostomy. The Mustard and Senning procedures also are known as atrial switches. *(7:402–417)*

13. **(A)** Normally related great vessels course perpendicular to each other. Demonstration of this relationship rules out transposition of the great vessels. *(25:498)*

14. **(B)** The purpose of an atrial septostomy is to mix deoxygenated systemic venous return with oxygenated pulmonary venous return. In truncus arteriosus and tetralogy of Fallot, this mixing occurs through a large ventricular septal defect. In Ebstein anomaly of the tricuspid valve, blood flow sequence is normal, therefore, mixing is not desirable. *(7:399–400)*

15. (B) There is about a 15% incidence of coronary artery aneurysm formation in children with Kawasaki disease. *(65:269)*

16. (B) Kawasaki disease is a childhood disease. Infants seem to be more likely to develop aneurysms than other children. *(65:273)*

17. (E) All of the above that are available should be used. *(8:223; 18:157–171)*

18. (A) The right ventricular outflow obstruction of tetralogy of Fallot is a dynamic obstruction; therefore, it may increase when the patient is distressed. *(7:278)*

19. (E) Although the proximal portions are the most frequently involved, the coronary system should be evaluated from every available view because aneurysms may occur anywhere. *(65:269–273)*

20. (C) In coarctation of the aorta, the descending aortic flow pulsatility is blunted such that the Doppler signal shows a slow acceleration and deceleration. *(8:217–221)*

21. (D) In situs solitus, the aorta descends anterior and to the left of the spine and the inferior vena cava ascends to the right of the spine. In situs inversus, the opposite is true. In left atrial isomerism, the inferior vena cava is frequently interrupted. *(2:35–56)*

22. (B) An asymmetric closure line is suggestive of a bicuspid aortic valve. Gradual closure is suggestive of depressed left ventricular contractility. Ejection time may be prolonged in severe valvular aortic stenosis. *(31:380–386)*

23. (E) Reversal of flow during diastole, as shown in Fig. 4–1, may be seen in any of the other conditions. The characteristic PW Doppler pattern in the descending aorta is very different for coarctation of the aorta. *(8:217–228; 13:279–295)*

24. (B) From the ECG, we can see that this is an end-diastolic frame. The 2-D image shows closed aortic and pulmonary valves, confirming that this is an end-diastolic frame. Red color representing flow toward the transducer may be appreciated coming into the main pulmonary artery from the patent ductus arteriosus. *(28:161–162, 189–190)*

25. (C) The red jet seen traversing the interatrial septum represents flow coming toward the transducer, therefore, it is shunting from the left atrium to the right atrium. Portions of the superior and inferior interatrial septum may be seen in the 2-D image. *(29:548–550)*

26. (D) The mitral vale is open in Fig. 4–4A. A thick bank of tissue appears in place of a normal tricuspid valve. A ventricular septal defect may be appreciated at the top of the ventricular septum in this image. In Fig. 4–4B, flow through the ventricular septal defect into the right ventricle is demonstrated by color flow Doppler during systole. *(31:374–375)*

27. (B) Flow through an inflow ventricular septal defect would be visualized at the level of the mitral annulus. Flow through a doubly committed subarterial ventricular septal defect would be visualized just proximal to the pulmonary valve in this view. Flow through a muscular ventricular septal defect would be visualized in the muscular portion of the ventricular septum. This portion of the ventricular septum is visible from the parasternal short axis at the level of the mitral valve and more apically. *(31:155–161, 183–188)*

28. (D) The mitral valve is always higher on the ventricular septum in the absence of an inflow ventricular septal defect. In this case, the atrioventricular valve of the right-sided ventricle inserts higher on the ventricular septum than the atrioventricular valve of the left-sided ventricle. *(25:324–325)*

29. (C) The aortic valve is closed and does not appear thickened. There is an echogenic line that extends posteriorly from the ventricular septum just proximal to the aortic valve. This represents a discrete subaortic membrane. In idiopathic hypertrophic subaortic stenosis, the interventricular septum would be significantly thickened. *(25:424–427)*

30. (A) Valvular aortic stenosis would cause the velocity of flow to increase just distal to the valve. Supravalvular aortic stenosis would cause the velocity of flow to increase in the aortic root. Coarctation of the aorta would cause the velocity of flow to increase past the level of the left subclavian artery. *(31:382)*

31. (C) The left coronary artery appears mildly dilated, and the large circle noted in the right atrium is the right coronary artery (with aneurysmal dilatation) as it courses within the right atrioventricular groove. *(65:268–273)*

32. (D) The entire right ventricular outflow tract is small in caliber. *(25:434)*

33. (E) The pulmonary artery branches may be imaged from all of these views. *(56:767–782)*

34. **(B)** The thickness of the right ventricular free wall may not be proportionate to the increase in pulmonary artery pressure. The end-diastolic and not peak gradient of pulmonary regurgitation may be used. Acceleration and ejection time should be measured from the right ventricular outflow tract.   *(18:157–171)*

35. **(D)** The subclavian artery is used in the construction of the Blalock-Taussig shunt. In a central shunt, the pulmonary artery is connected to the aorta directly or via a conduit. In the Waterston shunt, the ascending aorta is connected to the right pulmonary artery, and in the Potts anastomosis, the descending aorta is connected to the pulmonary artery.   *(33:384–385)*

36. **(A)** $Q_p:Q_s$ is a comparison of pulmonary flow to systemic flow used to estimate the amount of blood flow through a systemic to pulmonary shunt. Flow is calculated by multiplying area by velocity of flow. This calculation must be done for the systemic circulation and for the pulmonary circulation. When the shunt is at the level of the ventricles, pulmonary flow may be calculated using the pulmonary valve or the mitral valve (i.e., pulmonary venous return). The systemic flow may be calculated by using the aortic valve or tricuspid valve (i.e., systemic venous return). The calculation is done to determine how much more blood is going through the pulmonary vasculature than the systemic vasculature.   *(10:825–827; 12:339–344)*

37. **(B)** Because the atrial septal defect is the only outlet for the blood in the right atrium, it is an obligatory right to left shunt.   *(31:375)*

38. **(A)** Patients with Marfan syndrome are also at risk for aortic dissections, but only a limited amount of the aorta is visualized here. The other two abnormalities are not frequently associated with this syndrome.   *(7:792–793)*

39. **(D)** The echogenic line visualized in the left atrium in Fig. 4–11 is an interatrial baffle constructed to redirect blood flow in what is known as an "atrial switch."   *(25:552–557)*

40. **(E)** Because pulmonary venous flow returns directly to the right atrium, it will be dilated.   *(31:368–371)*

41. **(E)** Color flow aids tremendously in demonstrating the anomalous channels and connections.   *(71:341–347)*

42. **True.** Constriction of the ductus is physiologically delayed in this group.   *(7:209–218)*

43. **True.** Prostaglandin E may be administered to keep the ductus arteriosus patent in infants with severe right ventricular outflow obstruction or atresia or great vessel malformations.   *(7:221–222)*

44. **True.** The membrane inserts proximal to the left atrial appendage in cortriatriatum and distal to it in supravalvar mitral ring.   *(7:599–602)*

45. **False.** These children more commonly have the complete form of atrioventricular defect.   *(7:176)*

46. **False.** Significant cyanosis during infancy occur only when there is associated pulmonary stenosis.   *(7:507)*

47. **False.** There is a spectrum of severity in this malformation, and mild forms may remain asymptomatic.   *(23:142)*

48. **False.** It is very rare to have distal involvement in the absence of proximal aneurysm formation.   *(65:275)*

49. **True.** In severe cases, it may be difficult to obtain a reliable Doppler signal because of decreased flow through the area of obstruction. The Doppler derived gradient may be somewhat higher than the systolic pressure differences measured from the arm and thigh because peak systolic pressure occurs at slightly different times in these two areas; therefore, the blood pressure method yields a peak-to-peak pressure difference, whereas the Doppler method yields an instantaneous pressure difference.   *(8:217–219)*

50. **True.** Suprasternal coronal evaluation of the extracardiac vessel should be included in patients in whom this may be a concern for planning of surgical procedures.   *(69:137)*

51. **True.** This has traditionally been the most common position for evaluation of pulmonary valve stenosis.   *(56:765)*

52. **True.** The sound beam is angled anteriorly, and the transducer is moved to just below the left nipple.   *(57:844–848)*

53. **True.** The sound beam is angled anteriorly and slightly to the left.   *(56:765)*

54. **True.** In a few cases, this may be the only position from which a diagnostic Doppler signal can be obtained.   *(57:844–848)*

55. **False.** The area of the fossa ovalis appears to be intact.   *(7:173–174)*

56. **True.** The portion of atrial septum just above the level of the atrioventricular valves is absent.

(46:309–314)

57. **False.** There is a common atrioventricular valve with chordal insertions onto the ventricular septum.

(46:315–319)

58. **True.** The left ventricle is about one third the size of the right ventricle. The interventricular septum may be seen bowing into the left ventricle.

(46:319–330)

59. **False.** The diagnosis is an unbalanced complete atrioventricular septal defect. In Ebstein anomaly of the tricuspid valve, the tricuspid valve leaflets are adherent to the right ventricular walls.   *(25:293–305)*

60. **False.** The systolic murmur is probably caused by atrioventricular valve insufficiency.   *(7:181–187)*

REFERENCES

References appear on page 172.

CHAPTER 5

GENERAL ABDOMINAL SONOGRAPHY

Kerry E. Weinberg

Study Guide

Major Vessel Landmarks—Prevertebral vessels are used as landmarks to identify normal anatomy and pathology. All vessels are anechoic and are tubular shaped when imaged along their long axis and round or oval shaped in short axis. Most vessels follow a vertical course. It is important to know the location of the organ to help determine the long axis of the vessel. Fig. 5–1 demonstrates the prevertebral vessels.

Aorta—The aorta enters into the abdominal cavity through an orifice (opening) in the diaphragm at the level of the first lumbar vertebra (L1). It follows a vertical course anterior to the spine and slightly to the left of midline. An increased distance between the aorta and spine may indicate retroperitoneal pathology, such as adenopathy, fibrosis, or a hematoma.

The aorta bifurcates at the level of the umbilicus (L4) into the right and left common iliac arteries. The common iliac arteries branch into the internal iliac artery, which supply blood to the internal organs in the pelvis and to the external iliac arteries, which supplies blood to the lower extremities.

Measurements—The aorta decreases in size as it courses inferiorly. The normal AP dimension of the aorta lumen should be < 3 cm.

Thoracic:	2.5 cm
Diaphragm:	2.5–3.0 cm
Midabdomen:	2.0–2.5 cm
Renals:	1.8–2.0 cm
Bifurcation:	1.5–1.8 cm
Common iliac:	1.0–1.3 cm

Branches of the Aorta—superior to inferior

Celiac—the celiac axis or trunk branches off the anterior border of the aorta. It is approximately 2–3 cm long and trifurcates into:

1. ***The common hepatic artery,*** which follows a horizontal course to the right. The gastroduodenal artery is a branch of the common hepatic artery and follows a vertical course and is used as the landmark for the anterior lateral aspect of the head of the pancreas. After the gastroduodenal artery branch the common hepatic artery becomes the proper hepatic artery and enters the liver at the level of the porta hepatis. The hepatic artery courses anteriorly to the portal vein and adjacent to the common bile duct. Once the hepatic artery is intrahepatic it branches into the right, left, and middle hepatic arteries.
2. ***The left gastric artery*** is usually not visualized on ultrasound.
3. ***The splenic artery*** follows a tortuous horizontal course along the anterior superior border of the pancreas. It enters the spleen at the splenic helium.

Superior mesenteric artery (SMA) branches from the anterior border of the aorta and follows a vertical course anterior and parallel to the aorta. The SMA is posterior to the body of the pancreas.

Renal arteries branch from the posterior–lateral border of the aorta and course horizontally to the hilum of the kidneys. The right renal artery courses posteriorly to the inferior vena cava (IVC). The left renal artery courses directly into the renal hilum.

Gonadal arteries are small vessels that arise off the anterior border of the aorta and course vertically. They are not routinely visualized by ultrasound.

The ***inferior mesenteric artery*** is a small artery that branches off the anterior aspect of the aorta. It follows a vertical course and is slightly to the left of midline. It is not routinely imaged on an ultrasound examination. Doppler blood flow of the vessels is included in Chapter 6.

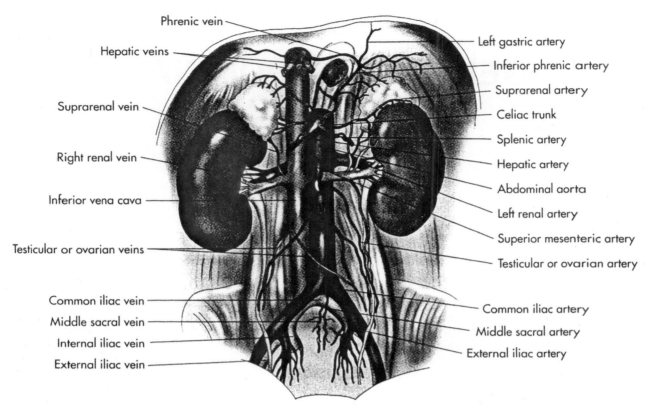

Figure 5–1. The abdominal aorta and its tributaries. *(Reprinted with permission from Hagen-Ansert S. Textbook of Diagnostic Ultrasonography. 5th ed. St. Louis: Mosby; 2001, 74.)*

PATHOLOGY OF ARTERIES

Arteriosclerosis—is primarily an arterial disease in which the vessel wall loses its elasticity and becomes hardened. Atherosclerosis is the most common form in which lipid deposits occur in the inner lining of the artery wall (tunica intima). These deposits may lead to fibrosis and calcifications.

Aneurysm is the dilatation of a segment of a vessel wall caused by a weakness of all three layers of the vessel wall. They are more common in arteries than veins. The most common cause of aneurysms is arteriosclerosis and associated hypertension. Other causes include: congenital weakness of a vessel wall, trauma, untreated syphilis, or infections, especially those resulting from bacterial endocarditis. Marfan syndrome is associated with aneurysms in the ascending portion of the aorta extending up to the aortic valve.

Aortic aneurysm is diagnosed when the aortic A/P diameter is > 3 cm. The aorta is measured from outer border to outer border. In addition, the size of the lumen is also measured when plaque or calcifications are present. Any aneurysm greater than 7 cm is at a great risk of rupturing. A ruptured aortic aneurysm has a 100% mortality rate. The location of the aneurysm is important to document, especially to note if the aneurysm is at the level of the renal arteries. The majority of aneurysms are located below the level of the renal arteries.

Aneurysms are classified as true, dissecting, or pseudo (false).

True aneurysm have dilatation of all three layers of the vessel wall (tunica intima, tunica media, tunica adventitia). Clinical findings include; palpable pulsitile abdominal mass of physical examination and back or leg pain. The following lists types of true aneurysms:

1. Fusiform: the most common type of aortic aneurysms characterized by an elongated spindle-shaped dilation of the artery
2. Saccular: characterized by a focal outpouching of the vessel wall. They are primarily caused by trauma or infection.
3. Berry: small round outpouchings 1–1.5 cm in diameter and are typically found within the cerebral vascular system. Rupture usually causes death.

Dissecting aneurysm (not a true aneurysm) occurs when there is a tear of the intima layer of the vessel wall causing blood to collect between the intima layer and media layer. The artery will have two lumens, a true lumen and a false lumen. Dissecting aneurysms are most commonly seen in people with hypertension or Marfan syndrome.

Clinical findings include severe pain over the site of the aneurysm and, in cases where the dissection is at the level of the ascending aorta, the pain may mimic a myocardial infarction (MI). Sonographic appearance may include the demonstration of two lumens with a pulsating intimal flap.

Pseudo aneurysm results from a tear in the vessel wall that permits blood to escape into the surrounding tissue. The blood becomes walled off from the vessel and presents as a mass adjacent to the vessel wall. Color Doppler is used to diagnose a pseudo aneurysm; the site of communication between the true lumen and false lumen may be demonstrated, and the blood flow in the false lumen is turbulent. The major causes are from either an arterial catheterization or trauma.

Inferior Vena Cava—The inferior vena cava (IVC) is formed at the confluence of the right and left common iliac veins at the level of the umbilicus (L5). The IVC lies slightly to the right of midline and courses anteriorly as it ascends into the right atrium of the heart. The IVC varies in size with respiration, increases with exhalation and held inspiration, and decreases with a Valsalva maneuver.

Major Branches into the IVC

Hepatic Veins—see section under liver.

Renal Veins—The right renal vein follows a short course from the hilum of the right kidney into the IVC. The left renal vein follows a course anterior to the aorta and posterior to the superior mesenteric artery before entering into the IVC.

Gonadal Veins—The right gonadal vein empties directly into the IVC. The left gonadal vein empties into the left renal vein, which drains into the IVC.

Pathology that Affects the Size of the IVC

The IVC is dilated with hepatomegaly, pulmonary hypertension, congestive heart failure (CHF), constrictive pericarditis, right atria myxoma, atherosclerotic heart disease, and right ventricular failure.

The most common tumor that involves the IVC is renal cell carcinoma. Renal cell carcinoma may invade the renal vein and IVC. This is more common with the right kidney because of the short distance the right renal vein has to travel to enter into the IVC. Thrombus may also be identified as low-level echoes within the IVC. Thrombus in the IVC may cause Budd–Chairi disease.

Causes of IVC Displacement

Lymphadenopathy
Mass in posterior, caudate, or right hepatic lobe of the liver
Right renal mass
Right adrenal mass
Tortuous aorta

Retroperitoneal tumors; retroperitoneal liposarcoma, leiomyosarcoma, osteosarcoma, rhabdomyosarcoma

Portal System—see liver section

LIVER

Gross anatomy of the liver—The liver is the largest organ in the body. The right lobe is five to six times larger than the left lobe. A longitudinal measurement of the right lobe greater then 15–17 cm is considered hepatomegaly. A Riedel's lobe is a normal variant of the right lobe of the liver, which is more common in women. The right lobe of the liver extends inferiorly and may be mistaken for a hepatomegaly or a tumor.

The liver is completely covered by Glisson's capsule. It is mostly an intraperitoneal organ except for the bare area posterior to the dome of the liver, porta hepatis region, and the gallbladder fossa region.

Parenchymal Architecture

The normal liver parenchyma is homogenous in texture, and its echogenicity may be compared to other abdominal organs. The following is going from the most echogenic to the least echogenic:

renal sinus > pancreas > liver $\geq$ spleen > renal cortex > renal medullary pyramids

Methods for Liver Division—Lobes, Ligaments, and Fissures (Figs. 5–2 and 5–3)

A number of different methods are used for liver division: hepatic veins, fissures, ligaments, and portal veins. Ligaments and fissures are used as landmarks in the more caudad liver sections. Couinaud's system (used for hepatic lesion localization) divides the liver into eight segments and uses both hepatic veins and portal veins as landmarks.

Lobes

Liver is subdivided by a number of methods. Anatomically, the liver is subdivided into three lobes: right—anterior and posterior segments; left—medial (quadrate) and lateral segments; and the caudate lobe—lies on the posteriosuperior surface of the left lobe. The hepatic veins are intersegmental and are used as sonographic landmarks on the superior aspect of the liver:

Middle Hepatic Vein—divides the liver into right and left lobes

Right Hepatic Vein—divides the right lobe of the liver into anterior and posterior segments

Left Hepatic Vein—divides the left lobe of the liver into medial and lateral segments

Both the right and left hepatic veins drain blood from the caudate lobe.

Ligamentum Venosum—The ligamentum venosum is a remnant of the fetal ductus venosus. It divides the

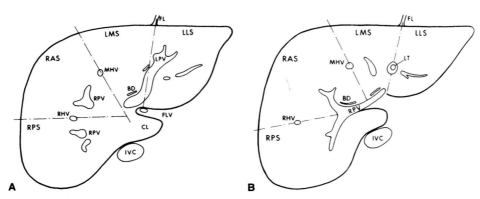

Figure 5–2. (A) Graphic representation. IVC = inferior vena cava; RPS, RAS = right lobe posterior and anterior segments; LMS, LLS = medial and lateral segments of left lobe; FLV = fissure of ligamentum venosum; RPV = right vein branch; RHV, MHV = right and middle hepatic veins; BD = bile duct. **(B)** LMS, LLS = medial and lateral segments of left lobe; FL = falciform ligament; LT = ligamentum teres. *(Reprinted with permission from Sexton CC, Zeman RK. Correlation of computed tomography, sonography and gross anatomy of the liver. AJA. 1983; 141:711–718.)*

caudate lobe from the left lobe. It may be visualized sonographically on either a longitudinal or transverse scan as an echogenic line extending transversely from the porta hepatis.

Ligamentum Teres (Round Ligament)—The ligamentum of teres is contained in the falciform ligament. It is a remnant of the fetal umbilical vein. It courses within the left intersegmental fissure, dividing the left lobe into medial and lateral segments. Sonographically, it is best visualized on a transverse view as a round echogenic structure just to the right of midline.

Falciform Ligament—The falciform ligament contains the ligamentum of teres. It extends from the umbilicus to the diaphragm and attaches the liver to the anterior abdominal wall and diaphragm. It divides the right and left lobe of the liver on the diaphragmatic surface.

Coronary Ligament—The coronary ligament is contiguous with the falciform ligament. It connects the posterior surface of the liver to the diaphragm.

Main Lobar Fissure (Middle Intersegmental Fissure)—The main lobar fissure separates the right and left lobes of the liver. It is visualized sonographically as an echogenic linear line extending from the portal vein to the neck of the gallbladder. Table 5–1 is a guide to the anatomic structures useful in defining segmental anatomy.

Couinaud's Anatomy—Each segment has it's own blood supply with a branch of the portal vein in the center bounded by a hepatic vein. The liver is divided horizontally into four (4) segments by the hepatic veins and each segment is divided transversely by either the right or left portal vein (Table 5–2) (Figure 5–4).

Liver Vessels—Hepatic Veins, Portal Vein, Hepatic Artery (Table 5–3)

The liver has a dual blood supply system. It receives blood from both the hepatic artery and portal vein. The main portal vein blood carries nutrients from the gastrointestinal tract, gallbladder, pancreas, and spleen. The majority of the total blood supplied to the liver is from the main portal vein.

Hepatic Veins—There are three hepatic veins: right, middle, and left. They follow a superior posterior course and drain deoxygenated blood into the inferior vena cava (IVC). Hepatic veins are nonpulsatile, increase in size as they course superiorly toward the IVC, and the walls are less echogenic than the portal veins.

Portal Vein—The portal vein is formed posterior to the pancreatic neck by the confluence of the splenic vein and superior mesenteric vein. It follows a cephalic right oblique course and enters into the liver at the porta hepatis also known as the portal triad. The main portal vein lies anterior to the IVC, cephalic to the head of the pancreas, and caudal to the caudate lobe. The main portal vein bifurcates in the liver into the right and left portal veins.

Right Portal Vein—The right portal vein is larger than the left portal vein. It follows a posterior caudad course and further divides into anterior and posterior branches.

Left Portal Vein—The left portal vein follows a cephalic anterior course to supply blood to the left lobe of the liver. It is the umbilical portion of the portal vein.

Hepatic Artery—The hepatic artery originates from the celiac axis and courses transversely. The hepatic artery and the common bile duct are anterior to the portal vein as they enter the liver at the portal hepatis, with the common bile duct slightly more lateral. The hepatic artery is at the same level as the hepatoduodenal ligament and is superior to the head of the pancreas.

The portal triad consists of the portal vein, which lies posterior to the hepatic artery and common bile duct. They all course together in a collagenous sheath and extend throughout the liver.

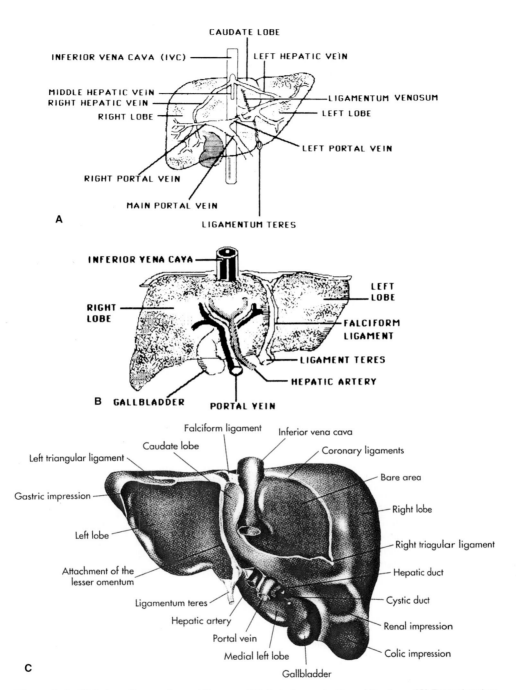

Figure 5–3. (A) Lobes, ligaments, and fissures. **(B)** Anterior projection of the liver. **(C)** Posterior view of the diaphragmatic surface of the liver. The caudate lobe is located on the posterosuperior surface of the right lobe, opposite the tenth and eleventh thoracic vertebrae. *(Reprinted with permission from Hagen-Ansert S. Textbook of Diagnostic Ultrasonography. 5th ed. St. Louis: Mosby; 2001, 113.)*

Common Bile Duct—The common bile duct is formed by the confluence of the common hepatic duct and the cystic duct. The superior portion of the biliary duct, which is anterior to the right portal vein is the common hepatic duct. The common bile duct follows an oblique posterocaudal course and travels along the dorsal aspect of the pancreatic head before it joins with the main pancreatic duct, and together they enter into the second portion of the duodenum.

Liver Function Tests

1. Aspartate aminotransferase (AST), formerly known as serum glutamic-oxaloacetic transaminase (SGOT): This is increased with hepatocellular

TABLE 5–1. INTERSEGMENTAL FISSURES

Fissures	Location	Landmark
Right intersegmental	Divides the right lobe into anterior and posterior segments	Right hepatic vein
Left intersegmental	Divides the left lobe into medial and lateral segments	Left hepatic vein Ligament of Teres Left portal vein Middle hepatic vein
Middle intersegmental (Main lobar fissure)	Divides the liver into right and left lobes	Oblique plane connecting gallbladder fossa and IVC

disease and is useful in detecting acute hepatitis before jaundice occurs and following in the course of hepatitis. It is not increased in cases of such chronic liver disease as cirrhosis or obstructive jaundice. It is increased in liver cell necrosis due to: viral hepatitis, toxic hepatitis, and other forms of acute hepatitis.

2. Alanine aminotransferase (ALT), formerly known as serum glutamic pyruvic transaminase (SGPT): This enzyme is increased with hepatocellular disease and is used to assess jaundice. It rises higher than AST in cases of hepatitis and takes 2–3 months to return a normal level.

3. Alkaline phosphatase (ALP): Normally found in serum. Its level rises in liver and biliary tract disorders when bile excretion is impaired. Obstruction of bile can be caused by either a biliary or liver disorder such as; obstructive jaundice, biliary cirrhosis, acute hepatitis, and granulomatous liver disease.

4. Ammonia: Normally metabolizes in the liver and is excreted as urea; increased in hepatocellular disease

TABLE 5–2. COUINAUD'S ANATOMY

Segments	Location	Supplied by Branches of
I	Caudate lobe	R & L portal veins
II	Lateral segment of left lobe–superior	Ascending segment of LPV
III	Lateral segment of left lobe–inferior	Descending segment of the LPV
IV	Medial segment of the left lobe–quadrate	Horizontal segment of the LPV
V	Anterior segment of the right lobe	Anterior branch of the RPV
VI	Posterior segment of the right lobe–inferior	Posterior branch of the RPV
VII	Posterior segment of the right lobe–superior	Posterior branch of the RPV
VIII	Anterior segment of the right lobe–superior	Anterior branch of the RPV

5. α-Fetoprotein (AFP): A protein normally produced by the fetal liver and yolk sac, GI tract, scrotal and hepatocellular (hepatomas) germ cell neoplasms, and other cancers in adults. AFP level is used to monitor chemotherapy treatment and prenatal diagnosis neural tube defects in the fetus; rarely in other cases.

6. Bilirubin: Derived from the break down of red blood cells into hemoglobin. Excreted by the liver in bile (main pigment). When destruction of red blood cells increases greatly or when the liver is unable to excrete normal amounts, the bilirubin concentration in the serum increases. If it is increased too high, jaundice may occur. Levels of indirect and direct bilirubin may determine intrahepatic and extrahepatic obstruction.

   Direct bilirubin (conjugated bilirubin): It is elevated when there is an obstruction of the biliary system—obstructive jaundice.

   Indirect Bilirubin (unconjugated bilirubin): Excessive destruction of red blood cells/hemolysis associated with anemias and liver disease; elevation of the total bilirubin occurs with hepatitis, hepatic metastasis.

7. Hematocrit: Volume percentage of erythrocytes in the whole body; a drop in hematocrit can indicate a hematoma due to liver trauma or bleeding elsewhere in the body.

8. Leukocytosis: A substantial increase in white blood cells above the normal range indicates an inflammatory process or abscess.

9. Prothrombin Time (PT): Prothrombin is converted to thrombin in the clotting process by action of vitamin K that is absorbed in the intestines and stored in the liver. When liver function is compromised by liver disease prothrombin is decreased and can cause uncontrolled hemorrhage.

10. Urinary Bile and Bilirubin: Bile and bilirubin are not normally found in the urine. There may be spillover into the blood when there is obstructive liver disease and excessive red cell destruction. Bile pigments are found in the blood when there is a biliary obstruction. Bilirubin is found alone when there is an excessive amount of red blood cell destruction.

11. Urinary Urobilinogen: This test is used to differentiate between a complete obstruction of the biliary tract vs. an incomplete obstruction of the biliary tract.

   Urobilinogen is a product of hemoglobin breakdown and can be elevated in cases of: liver disease, hemolytic disease or with severe infections. Urobilinogen does not increase or there is no excess amount found in urine in cases of complete biliary obstruction.

12. Fecal Urobilinogen: Traces of urobilinogen is normally found in fecal matter, but an increase or decrease in normal amounts may indicate hepatic digestive abnormalities. An increase may suggest

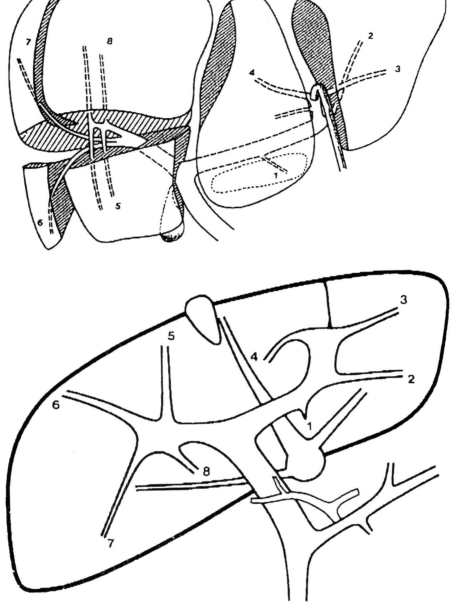

Figure 5–4. Couinaud's anatomy.

TABLE 5–3. DIFFERENTIATE BETWEEN THE PORTAL VEIN AND HEPATIC VEINS

Portal Veins	Hepatic Veins
Walls are more echogenic because of collagen within the wall	Caliper changes in size with respiration
Branches horizontally and orientated toward the portal hepatis	Branch vertically and orientated toward the IVC
Decreases in caliper as it courses away from the portal hepatis	Increases in caliper as it courses toward the IVC

an increase in hemolysis. A decrease is seen with complete obstruction of the biliary system.

Diffuse Hepatocellular Disease—There is a decrease in liver function with an increase in the liver enzymes, the increase in the liver enzymes is directly related to amount of hepatocytes necrosis. Total bilirubin levels may be elevated with increase prothrombin time (blood clotting factor). Diffuse liver disease has a varied sonographic appearance depending on if it is acute or chronic (Tables 5–4, 5–5).

TABLE 5–4. DIFFUSE LIVER DISEASE

Diffuse Liver Disease	Clinical Findings/Etiology	Laboratory Data	Sonographic Appearance
Fatty liver—accumulation of fat within the hepatocytes	ETOH abuse, steroids, malignancy, diabetes mellitus, protein malnutrition, hepatitis	Increased LFTs because of hepatocellular disease	Progressive disease—enlarged left and caudate lobe, increase liver echogenicity with decrease through transmission as the disease progresses, decrease visualization of vessel walls
Acute viral hepatitis—diffuse inflammatory process of the liver, most common types HAV, HBV, and HCV	Malaise, nausea, fever, pain, may be jaundiced, enlarged tender liver	Increased bilirubin, ALT higher levels than AST, alkaline phosphatase	Hepatosplenomely, hypoechoic liver parenchyma, renal cortex more echogenic than the liver, increased echogenicity of portal vein walls, thicken gallbladder wall
Chronic viral hepatitis most common types HBV and HCV	Malaise, nausea, fever, pain, may be jaundiced, enlarged tender liver in the early stages	Increase—bilirubin, ALT, AST, alkaline phosphatase	Liver parenchyma is coarse and echogenic, the walls of the portal system blend with the liver echogenicity
Cirrhosis—diffuse fibrotic process that involves the entire liver, most commonly caused ETOH abuse, HBV or HBC	Fatigue, weight loss, diarrhea, dull RUQ pain, increased abdominal girth if ascites is present	LFTs depend upon the stage and function of the liver, the following values are increased: ALT, AST, alkaline phosphatase, serum and urine conjugated bilirubin values	Late features—small nodular echogenic liver with decreased through transmission, caudate lobe may be sparred in severe cases—ascites, portal hypertension, collateral vessels, patent umbilical vein
Chronic (passive) hepatic congestion	History of heart failure, acute phase causes RUQ pain	Normal or slightly abnormal LFTs	Acute disorder—hepatomegaly, dilatation of IVC, hepatic veins—reverse flow during systole, slightly pulsatile portal vein
Glycogen storage disease—autosomal recessive disorder of carbohydrate metabolism, Von Gierke's disease is the most common type	Usually occurs in infancy or young childhood, hypoglycemia	Decreased glucose-6-phosphatase	Hepatomegaly, fatty liver infiltration with diffuse increase liver echogenicity

Causes of Jaundice
Medical Jaundice (Nonobstructive)

Hepatocellular Diseases—Disturbances within the liver cells that interfere with excretion of bilirubin:
  Hepatitis
  Drug-induced cholestasis
  Fatty liver (most common cause ETOH abuse)
  Cirrhosis

Hemolytic Disease—An increase in red blood cell destruction that results in the increase of indirect bilirubin (nonobstructive jaundice):
  Sickle-cell anemia
  Cooley's anemia

Surgical Jaundice (Obstructive)—Interference with the flow of bile caused by obstruction of the biliary tract. There are many causes of obstruction, some of the causes are:
  Choledocholithiasis
  Pancreatic pseudocyst
  Mass in the head of the pancreas
  Hepatoma
  Metastatic carcinoma
  Cholangiocarcinoma

Mass in the porta hepatis
Enlarged lymph nodes at the level of the porta hepatis

Vascular Abnormalities Within the Liver
Portal Hypertension—
Etiology:
  Intrahepatic—Most common cause is cirrhosis, Budd–Chiari syndrome
  Extrahepatic—thrombosis, occlusion and compression of portal or splenic veins, congestive heart failure

Clinical Findings:
  Formation of collateral venous channels
  Splenomegaly
  Gastrointestinal bleeding caused by opening of low pressure vascular channels
  Ascites

Sonographic Findings:
  Dilatation of the portal vein (> 13 mm)
  Dilatation of SMV and splenic vein (> 10 mm)
  Formation of collaterals (portal vein, splenic vein, SMV can be normal size)
  Varices—esophageal, splenorenal, gastrorenal, intestinal

TABLE 5–5. FOCAL DISEASE OF THE LIVER

Tumors	Clinical Findings	Laboratory Values	Sonographic Appearance
Cysts, congenital	Usually asymptomatic—if cysts become large hepatomegaly and jaundice may occur	Normal LFTs	Round, smooth thin walls, anechoic, increased through transmission
Polycystic disease	More than 50% associated with renal cystic disease	Normal LFTs	Multiple cysts of various sizes in the liver parenchyma
Acquired cysts Echinococcal cyst (hydatid)— caused by a parasite	Usually asymptomatic—may cause pain if cysts become large	Jaundice and increased alkaline phosphatase if cysts cause biliary obstruction	Depends on the level of maturity— solitary cysts which may have thick or calcified walls, mother daughter cysts, honey comb appearance or solid in appearance
Infection Abscess (pyogenic)	Fever, pain, nausea, vomiting, diarrhea, pleuritic pain	Leukocytosis, elevated LFTs, anemia	Usually found in the right lobe, solitary, variable size, anechoic to echogenic or complex may have calcifications or shadowing from gas
Fungal infection—Candidiasis	Immunocompromised; i.e., AIDS, organ transplant, malignancy; RUQ pain, fever	Varied—depending on the cause	Hepatomegaly, fatty infiltrations, focal lesions—"wheel within a wheel,"[1] becomes more hypoechoic
Hematoma	RUQ pain, hypotension	Decreased hematocrit, leukocytosis	Varied depending on age—mostly cystic (fresh blood), echogenic, mixed appearance, irregular shape
Benign solid tumors Cavernous hemangioma (most common)	Usually asymptomatic, more prevalent in women	Normal LFTs	Varied—usually small, round in the right lobe, subcapsular, usually homogeneous with increased through transmission
Focal nodular hyperplasia (FNH)	Usually asymptomatic, increase incidence in women on oral contraceptives	Normal LFTs	Varied—usually echogenic, usually found in the right lobe, similar in appearance as adenomas, hepatomas
Liver cell adenoma	Usually asymptomatic, or as a palpable mass, increase incidence in women on oral contraceptives or men on steroids	Normal LFTs	Varied—most often found in the right lobe, subcapsular, hyperechoic may have areas of hemorrhage
Infantile hemangioendothelioma	Usually occurs before 6 months of age, abdominal mass, congestive heart failure secondary to arteriovenous shunting	Normal AFP excludes the mass being malignant	Varied—hyperechoic, hypoechoic or mixed echogenicity
Malignant tumors Hepatocelluar carcinoma (HCC) hepatoma-associated with longstanding cirrhosis Hepatic angiosarcoma (rarely seen in people 60–80 years of age)	Acute—palpable mass, rapid liver enlargement, jaundice, weight loss, Chronic—, portal hypertension, ascites, splenomegaly, Budd-Chiari syndrome	Increased AST, ALT, alkaline phosphatase, 70% of the time AFP will be present	Varied—hypoechoic in early stage and becomes hyperechoic, may be singular or multiple
Hepatoblastoma—usually found during infancy or childhood	Abdominal enlargement, hepatomegaly, weight loss, nausea, vomiting, precocious puberty	Abnormal LFTs, elevated AFP	Varied—heterogeneous, hyperechoic or cystic with internal septations
Metastatic lesions—more common than primary malignancies	Primary sites—gastrointestinal tract, breast, lungs Causes symptoms 50% of the time	LFTs usually abnormal, increased in total bilirubin, alkaline phosphatase	Varied—hyperechoic, hypoechoic, complex, target lesions, anechoic

[1]Jeffrey RB, Rallas PW: New York: Raven Press; 1995.

Portafugal (reversal) blood flow
Splenomegaly
Recanalization of the umbilical vein > 3mm

Portal Vein Obstruction—
Etiology:
Thrombosis, invasion of the portal vein by tumor

Clinical Findings:
Hepatocellular carcinoma, pancreatic or GI cancer or lymphoma

Sonographic Findings:
Nonvisualization of the portal vein
Echoes within the portal vein
Dilatation of the splenic and superior mesenteric vein (proximal to the level of obstruction)

Budd–Chiari Syndrome—
Etiology:
Obstruction of the hepatic veins caused by thrombosis or compression from a liver mass

Clinical Findings:
Abdominal pain
Jaundice
Abnormal liver function tests
Hepatomegaly
Ascites

Sonographic Findings:
Reduced or nonvisualization of the hepatic veins
Hepatic veins proximal to the obstruction may be dilated
Large and hypoechoic caudate lobe
Ascities
Abnormal Doppler blood flow

GALLBLADDER

Gross Anatomy
The gallbladder is mostly intraperitoneal and is located in the gallbladder fossa, which is on the visceral surface of the liver. It lies between the right and left lobes of the liver and posterior and caudal to the main lobar fissure. The gallbladder is a pear-shaped structure with a thin wall that is less than 3 mm. It is approximately 8 cm in length, with a transverse diameter less than 5 cm. The gallbladder is divided into three main segments: fundus, body, and neck. The fundus is the most anterior segment, while the neck has a fixed anatomic relationship to the right portal vein and main lobar fissure. The neck tapers to form the cystic duct. The spiral valves of Heister are located in the cystic duct, and stones may collect here.

The right and left hepatic ducts join together to form the common hepatic duct whose function is to transport bile to the gallbladder. Bile enters and exits the gallbladder via the cystic duct. The cystic duct unites with the common bile duct to transport concentrated bile to the second portion of the duodenum.

Function
The three main functions of the gallbladder are to concentrate bile, store the concentrated bile, and transport the bile to the duodenum. The release of the hormone cholecystokin is stimulated when food enters into the stomach, especially fatty foods and dairy products. Cholecystokinin stimulates the gallbladder to contract and the sphincter of Oddi to relax and open. The intraductal pressure decreases with the contraction of the gallbladder and the opening of the sphincter of Oddi. The bile flows to the small intestine, which aids in the digestion of food by breaking down fatty foods and dairy products.

Gallbladder Variants and Anomalies
Junctional fold—Is the most common variant, and is a fold or septum located on the posterior gallbladder wall between the body and neck.

Phrygian cap—A fold located in the fundal portion of the gallbladder.

Hartman's pouch—A small sac located between the junctional fold and the neck of the gallbladder. It is an area where stones may collect.

Septations—Folds that protrude into the lumen of the gallbladder. There may be multiple folds located in a gallbladder.

Congenital anomalies are rare; the gallbladder can have an ectopic location and be found intrahepatic.

Laboratory Values of Biliary Tract Disease
White Blood Count (WBC)—increased in cases of infection, acute cholecystitis, chronic cholecystitis, cholangitis

Serum Bilirubin—increased in cases where the biliary system becomes obstructed, gallbladder carcinoma

Abnormal liver function tests

Serum alkaline phosphatase (ALP)—increased in cases of posthepatic jaundice

Prothrombin time (PT)—The clotting time is longer in patients with acute cholecystitis, carcinoma of the gallbladder, and prolonged CBD obstruction.

Aspartate amniotransferase (AST) and alanine amniotransferase (ALT) are abnormal in cases of cholecystitis, choledocholithiasis, and any injury to the bile ducts.

Sonographic Nonvisualization of the Gallbladder—The most common reason for not visualizing the gallbladder on a sonogram is normal physiological contraction of the gallbladder caused by the patient not being NPO. The gallbladder may not be identified in patients who have had a cholecystectomy, ectopic gallbladder, chronic cholecystitis with the gallbladder lumen filled with gallstones, solid mass obliterating the GB, intrahepatic obstruction, or a porcelain gallbladder. Agenesis of the gallbladder is very rare. When the GB in not identified on ultrasound, the gallbladder fossa should be documented. This can be accomplished by locating the right portal vein and following the main lobar fissure from the right portal vein to the GB fossa region.

Causes of a Large Gallbladder (Hydrops)—A large gallbladder can be caused by prolonged fasting, IV hyperalimentation, a cystic obstruction, or obstruction of the common bile duct. A Courvoisier gallbladder is a large gallbladder caused by an obstruction at the distal portion of the common bile duct. The patient has "painless" jaundice, elevated serum bilirubin, and abnormal liver function tests. The obstruction is usually caused by a malignancy in the area of the distal CBD (pancreatic head carcinoma, common duct carcinoma, duodenal carcinoma, ampulla of Vater carcinoma) or diabetes and postvagotomy.

Causes of a Small Gallbladder—A common cause of a small GB is that the patient has eaten. Other causes include: intrahepatic biliary obstruction (bile is unable to enter into the GB) chronic cholecystitis; liver disease that destroys the liver parenchyma and, therefore, decreases the production of bile; and in extremely rare cases, congenital hypoplasia of the GB.

Causes of Low Level Echoes in the Gallbladder Lumen/With Mobility

Sludge. The most common cause of sludge is stasis of bile attributable to cholecystitis, extrahepatic obstruction, hyperalimentation, or in patients who have been NPO for a long period of time. Sludge is a common precursor to gallstones. Sludge appears as low-level nonshadowing echoes in the dependent portion of the gallbladder that moves with a change in the patient position. Other causes of mobile low level echoes within the gallbladder lumen include; blood, pus and viscous bile. Intraluminal echoes that do not shadow or are nonmobile include: polyps, cholesterosis, artifacts, septi (junctional fold), and gallbladder carcinoma.

Pathology of the Gallbladder

Reasons for Gallbladder Wall Thickening Greater than 3 mm (Table 5–6)

Cholelithiasis (gallstones)—Patients may present a symptomatic or with right upper quadrant pain (RUQ) and a history of nausea and vomiting after eating. Cholecystitis is often present. Three characteristics of gallstones that must be present to diagnose gallstones

1. Echogenic foci—Echogenic due to the acoustic mismatch between the stones and bile
2. Posterior acoustic shadowing—Most of the sound is absorbed (attenuated), producing a shadow.
3. Gravity dependent—Stones are gravity dependent and move to the most dependent portion of the GB when the patient position is changed.

Structures That Can Mimic Gallstones

Gas in the duodenum

TABLE 5–6. REASONS FOR GALLBLADDER WALL THICKENING GREATER THAN 3 MM

Diffuse Thickening	Focal Thickening	Pseudo Thickening
Physiological due to eatin	Adenomyomatosis	Gain setting too high
Ascites	Polyps—cholesterol, papillary	TGC set inappropriate
Acute hepatitis	Gallbladder carcinoma—	Beam averaging artifact
Congestive heart failure	primary and secondary	Sludge
Cholecystitis	Metastatic wall masses	
Hypoalbuminemia		
AIDS		
Sepsis		

Shadowing from the spiral valves of Heister—refraction artifact from the cystic duct

Bowel—usually not a clean shadow

Air in the biliary tree—from previous surgery or GB fistula

Postcholecystectomy clips

Low-level echoes in the gallbladder lumen—no shadowing

Porcelain Gallbladder—calcium deposit on the wall of the gallbladder (usually attributable to chronic cholecystitis)

Polyps—are not gravity dependent, do not move with changing patient position

Adenomyomatosis—Hyperplastic change in the gallbladder wall (see page 198).

Causes of gallstones in children include hemolysis; for example, sickle cell disease, cystic fibrosis, malabsorption syndrome (Crohn's disease), hepatitis, and congenital biliary anomalies (choledochal cyst, biliary atresia).

Mirizzi Syndrome—Stone obstructing the cystic duct. Dilatation of the common hepatic duct and intrahepatic ducts with normal common bile duct.

Acute Cholecystitis—Acute cholecystitis is inflammation of the gallbladder wall with decreased gallbladder function. Acute cholecystitis is usually caused by an obstruction at the level of the cystic duct, bacterial infection in the biliary system, or pancreatic enzyme reflux. Clinically, the patients may present with acute RUQ pain positive Murphy's sign (point of pain over the gallbladder when compressed), jaundice, and fever. The laboratory findings can include elevated serum bilirubin and abnormal liver function tests (LFTs). Sonographic findings may include: diffuse gallbladder wall thickening > 3.0 mm; gallstones; 'halo' sign suggestive of subserosal edema; cystic artery along the anterior GB wall; transverse diameter > 5.0 cm; sludge; and pericholecystic fluid.

Complications of Acute Cholecystitis

Empyema—Pus in the Gallbladder—Clinically, the patient presents sicker than with acute cholecystitis, and sonographically, there will be low-level echoes in the GB lumen with thickening gallbladder wall.

Emphysematous Cholecystitis—Rare occurrence caused by gas forming bacteria in the wall of the gallbladder

Gangrene of the Gallbladder—Caused by absence of blood supply to the gallbladder

Perforation of the Gallbladder—Caused by infection and gallstones

Pericholecystic Abscess—Usually caused by perforation of the gallbladder

Ascending Cholangitis—Caused by spreading of the inflammation of the gallbladder

Acalculous Cholecystitis—Less than 5% of patients with cholecystitis will not have gallstones. The cause of acalculous cholecystitis is a combination of bile stasis and direct vascular changes. The etiology of this combination: trauma, patients who are NPO for long period of time

Chronic Cholecystitis—Caused by recurrent or chronic inflammatory changes of the gallbladder. It is the most common cause of symptomatic gallbladder disease and is associated with gallstones in 90% of the cases. Clinically, the patient presents with intermittent RUQ pain and intolerance to fatty and fried foods. Laboratory findings can include elevated AST, ALT, alkaline phosphatase, and increase of direct serum bilirubin. The sonographic appearance includes small or normal size gallbladder, gallstones, sludge, and thicken echogenic gallbladder wall. A positive WES sign may be imaged: the double arc and shadowing are caused by: W-echo from the gallbladder wall, E-echo from the gallstone, S-shadowing from gallstones.

Complications:
Bouveret's syndrome
Mirizzi syndrome
Fistula between the gallbladder and duodenum

Causes of pericholecystic fluid include: acute cholecystitis, pericholecystic abscess, ascites, pancreatitis, peritonitis, and acquired immunodeficiency syndrome (AIDS)

Porcelain Gallbladder—Porcelain gallbladder is the calcification of the gallbladder wall. The etiology is unknown. It is associated with gallstones and an increased incidence of gallbladder carcinoma. The sonographic appearance:
Curvilinear echogenic structure in the gallbladder fossa with posterior acoustic shadowing
Echogenic anterior and posterior with some shadowing
Irregular gallbladder wall with areas of echo densities and shadowing

Benign Tumors of the Gallbladder—Benign tumors of the gallbladder are rare. They represent over growth of the epithelial lining. Patients are usually asymptomatic.

Adenoma—The most common of the benign gallbladder tumors. They are frequently located in the fundus portion of the gallbladder and less than 1 cm in size. Sonographically they appear as low-level echo masses that do not shadow or move to the dependent portion of the gallbladder.

Adenomyomatosis—(a form of hyperplastic cholecystosis) Characterized by:
Hyperplasia of the epithelial and muscular surfaces of the gallbladder wall
Epithelial and intramural diverticula (Rokitansjy–Aschoff sinuses)
There are various types and the most common type is usually located at the fundus. They may also be annular or they can be either diffuse or segmental

Sonographic appearance:

Diffuse or segmental wall thickening

Intraluminal diverticula (RS sinuses) may be filled with bile, sludge or stones and appear either as anechoic or echogenic with distal shadowing or comet tail artifact. The reverberations are the sonographic appearance that differentiates this disease from an adenoma.

Cholesterolosis (strawberry gallbladder)—A form of hyperplastic cholecystosis. The gallbladder usually appears normal on ultrasound.

Polyps—Small echodensities attached to the gallbladder wall by a stalk; they do not shadow or move to the dependent portion of the gallbladder.

Carcinoma of the Gallbladder—The most common biliary malignancy. Pancreatic CA is the most common malignant cause to obstruct the biliary tree. Most of carcinomas of the gallbladder are adenomas. They usually do not occur until the sixth or seventh decade and are more common in women than men. Previous gallbladder disease; for example, inflammatory disease or gallstones are often precursors. Gallstones are usually present. Most patients have direct extension into the liver and surrounding structures (lymphatic). Signs and symptoms are similar to chronic cholesystitis (may be asymptomatic, loss of appetite, nausea, vomiting, intolerance to fatty foods and dairy products.) Sonographic appearance usually includes gallstones in addition to:

Solid mass filling the gallbladder lumen (most common type)

Localized thickened gallbladder wall with a small gallbladder lumen

Fungating mass projecting from the gallbladder wall into the lumen

Secondary findings
    Liver metastasis
    Regional lymphadenopathy

BILE DUCTS

Gross Anatomy

The intrahepatic radicles converge to form the main right and left hepatic ducts at the porta hepatis. The right and left hepatic ducts unite to form the common hepatic duct.

The common hepatic duct joins the cystic duct to form the common bile duct. The common bile duct courses along the hepatoduodenal ligament (ligament that attaches the liver to the duodenum), behind the duodenal bulb and posterior aspect of the pancreatic head to enter the second portion of the duodenum. The common bile duct joins with the main pancreatic duct at the ampulla of Vater (Fig. 5–5).

The common hepatic duct is always anterior to the right portal vein. The normal common bile duct lumen measures ≤ 8 mm, the walls are not included in the measurement. The normal diameter of the common bile duct may increase 1mm per decade starting at the sixth decade. This is due to the common bile duct becoming ecstatic with age. An enlarged common bile duct after a cholecystectomy is normal; if a patient is symptomatic (jaundiced and/or RUQ pain), a retained stone or a postoperative stricture must be ruled out.

Bile Duct Measurements in a Fasting Patient
    Common Hepatic Duct (CHD) ≤ 4 or 5 mm
    Common Bile Duct (CBD) ≤ 8 mm

Sonographic Appearance of the Biliary System. The cystic duct and intrahepatic ducts (right and left hepatic ducts) are not usually visualized on ultrasound unless they are dilated. The extrahepatic ducts, (common hepatic duct (CHD), and common bile duct (CBD), which are also known as the common duct), are routinely visualized on ultrasound.

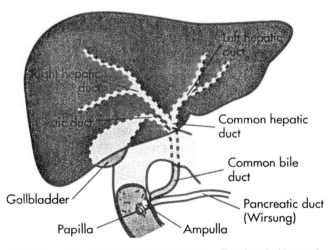

Figure 5–5. The common bile duct anatomy. *(Reprinted with permission from Gill, K. Abdominal Ultrasound A Practitioner's Guide. 1st ed. Philadelphia: WB Saunders Company, 2001, p. 125.)*

Sonographic Criteria for Intrahepatic Dilatation

The bile duct courses anterior to the portal veins. When dilated, a parallel channel sign (double-barrel shotgun sign) is imaged.

Increased number of tubular structures are imaged in the periphery of the liver.

Stellate formation of the tubes near the porta hepatis.

Posterior acoustic enhancement distal to the ducts.

The sonographic appearance of the biliary system varies depending upon the level of obstruction. Ducts dilate proximal to the level of obstruction. Intrahepatic dilation may be the only sonographic indication of an obstruction (Table 5–7). There may be intrahepatic dilation with common bile duct dilation with a normal gallbladder or intrahepatic and common bile duct dilation with a small gallbladder (Table 5–8). The cause of the later is chronic cholecystitis.

Biliary Atresia—The most common fatal liver disorder in children in the United States. There are two forms. In atresia of the intrahepatic radicles, there is non-visualization of the biliary radicles and gallbladder. In atresia of the extrahepatic radicles, there is an anastomosis of the biliary tree to the jejunum (second part of the small intestine), there will be dilatation of the intrahepatic radicles, and occasionally, the gallbladder will also be imaged. It is difficult to differentiate between biliary atresia and neonatal hepatitis. A nuclear medicine scan and hepatic biopsy may be needed to make a definite diagnosis.

Caroli's Disease—Caroli's disease is a genetic trait characterized by a segmental saccular dilatation of the intrahepatic ducts. Caroli's disease leads to bile stasis, bacterial growth, abscesses, cholangitis, formation of stones, and decreased liver function caused by the compression of the hepatocytes.

Sonographically, the liver will have multiple cystic structures that communicate with the intrahepatic ducts. Stones and echoes may appear within the bile ducts.

Choledochal Cyst—Choledochal cyst is characterized as a cystic dilatation and outpouching of the common duct wall. The signs and symptoms are intermittent jaundice, RUQ pain, RUQ mass, and failure to thrive. Sonographically, the dilated common bile duct is imaged entering into the cystic mass, and the gallbladder is

TABLE 5–7. TYPES OF BILIARY OBSTRUCTION

Biliary Obstruction without Dilatation	Dilatation without Biliary Obstruction
Obstruction occurred within 12–24 hours before exam—ducts may not be dilated yet	Post-op cholecystectomy
	Stone in biliary tree has passed

TABLE 5–8. LEVEL OF OBSTRUCTION CAUSING INTRAHEPATIC DILATATION

Common Bile Duct and GB normal size	Common Bile Duct— Dilated with Enlarged GB
Bile duct tumor (cholangiocarcinoma, Klastkin tumor)	Stones in the common bile duct
Sclerosing cholangitis	Chronic pancreatitis
Biliary atresia	Mass of the head of the pancreas (carcinoma)
Choledochal cyst	

imaged as a separate cystic structure. The intrahepatic radicles may be dilated.

Biliary System Pathology

Cholangitis—Inflammation of the biliary tract caused by bacterial infection of the biliary tract. Cholangitis is associated with biliary stasis caused by obstruction; for example, choledocholithiasis, biliary stricture, and neoplasm. The signs and symptoms are fever, jaundice, and upper abdominal pain. Abnormal laboratory tests include leukocytosis, increased serum bilirubin, and increased serum alkaline phosphatase. Sonographic appearance may include air in the biliary system, dilatation of the extrahepatic ducts, and the gallbladder may be enlarged.

Sclerosing cholangitis—Inflammation and fibrosis of bile duct commonly associated with intrahepatic calculi complications.

Choledocholiths—Stones in the common bile duct, which may cause common bile duct obstruction. The stones usually originate in the gallbladder. The signs and symptoms are biliary colic and jaundice. Patients may also present with gallstones and cholangitis. Laboratory tests show an increased serum bilirubin, increased alkaline phosphatase, and bacteremia. Sonographically, stones in the common bile duct are difficult to image because of the deep position of the duct, overlying bowel gas and a very small amount of fluid surrounding the stone, a stone may be positioned more posterior than the focal zone of the transducer. The common bile duct may be dilated with an echogenic focus and posterior acoustic shadowing.

Primary Malignant Tumors of the Biliary Tree

Adenocarcinoma and Squamous Cell Carcinoma—
All branches of the biliary tree may be affected, with the common bile duct being the most common site. Predisposing factors associated with carcinoma of the biliary tree are inflammation, cholelithiasis, and chronic ulcerative colitis. Signs and symptoms are anorexia, weight loss, RUQ pain, and jaundice. Sonographically, intraluminal soft-tissue echoes marked dilation with a normal pancreatic head, focal biliary stricture, or abrupt termination of the duct.

Klatskin Tumor—A Klatskin tumor is a carcinoma that arises at the union of the right and left hepatic ducts. This type of tumor has the worst prognosis because the patient typically does not have any symptoms and, therefore, does not get diagnosed until there is liver involvement. Sonographically, it presents as a solid mass at the junction of the right and left hepatic ducts. There is intrahepatic duct dilation without extrahepatic duct dilatation.

PANCREAS

Gross Anatomy

The pancreas lies transversely in the retroperitoneal cavity. It extends from the C-loop of the duodenum to the splenic helium and is divided into four parts: head, neck (sometimes included with the head), body, and tail. The size and shape of the pancreas may vary in size depending upon the age and body habitus of the patient. The anteroposterior measurements of the pancreas are approximately: head 3.0 cm, body 2.0 cm, and tail 2.0 cm. The pancreas has no capsule and is generally dumbbell or sausage shaped. Figure 5–6 Demonstrates the pancreas and its related landmarks.

The pancreas is difficult to visualize on ultrasound, and vascular landmarks are used to identify the pancreas and the pancreatic region. The head is anterior to the inferior vena cava and right renal vein. The common bile duct can be seen at the posterior lateral margin of the pancreatic head. The gastroduodenal artery may be visualized at the anterior lateral margin. Both structures are imaged as anechoic round structures that appear to be within the head of the pancreas.

The uncinate process is a tongue-like extension of the pancreatic neck. A prominent uncinate process will displace the superior mesenteric artery and vein anterior to the pancreas.

The body of the pancreas is the largest portion of the gland. The splenic vein is the most reliable landmark used to visualize the pancreas. The splenic vein courses along the posterior margin of the pancreas and joins with the superior mesenteric vein to form the portal vein. The portal confluence is posterior to the neck of the pancreas. The body is anterior to the superior mesenteric artery, superior mesenteric vein, splenic vein, left renal vein and aorta. The left renal vein, is imaged posterior to the superior mesenteric artery and anterior to the aorta.

The tail of the pancreas lies anterior to the left kidney and medial to the splenic helium. The splenic artery courses along the superior anterior border, and the splenic vein courses along the posterior border.

The main pancreatic duct, also called the Wirsung's duct, courses the entire length of the pancreas. It extends from the tail of the pancreas and joins with the common bile duct at the ampulla of Vater before entering into the second portion of the duodenum. The accessory duct, or Santorini's duct, courses diagonally through the head of the pancreas and enters into the duodenum separately.

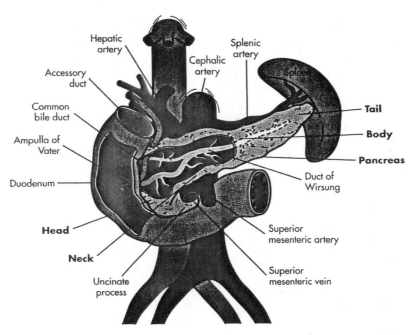

Figure 5–6. Anatomy of the pancreas. *(Reprinted with permission from Gill, K. Abdominal Ultrasound A Practitioner's Guide. 1st ed. Philadelphia: WB Saunders Company, 2001; 125, 151.)*

Table 5–9 lists the landmarks used for visualizing the pancreas on a sonographic examination.

Sonographic Appearance. The pancreas is a homogeneous organ with either the same echogenicity as the liver or slightly more echogenic than the normal liver. In children, the pancreas is less echogenic and relatively larger than in the adult. The pancreas is more difficult to visualize as people get older. The pancreas, which has no true capsule and becomes more echogenic, tends to blend in with the surrounding retroperitoneal fat. The main pancreatic duct may be seen as a tubular structure coursing from the tail of the pancreas to the head. The normal caliber varies from 2 to 3 mm, the largest diameter being in the head of the pancreas.

Function. The pancreas has an endocrine and exocrine function. The islets cells of Langerhans has three different types of cells, and each cell secretes a different type of hormone. The alpha cells secrete glucagon; beta cells secrete insulin; and delta cells secrete somatostatin.

The exocrine function of the pancreas secretes; amylase, lipase, and trypsin. These enzymes aid in digestion and are produced in the pancreas and travel to the duodenum through the pancreatic duct.

Pancreatic Diseases (Table 5–10)
Pancreatitis. Pancreatitis is a diffuse inflammatory process of the pancreas in which the pancreatic enzymes autodigest the pancreatic tissue. There are a number of

TABLE 5–9. LANDMARKS FOR VISUALIZING THE PANCREAS

Head	Neck	Body	Tail
Anterior to the inferior vena cava (IVC)	Anterior to the superior mesenteric vein (SMV)	Anterior to the aorta	Anterior to the splenic vein
Medial to the second portion of the duodenum	Anterior to the confluence of the SMV and splenic vein (portal confluence)	Anterior to the superior mesenteric artery (SMA)	Anterior to the left kidney
Right of the superior mesenteric artery (SMA)		Anterior to the left renal vein	Posterior to the stomach
Medial and anterior to the common bile duct (CBD)		Anterior to the splenic vein	Medial to the spleen
Medial and posterior to the gastroduodenal artery		Posterior to the antrum of the stomach	Posterior to the splenic artery

TABLE 5–10. DISEASES OF THE PANCREAS

Disease	Etiology	Signs and Symptoms	Laboratory Values	Sonographic Appearance	Complications
Acute pancreatitis	Alcohol abuse, biliary disease	Abdomen pain radiating to the back, nausea and vomiting, abdominal distension	Increased serum amylase and lipase	Enlarged, deceased echogenicity, extrapancreatic fluid, may have dilated pancreatic duct	Pseudocyst, abscess, hemorrhage, phlegmon, biliary and duodenal obstruction
Chronic pancreatitis	Alcohol abuse, biliary disease	Same as in acute pancreatitis, weight loss	Amylase and lipase level are not useful, fat in feces	Normal or smaller in size, heterogeneous, increased echogenicity, dilated pancreatic duct may have stones, dilated common bile duct	Pseudocyst, dilation of the biliary system, thrombosis of splenic and/or portal vein

mechanisms that cause the pancreatic enzymes to become activated within the pancreas. The most common causes in older adults include alcohol, biliary tract disease, trauma, surgery, perforated peptic ulcer disease, and drugs.

Causes of pancreatitis in younger patients include infectious agents—mumps and mononucleosis. Hereditary causes include cystic fibrosis and congenital pancreatitis (rare). Pancreatitis can either be classified as acute with or without complications or chronic.

Acute Pancreatitis. Patients present with abdominal pain characteristically in the epigastrium or periumbilical region with nausea and vomiting. The pain usually radiates to the back and commonly occurs following a large meal or alcohol binge. There is abdominal distension attributable to the decrease in gastric and intestinal motility and chemical peritonitis. The entire gland is usually affected, and sonographically, the pancreas may appear normal or is less echogenic.

Laboratory Values. Serum amylase will increase within the first 24 hours and remain elevated for 48 to 72 hours. Serum lipase will remain elevated for 5 to 14 days. There will also be an elevated white count, and if biliary obstruction occurs, an elevation in serum bilirubin will also be present. Complications of pancreatitis may include: pseudocyst, abscess, hemorrhage, phlegmon, and biliary and duodenal obstruction.

Edematous form occurs when the pancreas goes through inflammatory changes and interstitial edema. The gland becomes enlarged and is less echogenic on ultrasound. Acute pancreatitis may also be associated with intraperitoneal or retroperitoneal fluid.

Hemorrhagic pancreatitis occurs when there is a rapid progression of the disease caused by autodigestion of the pancreatic tissue, which causes areas of fat necrosis. This leads to rupture of the vessels in the pancreas and hemorrhage. Sonographically, the appearance will vary depending upon when the bleeding occurred. A mass may appear as homogeneous, cystic with debris, or heterogeneous. The pancreatic duct may be dilated.

Phlegmonous pancreatitis is a severe form of acute pancreatitis where the inflammation may extend to outside the pancreas. Sonographically, the pancreas is hypoechoic.

Pancreatic pseudocyst is the most common complication associated with acute pancreatitis. They are not true cysts because they do not have an epithelial covering. Pancreatic enzymes and blood escape from the pancreas tissue and become encapsulated form a pseudocyst. They are most commonly found in the lesser sac (anterior to the pancreas and posterior to the stomach) and may also be found in the pararenal space and transverse mesocolon. Sonographically, they are round, smooth thin-walled, and primarily anechoic and may be either singular or multiple. The fluid usually reabsorbs into the body; a small percentage may rupture.

Chronic pancreatitis occurs from continued destruction of the pancreatic parenchyma usually from repeated bouts of acute pancreatitis. Sonographically, the pancreas is either normal or small in size, with an irregular contour. The parenchyma is heterogeneous with increased echogenicity, and in 50% of cases, patients with malabsorption syndromes will have calcifications. With dilation of the pancreatic duct, stones may be imaged within the dilated duct. The common bile duct may also be dilated.

Benign Neoplasms may originate from endocrine or exocrine tissue. These focal lesions include: islet cell tumors, cystadenoma, and papilloma of the duct. Pancreatic cysts, abscesses, metastatic diseases to the pancreas, and lymphomas have the same sonographic appearances as when they are visualized in other areas of the body (Table 5–11).

Malignant Tumors. Pancreatic carcinoma can be subdivided into adenocarcinoma, cystadenocarcinoma, and such endocrine tumors as islet cell carcinoma. Adenocarcinoma is the most common, and it is usually located within the head. Sonographically, the pancreas is enlarged with irregular borders, the parenchymal pattern changes and becomes less echogenic. Dilation of the pancreatic duct. Associated

TABLE 5–11. FOCAL LESIONS OF THE PANCREAS

Growth	Signs and Symptoms	Laboratory Values	Clinical Pathology	Sonographic Appearance
Cysts True cysts	Usually asymptomatic		Have epithelial lining, may be continuous with the duct or arise from pancreatic tissue, most often found in the head	Smooth, thin wall, anechoic, increased through posterior transmission
Pseudocyst	Asymptomatic or may have the same symptoms as in acute pancreatitis, if pseudocyst is large may have pain	Increased serum amylase and lipase	Pancreatic enzymes that escape the pancreatic duct can tract anywhere, fluid may spontaneously reabsorb, or the pseudocyst may rupture	Round or takes the shape of the potential space; thick walls, usually anechoic, but may have debris; increased through posterior transmission
Benign Tumors Cystadenoma (microcytic adenoma)	No clinical symptoms	Increased serum amylase	More common in females	Found most commonly in the body and tail; anechoic masses with increased posterior enhancement; irregular margins, may have internal echoes
Islet cell tumor Insulinoma	Hypoglycemia	Elevated plasma insulin levels	Arises from the B cells of the islets of Langerhans; usually found in the tail and body	Small (1–2 cm) homogeneous solid masses; usually hypoechoic; may have areas of cystic degeneration
Malignant Tumors Adenocarcinoma	Symptoms occur late in the disease process, pain, weight loss, painless jaundice	Increased serum amylase, bilirubin; increased alkaline phosphatase (liver metastases); increased AST (SGOT)	Arises from the exocrine tissue; accounts for the majority of all malignant pancreatic tumors; usually found in the head	Focal mass with irregular ill-defined borders; decreased echogenicity; Courvoisier's sign (enlarged gallbladder); ascites; metastases
Cystadenoma-carcinoma	Epigastric pain		Rare malignant tumor; usually found in the body or tail	Cystic mass with irregular borders; thick walls, and may have solid components

findings include: dilatation of the common bile duct secondary to enlargement of the pancreatic head; liver metastases; nodal metastases; portal vein involvement; compression on the IVC; and Courvoisier's sign (Table 5–11).

Cystadenocarcinoma is visualized sonographically as an irregular cystic lobulated mass with thick walls. It is more commonly seen in the body or tail.

Islet Cell Carcinomas are usually small and well circumscribed and found in the body and tail. One-third of all islet cell tumors are nonfunctioning tumors, and 92% of these are malignant.

With any type of pancreatic carcinoma, clinically, they are associated with increase in alkaline phosphatase and bilirubin secondary to biliary obstruction. Metastasis to the liver, portal vein, and lymphadenopathy may also be seen.

SPLEEN

Gross Anatomy
The spleen is the largest mass of reticuloendothelial tissue in the body. It normally measures approximately 12–14 cm in length, 7 cm in width, and 3 cm in anteroposterior dimension. It is located in the left upper quadrant, left hypochondriac region, inferior to the diaphragm, and posterolateral to the stomach. The tail of the pancreas is medial to the splenic hilum. The left kidney is medial and posterior to the spleen; the stomach and left colic flexure are both medial to the spleen.

The spleen is an intraperitoneal organ except for the hilum area. The capsule is fibroelastic and is composed of small fibrous bands that gives the spleen its frame work and permits it to expand in size. The splenic artery, which is a branch of the celiac axis, courses along the anterior superior border of the pancreas and enters into the spleen at the splenic hilum. The splenic artery divides into six branches once it enters into the spleen. The splenic vein exits at the splenic hilum and courses transversely across along the posterior aspect of the pancreas and joins with the superior mesenteric vein to form the portal vein.

The spleen is not essential to life, but is has important functions especially during the fetal period. It is the main component of the reticuloendothelial system and its' functions include: the breakdown of hemoglobin and the formation of bile pigment; formation of antibodies, production of lymphocytes and plasma cells; a reservoir for blood; and blood formation in the fetus (erythrocytes) or when there is severe anemia.

The spleen is a homogenous organ and is either slightly less echogenic or isoechoic to the normal liver. The spleen is crescent shaped with a convex superior lateral border and concave medially. The inferior portion is tapered.

Congenital Anomalies–The most common congenial anomaly is the accessory spleen. Splenic tissue separate from the spleen is usually found near the splenic hilum or adjacent to the tail of the pancreas. Accessory spleens are typically small and round and have the same echogenicity as the spleen. They are difficult to demonstrate on ultrasound and must be differentiated from lymphadenopathy.

A *wandering spleen* is a spleen in an ectopic location usually found in the pelvis. The patient usually presents with an abdominal or pelvic mass and intermittent pain. Splenic torsion may occur and color Doppler is used to document the vascularity.

Asplenia is rare and often associated with congenital heart disease and other anomalies.

Aplasia is failure of the spleen to develop.

Neoplasms of the Spleen

The spleen is seldom the site for primary disease but often the site for secondary disease. Benign and malignant tumors are rare.

Benign Neoplasms of the Spleen. These include congenital cysts, cysts associated with polycystic disease, hemangiomas (most common primary tumor of the spleen), and lymphangioma (Table 5–12).

Trauma. Blunt trauma (motor vehicle accident, sports injury) to the spleen are common causes for trauma to the spleen. A subcapsular hematoma may form, grow, and cause the spleen to rupture. Spontaneous rupture of the spleen may also occur in certain disease states (i.e., leukemia), when the spleen is massively enlarged and soft.

Malignant Tumors of the Spleen

Primary malignant tumors arise from the capsule (sarcoma) the most common one being angiosarcoma or they may come from the splenic tissue (lymph), lymphoma. Secondary malignant tumors of the spleen are metastatic from the breast, malignant melanoma, or the ovaries (Table 5–12).

Pathologies of the Spleen

The pathological sonographic appearance of the spleen can be divided into two categories, focal and diffuse. Diffuse splenomegaly can be caused by: congestive splenomegaly (i.e., cirrhosis, portal hypertension, and heart failure); infections (i.e., hepatitis, HIV/AIDS, tuberculosis); storage disease (i.e., Gaucher disease, diabetes mellitus, and Niemann Pick disease); and hemodialysis. It is important to remem-

TABLE 5–12. FOCAL AND DIFFUSE PATHOLOGY OF THE SPLEEN

Sonolucent Focal Pathology
  Splenic cysts
  Abscess
  Hematoma
  Lymphoma
  Metastases
  Infarction
  Cystic lymphangioma
Echogenic Focal Pathology
  Metastases
  Cavernous hemangioma
  Hamartoma
Varied Focal Echogenicity
  Infarction
  Abscess
Diffuse Pathology—Decreased Echogenicity
  Congestion
  Multiple myeloma
  Lymphopoiesis
  Granulocytopoiesis (e.g., acute or chronic infection)
  Erythropoieses (e.g., sickle cell disease, hemolytic anemia, thalassemia)
Diffuse Pathology—Increased Echogenicity
  Leukemia
  Lymphoma

ber that diseases go through different stages and the sonographic appearance will vary depending upon the stage of the disease (Table 5–13).

Some disease processes that affect the spleen will not produce any focal lesions or changes in the echogenicity of the spleen. They will affect the splenic size by either causing atrophy or enlargement of the spleen (Table 5–13).

Atrophy of the spleen is seen less commonly than splenomegaly. Myelofibrosis and sickle cell disease cause destruction of the splenic parenchyma. The spleen decreases in size and sonographically, becomes echogenic. In many cases, an atrophic spleen is not visualized on ultrasound.

Splenic Size. The size of the spleen varies with energy and nutritional state of the person. It also varies at different

TABLE 5–13. CAUSES OF SPLENOMEGALY

Minimal	Moderate	Massive
Acute splenitis	Acute leukemia	Chronic leukemia
Acute splenic congestion (CHF, portal hypertension)	Infectious mononucleosis	Lymphoma
	Cirrhosis with portal hypertension	Hodgkin's disease
		Parasitic infections
Acute febrile disorders (systemic toxemias, intraabdominal infections)	Chronic splenitis	Primary tumors of the spleen
	Storage diseases (e.g., Gaucher's disease, amyloidosis)	
	Tuberculosis	
	Chronic congestion	

states in life—at birth, it has the same proportion to the total body weight as in the adult. The relationship of the spleen to body size and nutritional state of the individual is important.

KIDNEY

Gross Anatomy

The paired kidneys and ureters are retroperitoneal, lying anterior to the deep muscles of the back (psoas major muscle). The kidneys have three layers for protection and support. The true capsule or fibrous capsule is the most inner layer and is imaged sonographically as an echogenic reflector surrounding the renal cortex. Surrounding the true capsule is a layer of fat (adipose) called the perirenal fat. The adrenal gland is located anterior, superior, and medial to the each kidney and is separated from the kidney by the layer of perirenal fat. Gerota's fascia is a fibrous sheath that encloses both the adrenal gland and the kidney.

The kidney is divided into two regions, the renal sinus and the parenchyma. The renal parenchyma is measured from the margin of the renal sinus to the border of the kidney. The average adult kidney size is 11.5 cm in length, 6 cm in width, and 3.5 cm in thickness. In children, renal size varies with age.

Sonographically, the kidney parenchyma has two distinct areas: the outer cortex and the inner medullary pyramids, which surround the renal sinus. The cortex is homogenous with relativity low-level echoes that are slightly less echogenic than the normal liver. The medullary pyramids are relatively hypoechoic round or triangular areas between the cortex and the renal sinus. These are separated from each other by bands of cortical tissue, called columns of Bertin, that also extend inward to the renal sinus. The intense specular echoes at the corticomedullary junction are from the arcuate arteries.

The inner echogenic portion of the kidney consists of the renal sinus. The renal sinus contains fat, calyces, infundibula, renal pelvis, connective tissue, renal vessels, and lymphatics. The renal hilum is where blood vessels, nerves, lymphatic vessels, and the ureter enter or exit the renal sinus.

The superior end of the ureter is expanded and forms a funnel-shaped sac called the renal pelvis, which is located within the renal sinus. The renal pelvis is divided into two or three tubes called major calyces, and they are divided into 8 or 18 minor calyces. The apex of the medullary pyramid called the renal papilla indents each minor calyx.

The infundibula (funnel portion of the calyces) are collapsed and not seen within the echogenic renal sinus in a subject that has restricted fluid intake. During diuresis, the narrow channels traversing the sinus can be identified. In patients with an extrarenal pelvis, a fluid-filled structure extending medially to the kidney can be identified. Placing the patient in a prone position will compress the extrarenal pelvis and assist in making the diagnosis.

Maternal pyelocaliectasis without mechanical obstruction is commonly observed during pregnancy and seen more frequently in the right kidney. Fetal pyelectasis is also common in utero, and there are measurements used to distinguish it from hydronephrosis. Structures adjacent to the kidneys (Table 5–14).

Functions of the Kidneys

The kidneys serve in the excretion of inorganic compounds; for example Na^+, K^+, Ca^{++}; excretion of organic compounds; for example, creatinine; blood pressure regulation; erythrocyte volume regulation; and vitamin D and Ca^{++} metabolism.

The ultimate goals of the kidney functions are to:

1. Maintain salt and water balance
2. Regulate the fluid volume
3. Maintain acid and base balance

Laboratory Values

Blood and urine tests are performed to determine renal dysfunction. Renal function cannot be estimated by the use of ultrasound.

1. Serum creatinine is elevated with renal dysfunction. Renal dysfunction occurs when the functioning unit of the kidney (nephron) is destroyed.
2. Blood urea nitrogen (BUN) is elevated when there is acute or chronic renal disease or urinary obstruction. A decrease in BUN may occur with overhydration, liver failure, or pregnancy.

Renal Congenital Anomalies

Renal congenital anomalies include incorrect position, number, and shape. One of the most common anomalies is a duplex collecting system. There may be duplication of the ureters, which may enter into the bladder separately, or more commonly, they will join together and enter into the bladder as one ureter.

Position. Embryologically, the kidneys form in the pelvis in an anteroposterior orientation. They ascend and rotate to the adult position, so that the upper pole of each kidney is more medial than the lower pole. Kidneys not located in the renal fossa are called ectopic kidneys.

Pelvic kidney occurs when the kidney fails to ascend out of the pelvis.

TABLE 5–14. STRUCTURES ADJACENT TO THE KIDNEYS

Anterior to the Right Kidney	Anterior to the Left Kidney	Posterior to the Kidneys
Right adrenal gland	Left adrenal gland	Diaphragm
Liver	Stomach	Quadratus lumborum muscles
Duodenum	Spleen	Psoas muscle
Right colic (hepatic flexure)	Pancreas	
Small intestine	Jejunum (2nd part of the small intestine)	

Horseshoe kidney is the most common form of fusion anomaly. The kidneys lie in an oblique transverse position in the lower abdomen. The kidneys are more commonly fused together at lower poles than at the middle or upper poles.

Number. Anomalies of kidney number would include a solitary kidney (single functioning kidney with the ipsilateral atrophied kidney), unilateral renal agenesis (absence of one kidney and ureter), and a supranumary kidney (duplication of the kidney, pelvis, and ureter).

Unilateral renal agenesis is frequently associated with other genital anomalies; for example, bicornuate uterus, unicornuate uterus, and uterine and vaginal septations. Bilateral renal agenesis is fatal.

Shape. Congenital variations include hypertrophied columns of Bertin (prominent cortical tissue in the medulla < 3 cm), fetal lobulation (lobulated renal surface), dromedary (splenic) hump (bulge of cortical tissue on the lateral aspect of the left kidney), renunculus, and fusion of the kidney (horseshoe kidney, cake kidney). All of the above, except the later, may mimic a mass on ultrasound. Congenital cystic diseases that distort the reniform shape are also included in this category, infantile polycystic kidney disease, adult polycystic kidney disease and multicystic kidney disease.

Polycystic Disease. Polycystic disease may be present at birth or may not manifest until adulthood.

Infantile Polycystic Kidney Disease (IPKD) or Autosomal Recessive Polycystic Disease (ARPKD) or (Potter Type I). This is the least common and most fatal of the three cystic diseases. It is an autosomal recessive trait and is more common in females (2:1). Sonographically, it presents as bilateral echogenic, enlarged kidneys with cysts (the cysts classically are too small to be resolved). If survival past infancy occurs, hepatic fibrosis becomes a complication, with death resulting from hepatic failure and/or bleeding from esophageal varices.

Adult Polycystic Kidney Disease (APKD) or Autosomal Dominant Polycystic Kidney Disease (ADPKD) or Potter Type III. This is an autosomal dominant disease and occurs relatively frequently. The disease may be latent for many years and not manifest itself until the 4th decade. Patients present with decreasing renal function, hypertension, and may have flank pain. Sonographically, APKD presents as bilateral large kidneys with randomly distributed cortical cysts of various sizes, and in the advanced stages, the kidneys loose the reniform shape. Associated finding include cysts in the liver, pancreas, and spleen. Destruction of the residual renal tissue in advance stages leads to renal failure.

Medullary Cystic Disease. It can be either dominant or recessive. Juvenile onset is autosomal recessive and adult onset is autosomal dominant. Clinically, patients present with renal failure. Sonographically, there are small cysts in the medullary portion of both kidneys with a

decreased definition between the cortical/medulla junctions. Hydronephrosis is caused by an obstruction of the outflow of urine. The renal pelvis and calyces become dilated and compress the renal parenchyma causing renal insufficiency. The dilatation may be unilateral or bilateral depending upon the level of the obstruction. The amount of dilation determines if it is mild (Grade 1), moderate (Grade II) or severe (Grade III). The absence of a renal jet and an RI of less than 0.70 will substantiate the diagnosis of renal obstruction.

Hydronephrosis. There are two major classifications of hydronephrosis: intrinsic and extrinsic.

Intrinsic Hydronephrosis. This may be the result of:
  Stricture
  Renal calculi
  Bleeding or blood clot
  Ureterocele
  Pyelonephrosis
  Tuberculosis

Extrinsic Hydronephrosis. This may be the result of:
  Pregnancy (usually involves the right kidney)
  Pelvic masses (e.g., ovarian or fibroids)
  Bladder neck obstruction
  Trauma
  Retroperitoneal fibrosis
  Prostatic hypertrophy
  Urethritis
  Inflammatory lesions—pelvis, gastrointestinal, retroperitoneal
  Neurogenic bladder

Congenital Hydronephrosis. This is present and existing from the time of birth. This may present as:
  Ureteropelvic (UPJ) obstruction
  Ectopic ureterocele usually caused by a duplex collecting system
  Retrocaval ureter
  Posterior urethral valve (PUV)

False-Positive Hydronephrosis. This denotes a test result positive for hydronephrosis when there is no hydronephrosis present. Sonographically, the following may mimic hydronephrosis (dilatation of the collecting system).
  Normal diuresis
  Overdistended bladder
  Parapelvic cyst
  Renal sinus lipomatosis
  Extra renal pelvis
  Reflux—vesicoureteral
  Diabetes insipidus

False-Negative Hydronephrosis. This denotes a test result that wrongly excludes the diagnosis of hydronephrosis. Patients suffering from severe dehydration or intermittent obstruction may have hydronephrosis without dilatation of the collecting system.

Severe dehydration

Nephrolithiasis with intermittent obstruction

Tables 5–15 and 5–16 outline the clinical and sonographic findings associated with cystic and solid renal masses.

Nephrolithiasis (Renal Calculi)

Nephrolithiasis are more commonly found in men than women and typically in people who have urinary stasis. Nephrolithiasis may be composed of uric acid, cystine, or calcium. Sonographically, renal calculi appear as highly reflective echogenic foci. A high-frequency transducer with proper settings of the focal zones is necessary to document posterior shadowing. Using tissue harmonics can also assist in seeing posterior acoustic shadowing. The "twinkle sign" is a color artifact that has been seen with urinary stones. The "twinkle sign" is described as rapidly changing colors that are seen posterior to an echogenic reflector, that is, stones). A Staghorn calculus is large stones located in the central portion of the kidney, the collecting system, and takes the shape of the calyces. Renal obstruction may be secondary to stones located in the collecting system.

TABLE 5–15. RENAL CYSTIC MASSES

Cystic Masses	Clinical Findings	Sonographic Findings
Simple cyst	1. Seen in 50% of patients over the age of 55 2. Usually originates in the renal cortex 3. Asymptomatic unless they are large and obstruct the collecting system 4. Unilocular	1. Anechoic 2. Thin walls 3. Round 4. Increased through acoustical transmission
Atypical cyst	1. Septated or multilocular 2. Septations have no pathological significance	Fulfills all of the criteria for a simple cyst but, will have internal echogenic lines i.e. septations
Parapelvic cyst	1. Originates from renal parenchyma and is seen in the renal hilum 2. May present with hypertension and pain	1. Fulfills the criteria for a simple cyst but located within the renal pelvis 2. Solitary and large 3. Does not communicate with the collecting system
Peripelvic cysts	1. Originates in the renal pelvis 2. May develop from the lymphatic system or obstruction	1. Small, multiple, and irregular shape 2. May appear as dilated renal pelvis 3. Does not communicate with the collecting system
Inflammatory cysts	1. Simple cysts that have become infected 2. An increase in leukocytosis 3. Pain	1. Complex pattern of internal echoes from inflammatory debris 2. Slightly thicken walls, not as thick as chronic abscess
Hemorrhagic cysts	1. 6% of all renal cysts will hemorrhage 2. Increase incidence in polycystic disease	Complex echo pattern dependent upon state of hemorrhage
Calcified cysts	2% of all cysts will calcify	1. Anechoic 2. Smooth round borders that are echogenic or have echogenic foci 3. calcified walls attenuate sound making it difficult to visualize the complete cyst
Renal abscess (carbuncle)	1. Fever, chills, flank pain 2. Elevated white blood count	1. May appear solid early in the course 2. Complex echo pattern due to debris 3. Walls are thicken and irregular 4. Gas may produce a dirty shadow
Hydronephrosis	Obstruction a. Intrinsic—within the collecting system by a stone or stricture b. Extrinsic—a mass compresses the ureter or bladder outlet	The calices, infundibula and renal pelvis dilate due to the obstruction of urine flow. Minor dilatation (Grade 1)—slight splaying of the collecting system Moderate dilatation (Grade 2)—increased dilation of the collecting system with thinning of the parenchyma Severe dilatation (Grade 3)—huge anechoic collecting system with lose of shape and very little parenchyma
Pyonephritis	Pus in the dilated collecting system complication of hydronephrosis that occurs secondary to urinary stasis and infection	Dilated pelvocaliceal system filled with internal echoes, shifting urine-debris level, may have shadowing caused by gas-forming organisms
Renal Sinus Disease Renal sinus lipomatosis	More common in older patients; may be secondary to chronic calculus disease and inflammation. The renal sinus is replaced by fatty tissue.	In replacement lipomatosis, the kidney is enlarged, the renal sinus appears hypoechoic because of fat (one of the few times that fat appears hypoechoic instead of echogenic).

TABLE 5–16. SOLID RENAL MASSES

Tumors	Clinical Findings	Sonographic Findings
Benign Solid Tumors		
Angiomyolipoma, also called renal hamartoma (tumor composed of fat, muscle, and blood vessels)	More common in women than men (2:1). Symptoms are flank pain, hematuria, and hypertension	Discrete highly echogenic mass found in the cortex
Adenomas (benign counter part of renal cell carcinoma)	Asymptomatic or painless hematuria, usually found on autopsy	Small well-define isoechoic or hypoechoic mass found in the cortex
Connective tissue tumors 1. Hemangiomas 2. Fibromas 3. Myomas 4. Lipomas	Gross hematuria	These tumors present as homogenous echogenic lesions relating to their vascularity and fat content
Malignant Solid Tumors		
Hypernephroma (also known as adenocarcinoma, renal cell carcinoma (RCC), and von Grawitz tumor)	1. Affect males more than females (2:1) commonly after the age of 50 2. Hematuria 3. An arteriogram of the kidney demonstrates a mass with increased vascular supply with irregular branching 4. Metastases to bone, heart, and brain	1. Unilateral, solitary and encapsulated 2. Varied echogenicity from hypoechoic to echogenic 3. Look for metastases via the blood stream infiltrating the renal vein and IVC 4. Look for metastases to the contralateral kidney, ureter, peritoneum, liver, and spleen
Transitional cell carcinoma (affects the urothelium and may be located anywhere within the urinary system)	1. Occurs in the renal pelvis 2. Usually asymptomatic, may have pain or palpable mass 3. Painless hematuria 4. Known to be invasive	1. Invasive tumor not well-defined or encapsulated within the renal pelvis 2. Occasional appears as a bulky discrete mass 3. Hypoechoic or isoechoic
Renal lymphoma	1. Relatively common in patients with widely disseminated lymphomatous malignancy	1. Solid mass with low-level internal echoes 2. May appear similar to renal cysts but will not demonstrate increased through acoustic transmission
Wilms' tumor (nephroblastoma)	1. Most common malignancy of renal origin in children 2. Abdominal mass, hypertension, nausea 3. Hematuria	1. Early on encapsulated later on it may extend into the perirenal area 2. Varied sonographic appearance depending upon the amount of necrosis and/or hemorrhage

Laboratory Values. In cases of chronic obstruction, there is an increase in serum creatinine and BUN levels. In acute obstruction, there are no specific lab values. Urine may show hematuria and/or bacteria.

Signs and Symptoms. Renal colic, flank pain, nausea, and vomiting.

Renal Failure

Renal failure is the kidneys' inability to filter metabolites from the blood resulting in decreased renal function, which may be either acute or chronic. Laboratory findings are increased serum BUN and serum creatinine levels.

Etiology.

Prerenal Causes. Renal hypoperfusion secondary to a systemic cause can occur as a result of vascular disorders leading to renal failure and includes the following conditions.

Nephrosclerosis. Arteriosclerosis of the renal arteries, resulting in ischemia of the kidney. Nephrosclerosis develops rapidly in patients with severe hypertension.

Infarction. This may result from occlusion or stenosis of the renal artery.

Renal Artery Stenosis. Any narrowing of the renal artery will affect the blood flow to the kidney, resulting in atrophy of the kidney and decreased renal function.

Congestive Heart Failure. This may cause renal hypo-perfusion secondary to heart failure.

Thrombosis. Thrombosis of the renal vein will increase the intravascular pressure and, thus, decrease blood flow to the kidney.

Sonography. Doppler of the renal artery is employed to detect arterial blood flow patterns either directly from the renal artery or indirectly from parenchyma flow patterns.

Renal Parenchymal Disease—Infection and Inflammatory Disease

Acute Tubular Necrosis (ATN). Of the acute renal medical diseases, this is the most common cause of acute renal failure. The destruction of the tubular epithelial cells of the proximal and distal convoluted tubules may occur as a result of ingestion or inhalation of toxic agents, ischemia caused by trauma, hemorrhage, acute interstitial nephritis, cortical necrosis, and diseases of the glomeruli.

Pyelonephritis. Infection is the most common disease of the urinary tract, and the combination of parenchymal, caliceal, and pelvic inflammation constitutes pyelonephritis. Bacteria ascending from the urinary bladder or adjacent lymph nodes to the kidney usually cause infection of the kidney.

Glomerulonephritis. Etiology is unknown, but it frequently follows other infections.

Metabolic Disorders. Diabetes mellitus, amyloidosis, gout, and nephrocalcinosis (deposit of calcium in the renal parenchyma) are metabolic disorders associated with renal failure.

Chronic Nephrotoxicity. This caused by exposure to radiation, heavy metals, industrial solvents, and drugs.

Sonography. In acute renal failure, the kidney may be normal sized or enlarged. There may be decreased definition between the medullary/cortical junctions. As the case progresses from acute to chronic, the echogenicity will increase. There is no definite correlation between the echogenicity of the kidney, the kidney size, and degree of decreased renal function. Patients in end stage renal failure will have small echogenic kidneys that are difficult to image sonographically.

Postrenal Causes. These include urinary tract obstruction, which cause hydronephrosis, and may be congenital or acquired intrinsically and extrinsically.

Sonography. There are varying degrees of the dilation of the renal sinus, calyces, infundibulum, and pelvis.

Renal Medical Diseases (Table 5–17)

Type I. There is increased cortical echogenicity with a decrease in corticomedullary differentiation. Type I diseases are those caused by glomerular infiltrate, such as acute and chronic glomerulonephritis, acute lupus nephritis, nephrosclerosis, any type of nephritis, and renal transplant rejection. All these disorders can cause the echogenicity of the renal cortex to be greater than the liver and spleen. As the disease progresses to the chronic state, the kidney becomes smaller, the cortex becomes more echogenic, and eventually the medulla will come equally echogenic.

TABLE 5–17. RENAL MEDICAL DISEASES

Disease	Clinical Findings	Sonographic Appearance
Acute pyelonephritis	Ninety percent are female, dysuria, urinary frequency, fever, leukocytosis, bacteriuria	Normal or enlarged kidneys, may have mild hydronephrosis; enlarged corticomedullary area with decreased echogenicity and loss of definition between the cortex and medulla; low level echoes may be produced by multiple small abscesses and areas of necrosis in the cortex and medulla
Chronic pyelonephritis	Affects male and females; usually caused by recurrent urinary tract infection or inadequately treated pyelonephritis; proteinuria	Normal or small kidneys; parenchymal thinning; increased echogenicity due to fibrosis
Acute lobar nephronia (acute focal bacteria nephritis)	Inflammatory mass without drainable pus results from gram-negative bacteria that ascends from ureteral reflux; fever, chills, flank pain	Poorly defined cystic mass containing echoes that may disrupt the corticomedullary junction; unable to differentiate from an abscess
Xanthogranulomatous pyelonephritis	Rare form of inflammatory disease found in patients with long-standing renal calculi	Enlarged kidneys with multiple anechoic or hypoechoic areas
Glomerulonephritis	Glomerular disease results from an immunological reaction in which antigen-antibody complexes in the circulation are trapped in the glomeruli. It is the most common cause of renal failure. In the acute stage—oliguria, edema, increased BUN, increased creatinine and increased serum K. In the chronic state—polyuria, proteinuria to such a high extent that 50% of patients develop nephritic syndrome.	Increased echogenicity of the renal cortex with a decrease of the renal size as the disease progresses
Acute tubular necrosis (ATN)	Most common cause of acute renal failure may result from ischemia, decreased blood flow to and from the kidney, renal transplant. It may be toxin induced or from trauma/surgery.	Enlarged kidney, especially in the anteroposterior diameter; normal renal parenchyma; renal medullary pyramids will appear more prominent and anechoic

Type II. There is distortion of normal anatomy involving cortex and medullary pyramids; sonographically, there is a decrease in the corticomedullary differentiation in either a focal or diffuse manner. The type II pattern is seen with such focal lesions as cysts, abscesses, hematomas, bacterial nephritis (lobar nephronia), infantile polycystic disease, adult polycystic disease, chronic pyelonephritis, and chronic glomerulonephritis.

Renal Transplants

The transplanted kidney is placed within the iliac fossa. A baseline sonogram is performed within 48 hours post operatively to document the exact location, size, and sonographic appearance of the transplanted kidney. The most serious sign of transplant rejection is renal failure. Clinical signs of renal rejection include, fever, pain, and decreased urine output. The laboratory results are the same as renal failure, elevated BUN, and serum creatinine.

Acute rejection of the transplanted kidney may be caused by acute tubular necrosis (ATN), or arterial obstruction. Differentiating between the different causes of renal failure is important to ensure proper treatment is administered.

In cases of acute rejection, the kidney appears sonographically as an enlarged kidney with increased cortical echogenicity, decreased renal sinus echogenicity, irregular sonolucent areas in the cortex, enlarged and decreased echogenicity of the pyramids, distortion of the renal outline, and indistinct corticomedullary junction.

Rejection caused by acute tubular necrosis usually results in a normal sonogram. In rejection caused by acute renal arterial occlusion, the sonographic appearance seems grossly normal. However, duplex Doppler studies may reveal an absence or decreased diastolic flow.

Perinephric fluid collections, commonly associated with the transplanted kidneys, are lymphocele, urinoma, abscess, and hematoma (Table 5–18).

URETERS

The ureters are located in the retroperitoneal cavity and course along the anterior surface of the psoas muscle along the medial side. The ureters are approximately 6 mm in diameter. The three most common places for obstruction to occur are: at the ureteropelvic junction (UPJ); as they cross over the pelvic brim; and at the junction into the bladder. In the pelvis, the ureters are anterior to the iliac vessels.

Urine can be imaged entering into the urinary bladder with the use of color Doppler. Color Doppler is used because the ureteral jet will cause a Doppler shift because of the continued changes in the turbulent flow in the urine. If the bladder has recently been overly distended, ureteral jets may not be imaged because of the specific gravity of the urine in the ureters and in the bladder being similar, thus causing no Doppler shift. Ureteral jets occur at regular intervals, approximately every 2–3 seconds. They appear as bursts of color entering from the base of the bladder flowing toward the center of the bladder and lasting for a fraction of a second. The absence or decrease of a ureteral jet indicates the presence of an obstruction.

Congenital Anomalies of the Ureters

These include double or bifid ureter, narrowing, strictures, diverticuli, and hydroureter caused by a congenital defect, as in polycystic kidney, or acquired, as in a low ureteral obstruction.

Megaureter in Childhood (Primary-Nonobstructive, Nonrefluxing Megaureter)

This includes prune belly syndrome (Eagle–Barrett syndrome), deficiency of the abdominal musculature, and urinary tract abnormalities (large hypotonic bladder, undescended testes, hydroureter), and retroperitoneal fibrosis, which fixes the ureter and prevents peristalsis, leading to functional obstruction.

Secondary Megaureter

This is caused by reflux of urine or obstruction.

Ureteral abnormalities are viewed in Table 5–19.

BLADDER

Gross Anatomy

The urinary bladder is a thin wall triangular structure that is located directly posterior to the pubic bone. The apex of the bladder points anteriorly and is connected to the umbilicus by the median umbilical ligament, the remains of the

TABLE 5–18. PERINEPHRIC FLUID COLLECTIONS

Type	Clinical Findings	Sonographic Appearance
Abscess (Renal carbuncle is a confluence of several small abscesses.)	Flank pain, high white blood count, fever	Usually echogenic with irregular thicken walls, may have shadowing within caused by gas
Hematoma	Drop in hematocrit	Same sonographic appearance as an abscess depending upon the age and amount of clot/liquification
Urinoma	An encapsulated collection of extravasated urine	Usually anechoic, may have low level echoes if superimposed with infection
Lymphocele	Collection of lymphatic fluid	Usually anechoic, may have low level echoes if superimposed with hemorrhage

Abscess, hematoma, urinoma, and lymphocele are commonly associated with renal transplant, although it is not exclusive.

TABLE 5–19. URETERAL ABNORMALITIES

Abnormality	Clinical Finding	Sonographic Appearance
Posterior urethral valves syndrome (PUV): A flap of mucosal tissue covers the opening in the area of the prostatic urethra, causing a urinary outlet obstruction.	Most common cause of urinary obstruction in the male infant and are the second most common cause of hydronephrosis in the neonate. Decreased urine output, failure to thrive and severe cases renal failure in infants. Older patients will experience decreased urine output, dysuria, and urinary tract infections (UTIs).	Distended bladder with a thickened wall bilateral hydroureters seen medial and posterior to the bladder and in severe cases hydronephrosis. The bladder may have a "key hole" appearance with dilation of the proximal portion of the urethra.
Ureterocele: A cystic dilation of the distal portion of the ureter with narrowing of the ureteric orifice; can be either congenital or acquired.	Patients are usually asymptomatic and the cysts are usually small. Ureterocele's may cause obstruction and infection of the upper urinary tract. If large they may cause bladder outlet obstruction.	An anechoic thin-walled structure of variable size and shape projecting into the bladder.

fetal urachus. The ureters enter at a posteroinferior angle, and the urethra extends from the bladder neck to the exterior of the body. The trigone is the area of the bladder between the neck and apex. It contains three orifices, two for the ureters and the one for the urethra.

A normal distended urinary bladder on ultrasound is imaged as a midline symmetrical anechoic structure. On a longitudinal scan it has a "sausage" shape and on a transverse scan, it has a somewhat round appearance. The bladder wall is imaged as a thin, smooth, echogenic line that measures between 3 to 6 mm in thickness. The normal bladder volume varies and can usually reach 500 mL without any major discomfort.

Bladder stones can develop in the bladder or may form in the kidney and pass to the bladder via the ureter. Patients passing a urinary tract stone present with renal colic, flank pain, and hematuria. Sonographically, the bladder stone appears as an echogenic focus with posterior acoustic shadowing. Calculi are gravity dependent (calculi moves to the dependent portion of the bladder when the patient is placed in a decubitus position). Ureteral jets are usually normal; rarely do the calculi obstruct the ureter.

During a pelvic ultrasound examination, the bladder wall thickness, irregularities of the wall, bladder shape, and lumen should be evaluated. There may be an extrinsic mass; for example, a fibroid or enlarged prostate, compressing the bladder and causing bladder distortion. Table 5–20 reviews abnormalities that will distort the wall and shape of the bladder.

ADRENAL GLANDS

Gross Anatomy
The adrenal glands are part of the endocrine system and consist of two distinct regions: the medulla, which is surrounded by the cortex. The adrenal glands are triangular-shaped structures located superior and anteromedial to the upper pole of the kidney. They measure 5 × 5 × 1 cm, but at birth, are proportionately much larger. Gerota's fascia encloses the kidneys, adrenals, and perinephric fat.

The right adrenal gland lies posterior and lateral to the inferior vena cava, lateral to the right crus of the diaphragm, and medial to the right lobe of the liver. To image the right adrenal gland the patient is typically placed in a left lateral decubitus position (right side up). The right adrenal gland is located between the right lobe of liver, IVC, and right kidney.

The left adrenal gland lies medial to the spleen, lateral to the aorta, and posterior to the tail of the pancreas. Sonographically, the normal adrenal glands in adults are difficult to visualize because of their small size and the echo texture being similar to the surrounding retroperitoneal fat. To image the left adrenal gland, the patient lies in a right lateral decubitus position (left side up) the transducer is placed in a coronal position. The left adrenal glands lies between the spleen, aorta, and left kidney, and these structures are used as sonographic landmarks. A computed tomography (CT) is the imaging modality of choice. Adrenal tumors may be identified on a sonogram usually by their displacement and/or compression of adjacent structures. See Table 5–21 for adrenal gland malfunctions.

The Right Adrenal Pathology Will Displace—
Anteriorly	*Posteriorly*
The retroperitoneal fat line	The right kidney
The inferior vena cava	
The right renal vein	

Left Adrenal Pathology Will Displace—
Anteriorly	*Posteriorly*
The splenic vein	The left kidney

Adrenal Cortex
The adrenal cortex, which produces steroid hormones, is subdivided into three zones listed from outer to inner: (1) the zona glomerulosa, which produces mineralocorticoids (for the regulation of aldosterone to regulate electrolyte metabolism); (2) the zona fasiculata, which produces glucocorticoids (for the regulation of cortisol, which is an anti-stress and anti-inflammatory hormone); and (3) the zona

TABLE 5–20. BLADDER ABNORMALITIES

Abnormality	Clinical Findings	Ultrasound Findings
Urachal cysts: The urachus connects the apex of the bladder with the allantois (an embryological structure with no function after birth) through the umbilical cord. Normally, it fibroses at birth, but it may, in part or in whole, remain patent. The urachus lies in the space Retzius (anterior to the urinary bladder)	A urachal cyst remains clinical asymptomatic until an infection develops, then there is vague abdominal pain and/or urinary complaints	An anechoic tubular structure in the lower mid-abdominal anterior wall. It may extend from the umbilicus to the bladder.
Diverticuli of the bladder: Pouchlike envaginations of the bladder wall. They can either be congenital or acquired.	The diverticula constitute a site of urinary stasis that tends to become infected	Diverticula vary greatly in size and may appear separate from the bladder. They are round, well-defined, thin-walled cystic masses. To help delineate it from an adnexal mass, have the patient void; it should disappear.
Reduplication: Complete reduplication of the bladder is rare	Unilateral reflex, obstruction or infection	Two bladders will be visualized separated by a peritoneal fold with two urethras and two external openings.
Reflux: Vesicoureteral reflex is a common urinary tract abnormality in children secondary to anomalies such as ectopic, posterior urethral valves, prune belly syndrome, neurogenic bladder, and primary congenital abnormalities of the bladder	Reflux may be a cause of chronic renal failure with scarring and atrophic changes in the kidney	Cysto–Conray (20%) is injected into the bladder. Each kidney is scanned while the contrast is injected. With each increasing grade of reflux, there is increasing renal collecting system dilation.
Bladder Neck Obstruction: The lower portion continuous with the urethra is called the neck.	In the male bladder, neck obstruction commonly is secondary to benign prostatic hypertrophy (BPH) or carcinoma. With prolonged obstruction the bladder wall will become thickened and trabeculate.	A thickened and irregular-walled bladder
Cystitis: Infection or inflammation of the bladder. More common in females because of the shorter urethra.	Secondary to diverticula, urethral obstruction, fistulas, cystocele, bladder neoplasm, pyelonephritis, neurogenic dysfunction, bladder calculi, trauma, pregnancy, rectal/vaginal fistula	In cases of long-standing infection or inflammation (chronic), the bladder walls may show inflammatory changes and thickening. In cases of a neurogenic bladder low level echoes may be seen in the bladder producing a pus–urine fluid level.
Primary Benign Tumor (uncommon): papilloma, epithelial, leiomyoma, neurofibroma, adenoma (associated with cystitis)	Patients present with painless hematuria, dysuria, frequent urination	Ultrasound cannot distinguish between a benign or malignant tumor. Small to massive solid tumors are seen projecting from the bladder wall, some may evaginate the bladder wall and may be smooth or irregular in contour. May mimic benign prostatic hypertrophy or cystitis. Outflow obstruction and hydronephrosis also need to be evaluated.
Primary Malignant Tumor: 95% are transitional cell carcinoma (TCC); 5% are squamous cell carcinoma	Invasive growths, with 40% having metastases to lymph nodes and invasion of the prostate and seminal vesicles. They are usually not detected until they have metastasized. Patients present with hematuria, urinary frequency, dysuria	Ultrasound cannot distinguish between a benign or malignant tumor. Small to massive solid tumors are seen projecting from the bladder wall, some may evaginate the bladder wall, and may be smooth or irregular in contour. May mimic benign prostatic hypertrophy or cystitis. Outflow obstruction and hydronephrosis also need to be evaluated.

reticularis, which produces gonadocorticoids (for regulation for the secretion of androgens and estrogens, which are the sex hormones of an individual).

The adrenal cortical hormones are regulated by the adrenocorticotropic hormones (ACTH) of the anterior pituitary gland. A *decrease* in adrenal cortical function leads to an increased ACTH, which then stimulates the adrenal cortex. An *increase* in concentration of adrenal hormones leads to a drop in ACTH secretion, which leads a to a drop in the activity of adrenal cortex.

The adrenal cortex may be affected either by lesions that produce an excess of steroid hormones or by lesions that

TABLE 5–21. ADRENAL GLAND MALFUNCTIONS

Malformations	Clinical Findings	Sonographic Findings
Adrenal Cortex		
Adrenocortical hyperfunction Cushing's syndrome	Increased corticosteroid production produces diabetes mellitus, protuberant abdomen from muscle weakening and loss of elastic tissue, rounded faces, mild hypertension, cardiac enlargement, and edema.	Varied—the adrenal glands may appear normal, diffusely enlarged, solid, cystic, or complex, with focal areas of necrosis or hemorrhage.
Conn's syndrome—benign	Hyperaldosteronism caused by an increase of aldosterone producing sodium retention, which leads to essential hypertension, increased thirst, and urination.	Varied—the adrenal glands may appear normal, diffusely enlarged, solid, cystic, or complex with focal areas of necrosis or hemorrhage.
Adenomas—may be functional or nonfunctional	Benign tumors associated with Cushing's and Conn's syndrome. May present with hypertension, diabetes, hyperthyroidism, and renal cell carcinoma.	Round or oval in shape usually larger than 1 cm, hypoechoic.
Adrenocortical hypofunction Addison's disease—rare condition	Decreased hormonal production causing hypotension, malaise, weight loss, changes in skin pigmentation, loss of body hair, and menstrual irregularity. 80% are attributable to idiopathic destruction, probably autoimmune in nature, and 20% are caused by tuberculosis.	Varied normal or hyperechoic may be small because of the destruction of cortical tissue.
Adrenal Medulla		
Pheochromocytoma—rare vascular tumors	Paroxysmal or sustained hypertension, angina, cardiac arrhythmias, anxiety, nausea, vomiting, and headaches. These features are caused by the concentration of catecholamines released into circulation. Large tumors may lead to heart failure and death.	Well-defined large masses highly vascular masses that can be cystic, solid, or heterogeneous with calcifications.
Neuroblastoma	A highly malignant tumor that arises from the sympathetic nervous tissue or adrenal medulla. Children can be asymptomatic or have weight loss, fever episodes of tachycardia, sweats, and headaches with a palpable abdominal mass.	Varied presentation—large echogenic, heterogeneous mass with areas of cystic degeneration and focal calcifications. The kidney will be displaced posteriorly and inferiorly.
Adrenal Masses		
Adrenal metastases	Most commonly from bronchogenic CA, lung adenocarcinoma, breast or stomach carcinoma.	Metastases to the adrenals vary in size and echogenicity.
Adrenal cysts—rare	None-patient are usually asymptomatic	Round or oval in shape, anechoic with increased through acoustical transmission. Adrenal cysts tend to become calcified, which appear as an echo-free structure, with an echogenic back wall with posterior shadowing (no through acoustic transmission).
Adrenal hematomas	Most often seen in infants caused by trauma from birth, prematurity or hypoxia. In adults, it is caused by trauma or anticoagulant therapy.	Varies depending upon the age of the bleed initially the hematoma is echogenic, and then it becomes sonolucent to complex and then calcified.

produce a deficiency. The adrenocortical hormones levels may be abnormal (increased or decreased production) as a result of a pituitary tumor, which can cause the overproduction or underproduction of ACTH.

Adrenal Medulla

The adrenal medulla produces epinephrine (adrenalin) and norepinephrine. These hormones have a wide range of effects.

Epinephrine dilates the coronary vessels and constricts the skin and kidney vessels. It increases coronary output, raises oxygen consumption, and causes hyperglycemia.

Norepinephrine constricts all arterial vessels except the coronary arteries (which dilate). It is the essential regulator of blood pressure.

Epinephrine, in particular, is responsible for the flight-or-fight reaction. It stimulates the metabolic rate, allowing more available energy.

GASTROINTESTINAL TRACT (GI)

Sonography is not routinely used to image the gastrointestinal tract because of the air within the canal. Normal bowel patterns can be imaged and recognized during an abdominal sonographic examination. Knowledge of the GI tract is essential for identifying the location of the pathology.

Gross Anatomy

The GI tract is composed of the esophagus, the stomach, the small intestine, and the colon.

The esophagus is a tubular structure that extends from the pharynx to the stomach. Its main function is to bring food and water to the stomach. The gastroesophageal junction (GEJ) can be identified slightly to the left of midline on a sagittal scan. Sonographically, it appears round with an echogenic center with a hypoechoic rim also referred to as a "target sign" or "bull's-eye" located posterior to the left lobe of the liver and anterior to the aorta.

The stomach lies between the esophagus and the duodenum. The opening between the stomach and the duodenum is called the pyloric orifice. The main function of the stomach is to break down food to chyme, which then passes through to the duodenum. Sonographically, the fluid-filled stomach is imaged as an anechoic structure with echogenic foci and thin walls. The five layers of the gastrointestinal tract are imaged sonographically from internal to externally as: mucosa (hyperechoic); intramural (hypoechoic); submucosa (hyperechoic); muscularis propria (hypoechoic); and serosal layer (hyperechoic).

The small intestine lies between the stomach and the colon and is divided into three parts: duodenum, jejunum, and the ileum. The main function of the small intestine is to absorb food.

The ileocecal valve connects the distal portion of the ileum to the first section of the colon, the cecum. The appendix is usually located in the RLQ as a tubular structure that extends from the cecum. The ascending colon ascends from the cecum along the right side of the body to the posterior inferior surface of to the liver. The ascending colon bends to the left and forms the hepatic flexure. The transverse colon extends across the body from the hepatic flexure to the splenic flexure. The splenic flexure is located posterior and inferior to the spleen and bends inferiorly forming the descending colon, which courses along the left side to the body and terminates at the sigmoid colon.

The sigmoid is the narrowest portion of the colon, and the distal end forms the rectum. The anal canal is the distal end of the rectum, which expels solid waste products (feces) from the body.

The main functions of the intestines are to reabsorb liquid and to form solid waste products, which are expelled from the body via the anus (see Table 5–22, Bowel pathologies).

BREAST*

Gross Anatomy

The breasts are mammary glands and consist of three layers of tissue: the subcutaneous layer; the mammary layer; and the retromammary layer. The subcutaneous layer is the most superficial layer and consists mainly of fat tissue. The middle layer or mammary layer is also called the parenchymal layer and is the functional layer of the breast. It consists of 15–20 lobes of fibroglandular tissue. The lobes vary in size and are pyramidal in shape, with the apex pointing to the areola. The lobes also have lactiferous ducts that course toward the nipple. The lobes are separated by loose and dense connective tissue. Copper's ligament (connective tissue) provides support of the parenchyma and connects the anterior and posterior fascial planes. The retromammary layer is the layer closest to the chest wall and consists of fat. The major pectoral muscle lies posterior to the retromammary layer and surrounds the pectoral minor muscle.

The main function of the female breast is to produce and secrete milk. Milk production occurs in the acini tissue, which is glandular tissue located in the breast parenchyma. The male breast has some ductal elements that do not develop to produce to milk. The male ducts may hypertrophy during puberty and later in life with hormonal fluctuations, in some disease processes, or with medications. The hypertrophy of the milk ducts is a benign condition called gynecomastia.

Mammography is the gold standard for imaging the breast. Sonography is used to supplement the mammographic findings, especially in young women with dense breast tissue, pregnant women, evaluation of a palpable mass, clarification of an abnormal mammographic finding,

_____
*Disclaimer: Not intended for breast registry.

TABLE 5–22. GASTROINTESTINAL PATHOLOGY

Pathology	Clinical Signs and Symptoms	Ultrasound Appearance
Appendicitis—common cause of acute abdomen in young adults	RLQ pain with rebound tenderness, increased white blood count, fever, vomiting, nausea	RLQ "target sign," appendix greater than 6.0 mm in diameter, hypoechoic wall greater then 2.0 mm, increased vascularity, noncompressible, may have pericecal fluid
Hypertrophic pyloric stenosis (HPS)—thickened muscle of the pylorus causing elongation and narrowing of the pylorus, more common in first born	Failure to thrive, projectile vomiting, dehydration, palpable "olive shaped" mass in epigastric region	"Target" sign (echogenic center with hypoechoic outer ring) medial to GB, anterior to right kidney, transverse muscle greater than 4 mm, pyloric length greater than 18 mm, fluid-filled stomach with no fluid entering into duodenum
Gastric carcinoma—more common in males, most common is gastric carcinoma	Abdominal mass, weight loss	"Target sign," increased vascular flow, may have gastric wall thickening
Ventral hernia—bowel protruding through the ventral wall	May cause bowel obstruction, usually a soft palpable mass	High-frequency linear probe is used to document bowel going anteriorly through the fascial defect

mass classification of solid versus cystic, and for needle guidance.

Sonographically, the breast appearance varies because of the following: age; amount of fat; parenchymal tissue; and if the woman is lactating. Breast tissue is homogenous. Young women tend to have dense breasts, and as a woman ages, the mammary tissue is replaced with fat tissue. The nipple is homogenous with midlevel echoes and posterior acoustic shadowing posterior to the nipple. The normal skin surface appears as two thin echogenic linear lines with less than 2-mm distance between the layers. Copper's ligament appears curvilinear and echogenic surrounding the hypo-echoic fat tissue. Normal lymph nodes are not imaged on sonographic examinations. In patients with little breast tissue, acoustic shadowing may be seen posterior to the ribs, with the spaces between the ribs seen in regular intervals appearing oval with midlevel echoes (see Table 5–23 for breast masses characteristics and Table 5–24 for breast pathology).

TABLE 5–23. SONOGRAPHIC CHARACTERISTICS OF BREAST MASS

Benign Masses	Malignant Masses
Shape—round, oval	Shape—irregular, taller than wider
Margins—well-defined, may have edge artifact	Margins—poorly defined, microlobulations
Compresses tissue	Invades surrounding tissue
Homogenous—isoechoic or anechoic	Heterogeneous— may have calcifications
Distal acoustic enhancement	Acoustic shadowing
Normal skin thickness	Skin thickening
	Mass growing toward nipple

TABLE 5–24. BREAST PATHOLOGY

Pathology	Clinical Signs and Symptoms	Sonographic Appearance
Benign		
Simple cyst—most common mass, may vary in size with menstrual cycle, may be singular or multiple	Pain, tenderness, palpable, firm, smooth, mobile	Round, oval, anechoic, thin walls, increased posterior acoustic enhancement
Complex cyst	Pain, tenderness, palpable, firm, smooth, mobile	Round, oval, low-level internal echoes, increased posterior acoustic enhancement
Abscess	Pain, fever, skin reddening, palpable mass, enlarged, nipple discharge, history of mastitis, invasive intervention, often affects lactating women,	Irregular shape, thick walls, cystic with low-level internal echoes or septations
Hematoma	Usually caused by trauma, surgery, biopsy, pain, palpable mass	Varied due to the age of the hematoma, well-defined, smooth walls, usually increased through acoustic transmission
Fibroadenoma—most common benign mass of women of child bearing age, influenced by estrogen, may be singular or multiple	Nontender palpable mass, moveable, firm	Round or oval, smooth borders, lobulated, homogeneous with low- to midlevel echoes, occasionally has a complex appearance
Fibrocystic changes—common condition in women over the age of 55	Tender full breasts, pain varies with menstrual cycle	Round or oval, smooth thin walls, anechoic, increased through posterior transmission, usually multilocular
Cystosarcoma Phylloides—seen women between 40–70 years, usually benign, but can also be malignant mass	Palpable mass that can be large, painless, mobile	Well-defined, mostly solid, but may have some internal anechoic areas caused by necrosis, cystic degeneration, or hemorrhage
Ductal Ectasia—dilation of the lactiferous ducts, seen in menopausal women and women who have nursed for a long time	Nipple inversion, intermittent pain, thick discharge from nipple	Dilated anechoic ducts coursing toward the nipple, usually bilateral
Gynecomastia—common male breast enlargement	Enlarged breast with palpable mass behind the nipple	Dilated ducts coursing toward the nipple, increased echogenicity below nipple, nipple retraction, hyperechoic breast tissue
Malignant		
Infiltrating ductal carcinoma—approx. 80% of breast malignancies	Painless, hard, nonmobile	Irregular borders, invades surrounding parenchyma, solid, hypoechoic
Infiltrating lobar carcinoma—occurs in women from late 20s to mid 80s increase risk for contralateral breast involvement	Nonmobile mass, nipple retraction	Irregular shaped, hypoechoic, posterior acoustic enhancement
Medullary carcinoma—fast-growing mass, usually found in women under 50 years old	Palpable mass, may have enlarged lymph nodes	Well-defined solid mass with internal echoes, sonographic appearance similar to fibroadenomas or abscesses

THYROID

Gross Anatomy

The thyroid is an endocrine gland that secretes three major hormones: thyroxine, triidothyronine, and calcitonin. The thyroid is located in the neck and has two lobes connected anteriorly by a narrow band of tissue, referred to as the isthmus.

The common carotid artery and internal jugular vein lie posterior and lateral, defining the posterolateral margins of the thyroid. The "strap muscles" lie anterior to the lateral aspect of the thyroid defining the anterolateral margins of the thyroid.

Surrounding Musculature and Structures

Sternohyoid muscle—anterior and slightly lateral

Sternothyroid muscle—posterior to the sternohyoid

Longus colli muscle—adjacent to the trachea and is posterior to the thyroid and the common carotid arteries

Esophagus—slightly to the left of midline and posterior to the thyroid

Sonographically, the thyroid has a homogeneous echogenicity that is greater than the strap muscles.

Normal Measurements of the Thyroid

Size

Lobes	*Isthmus*
Length: 4–6 cm	Length: 2 cm
Width: 1.5–2 cm	Width: 2 cm
Height: 2–3 cm	Height: 2–6 cm

Physiologically, there are two basic conditions that occur with the thyroid, hypothyroidism or hyperthyroidism. The anterior pituitary gland produces a thyroid-stimulating hormone, which regulates the hormones secreted by the thyroid gland. Table 5–25 outlines the pathologies of the thyroid that can be imaged sonographically.

SCROTUM

Gross Anatomy

The scrotum is a sac that is continuous with the abdomen and is divided by a septum, the medial raphe. Each space contains a testis, and epididymis, a portion of spermatic cord, and the ductus deferens (Fig. 5–7). A thin, double layer of peritoneum, and the tunica vaginalis line the inner wall of the scrotum. This double layer of peritoneum normally contains a small amount of fluid.

The testicles are ovoid glands that measure approximately $4 \times 2 \times 3$ cm. A dense white fibrous capsule, tunica albiguina, encases each testicle and then enters the gland, separating the testes into approximately 200 cone-shaped lobules. Within these lobules, two primary functions occur: spermatogenesis (the production of spermatozoa);

and the secretion of testosterone by the interstitial cells (Leydig cells).

The secretions are carried through the lobules to the rete testis. A series of ducts, efferent ductules, drain the rete testis, piercing the tunica albuginea, and entering the head of the epididymis.

The epididymis consists of a single tightly coiled duct that drapes the posterior aspect of the testis. The most superior aspect of the epididymis is the head, followed by the body and tail. This duct continues as the ductus deferens (vas deferens), leaving the pelvis via the inguinal canal with the testicular artery, the draining veins of the scrotum, nerves, and lymphatics to form the spermatic cord. Each spermatic cord now extends over the top and down the posterior surface of the bladder, coming together to join the duct from the seminal vesicle to form the ejaculatory ducts. The ejaculatory ducts pass through the prostate gland to terminate in the urethra.

Normal Sonographic Anatomy of the Scrotum

The normal testicle has a homogeneous echo pattern of medium-level echogenicity. The skin is a thin, smooth, echogenic, linear structure measuring less than 2 mm. Posteriorly and superiorly capping the testis, the epididymial head is clearly distinguished because of its coarser, more echogenic pattern. The body of the epididymis is more difficult to differentiate because of its posterior position, and the tail is rarely seen. A bright echogenic band, representing the mediastinum testis is seen in the 9 o'clock position; on the left side, it is seen in the 3 o'clock position. Between the layers of the tunia vaginalis, a small amount of fluid is normally found.

The testicular artery and veins of the pampiniform plexus, which run along the posterior aspect of the testicle in the region of the epididymis, are not normally seen.

Scanning the testis transversely, comparing each testis and epididymis as to size, echogenicity, and vascularity, is the best guide for detecting lesions, enlargement, or torsion.

There are no specific laboratory tests used to identify scrotal pathology. A decrease in sperm count may occur in cases of male infertility (Table 5–26 outlines scrotal pathology associated clinical and sonographic finding).

DIAPHRAGM

Gross Anatomy

The diaphragm is dome-shaped muscle separating the thorax from the abdominal cavity. The diaphragm covers the superior and lateral border of the liver on the right side and the spleen on the left side. Sonographically, the diaphragm is identified as a thin, echogenic, curvilinear interface between the lungs and liver (spleen).

The *subphrenic space* is between the liver (or spleen) and the diaphragm and is a common site for abscess.

TABLE 5–25. THYROID PATHOLOGY

Pathology Imaged by Sonography	Sonographic Characteristics
Adenomas (benign). Most common nodule occurring in the thyroid. May be singular or multiple. Also commonly seen in the parathyroid glands.	Well-defined round or oval mass that varies in size from small to very large. Varied echogenicity from echogenic, isoechoic to a solid homogenous mass with few internal echoes, resembles a cystic structure. Usually are solid masses, which often have an anechoic halo, created by blood and edematous tissue compressing the surrounding parenchyma. A halo may also be seen with malignant masses.
Simple cyst. Usually developmental, such as thyroglossal duct (located midline anterior to the trachea and brachial cleft (located more laterally)	Anechoic, no internal echoes, smooth, thin well-defined walls, increased acoustic through transmission
Hemorrhagic cysts. Usually caused by trauma or degeneration of adenoma.	Cystic mass with irregular borders that may have multiple septations and/or low-level internal echoes.
Acute thyroiditis. Thyroiditis is usually found in middle-age women. Clinically, the thyroid is enlarged, tender, and the patient has a fever.	Diffuse enlargement with decreased echogenicity of the lobes. The enlargement of the lobes is not symmetrical, the right lobe is usually larger.
Subacute thyroiditis	Diffuse enlargement with decreased echogenicity of the gland
Hashimoto's thyroiditis. Most common cause of hypothyroidism in young or middle-age women. Characteristically, there is painless diffuse enlargement of the thyroid gland. Treatment includes thyroid hormones.	Inhomogeneous pattern with overall decreased echogenicity of the gland.
Goiter. A goiter consists of multiple adenomas and is associated with hyperthyroidism.	In its initial stages, the thyroid is enlarged and may have a normal sonographic pattern. In later stages, may have multiple discrete nodules or diffusely nodular with heterogeneous echo pattern and no normal tissue, nodes may have cystic degeneration and calcification within.
Graves' disease. An autoimmune disease characterized by thyrotoxicosis.	The thyroid is diffusely enlarged and hypoechoic with an increased vascularity identified by color Doppler.
Carcinoma—80% are papillary. They usually grow slow and are seen in adults. Patients may present with difficulty breathing and swallowing with a palpable neck mass.	Sonography cannot differentiate between a benign and a malignant lesion. Malignancies tend to have irregular borders or are poorly defined. The sonographic appearance is varied; the mass may appear small or large, usually singular and hypoechoic. Cystic degeneration and focal calcifications may be present.

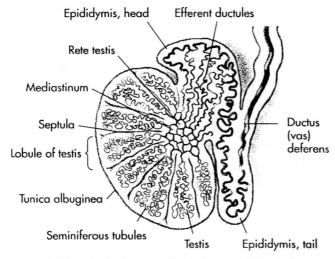

Figure 5–7. Longitudinal section of the testis and epididymis. (The size of the seminiferous tubules is exaggerated.) *(Reprinted with permission from Hagen-Ansert S. Textbook of Diagnostic Ultrasonography. 5th ed. St. Louis: Mosby; 2001, 410.)*

Crura of the Diaphragm

The diaphragmatic crura are right and left fibromuscular bundles that attach to the lumbar vertebra at the level of L3 on the right and L1 on the left. They act as anchors to the diaphragm.

The left crus can be visualized anterior to the aorta above the level of the celiac artery. Below the celiac artery, the crura extend along the lateral aspects of the vertebral columns. The right crus is visualized posterior to the caudate lobe and IVC.

FLUID COLLECTIONS

Ascites

Ascites is an abnormal accumulation of serous fluid in the peritoneum. It is always secondary to a pathological process. It may be:

- Transudative—anechoic/freely mobile usually benign, free-floating bowel in the abdomen

(list continued on p. 219)

TABLE 5–26. SCROTAL PATHOLOGY

Pathology	Clinical Findings	Sonographic Findings
Epididymis		
Acute epididymitis	Specific epididymitis stemming from gonorrhea, syphilis, mumps, and/or tuberculosis. Non-specific epididymitis is usually the result of a urinary tract infection. Traumatic epididymitis caused by strenuous exercise. Most common cause of acute scrotal pain that increases over a 1 to 2 day period, fever, and dysuria	The epididymitis is enlarged and more hypoechoic.
Chronic epididymitis	Specific epididymitis stemming from gonorrhea, syphilis, mumps, and/or tuberculosis. Non-specific epididymitis is usually the result of a urinary tract infection. Traumatic epididymitis caused by strenuous exercise	The epididymitis is thickened, very echogenic, and may contain calcifications.
Scrotal abscess	Most commonly preceded by epididymitis or orchitis. Characterized by fever, scrotal pain, and scrotal swelling	Sonolucent or complex mass with increased blood flow to the periphery and no blood flow in the mass
Spermatocele	A cystic mass of the epididymis containing spermatozoa	A cystic structure found superior to the testis, may be loculated and contain low-level echoes
Testis		
Orchitis	Inflammation of a testis caused by trauma, metastasis, mumps, or infection (chlamydia)	The testis is enlarged and is less echogenic than the normal testis. An abscess of the testis appears as localized heterogeneous areas.
Seminoma (malignant)	Most common but the least aggressive testicular malignant tumor found in men between the ages of 30 and 40. Usually found in the tunica albuginea. Patients have elevated follicle-stimulating hormone levels.	Usually a solid homogeneous hypoechoic mass that may have hyperechoic areas.
Teratoma	This tumor is usually benign, but may become malignant if not treated. Found in young men between the ages of 25 and 35.	Well-defined complex mass with areas of hemorrhage, necrosis, and calcifications.
Testicular torsion (spermatic cord torsion)	Usually occurs in prepubertal boys. There is torsion of the spermatic cord, which causes strangulation of the blood supply to the testis, which causes edema. Acute scrotal pain with nausea and vomiting.	Varied nonspecific appearance, initially the testicle and epididymal head are enlarged and hypoechoic because of edema. The scrotal wall may become thickened, and a hydrocele may be found. If the torsion is partial, there will be reduced blood flow with increased blood flow to the peritesticular soft tissue. If the torsion is complete, there will be no blood flow. In chronic torsion, the testicle is small and heterogeneous because of areas of infarcts and necrosis. Comparison of blood flow in the contralateral testicle is necessary for a diagnosis.
Intratesticular hemorrhage		Echogenic mass
Pampiniform Plexus		
Varicocele	Enlargement of the veins of the spermatic cord, commonly occurring on the left side because of drainage into the left renal vein. A right side varicocele is associated with a renal tumor.	Numerous anechoic tortuous structures lying posterior to the testis and extending superiorly past the epididymis. Increasing the venous pressure by having the patient perform a Valsalva maneuver or having the patient stand will cause dilatation of the veins.
Scrotum		
Hydrocele	Abnormal amount of serous fluid between the parietal and visceral layers of the tunica vaginalis of the scrotum. Usually caused by epididymitis but may also be caused by orchitis, torsion or trauma may also be congenital. Often found in male infants, and the fluid will reabsorb within the first year of life.	The testis and epididymis are surrounded by fluid.
Inguinal hernia	Herniation of the abdominal contents into the scrotal sac	Peristalsis of the mass will be visualized sonographically. Echogenic foci with a dirty shadow representing air within the loops of bowel will be seen
Undescended testicles (cryptorchidism)	The testicle or testis is not located in the scrotal sac. 80% are found in the inguinal canal and are palpable.	Difficult to identify testicles in the abdominal cavity.

- Exudative—internal echoes/loculated—associated with infection and malignancy
- Bowel matted or fixed to posterior abdominal wall—associated with malignancy
- Nonmobile fluid associated with coagulated hematoma (trauma)

Pathology Associated With Ascites
- Congestive heart failure
- Infection (inflammatory process)
- Kidney failure
- Liver failure/disease—end-stage fatty liver, cirrhosis
- Malignancy
- Ruptured aneurysm
- Pyogenic peritonitis
- Tuberculosis
- Portal venous system obstruction
- Obstruction of lymph nodes
- Obstruction of vessels—Budd–Chiari
- Acute cholecystitis
- Ectopic gestation
- Postoperative

Clinical Presentation
The clinical presentation of ascites is a distended abdomen. In cases of massive ascites respiratory distress will also be present.

Sonographic Findings
Accumulations occur (supine position) in the following order:

1. inferior tip—right lobe liver
2. superior portion—right flank
3. pelvic cul-de-sac
4. right paracolic gutter—lateral and anterior to liver
5. Morrison's pouch

   - Ascites is found inferior to the diaphragm
   - Gross (massive) ascites—extrahepatic portion falciform ligament seen attaching liver to anterior abdominal wall
   - Ascites may cause a downward displacement of the liver
   - May cause gallbladder wall to appear to thicken
   - Liver may appear more echogenic
   - May see patent umbilical vein
   - Changing patient's position to observe fluid movement may be useful
   - Disproportional accumulation in lesser sac suggestive of adjacent organ pathology (i.e., acute pancreatitis, pancreatic CA)

Abscess
An abscess is an encased collection of pus (acute/chronic). A cavity formed by liquefactive necrosis within solid tissue.

Pathology Associated with Abscesses
- Penetrating trauma (wounds)
- Postsurgical procedures
- Retained products of conception
- Pelvic inflammatory disease (PID)
- Chronic bladder disease
- Sepsis—blood-borne bacterial infection
- Long-standing hematomas
- Postcholecystectomy—site of the gallbladder fossa
- GI tract—peptic ulcer perforation; bowel spill during surgery (peritonitis)
- Urinary tract infection (UTI)
- Infected ascites with septa/debris
- Amebic abscess—may be densely echogenic

Clinical Presentation. Pain, spiking fever, chills, elevated white blood cell count, solitary or multiple sites, tenderness.

Hepatic Abscess
Intrahepatic
Abscesses are most often associated in the Western hemisphere with cholangitis also seen with sepsis and penetrating trauma to liver.

- Location: within liver parenchyma
- Differential diagnosis: solid tumor, usually round lesion with scattered internal echoes, variable through transmission

Subhepatic
Abscess associated with cholecystectomy

- Location: inferior to liver; fluid collection anterior to right kidney (Morison's pouch); GB fossa (postcholecystectomy)

Subphrenic
Abscess associated with bacterial spill into peritoneum during surgical procedure; bowel rupture; peptic ulcer perforation; trauma

- Location: fluid collection superior to the liver, inferior to diaphragm; transmission variable; gas (dirty shadowing)

General Sonographic Findings. A variable, complex, solid, cystic lesion with septa, debris, and scattered echoes; through transmission may be good; mass/cyst with shaggy/thick irregular walls; mass displacing surrounding structures; complex mass with dirty shadowing from within. *Presence of gas within a mass suggests an abscess (may also be attributable to fistulous communication with bowel or airway or outside air).*

General Differential Diagnosis. Necrosing tumor with fluid center (these usually have thicker walls and *no gas*).

Ascites Versus Abscess
A localized area of ascites may be mistaken for an abscess. Place the patient in the erect or Trendelenburg position; ascites will shift to the dependent portion, but an abscess will not, unless it contains air; the air/fluid level will shift.

Pleural Effusion

Pleural effusions are nonspecific reactions to an underlying pulmonary or systemic disease such as cirrhosis. Obtaining fluid for analysis may allow a more specific diagnosis.

Sonographic appearance shows a pleural effusion usually as an echo-free (anechoic), wedge-shaped area that lies posteromedial to the liver and posterior to the diaphragm. Occasionally, pleural effusions contain internal echoes, sometimes indicating the presence of a neoplasm. These echoes may be caused by blood or pus (empyema), especially when the collection is loculated. Loculated effusions do not always lie adjacent to the diaphragm and may be loculated anywhere on the chest wall. Sometimes effusions lie between the lung and the diaphragm and are known as subpulmonic. Right-sided pleural effusions can be assessed easily on a view demonstrating the diaphragm and the liver. Effusions on the left side are more difficult to see in the supine position but can be seen more readily with the patient in an oblique position and imaging through the spleen.

RETROPERITONEUM

The retroperitoneum is the area between the posterior portion of the parietal peritoneum and the posterior abdominal wall, extending from the diaphragm to the pelvis.

Divisions

The retroperitoneum is divided into three areas by the renal fossa (Gerota's fascia): Fig. 5–8 demonstrates the division of the retroperitoneum into anterior perirenal and posterior perirenal spaces (Koenigsberg M. Sonographic evaluation of the retroperitoneum. *Semin Ultrasound CT MRI.* 1982;3:2)

– The anterior perirenal space contains the retroperitoneal portion of the intestines and the pancreas

– The perirenal space contains the kidneys, ureters, adrenal glands, aorta, IVC, and retroperitoneal nodes

– The posterior perirenal space contains the posterior abdominal wall, iliopsoas muscle, and quadratus muscle

Pathology

The retroperitoneal area is subject to infection, bleeding, inflammation, and tumors.

Anterior Perirenal Space. Pancreatic pathology, carcinoma of the duodenum, ascending and descending colon causing bowel thickening or infiltration resulting in a "bull's-eye."

Perirenal Space. Kidney diseases, adrenal diseases, invasion or displacement of IVC, aortic aneurysms, ureteral abnormalities, sarcoma, liposarcoma, aortic, and retroperitoneal adenopathy.

Posterior Perirenal Space. Renal transplant is usually performed in this extraperitoneal space within the iliac fossa, using the iliac vessels for anastomosis.

Primary Retroperitoneal Tumors

Primary retroperitoneal tumors are mostly malignant; rapidly growing; and larger tumors are more likely to show

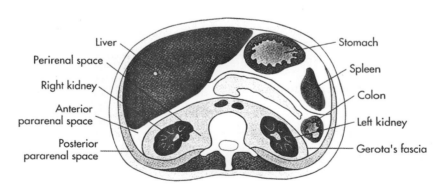

Figure 5–8. Anatomy of the retroperitoneal compartments. Diagram of a right parasagittal view demonstrates the lumbar and iliac fossae. The lumbar fossa extends from the diaphragm (1) to the ilium (10). The anterior pararenal space is limited anteriorly by the peritoneum (15) and posteriorly by the anterior renal foscia (4). The perirenal space is contained between the anterior (4) and posterior (8) renal fascia (14) that continues about the entire abdomen. The retrofascial muscles (quadratus lumborum [17], psoas [12], and iliacus [13]) are also demonstrated. Note that the lumbar compartments are open inferiorly and merge as they enter the iliac fossa. 2 = liver, 3 = bare area of liver, 5 = kidney, 6 = duodenum, 9 = ascending colon, 11 = retrocecal appendix, 16 = ureter, 17 = iliac vessels.

evidence of necrosis and hemorrhage. Concurrence of mass with ascites indicates invasion of peritoneal surfaces.

Liposarcoma. Originates from fat. Liposarcoma has a complex echogenic pattern with thick walls.

Fibrosarcoma. Originates from connective tissue. Fibrosarcoma has a complex mostly sonolucent pattern, invading surrounding tissues.

Rhabdomyosarcoma. Originates from muscle. It occurs as a solid, complex, or homogeneous echogenic mass, invading surrounding tissue.

Leiomyosarcoma. Originates from smooth muscle. It occurs as a complex echodense mass that may have areas of necrosis and cystic degeneration.

Teratoma. Originates from all three germ cell layers. Most teratomas occur in the area of the upper pole of the left kidney. Ninety percent are benign. They are complex with echogenic and cystic areas. Fifty percent occur in children.

Neurogenic Tumors. Originate from nerve tissue and occur mostly in the paravertebral region. They are heterogeneous and echogenic.

Secondary Retroperitoneal Tumors

Secondary retroperitoneal tumors are primary recurrences from previously resected tumors or recurrent masses from previous renal carcinoma.

Ascitic fluid along with a retroperitoneal tumor usually indicates seeding or invasion of the peritoneal surface. Evaluation of the para-aortic region should be made for extension to the lymph nodes. The liver should also be evaluated for metastatic involvement.

Retroperitoneal Fibrosis

Retroperitoneal fibrosis is the formation of thick sheets of connective tissue extending from the perirenal space to the dome of the bladder. It encases, rather than displaces, the great vessels, ureters, and lymph channels, causing obstruction. Severe uropathy may ensue. The etiology of retroperitoneal fibrosis is usually idiopathic, but it may sometimes be associated with aortic aneurysm.

Clinical Findings. The clinical findings in retroperitoneal fibrosis include hydronephrosis, hypertension, anuria, fever, leukocytosis, anemia, nausea and vomiting, weight loss, malaise, palpable abdominal or rectal mass, and abdominal, back, or flank pain. It is more frequent in males than females, and it most common at ages 50 through the 60s.

Sonographic Findings. Retroperitoneal fibrosis appears as thick masses anterior and lateral to the aorta and IVC, extending from renal vessels to the sacral promontory. The anterior to hypoechoic sheets have smooth, well-defined anterior margins and irregular, poorly defined posterior margins. The differential diagnosis includes lymphoma, nodal metastases, and retroperitoneal sarcoma or hematoma.

Retroperitoneal Fluid Collections. Collections of fluids in the retroperitoneum include abscesses, hematomas, urinomas, lymphoceles, and cysts.

LYMPHATIC SYSTEM

Gross Anatomy

The lymphatic system arises from veins in the developing embryo and is closely associated with veins throughout most parts of the body. Lymphatic vessels assist veins in their function by draining many of the body tissues and, thus, increasing the amount of fluid returning to the heart. The lymph vascular network does not form a closed-looped system such as the blood vascular system. Lymph vessels begin as tiny, colorless, unconnected capillaries in the connective tissues. These merge to form progressively larger vessels that are interrupted at various sites by small filtering stations called lymph nodes. The lymph fluid from the entire body ultimately drains into the IVC.

This lymphatic network has tremendous clinical significance. Interruption of lymph drainage in an area generally creates considerable swelling (edema) owing to the accumulation of fluids. In addition, the lymph vessels offer a variety of routes for cancer cells to move from one site to another (metastasis).

Lymph Nodes

Lymph nodes contain lymphocytes and reticulum cells, their function being one of filtration and production of lymphocytes and antibodies. All the lymph passes through nodes, which act as filters not only for bacteria but also for cancer cells. Enlargement of lymph nodes is a usual sign of an ongoing bacterial or carcinogenic process. Normal lymph nodes measure less than 1 cm in size. The parietal nodes follow the same course as the prevertebral vessels, while the visceral nodes are more superficial and generally follow the same course as the organ specific vessels follow. Sonographically, we can evaluate lymph nodes in the pelvis, retroperitoneum, portahepatis, perirenal, and prevertebral vasculature.

Function. The lymph nodes function in (1) the formation of lymphocytes, (2) the production of antibodies, and (3) the filtration of lymph.

Sonographic Appearance. To visualize lymph nodes they must be at least 2 cm in size. They are very homogeneous. Lymph nodes are typically hypoechoic, but there is not through transmission. Lymphomas have a nonspecific appearance but in general:

- adenopathy secondary to lymphoma are usually sonolucent

- adenopathy secondary to metastatic disease is usually complex
- posttherapy enlarged nodes are usually very echogenic but may develop cystic areas secondary to necrosis

Periaortic nodes have specific characteristics: They may drape the great vessels anteriorly (obscuring sharp anterior vascular border); may have a lobular, smooth, or scalloped appearance; and with mesenteric involvement, they may fill most of the abdomen in an irregular complex necrosis.

Para-aortic nodes may displace the celiac axis and superior mesenteric artery anteriorly. Enlarged nodes posterior to the aorta or will displace the great vessels away from the spine, this is referred to as the floating aorta sign. The "sandwich" sign occurs when nodes surround the mesenteric vessels.

Sonographic Technique. Concentrate on prevertebral vessels, aorta, IVC; portahepatic (can produce *biliary obstruction*); spleen size; iliopsoas muscles; urinary bladder contour; perirenal; retroperitoneum; and pelvis.

Para-aortic lymph nodes are involved with lymphoma in 25% of cases and 40% with Hodgkin's disease. The sonographic appearance of these lymphomatous nodes varies from hypoechoic to anechoic with no increased through transmission. Occasionally, anechoic nodal masses may resemble cystic structures. Nodal enlargement secondary to other neoplasms or inflammatory processes, such as retroperitoneal fibrosis, may be indistinguishable from lymphomatous lymphadenopathy. Para-aortic or para-caval nodes frequently obscure the sharp anterior vascular border or compress the aorta or IVC. Placing a patent in a decubitus position demonstrating the aorta and IVC facilitates sonographic imaging of the retroperitoneal area down to the aortic bifurcation.

Tumors of Lymphoid Tissue
Lymphomas (Tumors of Lymphoid Tissue). *Hodgkin's disease* (40%) is a malignant condition characterized by generalized lymphoid tissue enlargement (e.g., enlarged lymph nodes and spleen). Twice as many males as females are affected. It usually occurs between the ages of 15 and 34 or after 50. Histopathologic classification: Reed–Sternberg cells (RS) and multinucleated cells are present.

Non-Hodgkin's disease (60%) is further subdivided into nodular and diffuse histopathologies. It is a heterogeneous group of diseases that consists of neoplastic proliferation of lymphoid cells that usually disseminate throughout the body. It occurs in all age groups with the incidence increasing with age.

Mesenteric nodal involvement in less than 4% in patients with Hodgkin's disease but more than 50% in non-Hodgkin's patients. Lymphomatous cellular infiltration of the greater omentum may be seen as a uniformly thick, hypoechoic band-shaped structure. The appearance of mesenteric nodes can resemble that of retroperitoneal nodes.

Mesenteric masses may also appear as multiple cystic or separated masses that may resemble fluid-filled bowel loops. Perihepatic nodes, celiac axis nodes, splenic-hilar, and renal-hilar nodes may also be demonstrated sonographically. Although most are hypoechoic to anechoic, inhomogenous areas of increased echogenicity can be found in areas of focal necrosis within large nodes. Nodes can encase or invade adjacent organs and produce significant organ displacement; whereas, portal nodes produce biliary obstruction.

Extranodal Lymphoma. The liver, kidneys, GI tract, pancreas, and thyroid may show lymphomatous involvement.

Hepatic Lymphoma. Hepatic lymphomatous involvement presents as multiple hypoechoic or anechoic focal parenchymal defects. Although these anechoic lesions may resemble cystic structures, they rarely demonstrate enhanced posterior acoustic transmission or peripheral refractory shadowing. Hepatic abscesses, metastases from sarcomas or melanomas, focal areas of cholangitis, radiation fibrosis, and extensive hemosiderosis have presented with findings sonographically indistinguishable from hepatic lymphoma.

Renal Lymphomas. Less than 3% of all non-Hodgkin's lymphomas present with renal involvement, mainly Burkitt's lymphoma or diffuse histiocystic lymphomas.

Gastrointestinal Lymphoma. Fifteen percent of non-Hodgkin's lymphomas may present with gastrointestinal involvement. Sonographic features include a relatively hypoechoic mass with central echogenic foci. The sonographic appearance is nonspecific for lymphomatous involvement gastric carcinoma or gastric wall edema may have the same sonographic appearance.

Pancreatic Lymphoma. Ten percent of non-Hodgkin's patients present with pancreatic involvement—portions of tissue represented by focal hypoechoic or anechoic masses.

Thyroid Lymphoma. Lymphomatous thyroid masses also present in the same manner.

Inflammatory Conditions
There are three inflammatory conditions of the lymphatic system: acute and chronic lymphadenitis and infectious mononucleosis.

Common primary tumors with metastases to lymph are those of the breast, lung, melanoma, prostate, cervix, and uterus.

Sonographic Pitfalls
1. Enlarged nodes can mimic aortic aneurysm at lower gain settings on longitudinal scans; transverse scans are needed to differentiate.

2. Aneurysms enlarge fairly symmetrically; whereas, enlarged nodes tend to drape over prevertebral vessels.
3. Bowel can mimic enlarged nodes so check for peristalsis; nodes are reproducible, bowel is not.

RETROPERITONEAL VERSUS INTRAPERITONEAL MASSES

The retroperitoneal location of a mass is confirmed when there is:

- anterior renal displacement
- anterior displacement of dilated ureters
- anterior displacement of the retroperitoneal fat ventrally and often cranially; whereas, hepatic and subhepatic lesions produce inferior and posterior displacement. The direction of displacement may permit diagnosis of the anatomical origin of right upper quadrant masses.
- anterior vascular displacement—aorta, IVC, splenic vein, superior mesenteric vein

Questions

1. The renal parenchyma is separated into the cortex and medulla by the

   (A) glomeruli
   (B) renal fat
   (C) arcuate vessels
   (D) renal pelvis
   (E) renal calyces

2. A 2-year-old boy presents with hematuria and a palpable left flank mass. An ultrasound examination is performed, and a solid renal mass is identified. This finding is most characteristic of

   (A) hypernephroma
   (B) Wilm's tumor
   (C) neuroblastoma
   (D) infantile polycystic kidney disease
   (E) renal infarction

3. A patient presents with ampulla of Vater obstruction, distension of the gallbladder, and painless jaundice. This is associated with

   (A) hydropic gallbladder
   (B) choledochal cyst
   (C) Courvoisier's sign
   (D) Hartmann's pouch
   (E) Kehr's sign

4. Long-standing cystic duct obstruction will give rise to

   (A) porcelain gallbladder
   (B) hydropic gallbladder
   (C) septated gallbladder
   (D) gallbladder septations
   (E) gallbladder contraction

5. While performing an ultrasound examination, the sonographer finds that both kidneys measure 5 cm in length. They are very echogenic. One should consider the possibility of all of the following *except.*

   (A) chronic glomerulonephritis
   (B) chronic pyelonephritis
   (C) renal vascular disease
   (D) renal vein thrombosis

6. Staghorn calculus refers to a large stone within the

   (A) pancreas
   (B) urinary bladder
   (C) renal pelvis of the kidney
   (D) neck of the gallbladder
   (E) hepatic duct

7. Identify the gastrointestinal peptide hormone, which stimulates gallbladder contraction

   (A) gastrin
   (B) insulin
   (C) lipase
   (D) cholecystokinin
   (E) alkaline phosphatase

8. The portion of the liver that is not covered by the peritoneum is termed

   (A) quadrate lobe
   (B) caudate lobe
   (C) Riedel's lobe
   (D) bare area
   (E) left lobe

9. The normal thickness of the gallbladder wall

   (A) 15 mm
   (B) 10 mm
   (C) 7 mm
   (D) 5 mm
   (E) 3 mm

10. The pancreatic head lies

   (A) caudad to the portal vein and medial to the superior mesenteric vein
   (B) cephalad to the portal vein and medial to the superior mesenteric vein
   (C) caudad to the portal vein and anterior to the inferior vena cava

(D) cephalad to the portal vein and anterior to the inferior vena cava

11. Identify the sonographic pattern that best describes hydronephrosis

(A) distortion of the reniform shape
(B) multiple cystic space masses throughout the kidneys
(C) fluid-filled pelvocaliceal collecting system
(D) fluid-filled pararenal space
(E) echogenic renal cortex

12. A patient presents with a dilated interhepatic duct, dilated gallbladder, and a dilated common bile duct. Identify the level of obstruction this is most characteristic of

(A) proximal common bile duct
(B) distal common bile duct
(C) distal common hepatic duct
(D) cystic duct
(E) neck of the gallbladder

13. The most common location of pancreatic pseudocyst

(A) lesser sac
(B) porta hepatis area
(C) groin
(D) splenic hilum
(E) mediastinum

14. The extrahepatic portion of the falciform ligament

(A) courses between the inferior vena cava and the gallbladder
(B) is visualized when massive ascites is present
(C) connects the liver to the lesser sac
(D) is visualized when peritonitis is present
(E) is visualized when there is recanalization of the umbilical vein

15. The superior mesenteric artery arises 1 cm below the celiac trunk and courses

(A) 1 cm before it bifurcates
(B) inferiorly and lateral to the head of the pancreas
(C) anterior and parallel to the aorta
(D) transversely and caudad
(E) posterior to the inferior vena cava

16. The division by using Couinaud's sections into right and left lobes of the liver is

(A) main lobar fissure
(B) ligamentum venosum
(C) falciform ligament
(D) hepatoduodenal ligament

17. The portion of the pancreas that lies posterior to the superior mesenteric artery and vein is the

(A) head
(B) neck
(C) uncinate process
(D) body
(E) tail

18. The vessel that courses along the posterior surface of the body and tail of the pancreas is the

(A) superior mesenteric artery
(B) left renal vein
(C) aorta
(D) splenic artery
(E) splenic vein

19. Sonographically, the gastroesophageal junction can be visualized

(A) anterior to the inferior vena cava and posterior to the right lobe of the liver
(B) anterior to the aorta and posterior to the left lobe of the liver
(C) lateral to the head of the pancreas
(D) anterior to the stomach and medial to the spleen
(E) posterior to the left lobe of the liver and medial to the stomach

20. Adenomyomatosis of the gallbladder is

(A) a congenital anomaly that presents itself in the fourth or fifth decade
(B) an inflammation of the gallbladder and biliary ducts
(C) associated with chronic hepatitis
(D) proliferation of the mucosal layer which extends into the muscle layer
(E) a malignant process that involves the gallbladder wall and lumen

21. A common cause of acute pyelonephritis

(A) hypertension
(B) pyogenic bacteria
(C) renal cell carcinoma
(D) hydronephrosis

22. A renal sonogram is performed and an echogenic well-defined mass is identified in the renal cortex. This is characteristic of

(A) angiomyolipoma
(B) column of Bertin
(C) adenocarcinoma
(D) pyonephrosis
(E) renal stone

23. The gastroduodenal artery is a branch of the

(A) aorta
(B) celiac axis
(C) common hepatic artery

(D) left gastric artery
(E) duodenal artery

24. The largest zone of the prostate is the

(A) peripheral zone
(B) transition zone
(C) periurethral zone
(D) central zone

25. Identify the vessel that is seen anterior to the aorta and posterior to the superior mesenteric artery.

(A) splenic vein
(B) common hepatic artery
(C) gonadal artery
(D) gastric vein
(E) left renal vein

26. The liver is covered by a thick membrane of collagenous fibers intermixed with elastic elements. This membrane is called

(A) Glission's capsule
(B) Gerota's fascia
(C) Bowman's capsule
(D) Adipose capsule
(E) Crosby's capsule

27. Anterior displacement of the splenic vein can be caused by

(A) pancreatitis
(B) pseudocysts
(C) left adrenal hyperplasia
(D) aneurysm
(E) inferior vena cava thrombi

28. The vessel that originates from the celiac axis and is very tortuous is the

(A) splenic artery
(B) hepatic artery
(C) right gastric artery
(D) gastroduodenal artery
(E) gondal artery

29. When accessory spleens are present, they are usually located

(A) at the superior margin of the spleen
(B) on the posterior aspect of the spleen
(C) near the kidney
(D) near the splenic hilum
(E) near the left diaphragm

30. A fold at the fundal portion of the gallbladder is usually called

(A) Hartman's pouch
(B) junctional fold
(C) valves of Heister

(D) Phrygian cap
(E) pouch of Douglas

31. The inferior vena cava forms at the confluence of the

(A) right and left carotid veins
(B) right and left common iliac veins
(C) right and left lumbar veins
(D) right and left renal veins
(E) right atrium

32. Diffuse thickening of the gallbladder wall can be seen sonographically in all of the following *except*

(A) acute cholecystitis
(B) hepatitis
(C) congestive heat failure
(D) ascites
(E) portal hypertension

33. A gallbladder sonographic examination is performed, and a small gallbladder with intrahepatic dilatation is seen, this may indicate that the level of obstruction is at the level of the

(A) neck of the gallbladder
(B) common bile duct
(C) cystic duct
(D) common hepatic duct

34. The maximum inner diameter of the main pancreatic duct in young adults is

(A) 10 mm
(B) 8 mm
(C) 6 mm
(D) 4 mm
(E) 2 mm

35. The endocrine function of the pancreas produces

(A) insulin
(B) lipase
(C) amylase
(D) trypsin
(E) chymotrypsin

36. Identify the laboratory test used to access renal function

(A) serum creatinine
(B) serum bilirubin
(C) PSA 125
(D) hematocrit
(E) serum amylase

37. Adult polycystic disease may be characterized by all of the following *except*

(A) it is autosomal dominant disease
(B) it may be associated with cysts in the liver, pancreas, and spleen

(C) bilateral small and echogenic kidneys

(D) usually does not produce any symptoms until the third or fourth decade of life

(E) the kidneys lose their reniform shape

38. The best sonographic window to image the left hemi-diaphragm is the

(A) liver
(B) spleen
(C) stomach
(D) left kidney
(E) left lung

39. A patient in the late stages of sickle cell anemia will have a spleen that is

(A) enlarged and lobulated
(B) enlarged and echogenic
(C) small and hypoechoic
(D) small and echogenic

40. Bilateral hydronephrosis frequently occurs in patients with

(A) a renal calculi
(B) ureteropelvic junction obstruction (UPJ)
(C) pregnancy
(D) transplanted kidney
(E) prostate enlargement

41. In a patient with acute hepatis, the liver parenchyma sonographically appears as

(A) hypoechoic
(B) echogenic
(C) complex
(D) normal

42. A hypertrophied column of Bertin is a

(A) benign tumor of the kidney
(B) malignant tumor of the lower urinary tract
(C) renal variant
(D) a common cause of hydronephrosis
(E) complication of a renal transplant

43. A ureterovesical junction is

(A) junction between the renal pelvis joins the proximal ureter
(B) junction between the distal ureter and the base of the bladder
(C) junction between the renal pyramids and the distal calyces
(D) junction between the ejaculatory ducts and urethra

44. The landmark for the posterolateral border of the thyroid is

(A) trachea
(B) esophagus
(C) strap muscle
(D) common carotid artery
(E) superior thyroid artery

45. Clinical signs of renal disease includes all of the following *except*

(A) oliguria
(B) palpable flank mass
(C) generalized edema
(D) hypertension
(E) jaundice

46. Acute hydroceles may be caused by all of the following *except*

(A) infarction
(B) tumor
(C) testicular torsion
(D) trauma
(E) infection of the testis or epididymis

47. The most common location for a spermatocele is

(A) head of the epididymis
(B) body of the epididymis
(C) tail of the epididymis
(D) tunica vaginalis
(E) mediastinum testis

48. A 60-year-old man presents with hematuria and nocturnal urination. The ultrasound findings include an enlarged symmetrical homogeneous prostate. This is most characteristic of

(A) seminal vesicle disease
(B) acute prostatitis
(C) benign prostatic hyperplasia (BPH)
(D) carcinoma of the prostate
(E) normal prostate

49. The most common malignancy of the adrenal gland in children is

(A) adrenal adenoma
(B) adrenal neuroblastoma
(C) adrenal cyst
(D) pheochromocytoma
(E) lymphoma

50. If a mass in the area of the pancreatic head is found, what other structure should be examined sonographically?

(A) the liver
(B) the inferior vena cava
(C) the spleen
(D) the kidney
(E) the bowel

51. The most common primary carcinoma of the pancreas

    (A) insulinoma
    (B) cystadenocarcinoma
    (C) adenocarcinoma
    (D) pancreatic pseudocyst
    (E) lymphoma

52. The ligament of venosum separates which two lobes of the liver?

    (A) right and left lobe
    (B) medial portion of the left lobe and the lateral portion of the left lobe
    (C) caudate lobe and left lobe of the liver
    (D) anterior portion of the right lobe and the posterior portion of the right lobe

53. The most common benign neoplasm of the liver is

    (A) hemangioma
    (B) angiomyolipoma
    (C) focal nodular hyperplasia
    (D) abscess
    (E) adenoma

54. Patients with right-sided heart failure and elevated systemic venous pressure may develop

    (A) fatty liver
    (B) portal-systemic anastomoses
    (C) focal liver lesions
    (D) dilatation of the intrahepatic veins
    (E) hematomas

55. The right and left lobe of the liver are separated by the

    (A) round ligament
    (B) main lobar fissure
    (C) falciform ligament
    (D) ligament of venosum
    (E) right intersegmental fissure

56. Which of the following is not a retroperitoneal structure?

    (A) kidney
    (B) pancreas
    (C) aorta
    (D) spleen
    (E) psoas muscle

57. Identify the statement that is true about the portal vein

    (A) It is formed by the union of the common hepatic duct and the cystic duct.
    (B) It is only imaged sonographically when there is liver pathology.
    (C) It is formed by the union of the splenic vein and superior mesenteric vein.

    (D) It is very pulsatile.
    (E) It is commonplace for stones to form.

58. The common bile duct is joined by the pancreatic duct as they enter the

    (A) first portion of the duodenum
    (B) second portion of the duodenum
    (C) third portion of the duodenum
    (D) fourth portion of the duodenum
    (E) pylorus of the stomach

59. A patient presents with empyema of the gallbladder, the sonographer should expect to find

    (A) pus within the gallbladder
    (B) common bile duct obstruction
    (C) stones within the gallbladder
    (D) abscess surrounding the gallbladder
    (E) duplication of the gallbladder

60. Identify the laboratory value which is specific for a hepatoma of the liver

    (A) alkaline phosphatase
    (B) alpha-fetoprotein
    (C) serum amylase
    (D) bilirubin
    (E) serum albumin

61. If the prostate is found to be enlarged, one should also check the

    (A) spleen for enlargement
    (B) scrotum for hydroceles
    (C) kidneys for hydronephrosis
    (D) liver for metastases
    (E) gallbladder for stones

62. The body of the pancreas is bound on its anterior surface by the

    (A) atrium of stomach
    (B) greater sac
    (C) splenic vein
    (D) common bile duct
    (E) duodenum

63. On a transverse scan, the portal vein is seen as a circular anechoic structure

    (A) anterior to the inferior vena cava
    (B) posterior to the aorta
    (C) medial to the head of the pancreas
    (D) inferior to the head of the pancreas
    (E) anterior to the common bile duct

64. Hyperthyroidism associated with a diffuse goiter is associated with

    (A) papillary carcinoma
    (B) Grave's disease

(C) Hashimoto's thyroiditis

(D) adenoma

65. Identify the part of the pancreas that lies anterior to the inferior vena cava and posterior to the superior mesenteric vein.

(A) head

(B) neck

(C) body

(D) uncinate process

(E) tail

66. In a dissecting aneurysm, the dissection is through

(A) the adventia

(B) the media

(C) the intima

(D) all three layers

67. The adrenal gland can be divided into

(A) pelvis and sinus

(B) cortex and medulla

(C) major and minor calices

(D) head and tail

(E) fundus and body

68. A patent umbilical vein may be found in the

(A) ligamentum venosum

(B) main lobar fissure

(C) ligamentum teres

(D) intersegmental ligament

(E) gallbladder fossa

69. All of the following are characteristic for dilated intrahepatic bile ducts *except*

(A) the parallel channel sign

(B) irregular borders to dilated bile ducts

(C) echo enhancement behind dilated ducts

(D) decreasing size as they course toward the porta hepatis

(E) do not fill with color

70. A retroperitoneal abscess may be found within in all of the following *except*

(A) rectus abdominus muscle

(B) psoas muscle

(C) iliacus muscle

(D) quadratus lumborum muscle

71. Dilation of the intrahepatic biliary ducts without dilatation of the extrahepatic ducts may be caused by all of the following *except*

(A) Klatskin tumor

(B) enlarged portal lymph nodes

(C) cholangiocarcinoma

(D) pancreatic carcinoma

72. A 42-year old female presents postcholecystectomy with right-upper quadrant pain, elevated serum bilirubin (mainly conjugated), and bilirubin in her urine. This is best characteristic of

(A) hepatitis

(B) stone, tumor, or stricture causing obstruction of the bile duct

(C) small common duct stone less then 5 mm in diameter

(D) alkaline phosphatase will be normal

(E) pancreatic pseudocyst

73. A cause of a small gallbladder is

(A) prolonged fasting

(B) insulin-dependent diabetes

(C) chronic cholecystitis

(D) hydrops

(E) ascites

74. Identify the vessel that is located superior to the pancreas

(A) inferior vena cava

(B) superior mesenteric artery

(C) splenic vein

(D) celiac axis

(E) left renal vein

75. A retroperitoneal tumor will cause _____ displacement of organs.

(A) anterior

(B) posterior

(C) medial

(D) lateral

(E) not

76. Anterior displacement of the abdominal aorta may be caused by

(A) enlarged adrenal gland

(B) kidney mass

(C) aortic aneurysm

(D) enlarged lymph nodes

(E) inferior vena cava thrombus

77. Sonographically, enlarged lymph nodes most commonly appear as

(A) solid masses

(B) complex masses

(C) cystic masses with increased through transmission

(D) hypoechoic masses with no increased through transmission

(E) irregular shaped masses with small focal areas of calcification

78. Portal fugal blood flow is best described as

(A) reversal of blood flow

(B) turbulent blood flow

(C) intermittent blood flow
(D) no blood flow
(E) normal blood flow

79. Anatomic landmarks for sonographically locating the left adrenal gland are

(A) aorta, stomach, and spleen
(B) aorta, spleen, and left kidney
(C) inferior vena cava, spleen, and left kidney
(D) inferior vena cava, stomach, and left kidney
(E) stomach, pancreas, and left kidney

80. Nonshadowing, nonmobile, echogenic foci imaged within the gallbladder lumen are most likely

(A) polyps
(B) calculi
(C) biliary gravel
(D) sludge balls
(E) thin bile

81. Hydrops of the gallbladder is

(A) a small contracted gallbladder
(B) a gallbladder with a thicken wall
(C) a thick wall gallbladder filled with stones
(D) congenital duplication of the gallbladder
(E) an enlarged gallbladder

82. Jaundice in a pediatric patient is most likely caused by

(A) hepatitis
(B) fatty infiltration
(C) biliary atresia
(D) cirrhosis
(E) portal hypertension

83. The majority of primary retroperitoneal tumors are malignant. Identify an example of a primary retroperitoneal tumor.

(A) hepatoma
(B) hypernephroma
(C) leiomyosarcoma
(D) adenocarcinoma
(E) hematoma

84. Compare the echogenicities of the following structures and place them in increasing echogenic order.

(A) renal sinus < pancreas < liver < spleen < renal parenchyma
(B) renal sinus < liver < spleen < pancreas < renal parenchyma
(C) pancreas < liver < spleen < renal sinus < renal parenchyma
(D) renal parenchyma < liver < spleen < pancreas < renal sinus
(E) renal parenchyma < pancreas < renal sinus < spleen < liver

85. In comparison to the normal adult, the pancreas in children will be relatively

(A) more echogenic
(B) less echogenic
(C) the same echogenicity
(D) larger and less echogenic
(E) complex

86. The kidneys, the perinephric fat, and the adrenal glands are all covered by

(A) a true capsule
(B) Gerota's fascia
(C) peritoneum
(D) Glission's capsule
(E) quadratus lumborum muscle

87. The largest major visceral branch of the inferior vena cava is the

(A) portal vein
(B) hepatic veins
(C) renal veins
(D) inferior mesenteric vein
(E) gonadal veins

88. The spleen is variable in size, but it is considered to be

(A) concave superiorly and inferiorly
(B) convex superiorly and concave inferiorly
(C) concave superiorly and convex inferiorly
(D) convex superiorly and inferiorly

89. A malignant solid renal mass can be all of the following *except*

(A) renal cell carcinoma
(B) adenocarcinoma of the kidney
(C) oncocytoma
(D) transitional cell carcinoma

90. The most common neoplasm of the prostate

(A) adenocarcinoma
(B) congenital cyst
(C) benign cystic teratoma
(D) seminoma
(E) abscess

91. Identify the statement, that correctly describes the anatomic location of structures adjacent to the spleen.

(A) The diaphragm is superior, lateral, and inferior to the spleen.
(B) The fundus of the stomach and lesser sac are medial and posterior to the splenic helium.
(C) The left kidney lies inferior and medial to the spleen.
(D) The pancreas lies anterior and medial to the spleen.
(E) The adrenal gland is anterior, superior, and lateral to the spleen.

92. The sonographic findings that are associated with hematoceles include

    (A) a cyst along the course of the vas deferens
    (B) blood filled sac that surrounds the testicle, secondary to trauma or surgery
    (C) dilated veins caused by obstruction of the venous return
    (D) a condition in which the testicles have not descended
    (E) a solid mass outside the testes

93. When scanning a 22-year-old patient to rule out cholelithiasis, a single echogenic lesion is seen within the liver. This most characteristic of

    (A) a cavernous hemangioma
    (B) a hematoma
    (C) a hepatic cyst
    (D) an abscess
    (E) lipoma

94. Normal measurements of the thyroid gland are

    (A) 3–4 cm in anteroposterior and length dimensions
    (B) 2–3 cm in anteroposterior dimensions and 4–6 cm in length
    (C) 1–2 cm in anteroposterior dimensions and 4–6 cm in length
    (D) 3–5 cm in anteroposterior dimensions and 6–8 cm in length
    (E) 4–6 cm in anteroposterior dimensions and 8–10 cm in length

95. A 15-year-old boy presents with sudden intense right scrotal pain, nausea, and vomiting. A sonogram is performed, and an enlarged hypoechoic right scrotum with decrease arterial flow is documented. The left scrotum is normal. This is most consistent with

    (A) testicular rupture
    (B) varicocele
    (C) spermocele
    (D) torsion
    (E) hydrocele

96. Ascites can be caused by all of the following *except*

    (A) malignancy
    (B) nephritic syndrome
    (C) congestive heart failure
    (D) tuberculosis
    (E) adenomyomatosis

97. The best way of delineating a dissecting aneurysm on sonography is to

    (A) Begin scanning in the transverse section and document serial scans.
    (B) Show an intimal flap pulsating with the flow of blood.
    (C) Scan the patient in a decubitus position to document the aorta and inferior vena cave simultaneously.
    (D) Document the renal arteries.
    (E) Have the patient perform a Valsalva maneuver to dilate the aorta.

98. Obstructive jaundice may be diagnosed sonographically by demonstrating

    (A) a mass of the head of the pancreas with a dilated common bile duct
    (B) an enlarged liver
    (C) a fibrotic and atrophic liver
    (D) cholangitis
    (E) portal hypertension

99. In patients with uncomplicated acute epididymitis

    (A) There is enlargement of the scrotum with focal or generalized thickening of the epididymis.
    (B) The epididymis is uniformly enlarged and more anechoic than usual.
    (C) a located fluid collection with low-level echoes cephalad to the testis
    (D) There is a decrease of blood flow to the epididymitis.
    (E) The epididymitis is too tender to be touched and cannot be scanned.

100. A subhepatic abscess would be located

    (A) superior to the liver
    (B) inferior to the liver, anterior to the right kidney
    (C) inferior to the liver, posterior to the right kidney
    (D) adjacent to the porta hepatis
    (E) inferior to the pleura and superior to the liver

101. Which of the following is *not* a remnant of the fetal circulation

    (A) ligamentum teres
    (B) ligamentum venosum
    (C) falciform ligament
    (D) coronary ligament

102. A major branch of the common hepatic artery is the

    (A) gastroduodenal artery
    (B) coronary artery
    (C) esophageal artery
    (D) left gastric artery
    (E) duodenal artery

103. A 44-year-old patient presents with painless jaundice and a palpable right upper quadrant mass. This is most characteristic of

    (A) acute hepatitis
    (B) cirrhosis
    (C) porcelain gallbladder
    (D) Courvoisier gallbladder
    (E) Klatskin tumor

104. A common anatomical variant is a bulge of the lateral border of the left kidney. This is called a

    (A) junctional parenchymal defect
    (B) phrygian cap
    (C) column of Bertin
    (D) Bowman's capsule
    (E) dromedary hump

105. One can image all of the following in a case of end-stage liver disease *except*

    (A) ascites
    (B) small atrophied liver
    (C) biliary dilatation
    (D) portal hypertension
    (E) echogenic nodular liver

106. The head of the pancreas is located anterior to the

    (A) inferior vena cava
    (B) aorta
    (C) superior mesenteric artery
    (D) splenic vein
    (E) portal vein

107. The lesser sac is located between

    (A) pancreas and the inferior vena cava
    (B) stomach and pancreas
    (C) abdominal wall and stomach
    (D) liver and right kidney
    (E) stomach and spleen

108. The renal pyramids are found in the

    (A) cortex
    (B) medulla
    (C) renal pelvis
    (D) renal sinus
    (E) loop of Henle

109. On a longitudinal scan of the scrotum, the most superior portion is the

    (A) ductus deferens
    (B) rete testis
    (C) head of the epididymis
    (D) tunical albuginea
    (E) spermatic cord

110. Chronic renal disease is associated with

    (A) an enlarged kidney with a small contralateral kidney
    (B) unilateral hydronephrosis
    (C) small echogenic kidneys
    (D) renal carbunical
    (E) an ectopic kidney

111. A 50-year-old female with a long history of alcoholism presents with increased abdominal girth. A sonogram of the abdomen is performed and the most probable finding is

    (A) liver metastases
    (B) massive ascites with a small echogenic liver
    (C) hepatoma
    (D) gallstones with a mass in the lumen of the gallbladder
    (E) dilated intrahepatic biliary ducts

112. Chronic active hepatitis is a progressive destructive liver disease that eventually leads to

    (A) liver cysts
    (B) hepatoma
    (C) cirrhosis
    (D) pancreatitis
    (E) liver metastases

113. The seminal vesicles

    (A) produce sperm located within the prostate
    (B) produce sperm located posterior to the urinary bladder
    (C) are the reservoir for sperm and are located posterior to the urinary bladder
    (D) are the reservoir for sperm and are located between the mediastinum testes and the pampiniform plexus
    (E) are the reservoir for sperm and located in the peripheral zone of the prostate

114. A 6-year old child presents with recurrent fever, right upper quadrant pain, and jaundice. An abdominal sonogram is performed. The liver and gallbladder appear normal, but a 2-cm cyst is seen communicating with the common bile duct. This cystic structure most likely represents

    (A) a choledochal cyst
    (B) a pseudocyst
    (C) an aortic aneurysm
    (D) a mucocele
    (E) hydatid cyst

115. A 35-year-old woman presents with a tender neck, and on physical exam an enlarged thyroid is found. An enlarged inhomogeneous thyroid with irregular borders is seen on the sonogram. This is most characteristic of

    (A) a malignant lesion
    (B) Grave's disease
    (C) cyst
    (D) adenomatous hyperplasia
    (E) Hashimoto's thyroiditis

116. Calcification of the gallbladder wall is called

    (A) cholesterolosis
    (B) Courvoisier gallbladder
    (C) hydropic gallbladder
    (D) porcelain gallbladder

117. A 60-year-old man presents with an abdominal pulsatile mass and high blood pressure. This is most characteristic of

(A) an aneurysm
(B) a mesenteric cyst
(C) gallstones
(D) Budd-Charai
(E) portal hypertension

118. Identify the vessel that may be imaged posterior to the inferior vena cava.

(A) right renal vein
(B) right renal artery
(C) left renal vein
(D) left renal artery
(E) no vessels course posterior to the inferior vena cava

119. The retroperitoneal space is defined as the area between

(A) posterior portion of the parietal peritoneum and the posterior abdominal wall muscles
(B) anterior portion of the parietal peritoneum and the posterior abdominal wall muscles
(C) anterior portion of the parietal peritoneum and the posterior portion of the parietal peritoneum
(D) anterior abdominal wall and the posterior parietal peritoneum
(E) posterior to the great vessels and anterior to the lumbar spine

120. An abdominal sonogram is performed, and there is a suggestion of a mass in the head of the pancreas. Identify the other structures that should be evaluated.

(A) the biliary system and gallbladder to evaluate biliary obstruction
(B) the hepatic artery and splenic artery to document dilatation
(C) the kidney to evaluate renal obstruction
(D) liver to evaluate focal masses
(E) spleen to document size

121. On a sonographic examination, a seminoma of the testicle may appear as a

(A) solid, homogeneous mass
(B) large, multilocular cystic mass
(C) small, simple cyst
(D) diffuse enlargement of the testicle
(E) small, complex mass

122. On a sonographic examination, thyroiditis will appear as

(A) multiple cysts within the thyroid
(B) diffuse enlarged thyroid with decrease echogenicity

(C) small, echogenic thyroid
(D) multiple complex masses within the thyroid
(E) fluid collection surrounding an enlarged thyroid

123. A pheochromocytoma is a benign hormone producing tumor of the

(A) thyroid
(B) kidney
(C) testicle
(D) pancreas
(E) adrenal gland

124. Identify the laboratory values, which are most consistent for a patient with acute pancreatitis.

(A) Creatinine and BUN will both rise, but creatinine remains higher for a longer period of time.
(B) Amylase and alkaline phosphatase will both rise, but amylase remains higher for a longer period of time.
(C) Amylase and lipase rise at the some rate, but lipase remains higher for a longer period of time.
(D) Insulin and glucose will both rise, but glucose will remain higher for a longer period of time.
(E) Epinephrine an norepinephrine will both rise and stay elevated for the same period of time.

125. When hypertrophic pyloric stenosis is imaged in the short axis the muscle wall measures at least

(A) 2 mm
(B) 4 mm
(C) 6 mm
(D) 8 mm
(E) 12 mm

126. A malignant tumor of the adrenal gland found in children is called

(A) nephroblastoma
(B) neuroblastoma
(C) hepatoma
(D) lymphoma
(E) sarcoma

127. Lymph nodes may be confused sonographically with all of the following *except*

(A) an abdominal aortic aneurysm
(B) chronic pancreatitis
(C) the crus of the diaphragm
(D) bowel

128. An abdominal sonogram is performed on a 35-year-old male with a history of primary cancer of the liver now presents with abdominal pain and increasing abdominal girth. This is most consistent with

(A) cholecystitis
(B) pancreatitis

(C) portal hypertension
(D) Budd-Chiari syndrome
(E) renal failure

129. During an abdominal sonogram, recannalization of the umbilical vein is identified. This may be associated with

(A) ascites
(B) an abscess
(C) a hematoma
(D) hepatoma
(E) portal hypertension

130. A pelvic kidney has

(A) an abnormal appearance in a normal location
(B) a normal appearance in an abnormal location
(C) a normal appearance in a normal location
(D) an irregular shape
(E) twice the renal volume

131. The ureteropelvic junction is located between the

(A) renal pelvis and the proximal portion of the ureter
(B) distal ureter and base of the bladder
(C) urethra and the bladder
(D) medulla and the cortex
(E) apex and the base of the bladder

132. One method to diagnosis renal obstruction is to document the resistive index (RI) greater than

(A) 0.07
(B) 0.09
(C) 0.30
(D) 0.50
(E) 0.70

133. Identify the syndrome that is associated with an adrenal mass.

(A) Murphy's syndrome
(B) Budd-Chiari syndrome
(C) Cushing's syndrome
(D) Frohlich's syndrome
(E) Graves' syndrome

134. Islet cell tumors of the pancreas are most likely to be located in the pancreatic

(A) head and neck
(B) neck and tail
(C) uncinate process
(D) body and tail
(E) head and body

135. The celiac axis branches consist of

(A) common hepatic, splenic, and right gastric arteries

(B) common hepatic, gastroduodenal, and left gastric arteries
(C) common hepatic, left gastric, and splenic arteries
(D) common hepatic, coronary, and phrenic arteries
(E) common hepatic, right, and left gastric arteries

136. The most common benign mass of the spleen is a

(A) cavernous hemangioma
(B) angiosarcoma
(C) congenital cyst
(D) lymphoma
(E) hematoma

137. The membrane that lines the abdominal cavity is the

(A) visceral peritoneum
(B) parietal peritoneum
(C) pleura
(D) endometrial lining
(E) serosal lining

138. Sonography of a normal functioning transplanted kidney will appear

(A) more echogenic than a normal kidney
(B) with a thin renal cortex and prominent medullary pyramids
(C) the same as a normal kidney
(D) twice the size as a normal kidney
(E) with the renal sinus and renal cortex being isoechoic

139. When performing a gallbladder examination, the patient is asked to be NPO (nothing by mouth) for approximately 6 hours before the examination because this will

(A) eliminate any overlying bowel gas
(B) make the patient more cooperative
(C) dehydrated, which will make the patient easier to scan
(D) cause bile to collect in the gallbladder
(E) cause the bile ducts to dilate

140. Transplanted kidneys are usually placed

(A) within the renal fossa
(B) in the pelvis along the iliopsoas margin
(C) in the pelvis anterior to the bladder
(D) within the abdominal rectus sheath
(E) in Morrison's pouch

141. Klatskin tumors cause

(A) dilatation of intrahepatic ducts
(B) dilatation of extrahepatic ducts
(C) gallstones
(D) pancreatitis
(E) porcelain gallbladder

142. Which of the following is *not* located in the peritoneal cavity

(A) gallbladder
(B) liver
(C) spleen
(D) pancreas
(E) hepatic veins

143. The splenic artery

(A) originates from the anterior abdominal aorta
(B) lies posterior to the inferior vena cava
(C) is tortuous, and courses along the superior aspect of the body and tail of the pancreas
(D) is the first branch of the abdominal aorta
(E) courses along the posterior aspect of the body and tail of the pancreas

144. Artifactual echoes may occur within cysts owing to each of the following *except*

(A) slice thickness artifacts
(B) side-lobe artifacts
(C) edge artifacts
(D) reverberation artifacts

145. In which of the following ways does ascites sonographically affect the liver?

(A) There will be no effect.
(B) The liver will appear more echogenic.
(C) The ascites will attenuate the liver, resulting in decreased echoes.
(D) The ascites will cause the liver to appear inhomogenous.

146. If the ultrasound beam passes through a fatty tumor within the liver, and we know that the speed of sound in fat is lower than in soft tissue, where will this fatty tumor be placed?

(A) farther away than it really is
(B) closer than it really is
(C) its true position
(D) smaller is size than it really is
(E) can be any of the above, depending upon the frequency of the transducer

147. A post trauma fluid collection located between the diaphragm and the spleen may represent

(A) ascites
(B) a pleural effusion
(C) a subcapsular hematoma
(D) a subphrenic abscess
(E) retroperitoneal fibrosis

148. A retroperitoneal sarcoma may displace the

(A) kidney posteriorly
(B) spleen anteriorly
(C) pancreas posteriorly
(D) diaphragm inferiorly
(E) aorta posteriorly

149. Splenomegaly may be caused by all of the following *except*

(A) an inflammatory process
(B) portal vein thrombus
(C) a left subphrenic abscess
(D) polycythemia vera
(E) chronic leukemia and lymphoma

150. The causes of a large gallbladder include all of the following *except*

(A) adenomyomatosis
(B) pancreatic carcinoma
(C) diabetes mellitus
(D) a fasting patient
(E) common duct obstruction

151. The quadratus lumbordum muscles are located

(A) medial to the lumbar spine
(B) in the anterior abdominal wall
(C) between the kidneys and the adrenal glands
(D) posterior to the kidneys
(E) perirenal

152. All of the following are associated with cirrhosis *except*

(A) ascites
(B) splenomegaly
(C) jaundice
(D) hepatomegaly
(E) collateral vessel development

153. Absence of an ureteral jet is consistent with

(A) pyelonephrosis
(B) parapelvic renal cyst
(C) obstructive hydronephrosis
(D) posterior urethral values
(E) renal cell carcinoma

154. A cystic mass that extends from the renal pelvis to outside the renal capsule is

(A) a parapelvic cyst
(B) an extrarenal pelvis
(C) a renal artery aneurysm
(D) a grade II hydronephrosis
(E) duplex collecting system

155. Fig. 5–9 is a longitudinal scan to the left of midline. The linear anechoic structure is the

(A) gallbladder
(B) aorta

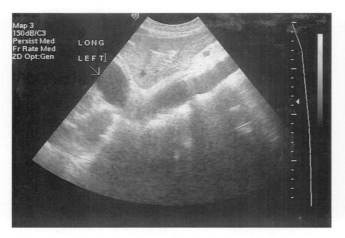

Figure 5–9. Longitudinal sonogram of the upper abdomen.

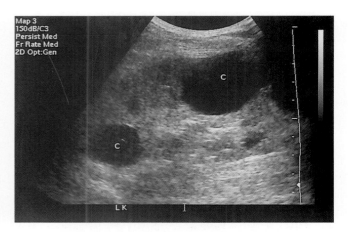

Figure 5–11. Longitudinal view of the left kidney.

(C) inferior vena cava

(D) hepatic veins

(E) heart

156. The arrow in Fig. 5–9 is pointing to

(A) the diaphragm

(B) ascites

(C) abscess

(D) pleura effusion

(E) heart

157. Fig. 5–10 is a transverse view of the upper abdomen. The arrow is pointing to

(A) aorta

(B) inferior vena cava

(C) portal vein

(D) spine

(E) enlarged lymph node

158. A patient with normal renal function tests presents for a sonogram of the kidneys. Fig. 5–11 is a longitudinal image of the left kidney, this image most likely represents

(A) polycystic kidneys

(B) infected cysts

(C) hydronephrosis

(D) parapelvic renal cysts

(E) two simple cysts

159. A 35-year-old male with a history of diabetes presents with an increase of ALT and AST and vague abdominal pain. The longitudinal and transverse images Fig. 5–12A and Fig. 5–12B most likely represents

(A) fatty liver

(B) severe hepatitis

(C) cirrhosis

(D) metastases

(E) Budd-Chiari syndrome

160. The finding in Fig. 5–13 is most characteristic of a liver

(A) abscess

(B) cavernous hemangioma

(C) hematoma

(D) hydatid cyst

(E) metastatic lesion

161. A 35-year-old female presents with right upper quadrant pain, nausea, and vomiting. The findings in Fig. 5–14 are most consistent with

(A) acute cholecystitis

(B) chronic cholecystitis

(C) adenomyosis

(D) a gallbladder of a patient who has just eaten

(E) a normal gallbladder

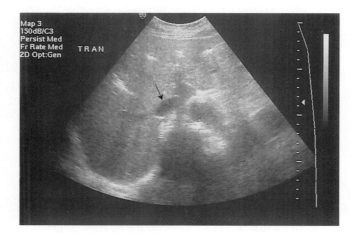

Figure 5–10. Transverse sonogram of the upper abdomen.

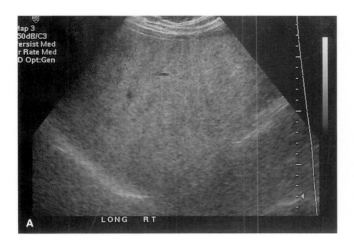

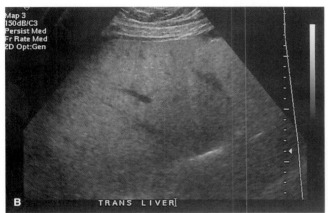

Figure 5–12. (A) Longitudinal sonogram through the liver. **(B)** Transverse sonogram through the liver.

162. The arrow in Fig. 5–14 is pointing to

    (A) pericholecystic fluid collection
    (B) loop of bowel

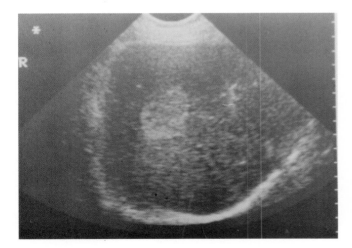

Figure 5–13. Longitudinal sonogram through the right lobe of the liver.

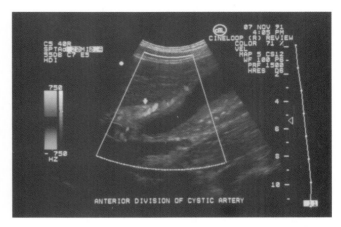

Figure 5–14. A longitudinal sonogram at the level of the gallbladder.

    (C) cystic artery
    (D) gastroduodenal artery
    (E) portal vein

163. The finding in Fig. 5–15A and Fig. 5–15B are characteristic of

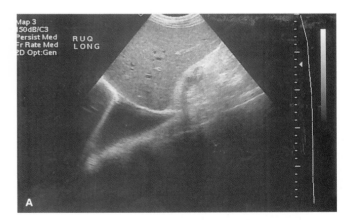

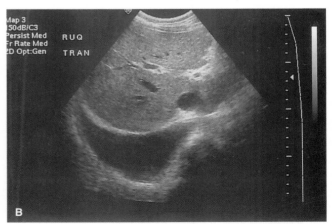

Figure 5–15. (A) Longitudinal sonogram through the upper abdomen. **(B)** Transverse sonogram through the upper abdomen.

(A) pleural effusion
(B) pleural abscess
(C) ascites
(D) dissecting aneurysm
(E) fatty liver

164. Fig. 5–16 is a transverse scan at the level of the liver and right kidney. The liver abnormality is most consistent with

(A) hydatid cyst
(B) hematoma
(C) metastatic lesions
(D) cavernous hemangioma
(E) infected cysts

165. The arrow in Fig. 5–17 is pointing to the

(A) main portal vein
(B) hepatic vein
(C) right portal vein
(D) phrenic vein
(E) free fluid

166. The arrow in Fig. 5–18 is pointing to

(A) the right crus of the diaphragm
(B) the right renal artery
(C) the right adrenal gland
(D) the right renal vein
(E) the right portal vein

167. The arrow in Fig. 5–19 is pointing to

(A) levator ani muscle
(B) quadratus lumborum muscle
(C) psoas muscle
(D) internal oblique muscle
(E) rectus abdominis muscle

168. The patient in Fig. 5–20 presented with massive ascites. The arrow is pointing to

(A) ligamentum teres
(B) ligamentum venosum

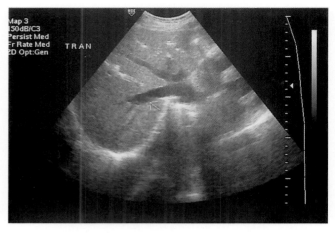

Figure 5–17. Transverse scan of the upper abdomen.

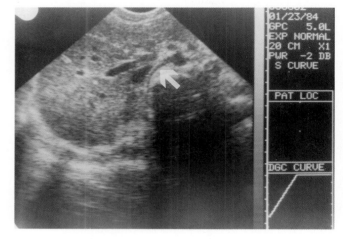

Figure 5–18. Transverse scan of the abdomen.

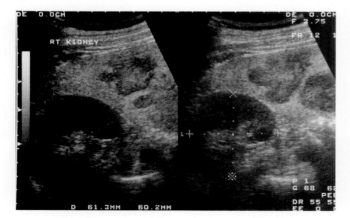

Figure 5–16. A transverse view of the right kidney.

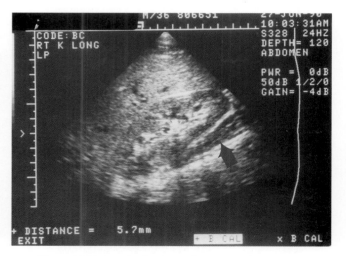

Figure 5–19. Longitudinal scan through the right kidney.

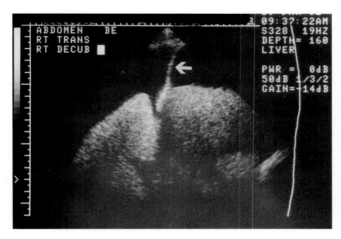

Figure 5–20. Transverse scan through the liver.

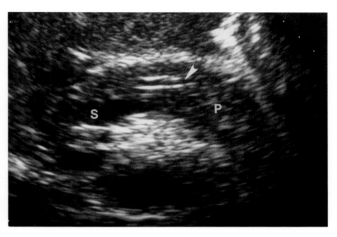

Figure 5–21. Transverse scan through the pancreas.

(C) falciform ligament
(D) coronary ligament
(E) splenorenal ligament

169. A 1-week-old male infant presents with a left flank mass. An IVP demonstrates a normal right kidney, but there is no visualization of the left kidney. A sonogram is performed and numerous noncommunicating round cystic structures are demonstrated in the left renal fossa, the largest of which is located laterally. No renal parenchyma is identified. The right kidney is normal. This most probably represents

(A) severe hydronephrosis
(B) polycystic kidneys
(C) a multicystic kidney
(D) nephroblastoma
(E) unilateral renal agenesis

170. Which of the following is an echogenic linear line extending from the portal vein to the neck of the gallbladder?

(A) cystic duct
(B) right hepatic vein
(C) left portal vein
(D) main lobar fissure
(E) round ligament

171. The most common primary neoplasm of the pancreas is a(n)

(A) adenocarcinoma
(B) insulinoma
(C) pseudocyst
(D) cystadenoma
(E) congenital cyst

172. A patient presents with epigastric tenderness, fever, and an increase in serum amylase and lipase. The arrowhead in Fig. 5–21 is pointing to the

(A) splenic artery
(B) splenic vein
(C) antrium of the stomach
(D) hepatic artery
(E) pancreatic duct

173. The diagnostic possibilities in the patient in Fig. 5–21 include

(A) acute pancreatitis
(B) phlegmonous pancreatitis
(C) hemorrhagic pancreatitis
(D) chronic pancreatitis
(E) normal pancreas

174. A 65-year-old patient with a history of hypertension and a palpable pulsatile mass on physical. The finding in Fig. 5–22A–D are most likely

(A) cholecystitis with a gallstone
(B) hematoma
(C) aortic aneurysm
(D) abscess
(E) hemorrhagic pseudocyst

175. The arrow in Fig. 5–23 is pointing to

(A) splenic vein
(B) superior mesenteric artery
(C) celiac artery
(D) splenic artery
(E) gondal artery

176. The findings in Fig. 5–24 represent

(A) acute pancreatitis
(B) pancreatic pseudocyst
(C) chronic pancreatis
(D) adenocarcinoma of the pancreas
(E) normal pancreas

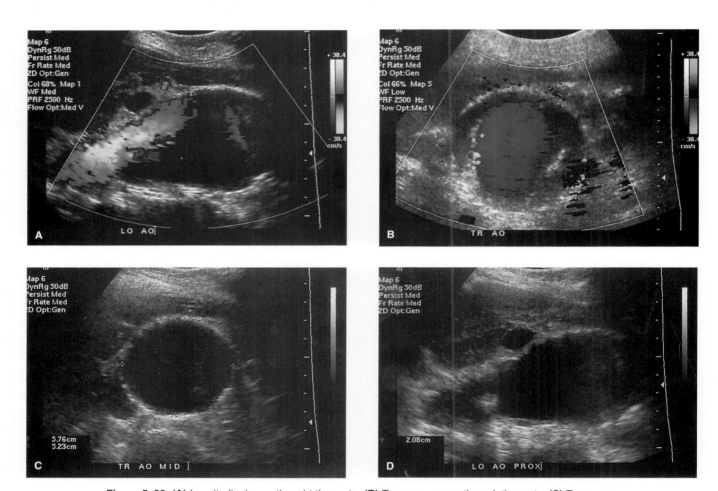

Figure 5–22. (A) Longitudinal scan thought the aorta. **(B)** Transverse scan through the aorta. **(C)** Transverse sonogram through midabdomen aorta. **(D)** Longitudinal sonogram through the proximal section of the aorta.

177. The arrow in Fig. 5–25 points to

(A) a medullary pyramid
(B) a renal cyst
(C) diverticula of the calyce
(D) a parapelvic cyst
(E) renal artery aneurysm

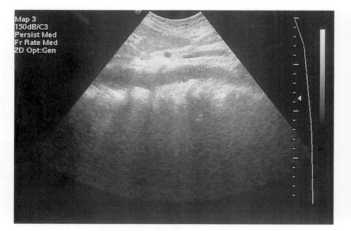

Figure 5–23. Longitudinal scan through the midline of the abdomen.

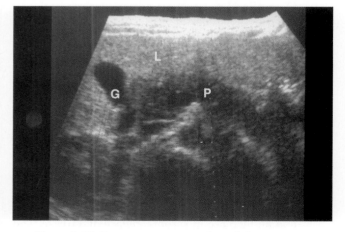

Figure 5–24. Transverse sonogram through the pancreas.

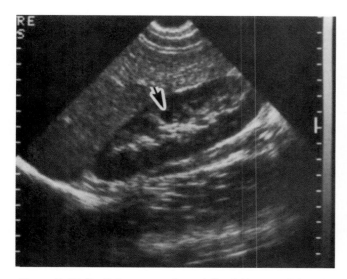

Figure 5–25. Sagittal sonogram through the right upper abdomen.

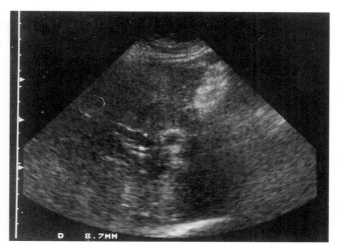

Figure 5–27. Oblique view through the right upper quadrant.

178. The arrow in Fig. 5–26 is pointing to

(A) sludge
(B) polyp
(C) calculi
(D) metastatic neoplasm
(E) normal gallbladder

179. The artifact on Fig. 5–26 is called

(A) reverberation
(B) edge artifact
(C) scattering
(D) acoustic shadowing
(E) posterior acoustic enhancement

180. The linear anechoic structure, which the calipers are measuring in Fig. 5–27 is the

(A) left portal vein
(B) main portal vein
(C) middle hepatic vein
(D) patient umbilical vein
(E) common bile duct

181. The structure in Fig. 5–27, which the caliper is measuring is

(A) normal in caliber
(B) small in caliber
(C) large in caliber
(D) unable to determine

182. The findings in Fig. 5–28 are characteristic of

(A) intrahepatic dilatation
(B) pneumobilia
(C) acute hepatitis
(D) chronic hepatitis
(E) hepatocellular carcinoma

183. The abnormal findings in Fig. 5–29 include

(A) hydrated disease
(B) fatty liver
(C) cavernous hemangioma

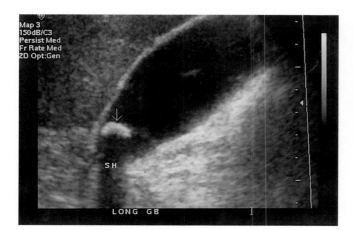

Figure 5–26. Longitudinal sonogram through the gallbladder.

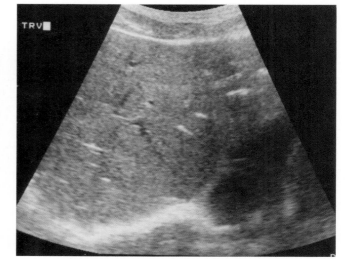

Figure 5–28. Transverse sonogram through the upper abdomen.

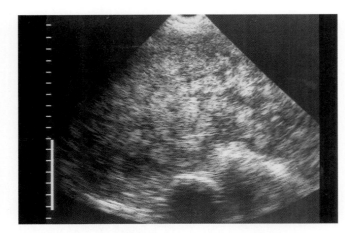

Figure 5–29. Transverse scan through the liver.

(D) multiple abscesses

(E) liver metastasis

184. The sonographic findings in Fig. 5–30 include

(A) splenomegaly

(B) a subphrenic abscess

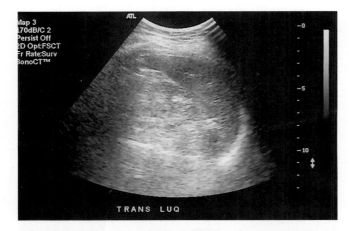

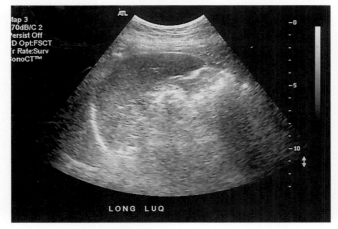

Figure 5–30. Coronal image through the left upper quadrant.

(C) subcapsular hematoma

(D) normal appearing spleen

(E) metastasis within the spleen

185. The common bile duct is formed by the

(A) right and left hepatic ducts joining the cystic duct

(B) cystic duct joining the right hepatic duct

(C) common duct joining the cystic duct

(D) common duct joining the neck of the gallbladder

(E) common duct joining the pancreatic duct

186. An aneurysm is usually the result of

(A) degenerative joint disease

(B) atherosclerosis

(C) hypertension

(D) diabetes

(E) cystic fibrosis

187. The arrow in Fig. 5–31 is pointing to

(A) common hepatic duct

(B) hepatic artery

(C) common bile duct

(D) portal vein

(E) hepatic vein

188. The sonographic findings in Fig. 5–32 are consistent with

(A) column of Bertin

(B) prominent renal pyramid

(C) junctional parenchymal defect

(D) duplex collecting system

(E) sinus lipomatosis

189. The arrow in Fig. 5–33 is pointing to

(A) calculi in common bile duct

(B) calculi in neck of gallbladder

(C) air in bile system

(D) Klatskin tumor

(E) sludge

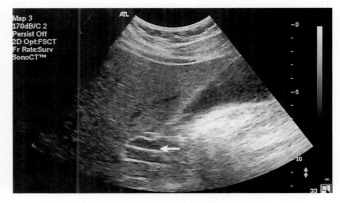

Figure 5–31. Magnified sagittal sonogram of the portal hepatis area.

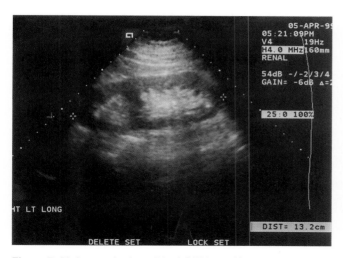

Figure 5–32. Long axis view of the left kidney. *(Courtesy of Sheptim Telegrafi, MD, New York University.)*

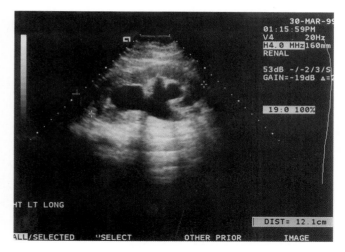

Figure 5–34. Long axis scan through the left kidney. *(Courtesy of Sheptim Telegrafi, MD, New York University.)*

190. A renal ultrasound is performed on a 30-year-old patient with right flank pain, elevated BUN, and creatinine. The findings in Fig. 5–34 are consistent with all of the following *except*

(A) stone in ureter
(B) enlarged prostate
(C) gallstones
(D) posterior urethra valve (PUV)
(E) bladder mass

191. Fig. 5–35 suggests that the patient has a

(A) horseshoe kidney
(B) unilateral renal agenesis
(C) three kidneys
(D) pelvic kidney
(E) cross ectopic kidney

192. A patient presents with a history of epigastric pain and elevated lipase. The arrows in Fig. 5–36 are pointing to

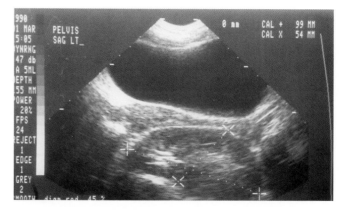

Figure 5–35. Sagittal sonogram through the pelvis.

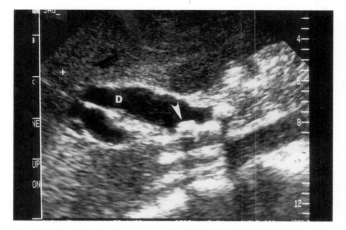

Figure 5–33. Magnified oblique sonogram of the portal hepatis area.

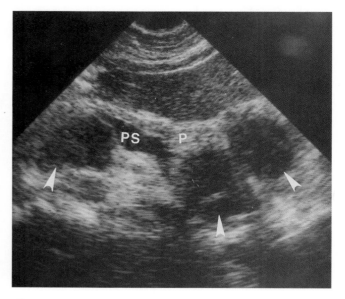

Figure 5–36. Transverse sonogram through the pancreatic region.

(A) lymph nodes
(B) mesenteric cysts
(C) pseudocysts
(D) abscesses
(E) normal vessels

193. The arrow in Fig. 5–37 is pointing to

(A) pseudocyst
(B) perirenal fluid
(C) dromedary hump
(D) pleura effusion
(E) renal cyst

194. The findings in Fig. 5–38 are consistent with

(A) patient who has just eaten
(B) porcelain gallbladder with gallstones
(C) gallbladder carcinoma
(D) adenomyomatosis
(E) acute cholecystitis with gallstones

195. Identify the artifact to which the arrow in Fig. 5–39 is pointing

(A) comet tail
(B) noise
(C) slice thickness
(D) refraction
(E) side lobes

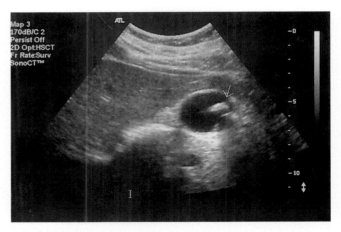

Figure 5–38. Left decubitus scan through the upper abdomen.

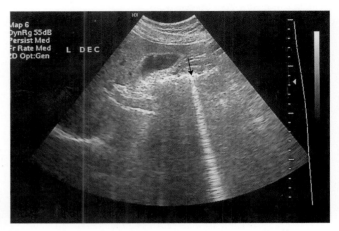

Figure 5–39. Left decubitus scan through the upper abdomen.

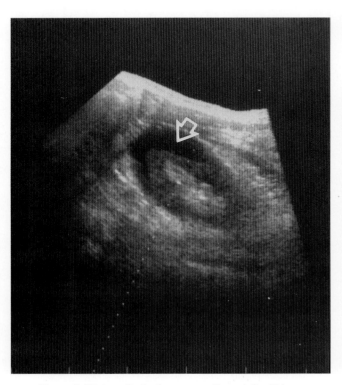

Figure 5–37. Longitudinal sonogram through the kidney.

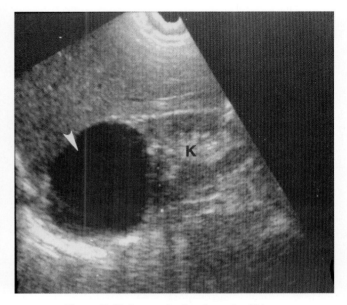

Figure 5–40. Long axis view through a kidney.

196. The arrow in Fig. 5–40 is pointing to

    (A) gallbladder
    (B) upper pole hydronephrosis
    (C) renal cyst
    (D) aneurysm
    (E) dilated ureter

197. The patient in Fig. 5–40 will most likely present with

    (A) flank pain
    (B) fever
    (C) nausea and vomiting
    (D) no symptoms
    (E) jaundice

198. The calipers in Fig. 5–41 is measuring

    (A) antrium of stomach
    (B) lymph node
    (C) pancreatic pseudocyst
    (D) body of pancreas
    (E) aorta filled with thrombus

199. A 35-year-old male presents with right upper quadrant pain and recurrent attacks of pancreatitis. His laboratory results could indicate a(n)

    (A) increase in blood urea nitrogen (BUN)
    (B) decrease in serum amylase
    (C) increased lipase
    (D) increase in indirect bilirubin
    (E) increase in alkaline phosphatase

200. Sonographically, one can recognize fatty infiltration of the liver by all of the following *except*

    (A) hepatomegaly
    (B) parenchymal echoes are echogenic
    (C) decreased vascular structure
    (D) decreased through transmission
    (E) a focal mass

201. Obstruction of the common bile duct by a mass in the head of the pancreas will lead to?

    (A) dilated gallbladder with dilated biliary radicles
    (B) contracted gallbladder with dilated biliary radicles
    (C) dilated biliary radicles with normal or shrunken gallbladder
    (D) portal hypertension
    (E) cirrhosis

202. A 41-year-old male presents with epigastric pain and a history of alcoholism. The findings in Fig. 5–42 include

    (A) fatty pancreas
    (B) adenocarcinoma
    (C) metastatic disease to the pancreas
    (D) chronic pancreatitis
    (E) normal

203. A 50-year-old women presents with painless hematuria. A longitudinal view of the left kidney is imaged in Fig. 5–43. The findings are most consistent with

    (A) transitional cell carcinoma
    (B) renal cell carcinoma
    (C) adenoma
    (D) angiolipoma
    (E) oncocytoma

204. What is the most common medical disease that causes acute renal failure?

    (A) acute tubular necrosis
    (B) renal infarction
    (C) diabetes
    (D) hypertension
    (E) nephrocalcinosis

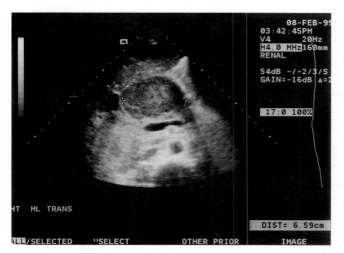

Figure 5–41. Transverse sonogram of the upper abdomen. *(Courtesy of Sheptim Telegrafi, MD, New York University.)*

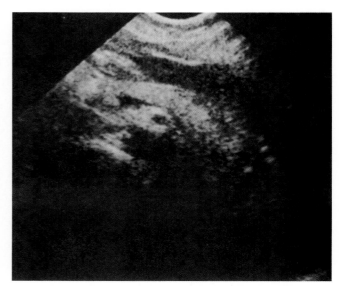

Figure 5–42. Transverse sonogram of the upper abdomen.

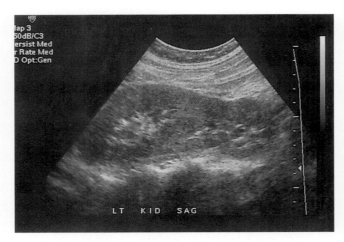

Figure 5–43. A longitudinal sonogram of the left kidney.

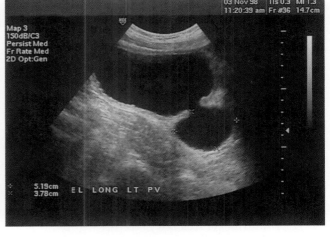

Figure 5–45. Left sagittal sonogram of the pelvis.

205. Fig. 5–44 is consistent with

(A) adult polycystic kidneys
(B) hydronephrosis
(C) medullary sponge kidney
(D) medullary cystic disease
(E) acquired cystic disease found in dialysis

206. A pelvic sonogram is performed. Fig. 5–45 is consistent with

(A) enlarged prostate
(B) cystitis
(C) bladder carcinoma
(D) bladder cyst
(E) diverticula

207. The arrows in Fig. 5–46 are pointing to

(A) thrombus
(B) polyp
(C) bowel
(D) calculi
(E) parapelvic cyst

208. Fig. 5–47 is a midline longitudinal scan of the abdomen. The abnormality is

(A) an ectopic gallbladder
(B) aneurysmal dilatation of the distal abdominal aorta
(C) occlusion of abdominal aorta by thrombus
(D) dissecting aneurysm
(E) enlarged psoas muscle

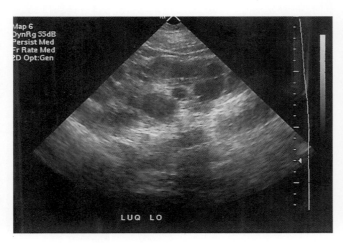

Figure 5–44. Longitudinal sonogram of the kidney.

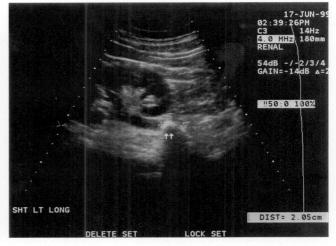

Figure 5–46. Longitudinal scan of the left kidney. *(Courtesy of Sheptim Telegrafi, MD, New York University.)*

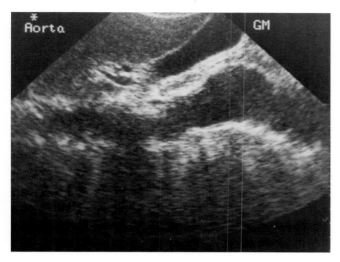

Figure 5–47. Midline longitudinal scan of the abdomen.

209. Onset of pain while scanning over the gallbladder is termed

   (A) Kehr's sign
   (B) candle sign
   (C) Murphy's sign
   (D) Chandelier's sign
   (E) Courvoisier gallbladder

210. The most likely diagnosis in Fig. 5–48 is

   (A) biliary obstruction caused by cholelithiasis
   (B) biliary obstruction caused by pancreatitis
   (C) distended portal vein caused by portal hypertension
   (D) distended hepatic vein caused by chronic congestive heart failure
   (E) obstruction of the distal common duct caused by a pancreatic tumor

211. All of the following statements concerning the sonographic patterns of periaortic lymph nodes are correct *except*

   (A) They may drape or mantle the great vessels anteriorly.
   (B) They may displace the superior mesenteric artery posteriorly.
   (C) They may displace the great vessels anteriorly.
   (D) They may have lobar, smooth, or scalloped appearance.
   (E) As mesenteric involvement occurs, the adenopathy may fill most of the abdomen in an irregular complex pattern.

212. The findings in Fig. 5–49 are associated with all of the following *except*

   (A) diabetes
   (B) hepatitis
   (C) malignancy
   (D) chronic pancreatitis
   (E) portal caval shunts

213. The blood flow in Fig. 5–50 is consistent with

   (A) right sided heart failure
   (B) cirrhosis
   (C) Budd-Chiari syndrome
   (D) cavernous transformation of the portal vein
   (E) normal blood flow in the hepatic and portal veins

214. The arrow in Fig. 5–51 is pointing to

   (A) a mass in the head of the pancreas
   (B) c-loop of duodenum
   (C) bowel mass
   (D) calculi
   (E) loculated fluid with debris

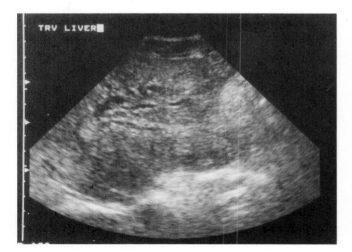

Figure 5–48. Transverse sonogram of the liver.

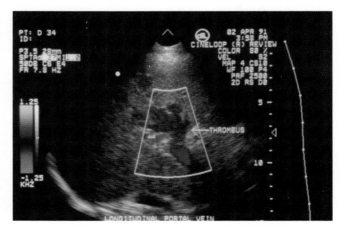

Figure 5–49. Longitudinal sonogram of the portal vein.

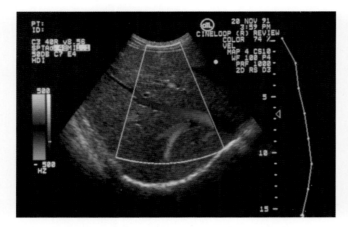

Figure 5–50. Transverse sonogram of the upper liver.

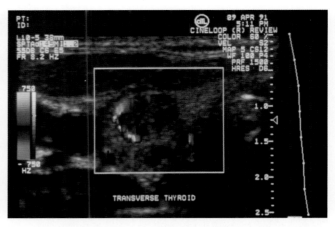

Figure 5–52. Transverse sonogram through the thyroid.

215. The calipers in Fig. 5–51 are measuring

(A) common hepatic duct
(B) common bile duct
(C) main portal vein
(D) hepatic vein
(E) inferior vena cava

216. The findings in Fig. 5–51 are consistent with

(A) mass in the head of the pancreas
(B) intrahepatic obstruction
(C) choledocholithiasis
(D) liver trauma
(E) liver cell carcinoma

217. Fig. 5–52 is a transverse sonogram through the right lobe of the thyroid. The findings are consistent with

(A) Grave's disease
(B) thyroiditis
(C) papillary carcinoma
(D) primary hyperplasia
(E) adenoma

218. The mostly likely diagnosis in the patient in Fig. 5–53 is

(A) testicular tumor
(B) testicular torsion
(C) epididymitis

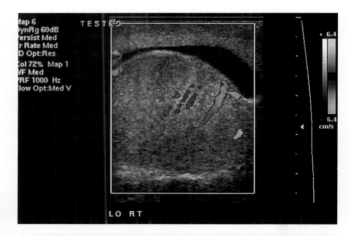

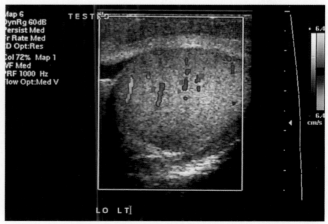

Figure 5–53. Longitudinal sonogram of the right hemiscrotum.

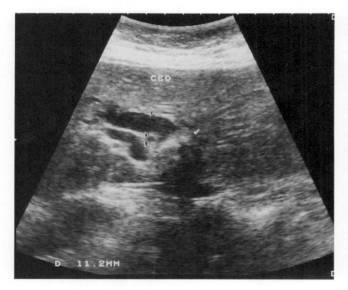

Figure 5–51. Oblique sonogram of the liver.

(D) cryptorchidism

(E) normal testicle

219. The presenting symptom of a testicular malignant tumor may be

(A) para-aortic lymphadenopathy

(B) acute scrotal pain

(C) leukemia

(D) retroperitoneal lymphadenopathy

(E) all of the above

220. Fig. 5–54 is a parasagittal transrectal sonogram of the prostate rotated slightly from the midline. The abnormality is

(A) an atrophied prostate

(B) absence of the seminal vesicle

(C) a lesion in the peripheral zone

(D) dilated ejaculatory duct

(E) benign prostatic hypertrophy

221. The laboratory value used to evaluate the function of the prostate is

(A) sperm count

(B) prostatic specific antigen (PSA)

(C) CA 125

(D) amylase

(E) creatinine

222. The left testicular vein drains into the

(A) inferior vena cava

(B) left internal iliac vein

(C) common internal iliac vein

(D) left renal vein

(E) prostatic vein

223. Fig. 5–55 is a transverse sonogram of the left lobe of the liver. The arrow points to

(A) hepatic vessels

(B) hypoechoic lesions

(C) portal sinuses

(D) biliary radicles

(E) none of the above

224. Diagnostic possibilities in the findings in Fig. 5–55 include

(A) metastases

(B) hemangiomas

(C) infection foci

(D) abscesses

225. The arrow in Fig. 5–56 is pointing to

(A) coronary ligament

(B) ligamentum of Teres

(C) granuloma

(D) lesser omentum

(E) main lobar fissure

226. The findings in Fig. 5–57 are associated with all of the following *except*

(A) increase in alpha-fetoprotein level

(B) increase in direct bilirubin

(C) increase in alkaline phosphatase

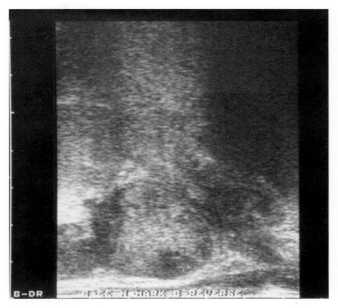

Figure 5–54. Parasagittal transrectal sonogram of the prostate rotated slightly from the midline.

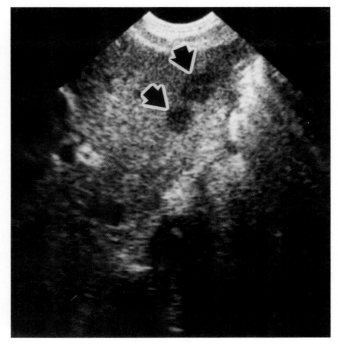

Figure 5–55. Transverse sonogram of the left lobe of the liver.

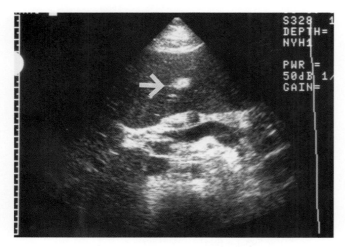

Figure 5–56. Transverse scan of the liver.

(D) jaundice

(E) none of the above

227. The findings in Fig. 5–57 are consistent with

(A) Budd-Chiari syndrome

(B) portal hypertension

(C) right-sided heart failure

(D) carcinoma of the common bile duct

(E) gallstones

228. The findings in Fig. 5–58 are associated with all of the following *except*

(A) hypoproteinemia

(B) congestive heart failure

(C) acute hepatitis

(D) cholecystitis

(E) choledocholithiasis

229. The findings in Fig. 5–59 are suggestive of

(A) acute hepatitis

(B) fatty liver

(C) metastatic disease of the liver

(D) multiple hematomas

(E) cirrhosis

230. The laboratory findings of renal failure include

(A) creatinine and alkaline phosphatase

(B) creatinine and blood urea nitrogen

(C) serum amylase and lipase

(D) serum amylase and creatinine

(E) alkaline phosphatase and alpha-fetoprotein

231. The head of the pancreas is located to the right of the

(A) celiac axis

(B) inferior vena cava

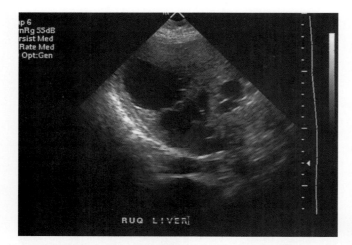

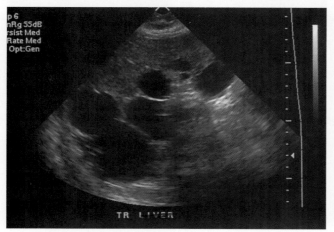

Figure 5–57. Longitudinal scan of the right lobe of the liver.

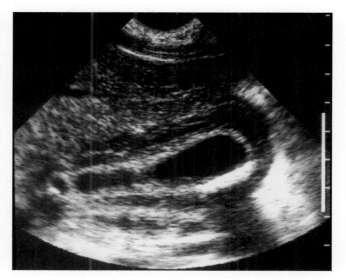

Figure 5–58. Longitudinal magnified sonogram of the gallbladder.

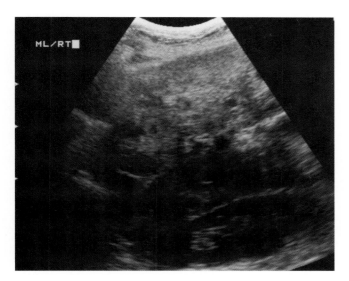

Figure 5–59. Longitudinal sonogram of the right lobe of the liver.

(C) gastroduodenal artery
(D) common bile duct
(E) portal splenic confluence

232. Crohn's disease is

(A) a mass in the stomach
(B) a parasitic condition
(C) an inflammation of the bowel
(D) loculated fluid in the peritoneal cavity
(E) a mass relating to the pancreas and biliary system

233. A resistive index (RI) greater than 0.70 in a kidney is consistent with early

(A) obstructive jaundice
(B) obstructive hydronephrosis
(C) renal cell carcinoma
(D) benign renal cyst
(E) polycystic renal disease

234. A postrenal transplant perirenal fluid collection can be all of the following *except*

(A) parapelvic cyst
(B) urinoma
(C) lymphoma
(D) hematoma
(E) abscess

235. The Doppler characteristic of the venous blood flow in a varicocele is

(A) increased blood flow
(B) irregular waveform
(C) triphasic flow
(D) no change in flow
(E) no blood flow

236. A 40-year-old patient presents with epigastric pain and jaundice. Fig. 5–60 is a transverse scan through the midabdomen. The crossbars delineate the area of interest. It is consistent with

(A) bowel mass
(B) liver mass
(C) omental mass
(D) pancreatic mass
(E) normal finding

237. A 60-year-old male presents for a pelvic ultrasound. The findings in Fig. 5–61A and Fig. 5–61B are consistent with

(A) foley catheter
(B) cystitis
(C) bladder carcinoma
(D) polyp
(E) enlarged prostate

238. The arrow in Fig. 5–62 is pointing to

(A) ascites
(B) pleura effusion
(C) an abscess
(D) a hematoma
(E) a cyst

239. Fatty infiltration of the liver can be assessed sonographically by visualizing

(A) echogenic vessel walls seen throughout the liver
(B) hypoechoic diaphragm
(C) increase liver echogenicity
(D) multiple echogenic focal masses
(E) small nodular liver

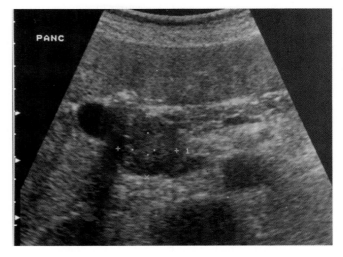

Figure 5–60. Transverse sonogram at the level of the pancreas.

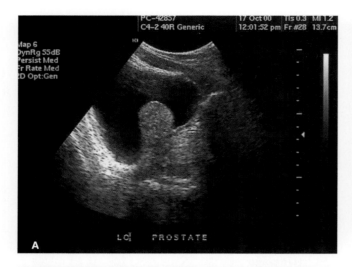

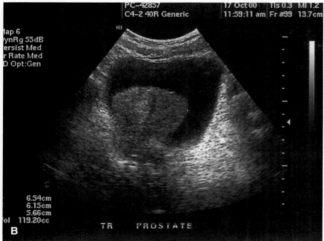

Figure 5–61. (A) Longitudinal transabdominal scan at the level of the bladder. **(B)** Transverse transabdominal scan of the bladder.

240. In the subacute phase of testicular torsion the testes appear

(A) anechoic areas in testes with decreased blood flow
(B) small and echogenic
(C) enlarged with increased blood flow
(D) normal size with decrease in size of the epididymis

241. The most likely diagnosis of Fig. 5–63 is

(A) hematoma
(B) metastases
(C) abscess
(D) hemangioma
(E) hydrated cysts

242. A patient who has blunt trauma to the abdomen earlier in the day presents with left upper quadrant pain

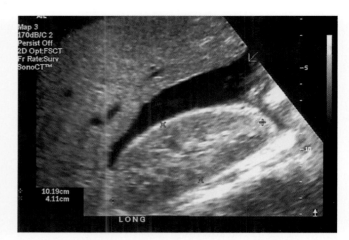

Figure 5–62. Sagittal sonogram obtained through the right upper abdomen.

and a decrease in hematocrit. An echogenic mass is seen in the spleen. This is consistent with

(A) abscess
(B) lymphoma
(C) infection
(D) hematoma
(E) leukemia

243. Hemangiomas can be diagnosed by

(A) needle biopsy
(B) a tagged red blood cell liver scan
(C) a computed tomographic (CT) scan
(D) a magnetic resonance imaging (MRI) scan
(E) all of the above

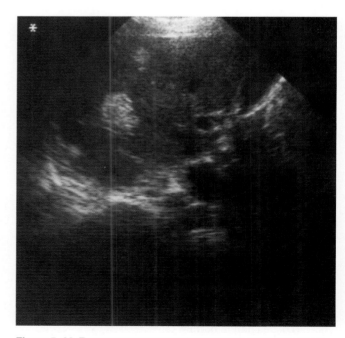

Figure 5–63. Transverse sonogram throughout the right hepatic lobe.

244. The most likely diagnosis in the patient in Fig. 5–64 is

(A) cirrhosis
(B) pyonephritis
(C) acute glomerulonephritis
(D) chronic renal disease
(E) renal agenesis

245. Fig. 5–65 is a transverse sonogram of the right and left scrotum. This image is consistent with

(A) torsion
(B) orchiectomy
(C) cryptorchidism
(D) epididymitis
(E) normal testicles

246. Fig. 5–66 is a duplex Doppler sonogram obtained in the upper hemiscrotum. The abnormality is

(A) dilated spermatic duct
(B) dilated vessels near the head of the epididymis
(C) extratesticular vascular tumor
(D) pampinform venous plexus
(E) dilated deferential artery

247. The most likely diagnosis from the findings in Fig. 5–66 is

(A) varicocele
(B) hydrocele
(C) testicular torsion
(D) spermatocele
(E) testicular infarct

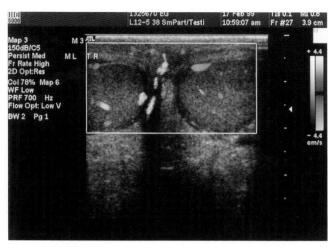

Figure 5–65. Transverse sonogram of the right and left testicles.

248. The muscle that lies posterior to the breast is the

(A) Cooper's muscle
(B) pectoralis muscle
(C) levator ani muscle
(D) rectus muscle
(E) transverse muscle

249. What is the most common benign breast mass in women during their reproductive years?

(A) cyst
(B) abscess
(C) fibroadenoma
(D) enlarged lymph nodes
(E) hyperplasia

250. The findings in Fig. 5–67 are consistent with

(A) gallbladder carcinoma
(B) adenomyomatosis

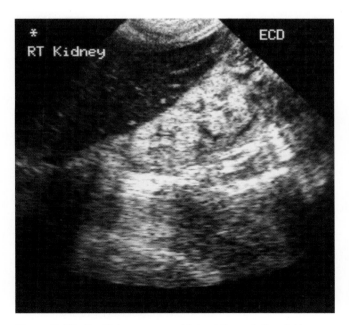

Figure 5–64. Sagittal sonogram obtained through the right upper quadrant.

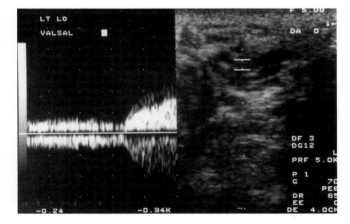

Figure 5–66. Duplex Doppler sonogram obtained in the right upper hemiscrotum.

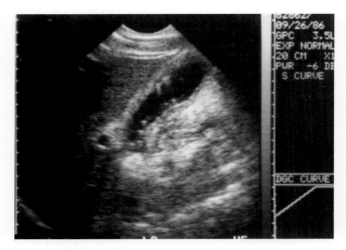

Figure 5–67. Longitudinal scan of the gallbladder.

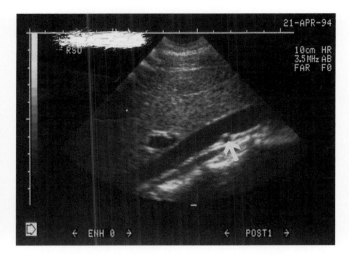

Figure 5–68. Longitudinal scan of the upper abdomen.

(C) cholecystitis
(D) gallbladder polyp
(E) metastasizes to the gallbladder

251. A jaundiced male child with a hemolytic disorder may be found to have a(n)

(A) increase in direct bilirubin
(B) increase in indirect bilirubin
(C) increase in alphafetoprotein
(D) increase in prothrombin time
(E) normal liver function tests

252. Which of the following statements are true?

(A) Bowman's capsule is the fibrous capsule around the kidney.
(B) A glomerulus, Bowman's capsule, and renal tubules together constitute a nephron.
(C) Nephrons are the only structures, in which active transport of substances through cell membrane does not occur.
(D) The renal cortex secretes hormones called corticoids.
(E) Nephrons are not an important part of the production of urine.

253. Fig. 5–68 is a longitudinal scan through the abdomen. The linear longitudinal vessel which is being imaged is the

(A) aorta
(B) inferior vena cava
(C) main portal vein
(D) none of the above

254. In Fig. 5–68 the arrow is pointing to

(A) psoas muscle
(B) left renal vein

(C) superior mesenteric artery
(D) right renal artery
(E) phrenic artery

255. Fig. 5–69 is a transverse sonogram obtained through the urinary bladder. This image is consistent with

(A) a thickened posterior bladder wall
(B) bladder stone
(C) reverberation artifact
(D) bladder diverticula
(E) an ectopic ureter

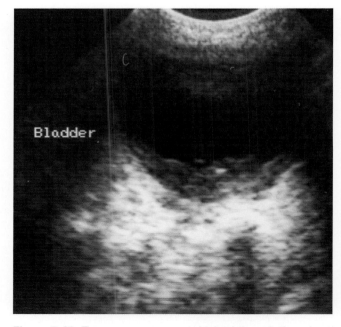

Figure 5–69. Transverse sonogram obtained through the urinary bladder.

256. The most likely diagnosis in the patient in Fig. 5–69 is

   (A) bladder tumor
   (B) over distended bladder
   (C) cystitis
   (D) ureterocele
   (E) foley catheter

257. A longitudinal scan is performed on the right side of the abdomen. The arrow in Fig. 5–70 is pointing to a small fluid collection in the

   (A) pleura cavity
   (B) lesser sac
   (C) right paracolic gutter
   (D) subhepatic space
   (E) right subphrenic space

258. A transverse scan of the upper abdomen is performed. The arrow in Fig. 5–71 is pointing to

   (A) the heart
   (B) pleural effusion
   (C) pericardial effusion
   (D) hemangioma
   (E) hydatid cyst

259. The liver in Fig. 5–71 is consistent with

   (A) fatty infiltrations
   (B) hepatitis
   (C) hepatocellular carcinoma
   (D) diabetes mellitus
   (E) normal finding

260. A normal variant of the liver in which the right lobe of the liver extends below the lower pole of the right kidney is called

   (A) Murphy's lobe
   (B) quadrate lobe

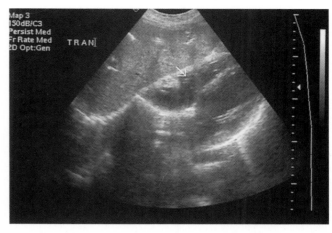

Figure 5–71. Transverse scan through the upper abdomen.

   (C) duplication of the right lobe
   (D) Reidel's lobe
   (E) extra lobe

261. Fig. 5–72 longitudinal scan through the right lower quadrant. This image is consistent with

   (A) appendicitis
   (B) bowel obstruction
   (C) Crohn's disease
   (D) intersuppection
   (E) volvulus

262. Fig. 5–73 is a long axis view of the gallbladder. The abnormality is

   (A) a distended gallbladder with thickened walls
   (B) a positive WES sign

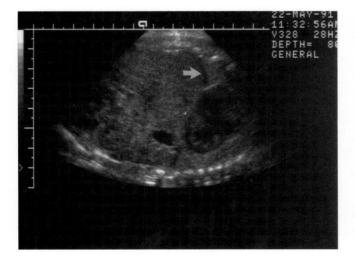

Figure 5–70. Longitudinal scan through the right upper abdomen.

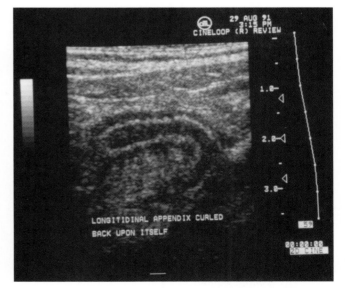

Figure 5–72. Longitudinal sonogram of the right lower quadrant.

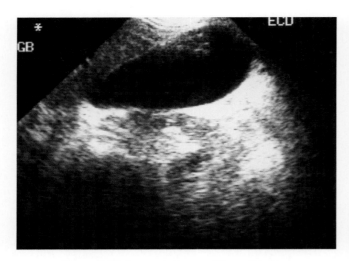

Figure 5–73. Long axis image of the gallbladder.

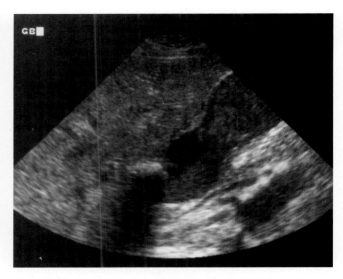

Figure 5–74. Longitudinal magnified sonogram through the right upper quadrant.

(C) multiple floating, low-level echoes

(D) an hydropic gallbladder

(E) porcelain gallbladder

263. The most likely diagnosis in the patient in Fig. 5–73 is

(A) obstruction of the cystic duct

(B) Klatskin tumor

(C) acalculus cholecystitis

(D) gallbladder carcinoma

(E) adenoma of the gallbladder

264. Hydrops of the gallbladder may be secondary to all of the following *except*

(A) sludge

(B) mass in the head of the pancreas

(C) obstruction of the distal common bile duct by a mass of the ampulla of vater

(D) stones in Hartman's pouch

(E) surgery

265. Fig. 5–74 is a longitudinal view of the gallbladder in a patient with history of gallbladder disease. This image is most consistent with

(A) chronic cholecystitis

(B) hepatitis

(C) metastasizes to the gallbladder

(D) gallbladder carcinoma

(E) a patient who just ate a fatty meat

266. Fig. 5–75 is a magnified picture of a neonatal abdomen. The arrow is pointing to

(A) a small kidney

(B) a compressed loop of bowel

(C) enlarged adrenal gland

(D) contracted gallbladder

267. A longitudinal scan of the right lobe of the liver is performed in a post operative patient. The most likely diagnosis in the patient in figure Fig. 5–76 is

(A) subphrenic collection

(B) subcapsular collection

(C) subhepatic collection

(D) loculated ascites

(E) perigastric collection

268. The patient in Fig. 5–76 has a fever and a low hematocrit. The patient was placed in a decubitus position and the low-level echoes within the collection did not move. This is most diagnostic of

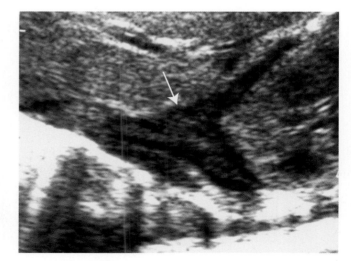

Figure 5–75. Magnified longitudinal sonogram of a neonatal abdomen.

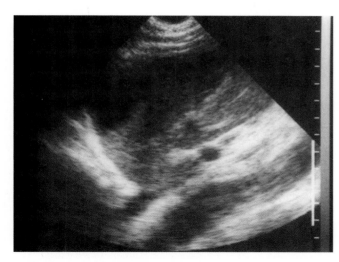

Figure 5–76. A longitudinal scan of the right lobe of the liver.

(A) abscess
(B) hematoma
(C) infected cyst
(D) hemorrhagic cyst
(E) malignant fluid

269. Fig. 5–77 is a transverse scan at the level of the pancreas. The arrows are pointing to the

(A) bowel
(B) stomach
(C) lesser sac
(D) duodenum
(E) pancreas

270. The patient in Fig. 5–77 presents with normal laboratory values and persistent epigastric pain. What pathology is this image consistent with

(A) chronic pancreatitis
(B) acute pancreatitis
(C) complicated pancreatic pseudocyst
(D) bowel mass
(E) insulinoma

271. Fig. 5–78 is a coronal image through the left upper quadrant of the abdomen. The arrow is pointing to

(A) left kidney
(B) the normal left adrenal gland
(C) stomach
(D) the left crus of the diaphragm
(E) the splenic flexure

272. The longitudinal anechoic structure in Fig. 5–78 is

(A) right renal vein
(B) left renal artery
(C) aorta
(D) inferior vena cava
(E) artifact

273. A condition that may affect the adrenal gland

(A) neonatal hypotension
(B) severe fulminant tuberculosis infection
(C) malignant lung carcinoma
(D) breast carcinoma
(E) all of the above

274. Fig. 5–79 is a transverse scan obtained through the abdomen of a child with a palpable mass.

(A) a complex mass with areas of septations and debris

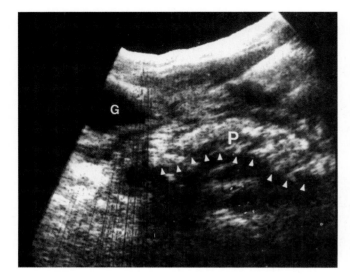

Figure 5–77. A transverse scan at the level of the pancreas.

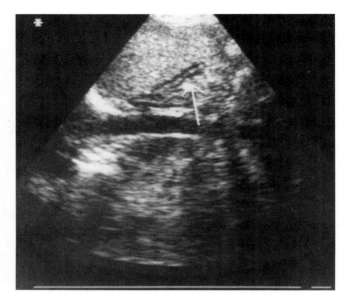

Figure 5–78. Coronal image through the left upper quadrant.

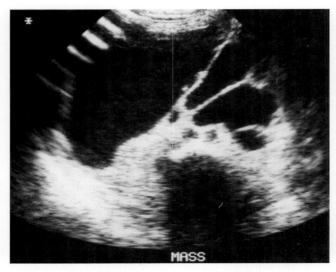

Figure 5–79. Transverse scan obtained through the abdomen of a child with a palpable mass.

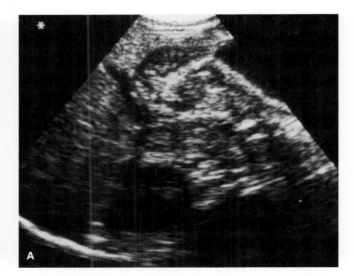

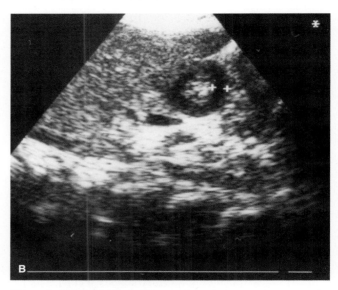

Figure 5–80 (A) Longitudinal image through the gastric antrum of a child. **(B)** Transverse scan through the gastric antrum of a child.

(B) a cystic mass appears to displace bowel and mesentery
(C) free fluid within the abdomen
(D) loculated fluid collection

275. The most likely diagnosis in the patient in Fig. 5–79 is

(A) mesenteric cyst
(B) complicated ascites
(C) ovarian carcinoma
(D) abscess

276. Fig. 5–80A and Fig. 5–80B are long and short axis sonograms through the gastric antrum of a child. How would you describe the image?

(A) atrophy of the antrum wall
(B) mass of the antrum wall
(C) thickened antrum wall and increase length
(D) shorten pyloric canal and shorten length
(E) normal

277. The most likely diagnosis in the patient in Fig. 5–80A and Fig. 5–80B is

(A) normal stomach
(B) hypertrophic pyloric stenosis
(C) duodenal tumor
(D) mass in the lesser sac
(E) infected lymph nodes

278. Fig. 5–81 is a transverse sonogram through the upper abdomen. This image is most consistent with

(A) chronic pancreatitis
(B) gastric outlet obstruction
(C) insulinoma
(D) portal hypertension
(E) normal pancreas

279. What portion of the pancreas is anterior to the formation of the portal vein?

(A) head
(B) neck
(C) isthmus
(D) body
(E) tail

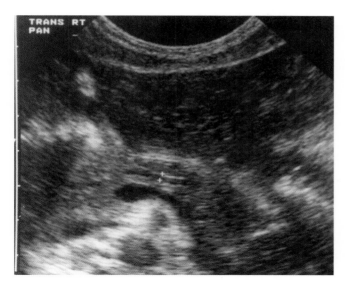

Figure 5–81. Transverse image obtained in the upper abdomen.

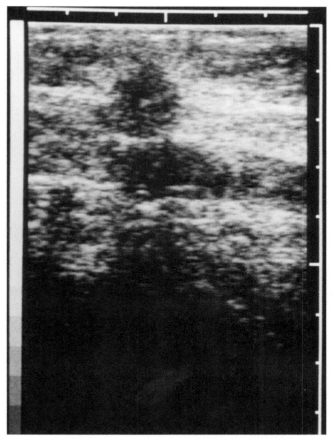

Figure 5–82. Long axis sonogram at 10:00 of the right breast.

280. What is the most common islet cell tumor?

    (A) adenocarcinoma
    (B) pseudocyst
    (C) true cyst
    (D) insulinoma
    (E) gastrinoma

281. Fig. 5–82 is a longitudinal image at ten o'clock of the right breast. The abnormality is a

    (A) cystic lesion within the breast
    (B) complex mass within the breast
    (C) solid lesion with irregular borders
    (D) solid lesion with well-circumscribed borders
    (E) normal dense tissue

282. The most likely diagnosis in the patient in Fig. 5–82 is

    (A) cyst
    (B) fibroadenoma
    (C) carcinoma
    (D) mastitis
    (E) normal dense breast tissue

283. The sonographic appearance of a benign breast mass includes all of the following *except*

    (A) well-circumscribed borders
    (B) round or oval in shape
    (C) smooth borders
    (D) taller in size than wider
    (E) homogeneous with moderate low level echoes

284. The arrow in Fig. 5–83 is pointing to

    (A) major lobar fissure
    (B) ligamentum of Teres
    (C) ligamentum of venosum
    (D) air in bile duct
    (E) cholecystectomy clip

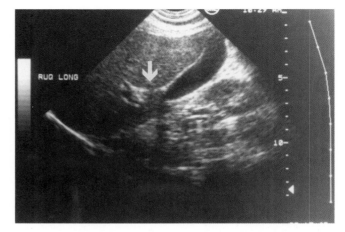

Figure 5–83. Longitudinal scan of the right upper quadrant.

285. The findings in Fig. 5–84 are associated with the following *except*

(A) alkaline phosphatase
(B) serum glutamic–oxaloacetic transaminase
(C) direct bilirubin
(D) alpha-fetoprotein
(E) jaundice

286. The findings in Fig. 5–85 is consistent with

(A) Budd-Chiari
(B) hepatitis
(C) dilated biliary radicles
(D) gallstones
(E) fatty infiltrations

287. The findings in Fig. 5–86 are consistent with

(A) portal hypertension
(B) congestive heart failure
(C) fatty liver disease
(D) cirrhosis
(E) normal scan

288. Which of the following ligaments are visualized in Fig. 5–87

(A) middle lobar ligament
(B) ligament venosum
(C) coronary ligament
(D) round ligament
(E) gastroduodenal ligament

289. Fig. 5–88 is an upright coronal image of the lower left hemithorax of a 12-year-old child with a fever. The abnormality is

(A) loculated pleural effusion
(B) nonloculated pleural effusion
(C) hydronephrotic kidney
(D) herniated bowel

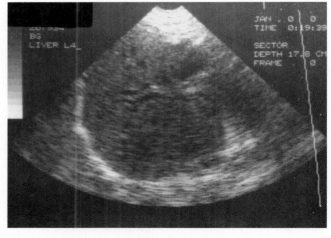

Figure 5–85. Longitudinal scan of the liver.

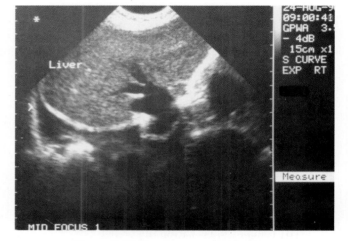

Figure 5–86. Transverse scan of the liver.

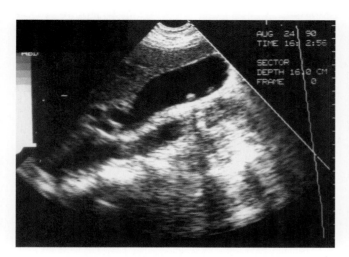

Figure 5–84. Longitudinal scan of the gallbladder.

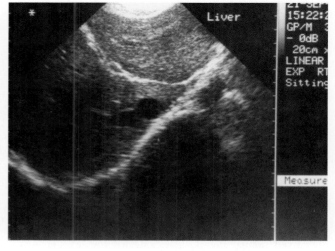

Figure 5–87. Transverse scan of the liver.

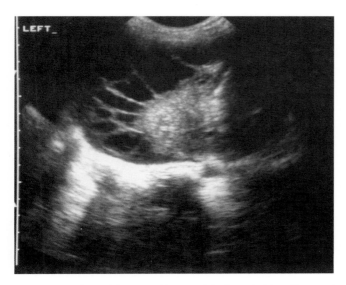

Figure 5–88. An upright coronal image of the lower left hemithorax of a 12-year-old child with a cough and fever.

290. The most likely diagnosis in the patient in Fig. 5–88 is

(A) simple effusion
(B) cystic lung mass
(C) obstructed bowel
(D) empyema
(E) obstructed kidney

291. A patient presents with right upper quadrant pain, fever, nausea, and leukocytosis. The findings in Fig. 5–89 are most consistent with

(A) gallbladder carcinoma
(B) chronic cholecystitis

(C) adenomyomatosis
(D) acute cholecystitis
(E) postprandial gallbladder contraction

292. The findings shown in Fig. 5–90 are consistent with

(A) chronic cholecystitis with cholelithiasis
(B) adenomatosis
(C) postprandial gallbladder contraction
(D) duodenal bulb
(E) post cholecystectomy clip

293. A patient presents with an increase in direct bilirubin, alanine aminotransferase (ALT), and alkaline phosphatase. The findings in Fig. 5–91 are suggestive of

(A) liver metastases
(B) hepatoma
(C) cirrhosis
(D) fatty infiltrations
(E) hematomas

294. A patient presents with vague right upper quadrant pain and normal liver function laboratory results. The echogenic mass in Fig. 5–92 is suggestive of a liver

(A) abscess
(B) hematoma
(C) hepatoma
(D) echinococcal cyst
(E) hemangioma

295. The echogenic mass in Fig. 5–92 is located in the

(A) posterior segment of the right lobe
(B) anterior segment of the right lobe
(C) anterior segment of the left lobe
(D) medial segment of the right lobe
(E) medial segment of the left lobe

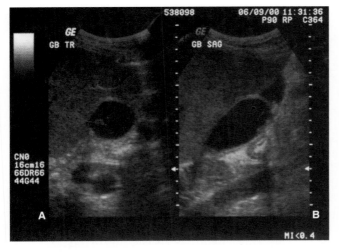

Figure 5–89. (A) Transverse image of the gallbladder. **(B)** Long axis image of the gallbladder.

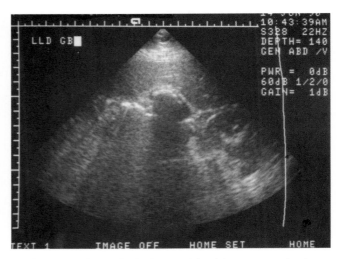

Figure 5–90. Longitudinal scan of the right upper quadrant.

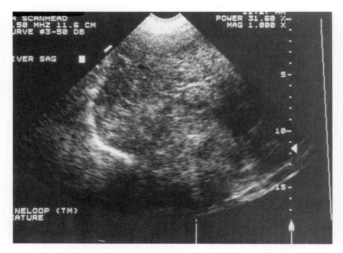

Figure 5–91. Longitudinal scan of the liver.

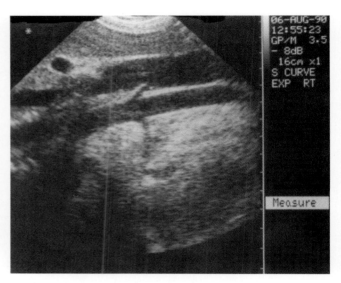

Figure 5–93. Coronal scan of the midabdomen.

296. The malformation variant in the gallbladder that involves an acutely angulated pouch of the fundus is termed

    (A) phyragian cap
    (B) duplication of the gallbladder
    (C) Hartman's pouch
    (D) junctional fold
    (E) Murphy's cap

297. Identify the vessels being imaged in Fig. 5–93 in the order that they appear (anterior to posterior)

    (A) inferior vena cava, portal vein, left renal vein, right renal vein
    (B) inferior vena cava, aorta, right hepatic artery, splenic artery
    (C) inferior vena cava, aorta, left renal vein, right renal vein

    (D) inferior vena cava, aorta, right renal artery, left renal artery
    (E) inferior vena cava, portal vein, right hepatic vein, left hepatic vein

298. The portal veins can be differentiated from the hepatic veins by all of the following *except*

    (A) portal veins becomes larger as they approach the diaphragm
    (B) portal veins have echogenic borders
    (C) portal veins bifurcate into the right and left branches
    (D) the main portal vein is part of the portal triad

299. Horseshoe kidney may be confused sonographically with which of the following?

    (A) carcinoma of the head of the pancreas
    (B) lymphadenopathy
    (C) hypernephroma
    (D) gastric mass
    (E) aortic aneurysm

300. A 53-year-old man with a history of liver cirrhosis presents with increased abdominal girth. Fig. 5–94 demonstrates a thickened gallbladder wall is most likely associated with

    (A) calculous cholecystitis
    (B) pancreatitis
    (C) portal hypertension
    (D) adjacent ascites
    (E) loss of appetite

301. The arrow in Fig. 5–95 is pointing to the

    (A) inferior vena cava
    (B) superior mesenteric artery

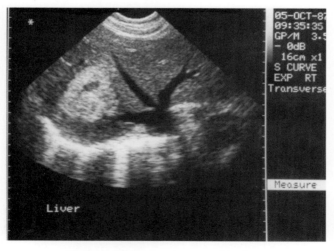

Figure 5–92. Transverse scan of the liver.

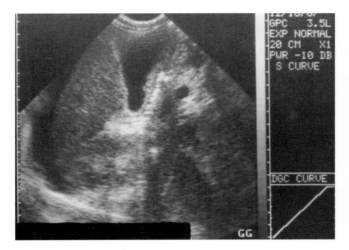

Figure 5–94. Longitudinal scan of the liver and gallbladder.

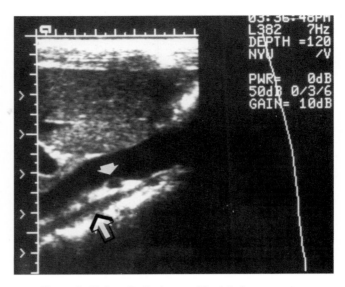

Figure 5–96. Longitudinal scan of the inferior vena cava.

(C) celiac
(D) right crus of the diaphragm
(E) psoas muscle

302. The left crus of the diaphragm may get confused with the

(A) left adrenal gland
(B) aorta
(C) splenic vein
(D) superior mesenteric artery
(E) accessory spleen

303. The arrow in Fig. 5–96 is pointing to

(A) inferior vena cava
(B) psoas muscle
(C) lumbar artery
(D) right crus of diaphragm
(E) right adrenal gland

304. The arrowhead in Fig.5–96 is pointing to

(A) right renal vein
(B) right renal artery
(C) left renal vein
(D) left renal artery
(E) celiac axis

305. The arrow Fig. 5–97 is pointing to

(A) hepatic artery
(B) common duct
(C) portal vein
(D) hepatic vein
(E) main lobar fissure

306. The shadowing from the region of the gallbladder neck in Fig. 5–97 is most likely due to

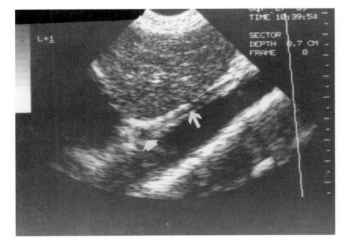

Figure 5–95. Longitudinal scan of the aorta.

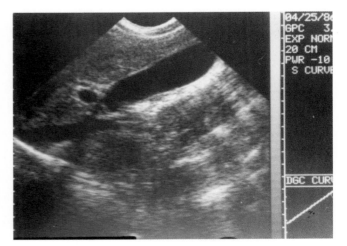

Figure 5–97. Longitudinal scan of the gallbladder.

(A) stones in Hartman's pouch
(B) cystic duct stone
(C) valves of Heister
(D) air
(E) refraction

307. There appears to be two echogenic masses in Fig. 5–98. One is anterior to the diaphragm(indicated by the calipers), and the other one is posterior to the diaphragm (indicated by the arrow). This phenomenon is usually caused by

(A) slice-thickness artifact
(B) reflection
(C) mirror-image artifact
(D) refraction
(E) side lobe artifact

308. A 38-year-old male, who is an intravenous drug abuser, with a known mediastinal mass is seen in Fig. 5–99A and Fig. 5–99B. Fig. 5–99A demonstrates

(A) a mass near the head of the pancreas
(B) periportal lymphadenopathy
(C) chronic cholecystitis
(D) Klatzkin tumor
(E) liver mass

309. Fig. 5–99B demonstrates

(A) a normal kidney
(B) a kidney consistent with acute renal insufficiency
(C) a kidney consistent with chronic renal insufficiency
(D) renal cell carcinoma
(E) an adrenal gland in the renal fossa

310. A sonogram is performed on a 32-year-old women with a history of pancreatic carcinoma. The scan in Fig. 5–100 most likely represents

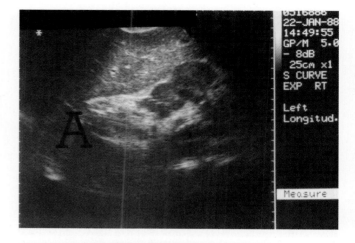

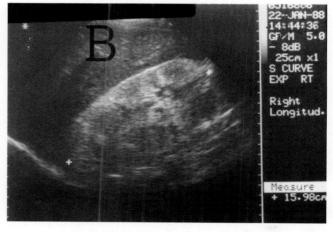

Figure 5–99. (A) Sagittal scan of the right upper quadrant. (B) Sagittal scan through the right kidney.

(A) celiac nodes
(B) an aortic aneurysm
(C) horse shoe kidney
(D) gastric lesion
(E) lesser sac mass

311. What type of aneurysm is demonstrated Fig. 5–101?

(A) fusiform
(B) saccular
(C) cylindrical
(D) berry
(E) dissecting

312. The arrow in Fig. 5–102 is pointing to the

(A) right renal artery
(B) right renal vein
(C) left renal artery
(D) left renal vein
(E) gastroesophageal junction

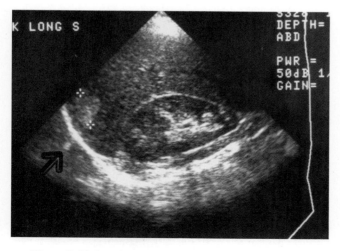

Figure 5–98. Longitudinal scan of the right upper quadrant.

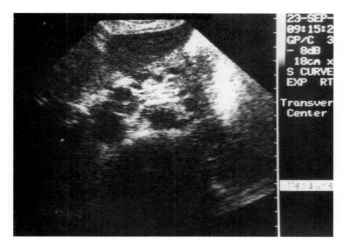

Figure 5–100. Transverse scan of the abdomen.

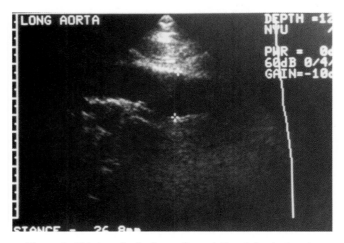

Figure 5–101. Longitudinal scan through the abdominal aorta.

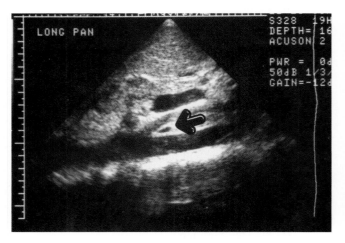

Figure 5–102. Longitudinal scan through the abdominal aorta.

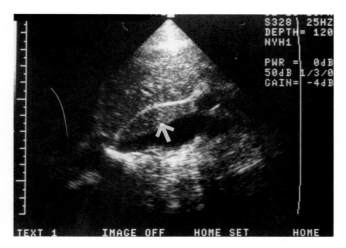

Figure 5–103. Sagittal scan through the right upper quadrant.

313. The arrow in Fig. 5–103 is pointing to

   (A) head of the pancreas
   (B) body of the pancreas
   (C) caudate lobe of the liver
   (D) medial aspect of the left lobe
   (E) right lobe of the liver

314. The thin black arrow in Fig. 5–104 is pointing to

   (A) celiac axis
   (B) superior mesenteric artery
   (C) portal vein
   (D) left gastric artery
   (E) hepatic artery

315. The white arrowhead in Fig. 5–104 is pointing to

   (A) celiac axis
   (B) superior mesenteric artery
   (C) portal vein
   (D) left gastric artery
   (E) hepatic artery

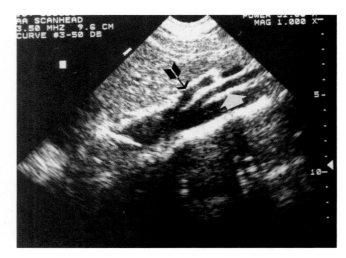

Figure 5–104. Sagittal scan through the right upper quadrant.

316. The vessel that lies posterior to the pancreas in Fig. 5–104 is the

(A) splenic vein
(B) aorta
(C) portal vein
(D) left renal vein
(E) hepatic vein

317. The arrow in Fig. 5–105 is pointing to

(A) normal head of pancreas
(B) normal body of pancreas
(C) C-loop of the duodenum
(D) caudate lobe of the liver

318. The arrow in Fig. 5–106 is pointing to

(A) normal head of pancreas
(B) normal body of pancreas
(C) caudate lobe of liver
(D) splenic flexure

319. The arrow in Fig. 5–107 is pointing to

(A) gastroduodenal artery
(B) common bile duct
(C) portal vein
(D) superior mesenteric vein
(E) hepatic artery

320. The structure that defines the anterolateral aspect of the head is the

(A) superior mesenteric artery
(B) inferior vena cava
(C) splenic vein
(D) common bile duct
(E) gastroduodenal artery

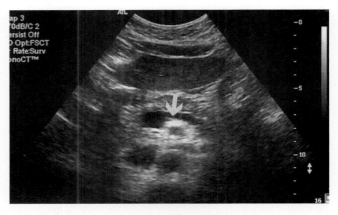

Figure 5–106. Transverse sonogram through the pancreas.

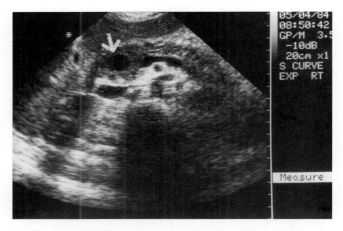

Figure 5–107. Transverse sonogram through the pancreas.

321. The arrows in Fig. 5–108 are pointing to

(A) peripelvic cysts
(B) extrapelvic cysts
(C) parapelvic cysts
(D) renal pyramids
(E) dilated calyces

322. The arrow in Fig. 5–109 the arrow is pointing to

(A) dilated loop of bowel
(B) dilated ureter with stone
(C) internal iliac vessel with thrombus
(D) appendix
(E) granuloma

323. What pathology will most likely be seen in the urinary bladder of the patient in Fig. 5–109?

(A) absence of the ureteral jet
(B) thickened Foley catheter
(C) focal thickening bladder wall
(D) bladder carcinoma
(E) debris in the bladder

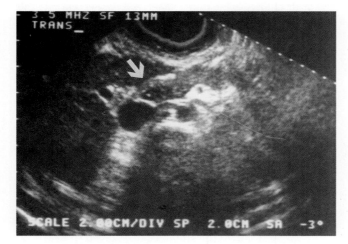

Figure 5–105. Transverse scan through the pancreas.

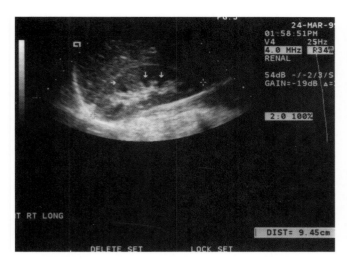

Figure 5–108. Long axis image of the right kidney. *(Courtesy of Sheptim Telegrafi, MD, New York University.)*

324. Ureteral jets will be seen in all of the following *except*

(A) extrapelvic cyst
(B) obstructive hydronephrosis
(C) renal artery aneurysm
(D) parapelvic cyst
(E) transient diuresis

325. A 30-year-old patient with a history of biliary disease presents with fever, pain, leukocytosis. An abdominal sonogram is performed. The areas labeled A in Fig. 5–110 is area consistent with

(A) hematomas
(B) complicated cysts
(C) abscesses

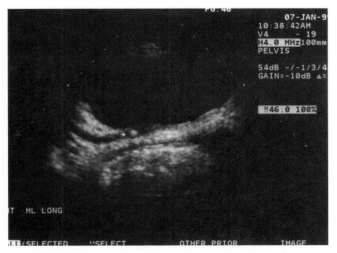

Figure 5–109. Long axis sonogram through the urinary bladder. *(Courtesy of Sheptim Telegrafi, MD, New York University.)*

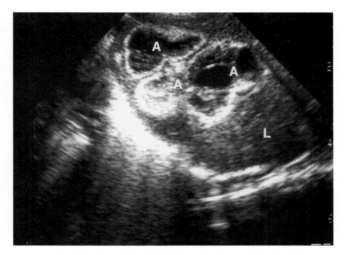

Figure 5–110. Longitudinal sonogram of the liver.

(D) echinococcal disease
(E) metastatic lesions

326. A patient presents with polycystic liver disease. What other organ should also be evaluated by sonogram?

(A) spleen
(B) pancreas
(C) gallbladder
(D) adrenal glands
(E) kidneys

327. Identify the vessel with a postprandial low-resistive blood flow.

(A) celiac artery
(B) hepatic artery
(C) splenic artery
(D) superior mesenteric artery
(E) aorta

328. The arrows in Fig. 5–111 are pointing to

(A) ascites
(B) perinephric fluid
(C) pleura effusion
(D) fluid in Morrison's pouch
(E) normal renal cortex

329. Fig. 5–112 is a transverse view of the bladder. The arrow is pointing to

(A) bladder stone
(B) bladder diverticula
(C) bladder mass
(D) foley catheter
(E) ureteral jet

330. The arrow in Fig. 5–113 is pointing to

(A) antrum of the stomach
(B) head of the pancreas

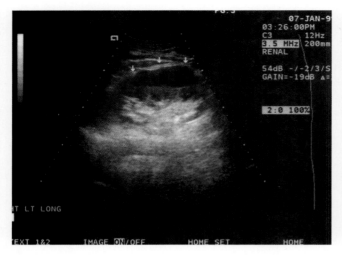

Figure 5–111. Longitudinal sonogram of the left kidney. *(Courtesy of Sheptim Telegrafi, MD, New York University.)*

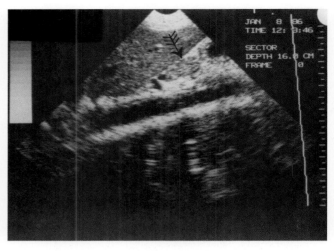

Figure 5–113. Longitudinal scan of the inferior vena cava.

(C) caudate lobe of the liver
(D) body of the pancreas
(E) adrenal gland

331. Fig. 5–114 is consistent with

(A) chronic pancreatitis
(B) acute pancreatitis
(C) adenocarcinoma
(D) islet cell tumor
(E) normal scan

332. A 37-year-old man with a history of repeated episodes of pancreatitis due to alcoholism presents with epigastric mass. Fig. 5–115 is suggests

(A) negative study
(B) adenocarcinoma

(C) pancreatic pseudocyst
(D) acute pancreatitis
(E) chronic pancreatitis

333. The most common complication of a pancreatic pseudocyst is

(A) infection
(B) reabsorption
(C) calcification
(D) hemorrhage
(E) rupture

334. A sonogram of the abdominus rectus muscle is ordered. The most appropriate transducer to use to obtain optimal images is

(A) 2.5 MHz curve linear
(B) 5.0 MHz curve linear

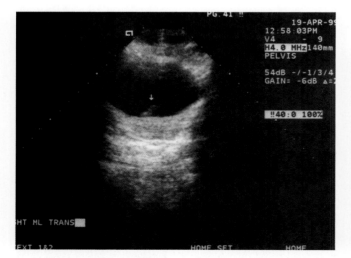

Figure 5–112. Transverse scan of the urinary bladder. *(Courtesy of Sheptim Telegrafi, MD, New York University.)*

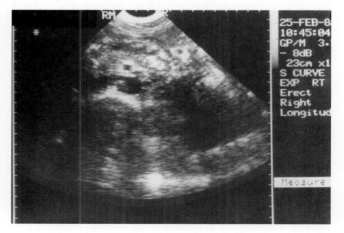

Figure 5–114. Transverse sonogram through the pancreas.

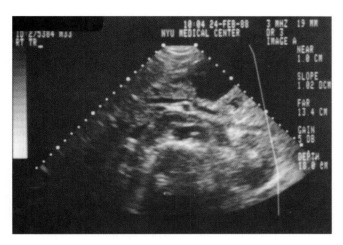

Figure 5–115. Transverse sonogram through the pancreas.

(C) 3.5 MHz mechanical sector
(D) 5 MHz linear
(E) transrectal probe

335. The area anterior to the right kidney and posterior to the right lobe of the liver is called

(A) pouch of Douglas
(B) Morison's pouch
(C) Hartman's pouch
(D) lesser sac
(E) greater sac

336. A 34-year-old male presents with flank pain. The ureteral jets are normal. Fig. 5–116 is suggestive of

(A) renal cell carcinoma
(B) pyonephrosis
(C) pyelocaliectasis

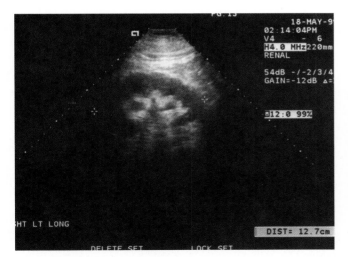

Figure 5–116. A longitudinal sonogram through the left kidney. *(Courtesy of Sheptim Telegrafi, MD, New York University.)*

(D) pyelonephrosis
(E) renal transplant

337. The renal transplant patient in Fig. 5–117 was referred for a sonogram. The perirenal fluid collection may be associated with all of the following *except*

(A) abscess
(B) hematoma
(C) ascites
(D) urinoma
(E) lymphocele

338. A postrenal transplant patient presents with fever, flank pain, localized tenderness, and leukocytosis. A renal sonogram is performed, and a perinephric fluid collection is documented. These finding are most consistent with

(A) abscess
(B) hematoma
(C) lymphocele
(D) renal cyst
(E) urinoma

339. In Fig. 5–118, the anechoic structures visualized within the liver are

(A) normal bile ducts
(B) dilated bile ducts
(C) hepatic arteries
(D) hepatic veins
(E) portal veins

340. In Fig. 5–119, the organ that the arrow is pointing to is consistent with

(A) normal pancreas
(B) acute pancreatitis
(C) chronic pancreatitis
(D) adenocarcinoma
(E) islet cell tumor

341. A 38-year-old man presents with a history of enuresis presents for a pelvic sonogram. Fig. 5–120 is most consistent with

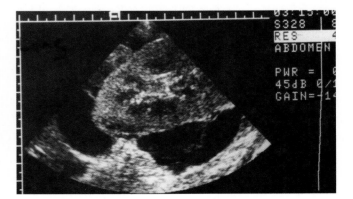

Figure 5–117. Longitudinal scan though the kidney.

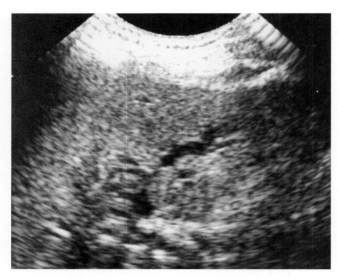

Figure 5–118. A magnified view through the liver.

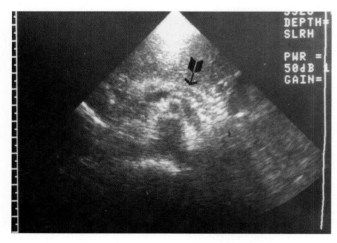

Figure 5–119. Transverse scan through the pancreas.

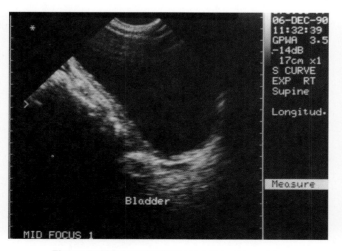

Figure 5–120. Longitudinal scan of a male pelvis.

(A) a normal pelvic sac
(B) an enlarged prostate
(C) diffuse bladder wall thickening
(D) bladder outlet obstruction
(E) endometriosis of the bladder wall

342. Fig. 5–121 is most consistent with

(A) hepatitis
(B) cirrhosis
(C) pyelonephritis
(D) pyelocaliectasis
(E) chronic renal failure

343. Identify the laboratory values that would most likely be elevated in the patient in Fig. 5–121.

(A) alanine aminotransferase (ALT) and aspartate aminotransferase (AST)
(B) alkaline phosphatase and bilirubin
(C) amylase and lipase
(D) creatinine and blood urea nitrogen (BUN)
(E) acid phosphatase and white blood count (WBC)

344. Internal echoes inside the renal cyst, shown in Fig. 5–122 may be due to all of the following *except*

(A) reverberation
(B) beam width artifact
(C) refraction
(D) attenuation
(E) side lobe artifact

345. The findings in the transverse scan in Fig. 5–123 of the right kidney is most consistent with

(A) parapelvic cyst
(B) ureteropelvic junction obstruction (UPJ)
(C) nonobstructive hydronephrosis
(D) adult polycystic kidney disease
(E) infantile polycystic kidney disease

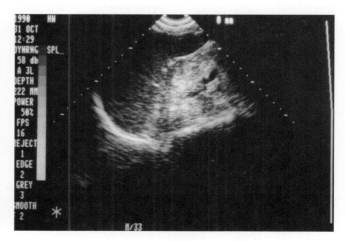

Figure 5–121. Longitudinal scan of the left kidney.

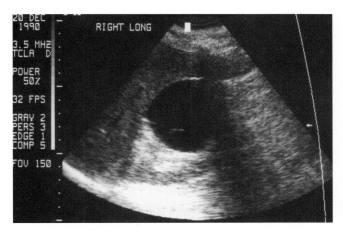

Figure 5–122. Longitudinal scan of the right kidney.

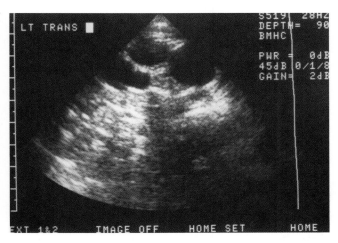

Figure 5–124. Transverse scan of the left kidney of a newborn.

346. The neonate in Fig. 5–124 presented with a palpable abdominal mass. The sonogram is most suggestive of

(A) multicystic dysplastic kidney
(B) pyonephrosis
(C) infantile polycystic disease
(D) peripelvic cysts
(E) extrapelvic cysts

347. Fig. 5–125 suggests that this patient may have all of the following *except*

(A) normal kidney
(B) benign prostate hyperplasia
(C) prostatitis
(D) calculi
(E) retroperitoneal fibrosis

348. A scrotal scan was performed on a 69-year-old man. The findings in Fig. 5–126 are consistent with

(A) epididymitis
(B) hydrocele

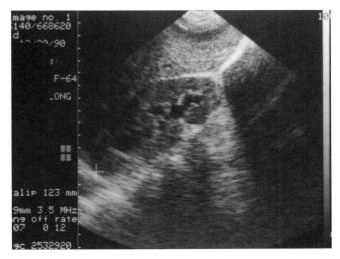

Figure 5–125. Longitudinal scan of the right kidney.

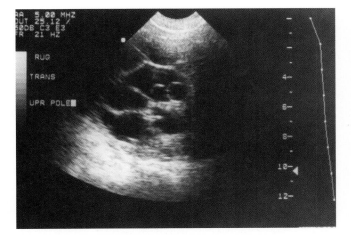

Figure 5–123. Transverse scan of the right kidney.

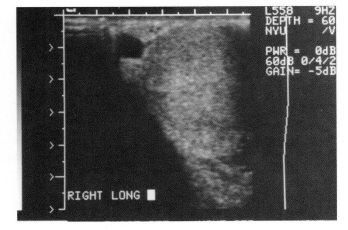

Figure 5–126. Longitudinal scan through the right testis.

(C) seminoma
(D) varicocele
(E) spermatocele

349. A scrotal scan was performed on a 78-year-old man. The arrow in Fig. 5–127 is pointing to

(A) a fractured testicle
(B) normal head of epididymis
(C) the mediastinum
(D) seminoma
(E) testicular torsion

350. Fig. 5–128 is a longitudinal scan through a male pelvis. The arrow is pointing to

(A) prostate
(B) seminal vesicle
(C) prostatic urethra
(D) membranous urethra
(E) urethra

351. A young male patient presents with right testicular pain. A scan of his testicles is performed. The arrow in Fig. 5–129 is pointing to

(A) spermatocele
(B) epididymal cyst
(C) cryptorchism
(D) varicocele
(E) mediastinum

352. The longitudinal scan of the right kidney in Fig. 5–130 is consistent with

(A) acute pyelonephritis
(B) acute tubular necrosis
(C) tubular sclerosis
(D) acute focal bacteria nephritis
(E) duplex collecting system

353. A transverse scan of the upper abdomen. The arrow in Fig. 5–131 is pointing to

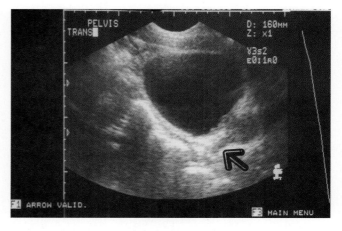

Figure 5–128. Longitudinal scan through a normal male pelvis.

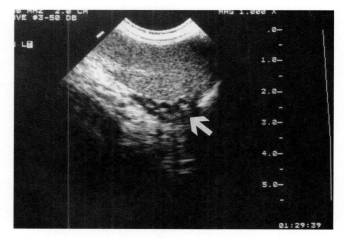

Figure 5–129. Longitudinal scan through the right testis.

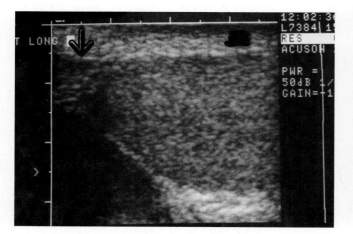

Figure 5–127. Magnified longitudinal scan of the right testis.

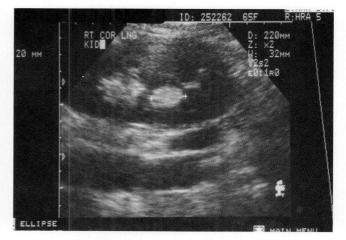

Figure 5–130. Coronal scan of the right kidney.

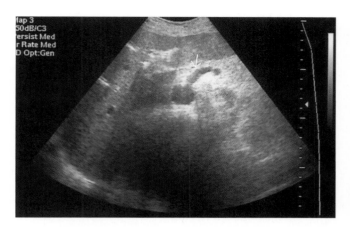

Figure 5–131. Transverse scan of the upper abdomen.

(A) hepatic vein
(B) splenic artery
(C) celiac axis
(D) hepatic artery
(E) portal confluence

354. Fig. 5–132 is an abdominal longitudinal scan of a 14-day-old baby boy born 2 weeks prematurely. The arrow is pointing to

(A) normal adrenal gland
(B) perirenal hemorrhage
(C) retroperitoneal fat
(D) neuroblastoma
(E) pheochromocytoma

355. Fig. 5–133 is a coronal scan of the left kidney. This image suggests

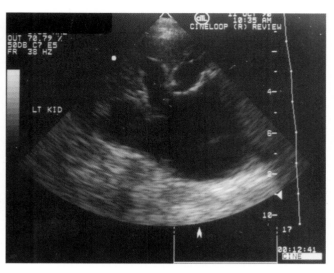

Figure 5–133. Coronal scan of the kidney.

(A) an extrapelvic cyst
(B) hydronephrosis
(C) pyonephrosis
(D) urinoma
(E) renal infarct

356. A longitude scan of the right kidney is performed. The thin black arrow in Fig. 5–134 is pointing to

(A) the renal sinus
(B) arcuate arteries
(C) renal medullary pyramids
(D) simple renal cysts
(E) renal stone

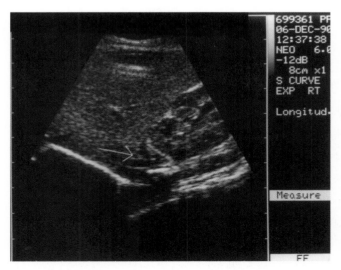

Figure 5–132. Longitudinal sonogram of a neonate through the area of the right kidney.

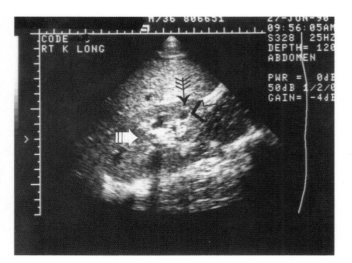

Figure 5–134. Longitudinal scan of the right kidney.

357. The open arrowhead in Fig. 5–134 is pointing to

(A) the renal sinus
(B) arcuate arteries
(C) renal medullar pyramids
(D) simple renal cyst
(E) renal stones

358. The larger black arrow in Fig. 5–134 is pointing to

(A) renal column of Bertin
(B) an angiomyolipoma
(C) dromedary hump
(D) bifod collecting system
(E) the renal pelvis

359. A patient presents with vague abdominal pain and an elevated bilirubin and liver function tests. The finding in Fig. 5–135 may be initiated by all of the following *except*

(A) stone in the common bile duct
(B) mass in the head of the pancreas
(C) mass in the ampullary of Vater
(D) diffuse metastatic disease of the liver
(E) cirrhosis

360. A patient presents with a spleen that is palpable on physical examination. Fig. 5–136 is a transverse image of the spleen. The finding may be initiated by all of the following *except*

(A) lymphoma
(B) portal hypertension
(C) infectious disease
(D) myeloproliferation
(E) neuroblastoma

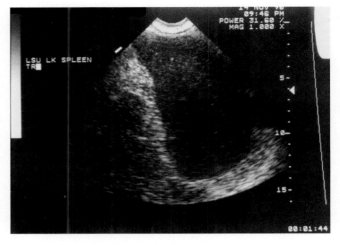

Figure 5–136. Longitudinal scan of the spleen.

361. A 25-year-old women presents for an abdominal sonogram. A longitudinal scan of the liver is performed. The two cystic structures in Fig. 5–137 are most likely

(A) liver metastases
(B) hydatid cysts
(C) simple benign cysts
(D) lymphoma
(E) polycystic liver disease

362. A 70-year-old man with a history of weight loss, abdominal pain, and anorexia. Figs. 5–138A–C suggest

(A) negative study
(B) pancreatic pseudocyst
(C) acute pancreatitis
(D) chronic pancreatitis
(E) pancreatic adenocarcinoma

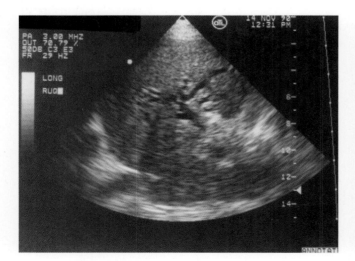

Figure 5–135. Longitudinal scan of the liver.

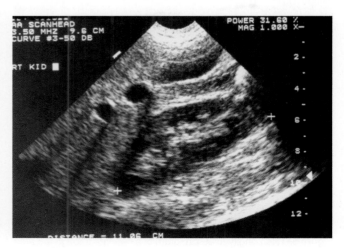

Figure 5–137. Longitudinal scan through the right upper quadrant.

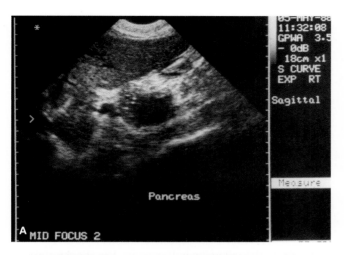

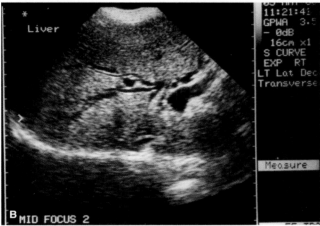

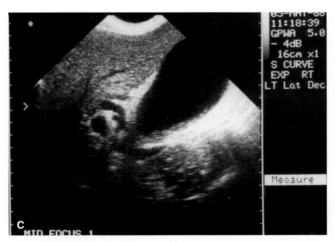

Figure 5–138. (A) Sagittal scan through the head of the pancreas. **(B)** Sagittal scan through the liver. **(C)** Sagittal scan through the gallbladder.

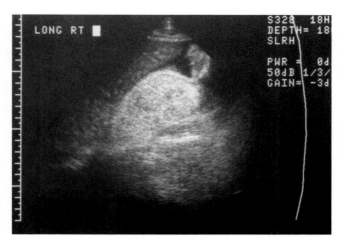

Figure 5–139. Longitudinal scan through the right kidney.

(C) tubular sclerosis

(D) chronic glomerulonephritis

(E) medullary cephrocalcinosis

364. Fig. 5–140 is a sagittal transrectal sonogram of the prostate. What laboratory value would most likely be elevated?

(A) prostatic-specific antigen (PSA)

(B) creatinine

(C) white blood cell count

(D) estrogen

(E) amalase

363. Fig. 5–139 is most consistent with

(A) acute pyelonephritis

(B) acute tubular necrosis

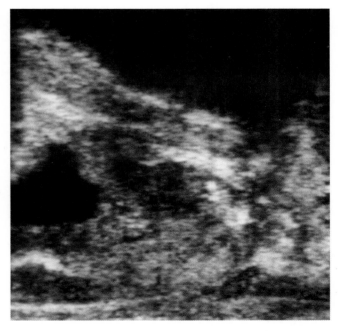

Figure 5–140. Midline sagittal transrectal sonogram of the prostate.

365. Hashimoto's disease is a type of chronic

(A) gastroenteritis
(B) thyroiditis
(C) orchitis
(D) prostatitis
(E) hepatitis

366. The two lobes of the thyroid are connect by the

(A) sternothyroid muscle
(B) common carotid artery
(C) trachea
(D) isthmus
(E) lower poles

367. A type of a malignant adrenal mass is a(n)

(A) adenoma
(B) myelolipoma
(C) cyst
(D) pheochromocytoma
(E) neuroblastoma

368. An enlarged right adrenal gland will displace the inferior vena cava

(A) anteriorly
(B) posteriorly
(C) medially
(D) laterally
(E) no displacement

369. The cursors labeled 2 in Fig. 5–141 are measuring

(A) an angiomyolipoma
(B) a column of Bertin
(C) a renal cyst
(D) a pancreatic pseudocyst
(E) an adrenal cyst

370. The laboratory value in the patient in Fig. 5–141 will most likely be

(A) elevated creatinine
(B) decreased blood urea nitrogen (BUN)
(C) elevated amylase
(D) elevated uric acid
(E) normal

371. Fig. 5–142 is a sonogram of the right kidney. This image is consistent with

(A) chronic renal failure
(B) obstructive uropathy
(C) calculi
(D) column of Bertin
(E) renal pyramid

372. All of the following will increase the chance of documenting shadowing posterior to a small renal stone *except*

(A) decrease gain
(B) focal zone set at the level of the calculi
(C) increase the transducer frequency
(D) use a linear probe
(E) tissue harmonics

373. Fig. 5–143 of the left kidney is consistent with

(A) hydronephrosis
(B) hydroureter
(C) pyonephrosis
(D) vesicoureteral obstruction
(E) hypernephroma

374. Fig. 5–144 is a longitudinal scan of the right upper quadrant. The abnormality is

(A) a hypoechoic texture of the renal parenchyma
(B) an echogenic liver texture

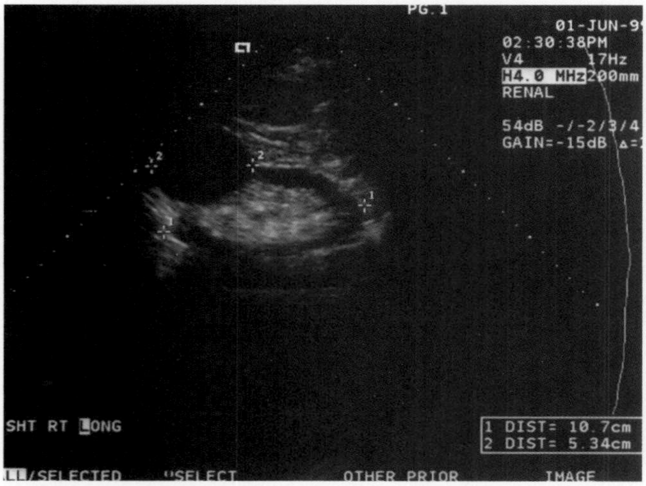

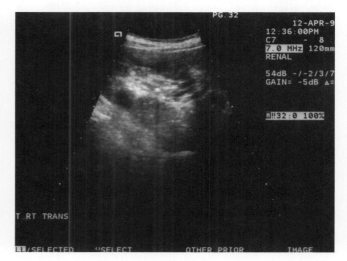

Figure 5–141. Long axis scan of the right kidney. *(Courtesy of Sheptim Telegrafi, MD, New York University.)*

Figure 5–142. Scan through the right kidney. *(Courtesy of Sheptim Telegrafi, MD, New York University.)*

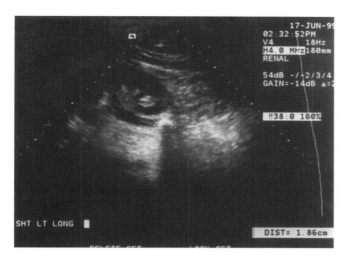

Figure 5–143. Coronal scan through the left kidney. *(Courtesy of Sheptim Telegrafi, MD, New York University.)*

(C) atrophy of the kidney
(D) metastases
(E) none—inappropriate technical settings

375. Fig. 5–144 is consistent with all of the following *except*

(A) glycogen storage disease
(B) fatty metamorphosis
(C) echinococcal disease
(D) severe hepatitis
(E) hemochromatosis

376. To optimize a sonogram all of the following must be taken into consideration *except*

(A) change over all gain
(B) time gain compensation (TGC)

(C) depth and focus
(D) transducer frequency and type
(E) speed of sound

377. Fig. 5–145 is a duplex color Doppler sonogram of the right kidney. The Doppler finding is consistent with a

(A) normal kidney
(B) obstructive uropathy
(C) pelviectasis
(D) renal artery stenosis
(E) hypertension

378. Splenomegaly is diagnosed when the spleen is greater than

(A) 8 cm
(B) 11 cm
(C) 13 cm
(D) 15 cm
(E) 18 cm

379. Fig. 5–146 is a long axis sonogram of the right upper quadrant of the abdomen. The image is best described as a

(A) contracted gallbladder filled with stones
(B) contracted gallbladder without stones
(C) postcholecystectomy
(D) heterogeneous liver
(E) echogenic focal mass

380. The most likely diagnosis of the patient in Fig. 5–146 is

(A) cholecystectomy
(B) gastric mass
(C) acalculous cholecystitis
(D) calculous cholecystitis
(E) normal abdomen

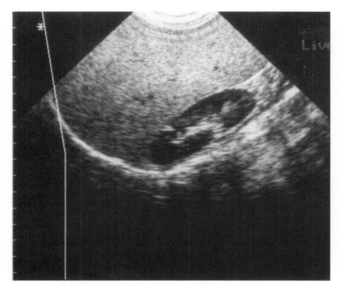

Figure 5–144. Longitudinal scan of the right upper quadrant.

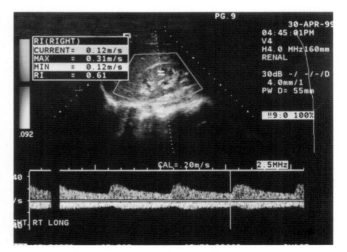

Figure 5–145. Long axis view of the right kidney. *(Courtesy of Sheptim Telegrafi, MD, New York University.)*

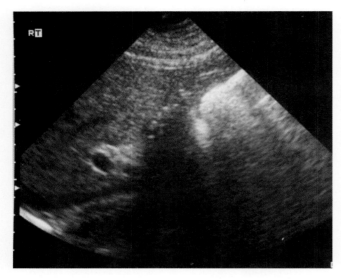

Figure 5–146. Long axis sonogram of the upper abdomen.

381. The laboratory finding in the patient in Fig. 5–146 would most likely be consistent with

(A) increase in amylase
(B) increase in creatinine
(C) decrease in prothrombin time
(D) decrease in indirect bilirubin
(E) increase in alkaline phosphatase

382. Fig. 5–147 is a transverse image of the right side of the neck at the level of the common carotid artery. The abnormality is

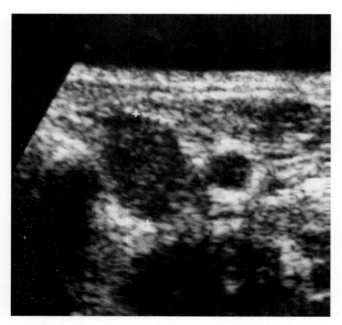

Figure 5–147. Transverse image of the right side of the neck at the level of the common carotid artery.

(A) thrombosis of the common carotid artery
(B) a parathyroid mass
(C) a thyroid mass
(D) a mass of the strap muscle
(E) enlarged lymph node

383. The most likely diagnosis of the patient in Fig. 5–147 is

(A) parathyroid adenoma
(B) thyroid adenoma
(C) lymph node
(D) normal neck tissue

384. Parathyroid adenomas may be associated with

(A) hypercalcemia
(B) hypertension
(C) bloating
(D) acne
(E) headaches

385. The spiral values of Heister are located in the

(A) ampulla of Vater
(B) junction of the cystic duct and common duct
(C) junction of the right and left common hepatic duct
(D) proximal portion of the cystic duct
(E) fundus of the gallbladder

386. Identify the pre-existing condition that occurs in patients with hepatomas.

(A) hematomas
(B) abscesses
(C) gallstones
(D) developmental cysts
(E) cirrhosis

387. A 3-year-old child with a clinical history of intermittent pain, jaundice, and a palpable mass presents for an abdominal sonogram. A cystic dilation of the common bile duct is seen in the liver. This is most characteristic of

(A) biliary atresia
(B) hepatitis
(C) choledochal cyst
(D) hypertrophy pyloric stenosis
(E) normal liver finding

388. Carcinoma of the gallbladder would most likely appear as a(n)

(A) thin-walled gallbladder
(B) small gallbladder with thickened walls
(C) large gallbladder with a halo surrounding it
(D) diffusely thickened gallbladder with gallstones
(E) echogenic mass with no distinguishing features of a gallbladder

389. A baker cyst is usually located

   (A) adjacent to the thyroid
   (B) behind the nipple in a breast
   (C) within the rectus abdominis muscle
   (D) posterior to the uterus
   (E) behind the knee

390. What is the most common congenital cause of urinary tract obstruction in males?

   (A) ureteropelvic junction obstruction (UPJ)
   (B) posterior urethral valve (PUV)
   (C) infantile polycystic kidney disease
   (D) undescended testis
   (E) duplex collecting system

391. What is a Reidel's lobe?

   (A) elongation of the left lobe
   (B) a duplication of the caudate lobe
   (C) tongue like extension of the right lobe
   (D) a small right lobe
   (E) transposition of the liver lobes

Answers and Explanations

At the end of each explained answer there is a number combination in parentheses. The first number identifies the reference source; the second number or set of numbers indicates the page or pages on which the relevant information can be found.

1. **(C)** Arcuate vessels separate renal parenchyma into cortex and medulla. Sonographically, they may be imaged as intense specular echoes within the cortico-medullary junction. *(1:247, 254)*

2. **(B)** Wilm's tumor is the most common solid renal mass in young children. The tumor may spread through the renal capsule and invade the renal vein. *(1:275)*

3. **(C)** Courvoisier's sign. Courvoisier law is enlargement of the gallbladder caused by an obstruction of the common bile duct from outside the biliary system. The obstruction usually results from carcinoma of the head of the pancreas and not from a stone in the common duct. The latter produces little or no dilatation of the gallbladder because the gallbladder is usually scarred from infection. Classically, patients present with painless jaundice and a gallbladder palpable on physical exam. *(1:175)*

4. **(B)** Hydropic gallbladder. Complete obstruction of the neck of the gallbladder or the cystic duct leads to hydrops or mucocele of the gallbladder. In this condition, the bile within the gallbladder is absorbed and replaced by a mucoid secretion from the lining of the gallbladder. *(5:130)*

5. **(D)** Renal vein thrombosis in the acute stage is associated with enlarged kidneys with a dilation of the renal vein proximal to the obstruction. There will either be a decreased or no blood flow on Doppler. Bilateral small kidneys are associated with end-stage renal disease. The normal adult kidneys range from 9 to 12 cm in length. The renal parenchyma is normally less echogenic when compared to the liver parenchyma. In cases of end-stage renal disease, the kidneys become more echogenic. End-stage renal disease may be caused by chronic glomerulonephritis, pyelonephritis, and renal vascular disease. *(1:98–99)*

6. **(C)** A staghorn calculus is a large stone located within the renal pelvis of the kidney. *(4:375)*

7. **(D)** Cholecystokinin, a hormone released by the intestinal mucosa, stimulates the release of bile from the gallbladder and pancreatic enzymes from the pancreas. *(1:164)*

8. **(D)** The liver is an intraperitoneal structure. The portion of the liver that is not covered by peritoneum is termed the bare area. The bare area is located between the right and left triangular ligaments. *(1:112)*

9. **(E)** The normal thickness of the gallbladder wall is 3 mm. Thicker walls suggest a pathologic condition that may be biliary in nature. *(1:175)*

10. **(C)** The pancreatic head lies caudad to the portal vein and anterior to the inferior vena cava. *(1:208)*

11. **(C)** Hydronephrosis is a fluid-filled pelvocaliceal collecting system. Sonographically, hydronephrosis has varied appearances from a mildly distended pelvocaliceal collecting system to moderately distended fluid-filled pelvocaliceal collecting system, and in the most severe form, the kidneys appear cystic with very little renal cortical tissue. *(1:284–285)*

12. **(B)** On a sonographic examination dilatation of the interhepatic ducts, common bile duct, and gallbladder (the gallbladder enlarges before the biliary tree because it has the greatest surface area) is imaged, one should expect the obstruction to be at the distal common bile duct. *(1:189)*

13. **(A)** The most common location of a pancreatic pseudocyst is in the lesser sac, which is located anterior to the pancreas and posterior to the stomach. *(1:216)*

14. **(B)** The extrahepatic portion of the falciform ligament can be visualized when there is massive ascites. The falciform ligament contains the ligamentum of teres and will appear sonographically as an echogenic linear band attaching the bare area of the liver to the anterior abdominal wall. *(1:114)*

15. **(C)** Anterior and parallel to the aorta. *(4:55)*

16. **(A)** The division by using Couinaud's sections into right and left lobes of the liver is by the imaginary plane, the main lobar fissure. *(5:94)*

17. **(C)** A prominent uncinate process of the pancreas lies posterior to the superior mesenteric artery and vein. *(1:208, 4:55)*

18. **(E)** The splenic vein courses transversely across the body along the posterior portion of the body and tail of the pancreas. *(5:151)*

19. **(B)** The gastroesophageal junction can sonographically be visualized anterior to the aorta and posterior to the left lobe of the liver. *(1:231)*

20. **(D)** Adenomyomatosis is a benign proliferation and thickening of the muscle layer and glandular layer of the gallbladder with formation of intramural diverticula called Rokitansky–Aschoff sinuses (RAS). There are three forms: diffuse, segmental, and localized. It is more common in women, with increasing incidence after the age of 40. *(5:134–135)*

21. **(B)** Acute pyelonephritis is caused by pyogenic bacteria, which invade the renal tissue. It is more common in women. *(10:142)*

22. **(A)** Angiomyolipoma is an uncommon benign renal mass, which is composed of blood vessels, fat, and muscle. They appear on ultrasound as an echogenic well-defined mass located in the renal cortex. When the mass is small, the patient is usually asymptomatic. Symptoms usually do not appear until the mass enlarges and bleeds, which causes severe flank pain and hematuria. *(10:152)*

23. **(C)** The gastroduodenal artery is a branch of the common hepatic artery. It is a landmark for the anterior lateral aspect of the head of the pancreas. *(4:241)*

24. **(A)** Two-thirds of the prostate is glandular tissue. The glandular tissue is divided into four zones and the peripheral zone accounts for approximately 70% of the glandular tissue. It is located along the posterior, lateral, and apical portions of the gland. *(4:449)*

25. **(E)** The left renal vein courses transversely across the body to enter into the inferior vena cava. It may be identified sonographically as a tubular anechoic structure between the aorta and superior mesenteric artery. *(9:183)*

26. **(A)** Glisson's capsule is a dense fibroelastic membrane that completely surrounds the liver and encloses the portal vein, hepatic artery, and bile ducts within the liver. *(4:117)*

27. **(C)** Left adrenal hyperplasia may cause anterior displacement of the splenic vein and posterior or inferior displacement of the left kidney. *(4:489)*

28. **(A)** The celiac axis has three branches, the common hepatic artery, left gastric artery, and splenic artery. Sonographically, only a short section of the splenic artery can be seen because of its tortuous course. *(5:72–73)*

29. **(D)** Accessory spleens are the most common congenital anomaly of the spleen. They are difficult to image sonographically, but when imaged they are most often seen at the hilum of the spleen. *(1:312)*

30. **(D)** A congenital fold between the body and fundus of the gallbladder is called a Phrygian cap. *(5:126)*

31. **(B)** The inferior vein cava forms at the confluence of the right and left common iliac veins, and it empties into the right atrium of the heart. *(5:75)*

32. **(E)** Diffuse thickening of the gallbladder wall is a nonspecific finding frequently seen when there is no primary gallbladder disease. It can be seen with acute and chronic cholecystitis but may also be secondary to right-sided heart failure, hepatitis, and benign ascites. In a patient not being NPO, physiologic contraction of the gallbladder has occurred and is one of the most common causes of diffuse thickening of the gallbladder wall. *(4:217)*

33. **(D)** If on a sonographic examination, one finds dilated intrahepatic ducts and a small gallbladder, the obstruction will usually be at the level of the common hepatic duct above the entry of the cystic duct. Bile will not be able to pass through the level of obstruction to fill the gallbladder. *(4:220)*

34. **(E)** The maximum inner diameter of the main pancreatic duct in a young adult patient measures 2 mm. *(5:152)*

35. **(A)** The endocrine function of the pancreas is to produce insulin, glucagon, and somatostatin. The exocrine function of the pancreas is to produce lipase, amylase, trypsin, and chymotrypsinogen. *(5:149–159)*

36. (A) Creatinine and blood urea nitrogen (BUN) are commonly used to measure renal function. Creatinine is normally filtered out of the blood by the kidneys and removed from the body via the urine. *(1:426)*

37. (C) Adult polycystic renal disease is an autosomal dominate disease, which usually does not produce symptoms until the third or forth decade of life. It is also associated with cysts in the liver, pancreas, spleen, and testes. Sonographically, the kidneys are enlarged with multiple cysts of varied size. The kidneys lose their reniform shape as the cysts enlarge. *(1:264)*

38. (B) The spleen is the best sonographic window to use to image the left hemidiaphragm. *(5:225)*

39. (D) Patients in the sickle cell crisis (early stages of the disease) will have an enlarged spleen. In the later stages, the spleen becomes fibrotic and atrophies. When the spleen is not imaged, it is referred to as autosplenectomy. *(5:233)*

40. (E) Bilateral hydronephrosis occurs when the cause of the obstruction is in the lower urinary system i.e., enlarged prostate, bladder tumor, posterior urethral valve syndrome (PUV). *(5:186)*

41. (D) The amount of liver damage in patients with acute hepatitis varies from mild to severe. The liver parenchyma may appear normal in a patient with acute hepatitis. *(1:138–139)*

42. (C) A hypertrophied column of Bertin is a normal variant of the kidney where there is an indentation of cortical tissue into the renal sinus. *(1:257)*

43. (B) The ureterovesical junction is the junction between the distal ureter and the base of the bladder. *(5:172)*

44. (D) Posterolateral to the thyroid is the common carotid artery, internal jugular vein, and the vagus nerve. *(1:397)*

45. (E) Signs of renal failure included: oliguria, palpable flank mass, generalized edema, pain, fever, hypertension, and muscle weakness are some of the clinical signs of acute renal failure. *(4:392–393)*

46. (C) A hydrocele is a common cause of scrotal pain. It can be either congenital or caused by trauma, mass, infarction, inflammation, or trauma. *(1:418)*

47. (A) The most common location of a spermatocele is the head of the epididymis. Spermatoceles is a retention cyst that may occur following vasectomy, scrotal surgery, or epididymitis. *(4:748)*

48. (C) A common problem in older men is benign prostatic hyperplasia. Patients present with urinary tract infections, increased resistance, and frequent urination. Sonographically, the prostate appears homogeneous, symmetrically enlarged with a continuous border. *(1:426)*

49. (B) Adrenal neuroblastoma is the most common malignancy of the adrenal gland found in children. *(1:343)*

50. (A) When a mass is visualized in the area of the head of the pancreas, one should check the liver for metastasis and dilation of the intrahepatic ducts. The common bile duct and main pancreatic duct may be dilated secondary to obstruction caused by enlargement of the mass. *(2:218–219)*

51. (C) Adenocarcinoma is the most common primary carcinoma of the pancreas. It is most frequently found in the head of the pancreas. The clinical systems are weight loss, painless jaundice, nausea, and pain radiating to the back. *(1:218)*

52. (C) The ligamentum of venosum separates the anterior portion of the caudate lobe from the left lobe of the liver. *(5:95)*

53. (A) The most common benign neoplasm of the liver is a hemangioma, which is also called a cavernous hemangioma. They can be either single or multiple, and are more commonly found in women and in the right lobe of the liver. *(5:103–104)*

54. (D) Blood from the hepatic veins drain into the inferior vena cava, which delivers deoxygenated blood to the right atrium of the heart. Right-side heart failure will produce venous congestion of the liver, which will lead to marked dilation of the intrahepatic veins. *(4:155)*

55. (B) The main lobar fissure separates the right and left lobes of the liver. *(4:121)*

56. (D) The spleen is an intraperitoneal structure. Retroperitoneal structures include the kidney, pancreas, great vessels, adrenal glands, psoas muscles, and duodenum. *(4:507)*

57. (C) The splenic vein and superior mesenteric vein join together to form the portal vein. The junction of the splenic vein and superior mesenteric vein occurs posterior to the neck of the pancreas. *(5:78)*

58. (B) The common bile duct unites with the main pancreatic duct just before entering the second portion of the duodenum. *(1:197)*

59. (A) Empyema of the gallbladder is a complication of acute cholecystitis. The patient presents with high spiking fever, chills, and leukocytosis. The walls of the gallbladder are thickened, and the lumen is filled with pus and debris. There may be a "dirty" shadow caused by the gas, which is formed by the bacteria. *(4:216)*

60. (B) A cause of an increase in alpha-fetoprotein in a nonpregnant patient is a hepatoma of the liver.
(1:148)

61. (C) If the prostate is found enlarged, one should check the kidneys for hydronephrosis. An enlarged prostate gland is a common cause of bladder neck obstruction in older men. *(4:419)*

62. (A) The anterior wall of the body of the pancreas is the posterior wall of the antrum of the stomach.
(1:196)

63. (A) On a transverse scan the portal vein is seen as a circular structure anterior to the inferior vena cava and superior to the head of the pancreas. *(1:87)*

64. (B) The most common cause of hyperthyroidism is Grave's disease. Grave's disease is an autoimmune disease where the immune system attacks the thyroid and causes diffuse enlargement of the thyroid gland. *(5:277)*

65. (D) A prominent uncinate process is anterior to the inferior vena cava and posterior to the superior mesenteric vein. *(1:196)*

66. (C) A dissecting aortic aneurysm is when there is a tear through the intima layer and a blood-filled channel forms within the aortic wall. Patients are usually hypertensive males and have a known aneurysm.
(1:91–92)

67. (B) The adrenal glands can be divided into the cortex and medulla. The cortex has three zones, and each zone secretes a different type of steroid hormone, while the medulla secretes epinephrine and norepinephrine. *(1:336)*

68. (C) The ligament of teres is formed embryologically from the portal sinus branch of the umbilical vein. This canal closes after birth. Recanalization of the umbilical vein is associated with end-stage cirrhosis and portal hypertension. *(5:97, 111)*

69. (D) The parallel channel sign, irregular borders, and echo enhancement posterior to the dilated ducts are all characteristic of dilated intrahepatic bile ducts. It is common bile duct near the porta hepatis that is the first to dilate and is greatest in size.
(4:227–229)

70. (A) The rectus abdominus muscle arises from the pelvis lines, but it lines the anterior abdominal wall; therefore, it is not located in the retroperitoneal cavity. *(4:19)*

71. (D) A Klatskin tumor originates at the junction of the right and left hepatic ducts. Cholangiocarcinoma is a primary adenocarcinoma located in the intrahepatic ducts. A Klatskin tumor, cholangiocarcinoma, and enlarged portal lymph nodes will only cause intrahepatic obstruction. Pancreatic carcinoma will initially obstruct the common bile duct before intrahepatic dilatation occurs. *(1:189)*

72. (B) Direct or conjugated bilirubin elevated levels are seen in cases of obstructive jaundice. The laboratory results suggest obstructive jaundice, and one must check for the causes of the obstruction. *(4:199)*

73. (C) Prolonged fasting and diabetes, especially in one who is insulin dependent, are causes of enlarged gallbladder. Ascites is a nonbiliary cause of diffuse thickening of the gallbladder wall. Chronic cholecystitis is a cause of a small gallbladder. *(4:217, 220)*

74. (D) The celiac axis originates within the first 2 cm of the abdominal aorta; therefore, it is located superior to the pancreas. All of the vessels listed are used as landmarks for locating and imaging the pancreas.
(5:150–151)

75. (A) Retroperitoneal masses tend to cause anterior and cranial displacement of surrounding organs. The direction of the displacement is one way to distinguish between a retroperitoneal mass versus a peritoneal mass. *(1:343)*

76. (D) Enlarged paraspinal lymph nodes may displace the aorta anteriorly, causing the aorta to appear to be "floating." *(1:339)*

77. (D) Sonographically, enlarged nodes appear as anechoic masses with no demonstration of through transmission on account of its composition.
(1:340–341)

78. (A) Portafugal (hepatofugal) blood flow is the reversal of blood flow, blood flow toward the spleen. This may be caused by portal hypertension or liver disease.
(3:10–11)

79. (B) Anatomical landmarks helpful in locating the left adrenal gland are the aorta, spleen, left kidney, and left crus of the diaphragm. *(1:331)*

80. (A) Gallbladder polyps can be distinguished from calculi by the absence of shadowing and movement.
(1:176–177)

81. (E) Hydrops is dilatation of the gallbladder, which may be caused by an obstruction in the cystic duct. The gallbladder is palpable, and the patient may be asymptomatic or may present with pain, nausea, and vomiting. The intrahepatic and extrahepatic ducts are not dilated. *(5:130)*

82. (C) The most common cause of jaundice in the pediatric patient is biliary atresia, a narrowing and obstruction of the intrahepatic bile duct.   *(4:204)*

83. (C) Examples of primary retroperitoneal tumors imaged sonographically are leiomyosarcomas, neurogenic tumors, fibrosarcomas, rhabdomyosarcomas, and teratomatous tumors.   *(1:344)*

84. (D) A series of relative echogenicity has been established. Going from least echogenic to most, renal parenchyma < liver < spleen < pancreas < renal sinus.   *(5:153, 4:328)*

85. (D) The pancreas in children will be relatively less echogenic and larger in size relative to the body size. The echogenicity of the pancreas increases with age because there is an increase in body fat deposition, which increases the amount of body fat within the parenchyma of the pancreas.   *(5:153)*

86. (B) The kidneys are covered by three layers: the true capsule is the most internal layer that covers just the kidney; the perinephric fat is the middle layer, which is between the kidney and adrenal gland; and Gerota's fascia surrounds the kidneys, perinephric fat, and the adrenal glands.   *(1:248)*

87. (B) The middle, right, and left hepatic veins originate in the liver and drain directly into the inferior vena cava at the level of the diaphragm. They are the largest major visceral branches of the inferior vena cava.   *(5:76)*

88. (B) The spleen is variable in size but it is considered to be convex superiorly and concave inferiorly.   *(5:225)*

89. (C) Hypernephroma is a malignant solid renal tumor, which is also called renal cell carcinoma or adenocarcinoma of the kidney. Transitional cell carcinoma is the most common tumor to the collecting system. Oncocytoma is a rare benign renal tumor.   *(1:273, 3:71–72)*

90. (A) Adenocarcinoma is the most common malignant tumor of the prostate. Patients are usually asymptomatic or may present with urgency and hesitation of urination.   *(1:426–427)*

91. (C) The left kidney lies inferior and medial to the spleen. The diaphragm is superolateral, and posterior to the spleen, and the stomach, tail of the pancreas; splenic flexure is medial to the spleen.   *(1:311)*

92. (B) A hematocele is a condition in which blood fills the scrotal sac. Sonographically, an acute hematocele appears with thickened scrotal walls and fluid within the scrotal sac without increased through transmission. It is usually a result of trauma or surgery.   *(4:752–753)*

93. (A) A cavernous hemangioma is the most common benign hepatic neoplasm, and the most common sonographic appearance is an echogenic round or oval with well-defined borders.   *(1:147)*

94. (C) The normal thyroid gland measures 1–2 cm in anteroposterior dimension and 4–6 cm in length.   *(1:396)*

95. (D) Torsion is more common in children or teenage boys. It is a weakening in the attachment of the mesentery from the spermatic cord to the testicle. Clinically, the patient presents with a sudden extreme pain in the scrotum. Treatment must occur within 5 or 6 hours of onset to save the testicle. The sonographic appearance varies according to the length of time that diagnosis is made. Acute torsion occurs within the first 24 hours. In the early stages, there is a decrease in the arterial flow to the testis. An enlarged epididymis and enlarged hypoechoic testis is imaged. There may be thickening of the scrotal skin and/or the formation of a hydrocele.   *(5:333)*

96. (E) Ascites is always secondary to a primary disease process. Some of the causes of ascites include congestive heart failure, nephritic syndromes, infections; i.e., tuberculosis, trauma, and malignancy. Adenomyomatosis is a benign gallbladder condition, where there proliferation of the mucosal lining of the gallbladder into the muscle layer. Diverticulum of the muscle layer occurs and bile may collect there and cause ring-down artifacts.   *(4:46, 5:134–135)*

97. (B) Sonographically, the best way to diagnosis a dissecting aneurysm is to document the intimal flap moving with the pulsations of blood through the aorta.   *(4:70–71)*

98. (A) A mass in the head of the pancreas with a dilated common bile duct is suggestive of obstructive jaundice.   *(1:189)*

99. (B) In patients with uncomplicated acute epididymitis there will be enlargement of the epididymal head or the entire epididymis. The epididymis has a decrease in echogenicity, and there may be increased blood flow with a reactive hydrocele.   *(1:413–415)*

100. (B) A subhepatic abscess would be located inferior to the liver and anterior to the right kidney. This space is also referred to as Morrison's pouch. Other common sites for abscesses are the subphrenic, perinephric, intrarenal, intrahepatic, pelvic, and around lesions at the site of surgery.   *(5:255)*

101. (D) The ligamentum venosum is a remnant of the fetal ductus venosus; the ligament of teres and the falciform ligament are remnants of the fetal umbilical vein. The coronary ligaments define the bare area of the liver. *(1:114, 5:95)*

102. (A) The gastroduodenal artery is a major branch of the common hepatic artery. *(5:73)*

103. (D) Patients with Courvoisier gallbladder present with painless jaundice and a palpable right upper quadrant mass. The obstruction of the common bile duct is usually caused by enlargement of the head of the pancreas. Patients with acute hepatitis and cirrhosis do have painless jaundice. The jaundice is not caused by obstruction of the biliary system. It is caused by destruction of the liver parenchyma. Porcelain gallbladder is calcification of the gallbladder wall. *(5:109–111, 137)*

104. (E) A dromedary hump is a cortical bulge of the lateral border of the left kidney. A junctional parenchymal defect is a distinct division between the upper and lower pole of the kidney. A column of Bertin is prominent indentations of the renal sinus. All of these variants have a mass effect on ultrasound. A Phrygian cap is a fold between the fundus and body of the gallbladder. *(1:256–257)*

105. (C) Ascites, small liver, portal hypertension, and nodular liver borders may all be present with end-stage liver disease. The bile ducts will not be dilated because of the fibrotic liver parenchyma. *(1:139)*

106. (A) The head of the pancreas is located anterior to the inferior vena cava. *(1:196)*

107. (B) The lesser sac is located between the stomach and pancreas. *(1:216)*

108. (B) The renal pyramids are located in the medulla of the kidney. *(1:248)*

109. (C) The head of the epididymis is located superior to the testes. The rest of the epididymis courses along the posterior margin of the testicle inferiorly. *(4:721–722)*

110. (C) In chronic renal disease, both kidneys are small and echogenic. *(1:268)*

111. (B) A long history of alcoholism is a major cause of cirrhosis and ascites often is seen secondary to cirrhosis. *(4:149, 152)*

112. (C) Chronic active hepatitis may progress to cirrhosis. The etiology of chronic active hepatitis is usually idiopathic but may be viral or immunological. *(1:148)*

113. (C) The seminal vesicles are reservoirs for sperm and located posterior to the urinary bladder. *(1:408)*

114. (A) Choledochal cyst is a rare focal cystic dilatation of the common bile duct caused by an anomalous junction of the common bile duct with the main pancreatic duct. The reflux of the pancreatic enzymes causes a weakness of the common bile duct wall and an out-pouching of the wall. Choledochal cysts may be associated with gallstones, cirrhosis, and pancreatitis. Clinically, the patient present with pain, fever, abdominal mass, or jaundice. *(1:177)*

115. (E) Hashimoto's thyroiditis is chronic inflammation of the thyroid. It is a common cause of hypothyroidism in regions where there is a lack of iodine. The entire thyroid gland is involved, and sonographically, the thyroid is enlarged with irregular borders with decreased heterogeneous echoes. People with Graves disease present with hyperthyroidism, bulging eyes, and skin thickening. The thyroid is enlarged with increase vascularity. Malignant tumors of the thyroid are rare and have varied appearance on ultrasound from a single small solid nodule to hypoechoic to being isoechoic with the thyroid tissue. In 50% of cases, there will be calcification. *(1:402)*

116. (D) Calcification of part or the entire wall of the gallbladder is called a porcelain gallbladder. It is associated with chronic cholecystitis and gallstones. These patients have a higher risk of carcinoma of the gallbladder. *(1:185)*

117. (A) Patients typically are diagnosed with an aortic aneurysm by a pulsatile mass noted on physical examination. They usually have a history of smoking and vascular disease, such as hypertension. On ultrasound, it is important to measure the diameter of the lumen and the location of the aneurysm in reference to the renal arteries. *(1:90–91)*

118. (B) The right renal artery courses posterior to the inferior vena cava and may be imaged as a round anechoic structure posterior to the inferior vena cava on a longitudinal scan. *(1:84)*

119. (A) The retroperitoneal space is the area between the posterior portion of the parietal peritoneum and the posterior abdominal wall muscle. *(1:238)*

120. (A) When there is extrinsic pressure and obstruction of the common bile duct (i.e., a mass in the head of the pancreas), the gallbladder and biliary tree will be enlarged. *(5:159–162)*

121. (A) A seminoma is a solid malignant mass of the testicles that is usually unilateral and appears hypoechoic on a sonographic examination. *(5:338)*

122. (B) Thyroiditis appears sonographically as a diffuse enlargement of the thyroid with a decrease in echogenicity.   *(5:279)*

123. (E) Pheochromocytoma is a benign adrenal tumor of the medulla. It secretes both epinephrine and norepinephrine.   *(4:502–503)*

124. (C) The serum amylase and lipase both elevate upon the onset of pancreatitis, but amylase reaches its maximum value within 24 hours. Lipase remains elevated for a longer period of time.   *(4:249)*

125. (B) Hypertrophic pyloric stenosis (HPS) is more commonly seen in males between the ages of 1 week and 6 months. The pylorus is the channel between the stomach and duodenum. When the muscle of the pylorus is thickened, it prevents food from entering the stomach. The child typically presents with projectile vomiting, dehydration, and a palpable olive size mass in the epigastric region. The diagnosis of HPS is made if the length of the pylorus is greater than 18 mm, the anterior to posterior diameter is greater than 15 mm or the muscle thickness is greater than 4 mm.   *(4:587–588)*

126. (B) Neuroblastoma is a malignant tumor of the adrenal medulla that is found in children.   *(4:503)*

127. (B) Enlarged lymph nodes are hypoechoic with no increase in through transmission. Aortic aneurysm, crus of the diaphragm, and bowel may all appear sonographically as hypoechoic. Chronic pancreatitis is imaged as echogenic.   *(4:512)*

128. (D) Budd-Chiari syndrome is caused by thrombus in the hepatic veins or in the inferior vena cava causing obstruction of blood flow to the heart. The obstruction may be congenital or acquired. Budd-Chiari is associated with renal cell carcinoma, primary carcinoma of the liver or prolonged usage of oral contraceptives. It is characterized by abdominal pain, massive ascites, and hepatomegaly. Sonographically, the right lobe of the liver may be small with normal or enlarged caudate lobe. There will either be absence of blood flow in the hepatic veins and inferior vena cava or abnormal blood flow pattern on Doppler.   *(4:160–161)*

129. (E) In response to the increased pressure in the portal vein, which is associated with portal hypertension, there may be recanalization of the umbilical vein, which is located within the ligamentum of teres.   *(1:154–155)*

130. (B) A pelvic kidney is kidney that has failed to ascend to the renal fossa. It is located in the pelvis but has the same sonographic appearance as a kidney located in the renal fossa.   *(5:173)*

131. (A) The ureteropelvic junction (UPJ) is where the renal pelvis narrows and joins the proximal portion of the ureter.   *(5:172)*

132. (E) According to Platt et al. an RI of the renal artery greater than 0.70 is 90% accurate in diagnosing renal obstruction.   *(5:211)*

133. (C) Cushing's syndrome is an adrenal disease where there is over secretion of glucocorticoids.   *(1:343)*

134. (D) Islet cell tumors of the pancreas are well-circumscribed solid masses with low-level echoes and are frequently found in the body and tail of the pancreas and rarely in the head of the pancreas.   *(1:219, 223)*

135. (C) The celiac artery has three branches the common hepatic artery, left gastric artery and the splenic artery.   *(5:72)*

136. (A) The most common benign mass of the spleen is a cavernous hemangioma. The most common malignant tumor of the spleen is an angiosarcoma. Congenital cysts of the spleen are rare, and lymphomas are not benign masses.   *(5:234)*

137. (B) The parietal peritoneum lines the abdominal cavity. Organs are intraperitoneal if they are surrounded by peritoneum; or retroperitoneal if only their anterior surface is covered.   *(4:35–37)*

138. (C) A normally functioning transplanted kidney will have the same sonographic appearance as a normal kidney located in the renal fossa.   *(4:400)*

139. (D) When food-containing fat enter the small intestines, cholecystokinin is released into the blood stream, which activates the contraction of the gallbladder and the relaxing of the sphincter of Oddi.   *(4:198)*

140. (B) A transplanted kidney is usually placed in the pelvis along the iliopsoas margin and anterior to the psoas muscle. The ureter of the donor kidney is anastomosed to the bladder. The donor renal artery is anastomosed to the external iliac artery, while the renal vein is connected to the internal iliac vein.   *(4:399)*

141. (A) Klatskin tumors arise at the junction of the right and left hepatic ducts and causes dilation of the intrahepatic ducts with no dilatation of the extrahepatic ducts.   *(5:141–142)*

142. (D) The liver, spleen, hepatic veins, and gallbladder are located in the peritoneal cavity. The great vessels, pancreas, adrenal glands, and kidneys are not surrounded by peritoneum; therefore they are located in the retroperitoneal cavity. *(1:328)*

143. **(C)** The splenic artery originates from the celiac axis and courses along the superior aspect of the pancreas body and tail. *(5:72)*

144. **(C)** Artifacts result from a variety of sources including thickness and side-lobe artifacts, reverberation artifacts, electronic noise, and range ambiguity effects. Edge effects cause acoustic shadowing owing to reflection and refraction of sound. *(5:12–13)*

145. **(B)** When ascites is present it acts as an acoustic window. Therefore, the liver will appear more echogenic. There is always posterior acoustic enhancement when the sound travels through fluid. *(5:11)*

146. **(A)** All ultrasound equipment is calibrated at 1540 m/s, the speed of sound in soft tissue. When the ultrasound beam goes through a fatty tumor with a lower propagation speed, the tumor will appear *farther* away than its actual distance. *(5:13)*

147. **(D)** A fluid collection located between the diaphragm and the spleen may represent a subphrenic abscess. *(1:348)*

148. **(B)** If a mass is solid, displacement of adjacent organs will aid in helping to evaluate the origin of the mass. In a retroperitoneal sarcoma, the kidney, spleen, and pancreas would be displaced anteriorly. *(1:348–349)*

149. **(C)** Splenomegaly may be caused by congestion, i.e., portal thrombosis, trauma, infection, Hodgkin's disease, lymphoma, neoplasms, storage diseases, and polycythemia vera. *(1:318–319)*

150. **(A)** Adenomyomatosis is a benign infiltrative disease that causes a diffuse thickening of the gallbladder wall. It does not cause enlargement of the gallbladder. *(5:134–135)*

151. **(D)** Posterior to the kidneys are the quadratus lumborum muscle, diaphragm, psoas muscle, and twelfth rib. *(5:248)*

152. **(D)** Patients with chronic cirrhosis will have a small nodular fibrotic liver, which impedes blood flow through the liver causing collateral vessel development and portal hypertension. Ascites, peripheral edema, and splenomegaly are usually secondary to the increase in pressure in the portal vein. Liver failure causes jaundice and an increase in the clotting time. Sonographically, the liver is small and echogenic. *(4:151)*

153. **(C)** Ureteral jets are not p. obstructive hydronephrosis. A terior urethra valves may obstru the body. In cases of severe obstru pressure in the urinary bladder ma and renal collecting system to dilate usually does not cause hydronephrc

154. **(B)** An extrarenal pelvis extends i pelvis to outside the renal capsule. O ferentiate an extrarenal pelvis from hy is to place the patient prone. The press lapse the extrarenal pelvis.

155. **(B)** The linear anechoic structure slightly ι of midline is the aorta.

156. **(E)** The arrow is pointing to the heart, wl superior to the diaphragm.

157. **(B)** The arrow is pointing to a round anechoic stι ture anterior and slightly to the left of the spine. *(5:7.*

158. **(E)** Simple cysts are present in 50% of all adults over the age of 50. They are usually of no clinical significant and may be located anywhere in the kidney. Fig. 5–11 of the left kidney documents a small upper pole cyst with a larger cyst of the lower pole. *(1:263)*

159. **(A)** The most common causes of a fatty liver are alcohol abuse and obesity. Diabetes, chemotherapy, cystic fibrosis, and tuberculosis are other causes of fatty liver infiltration. The liver varies in appearance depending upon the severity of the fatty changes. The liver parenchyma will have an increase in echogenicity with a decrease in acoustic penetration. In cases of severe fatty infiltration, there will be a decrease in the echogenicity of the portal vessel walls caused by the increase in the echogenicity of the liver parenchyma. There may be difficulty in visualization of the diaphragm because of the increase of the liver parenchyma. *(4:145)*

160. **(B)** Cavernous hemangioma is a common benign tumor of the liver. Patients usually are asymptomatic unless the tumor starts to bleed, causing right upper abdominal pain. Sonographically, hemangiomas typically appear as echogenic, round, well-defined masses with posterior acoustic enhancement. They may be either singular or multiple. *(1:147)*

161. **(A)** Acute cholecystitis is usually associated with gallstones. Sometimes there may be cholecystitis without gallstones, which is referred to as acalculous cholecystitis (AAC). The sonographic appearance will be the same except for the presence of

echogenic foci with posterior shadowing within the gallbladder lumen. *(5:213)*

. **(C)** The sonographic characteristics of acute cholecystitis include: an enlarged gallbladder with a transverse diameter greater than 5 cm, gallbladder wall greater than 5 mm, pericholecystic fluid, a positive Murphy's sign, and an enlarged cystic artery. Not all of the sonographic criteria will be present in every case of cholecystitis. *(5:213, 216)*

163. **(A)** The pleural sac surrounds the lungs. The internal pleural (visceral pleura) lines the lungs, while the external pleura (parietal pleura) lines the inner surface of the chest wall. A pleural effusion is fluid superior to the diaphragm in the pleural sac. The diaphragm must be identified to differentiate fluid in the pleural space verses fluid in the abdominal cavity (ascites). *(1:552)*

164. **(C)** The liver is a common site for metastatic involvement. The most common primary sites include the colon, breast, and lungs. Metastatic lesions to the liver have varied sonographic appearances. They may be hypoechoic, echogenic, well defined, or cause a diffuse echogenic hepatic pattern. *(1:152–153)*

165. **(B)** The arrow is pointing to a normal hepatic vein, which drains into the inferior vena cava. *(5:76)*

166. **(B)** The arrow is pointing to the right renal artery, which lies posterior to the inferior vena cava. *(5:74)*

167. **(B)** The quadratus lumborum muscle is posterior to the kidney and courses lateral to the psoas muscle. It protects the posterior and lateral abdominal wall. *(4:19,324)*

168. **(C)** The falciform ligament extends from the umbilicus to the diaphragm and can only be imaged sonographically when massive ascites is present. *(1:114)*

169. **(C)** A multicystic (dysplastic) kidney is a common cause of a palpable neonatal mass. It is usually unilateral. Bilateral multicystic pathology is not compatible with life. *(1:270)*

170. **(D)** The main lobar fissure is a landmark used to document the gallbladder fossa when there is nonvisualization of the gallbladder. It appears sonographically as an echogenic linear structure that extends from the portal vein to the neck of the gallbladder. *(1:114)*

171. **(A)** The most common primary neoplasm of the pancreas is an adenocarcinoma. *(1:218)*

172. **(E)** The arrowhead is pointing to an enlarged pancreatic duct. The normal measurement of the pancreatic duct is less than 2 mm. *(4:244)*

173. **(A)** Sonographically acute pancreatitis may appear normal or diffusely enlarged with a decrease in echogenicity. The pancreatic duct may be enlarged. Hemorrhagic pancreatitis appearance depends upon the age of the hemorrhage. Usually there will be a well-defined mass in the head of the pancreas. Phlegmonous pancreatitis typically has an ill-defined hypoechoic mass on ultrasound. Chronic pancreatitis on a sonogram is usually atrophied and is very echogenic. There may be dilation of the main pancreatic duct secondary to a stone in the duct.

174. **(C)** Aortic aneurysm with a small thrombus in the proximal aorta and partial occlusion documented by color Doppler on both a transverse and longitudinal view. *(4:66)*

175. **(B)** The superior mesenteric artery is a ventral branch of the aorta. It courses parallel and anterior to the abdominal aorta. *(9:44)*

176. **(A)** The sonographic appearance of acute pancreatitis varies depending upon the severity of the inflammation. The echogenicity is hypoechoic and usually less than the liver. The pancreas may be enlarged with a dilated pancreatic duct. *(10:88–89)*

177. **(A)** The arrow is pointing to a medullary pyramid. *(1:255)*

178. **(C)** Most gallstones (calculi) sonographically appear as mobile echogenic foci with posterior shadowing. A percentage of gallstones appear as echogenic foci without acoustic shadowing. *(10:59)*

179. **(D)** Acoustic shadowing.

180. **(E)** The common bile duct is a sonolucent tubular structure that is imaged anterior to the portal vein. *(10:53)*

181. **(C)** The upper limits of normal of the common bile duct (CBD) is 8 mm. The CBD diameter increases in size after the age of 50 by approximately one mm per decade. *(10:53)*

182. **(B)** Pneumobilia is air in the biliary tract. Air in the biliary tract may be caused from chronic cholecystitis, biliary-enteric fistula or a surgical complication. Sonographically pneumobilia appears as echogenic foci usually found in the region of the porta hepatis. There may be motion and weak posterior acoustic shadowing of the foci. *(10:80)*

183. (E) Liver metastatic disease has various sonographic appearances. It may present as multiple echogenic masses of varying sizes. Malignant masses tend to have irregular borders and invade the surrounding tissue. Metastasis of the liver may present as a well-defined mass, hypoechoic mass, or a cystic lesion. Primary sites include the colon and breast.   *(10:34)*

184. (D) The spleen appears normal.   *(9:139)*

185. (C) The common bile duct is formed from the confluence of the common hepatic duct and the cystic duct.   *(9:92)*

186. (B) Atherosclerosis is the most common cause of an aneurysm.   *(1:90)*

187. (C) The arrow is pointing to the common bile duct, which is located anterior to the portal vein. The main portal vein, common bile duct, and hepatic artery form the porta hepatis.   *(9:82)*

188. (D) A duplex collecting system is a common renal variant. The echogenic renal sinus is separated by renal parenchyma. A duplex collecting system can mimic a mass occupying part of the renal sinus.   *(1:257)*

189. (A) An echogenic foci with posterior acoustic shadowing is the sonographic appearance of a calculi. A calculi in the common bile duct may cause dilation of the duct.   *(1:86)*

190. (C) Hydronephrosis may be unilateral or bilateral. An enlarged prostate, posterior urethra valve, pelvic mass, or a mass in the urinary bladder may cause bilateral renal obstruction. A stone in the ureter may cause unilateral hydronephrosis. Gallstones do not cause compression on the urinary system and have no effect on the urinary system.   *(4:368–369)*

191. (D) Kidneys normally migrate to the renal fossa during the embryonic period. Any kidney not located in the renal fossa is an ectopic kidney. A pelvic kidney may mimic an adnexal mass and is associated with other abnormalities, vesicoureteral reflux and genital.   *(1:258)*

192. (C) Pancreatic pseudocysts are fluid-filled structures that may be a complication of acute pancreatitis. They are usually filled with pancreatic enzymes, but they may also have blood or pus within. Pseudocysts have various sonographic appearances. They may appear cystic with or without debris, or they may appear solid. They are most often found in the region around the pancreas, lesser sac, or by the tail.   *(4:251)*

193. (B) The retroperitoneum has three potential spaces where fluid collections and space occupying lesions (abscesses and hematomas) can be found, the anterior pararenal space, the posterior pararenal space, and the perirenal space. The perirenal space is located is located within Gerota's fascia. The kidneys, adrenal glands, lymph nodes, blood vessels, and perirenal fat are located within Gerota's fascia.   *(1:40)*

194. (E) In the majority of cases with acute cholecystitis, there will also be gallstones. Symmetrical gallbladder wall thickening greater than 3 mm is a nonspecific sign of acute cholecystitis. Gallbladder wall thickening is also seen in patients with ascites, hepatitis, hypoproteinemia, hypoalbuminemia, heart failure, renal disease, systemic venous hypertension, and in patients who have eaten.   *(1:175)*

195. (A) Ring down artifact is also called comet tail artifact. A ring down artifact is a series of reverberations that appear as linear lines posterior to a strong interface. In Fig. 5–39, the gas in the bowel caused the reverberations.   *(7:505)*

196. (C) Renal cysts are commonly seen in over 50% of people over the age of 50. Cysts are anechoic, round or oval in shape with increased through transmission. They can be either singular or multiple and located anywhere in the kidney.   *(1:263)*

197. (D) Renal cysts usually affect renal function and patients are typically asymptomatic unless the cyst is very large or compresses the collecting system causing hydronephrosis.   *(1:263)*

198. (B) Lymph nodes are only visualized on a sonographic examination if they are enlarged greater than 1 cm. Common sites to image enlarged lymph nodes include around the great vessels (paraortic and paracaval), peripancreatic, renal hilum, and mesenteric region. Sonographically, lymph nodes are seen round, echo poor, homogeneous masses with no increase in the posterior through transmission.   *(1:332, 338–339)*

199. (C) A rise in lipase level indicates acute pancreatitis or pancreatic carcinoma. Amylase levels will also rise with acute pancreatitis but do not stay elevated as or as specific as lipase levels.   *(1:204–205)*

200. (E) Fatty infiltration of the liver usually causes a diffuse hyperechoic pattern not a focal pattern.   *(4:145)*

201. (A) Courvoisier's law states, obstruction of the common bile duct because of pressure from the outside the biliary system will lead to an enlarged gallbladder with dilatation of the biliary radicles.   *(1:218)*

202. **(D)** Chronic pancreatitis occurs after repeated bouts of acute pancreatitis, which is usually caused by biliary disease or alcoholism. The pancreatic tissue becomes fibrotic from chronic inflammation. The fibrotic and fatty changes cause the pancreas to appear more echogenic on a sonogram than normal. The borders may be irregular and dilatation of the pancreatic duct may be secondary to stone formation, causing dilatation of the pancreatic duct. As people get older, the pancreas becomes more echogenic, it is a normal part of the aging process. *(1:214)*

203. **(B)** Renal cell carcinoma is the most common renal tumor. It is more common in males, and there is an increase incidence of renal cell carcinoma in patients who are on long-term renal dialysis or have Von Hippel–Lindau disease. The sonographic appearance varies depending upon the stage of the mass. In stage one, the mass has not metastasized outside the true capsule of the kidney. Angiolipoma, adenoma, and oncocytoma are benign tumors of the kidney. *(1:266, 272)*

204. **(A)** Acute tubular necrosis is the most common medical cause of renal disease. Renal infarction is occlusion of a vessel caused by thrombus; it usually occurs in the periphery of the kidney. Patients with diabetes may have small echogenic kidneys, which is the sonographic appearance of chronic renal disease. Nephrocalcinosis disease sonographically appears as echogenic renal pyramids with or without shadowing. *(1:289)*

205. **(A)** Adult polycystic kidney disease is an inherited autosomal dominant disease that most often manifests in the fourth decade. It manifests by cystic dilatation of the proximal convoluted tubules, Bowman's capsule, and the collecting tubules. It is mostly a bilateral process, with associated cysts in the liver, pancreas, lungs, spleen, thyroid, bladder, ovaries, and testes. The kidneys are enlarged with cysts in the renal cortex and the kidney may lose its reniform shape. *(4:349–350)*

206. **(E)** A bladder diverticula is an out-pouching of the bladder wall. A diverticula may be congenital or acquired. An increase of the pressure within the bladder may be caused by a bladder outlet obstruction or a neurogenic bladder, which may lead to a weakening of the bladder wall leading to an out-pouching of the wall. A small connection between the bladder and diverticula may be seen on ultrasound, even after the patient has emptied his or her bladder. *(4:426)*

207. **(D)** A calculi in the proximal ureter. *(1:301)*

208. **(B)** A fusiform aneurysm is a uniform dilation of a vessel. The majority of aneurysms occur below the level of the renal arteries. *(4:65–66)*

209. **(C)** Murphy's sign is pain over the gallbladder region upon palpitation on physical examination. Kehr's sign is pain LUQ radiating to left shoulder. It is associated with a ruptured spleen. *(5:127)*

210. **(E)** This is an example of biliary duct obstruction of both the intra and extrahepatic ducts. A mass at the head of the pancreas may cause dilatation of both the intra and extrahepatic ducts in addition to an enlarged fluid filled gallbladder (Courvoisier's law). *(10:94)*

211. **(B)** Periaortic nodes will displace the superior mesenteric artery anteriorly *not* posteriorly. *(1:338–339)*

212. **(A)** Portal vein thrombus many be associated with various pathologies and conditions: hepatitis, chronic pancreatitis, trauma, malignancy, septicemia, pregnancy, portal caval shunts, and splenectomy. The development of collaterals is called cavernous transformation of the portal vein. *(5:115)*

213. **(E)** The image is of normal blood flow in the hepatic and portal veins. The color flow map on the left of the image is used to decipher the direction of blood flow. According to the color flow map, red is blood flow toward the transducer, and blue is blood flow away from the transducer. *(5:75–79)*

214. **(D)** The image is of calculi in the common bile duct causing dilatation of the duct. *(1:186)*

215. **(B)** The dilated common bile duct is located anterior to the portal vein. *(1:186)*

216. **(C)** Choledocholithiasis. Stones are usually produced in the gallbladder and the gallbladder should be evaluated for stones. Any obstruction of the common bile duct causes obstruction and dilatation of the duct. *(1:181)*

217. **(E)** An adenoma is a benign thyroid mass that compresses the surrounding tissue. Sonographically, it has varied appearances, from anechoic to echogenic. Commonly, a halo can be seen surrounding the adenoma. When there is hyperfunction, an increase of blood flow may be demonstrated around the mass. Grave's disease is associated with hyperthyroidism with a diffuse homogeneous appearance on ultrasound. Papillary carcinoma has a hypoechoic appearance with microcalcification on ultrasound. *(1:303)*

218. **(A)** The image is of a testicular tumor. The epididymis is enlarged in cases of testicular torsion and epididymitis. In cases of varicocele, there will be enlarged vessels, and a spermatocele produces a sonolucent lesion usually in the region near the head of the epididymis. The epididymis is normal on the image.   *(1:415,421)*

219. **(E)** Lymphadenopathy, leukemia, or acute scrotal pain may be a presenting symptom associated with a testicular tumor.   *(1:421, 423)*

220. **(C)** The transrectal sonogram demonstrates a hypoechoic lesion in the peripheral zone. The peripheral zone is the largest zone of glandular tissue, and it is the zone where most malignant tumors are found.   *(1:425–426)*

221. **(B)** The serum prostatic specific antigen (PSA) is used to evaluate the function of the prostate. An elevation of PSA over 4.0 ng/mL is indicative of prostatic disease. A PSA density greater than 0.12 to 0.15 is considered abnormal. An increase in PSA velocity greater than 20% in a year usually warrants a biopsy of the prostate. Creatinine is used to evaluate renal function; CA 125 is a nonspecific test for malignancy; and amylase is used to evaluate the pancreas; it is elevated early in acute pancreatitis.   *(1:426)*

222. **(D)** The left renal vein.   *(1:410)*

223. **(B)** The arrow points to hypoechoic lesions within the left lobe. Focal nodular hyperplasia can be either hypoechoic or hyperechoic focal masses.   *(4:168)*

224. **(C)** Hypoechoic lesions may be the result of infectious foci. It is very unusual to have metastases with hypoechoic echogenicity. Occasionally, lymphomas may appear as hypoechoic liver metastases. Hemangiomas are echogenic.   *(4:168)*

225. **(B)** The arrow is pointing to the ligamentum of Teres. The ligamentum of Teres is best visualized on a transverse scan of the liver. It divides the left lobe into medial and lateral segments.   *(1:111)*

226. **(A)** Alpha-fetoprotein level is elevated in cases of hepatocellular carcinoma and in pregnant women. In cases of biliary obstruction, the patient may be jaundiced, have elevated direct bilirubin, alkaline phosphatase, and pruritus.   *(1:139, 148)*

227. **(D)** Intrahepatic dilatation may be caused by carcinoma of common bile duct or a malignant invasion of the portal hepatis. Dilatation of the intrahepatic ducts is best imaged in the periphery of the liver.   *(1:139)*

228. **(E)** Choledocholithiasis appears as echogenic foci in the common bile duct with dilation of the duct. Chole-

cystitis, right-sided heart failure, and hypoproteinemia are some the causes of a thickened gallbladder wall.   *(3:38)*

229. **(C)** Metastases are neoplastic involvement in the liver, causing liver enlargement with multiple nodules of varying sonographic patterns. Metastases have been describes as hypoechoic, echogenic, bull's-eye, anechoic, and diffusely inhomogeneous. The patient typically presents with weight loss, decreased appetite, abnormal lever function tests, and hepatomegaly.   *(1:152–153)*

230. **(B)** Increased levels of creatinine and blood urea nitrogen are seen in renal failure.   *(1:251)*

231. **(E)** The head of the pancreas is to the right of the portal splenic confluence, anterior to the inferior vena cava, and medial to the c-loop of the duodenum.   *(1:196)*

232. **(C)** Crohn's disease is chronic inflammation of the bowel. It usually affects the ileum but may affect both the small and large intestine. It is most often seen in young adults.   *(4:296)*

233. **(B)** An early sign of obstructive hydronephrosis is the intrarenal vessels having an RI greater than 0.70. The RI returns to normal after 72 hours.   *(1:285)*

234. **(A)** A parapelvic cyst is located in the renal hilum. A hematoma, lymphoma, abscess, and urinoma are perirenal fluid collections that can readily be identified on ultrasound.   *(1:269, 292)*

235. **(A)** Increased flow within the dilated vessels can be seen with a Valsalva maneuver. Varicoceles are more common on the left side.   *(4:750)*

236. **(D)** Mass in the head of the pancreas.   *(10:94)*

237. **(E)** Enlarged prostate may be seen during a transabdominal pelvic examination indenting the base of the urinary bladder. An evaluation of the prostate gland is performed by transrectal sonography.   *(1:424)*

238. **(A)** Ascites is free fluid and appears anechoic on sonograms.   *(1:38, 352)*

239. **(C)** In cases of moderate to serve fatty infiltration, the echogenicity of the liver will be increased. The diaphragm and intrahepatic vessel borders may be difficult to seen because of the increase attenuation of the liver parenchyma.   *(1:134–135)*

240. (A) The testicle may have anechoic areas, and the epididymis has a complex appearance. Associated findings include an enlarged epididymis and a reactive hydrocele. Doppler and color Doppler are used to evaluate if the torsion is complete or incomplete. In cases of complete torsion, there will be no blood flow to the affected testicle.   *(5:333)*

241. (D) This is an echogenic focus within the liver most consistent with a hemangioma. Hemangiomas are the most common benign neoplasms of the liver.   *(5:103)*

242. (D) The spleen is common a site of blunt abdominal trauma. The hematoma will be contained in the spleen if there is no rupture of the splenic capsule. A decrease in hematocrit is an indication that there is blood loss from the cardiovascular system.   *(1:321)*

243. (E) A hemangioma has the same sonographic appearance as a live cell adenoma, focal nodular hyperplasia, hepatocellular carcinoma, and metastases to the liver. All of these are benign neoplasms that may appear echogenic on ultrasound. Other diagnostic tests can be used to make a definite diagnosis.   *(1:148)*

244. (D) Chronic renal disease is imaged as small echogenic kidneys. It may be unilateral or bilateral. Chronic renal disease has many causes such as parenchymal disease, hypertension, and renal artery stenosis.   *(1:289)*

245. (E) Normal testicles have a homogenous appearance. When performing color Doppler, the setting should be set as low as possible on the unaffected side and be compared with the affected side. Cryptorchidism is an undescended testicle; orchiectomy is removal of the testicle; and epididymitis is inflammation of the scrotum.   *(1:323)*

246. (B) This sonogram is diagnostic of varicocele, dilated vessels near the head of the epididymis.   *(5:329)*

247. (A) A varicocele appears as tortuous vessels near the head of the epididymis, mostly occurring on the left. The reason varicoceles occur more on the left side is that the left testicular vein courses into the left renal vein; whereas, the right testicular vein drains into the right spermatic vein.   *(5:329)*

248. (B) The pectoralis muscle lies directly posterior to the retromammary layer of breast tissue. The rectus muscle and transverse muscle are located in the ventral abdominal wall, and the levator ani muscle is located in the pelvis.   *(5:293)*

249. (C) Fibroadenomas are the most common benign breast masses in women between the ages of 15 and 40 years.   *(5:26)*

250. (B) This sonogram is a classic image of adenomyomatosis of the gallbladder. Sonographically, one should look for diffuse segmental thickening of the gallbladder wall with intramural diverticula protruding into the lumen.   *(4:224)*

251. (B) In hemolytic disease associated with abrupt breakdown of large amounts of red blood cells, the reticuloendothelial cells receive more bilirubin than they can detoxify. Therefore, one would present with an elevated indirect or unconjugated bilirubin.   *(1:122–124)*

252. (B) Bowman's capsule and glomerulus together are termed the renal corpuscle. Extending from Bowman's capsule is a renal tubule. Each tubule has three sections: a proximal tubule, a distal convoluted tubule, and a loop of Henle. Together the Bowman's capsule, glomerulus, and renal tubules constitute a nephron.   *(4:333–335)*

253. (B) The great vessel being imaged is the inferior vena cava. No vessel is imaged sonographically posterior to the aorta.   *(9:171)*

254. (D) The right renal artery is the only vessel located posterior to the inferior vena cava.   *(9:169)*

255. (A) The sonogram is consistent with a thickening of the posterior bladder wall.   *(4:433)*

256. (C) A focal thickening of the bladder wall may be due to cystitis. There are many causes of inflammation of the bladder wall including catheterization, bladder stone, bladder mass, renal disease, poor hygiene, and any disease state which causes stasis of urine in the bladder.   *(4:432)*

257. (D) The subhepatic space is located between the right lobe of the liver and the right kidney.   *(4:39)*

258. (A) The arrow is pointing to the heart.

259. (E) The liver in sonographic image is normal. The normal liver is homogeneous with midlevel echogenicity.   *(9:85)*

260. (D) Riedel's lobe is a normal variant of the right lobe of the liver. There is a tongue-like inferior projection of the right lobe. It extends below the lower pole of the right kidney during normal respiration.   *(9:86)*

261. (A) A patient with an acute appendicitis presents with right lower quadrant pain and rebound tenderness over McBurney's point, elevated white blood count, fever, nausea, and vomiting. Sonographically, the appendix wall will be thickened over 2 mm, and the outer diameter will be greater than 6 mm. The appendix will be noncompressible.   *(1:237–240)*

262. **(D)** This sonogram documents an enlarged gallbladder.   *(10:69)*

263. **(A)** Hydrops of the gallbladder may be related to obstruction at the level of the cystic or distal common bile duct.   *(10:69)*

264. **(A)** Sludge in the gallbladder does not cause hydrops of the gallbladder. Other causes of hydrops include: mucocutaneous lymph node syndrome (Kawasaki's disease), prolong biliary status, hyperalimentation, and hepatitis.   *(10:69)*

265. **(D)** Gallbladder carcinoma is rare. Patients who have had a history of gallbladder disease are at an increased risk of getting primary gallbladder carcinoma. Patients do not always have symptoms, and if they do, they are the same as other gallbladder diseases. Primary carcinoma of the gallbladder usually does not get diagnosed in the early stages; therefore, there is a high mortality rate. Gallbladder carcinomas have a number of different appearances on sonogram and are nonspecific. Gallstones with an interluminal mass is highly suggestive of gallbladder carcinoma. The sonographic appearance for adenomyosis, acute or chronic cholecystitis, blood clot, cholesterolosis, and papillary adenoma all may have the same sonographic appearance of gallbladder carcinoma.   *(10:71–72)*

266. **(C)** The adrenal glands are large and easily imaged in the neonate. The echogenic medulla surrounded by the more hypoechoic cortex is imaged as separate layers.   *(5:240)*

267. **(B)** Subcapsular collections are located inferior to the diaphragm, and they conform to the shape of the organ.   *(1:34)*

268. **(B)** Hematomas may be a complication from surgery. Most hematomas will resolve, but some will become infected and progress into an abscess. Patients may present with a decreased hematocrit and fever. One way to distinguish between a space-occupying lesion (hematoma, abscess) and ascites is to place the patient into a different position. A space-occupying lesion will not change its appearance; whereas, free fluid will shift to the most dependent portion of the body.   *(7:276)*

269. **(E)** The pancreas is echogenic with calcifications.   *(10:90)*

270. **(A)** Patients with chronic pancreatitis may present with chronic epigastric pain, or with right upper quadrant pain, which radiates to the back. The pain may be preceded by a large meal or alcohol consumption. Serum lipase, serum amylase, and bilirubin will be normal unless there is also acute inflammation of the pancreatic tissue. The sonographic appearance varies from a normal appearance to a heterogeneous echogenic pattern with areas of calcification. The main pancreatic duct may be dilated, and in some cases, there will be dilatation of the extrahepatic biliary ducts.   *(10:90–91)*

271. **(B)** Normal left adrenal gland.   *(1:337)*

272. **(C)** This sonogram demonstrates a normal left adrenal gland. The sonographic landmarks for imaging the left adrenal gland are the aorta and left kidney.   *(1:337)*

273. **(E)** All of the above are conditions may affect the adrenal gland. The primary malignancy that metastases to the adrenal gland can be from the lungs, breast, liver, bones, lymphoma, melanoma, and the gastrointestinal tract. A decrease in oxygen during delivery may cause hemorrhage to the adrenal glands during the neonatal period.   *(4:489–491)*

274. **(B)** A cystic mass appears to displace the bowel.   *(1:357)*

275. **(A)** The image is most consistent with a mesenteric cyst. The mesenteric cyst displaces the bowel and mesentery posteriorly. An ovarian cyst and free fluid do not displace bowel posteriorly.   *(1:357)*

276. **(C)** The longitudinal and transverse scan demonstrates marked thickening and lengthening of the antral muscle (pyloric canal and muscle).   *(1:462)*

277. **(B)** This is consistent with hypertrophic pyloric stenosis. The criteria for this diagnosis include wall thickness greater than 3.5 mm and pyloric length greater than 16 mm.   *(1:463)*

278. **(E)** The image is consistent with a normal pancreas. The main pancreatic duct may be visualized in a normal pancreas. The normal pancreatic duct measures less than 2 mm.   *(1:197)*

279. **(B)** The main portal vein is formed posterior to the neck of the pancreas.   *(1:201)*

280. **(D)** The most common functioning islet cell tumor is an insulinoma. Islet cell tumors can either be functional or nonfunctional, benign or malignant.   *(1:219)*

281. **(C)** This real time image of the breast demonstrates a solid mass with irregular borders.   *(1:381)*

282. **(C)** A biopsy was performed; this is a carcinoma.
(1:381)

283. **(D)** A benign breast mass is usually singular, homogeneous with moderate internal echoes, smooth walls, round or oval in shape, and with well-circumscribed walls. *(1:381)*

284. **(A)** The main lobar fissure is seen on a longitudinal scan as a linear echo coursing from the right portal vein to the neck of the gallbladder. It is also used as a landmark dividing the liver into right and left lobes. *(4:121)*

285. **(D)** In obstructive jaundice, alkaline phosphatase, and direct bilirubin will be very high with aspartate aminotransferase (AST) also being increased. Patients with hepatitis will also have an increase in alanine aminotransferase (ALT). Alpha-fetoprotein is elevated in nonpregnant adults when there is carcinoma of the liver. *(4:138)*

286. **(C)** The sonogram demonstrates dilated biliary radicles. Color Doppler may be used especially in the left lobe of the liver to distinguish the difference between dilated biliary radicles and port veins. *(4:229)*

287. **(B)** This sonogram shows dilated hepatic veins and a dilated inferior vena cava. Congestive heart failure and hypertension are two of the most common causes of general dilatation of the inferior vena cava. *(5:85)*

288. **(B)** The ligament venosum is imaged on the sonogram. The fissure for the ligament venosum also contains the hepatogastric ligament, which is used as a landmark It separates the caudate lobe from the left lobe of the liver. *(5:95)*

289. **(A)** The chest radiograph demonstrates a large amount of fluid density in the left hemidiaphragm. Pleural fluid is seen superior to the diaphragm.
(1:348)

290. **(D)** The sonogram demonstrates that the fluid density contains multiple septi causing loculations of the fluid, consistent with empyema. Empyema is a fluid collection filled with pus. *(1:348)*

291. **(D)** The clinical signs of acute cholecystitis are leukocytosis, fever, nausea, vomiting, and right upper quadrant pain that may be referred to the right shoulder if the inflammation irritates the diaphragm. Sonographically, the gallbladder is enlarged with a thickened wall greater than 5 cm, there may be pericholecystic fluid, which is secondary to the inflammation. *(4:212)*

292. **(A)** In chronic cholecystitis, the gallbladder is usually contracted with thicken walls and cholelithiasis. The WES sign, wall-echo-shadow, anterior wall of the gallbladder, echogenic foci, and shadowing caused by the stone is a consistent finding in patients with chronic cholecystitis. In cases of acute cholecystitis, the gallbladder is usually enlarged with thickened walls and cholelithiasis. *(4:217, 220)*

293. **(A)** The liver is enlarged and heterogeneous consistent with metastatic disease. Metastatic patterns within the liver have various sonographic appearances anechoic, hypoechoic, echogenic, complex or a 'bull's-eye' appearance. *(4:176)*

294. **(E)** Hemangioma is a common benign neoplasm of the liver. They are usually incidental findings on a sonogram. Sonographically, they are usually echogenic and may be either singular or multiple in the liver. Clinically, the patients do not have any symptoms unless they become very large and hemorrhage. *(4:168)*

295. **(B)** The hemangioma is located between the right and middle hepatic veins; therefore, it is in the anterior segment of the right lobe. The right hepatic vein separates the right lobe into anterior and posterior segments; the middle hepatic vein divides the liver into right and left lobes. *(4:121, 125)*

296. **(A)** A phrygian cap is a normal variant of the gallbladder. It consists of a fold in the fundal end of the gallbladder. There are no associated problems with a phrygian cap. *(5:126)*

297. **(D)** The patient is in a left lateral decubitus position (right side up) with the transducer placed along the longitudinal axis of the abdomen. The liver is used as a window to visualize the inferior vena cava anterior to the aorta. Sometimes the renal arteries may be visualized arising from the aorta. This view is used to rule out lymphadenopathy surrounding the great vessels. *(1:339)*

298. **(A)** The portal vein is the largest at the region of the porta hepatis, and the main portal vein branches into the right and left portal veins. The left portal vein follows a superior anterior course and supplies blood to the left lobe. The right portal vein is larger and follows a caudal posterior course supplying blood to the right lobe of the liver. The walls of the portal veins appear more echogenic than the walls of the hepatic veins. The hepatic veins course dorsomedial toward the inferior vena cava. The most accurate method to differentiate the portal veins from the hepatic veins is to follow the course of the vessels into the liver. *(1:117)*

299. **(B)** Lymphadenopathy. Horseshoe kidneys occur during fetal development with fusion usually of the lower poles of the kidneys. The fused poles and the isthmus drape over the spine and may be confused with lymphadenopathy. *(4:348)*

300. **(D)** Cirrhosis is a chronic progressive disease leading to liver cell failure, portal hypertension, hepatoma, and ascites. The thickened gallbladder wall is most likely related to hypoproteinemia and to the adjacent ascites that will make the gallbladder appear thickened. *(4:152)*

301. **(D)** The crura of the diaphragm are extensions (tendinous fibers) of the diaphragm that attach to the vertebral process of L3 on the right and L1 on the left. The right crus appears as a hypoechoic linear structure and can be visualized as it courses from posterior to the inferior vena cava to anterior to the aorta. *(1:331)*

302. **(A)** The left crus of the diaphragm is medial to the left adrenal gland. *(1:331)*

303. **(D)** The right crus of the diaphragm. The right crus is posteromedial to the inferior vena cava and anteromedial to the right adrenal gland. *(1:332)*

304. **(B)** The right renal artery courses posterior to the inferior cava and anterior to the right crus of the diaphragm. *(1:332)*

305. **(B)** The common duct courses anterior to the portal vein. *(4:132)*

306. **(E)** When an ultrasound beam having an oblique incidence (not on a perpendicular angle) is directed at an interface and travels between two media (liver and gallbladder) of different propagation speeds, refraction of the ultrasound beam will occur (Snell's law). There is beam refraction off the curve surface of the gallbladder wall. *(11:42)*

307. **(C)** The echogenic foci posterior to the diaphragm (arrow) is a mirror-image artifact. A mirror-image artifact is a duplication artifact secondary to the sound beam reflecting off a strong reflector in its path; i.e., the diaphragm. This strong reflector acts as a mirror, and the image will present as two reflected objects rather than one. The image further from the transducer will be the artifact. *(5:13, 49)*

308. **(B)** The sonogram demonstrates periportal lymphadenopathy, which is characterized by enlarged lymph nodes that are secondarily involved in almost all infections and neoplastic disorders. Lymph nodes consist of lymphocytes and reticulum cells, their function being filtration and production of lymphocytes. All lymph passes through these nodes that act as filters, not only for bacteria but also for cancer cells. Sonographically, we can evaluate lymph nodes in the pelvis, retroperitoneum, portal hepatis, and perirenal and prevertebral vasculature. The sonographic appearance of lymphomatous nodes varies from hypoechoic to anechoic with very good sound transmission. *(4:508)*

309. **(C)** There is no definite correlation between kidney size and echogenicity and the degree of renal function. As a general rule, if the renal parenchyma (cortex) is more echogenic than a normal liver, chronic renal insufficiency should be considered. *(4:388)*

310. **(A)** The sonogram demonstrates celiac nodes surrounding the celiac artery and its winglike configuration. Note the increase distance between the celiac artery and the aorta caused by these masses. *(4:508,512)*

311. **(A)** This sonogram depicts a fusiform aneurysm. The fusiform aneurysm typically dilates and tapers at the ends. A saccular aneurysm is a discrete round structure, and the ectatic aneurysm is a dilatation longitudinally producing lengthening of the expanded vessel in a uniform diameter. The aorta is considered aneurismal if it exceeds 3 cm. Surgery is not required until the aorta becomes greater than 6 cm because the chance of rupturing is low. *(5:80)*

312. **(D)** The left renal vein courses between the aorta and the superior mesenteric artery. *(5:77)*

313. **(C)** The caudate lobe is anterior to the inferior vena cava and posterior to the caudate lobe. *(5:95)*

314. **(A)** The celiac artery is the first branch of the abdominal aorta. It arises off the anterior aspect of the aorta at the level thoracic vertebra. *(5:72)*

315. **(B)** The superior mesenteric artery is the second branch of the abdominal aorta. *(5:74)*

316. **(A)** The splenic vein is posterior to the body of the pancreas. *(5:78)*

317. **(A)** Normal head of the pancreas, which lies anterior to the inferior vena cava. *(5:150)*

318. **(C)** Normal tail, which lies anterior to the splenic vein. *(5:151)*

319. **(B)** Common bile duct, which defines the posterolateral margin of the pancreas. *(5:150)*

320. **(E)** The gastroduodenal artery defines the anteriolateral margin of the pancreas. *(5:150)*

321. **(D)** The renal medulla pyramids are hypoechoic. They are located between the echogenic renal sinus and the less echogenic renal cortex. *(1:255)*

322. **(B)** The sonogram documents a stone obstructing the ureter causing dilation of the ureter. Any pathology that obstructs the ureterovesical junction may cause dilatation of the ureters. If the obstruction is complete there will be absence of the ureteral jet; if the obstruction is partial, the ureteral jet will be decreased flow. *(1:278, 285)*

323. **(A)** Obstruction of the ureter causes absence or decrease flow in the ureteral jet on the same side as the pathology. Color Doppler is usually used to document ureteral jets. *(1:285)*

324. **(B)** The only time that ureteral jet is not present in when there is obstructive hydronephrosis. A number of conditions can mimic dilatation of the calyces, such as an extrarenal pelvis, parapelvic cysts, transient diuresis, renal artery aneurysm, and megacalyces. Color Doppler can be used to document the presence of a renal artery aneurysm. *(1:285)*

325. **(C)** The clinical symptoms of a patient with a liver abscess include; pain, fever, right upper quadrant pain, and leukocytosis. Abscesses may appear sonographically as round, hypoechoic, with increased posterior acoustic enhancement, or they may be complex and irregular in shape. In pyogenic abscess, there may be gas present; and gas appears as hyperechoic with a dirty shadow. *(1:144–145)*

326. **(E)** Polycystic renal disease is associated in 60% of patients with polycystic liver disease. *(1:144)*

327. **(D)** The blood flow in the superior mesenteric artery in a fasting patient has a high-resistive index. Postprandially the blood flow changes to a low resistive index with an increase in the diastolic flow. *(1:100)*

328. **(B)** The perinephric space is surrounded by Gerota's fascia. *(1:329)*

329. **(E)** The arrow is pointing to a normal ureteral jet. One reason for not documenting ureteral jets is obstructive hydronephrosis. *(1:285)*

330. **(B)** The head of the pancreas lies anterior to the inferior vena cava. *(5:150)*

331. **(A)** Chronic pancreatitis is associated with a normal or small pancreas, irregular borders, and increased echogenicity caused by fibrotic changes, and calcification. There may be ductal dilatation with or without a stone in the duct. The laboratory values for chronic pancreatitis are usually normal. *(1:215)*

332. **(C)** A pancreatic pseudocyst is a fluid collection that arises as a complication of acute pancreatitis. The obstructed pancreatic duct increases in size until it ruptures, which causes the pancreatic enzymes to escape outside of the pancreas. The fluid localizes and becomes walled-off forming a pseudocyst. The most common location is in the lesser sac, but a pseudocyst may also be found in the pararenal space or extending into the pelvis or superiorly into the mediastinum. *(1:216)*

333. **(E)** The most common complication of a pancreatic pseudocyst is spontaneous rupture, which occurs in 5% of the patients. The fluid will drain half of the time into the peritoneal cavity and half of the time into the gastrointestinal tract. The former has a 50% mortality rate. *(1:216)*

334. **(D)** 5 MHz linear transducer. The rectus abdominis muscle courses from the anterior aspect of the symphysis pubis and pubis crest to the 5th, 6th and 7th costal cartilages and xiphoid process. It protects and covers the anterior abdominal wall, therefore, a high-frequency linear transducer is the best option because one does not need to penetrate deep to image the rectus abdominis muscle, and the linear array has a wide field of view. *(1:31, 5:15)*

335. **(B)** Morison's pouch is located anterior to the right kidney and posterior to the inferior right lobe of the liver. The lesser sac is anterior to the pancreas and posterior to the stomach. The pouch of Douglas is posterior to the uterus and anterior to the rectum. The greater sac extends from the diaphragm to the pelvis and contains most of the abdominal organs. *(1:36, 51)*

336. **(C)** Pyelocaliectasis is dilatation of the collecting system. The collecting system may be dilated because of overhydration, and it is a common finding in postrenal transplant patients. *(1:301, 4:405)*

337. **(C)** The perirenal fluid collection may be associated with lymphocele, a collection of lymph fluid caused by injury to the lymphatic channels during transplantation; hematoma, a collection of blood; and abscess, which are all associated with renal transplantation. It is difficult to differentiate one from the other. Urinoma is a collection of urine because of a urinary leak of an ureteropelvic or ureteroureter anastomosis. Abscess is a collection of pus caused by an inflammatory response. Ascites is not associated with a renal transplant. *(4:403–404)*

338. **(A)** Perinephric fluid collections are common in postoperative renal transplant patients. Fever, flank pain, and leukocytosis best correlates with an abscess. Because many fluid collections have the same sonographic appearance, the patient's clinical symptoms will help differentiate between them. Abscesses and hematomas tend to be more complex in appearance than urinomas and lymphoceles. Hematomas, abscesses, and urinoma usually develop earlier than lymphoceles. Lymphoceles typically do not develop until 4 to 8 weeks post op. A renal cyst is not associated with a renal transplant. *(4:403–404)*

339. **(B)** There are several sonographic criteria used to describe biliary dilatation. In this sonogram, we can recognize (1) tubular lucencies within the liver demonstrating posterior acoustic enhancement—bile opposed to blood increases transmission; (2) the tubules are irregular with jagged walls as opposed to veins and arteries that are straight—normal ducts are not visualized within the liver. *(4:229)*

340. **(C)** The arrow is point to an example of chronic pancreatitis. With chronic pancreatitis, the pancreas generally is diffusely smaller and more fibrotic than usual with areas of calcification and ductal dilatation. In acute pancreatitis, the pancreas is generally diffusely larger and less echogenic than normal. In adenocarcinoma and islet cell tumors, the pancreas is generally focally enlarged in the pancreatic head with the former and the tail in the latter. *(1:211)*

341. **(C)** There is irregular diffuse thickening of the bladder wall of unknown origin. The prostate is not enlarged, and there is no evidence of a bladder outlet obstruction that most commonly is secondary to benign prostatic hypertrophy or carcinoma. Enlarged endometrial tissue may be found penetrating the bladder wall and extending in the lumen in severe cases of endometriosis in premenopausal women. *(1:303)*

342. **(E)** Both kidneys in patients with chronic renal failure appear small and echogenic. It is a nonspecific finding and may result from hypertension, chronic inflammation, or chronic ischemia. *(1:289)*

343. **(D)** Serum creatinine and BUN (blood urea nitrogen) are elevated in kidney disease. *(1:250)*

344. **(D)** Attenuation is the decrease in amplitude and intensity as a wave travels through a medium. One of the criteria for a cyst is the posterior acoustic enhancement. A characteristic of fluid is that it does not absorb (attenuate) soundwaves. *(11:288)*

345. **(D)** Adult polycystic kidney disease is cystic dilatation of the proximal convoluted tubules, Bowman's capsule, and the collecting tubules. As the cysts grow in size, they compress the nephrons causing renal insufficiency, which usually manifests in the fourth decade of life. Cysts may also occur in the liver, spleen, pancreas, lungs, ovaries, or testes. Infantile polycystic disease in its most severe form is not compatible

with life. In less severe forms, the kidney will appear enlarged and echogenic because of the small cystic interfaces that occur in the kidney. Parapelvic cysts are cysts found around the renal pelvis region, they usually do not interfere with the renal function. Ureteropelvic junction (UPJ) is one of the most common congenital causes of hydronephrosis. Sonographically, it is seen as a dilatation of the collecting system and proximal portion of the ureter. *(1:270)*

346. **(A)** Multicystic displastic kidney disease is the most common cause of an abdominal mass in the newborn. It is usually unilateral, occurring more often in the left kidney. The contralateral kidney is at an increased risk for such abnormalities as ureteropelvic junction obstruction (UPJ). Sonographically, the cysts appear in varying sizes, with the largest cysts in the periphery, absence of the connections between the cysts, absence of an identifiable renal sinus, and absence of renal parenchyma surrounding the cysts. *(1:270)*

347. **(A)** This sonogram of the kidney is not normal. There is dilatation of the renal calyces. There are numerous causes for hydronephrosis; any pathology in the lower urinary system may cause bilateral hydronephrosis, while upper urinary pathology may cause unilateral hydronephrosis. Some of the causes of hydronephrosis include: congenital anomalies, as in posterior urethral valves (UPV), bladder neck obstruction; acquired causes, such as calculi, prostate enlargement, inflammation, bladder tumor; intrinsic causes, such as calculi, pyelonephritis, stricture, inflammation; and extrinsic causes, such as neoplasm and retroperitoneal adenopathy. *(1:279)*

348. **(E)** An extratesticular cyst is documented on the sonogram. This is consistent with a spermatocele, which is a cyst in the epididymis containing spermatozoa. An epididymis cyst would have the same sonographic appearance. A varicocele (enlargement of the veins of the spermatic cord) is also extratesticular but it is located on the posterior surface, more common of the left; and sonographically, it has a tubular shape. Seminoma is a malignant germ cell tumor within the testicle. *(5:331)*

349. **(B)** Normal head of the epididymis. *(1:410)*

350. **(B)** The arrow is pointing to the seminal vesicle, which is posterior to the bladder and superior to the prostate. *(1:424)*

351. **(D)** Varicocele is an enlargement of the veins of the pampiniform plexus, which course along the posterior aspect of the testicle and is more prominent on the left testicle. Venous dilatation occurs with an increase of pressure by either having the patient perform a Valsalva maneuver or by having the patient

stand. Spermatocele and epididymal cyst are found in the epididymis. Cryptorchism is another name for undescended testes. Mediastinum testis is found within the testis and connects the rete testis with the epididymis.   *(1:415)*

352. **(B)** Acute tuberous necrosis is the most common medical cause for renal failure. It is a reversible renal disease. Sonographically, the kidneys will appear enlarged with echogenic renal pyramids. Tuberous sclerosis involves numerous body systems. Sonographically, multiple cysts or angiomyolipomas are seen.   *(1:289)*

353. **(C)** The celiac axis is the first major branch of the aorta. It arises off the anterior aspect of the aorta before it trifurcates into the hepatic proper artery, splenic artery, and left gastric artery.   *(5:72)*

354. **(A)** The sonogram demonstrates a normal right adrenal gland. In utero and in the neonate, the adrenal glands are prominent, being one-third the size of the kidney.   *(4:622)*

355. **(B)** This decubitus coronal sonogram documents a severe dilatation of the renal collecting system extending into the renal pelvis, with marked thinning of the renal parenchyma. The low-level internal echoes are caused by artifact. Pyonephrosis is a collection of pus within the dilated collecting system. The pus is caused by long-standing stasis of urine. Sonographically, the dilated calyces will have internal echoes without increased posterior acoustic enhancement.   *(1:284, 289)*

356. **(B)** The arcuate arteries, which are arc-shaped vessels that separate the cortex from the medulla. They are imaged sonographically as small echogenic line above the renal pyramids.   *(1:247)*

357. **(C)** The open arrowhead is pointing to the renal medullary pyramids.   *(1:254)*

358. **(A)** Renal column of Bertin is composed of cortical tissue that extends into the medullary area between the pyramids.   *(1:257)*

359. **(E)** The sonogram documents dilated biliary radicles that are caused by obstructed biliary radicles. Dilation of biliary radicals may be secondary to a stone, mass lesions in the area of the head of the pancreas, a neoplasm, or metastatic lesions within the liver. Cirrhosis is related to "medical" jaundice, and there will be no evidence of biliary dilation.   *(1:189)*

360. **(E)** A neuroblastoma is an adrenal mass found in children. It will not cause splenomegaly.   *(1:476)*

361. **(C)** The patient was asymptomatic, it is most likely a simple benign hepatic cyst. Symptoms usually do not develop unless the cyst is large. Patients who have lymphoma, metastases, hydatid cysts, or polycystic liver disease will present with symptoms and elevated laboratory results.   *(1:142)*

362. **(E)** Adenocarcinoma is found most often in males, especially in black males. There is an increased incidence of adenocarcinoma in patients with a history of smoking, a high-fat diet, chronic pancreatitis, diabetes, or cirrhosis. Adenocarcinoma usually presents as a hypoechoic mass in the head of the pancreas (Fig. 5–139A). Associated findings include dilatation of the pancreatic duct, biliary dilatation (Fig. 5–139B), and an enlarged gallbladder (Courvoisier's gallbladder) (Fig. 5–139C).   *(4:255)*

363. **(D)** The sonogram documents a small echogenic kidney with a loss of distinction between cortex, medulla, and renal sinus. Chronic glomerulonephritis is the most common cause of chronic renal failure.   *(1:289)*

364. **(A)** Prostatic-specific antigen (PSA) is elevated in prostatic cancer, prostatitis, acute urinary retention, surgical manipulation, and benign prostatic hyperplasia (BPH). Creatinine is elevated in cases of renal insufficiency, amylase with pancreatitis, and white blood cell count with infections.   *(5:349)*

365. **(B)** There are different types of thyroiditis, and chronic thyroiditis is Hashimoto's disease. It is the most common cause of hypothyroidism. It usually occurs in young females. Sonographically, the thyroid is enlarged with either a heterogeneous or hypoechoic echo pattern.   *(5:279)*

366. **(D)** The two lobes of the thyroid are connected by isthmus, which is anterior to the trachea. The common carotid is located lateral to the thyroid and the sternothyroid muscle is anteriolateral to the thyroid.   *(5:272)*

367. **(E)** Neuroblastoma is a rare malignant mass found in children usually less than 8 years old. Adenoma, cyst, myelolipoma, and pheochromocytoma are benign adrenal masses. Infrequently, pheochromocytoma's may be malignant.   *(5:246)*

368. **(A)** The right adrenal gland is located posterior to the inferior vena cava. When the right adrenal gland enlarges, it may displace the inferior vena cava anteriorly.   *(5:240)*

369. **(C)** A simple renal cyst is common in people over the age of 30. They are found most frequently in the lower pole but can also be found on the upper pole.

The characteristics of a cyst are anechoic, thin walls, and increased through transmission.   *(5:177)*

370. **(E)** A simple renal cyst is usually an incidental findings and do not interfere with the function of the kidney, therefore the laboratory values are normal.   *(5:177)*

371. **(C)** Small renal calculi may be seen in the kidney without obstructing the collecting system.   *(4:375)*

372. **(D)** A linear transducer has a rectangular format, which allows a larger field of view. The large footprint of a linear transducer makes it difficult to scan intercostally because of the rib artifacts and does not increase resolution. The instrument settings of an ultrasound machine to produce the highest resolution are necessary to document posterior shadowing of small calculi. Factors that the sonographer can control to increase resolution include: use of a high-frequency transducer, decreasing gain (decreases scattering), place the focal zone at the area of interest, and the use of tissue harmonics.   *(5:15, 185)*

373. **(B)** A stone is obstructing the ureter causing a dilatation of the ureter, hydroureter.   *(1:278)*

374. **(B)** This sonogram demonstrates a marked increased echogenicity of the liver as compared with the kidney. The echogenicity of the liver should be compared with the kidney.   *(1:253)*

375. **(C)** In the adult, glycogen storage disease, fatty metamorphosis, chronic hepatitis, cirrhosis, hemochromatosis all present with an echogenic liver and decrease through penetration. In a child, this is frequently a complication of glycogen storage disease.   *(1:137)*

376. **(E)** The sonographer has no control over the speed of sound. To optimize a sonographic image, the sonographer is able to adjust and choose the overall gain, time gain compensation, transducer type and frequency, and the depth and focus control.   *(1:126)*

377. **(A)** A resistive index (RI) of less than 0.70 is considered normal.   *(1:284)*

378. **(C)** Splenomegaly is diagnosed when the spleen measures greater than 13 cm in the long axis. Sonographically, the left kidney will be compressed and displaced posteriorly.   *(1:314)*

379. **(A)** This image is of a gallbladder filled with stones.   *(1:180)*

380. **(D)** This sonogram demonstrates calculus cholecystitis. When the gallbladder is filled with calculi all that may be imaged on sonogram is the wall echo shadowing (WES) sign.   *(1:180)*

381. **(E)** The laboratory findings in patients with cholelithiasis are consistent with an increase in alkaline phosphatase. Other liver function tests may be abnormal (AST, ALT). Serum amylase may be elevated in patients with pancreatitis; increased creatinine is consistent with renal insufficiency; serum indirect bilirubin is elevated in patients with hepatocellular disease.   *(1:176)*

382. **(B)** A parathyroid mass. The parathyroid glands are located on the posterior medial surface of the thyroid glands. The sonogram documents a large mass adjacent to the thyroid and common carotid artery.   *(1:404)*

383. **(A)** The sonogram is an image of a parathyroid adenoma or carcinoma. Parathyroid adenomas are the most common cause of hyperparathyroidism. Sonographically, they are hypoechoic and usually round in shape.   *(1:405)*

384. **(A)** A patient with a parathyroid adenoma may present with hypercalcemia and low serum levels of phosphate.   *(1:405)*

385. **(D)** The valves of Heister are tiny valves located in the proximal portion of the cystic duct. They prevent the duct from kinking.   *(1:165, 166)*

386. **(E)** Patients with a history of cirrhosis have an increase incidence of developing hepatomas in the liver.   *(1:139)*

387. **(C)** A choledochal cyst is usually diagnosed in childhood and is more common in Asians. The most common sonographic appearance of a choledochal cyst is a cyst communicating with the common bile. If choledochal cysts are not diagnosed and treated early, the patient is at an increased risk of developing gallbladder carcinoma and cholangiocarcinoma.   *(5:137)*

388. **(D)** Primary gallbladder carcinoma is more commonly found in women and there is an increase incidence in people working in the textile, rubber, and automotive industries. Gallstones are present in the majority of cases, and a percentage of cases will present with a porcelain gallbladder. Sonographically, the gallbladder may also have a thickened wall, and a mass may be seen within the gallbladder lumen.   *(5:222)*

389. **(E)** A Baker cyst is located in the bursa posterior to the distal femur.   *(4:777)*

390. **(B)** Posterior urethra values is the most common cause of urethra obstruction in boys. The values located in the posterior urethra obstruct the urethra. Dilatation of the urethra, hydroureter, and hydronephrosis may occur secondary to the obstruction.   *(4:606)*

391. **(C)** A Reidel's lobe is an anatomic variation of the liver, where the right lobe of the liver has a tongue-like extension. It is more common in women, and on physical examination, the liver will give the impression of hepatomegaly.   *(4:126)*

REFERENCES

1. Hagen-Ansert SL. *Textbook of Diagnostic Ultrasonography.* 5th ed. St. Louis: CV Mosby; 2001.
2. *Stedman's Concise Medical Dictionary.* 3rd ed. Baltimore: Lippincott Williams & Wilkins; 1997.
3. *SDMS National Certification Review.* Dallas: Society of Diagnostic Medical Sonography; 2001.
4. Kawamura D. *Diagnostic Medical Sonography: A Guide to Clinical Practice: Abdomen and Superficial Structures.* 2nd ed. Philadelphia: Lippincott; 1992.
5. Gill K. *Abdominal Ultrasound A Practitioner's Guide.* Philadelphia: WB Saunders; 2001.
6. McGahan JP, Goldberg BB. *Diagnostic Ultrasound A Logical Approach.* Philadelphia: Lippincott; 1997.
7. Saunders RC, et al. *Clinical Sonography: A Practical Guide.* 3rd ed. Boston: Little Brown; 1998.
8. Fleischer AC, James AE. *Diagnostic Sonography Principles and Clinical Applications.* Philadelphia: WB Saunders; 1989.
9. Curry RA, Tempkin BB. *Ultrasonography: An Introduction to Normal Structure and Functional Anatomy.* Philadelphia: WB Saunders; 1995.
10. Krebs CA, Giyanani VL, Eisenberg RL. *Ultrasound Atlas of Disease Processes.* Norwalk, CT: Appleton & Lange; 1993.
11. Kremkau, F. *Diagnostic Ultrasound Principles and Instrumentation.* 6th ed. Philadelphia: WB Saunders; 2002.

CHAPTER 6

ABDOMINAL VASCULAR SONOGRAPHY

*Carol A. Krebs, Sandra L. Hughes, Karen K. Rawls,
and Thomas G. Hoffman*

Study Guide

INTRODUCTION

Abdominal ultrasound is a major part of most large ultrasound departments. The development of phased array and broad band width linear array transducer has made the real-time 2-D images exceptional in quality and contributes to the increasing demand for this noninvasive technology. With the addition of Doppler, duplex, and color flow Doppler, we are able to evaluate vascular physiology and pathophysiology as well. Color flow Doppler made a major impact in the evaluation of transplant patients in the 1980s that extended into the 1990s and the new millennium. This has led to the addition of many other abdominal vascular examinations. Suffice it to say, there were many obstacles in early abdominal vascular applications, including abdominal gas and inherent motion artifacts. Many of these problems have been overcome somewhat with motion suppressors and gas-inhibiting techniques, thus improving the quality and diagnostic value of the vascular examination.

To provide a comprehensive study of the abdominal vessels and the respective disease processes, we have categorized the study guide into sections: beginning with the vascular anatomy in normal text; followed by the sonographic and Doppler characteristics in boldface; and concluding with the various diseases for each entity. We hope this will provide an easy reference and study guide for the student sonographer.

Aorta, Celiac Axis (Hepatic Artery, Splenic Artery and Gastric Artery), Superior Mesenteric Artery, Inferior Mesenteric Artery, Common Iliac Arteries

The abdominal aorta is the continuation of the thoracic aorta beginning at the aortic hiatus of the diaphragm (Fig. 6–1). It runs parallel to the inferior vena cava slightly to the left of the midline and extends to the fourth lumbar, where it bifurcates into the right and left common iliacs.[1] The normal diameter of the aorta averages 2 cm in adults and varies with age, gender, race, and body size. The maximum diameter of the common iliac arteries is usually approximately, 1 cm, and the external iliac artery is slightly smaller.[2]

The abdominal aorta is best seen sonographically in the longitudinal image. The transverse image depicts the cross section of the aorta and provides the anterior–posterior (AP) diameter measurement. The aorta can be seen in the longitudinal plane from the superior portion just inferior to the diaphragm to the distal segment bifurcating into the common iliacs. Real-time imaging shows a tubular structure with smooth marinated echogenic walls. Color flow Doppler will demonstrate the lumen filled with color and some color changes caused by the high resistance. The spectral waveform shows a triphasic high-resistant waveform similar to the peripheral arteries. It has a rapid rise and sharp systolic peak followed by a rapid decline to the baseline during diastole (Fig. 6–2). It has a clear spectral window, and there may be absence of flow during diastole in the distal aorta because of increased peripheral resistance.[3]

The abdominal aorta has several branches that include; celiac axis (hepatic, gastric, splenic arteries), superior mesenteric artery, renal arteries and inferior mesenteric artery (Fig. 6–1). The celiac axis arises from the anterior surface of the abdominal aorta and is the first major branch. Approximately 1–2 cm from the origin, the celiac divides into the left gastric artery, common hepatic artery, and the splenic artery.

The celiac axis is best viewed in the transverse image. Real-time images demonstrate the classical "t"-shaped bifurcation, also termed the seagull appearance as the celiac artery branches into the hepatic artery and splenic artery.[2] The gastric artery is usually not seen on the ultrasound examination because of its location. It is the smallest of the

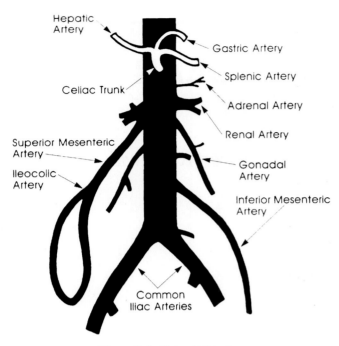

Figure 6–1. Abdominal aorta.

celiac branches and ascends to the left posterior to the omental bursa and the cardiac end of the stomach. The Doppler waveform of the celiac artery varies. It ranges from a relatively high-resistance pattern near the origin to a low-resistance pattern in the distal portion.[4] Continuous forward flow is present throughout diastole in the distal celiac artery because of the low resistance in the vascular beds of the liver and spleen. In the normal adult, it has a mean peak systolic frequency of 3.2 kHZ or 104 ± 18 cm/s.

The splenic artery is a terminal branch of the celiac artery and follows a tortuous course along the postero-superior margin of the pancreatic body and tail. The splenic

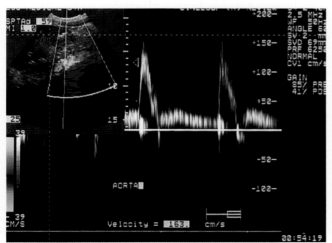

Figure 6–2. Spectral waveform of the aorta.

artery terminates by branching in the splenic hilum (Fig. 6–3).

Sonographically, the splenic artery can be seen in a transverse image underlying the body and tail of the pancreas. However, to visualize the splenic artery as it enters the splenic hilum, a left lateral position is necessary.[2] It has a low-resistance flow pattern with continuous forward flow throughout diastole. Because of the tortuous course of the splenic artery, the flow is turbulent with multiple color changes.[2]

The common hepatic artery arises as a terminal branch of the celiac trunk and runs a short distance to the right along the superior border of the pancreatic head before giving rise to the gastroduodenal artery. The gastroduodenal artery lies between the first portion of the duodenum and the anterior surface of the pancreatic head. After giving rise to the gastroduodenal artery, the common hepatic artery turns superior toward the porta hepatis and gives off the right gastric artery. At this point, the common hepatic artery becomes the proper hepatic artery, which terminates at the porta hepatis into the left and right hepatic arteries. The left and right branches subsequently divide within the liver into the segmental and subsegmental branches that parallel the bile ducts and the portal vein[4] (Fig. 6–4).

The hepatic artery can be traced with color flow imaging from its origin of the celiac axis to the right and left branches within the liver. A transverse image is used primarily with oblique views for the right and left branches. The spectral analysis shows a low-resistance flow characteristic with continuous forward flow throughout diastole.

The superior mesenteric artery (SMA) arises from the anterior surface of the aorta just below the celiac axis and runs parallel to the abdominal aorta just to the left of the midline. The SMA is comprised of a short anterior directed segment and a much longer inferior directed segment that ends in the vicinity of the ileocecal valve. The SMA lies posterior to the pancreas and anterior to the duodenum and left renal vein. The multiple branches of the SMA provide blood supply to the most of the duodenum, jejunum, ileum, cecum, ascending colon, and the transverse colon and may be referred to as the splanchnic arteries along with the celiac and the inferior mesenteric artery. Splanchnic means reference to the viscera.

The SMA is best seen in the longitudinal view. It appears on real-time imaging as an anechoic tubular structure sharply arising from the anterior abdominal aorta just below the celiac axis, left of the superior mesenteric vein, and posterior to the pancreas and splenic vein.[2] It descends parallel to the abdominal aorta in the sagittal plane. The Doppler waveform shows a high impedance flow pattern during fasting with turbulence at the origin. The diastolic waveform may be absent, and there may be turbulence at the origin, but it becomes more uniform distally. The blood flow will significantly increase following a meal, and the velocity may double. In the fasting state, there is an early diastolic flow reversal and the waveforms seem similar to the external carotid artery. The postprandial mean flow velocity is increased 1.8 times in 15 minutes, and 2.5 times at 45 minutes, depending upon the type of meal ingested.

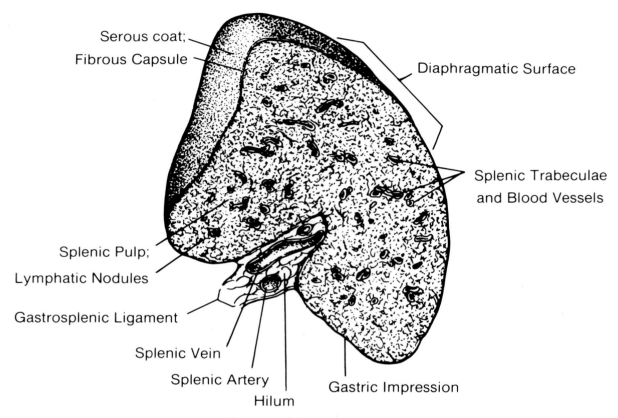

Serous coat;
Fibrous Capsule

Diaphragmatic Surface

Splenic Trabeculae
and Blood Vessels

Splenic Pulp;
Lymphatic Nodules

Gastrosplenic Ligament

Splenic Vein

Splenic Artery

Hilum

Gastric Impression

Figure 6–3. Splenic artery and vein.

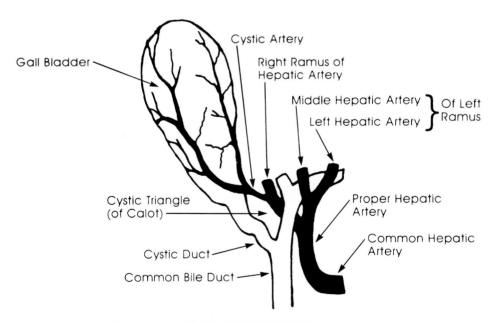

Gall Bladder

Cystic Artery

Right Ramus of
Hepatic Artery

Middle Hepatic Artery ⎫ Of Left
Left Hepatic Artery ⎭ Ramus

Cystic Triangle
(of Calot)

Proper Hepatic
Artery

Common Hepatic
Artery

Cystic Duct

Common Bile Duct

Figure 6–4. Hepatic artery.

Increases occur in peak systole, early and end diastole, and mean velocity. The postprandial blood flow pattern is increased with its maximal velocity occurring at 20 minutes postingestion of carbohydrates and at 45 minutes with fatty and mixed meals. The SMA flow increase is slightly lower-peaking at 90 min with a meal of protein only. A mean peak systolic frequency of 2.6 kHz or 140 ± 43 cm/s has been reported in the normal adult.

The inferior mesenteric artery is smaller than the superior mesenteric and supplies the left third of the transverse colon, the descending colon, sigmoid colon, and most of the rectum.[1] It is most often obscured by intestinal gas and not seen on the ultrasound examination.

DISEASE AND PATHOLOGY

Aneurysm

Aneurysm is defined as an abnormal dilatation of the vessel, usually focal in nature. A true aneurysm has the composite layers of the vessel wall intact, but stretched. A false aneurysm is described as having a hole in the arterial wall that permits escape of blood under pressure that generates a false aneurysm (pseudoaneurysm). The extravasated blood forms a hematoma. Atherosclerosis, trauma, or infection can cause[4] aneurysms. Males are affected more often, and symptoms may include: pulsatile mass, abdominal pain, backache, leg pain, or they may be asymptomatic.

There are several types of aneurysms based on their anatomical configuration which include:

- Saccular: a sac like or focal dilatation
- Fusiform: a spindle shaped lesion contiguous with the arterial lumen

There are also several physiological types of aneurysms, which include:

- False or pseudoaneurysm, which usually occurs secondary to vessel trauma. It is a sac-like structure communicating with the true arterial lumen; however, there is absence of all three layers of the arterial wall.
- Mycotic, which results from infectious process and involves the arterial wall
- Dissecting, which results from the separation of the vessel wall creating a true and false lumen

Ultrasound and color flow Doppler can identify aneurysms that may not be clinically apparent and provide a method of monitoring enlargement of the aneurysm. Measurements can be obtained of the internal and external lumen as well as any thrombus formation. An aortic aneurysm is considered when the distal aorta exceeds 3 cm in diameter or when the dilated segment is 1.5 times greater in diameter than the adjacent normal segment.[2] The aorta can be evaluated with real-time imaging, however, color flow Doppler better defines the complex aneurysm. The aneurysm will demonstrate turbulent blood flow with spectral broadening. The spectral analysis shows a damped bidirectional flow caused by the swirling blood within the aneurysm. Color flow Doppler shows a mixture of red and blue because of the bidirectional movement of blood with absence of flow in areas of thrombus. The SMA, renal arteries, and iliac arteries should also be evaluated in the presence of an aneurysm to determine if they are involved. This, in turn, determines the type of surgical reconstruction.[4]

A plain film of the abdomen may incidentally detect an aneurysm because of the calcified walls or displacement of surrounding structures. Computerized axial tomography (CT) and magnetic resonance imaging (MRI) are considered superior in demonstrating leakage or rupture of an aneurysm.[3]

Dissection

Dissection refers to the separation of the vessel wall. This creates a true and false lumen where blood can pass from the true lumen into the false. It is considered a disease of the media and usually occurs secondary to a tear in the intimal layer.[5] Risk factors include hypertension, cystic medial necrosis, Marfan syndrome, bicuspid aortic valve, coarctation of the aorta, giant cell arteritis, pregnancy, and some skeletal anomalies. It can also be secondary to trauma, aortic catheterization, and aortoiliac endarterectomy. An abrupt onset of pain reaching its peak immediately is very characteristic of an aortic dissection. Pain may vary according to the classification of the dissection. There are three classifications of aorta dissection according to DeBakey[3] (Fig. 6–5).

- Type 1. Dissection affects the ascending aorta, arch, and descending aorta.
- Type 11. Dissection only affects the ascending aorta.
- Type 111. Dissection involves the descending thoracic aorta and may extend into the abdominal aorta.

Real-time scanning shows two lumens separated by an echogenic intimal flap within the lumen of the abdominal aorta. The flap usually pulsates toward the true lumen. Doppler spectral analysis shows the rapid flow in the true lumen with turbulence and spectral broadening. There will be slow or absent flow in the false lumen. Color flow Doppler shows reversal of flow in the false lumen as a change in color. In some instances, the false lumen may be filled with echoes if thrombus is present, and there will be an absence of color flow.

Aortography is the most definitive diagnostic procedure that demonstrates the double lumen created by the dissection. CT with dynamic contrast technique or helical CT can demonstrate the filling of the true and false lumen.[3]

Stenosis and Occlusion of the Splanchnic (Visceral) Vessels

There are three main gastrointestinal arteries that arise from the aorta (celiac axis, superior mesenteric artery (SMA) and inferior mesenteric artery). As these major splanchnic arteries become critically narrowed, the other vessels dilate to carry more blood. There is a great propensity for collateralization with these vessels and, therefore, may delay the presence of symptoms. Normally, the splanchnic vascular bed receives 25–30% of the cardiac output and contains one-

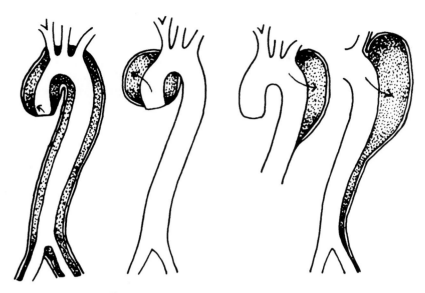

Figure 6–5. Classification of aortic dissection.

third of the total blood volume.[5] Stenosis of the splanchnic vessels is more often seen in older patients, especially those with atherosclerotic disease and primarily located at the origin of the vessels. However, it has been noted that functional stenosis of the celiac can be a result of compression by the diaphragm ligaments. Stenosis by compression can also be seen in the SMA because of the acute angle as the SMA arises from the aorta. Compression of the duodenum can occur as it lies between the aorta and the SMA, which causes partial intestinal obstruction, a condition referred to as "superior mesenteric artery compression syndrome." Patients' symptoms may include colicky abdominal pain, postprandial pain, weight loss, malabsorption, or epigastric bruit. Often these patients develop abdominal angina (food fear or delayed abdominal pain after eating and significant weight loss) in a slow insidious process that can lead to bowel infarction and serious sequelae. If the celiac artery is occluded, collateralization occurs through the pancreatico-duodenal arterial arcade, which is a network of small vessels surrounding the pancreas and duodenum. Sudden occlusion of the SMA is usually caused by embolus and usually has symptoms of extreme abdominal pain with vomiting, diarrhea, and then constipation; whereas, thrombus usually occurs with slow developing or chronic occlusion. Collateral blood supply to the SMA may delay symptoms and prevent bowel ischemia. The three principal collateral pathways are: the pancreaticoduodenal arcade, arch of Riolan, and the marginal artery of Drummond.[2]

Real-time imaging can demonstrate narrowing of the vessel and any calcified plaque secondary to atherosclerotic disease. The origin of the splanchnic arteries should always be depicted on the vascular abdominal examination. Color flow Doppler enhances the examination by making localization easier and clearly demonstrating any stenotic areas. Color flow Doppler usually shows turbulence and mixed colors at the origin; however, a significant stenosis will demonstrate an extreme mosaic pattern with narrowing of the vessel. Peak frequency of more than 3.5 times the peak aortic frequency suggests a stenosis. In cases of occlusion, there will be absence of flow in the arterial lumen.[3]

If there is a suspicion of mesenteric arterial disease, mesenteric angiograms with selective visceral lateral views are usually obtained. It is an excellent method of demonstrating any stenosis or occlusion of the splanchnic arteries and to determine the adequacy of the splanchnic circulation.[5]

Splenic Artery Aneurysms

Many times this is an incidental finding on the abdominal x-ray. There may be a bruit present in the left upper quadrant. The splenic artery aneurysm is one of the most common sites of intraabdominal aneurysm second to aortic aneurysm. It is more frequent in females and more commonly seen in patients with atherosclerosis (see characteristics under aneurysm).

Inferior Vena Cava (IVC)

The right and left common iliac veins join to form the IVC at the level of the fourth or fifth lumbar vertebra. It ascends superiorly toward the diaphragm along the right side of the spine, parallel to the abdominal aorta before draining into the right atrium. During its course, it receives venous blood from the vein and hepatic veins, renal veins right gonadal vein, right suprarenal vein, inferior phrenic lumbar veins (Fig. 6–6). Uncommon anomalies include duplication of the vena cava, absence of the vena cava, and a left-sided vena cava. Most anomalies of the IVC occur at and below the level of the renal veins. The most common anomaly is duplication (0.2–3.0%) or transposition (0.2–0.5%).[3]

On real-time images, the IVC is an anechoic tubular structure running parallel and to the right of the abdominal aorta. In patients with slow blood flow, representative intraluminal echoes may be seen. The IVC diameter rarely

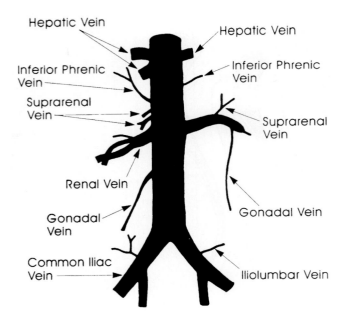

Figure 6–6. Inferior vena cava.

exceeds 2.5 cm, but the diameter is dependent on the patient size, stages of respiration, and right atrial pressure.[4] Dilatation of the IVC can occur with congestive heart failure, tricuspid regurgitation, or any condition associated with increased right atrial pressure. Deep inspiration limits venous return and markedly dilates the IVC. Doppler show a proximal pulsatile waveform with a wide spectrum of low frequencies. Color flow shows filling of the vessel lumen with color changes caused by pressure and respiratory motion. The spectral analysis is pulsatile near the heart, because of the reflected right atrial pulsations. Farther distally the flow pattern is phasic and similar to the pattern seen in extremity veins.[4]

Disease and Pathology

Thrombosis. This is the most common disorder of the vena cava usually caused by superior migration of thrombus from the lower extremity or pelvic thrombophlebitis. It can also be caused by dehydration, shock, hypercoagulable states, congestive heart failure, generalized sepsis, retroperitoneal infection, pelvic inflammatory disease, direct caval manipulation (filters and catheters), and iatrogenic (secondary to a surgical procedure in the lower extremity). Some malignant neoplasms may invade the inferior vena cava, such as renal carcinoma, adrenal carcinoma, pancreatic carcinoma, pheochromocytoma, hepatic carcinoma, Wilm's tumor, and lymphatic metastases from prostate and female gynecological malignancy. Symptoms may include swelling of the legs or signs and symptoms of an underlying primary neoplasm or asymptomatic.

On real-time imaging the inferior vena cava may be dilated, especially at the site of the thrombus. Acute thrombus tends to be more anechoic, and as it ages, it becomes more echogenic. It can be a partial or total occlusion of the lumen. The Doppler signal will be absent if the vessel is totally occluded. In partial occlusion, there will be a damped continuous waveform. Color flow Doppler is especially beneficial in identifying the anechoic thrombus and demonstrating the partial occlusion, with flow circumventing around the thrombus.

Radiographic procedures for evaluating the inferior vena cava include CT, MRI, and venocavography.

LIVER

Vascular Anatomy

Hepatic Artery. The hepatic artery, a branch of the celiac axis, is anatomically described above. It is the blood supply to the liver along with the portal vein with approximately 25% of blood coming from the hepatic artery and approximately 75% from the portal vein[5] (Fig. 6–7). This artery becomes of prime interest in liver transplant patients as well as portal hypertensive patients with either surgical or interventional stenting.

The hepatic artery is visualized normally on transverse scans at the level of the hepatoduodenal ligament (just cephalad to the head of the pancreas and adjacent to the porta hepatis). Both the common bile duct and the hepatic artery lie anterior to the portal vein at this level. The common bile duct lies lateral to the hepatic artery. The right and left branches can be seen using a transverse oblique plane. Color flow Doppler is preferred for ease of location to determine patency, especially in surgical patients where the vessel may deviate from its natural course. Color flow can also demonstrate any area of narrowing, kinking, or occlusion. The hepatic artery normally has a low resistance flow pattern with a large amount of continuous forward flow throughout diastole.

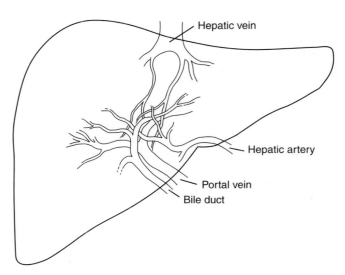

Figure 6–7. Vascular diagram of the liver.

Hepatic Veins. There are three major hepatic veins: right, middle, and left. They drain into the inferior vena cava and lie between the hepatic lobes. An accessory (inferior) right hepatic vein may be present, and, occasionally, one of the hepatic veins may be absent. The liver is divided into two lobes by the middle hepatic vein, which runs in the main interlobar fissure. The right hepatic vein divides the right lobe of the liver into the posterior and anterior segments. The left hepatic vein divides the left lobe of the liver into the medial and lateral segments.

The hepatic veins are best seen from an anterior subcostal approach or a right intercostal approach.[4] On real-time images, the hepatic veins are anechoic tubular structures increasing in size as they approach the diaphragm. There usual echogenic margins seen on the portal veins are absent on hepatic veins. The normal hepatic venous waveform is multiphasic with variations in the velocity and direction of flow. The waveform is influenced by pressure in the right atrium, compliance of the hepatic parenchyma and respiration[3] (Fig. 6–8).

Portal Vein. The portal vein provides 75–80% of the blood supply to the liver and 50% of the oxygen supply to that organ. The portal vein has an average length of 6.5 cm and average diameter of 0.8 cm. and is formed by the confluence of the splenic vein and the superior mesenteric vein. It courses cephalad and rightward into the porta hepatis, bifurcating into the right and left portal branches. The main undivided portal trunk lies immediately anterior to the inferior vena cava, just cephalad to the head of the pancreas and caudal to the caudate lobe. The portal vein enters at the hilus of the liver as the superior mesenteric and

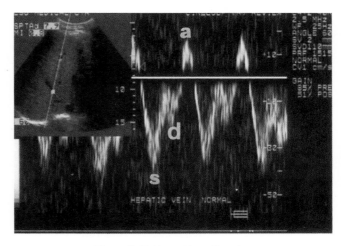

Figure 6–8. Normal hepatic veins.

splenic veins coalesce. The left portal vein is also the umbilical portion of the portal vein, which is of variable size. Organs of the gastrointestinal tract, the gallbladder, the pancreas, and the spleen are drained by the tributaries of the portal vein that enter the liver via the main portal vein to bring nutrients to the liver cells (Fig. 6–9). The portal triad is comprised of the portal vein, hepatic artery, and bile duct. They all travel together in a collagenous sheath (Glisson's capsule) extending throughout the liver.

The main portal vein is best seen sonographically in the transverse position at the level of the porta hepatis and can be followed from the confluence with the splenic vein into the main portal vein and subsequent right and left branches.

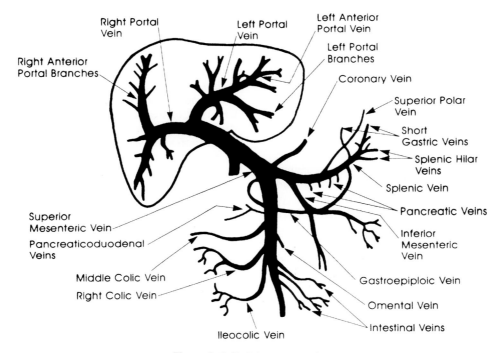

Figure 6–9. Portal venous system.

How does one differentiate sonographically between portal veins and hepatic veins?

1. Portal veins have brighter walls owing to collagen within the wall.
2. The branching angles have different orientation:
    a. Portal veins branch horizontally and are oriented toward the porta hepatis.
    b. Hepatic veins branch longitudinally and are oriented toward the inferior vena cava.
3. The caliber of a hepatic vein increases as it courses toward the diaphragm and inferior vena cava.
4. The caliber of the portal vein increases as it nears the porta hepatis.
5. Hepatic veins will vary in size during respiration.

Normal anterior posterior portal vein diameter should not exceed 13 mm with decrease in diameter during inspiration and increase in diameter during expiration or the Valsalva maneuver. Blood flow is regulated by the passive influence of the splanchnic arterial inflow and changes in systemic venous outflow related to respiration and right heart failure. There should be a normal antegrade (hepatopetal) flow. Respiration will produce slight alteration in the peak flow velocity. With inspiration, there is a slight deceleration, but persistence of antegrade flow. With expiration there is a slight increase in the velocity of forward flow. In normal fasting, supine individuals, the mean velocity is approximately 20–30 cm/s, while in fasting cirrhotic patients 10 cm/s is typical. There should be normal antegrade flow that sounds similar to a windstorm or the ocean. Respiration will create slight alterations in the peak flow velocity, but continuous forward flow (antegrade) should be present. Flow toward the liver is termed hepatopetal. With inspiration, there is a slight deceleration, but persistence of the antegrade flow with expiration there is a slight increase in velocity of the forward flow. The mean velocity is approximately 20–30 cm/s. Portal venous flow and velocity may decrease in response to exercise and is also affected by body posture. There may be a significant decrease in blood flow with a change in posture from the upright to the sitting position.

Disease and Pathology

Portal Vein Thrombosis. This condition may be associated with intra-abdominal abscess, dehydration, trauma, coagulation disorders, neonatal omphalitis, cirrhosis, blood dyscrasia, neoplastic processes, pancreatitis, endoscopic esophageal sclerotherapy, portal hypertension, infection or inflammation of the bowel, and portocaval shunts. Portal vein thrombosis can also occur with secondary to postpercutaneous injection of ethanol for hepatocellular carcinoma or liver transplantation.

Real-time imaging demonstrates an enlarged portal vein with intraluminal echoes. In patients with chronic thrombosis, the associated fibrosis causes an increased echogenicity. In acute portal vein thrombus, the thrombus tends to be hypoechoic or anechoic. Total obstruction of the portal vein will reveal an absence of the Doppler signal or color flow. Color flow Doppler is especially beneficial because it readily demonstrates the absence of color flow in the portal vein and the presence of color in any collaterals present. In cases of partial obstruction of the portal vein, color flow Doppler will show the flow around the thrombus with a partially patent vessel.

Correlating radiographic examinations include CT with contrast enhancement, MRI, and portal venography. Venography provides direct opacification of the portal venous circulation and determines portal venous pressure.

Cavernous Transformation of the Portal Vein. In this condition, there is thrombosis of the extrahepatic portal vein with the formation of periportal collaterals in the porta hepatis around the obstructed portal vein. This condition occurs in children and adults with an unknown etiology. In the neonate, it can be a result of omphalitis, generalized infection, umbilical vein catheter, dehydration, abdominal inflammation, or exchange transfusion. In the adult it can occur secondary to cirrhosis, pancreatitis, or a malignant process in the porta hepatis.[3]

The portal vein may be very difficult to define because of a decrease in size and the presence of high-level echoes in the lumen. Classically, multiple, tortuous, anechoic tubular structures are seen in the porta hepatis region, which represent periportal collaterals. There will be no Doppler flow in the portal vein, and the periportal collaterals will exhibit a characteristic phasic venous waveform. Color flow Doppler readily demonstrates the periportal collaterals with absence of color flow in the portal vein.

Portal venography is the procedure of choice for demonstrating portal vein occlusion with periportal collaterals in the porta hepatis. However ultrasound, CT, and MRI can be used to demonstrate this condition.

Portal Hypertension. Portal hypertension is defined as a portal venous pressure of more than 30 mm Hg. Normally the pressure in the portal venous system is quite low, only 2–3 mm Hg above the inferior vena cava pressure. As the resistance increases, the elevated venous pressure will rise. It does not usually exceed 33 mm Hg because the blood will be forced to travel in a retrograde fashion (hepatofugal) through pathways normally drained by the portal system. These pathways will become collaterals and enlarge. As the portal venous pressure continues to rise, other collaterals will come into existence. The major sites of collateral pathways are shown in Fig. 6–10.

Portal hypertension may be secondary to increased portal venous blood flow (hyperkinetic portal hypertension) which develops as a result of a congenital or acquired arterial portal fistula or shunt. It also occurs from an increase in resistance in the portal venous system. Portal hypertension caused by increased portal venous resistance can be classified into three categories: prehepatic, intrahepatic, and posthepatic. Prehepatic or presinusoidal portal hypertension is caused by thrombosis or obstruction of the extrahepatic portal vein (obstruction of the portal vein before it enters the liver).[3] Intrahepatic or sinusoidal portal hypertension is the most common and often secondary to cirrho-

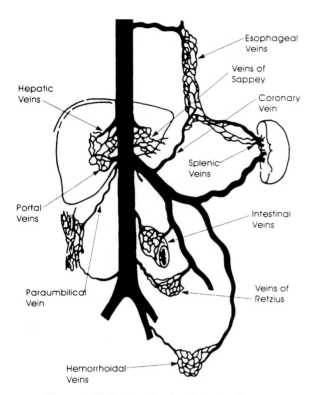

Esophageal
Veins

Veins of
Sappey

Hepatic
Veins

Coronary
Vein

Splenic
Veins

Portal
Veins

Intestinal
Veins

Paraumbilical
Vein

Veins of
Retzius

Hemorrhoidal
Veins

Figure 6–10. Portosystemic collateral pathways.

- Less than 20% increase in SMV or splenic vein diameter from quiet respiration and deep inspiration
- Portosystemic collaterals. (more common types listed below)
- Coronary vein dilatation greater than 5 mm
- Hepatofugal flow
- Pulsatile portal vein flow
- Decreased flow in the portal vein
- Altered response to drugs that affect portal venous flow
- Decreased volume flow in the portal vein
- Splenomegaly (>13 cm)
- Small liver size (<10 cm AP, <15 cm length, <20 cm width)
- Ascites
- Dilatation of superficial abdominal veins with multiple tubular tortuous vessels seen around the umbilical region (Caput medusae)
- The umbilical vein may be recanalized and dilated, which presents a bull's-eye appearance on the transverse scan view in the region of the falciform ligament.
- Splenorenal collateral may arise between the splenic vein and left renal vein.
- Splenocaval collateral may arise between the splenic hilum to the inferior vena cava.

Doppler and spectral analysis may reveal reversed portal venous flow (hepatofugal) or bidirectional flow. The Doppler sounds may be continuous without change during breathing or maneuvers. Portal venous flow can be greatly reduced by the diversion of flow through collateral channels. Decreased velocity (9.7 to 12.4 cm/s) is commonly seen in portal hypertensive patients. Color flow Doppler adds sensitivity to the examination and can easily demonstrate the direction of flow as well as define collateral flow patterns.

Contrast angiography is the gold standard for portal hypertension diagnosis. The procedure can determine the portal venous pressure and demonstrate the dilated portal vein with associated portosystemic collaterals. Angiography is also used in conjunction with embolization of varices and for intravenous shunting of the portal venous system.[3]

Transjugular Intrahepatic Portosystemic Shunt (TIPS)
In the presence of cirrhosis of the liver, the scarring and fibrosis of the liver provides resistance to the venous blood flood returning from the gastrointestinal tract through the portal vein and liver (portal hypertension). This results in increased venous pressure in the portal system that can result in bleeding from the gastrointestinal and the lower esophageal veins (esophageal varices).[6] The radiology interventional procedure, TIPS, decompresses the portal system and is an alternative to the surgically created shunts to reduce the venous pressure. It is primarily for treatment of recurrent gastrointestinal bleeding and refractory ascites in patients with portal hypertension. TIPS create a communication between the portal venous system and the hepatic venous system (Fig. 6–11). It maintains patency of

sis or any condition that increases the resistance to portal venous flow.[3] Posthepatic or postsinusoidal portal hypertension may occur secondary to hepatic venous outflow obstruction and can be seen with hepatic vein occlusion or suprahepatic inferior vena cava obstruction.

In patients with cirrhosis, a loss of respiratory velocity variability occurs, and the flow may appear flattened with a spectral waveform resembling a picket fence. With increasing portal hypertension, flow may become bidirectional (antegrade/hepatopetal and retrograde/hepatofugal). Hepatofugal or reversed venous flow is characteristic of portal hypertension. The portal vein enlarges with portal hypertension exceeding 13 mm in the AP diameter, and the diameter does not change diameter during inspiration, expiration, or Valsalva maneuvers. The portal vein may become comma shaped and surrounded by high-level echoes because of periportal fibrosis. Portal blood flow is usually reduced in patients with chronic liver disease and may be pulsatile in patients with congestive heart failure, tricuspid insufficiency, and any condition associated with elevated right atrial pressure. The splenic vein and superior mesenteric vein may be enlarged (over 10 mm in diameter), and there may be associated varices. The spleen may exceed 13 cm in length and have dilated veins in the splenic hilum. Ascites is a common finding.

Sonographic Characteristics of Portal Hypertension[3]
- Fatty infiltration of the liver
- Portal vein diameter greater than 13 mm

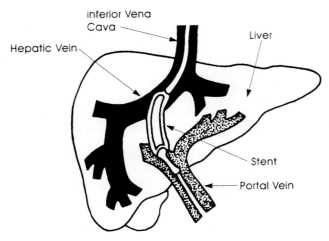

Figure 6–11. Transjugular intrahepatic portosystemic shunt (TIPS).

the portovenous system. The radiology interventional procedure consists of entry through the right internal jugular vein continuing to the superior vena cava and hepatic veins. The liver is punctured with subsequent stent placement between the hepatic vein and the portal vein. The stent is dilated to 8–10 mm with a balloon catheter, and a portogram is performed to evaluate the TIPS and denote any varices filling. Embolization of the gastroesophageal varices is done following the TIPS procedure if filling is seen on the portogram.[6]

Ultrasound is utilized for pre-TIPS, post-TIPS evaluation, and periodic monitoring of the shunt. The pre-TIPS examination provides a high-resolution gray scale scan survey of the abdomen with Doppler and color flow. Primarily to verify the portal hypertension characteristics, assess the size of the liver and spleen, locate any fluid collections, ascites, evaluate the portal venous system, and identify any collateral vessels. The Doppler and spectral analysis provides the portal venous flow characteristics and values that will be used as a baseline value for the post-TIPS examination. The post-TIPS examination evaluates the effectiveness of the shunt and helps to determine the management of the shunt. The examination is performed periodically at 1 day, 1 month, 3 months, 6 months, and 1 year thereafter and at any time the clinical exam or laboratory values are abnormal. In the post-TIPS exam, a gray scale survey is done with emphasis on the shunt to determine any narrowing or hyperplasia present within the shunt. The shunt will appear as a corrugated tubular structure extending from the portal vein to the hepatic vein. The stent normally measures 8–10 mm in the AP diameter. Color flow Doppler demonstrates patency of the shunt with color flow filling the shunt. Doppler spectral analysis is obtained in the portal vein, hepatic artery, the shunt (proximal, mid, and distal shunt), the hepatic veins, the inferior vena cava, and the splenic vein. Peak velocities in the shunt have ranged from 73 to 185 cm/s. An important factor is a comparison with the 1 day postop scan to note any changes. If the shunt begins to fail, portal flow

will decrease. As the portal flow decreases, the hepatic artery flow and resistive index (normal 0.60) will increase.

TIPS Complications

Acute Thrombus. Acute thrombus may be seen during the procedure or shortly afterward. Color flow Doppler will show a hypoechoic filling defect with color flow void and absence of Doppler signal in the area of the thrombus. In some cases, treatment can be initiated with an inflated occlusion balloon to dislodge the thrombus or suction embolectomy.[6]

Pseudointimal Proliferation (Hyperplasia). This condition is very common with stents and presents with stasis and debris buildup within the stent. It can occur early or late as a result of the growth of collagenous material between the stent and the endothelial surface of the stent lumen. The hyperplasia appears as hypoechoic echoes adjacent to the stent wall with narrowing of the lumen. There will be increased velocities on the spectral waveform proportional to the degree of stenosis. The stenosis can involve the stent or the hepatic vein.[6]

Stenosis. Stenosis can occur because of hyperplasia, technical positioning of the stent itself, or as a physiological consequence. The narrowed segment can be seen on real-time imaging with color flow Doppler exhibiting the mixed color pattern and increased velocities in the area of stenosis.[6] A stenosis does not produce hemodynamic changes until the diameter exceeds 50% narrowing. If the stenosis is hemodynamically significant it will cause elevation of the blood flow velocities and aliasing may occur. There will be decreased flow in the portal vein as the stent loses function.

Occlusion. In the preocclusive state, the stent will be seen on color flow Doppler with speckles of color in a lumen filled with gray echoes. The velocity will be greatly reduced throughout the stent at levels of 10–20 cm/s on the spectral analysis. There will also be a reduction in the portal flow with an increase in the hepatic artery flow. Total occlusion will show no color flow in the stent and no spectral waveform is obtained. The portal vein will have a decreased flow because of failure of the stent and varices can return if the stent fails.[6]

The venogram and portogram are primarily used during the procedure and for subsequent evaluation of the TIPS.

Budd–Chiari Syndrome. Hepatic veno-occlusive disease or Budd–Chiari is a rare disorder that results from high-grade stenosis or occlusion of the hepatic veins. This syndrome can be divided into primary and secondary types. The primary type usually occurs because of occlusion by a membrane or web, especially in the suprahepatic or intrahepatic portion of the inferior vena cava. The secondary type is usually related to trauma, pregnancy, neoplasm's medications, hypercoagulable conditions, or Behçet's syndrome. Pathological findings include parenchymal fibrosis, hemorrhage, congestion, and restricted hepatic veins secondary to fibrosis or thrombosis with a partially recanalized lumen in subacute and chronic stages. Symptoms include: enlargement of the liver, abdominal distension secondary to ascites, abdominal pain, edema, and superficial collateral veins. Some patients are asymptomatic.

On real-time imaging, the liver is usually enlarged and appears congested. It exhibits a mixed echogenic pattern, which is hyperechoic. The veins are frequently compressed and difficult to visualize because there is little or no flow. The vein walls may be thickened and an echogenic thrombus may be visualized. Ascites is present. Color flow Doppler will show no color flow in the occluded segments, and there may be minimal flow in other segments. Collaterals may be present.

There are several radiographic procedures that can demonstrate Budd–Chiari syndrome. A CT or MRI can demonstrate the decreased size or absence of the hepatic veins. The inferior vena cava may be narrowed or have low attenuation intraluminal echoes. Contrast venography will show the partial or complete occlusion of the veins and any involvement of the inferior vena cava with the venous collaterals.

Hepatic Tumors. Hepatic tumors, both primary and metastatic, are dependent on arterial circulation.[5] Doppler as well as contrast media has been used in the sonographic investigation of hepatic masses. The contrast media Levovist is one of the agents that has been used to demonstrate enhancement of the tumor vascularity.[2] Sonographic vascular characteristics of tumors are very variable depending on the type of tumor. Typically hemangiomas produce no Doppler signals, while primary hepatomas have a high-flow velocity as a result of direct arteriovenous communication.[7] It must also be noted that some benign conditions, such as focal nodular hyperplasia and adenomas, are also hypervascular. Color flow Doppler and power Doppler are often helpful in delineating the hepatic mass and demonstrating the vascularity. However, the definitive diagnosis is determined by a biopsy.

The majority of hepatic metastases are hypovascular. Primary hepatomas of the liver are often highly vascular, and this is easily demonstrated with color flow Doppler. If chemoembolization is performed, the hepatic artery can be monitored periodically to assess any possible recurrence. Ultrasound guidance for biopsy procedures is also frequently used in the diagnosis of hepatic tumors.

CT, MRI, radionuclide imaging, and ultrasound are all used for the evaluation of both benign and malignant lesions of the liver. Each modality has specific inherent capabilities that make it unique in imaging various entities. For example, computed tomography is preferred for evaluating traumatic lesions of the liver. It not only defines the extent of liver injury but any associated trauma to other organs. CT and ultrasound readily identify the benign cystic lesions; however, MRI is best at demonstrating the hemorrhage within the cyst. Likewise, angiography is superior in the detection of malignant lesions and demonstrating the vascularity of the mass. It can also demonstrate thrombosis within the vessels and collateral vessels present.

Liver Transplantation. Liver transplantation is the preferred treatment for end-stage liver disease. It improves the quality of life and increases the longevity of the patient. The transplant patient undergoes a preoperative sonogram and postoperative sonograms as well, when any abnormal condition arises. The ultrasound examination usually consists of a general survey of the abdomen for any masses or fluid collections. There is special emphasis on the size and tissue characteristics of the liver and spleen with appropriate measurements. The primary vessels are evaluated for patency and direction of flow they include: the hepatic artery (main, right and left branches), hepatic veins, portal venous system, superior mesenteric vein, portal-splenic confluence, splenic artery, splenic vein, and inferior vena cava. In the postsurgical examination, special emphasis is placed on the patency of the vessels and the anastomotic sites with a search for any postsurgical complications (see Fig. 6–12).

The examiner must be familiar with the transplant procedure and the reconstructed vascular anatomy for easy location of the vessels and anastomotic sites. The transplant graft may be an orthotopic cadaveric transplant (OLTX) where the recipient's liver and gallbladder are removed and a cadaveric donor liver is transplanted. There are at least three vascular anastomoses: extrahepatic portal vein, hepatic artery, and suprahepatic inferior vena cava and usually a fourth anastomoses of the infrahepatic inferior vena cava. Biliary drainage is performed with either a choledochostomy with a T-tube or a Rouxen-Y cholecystojejunostomy.[3] The other type of transplant is the heterotrophic transplantation where the recipient's original liver is retained, and part of a donor liver is inserted. Vascular anastomoses include the suprahepatic inferior vena cava, portal vein, and hepatic artery. Biliary drainage is via a choledochojejunostomy with a temporary drain.[3]

Complications of the Liver Transplant

Hepatic Artery Thrombosis. Demonstrating patency of the hepatic artery after transplantation is critical because it will lead to loss of the transplant and retransplantation. The hepatic artery preserves the integrity of the liver parenchyma as well as the intrahepatic and extrahepatic portions of the biliary tree. Real-time imaging demonstrates areas of infarction secondary to hepatic artery thrombosis. Color flow Doppler will show absence of color with no flow signal on the spectral analysis. If hepatic artery flow is not demonstrated, angiography should be performed.

Rejection is a common complication and is one of the main causes of post-procedure hepatic dysfunction.

Noninvasive tests cannot reliably determine rejection but can exclude other complications and demonstrate any parenchymal abnormalities. A definitive diagnosis is provided by a needle biopsy. Clinical signs include: fever, malaise, anorexia, and hepatomegaly. Laboratory findings include elevated serum bilirubin, alkaline phosphatase, and serum transaminase.[3]

Hepatic Artery Stenosis (HAT). A stricture or narrowing of the vessels can occur anywhere in the hepatic circulation

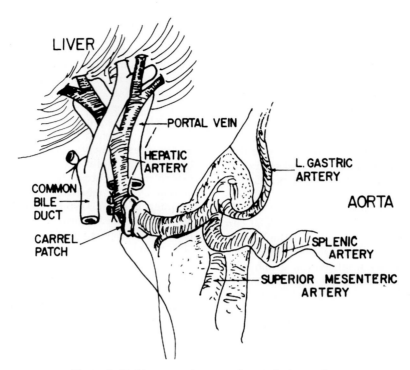

Figure 6–12. Liver transplant vascular surgical procedure.

of the recipient or in the transplant itself. Curling or coiling of the vessels may occur because of the excessive length of the reconstructed vessel. Spectral waveforms will show an elevated Doppler shift often with aliasing present. A peak velocity of more than 2 m/s or a systolic acceleration time greater than 0.8 s is suggestive of stenosis. Distal to the stenosis an RI of less than 0.5 indicates a significant proximal lesion. However, within the first 48 hours, the RI and systolic acceleration are unreliable. Color flow Doppler is the method of choice for localization and mapping the transplant vessels. Stenotic areas will have a narrowing with a mosaic color pattern in the area of the stenosis.

Portal Vein Thrombosis. Portal vein thrombosis can cause early graft failure and is associated with a high mortality rate. Real-time imaging will show the enlarged portal vein filled with echoes. Doppler and color flow will show an absence of flow or minimal flow in the portal vein. Collateral venous flow may be seen in close proximity to the occluded portal vein. In some instances there may be a difference in size of the portal vein in the donor and recipient that will mimic a stenosis but it will have no hemodynamic effects as seen with a true stenosis.

Portal Vein Stenosis. This is an uncommon anastomotic complication that occurs with a bandlike narrowing or irregularity. As time progresses, there may be associated aneurysmal dilation, significant pressure gradients, and possibly portal hypertension.

Inferior Vena Cava Stenosis and Thrombosis. Stenosis of the inferior vena cava is an uncommon complication usually related to a technical problem at the anastomotic site. It can also be secondary to compression from adjacent fluid collections or hematomas and has been reported possibly to occur in patients who had Budd–Chiari syndrome prior to surgery.

Biliary Complications. Biliary complications include obstruction, leaks, and generalized ductal changes. Strictures, nonfunctioning stent or T-tube, common duct redundancy, stones, and mucoceles of the cystic duct remnant can cause biliary obstruction. Strictures can be attributed to technical errors, ischemia, infection, and chronic rejection. Bile leaks can be seen on real time as sonolucent fluid collections in the biliary or drain area. Bilomas are irregular-shaped cystic structures with internal echoes and enhancement usually near the gallbladder fossa and porta hepatis region. Biliary obstruction is considered if the common duct exceeds 6 mm.

Pseudoaneurysms are not common but can occasionally be seen at the arterial anastomosis sites, and they may occur from infection or graft needle biopsy.

Multiple radiological imaging procedures used to evaluate the liver transplant which include:

- Radionuclide scintigraphy for liver perfusion, hepatocyte function, and bile excretion
- Hepatobiliary scintigraphy and ultrasound for the detection of bilomas and hepatic abscesses
- Cholangiography for the biliary system
- CT for biliary necrosis
- Angiography for patency of the vessels and perfusion of the organ

Pancreas

Pancreas Transplantation. More recently, the pancreas is transplanted in the abdomen and often accompanies a renal transplant. The arterial blood supply to the pancreas is the splenic artery and the superior mesenteric artery. The venous drainage of the pancreas can be via the portal vein of the donor into the iliac vein of the recipient or via an anastomosis between the donor portal vein and the superior mesenteric vein of the recipient. The success of pancreas transplantation has improved because of the improvements in organ recovery, refinement of the surgical procedure, better immunosuppression, and advanced critical care. The transplant may be performed for any of the following entities:

- Patients with end-stage renal disease secondary to diabetes, a combined kidney and pancreas transplant is performed
- Patients who have had a kidney transplant previously and have a pancreas transplant later
- Diabetic patients with evidence of secondary complications but who do not have renal failure receive only the pancreas transplant

Complication of Pancreas Transplant

Thrombosis. This condition can occur in the immediate post-transplantation period or later secondary to rejection or infection. Arterial thrombosis can occur at any of the anastomotic sites, whereas venous thrombosis tends to complicate the venous drainage and cause the pancreas to become edematous. It can also cause the artery to become thrombosed, ultimately leading to loss of the graft. There will be absence of color filling of the thrombosed vessel and no Doppler signal.

Pancreatitis. In most cases, some degree of pancreatitis occurs as a result of reperfusion injury. However, severe cases can lead to loss of the transplant.[3] Typically, pancreatitis presents on the real-time image with the pancreas slightly enlarged and more echolucent because of the associated edema. In chronic pancreatitis, the pancreas is fibrosed, and calcifications may be present.

Rejection. A common problem in transplant patients that has greatly improved in the last few years because of improvements in organ recovery, surgical procedures, and better immunosuppression therapy. Rejection is confirmed by a biopsy; however, ultrasound is used to rule out any other anomalies.

Intra-abdominal Abscess and Peritonitis. Duodenal leaks with abscess or peritonitis are a complication that results in graft loss. The most common organism is the candida albicans.

Renal

The renal arteries arise from the abdominal aorta and provide the blood supply to the kidneys (Fig. 6–13). They are usually single, but there may be multiple arteries on one or both sides. The right renal artery arises from the right anterolateral part of the abdominal aorta and runs posterior to the inferior vena cava and right renal vein and enters the hilum of the kidney. The left renal artery arises from the left posterolateral portion of the abdominal aorta and runs posterior to the left renal vein to enter the renal hilum. The main renal artery divides in the renal hilum into the anterior and posterior branches, which subdivide into the segmental arteries within the renal sinus echocomplex. The segmental arteries give rise to the interlobar arteries that run along side the renal pyramids. Arcuate arteries arise from the interlobar arteries and curve around the bases of the pyramids. The arcuate arteries give off multiple small vessels, the lobular arteries that supply the renal cortex[3] (Fig. 6–14).

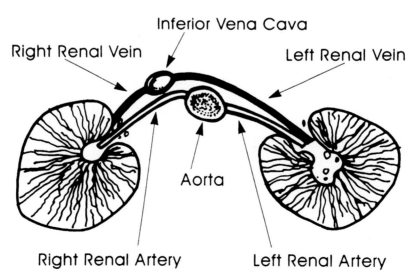

Figure 6–13. Cross section of the renal arteries.

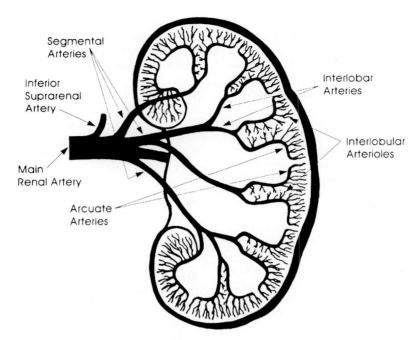

Figure 6–14. Renal arteries.

The renal arteries are best seen in a transverse image arising from the aorta or entering the renal hilum. They appear as sonolucent tubular structures coursing from the aorta to the renal hilum. Color flow imaging makes the length of the vessel easier to visualize. Normal renal artery flow is low impedance with continuous forward flow during diastole (Fig. 6–15). There will be a gradual decline in the systolic and diastolic amplitudes from the main renal artery to the intrarenal vessels. Peak systolic velocity in the normal renal artery is usually less than 100 cm/s. The RI from normal intrarenal arteries ranges from 9.58 to 0.64. A resistive index of 0.70 has been considered the upper limit of normal in the adult. These values are higher in premature infants, neonates, and children under the age of 4. The normal range would be 0.70–1.0.

Disease and Pathology
Renal Artery Stenosis. Renal artery stenosis often results in hypertension, which is defined as an increase in the sys-

tolic blood pressure of 140 mm Hg or above. Approximately 5–10% of hypertensive patients are caused by renal artery stenosis or intrinsic kidney disease. Renal artery stenosis can be caused by atherosclerosis, fibromuscular dysplasia, arteritis, middle aortic syndrome, aortic coarctation, neurofibromatosis, irradiation, renal artery aneurysm, congenital renal artery stenosis, emboli, thrombosis, congenital fibrous bands, vascular malformations and fistulas, pheochromocytoma, subcapsular and perirenal hematoma, traumatic occlusion, and neoplasms. The patient may be asymptomatic or present with hypertension, congestive heart failure, and renal failure. Real-time imaging may demonstrate a small kidney with the cortex decreased in thickness. Narrowing of the vessel at the site of the stenosis may be seen, as well as the presence of calcifications. There are two methods of evaluating renal artery stenosis: direct evaluation of the renal artery and evaluation of the distal intraparenchymal renal arteries. Doppler waveforms will show increased systolic velocity in the narrowed vessel, usually in the 100–180 cm/s range. If the systolic velocity is 3.5 times that of the aorta, it indicates a hemodynamically significant stenosis or greater than 60%. Acceleration time (interval from the beginning of the systolic flow to the peak systolic flow) greater than 0.1 indicates renal artery stenosis of more than 50%. Intrarenal arteries with a ratio of end diastolic to systolic velocity of under 0.23 is abnormal and characteristic of severe parenchymal vascular disease. An acceleration time of <0.07 seconds, an acceleration index of <3.78 kHz/S2/MHz, or loss of normal early systolic peak may indicate significant renal artery stenosis.[2] A tardus parvus waveform may be seen distal to a stenosis or occlusion. The RI exceeds 0.70% in renal artery stenosis. Color flow Doppler will provide easier localization of the

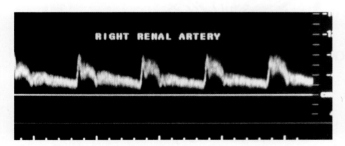

Figure 6–15. Normal renal artery spectral waveform.

stenotic area and demonstrate the area of narrowing with rapid mosaic color changes. Power Doppler is also beneficial in demonstrating the course of the renal artery and showing the perfusion of the kidney.[3] Other radiological examinations can detect renal artery stenosis and include: intravenous pyelography, radionuclide renography, and renal angiography. However, renal angiography is considered the gold standard.

Renal Vein Thrombosis. Renal vein thrombosis can occur in children and adults and is more common in the left renal vein. Clinical symptoms include flank pain, hematuria, flank mass, or pulmonary embolism. It has multiple causes, which include:

- Secondary to external compression or intrinsic pathology
- In the newborn, infection, dehydration, birth asphyxia, hypotension and maternal diabetes
- In the adult, primary renal disease such as nephrotic syndrome or membranous glomerulonephritis
- Systemic diseases, such as sickle cell anemia, diabetes mellitus, lupus erythematosis, and amyloidosis

Renal veins are seen on real-time imaging as a tubular anechoic structure extending from the kidney to the inferior vena cava. The right renal vein is shorter and lies superior to the right renal artery extending from the hilum to the right lateral wall of the inferior vena cava. The left renal vein runs from the left renal hilum to the inferior vena cava and lies anterior to the aorta and posterior to the superior mesenteric artery. The renal veins are characteristic of veins with a phasic flow moving with respiration. In cases of acute renal vein thrombosis, the kidney will be enlarged with hypoechogenicity. The renal sinuses become less echogenic, and the pyramids may be prominent with poor definition of the corticomedullary junction. The renal vein becomes enlarged, and the echogenic thrombus may be seen. However, in acute cases, often the thrombus can be anechoic, and color flow Doppler is ideal to demonstrate the filling void caused by occlusion. Spectral analysis will show absence of blood flow with complete obstruction, and in partial obstruction, there will be a continuous nonphasic flow around the thrombus.

Hydronephrosis. Hydronephrosis is abnormal dilatation of the renal calyces and renal pelvis. Most commonly caused by impaired renal function but may also occur on a functional or organic basis. Real-time imaging demonstrates the sonolucent fluid filled dilated pelvis and calyces. It has been noted that within 18 to 24 hours of renal obstruction there is intrarenal vasoconstriction, which results in reduced renal blood flow.[8] Obstructive hydronephrosis may also be associated with high impedance blood flow and reduced flow during diastole. The RI is greater than 0.70 in patients with obstructive hydronephrosis. Other causes of elevated resistive index include medical renal disease, perinephric and subcapsular hematoma, hypotension, and decreased heart rate.[3] The RI reflects the renal vascular resistance.

Renal Transplantation

Renal transplantation began in the early 1950s and has a high survival rate because of the success of the surgical procedure, improved care, and advances made in immunosuppressive therapy. Ultrasound is considered part of the routine protocol for evaluation of the renal transplant, beginning with the initial preoperative examination through the post-transplant period and periodically to evaluate the kidney. Real-time imaging provides the anatomical scan survey to identify the transplant kidney, provide accurate measurements, and to identify any perirenal or intrarenal anomalies. Color flow Doppler is the state of the art for ultrasound transplant examinations to identify patency of the vessels and provide hemodynamical information. Spectral analysis shows the flow characteristics and provides the resistive index or pulsatility index. A high resistivity index (RI) is associated with rejection, acute tubular necrosis, renal vein thrombosis, renal compression, pyelonephritis, and obstruction.[3]

The transplanted kidney is placed superficially within the ileopelvic region on the right side commonly (Fig. 6–16). In cases of retransplantation, the left side may be used. The iliac arteries and veins revascularize the transplant with the renal artery of the donor attached to the external iliac artery of the recipient. The venous anastomosis is made to the external or common iliac vein. A baseline sonogram should be obtained following the transplant to determine its exact location, size, and texture. This provides a comparison for all subsequent examinations.

On the real-time images, the renal transplant appears as a normal elliptical-shaped kidney in the iliac fossa. The ureter is anastomosed to the bladder via a ureteroneocystostomy and may sometimes be seen extending from the kidney to the bladder, especially in cases of obstruction. A

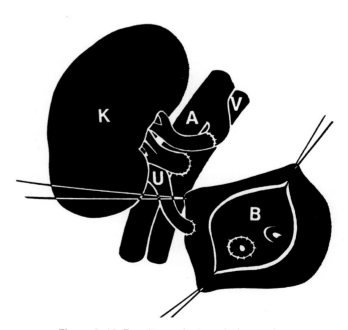

Figure 6–16. Renal transplant surgical procedure.

careful survey is performed of the lower abdomen to identify any perirenal masses, such as urinomas, lymphoceles, hematomas, or abscesses. Color Doppler demonstrates the renal artery and vein and anastomotic sites. They should be carefully evaluated for any kinks or stenosis. The intraparenchymal arteries and veins can also be demonstrated with perfusion views obtained with power Doppler. Spectral analysis shows the normal external iliac artery as a high-resistance triphasic waveform with a reverse component characteristic of a pulsatile peripheral artery. The renal artery has a steady waveform with a high continuous forward flow throughout diastole. The arterial anastomotic sites will show a higher velocity with turbulence. The main renal vein shows a spontaneous respiratory phasicity that tends to become more monophasic with the parenchymal veins. The normal RI is 0.5–0.7.

Renal Transplantation Complications

Rejection. Acute failure of the transplanted kidney may be produced by acute rejection, acute tubular necrosis, or arterial obstruction. It is important to differentiate between these complications for correct treatment to be administered.

Acute rejection sonographically appears as enlarged kidney with increased cortical echogenicity (58%); decreased renal sinus echogenicity; irregular sonolucent areas in the cortex (47%) enlarged and decreased echogenicity of the pyramids; distortion of the renal outline; and indistinct corticomedullary junction.

Rejection attributable to acute tubular necrosis usually results in a normal sonogram. In rejection attributable to acute due to acute renal arterial occlusion, the sonographic anatomy remains grossly normal. However, duplex Doppler studies may reveal an absence or reduction of diastolic flow.

Stenosis. This is a very common vascular complication and may develop early or later in the postoperative period. Kinking, torsion, and stenosis are complications that can be associated with the surgical procedure. Later, stenosis is caused by atherosclerosis or fibrosis. Clinical symptoms are hypertension, increased levels of serum creatinine, and a bruit in the region of the transplant. Color flow Doppler is used to evaluate the vasculature and will demonstrate any kinking or tortuosity in the artery with mixed color patterns and moderately increased velocities. Severe stenosis produces a turbulent flow pattern with a mosaic color pattern and narrowing of the lumen. The spectral analysis will show high velocities in the area of stenosis and a damped waveform throughout the distal parenchymal arteries. A ratio of renal artery to iliac artery peak systolic velocity greater that 3.0 indicates stenosis.[3]

Occlusion. Occlusion of the renal artery or vein, secondary to thrombosis, may occur in the immediate postoperative period because of surgical complications. Definitive diagnosis is imperative because this can lead to loss of the renal transplant. Arterial complications are usually associated with intimal or perfusion injuries. The vascular occlusive changes related to rejection may produce loss of renal function and infarction. Renal vein thrombosis can result from surgical complications or compression of the renal vein. Color Doppler is used to demonstrate patency of the vessels. Renal artery occlusion results in hyperechogenicity in the ischemic tissue. Power Doppler demonstrates the perfusion of the kidney with the absence of perfused flow in the infarcted segment. Renal vein thrombosis will show a swollen and congested kidney with a distended vein filled with echoes. There will be absence of the Doppler signal in the vessels. Renal vein thrombosis will alter the arterial signal and show an abrupt systolic Doppler shift and a blunted reversed diastolic flow in the renal artery.

Arteriovenous (AV) Fistulas. The AV fistulas are usually secondary to percutaneous needle biopsy. Some will regress spontaneously and are usually asymptomatic. However they can cause hypertension and massive bleeding. Color flow Doppler is required to identify the AV fistula. There will be a color jet with highly disorganized flow patterns in the area of the fistula between the artery and the vein. The spectral analysis shows extremely high velocities with irregular amplitudes in the feeding artery because of the high-pressure gradient and turbulent venous flow with arterial pulsations in the draining vein.

Pseudoaneurysms. This is another complication seen with percutaneous biopsy. The perforation of the arterial wall leads to the formation of the pseudoaneurysm whereby the blood moves back and forth during the cardiac cycle from the vessel to the pseudoaneurysm. The patient may be asymptomatic or the pseudoaneurysm may continue to enlarge and eventually rupture. The ultrasound characteristics were described in the previous text.

Radiographic imaging of the renal transplant include: radionuclide imaging for perfusion and functional status of the kidney, CT for preoperative and postoperative assessment, MRI for anatomic details with perfusion and functional information, angiography for vascular evaluation, and ultrasound for anatomical detail and vascular evaluation.

HEMODIALYSIS ACCESS GRAFTS

The most common indications for dialysis are uremic signs and symptoms, which become more prominent as the blood nitrogen (BUN) and creatinine levels rise. Other indications include: hyperkalemia (elevated blood level of potassium, which most often reflects defective renal excretion), fluid overload, and drug overdose.[8] Although it is recognized that renal transplantation is the preferred mode of replacement therapy for patients with end stage renal disease, it is also recognized that some patients are not suitable candidates for transplantation, which includes: poorly controlled diabetes, HIV infection, or cardiovascular disease. It is also common knowledge that the demand for kidneys has far outstripped the current number of suitable organs. Thus, dialysis is utilized for both acute and chronic renal failure.

The primary goal of the dialysis access is to maintain access to the circulation. There are several methods of dialysis, which include the following:

Peritoneal Dialysis

The peritoneum surrounding the abdominal cavity is used as a dialyzing membrane for the purpose of removing waste products or toxins as a result of renal failure. Dialyzing fluid is introduced into the peritoneal cavity via a catheter for a specified time and then allowed to drain.[9] The major disadvantage of this method is the possibility of recurrent peritonitis.[8]

Dialysis Catheters

Dialysis catheters are primarily used for acute hemodialysis. They provide quick access and are usually inserted percutaneously by surgical cutdown in the internal jugular or subclavian. Infection and thrombosis are major complications.

Autologous Arteriovenous Fistulas

These are surgical fistulas created with a native artery and vein. The most common being the Brescia–Cimino, which is surgically created between the radial artery and the cephalic vein (Fig. 6–17). Other types include the distal ulnar artery and basilic vein, brachial artery and cephalic vein, proximal radial artery and transposed basilic vein, and brachial artery and transposed basilic vein. This type of vascular access has a long longevity and resistance to infection and hyperplasia. However, one of the more common problems is the failure of the graft to mature.

Synthetic Arteriovenous Shunt Grafts

These are the most common type of grafts for chronic dialysis. However, they have a shorter longevity and a higher complication rate than the Brescia–Cimino fistulas. Usually placed in the upper extremity, they may be a loop shunt or straight shunt. Typical routing of the shunt includes: a straight shunt from the radial artery to the antecubital vein, a loop shunt between the brachial artery and the axil-

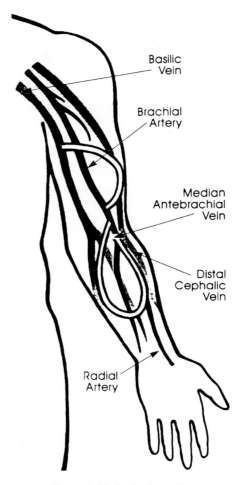

Figure 6–18. Synthetic grafts.

lary vein (Fig. 6–18). These grafts take approximately 5 to 10 days to mature. To mature, the native vein dilates to accommodate the volume outflow of the graft. Failure of the vein to dilate results in a restricted outflow and produces an outflow stenosis that eventually leads to graft failure. Because the graft is superficially located, it can easily be palpated. In fact, the "thrill" within the shunt verifies patency. The graft is originally placed in the nondominant arm of the patient. When it no longer functions, a new graft is placed in the opposite arm, and last the lower extremity. The lower extremity is more prone to increased risk of infection and symptomatic arterial steal.

Ultrasound plays a significant role in the management of the dialysis patient. Conventional duplex and color flow Doppler can demonstrate the patency of the graft and assess the hemodynamics. Graft abnormalities can be identified at an early stage, so treatment can be started and prevent graft loss. The graft is seen as an anechoic tubular structure with parallel echogenic lines that represent the synthetic graft wall. There will be focal dilatation in the native artery where the graft originates, and the outflow vein should be dilated. The graft can be traced with real-time and color flow Doppler from the feeding artery (inflow) to the draining vein

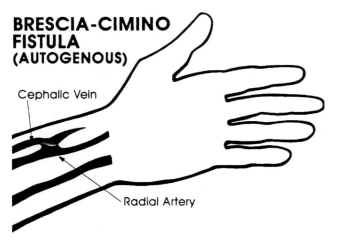

Figure 6–17. Brescia–Cimino fistula.

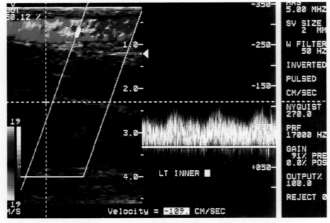

Figure 6–19. Normal graft spectral waveform with venous and arterial signals.

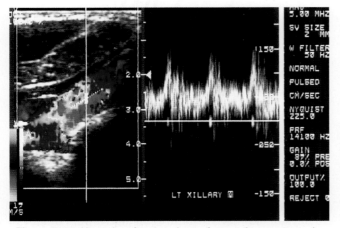

Figure 6–20. Normal graft spectral waveform at the anastomosis.

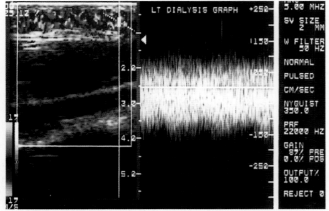

Figure 6–21. Normal graft venous outflow spectral waveform.

(outflow). Color flow Doppler shows patency of the shunt with a wide range of flow velocities and elevation of the velocity at the anastomotic sites (Figs. 6–19, 20, and 21). Doppler spectral waveforms demonstrate a monophasic waveform in the arteries that supply the graft. Peak systolic velocities range from 100 to 400 cm/s, with the anastomotic sites being the higher values. End diastolic velocities range from 60 to 200 cm/s. The draining veins have arterial pulsations with peak velocities of 30–100 cm/s. Spectral broadening may be seen because of the wide range of flow velocities.[3]

Dialysis Access Graft Complications

Graft Malfunction. Clinical indications of graft malfunction include: difficult needle placement, elevated venous pressure, abnormal lab values, recirculation, loss of thrill, swelling, and perigraft masses. Doppler flow velocities of less than 100 cm/s usually indicate a malfunctioning graft.[3]

Perigraft Masses. Perigraft masses include abscess, fluid leakage, hematomas, pseudoaneurysms, and hematomas. Real-time scan identifies any perigraft masses, however, it is often difficult to make a definitive diagnosis based on real time alone.

Color flow Doppler will identify any vascular mass, such as the pseudoaneurysm; however, hematomas, abscess, and fluid collections all give a similar appearance and require laboratory analysis.

Thrombosis. Thrombosis is more common with synthetic grafts and the most common cause of graft failure. There will be a decreased flow rate on dialysis of less than 250–300 mL/min with a recirculation rate greater than 15% or venous pressures in excess of 150 mm Hg, which indicate a failing graft. Subclavian or internal jugular hemodialysis catheters have a tendency for thrombus formation.[8] Real time shows the classic appearance of thrombus as an echogenic mass within the lumen of the vessel. Acute and newly formed thrombus appears anechoic, with the aging thrombus becoming more echogenic.

Stenosis. Most often graft failure results from stenosis of the venous limb followed by arterial limb stenosis. This is a common entity with access grafts and can occur as a result of various complications which include: formation of intimal hyperplasia, fibrosis that generally occurs at the anastomotic sites, failure of the graft to mature, and failure of the native vein to dilate, resulting in venous outflow stenosis. Real-time imaging can identify any narrowed segments, wall thickening, residual buildup, and calcifications. Color flow Doppler identifies the stenotic zone with mosaic color patterns. However, the access graft by nature has a high turbulent flow pattern, especially at the anastomotic. Spectral analysis demonstrates the stenosis with the focal elevation of velocities with low values on either end and usually accompanied by aliasing. A relative value of greater than 400 cm/s indicates a stenosis that should be compared to baseline values.

Occlusion. The graft is filled with echoes, and the walls appear collapsed. Color flow Doppler shows no flow. No Doppler signal can be obtained within the graft.

Infection. Synthetic grafts are more prone to infection. Symptoms of an infection or abscess include local erythema, induration, tenderness, and purulent drainage from incisional sites. Positive blood cultures may be present.[8] Ultrasound is used to identify any fluid collections or masses present but may be unable to differentiate such various entitie as abscess versus hematomas or complicated fluid collections. In these cases, biopsy or aspiration with lab confirmation makes the definitive diagnosis.

Aneurysms and Pseudoaneurysms. Aneurysms and pseudoaneurysms can be seen with synthetic grafts. They generally occur at puncture sites where subcutaneous hematomas accumulate and at the anastomotic sites. They are readily seen as pulsating masses on the real time with Color flow Doppler demonstrating the swirling changing color pattern in the aneurysm.[3,8]

Ischemic Steal Syndrome. Examination of the graft should always include bilateral blood pressures and a check for distal pulses to rule out ischemia and steal syndrome. Symptoms include: numbness of the fingers, paresis of the intrinsic muscles of the hands, and absent radial pulse.[8]

Doppler evaluation of the radial artery will show a reversal of flow due to being supplied (stealing) from the ulna artery. Compression of the ulna artery will cease the blood flow in the radial artery.

REFERENCES

1. Williams PL, Warwick R, Dyson M, et al. eds. *Gray's Anatomy.* 37th ed. New York: Churchill Livingstone; 1989.
2. Raymond HW, Zwiebel WJ, Swartz JD. *Semin Ultrasound CT MRI.* 1997;18.
3. Krebs CA, Giyanani VL, Eisenberg RL. *Ultrasound Atlas of Vascular Diseases.* Stamford, CT: Appleton & Lange; 1999.
4. Zwiebel WJ, Fruechte D. Basics of abdominal and pelvic duplex. Instrumentation, anatomy and vascular Doppler signatures. *Semin Ultrasound CT MRI.* 1992;13.
5. Schwartz SI, ed. *Principles of Surgery.* 4th ed. New York: McGraw-Hill; 1984.
6. Krebs CA. Transjugular intrahepatic portosystemic shunts (TIPS). *Vasc Ultrasound Today.* 1997; 2:42–46.
7. Syllabus, 1989. Conventional & Color-Flow Duplex Ultrasound Course. April 7–8, 1989, AIUM, Spring Education Meeting, Bethesda, MD.
8. Hallett JW, Brewster DC, Darling RC. *Handbook of Patient Care in Vascular Surgery.* New York: Little, Brown & Co; 1995.

Questions

1. Branches of the celiac axis include

   (A) hepatic, splenic, and gastric arteries
   (B) hepatic, superior mesenteric, and gastric arteries
   (C) hepatic, splenic, and renal artery
   (D) gastric, superior mesenteric, and inferior mesenteric arteries

2. The first branch of the abdominal aorta is the

   (A) superior mesenteric artery
   (B) inferior mesenteric artery
   (C) celiac artery
   (D) renal arteries

3. The sonographic term "seagull appearance" refers to

   (A) renal artery
   (B) superior mesenteric artery
   (C) gastroduodenal artery
   (D) celiac arteries

4. The splanchnic arteries comprises the

   (A) hepatic, splenic, and gastric arteries
   (B) celiac and renal arteries
   (C) celiac, superior mesenteric, inferior mesenteric arteries
   (D) renal, superior mesenteric, inferior mesenteric arteries

5. The term fusiform refers to a type of

   (A) aneurysm
   (B) pseudoaneurysm
   (C) dissection
   (D) arteriovenous malformation

6. A pulsating echogenic flap seen in the vessel lumen indicates

   (A) mycotic aneurysm
   (B) arterial dissection
   (C) false aneurysm
   (D) atherosclerotic disease

7. The presence of a low resistance waveform in the SMA or IMA in a fasting patient indicates

   (A) portal hypertension
   (B) pancreatitis
   (C) appendicitis
   (D) mesenteric ischemia

8. Stenosis of the renal arteries is indicated if

   (A) the peak systolic velocity is one-half the aortic peak systolic velocity
   (B) the peak systolic velocity is two times the aortic peak systolic velocity
   (C) the peak systolic velocity is three and one-half times the aortic peak systolic velocity
   (D) the peak systolic velocity remains unchanged

9. The radiology procedure recommended for diagnosing occlusion of the splanchnic arteries and demonstrating the collateral circulation is

   (A) MRI
   (B) ultrasound
   (C) Contrast enhanced computerized tomography
   (D) mesenteric angiogram with selective visceral views

10. The most common pathological condition of the inferior vena cava is

    (A) atherosclerotic disease
    (B) stenosis
    (C) occlusion
    (D) thrombosis

11. Which vessel supplies 75% of the blood to the liver?

    (A) hepatic artery
    (B) portal vein
    (C) inferior vena cava
    (D) hepatic veins

12. The portal vein is formed by the confluence of the

(A) splenic and superior mesenteric vein and, sometimes, the inferior mesenteric vein
(B) inferior mesenteric and superior mesenteric veins
(C) superior mesenteric and coronary vein
(D) splenic and inferior mesenteric vein

13. The portal triad is composed of

(A) portal vein, hepatic artery, superior mesenteric artery
(B) portal vein, hepatic artery, and bile duct
(C) portal vein, right hepatic artery, and left hepatic artery
(D) portal vein, hepatic vein, hepatic artery

14. Mycotic aneurysms occur secondary to

(A) surgery
(B) atherosclerotic disease
(C) infectious processes
(D) trauma

15. The predominate etiology for cirrhosis of the liver in the western hemisphere is

(A) alcoholism
(B) sclerosing cholangitis
(C) hepatitis
(D) hepatomas

16. A prominent venous collateral seen coursing along the abdominal wall from the portal vein to the umbilicus via the ligamentum teres and the falciform ligament is the

(A) caput medusae
(B) splenorenal
(C) coronary
(D) paraumbilical

17. The resistive index (RI) in the renal arteries should not exceed

(A) 0.02
(B) 0.05
(C) 0.07
(D) 1.00

18. The most common vascular pathway for tumor extension is the

(A) aorta
(B) inferior vena cava
(C) portal vein
(D) hepatic veins

19. Occlusion of the hepatic veins is termed

(A) Budd–Chiari
(B) Caput medusae
(C) sclerosing cholangitis
(D) congestive liver disease

20. Reversal of flow in the common hepatic artery indicates

(A) occlusion of the celiac artery origin
(B) occlusion of the SMA artery origin
(C) occlusion of the renal artery origin
(D) occlusion of the splenic artery origin

21. A collateral circulation for the splanchnic arteries does not include

(A) pancreaticoduodenal arcade
(B) arch of Riolan
(C) artery of Drummond
(D) gastroepiploic collaterals

22. Sonographic criteria for an abdominal aortic aneurysm does not include

(A) focal dilatation measuring 1.5 to 2 times greater than adjacent segment
(B) diameter of the vessel measuring more than 3 cm
(C) dilated focal segment exceeding 3 cm with thrombus present
(D) calcification in a focal segment without dilatation

23. Branches of the hepatic artery include

(A) splenic artery, gastric artery, gastroduodenal artery, right and left hepatic branches, cystic artery, and intrahepatic branches
(B) gastroduodenal artery, right gastric artery, right and left hepatic arteries, cystic artery, and intrahepatic branches
(C) celiac artery, superior mesenteric artery, right and left hepatic branches, and intrahepatic branches,
(D) gastric artery, right and left hepatic branches, cystic artery, and intrahepatic branches

24. In Fig. 6–22, the color flow Doppler shows a transverse view of the aorta and celiac and the respective waveform that illustrates

(A) normal celiac artery spectral analysis
(B) occlusion of the celiac artery
(C) stenosis of the celiac artery
(D) aneurysm of the celiac artery

25. In Fig. 6–23, the color flow Doppler with spectral analysis of a TIPS in the liver shows

(A) normal spectral analysis of the TIPS
(B) hyperplasia of the TIPS
(C) stenosis of the TIPS
(D) occlusion of the TIPS

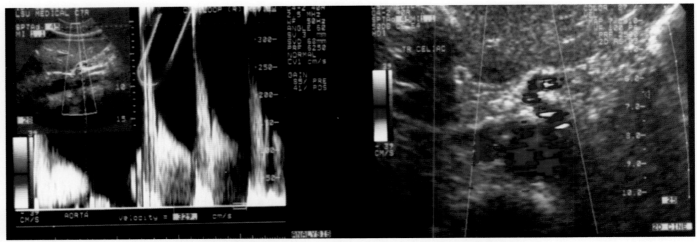

Figure 6–22. Color flow Doppler and spectral analysis of the celiac artery.

26. In Fig. 6–24, the real-time enlarged view of the portal vein shows

    (A) stenosis of the portal vein
    (B) normal portal vein
    (C) occlusion of the portal vein with periportal collaterals
    (D) aneurysm of the portal vein

27. In Fig. 6–25, the transverse real-time view of the aorta demonstrates

    (A) aneurysm with internal and external lumen measurements
    (B) dissecting aneurysm with internal membranes
    (C) leaking aneurysm with external hematoma
    (D) normal aorta

28. In Fig. 6–26, the longitudinal color flow Doppler of the liver shows

    (A) normal liver with entry of the SMV
    (B) cirrhosis of the liver with entry of the SMV
    (C) liver with TIPS placement
    (D) cirrhosis of the liver with paraumbilical collateral entering the falciform ligament

29. In Fig. 6–27, the spectral analysis of the anastomosis of a dialysis graft indicates

    (A) occlusion of the graft
    (B) occlusion of the native artery
    (C) high-grade stenosis at the anastomosis
    (D) pseudoaneurysm at the anastomosis

30. In Fig. 6–28, the color flow Doppler of the inferior vena cava shows

    (A) stenosis of the IVC
    (B) occlusion of the IVC
    (C) occlusion of the portal vein
    (D) stricture of the IVC

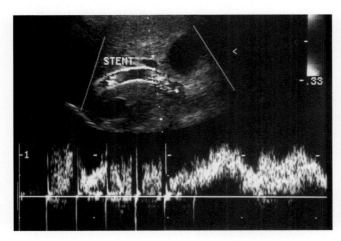

Figure 6–23. Color flow Doppler and spectral analysis of a TIPS.

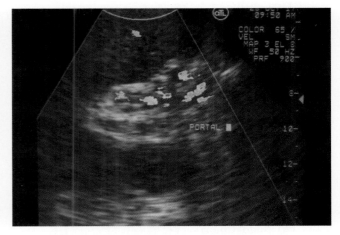

Figure 6–24. Real time view of the portal vein.

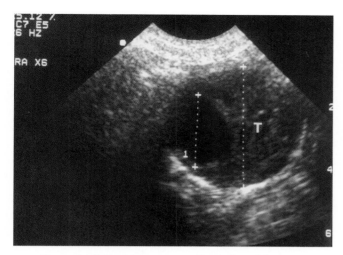

Figure 6–25. Real time cross sectional view of the aorta.

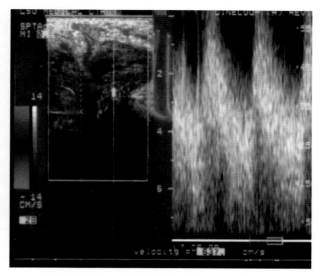

Figure 6–27. Spectral analysis of at the anastomosis site of a dialysis graft.

31. In Fig. 6–29, the color flow Doppler with spectral analysis of an intrarenal artery of a renal transplant indicates

    (A) occlusion of the main renal artery
    (B) high-grade stenosis in the proximal renal artery
    (C) high-grade stenosis in the distal renal artery
    (D) normal intrarenal arterial flow

32. In Fig. 6–30, the spectral analysis of the right renal artery indicates

    (A) normal renal arterial flow
    (B) occlusion of the renal artery
    (C) high-grade renal artery stenosis
    (D) moderate renal artery stenosis

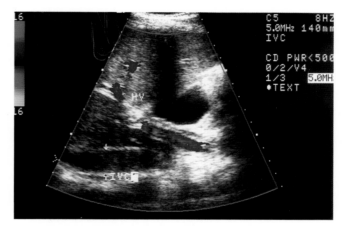

Figure 6–28. Color flow Doppler of the liver and inferior vena cava.

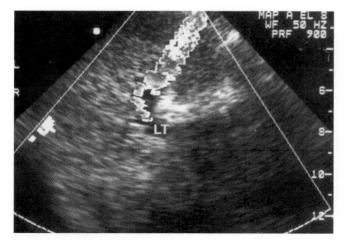

Figure 6–26. Longitudinal color flow Doppler of a patient with portal hypertension.

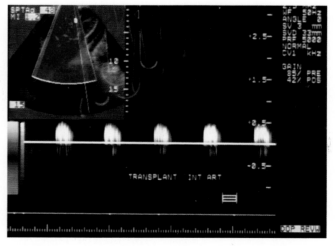

Figure 6–29. Spectral analysis of an intrarenal artery in a renal transplant patient.

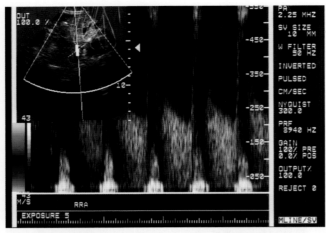

Figure 6–30. Spectral analysis of the right renal artery.

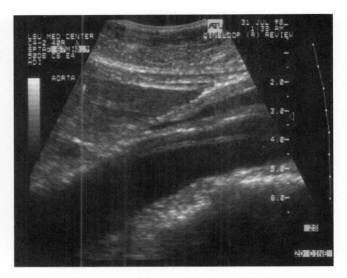

Figure 6–32. Real time image of the aorta.

33. In Fig. 6–31, the real-time image of the kidney in the transverse plane shows

   (A) renal hilum with normal vessels
   (B) renal collateral vessels
   (C) renal vein thrombosis
   (D) renal artery stenosis

34. In Fig. 6–32, the longitudinal real-time view of the abdominal aorta shows

   (A) aortic aneurysm
   (B) aortic dissection
   (C) aortic coarctation
   (D) aortic atherosclerotic disease with plaque

35. In Fig. 6–33, the real-time transverse view of the portal vein shows

   (A) enlarged portal vein secondary to cirrhosis
   (B) normal portal vein

   (C) portal vein with thrombus formation
   (D) total occlusion of the portal vein

36. In Fig. 6–34, the real-time longitudinal view of the abdominal aorta shows which branches?

   (A) celiac and inferior mesenteric arteries
   (B) hepatic and superior mesenteric arteries
   (C) celiac and inferior mesenteric arteries
   (D) celiac and superior mesenteric arteries

37. Which artery of the celiac axis is usually not seen on the ultrasound examination?

   (A) hepatic artery
   (B) splenic artery

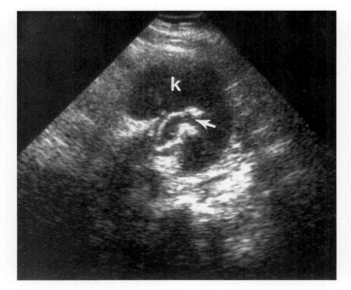

Figure 6–31. Real time image of the left kidney (k) and vessels (arrow).

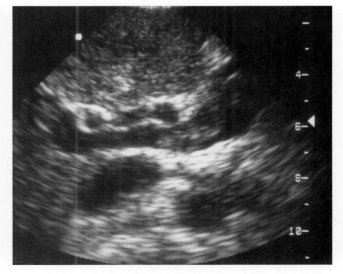

Figure 6–33. Real time image of the portal vein.

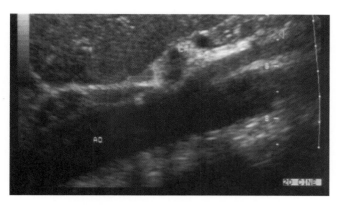

Figure 6–34. Real time image of the abdominal aorta.

(C) gastric artery
(D) renal artery

38. Which artery gives rise to the gastroduodenal artery?

(A) hepatic artery
(B) gastric artery
(C) splenic artery
(D) renal artery

39. Tributaries of the portal vein include

(A) splenic vein, superior mesenteric vein, coronary vein
(B) hepatic veins, splenic veins, gastric veins
(C) inferior vena cava, superior mesenteric veins
(D) superior mesenteric vein, splenic vein, para-umbilical vein, cystic vein, right gastric, left gastric

40. A patient in the supine resting position should have a portal vein measurement of no more than

(A) 7-mm in diameter
(B) 10-mm in diameter
(C) 13-mm in diameter
(D) 15-mm in diameter

41. Which veins enlarge as the approach the diaphragm?

(A) portal veins
(B) coronary veins
(C) hepatic veins
(D) splenic veins

42. Hepatic veins demonstrate what type of Doppler spectrum?

(A) chaotic, pulsatile phasic variations, and transmitted pulsations
(B) venous pattern with subtle phasic variations with respiration
(C) continuous high-pitched venous waveform
(D) low-pitch phasic flow variations

43. The gonadal veins drain the venous blood into the

(A) inferior vena cava
(B) renal veins
(C) inferior mesenteric vein
(D) iliac veins

44. Which of the following is not a surgical graft type for aortic aneurysms?

(A) simple aortic tube graft
(B) aortoiliac graft
(C) aortofemoral graft
(D) Brescia–Cimino

45. In a normal fasting patient, the SMA has which type of flow pattern?

(A) high-resistance
(B) low-resistance
(C) velocity exceeding 156 cm/s
(D) flow reversal

46. A venous collateral that arises from the portal vein approximately opposite of the superior mesenteric vein and seen on longitudinal images is the

(A) splenorenal
(B) gastroepiploic
(C) coronary vein
(D) umbilical vein

47. Which of the following is not characteristic of the right renal artery?

(A) It arises from the anterolateral aspect of the aorta.
(B) It passes posterior to the inferior vena cava from the aorta to the renal hilum.
(C) It has a low-resistance spectral waveform with forward flow throughout diastole.
(D) It lies anterior to the renal vein.

48. Which of the sonographic manifestations is not characteristic of rejection in a renal transplant?

(A) increased size of transplanted kidney
(B) prominence of renal pyramids
(C) decreased echogenicity of the renal sinus
(D) decreased flow resistance in the parenchymal arteries

49. The most common vascular complication of the renal transplant is

(A) renal artery occlusion
(B) renal artery stenosis
(C) arteriovenous fistula
(D) pseudoaneurysm

50. A pulsating abdominal mass slightly to the left of the midline suggests

(A) aortic occlusion
(B) acute mesenteric artery occlusion
(C) renovascular stenosis
(D) abdominal aortic aneurysm

51. The most common autologous AV fistula of the upper extremity for dialysis is

(A) loop forearm graft
(B) straight forearm graft
(C) upper arm loop graft
(D) Brescia–Cimino fistula

52. One of the most reliable clinical signs of patency in the dialysis graft is

(A) palpable thrill over the venous anastomosis
(B) pulses identified at the wrist
(C) absence of swelling, tenderness or erythema
(D) pulsating mass

53. Portal flow

(A) increases with expiration
(B) decreases with expiration
(C) increases with inspiration
(D) increases with exercise

54. Normal portal venous flow is

(A) hepatopetal (toward the liver)
(B) hepatofugal (away from the liver)
(C) bidirectional
(D) continuous high velocity

55. Cavernous transformation of the portal vein is

(A) thrombus in the intrahepatic portosystemic veins
(B) thrombus in the extrahepatic portosystemic veins
(C) obstruction of the hepatic veins
(D) obstruction of the inferior vena cava

56. Characteristics of portal hypertension does not include

(A) enlarged portal vein
(B) splenic enlargement
(C) portal flow may be reversed
(D) portal venous pressure less than 30 mm Hg

57. The term *caput medusae* means

(A) venous collaterals in the hemorrhoidal veins
(B) venous collaterals in the veins of Sappey
(C) coronary vein collaterals
(D) superficial multiple tubular anechoic structures in the umbilical region

58. Continuous venous flow indicates

(A) normal venous flow
(B) collateral venous flow
(C) portal venous flow
(D) hepatic venous flow

59. Increased portal pressure with decreased flow in the portal vein attributable to portal hypertension will

(A) decrease flow in the hepatic veins
(B) increase the portal venous flow
(C) decrease collateral venous flow
(D) increase collateral flow

60. A shunt between the left splenic vein and the left renal vein is

(A) splenocaval collateral
(B) pancreaticoduodenal varices
(C) splenorenal shunt
(D) periumbilical collateral

61. Which hepatic vein divides the liver into two lobes?

(A) right hepatic vein
(B) left hepatic vein
(C) middle hepatic vein
(D) portal vein

62. Transjugular intrahepatic portosystemic shunt (TIPS) is not

(A) surgical shunt for recurrent gastrointestinal bleeding
(B) a radiology interventional procedure
(C) treatment for recurrent gastrointestinal bleeding and refractory ascites in patients with portal hypertension
(D) placement of a metallic stent from the portal vein to the hepatic veins for reduction of venous pressure

63. Which is not a renal artery?

(A) segmental
(B) interlobar
(C) arcuate
(D) peroneal

64. The normal adult velocity range of the aorta is

(A) less than 70 cm/s
(B) 70–140 cm/s
(C) 100–150 cm/s
(D) 150–170 cm/s

65. The normal renal artery spectral waveform exhibits

(A) high impedance with absence of diastolic flow
(B) low impedance with continuous forward flow during diastole
(C) low impedance with negative flow during diastole
(D) high impedance with continuous forward flow during diastole

66. The renal veins are best seen on ultrasound in what position and plane?

(A) posterior in a longitudinal plane
(B) posterior in a transverse plane
(C) anterior in a longitudinal plane
(D) anterior in a transverse plane

67. A systolic blood pressure of 140 mm Hg or above is the definition for

(A) hydronephrosis
(B) hypertension
(C) chronic renal disease
(D) polycystic renal disease

68. If one kidney is much smaller than the other you would check for

(A) renal hydronephrosis
(B) renal mass
(C) renal artery stenosis
(D) occlusion of the renal vein

69. The acceleration time (AT) of the renal artery is defined as

(A) the interval from the onset of systolic flow to the initial peak systolic velocity
(B) the interval from the onset of diastolic flow to the initial peak systolic velocity
(C) the interval from the initial peak systolic velocity to the end of diastolic velocity
(D) the interval from the initial peak systolic velocity to the initial diastolic velocity

70. Tardus-parvus waveform refers to

(A) small partial pulse caused by proximal stenosis or occlusion
(B) small partial pulse caused by a distal stenosis or occlusion
(C) damped pulse caused by hydronephrosis
(D) damped pulse caused by a renal mass

71. In cases of renal artery stenosis the resistive index (RI)

(A) decreases
(B) remains approximately the same
(C) increases
(D) is variable

72. The term retroaortic renal vein means

(A) the left renal vein courses posterior to the abdominal aorta
(B) the left renal vein courses anterior to the abdominal aorta
(C) there are two left renal veins, one coursing anteriorly and one posteriorly
(D) the left renal vein runs posterior to the superior mesenteric artery

73. Clinical findings in cases of renal vein thrombosis do not include

(A) flank pain
(B) hematuria
(C) small sized kidney
(D) pulmonary embolism

74. The spectral waveform in the aorta

(A) rapid rise with a sharp systolic peak and rapid decline to the baseline during diastole
(B) low impedance with continuous forward flow during diastole
(C) sharp systolic peak with continuous forward flow during diastole
(D) high impedance with absence of diastole

75. Most of atherosclerotic aortic aneurysms occur at which level?

(A) at the level of the superior mesenteric and renal arteries
(B) below the level of the superior mesenteric and renal arteries
(C) above the level of the celiac axis
(D) between the celiac axis and the renal arteries

76. Which visceral artery changes its pattern and velocity after eating?

(A) splenic artery
(B) hepatic artery
(C) superior mesenteric artery
(D) renal artery

77. Which is the best imaging plane to demonstrate the celiac axis and its respective branches?

(A) longitudinal plane to the left of midline
(B) transverse plane just superior to the superior mesenteric artery
(C) transverse plane at the level of the renal arteries
(D) coronal plane depicting the aorta

78. Acute appendicitis would demonstrate

(A) increased vascularity
(B) decreased vascularity
(C) normal vascularity
(D) absence of blood flow

79. Blood flow to the appendix is via the

(A) superior mesenteric artery, ileocolic artery, appendicular artery
(B) inferior mesenteric artery, ileocolic artery, appendicular artery
(C) iliac artery, ileocolic artery, appendicular artery
(D) inferior mesenteric artery, iliac artery, appendicular artery

80. What renal transplant pathological condition has the same sonographic characteristics of rejection but differs in resistive index value?

   (A) occlusion of the renal artery
   (B) stenosis of the renal artery
   (C) presence of an arteriovenous malformation
   (D) acute tubular necrosis

81. Other than dialysis, what is another treatment for end-stage renal disease?

   (A) drug therapy
   (B) no treatment
   (C) transplantation
   (D) surgical removal of the diseased kidney

82. If a high-velocity jet is present at the site of stenosis in the renal artery, the color Doppler will show

   (A) laminar flow with slightly increased velocities in center stream
   (B) no change in the color in midstream
   (C) a mosaic color pattern representing turbulence and narrowing at the site of stenosis
   (D) an absence of color at the site of the high-velocity jet

83. The anastomosis site of the main renal artery in a renal transplant demonstrates a spectral waveform that wraps around with the peak appearing at the baseline. This is

   (A) aliasing because of exceeding the Nyquist limit
   (B) extreme turbulence with a forward and reverse flow pattern
   (C) an arteriovenous malformation with mixed arterial and venous patterns
   (D) a pseudoaneurysm with flow in and out of the aneurysm neck

84. An orthotopic liver transplant is

   (A) donor's organ is placed in an ectopic location
   (B) donor's organ placed in the normal location
   (C) portion of the donor's liver placed in an ectopic location
   (D) cadaver organ placed in an ectopic location

85. A complication of the liver transplant that is of critical importance is

   (A) rejection
   (B) mild biliary dilatation
   (C) portal vein narrowing
   (D) hepatic artery thrombosis

86. What type of dialysis access can be performed at home and is the least expensive

   (A) in-dwelling catheters
   (B) synthetic arteriovenous shunts

   (C) Brescia–Cimino fistula
   (D) peritoneal access

87. Color flow Doppler of the arteriovenous shunts shows

   (A) laminar flow pattern throughout the graft
   (B) mild turbulence at the anastomotic sites
   (C) no change in color patterns throughout the graft
   (D) mosaic pattern with turbulence throughout the graft

88. The synthetic dialysis access shunt in the arm will be located

   (A) in the forearm only
   (B) extend from the forearm to the upper arm
   (C) in the upper arm only
   (D) superficially

89. What provides the definitive diagnosis of a renal transplant perigraft mass or fluid collection?

   (A) ultrasound examination
   (B) angiography
   (C) aspiration/biopsy
   (D) scintigraphy

90. What is the most common cause of arteriovenous access shunt failure?

   (A) thrombosis
   (B) pseudoaneurysm
   (C) arteriovenous malformation
   (D) stenosis

91. Absence of color in the arteriovenous access shunt indicates

   (A) high-grade stenosis
   (B) occlusion
   (C) color settings set too low
   (D) color settings set too high

92. Gray scale imaging of the normal functional AV graft shows

   (A) two parallel echogenic walls with a sonolucent center
   (B) thin hypoechoic wall with an echogenic line in the center
   (C) two parallel echogenic walls with gray echoes in the center
   (D) absence of walls with an echogenic center

93. Which type of aneurysm typically has a "neck" with forward and reverse blood flow?

   (A) mycotic
   (B) saccular
   (C) fusiform
   (D) pseudoaneurysm

94. A noninvasive treatment for a pseudoaneurysm is

(A) ultrasound-guided compression repair
(B) angioplasty
(C) surgical reconstruction
(D) embolization

95. During an ultrasound-guided compression of the pseudoaneurysm, which lies adjacent to the common femoral artery, what vital sign is continuously monitored?

(A) common femoral arterial pulse
(B) iliac arterial pulse
(C) superficial femoral arterial pulse
(D) pedal pulse

96. In cases of acute arterial occlusion there is usually

(A) absence of collateral flow
(B) extensive collateral flow
(C) trickle flow
(D) intermittent flow

97. The etiology of the majority of arterial diseases is

(A) diabetes
(B) hypertension
(C) smoking
(D) atherosclerosis

98. The greatest risk of aortic aneurysms is

(A) dissection
(B) thrombus formation
(C) rupture
(D) extension into adjacent vessels

99. An abdominal bruit suggests

(A) presence of venous collaterals
(B) venous occlusion
(C) arterial aneurysm
(D) arterial stenosis or occlusive disease

100. The most common correctable cause of renal hypertension is

(A) genetic factors
(B) environmental factors
(C) chronic renal disease
(D) renal artery stenosis

101. The origin of the gastroduodenal artery is

(A) aorta
(B) superior mesenteric artery
(C) inferior mesenteric artery
(D) hepatic artery

102. Avascular is

(A) absence of vascular flow
(B) increased vascular flow

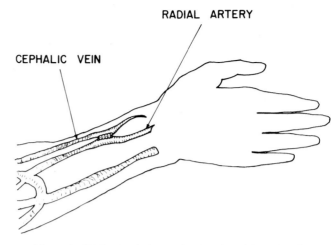

Figure 6–35. Anatomical vascular drawing of the extremity.

(C) intermittent vascular flow
(D) normal vascular flow

103. Fig. 6–35 is an anatomical drawing of

(A) straight graft
(B) loop graft
(C) Brescia–Cimino graft
(D) catheter

104. In Fig. 6–36, the longitudinal real-time scan of the aorta demonstrates

(A) saccular aneurysm
(B) fusiform aneurysm
(C) dissecting aneurysm
(D) pseudoaneurysm

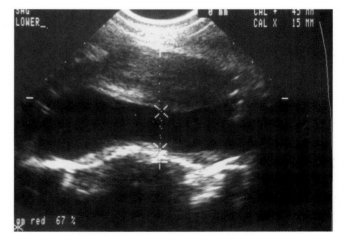

Figure 6–36. Longitudinal real time image of the aorta.

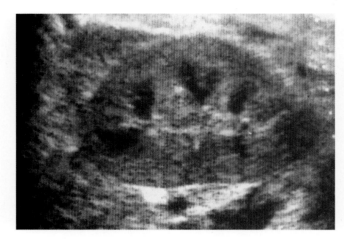

Figure 6–37. Renal transplant.

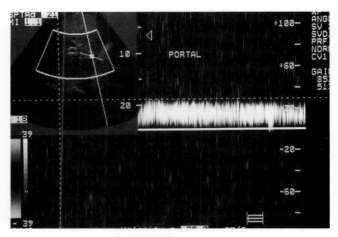

Figure 6–39. Spectral analysis of the portal vein.

105. In Fig. 6–37, the real-time scan of a renal transplant with clinical findings of pain and tenderness over the transplant and elevated serum creatinine levels indicates

(A) hydronephrosis
(B) perirenal mass
(C) rejection
(D) renal infarct

106. In Fig. 6–38, the longitudinal color flow Doppler of the spleen in a patient with bleeding esophageal varices shows

(A) splenic aneurysm
(B) splenorenal collaterals
(C) normal splenic vessels
(D) dilated splenic vein with varices

107. In Fig. 6–39, Doppler spectral analysis of the portal vein in a patient with portal hypertension demonstrates

(A) increased portal venous flow without respiratory changes

(B) continuous portal venous flow without respiratory changes
(C) biphasic portal venous flow without respiratory changes
(D) normal portal venous flow

108. Fig. 6–40 shows a transverse real-time image of the abdomen. Name the vascular structures.

109. Fig. 6–41 shows an angiography of the celiac axis. Name the three primary branches.

(A) hepatic, gastric, splenic
(B) hepatic, gastric, superior mesenteric
(C) gastric, splenic, superior mesenteric
(D) splenic, superior mesenteric, inferior mesenteric

110. Which of the three branches shown in Fig. 6–38 is usually not seen on the ultrasound examination?

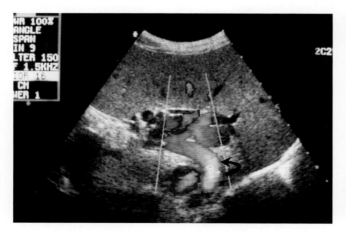

Figure 6–38. Color flow Doppler scan of the spleen.

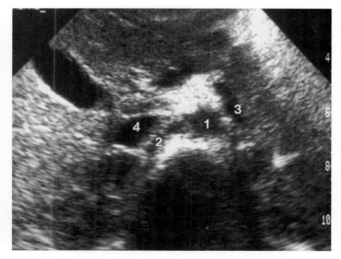

Figure 6–40. Transverse real time view of the abdomen.

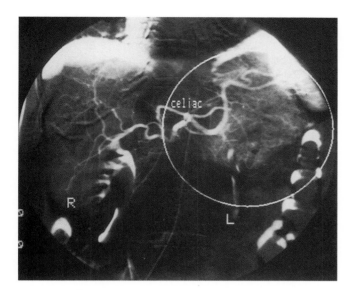

Figure 6–41. Angiogram of the celiac artery.

(A) hepatic
(B) gastric
(C) splenic
(D) superior mesenteric

111. In Fig. 6–42, spectral analysis of the superior mesenteric artery indicates

(A) fasting state
(B) postprandial state
(C) SMA stenosis
(D) SMA occlusion

112. The superior mesenteric artery is best seen on real-time examination in what plane?

(A) transverse
(B) longitudinal

(C) oblique
(D) lateral

113. In Fig. 6–43, the large vascular structure in the abdomen that runs parallel to the long axis of the body and slightly to the right of the midline is the

(A) aorta
(B) inferior vena cava
(C) superior mesenteric artery
(D) iliac artery

114. In Fig. 6–44, contrast venography of the abdominal vessels shows

(A) stenosis of the inferior vena cava
(B) occlusion of the inferior vena cava
(C) occlusion of the aorta
(D) stenosis of the aorta

115. The blood supply to the gallbladder is supplied by the

(A) left hepatic artery
(B) middle hepatic artery
(C) right hepatic artery
(D) cystic artery

116. In Fig. 6–45, color flow Doppler with spectral analysis of the renal transplant shows

(A) pseudoaneurysm
(B) renal artery stenosis
(C) arteriovenous malformation
(D) renal artery occlusion

117. In Fig. 6–46, angiogram of the liver transplant and spectral waveform analysis of the hepatic artery shows

(A) occlusion of the hepatic artery
(B) normal hepatic artery
(C) hepatic artery stenosis
(D) hepatic artery aneurysm

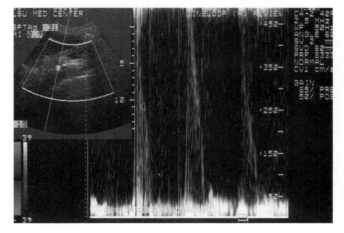

Figure 6–42. Spectral analysis of the superior mesenteric artery.

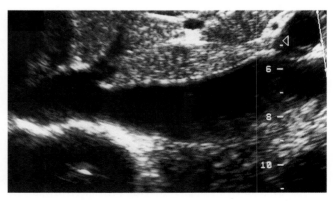

Figure 6–43. Real time image in a longitudinal plane just to the right of the midline.

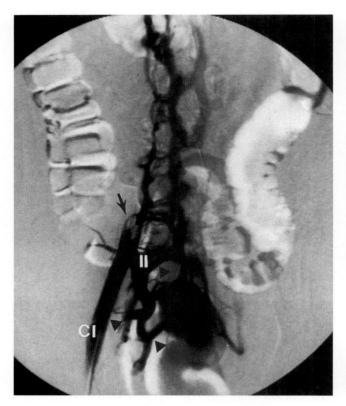

Figure 6–44. Contrast venography of the abdominal veins.

118. In Fig. 6–47, the angiogram shows which type of graft?

    (A) loop graft of the upper arm
    (B) straight graft of the upper arm
    (C) straight graft of the forearm
    (D) loop graft of the forearm

119. In Fig. 6–48, an interventional radiology technique seen in the figure to treat a mycotic aneurysm is

    (A) surgical reconstruction
    (B) ultrasound-guided compression
    (C) angiography and embolization
    (D) angiography with angioplasty

120. In Fig. 6–49, identify the numbered renal arteries in the digital angiogram.

121. What color flow Doppler technique shows the perfusion of the kidney but does not show speed or direction?

    (A) spectral waveform analysis
    (B) color flow Doppler imaging with spectral analysis
    (C) gray scale imaging
    (D) power Doppler

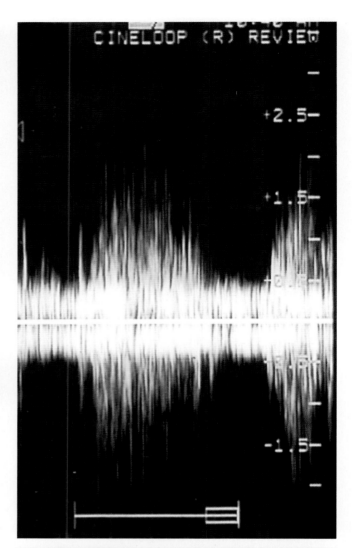

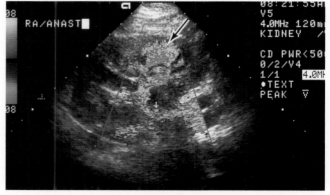

Figure 6–45. Color flow Doppler and spectral analysis of the renal transplant.

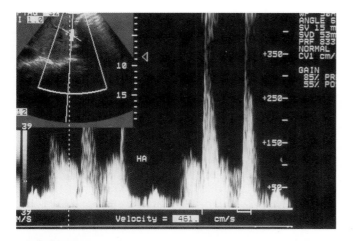

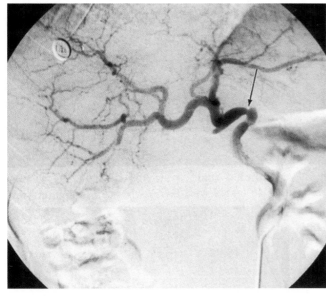

Figure 6–46. Angiogram and spectral analysis of the hepatic artery in a liver transplant.

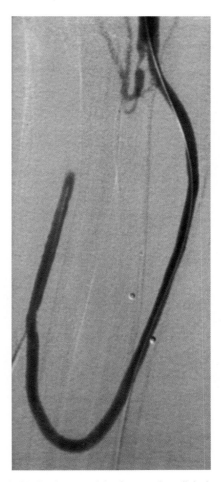

Figure 6–47. Angiogram of the forearm in a dialysis patient.

122. In Fig. 6–50, the spectral analysis of the normal renal artery is

    (A) high resistance with continuous forward flow in diastole

    (B) low resistance with an RI greater than 0.8

    (C) low resistance with continuous forward flow in diastole

    (D) high resistance at the origin and low resistance distally

123. Which is not correct? Distal to a renal artery stenosis the waveform shows

    (A) damping of intrarenal arteries

    (B) increase in systolic velocity

    (C) poststenotic turbulence

    (D) prolonged systolic acceleration time

    (E) absence of an early systolic peak

124. In Fig. 6–51, the real-time longitudinal scan of a renal transplant shows

    (A) hydronephrosis

    (B) perirenal mass

    (C) rejection

    (D) renal infarct

125. In Fig. 6–52, the color flow Doppler scan of the iliac and femoral arterial junction in a patient who has recently had heart catheterization shows

    (A) normal vessels

    (B) occlusion of the common femoral artery

    (C) common femoral artery stenosis

    (D) pseudoaneurysm

126. In Fig. 6–53, the real-time transverse scan at the level of the xiphoid process shows which vessels?

    (A) portal veins

    (B) hepatic artery

    (C) hepatic veins

    (D) renal arteries

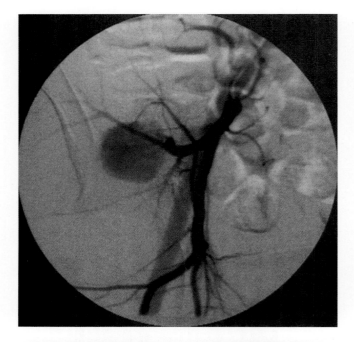

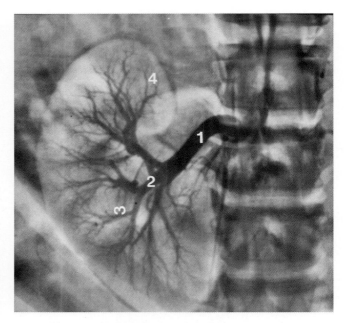

Figure 6–49. Digital subtraction of the renal arteries.

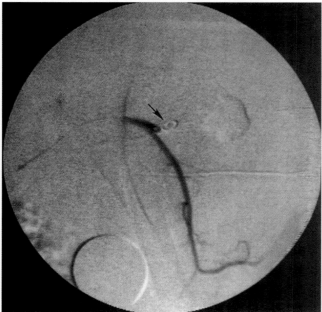

Figure 6–48. Angiogram and interventional procedure of the gluteal artery.

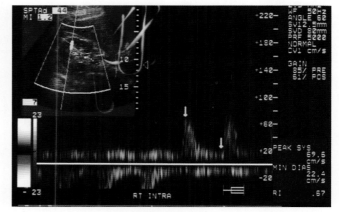

Figure 6–50. Spectral analysis of the renal artery.

127. In Fig. 6–54, the real-time transverse scan at the level of the xiphoid demonstrates

    (A) aortic aneurysm
    (B) portal vein thrombosis
    (C) thrombosis of the IVC extending into the hepatic veins
    (D) normal scan

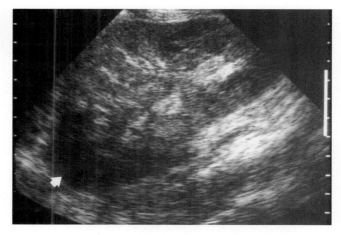

Figure 6–51. Real time image of the renal transplant.

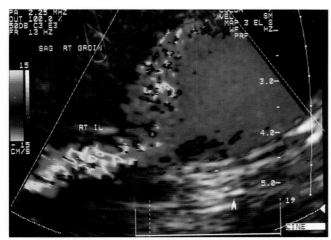

Figure 6–52. Color flow Doppler image of the iliac and common femoral arteries.

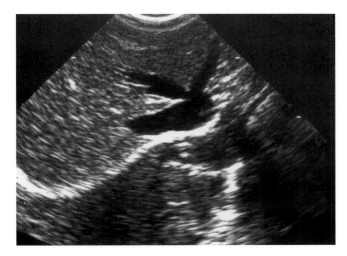

Figure 6–53. Real time transverse scan at the level of the xiphoid.

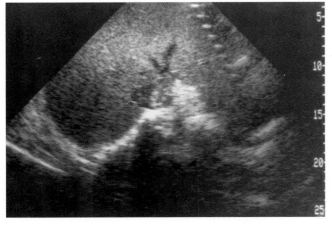

Figure 6–54. Real time transverse scan at the level of the xiphoid.

128. Transducer design for color flow Doppler of the abdomen includes

(A) mechanical sector
(B) phased array
(C) linear array
(D) A and B
(E) B and C
(F) all of the above

129. Which is not a transducer used for color flow Doppler applications?

(A) mechanical sector
(B) curvilinear array
(C) phased array
(D) continuous wave

130. Color flow Doppler uses the term "hue"; what is the meaning?

(A) amplitude information from the color signal
(B) saturation of the color signal
(C) brightness of the color signal
(D) perceived color dependent on frequency shift

131. To correct for aliasing of the spectral waveform you would not

(A) increase the frequency
(B) decrease the sample volume level
(C) adjust the baseline shift
(D) decrease the frequency

132. To ensure that low-level venous flow is detected we do not

(A) use high wall filters
(B) use low wall filters
(C) decrease the sampling rate (PRF)
(D) increase the color sensitivity

133. The most common type of liver transplant is

(A) orthotopic cadaver
(B) orthotopic partial
(C) heterotopic cadaver
(D) heterotopic partial

134. The abdominal aorta is considered aneurysmal if it exceeds

(A) 0.5 cm
(B) 1 cm
(C) 2 cm
(D) 3 cm

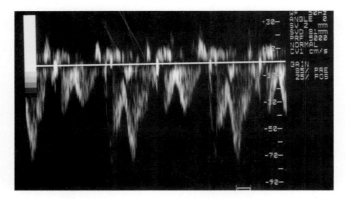

Figure 6–55. Spectral analysis of abdominal vein.

135. In Fig. 6–55, the spectral analysis waveform is characteristic of normal

(A) hepatic veins
(B) portal vein
(C) renal vein
(D) splenic vein

136. In Fig. 6–56, the color flow Doppler scan of the TIPS shows

(A) occlusion with absence of flow
(B) pre-occlusive with minimal flow
(C) stenosis with a color jet
(D) normal flow

137. Which vein courses in a transverse plane and underlies the body of the pancreas?

(A) superior mesenteric vein
(B) splenic vein
(C) portal vein
(D) superior and inferior mesenteric vein

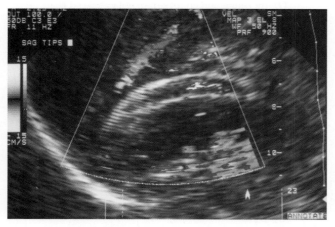

Figure 6–56. Color flow Doppler of the TIPS.

138. Which vessel is not included in a vascular examination of the renal transplant?

(A) iliac artery
(B) main renal artery
(C) intrarenal arteries (segmental, interlobar, intelobular, and arcuate)
(D) renal and iliac veins
(E) inferior vena cava

139. Which of the following scans is not routinely used to demonstrate the renal arteries?

(A) transverse scan of the aorta with origin of the renal arteries
(B) transverse scan of the renal artery at the hilum of the kidney
(C) longitudinal or transverse of the renal parenchyma for the intrarenal arteries
(D) transverse posterior scan of the renal hilum

140. Is the cystic artery of the gallbladder routinely seen on the abdominal color flow Doppler examination?

(A) yes
(B) no
(C) about 50% of the time
(D) about 75% of the time

141. What type of instrumentation is used with contrast agents?

(A) power angio
(B) continuous wave
(C) spectral waveform analysis
(D) harmonic imaging

142. Manifestations of portal hypertension caused by increasing venous pressure include

(A) bleeding esophageal varices
(B) ascites
(C) enlarge spleen
(D) all of the above

143. Which of the following is not true?

(A) Aortic aneurysms may be asymptomatic.
(B) Aortic aneurysms may be incidentally noted on an abdominal x-ray caused by calcifications in the aneurysm wall.
(C) usually occur below the level of the renal arteries
(D) may present as a pulsating mass
(E) usually have a membrane separating the true and false lumen

144. An acute appendix usually presents on color flow Doppler and real-time images as

(A) hypoechoic appendix with increased vascular flow

(B) hypoechoic appendix with decreased vascular flow

(C) is not seen on the ultrasound examination

(D) echogenic appendix with decreased vascular flow

145. Collateral vessels are

(A) secondary vessels that supply blood to circumvent obstructed vessels

(B) the main arterial blood supply

(C) have the same type of spectral waveform as the normal vessel

(D) have the same pathway as the normal vessel

146. Before scanning the transplant patient, it is of vital importance to know

(A) when the transplant was performed

(B) whether it is orthotopic or heterotopic

(C) what the patient's symptoms are

(D) the surgical procedure, how it was performed, and the anastomotic sites

147. Venous in-dwelling catheters have a propensity for

(A) infection

(B) displacement

(C) thrombus

(D) calcification

148. The key factor in management of a ruptured aortic aneurysm is

(A) obtain an angiogram

(B) obtain an ultrasound

(C) obtain an MRI

(D) expedite the patient to surgery

149. Complications of aortic graft surgery are

(A) hemorrhage or hematoma

(B) aneurysm or pseudoaneurysm

(C) stenosis or ischemia

(D) occlusion

(E) infection

(F) all of the above

150. Peripheral artery aneurysms occur more commonly in the

(A) aorta

(B) iliac

(C) femoral

(D) popliteal

(E) A and B

(F) all of the above

Answers and Explanations

At the end of each explained answer there is a number combination in parentheses. The first number identifies the reference source; the second number or set of numbers indicates the page or pages on which the relevant information can be found.

1. **(A)** The celiac artery has three branches; the common hepatic, splenic, and left gastric arteries.
(1:768; 2:379)

2. **(C)** The celiac artery also termed, celiac trunk or celiac axis, is the most cephalad visceral branch of the abdominal aorta. Followed by the superior mesenteric artery, the renal arteries, and the inferior mesenteric artery. *(2:379, 389)*

3. **(D)** The celiac trunk and two of its branches; the common hepatic artery and the splenic artery, appear as a "seagull" or "T configuration" in the transverse plane of the real-time or color flow Doppler scan. These vessels lie superior to the superior mesenteric, renal, and gastroduodenal arteries. *(3:204, 2:379)*

4. **(C)** Splanchnic arteries refer to the vessels that supply the bowel with blood. They are primarily the celiac artery, the superior mesenteric artery, and the inferior mesenteric artery. *(2:421)*

5. **(A)** There are several types of aneurysms which include: saccular, fusiform, false, mycotic, and dissecting. Saccular and fusiform are shapes of true aneurysms (dilatation of the arterial wall) with different anatomical configurations. The false or pseudoaneurysm is caused by a hole in the wall of a vessel and is not confined to the arterial wall. A dissection is where blood enters the medial of the vessel and dissects the vessel into a true and false lumen. The micotic aneurysm develops secondary to a septic emboli lodging in the arterial lumen.
(2:397, 398; 3:425)

6. **(B)** Classically, the dissecting aneurysm has two lumens separated by an echogenic intimal flap that can be seen on the real-time scan pulsating toward the true lumen. *(3:203)*

7. **(D)** In the normal fasting state, the superior mesenteric artery and inferior mesenteric arteries have a high resistance flow pattern. After the ingestion of a meal, the blood flow increases, and the high-resistance flow pattern changes to a low-resistance flow pattern. This is not true for the celiac artery, which the low-resistance pattern remains constant. *(2:422)*

8. **(C)** Renal artery stenosis is diagnosed by Doppler ultrasound when the peak systolic velocity in the stenosis is 180–200 cm/s or greater or when the peak systolic velocity of the renal artery is 3.5 times the peak systolic velocity of the aorta. This is the primary criterion. Other criteria include: damping of the distal waveform, and the acceleration index.
(2:461, 462; 4:8; 3:185, 186)

9. **(D)** Angiography is not only important to provide a definitive diagnosis for occlusion of the splanchnic arteries but also an important part of the successful management of acute intestinal ischemia. Angiography demonstrates the obstructing lesions as well as the collateral flow patterns and can provide such interventional procedures as thrombolytic therapy.
(5:239, 240)

10. **(D)** The most common pathological condition of the inferior vena cava is thrombosis followed by neoplasia or tumor. *(2:415, 416)*

11. **(B)** The portal vein supplies 75–80% of the blood supply to the liver and 50% of the oxygen. The hepatic artery supplies the remainder of the blood supply to the liver. In cases of portal hypertension where the portal venous flow is compromised, there is usually an increase in the hepatic artery flow to the liver. *(3:135)*

12. **(A)** The splenic and superior mesenteric veins and, in some cases, the inferior mesenteric vein join to form the portal vein posterior to the neck of the pancreas.
(3:135)

13. **(B)** The portal triad also termed the hepatic triad, which is defined as a group of three entities, objects,

or associations, includes the hepatic artery, portal vein, and bile duct, seen on the real-time image in the porta hepatis region.   *(7:1391)*

14. **(C)** Mycotic or infected aneurysm are caused by a growth of microorganisms in the vessel walls. They occur in multiple sites and are often seen as a complication of bacterial endocarditis. *(7:74; 3:425, 426)*

15. **(A)** Alcoholism is the most common cause of cirrhosis in the western hemisphere. Cirrhosis is one of the ten leading causes of death and the most common cause of cirrhosis in the United States. Cirrhosis is the end-stage manifestation of hepatocyte injury leading to tissue necrosis, fibrosis, and attempted regeneration of liver tissue.   *(6:941; 7:39; 2:439)*

16. **(D)** The umbilical or paraumbilical vein collateral is indicative of portal hypertension. It communicates with the superficial veins of the abdominal wall and connects freely with the superior and inferior epigastric veins. In advanced stages, it is called caput Medusae.   *(6:1282; 2:441; 7:742)*

17. **(C)** The renal artery spectral waveform exhibits a low-resistance flow pattern with continuous forward flow in diastole. A resistive index of 0.70 has been considered the upper limit of normal in adults.
(2:394; 3:177, 180)

18. **(B)** The common vascular pathway for tumor or thrombus extension is the inferior vena cava. Extrinsic tumors can compress or invade the inferior vena cava and include renal cell carcinoma, hepatocellular carcinoma, and a variety of other neoplasms that metastasize to the paracaval lymph nodes.
(2:416; 9:1076)

19. **(A)** Budd–Chiari disease or syndrome is defined as symptomatic obstruction or occlusion of the hepatic veins. It can be either acute or chronic with an unknown etiology. Possibly arising from neoplasms, strictures, liver disease, trauma, systemic infections, and hematologic disorders.   *(7:1289)*

20. **(A)** In patients with celiac artery occlusion at the origin, the collateral flow may be sufficient to produce normal Doppler signals in the hepatic and splenic arteries; however, the flow is reversed in the gastroduodenal and common hepatic arteries. *(2:421, 428)*

21. **(D)** Stenosis or occlusion of the splanchnic arteries can cause bowel ischemia. This is often prevented by collateralization through three main collateral channels; the pancreaticoduodenal arcade, the arch of Riolan, and the marginal artery of Drummond.
(2:421; 5:236)

22. **(D)** Classically the abdominal aortic aneurysm is dilated to 3 cm or more or 1.5 times the normal seg-

ment. The majority of abdominal aortic aneurysms are located in the infrarenal portion of the aorta and may extend into the iliac arteries. However, the renal arteries along with the iliac arteries are included in the sonographic examination to assist in the type of surgical reconstruction required.   *(2:397, 398; 3:197)*

23. **(B)** Branches of the hepatic artery include; the gastroduodenal, right gastric, right and left hepatic branches, cystic, intrahepatic branches, and occasionally the supraduodenal arteries. The splenic artery arises form the celiac artery and the celiac artery, arises from the aorta.   *(1:768)*

24. **(C)** The color scan view of the celiac demonstrates a turbulent mixture of colors. The spectral waveform analysis demonstrate a velocity of 329 cm/s, increased resistance, and spectral broadening, which indicates celiac artery stenosis. Celiac artery peak systolic velocity in normal fasting patients does not exceed 122 cm/s and end diastolic velocity ranges from 32 to 35 cm/s.   *(2:422; 10:337–342)*

25. **(A)** In the normal TIPS (Transjugular intrahepatic portosystemic shunts), color flow fills the stent from wall to wall with some turbulence present. The waveform is a phasic venous pattern that may be slightly pulsatile. Peak systolic velocity in the shunt normally ranges from 90 to 120 cm/s. Velocity ranges should be the same in both ends of the shunt. The portal vein is hepatopedal and increased compared to the preTIPS velocity. Portal vein velocity is at least 30 cm/s.   *(2:444; 11:1–7)*

26. **(C)** The gray scale real-time image demonstrates the occluded portal vein (P) filled with echoes. Superior to the portal vein multiple circular structures represent the periportal collaterals (arrows) The most important sonographic diagnostic signs of portal occlusion is the absence of portal flow and the lumen filled with echoes. Chronic portal vein thrombosis produces multiple tangles of tortuous vessels in the porta hepatis, which is termed cavernous transformation.   *(2:446)*

27. **(A)** Transverse plane of an aortic aneurysm with thrombus formation (T) and measurement of the internal and external lumen. Ultrasound is unique in that it demonstrates the patent internal lumen as well as thrombus and the external lumen. CT and MRI are superior to ultrasound in demonstrating leakage or rupture of an aneurysm. Contrast angiography identifies the site of origin and pattern of the aneurysm.   *(3:200)*

28. **(D)** Color Doppler liver in the longitudinal plane demonstrates an enlarged paraumbilical collateral vein entering the portal vein. It classically courses from the portal vein inferiorly through the falciform

ligament and continues superficially along the abdominal wall. This is a clinical hallmark of portal hypertension. The cirrhotic shrunken liver is also seen surrounded by ascites.   *(2:441–443; 9:943)*

29. **(C)** A high-grade velocity in excess of 637 cm/s at the anastomotic site of the native artery (inflow stenosis) and the dialysis graft. The waveform shows greatly increased velocities, increased diastolic flow, and spectral broadening. The velocity is always higher at the anastomotic sites; however, it should be no greater than 400 cm/s.   *(2:20; 3:412)*

30. **(B)** A longitudinal color flow Doppler scan approximately 2 cm the right shows the distended IVC completely filled with echoes, which rules out partial obstruction. There is no narrowing of the vessel as would be seen with a stricture or stenosis and no color flow as seen in the patent SMV and the hepatic vein.   *(2:415–416)*

31. **(B)** Distal to a high-grade stenosis the spectral waveform will be damped and monophasic. If there was occlusion of the main renal artery, there would be no flow. The normal renal artery is a low resistance triphasic waveform; however, distal to the stenosis it becomes grossly rounded, and monophasic.   *(2:462)*

32. **(C)** High-grade stenosis demonstrated on the spectral analysis with a systolic peak velocity of over 552 cm/s with aliasing. The normal peak systolic velocity in the normal renal arteries is 74 to 127 cm/s.   *(2:461)*

33. **(C)** The real-time image of the kidney (K) in the transverse plane at the level of the renal hilum shows an occluded distended vein filled with echoes (arrow). This is a common route for tumor or thrombus extension. Normal vessels would be smaller in size and sonolucent. Collateral vessels are variable in size and tortuous. To identify the absence of renal venous flow the Doppler cursor would be placed in the renal artery to identify the arterial waveform and then moved to the occluded vessel showing no venous flow.   *(9:1076)*

34. **(B)** Real-time imaging demonstrates the sonolucent aorta with an echogenic membrane that was pulsating toward the lumen, characteristic of an aortic dissection. It can be seen that the echogenic membrane divides the aorta into two lumens, one much smaller than the other. This is the false lumen (smaller) and the true lumen (larger). There is no dilatation, as with aneurysm, or narrowing, as with coarctation. The vessel is free from any calcifications or plaque formation associated with atherosclerotic disease.   *(3:203)*

35. **(C)** The transverse enlarged ultrasound view of the portal vein shows an echogenic thrombus in the lumen of the vessel. It is not totally occluded, and the remaining lumen is sonolucent. There is an area of focal dilatation in the region of the thrombosis, but overall, the portal vein is not enlarged. In cases where isolated thrombus is seen in the portal vein, a careful survey should be done to see any extension of the thrombus and to verify flow, partial flow, or occlusion.   *(2:446)*

36. **(D)** The real-time longitudinal scan obtained 1 cm to the left of the midline shows the abdominal aorta and two branches. The first shorter branch is the celiac, which is the first branch of the aorta, and the longer branch just inferiorly to the celiac is the superior mesenteric artery. This is an excellent view to see the origin of these vessels and to determine if there is any narrowing, plaque, or calcifications present.   *(2:379, 380)*

37. **(C)** The celiac artery has a right branch (hepatic artery), a left branch (gastric artery), which is usually not seen on the ultrasound, and splenic, which is a left branch. The hepatic artery and the splenic artery are identified as the "seagull appearance" or the "T configuration" on ultrasound.   *(2:379)*

38. **(A)** The first branch of hepatic artery is the gastroduodenal artery, and it courses between the duodenum and the neck of the pancreas. The gastroduodenal artery is located anterolateral to the head of the pancreas; the common bile duct is posterolateral to the inferior portion of the head of the pancreas. This landmark has long been used to identify the location of the common bile duct.   *(1:768, 769; 3:85)*

39. **(D)** The tributaries of the portal vein include: splenic, superior mesenteric, left gastric, right gastric, paraumbilical, and cystic veins. Those routinely seen on ultrasound include the splenic and superior mesenteric veins.   *(1:819)*

40. **(C)** The diameter of the portal vein should not exceed 13 mm and should vary with inspiration and expiration.   *(3:135; 2:390)*

41. **(C)** The hepatic veins enlarge as they approach the diaphragm, and the portal veins appear larger as they approach the porta hepatis. This has long been a method of differentiation of the hepatic veins and the portal veins.   *(8:17)*

42. **(A)** The hepatic veins venous flow is chaotic, with phasic variations and transmitted pulsations. They differ from the collateral venous vessels with continuous high-pitched Doppler waveforms and the low phasic flow seen in other venous structures. The pulsatile pattern is a result of the transmission of right atrial pulsations into the veins.   *(2:392)*

43. **(B)** The testicular veins and the ovarian veins which constitute the gonadal veins drain into the renal veins and subsequently the inferior vena cava. This is an important concept when determining patency of the gonadal veins. *(1:818)*

44. **(D)** The Brescia–Cimino fistula is an autogenous dialysis access graft. The others are aortic aneurysm surgical grafts named according to location of the graft and the arteries involved. *(4:20)*

45. **(A)** The superior mesenteric has a high-resistance flow pattern in the fasting patient. It may be turbulent at the origin, and there may be absent or reverse flow in diastole. Blood flow increases after eating. The normal peak systolic velocity in the fasting patient is approximately 140 cm/s and does not exceed 156 cm/s. *(2:389, 422; 3:209, 210)*

46. **(C)** The portosystemic collateral that arises from the portal at the level of the superior mesenteric is the coronary vein or left gastric vein. The normal coronary vein does not exceed 4 mm. In cases of portal hypertension, a search is made to identify this collateral vessel. *(2:441–443)*

47. **(D)** The right renal artery lies posterior to the renal vein. It is unique in that it passes posterior to the inferior vena cava as it courses from the hilum to the aorta. It arises from an anterolateral aspect of the aorta and has a low resistance waveform. *(2:455)*

48. **(D)** The classical gray scale characteristics of renal transplant rejection include: hypoechogenicity, enlargement of the renal pyramids, increased size of the transplant with diminished echogenicity of the renal sinus echo complex, and increased echogenicity of the cortex. The pulsatility index is greater than 1.8, and the resistivity index is greater than 0.9, indicating increased peripheral resistance. *(8:169, 170; 2:468)*

49. **(B)** In the renal transplant, renal artery stenosis is the most common vascular complication, while occlusion of the renal artery is less common. *(2:470–471)*

50. **(D)** A pulsating abdominal mass in the region of the aorta, slightly left of the midline would suggest an aortic aneurysm. In cases of stenosis or atherosclerosis, a systolic bruit is often heard. In the abdominal vessels, a bruit would be heard. In cases of occlusion of the abdominal arteries, pain and necrosis are generally the manifestations. *(6:901)*

51. **(D)** The Brescia–Cimino fistula is the most common autologous fistula for dialysis access. It is constructed between the cephalic vein and the radial artery. Other types are the antecubital between the basilic or cephalic veins and the brachial artery. For chronic dialysis, the most common type of dialysis access is the synthetic AV shunt grafts which may be loop or straight grafts, placed in the forearm or upper arm. *(5:285)*

52. **(A)** One of the most reliable signs of dialysis graft patency is a palpable thrill over the venous anastomosis and distal vein. Other clinical evaluations for patency include the listening of the machinery-type murmur with a stethoscope and checking the hand for any ischemic steal syndromes. *(5:288)*

53. **(A)** Portal venous flow has hepatopetal flow toward the liver that decreases with inspiration and increases with expiration. The normal velocity is approximately 20–30 cm/s. Flow also decreases with exercise and with chronic liver disease. *(3:135, 138)*

54. **(A)** Portal venous flow is toward the liver (hepatopetal); however, with chronic liver disease it may be reversed (hepatofugal) or bidirectional. *(3:135, 149)*

55. **(B)** Cavernous transformation of the portal vein occurs secondary to thrombosis of the extrahepatic portal vein. This leads to the formation of periportal collaterals in the porta hepatis around the obstructed portal vein. *(3:144)*

56. **(D)** Portal hypertension is defined as portal vein pressure of more than 30 mm Hg. Characteristics include: enlarged portal vein, splenic enlargement, reversed or bidirectional flow, patent venous collateral patterns, and decreased flow in the portal vein. *(3:148, 162)*

57. **(D)** *Caput medusae* is defined as dilated cutaneous veins around the umbilicus primarily seen in the newborn or patients with cirrhosis of the liver. This is a very striking clinical presentation. Usually, the patient with cirrhosis has a distended abdomen with multitudes of superficial collateral vessels seen around the belly button. *(7:217)*

58. **(B)** Normally venous flow is phasic with respiration. Continuous venous flow is seen with venous collaterals. Collateral venous flow is often high pitched and does not change with respiration. *(3:149; 12:293)*

59. **(D)** In cases of portal hypertension, where flow is restricted through the liver, alternate routes or portosystemic collaterals develop to conduct the blood to the heart. As portal flow decreases and pressure increases, the collateral flow will increase. *(2:441)*

60. **(C)** The splenorenal shunt is one of the portosystemic collaterals seen in portal hypertension. *(3:162, 163; 12:295, 296)*

61. (C) The middle hepatic vein divides the liver into two lobes. It runs in the main interlobar fissure. The right hepatic vein divides the right lobe of the liver into the posterior and anterior segments and the left hepatic vein divides the left lobe of the liver into medial and lateral segments.   *(3:154)*

62. (A) The TIPS procedure is a radiology interventional procedure that is an alternative to the surgically created shunt for treatment of the portal hypertensive patient.   *(3:160)*

63. (D) The renal artery and its corresponding branches include: main, segmental, interlobar, arcuate, and interlobular arteries. The peroneal is a continuation or branch of the popliteal artery.   *(3:179; 7:789)*

64. (B) The velocity of the aorta is normally in the range of 70–140 cm/s.   *(12:240; 3:196)*

65. (B) The renal arteries have a low resistance flow pattern with continuous forward flow during diastole. This is caused by the low resistance in the renal vascular bed and will be seen throughout the kidney.   *(2:394)*

66. (D) The renal veins are best seen in the transverse plane from the anterior. In children, a coronal plane from the lateral position is often used.   *(2:394)*

67. (B) Hypertension is defined as persistent high arterial blood pressure. The criteria include 140 mm Hg systolic and 90 mm Hg diastolic, and these can vary somewhat according to various authors.   *(7:635; 3:184)*

68. (C) If one kidney is much smaller than the other, you would automatically evaluate the renal arteries and evaluate for renal artery stenosis. In cases of renal vein occlusion, the kidney tends to enlarge because of venous congestion. In cases of renal masses, depending on the size of the mass, the kidney will increase in size with respect to the size of the mass. In cases of hydronephrosis, the kidney will enlarge as the collecting system of the kidney becomes increasing dilated.   *(3:184)*

69. (A) Acceleration time (AT) is defined as the interval from the onset of the systolic flow to the initial peak systolic velocity with the normal value 0.07–0.1 s.   *(3:185; 2:462)*

70. (A) Tardus-parvus is also referred to as a small pulse or partial, seen secondary to renal artery stenosis. It is seen distal to the renal artery stenosis in the intrarenal arteries. The "tardus" indicates a prolonged or delayed early systolic acceleration and the "parvus" means the diminished amplitude and rounding of the systolic peak.   *(2:463)(3:186)(13:26–29)*

71. (C) The resistive index as well as the acceleration time will increase with renal artery stenosis.   *(3:186)*

72. (A) The left renal vein courses anterior to the aorta and posterior to the SMA. However variants include: the left renal vein is circumaortic with separate veins passing anterior and posterior to the aorta and retroaortic where the renal vein courses posterior to the aorta.   *(2:394)*

73. (C) Clinical findings of renal vein thrombosis include pain, hematuria, and the possible complication of pulmonary embolism. The kidney is usually swollen due to the venous congestion. A small sized kidney is usually associated with renal artery stenosis or chronic renal disease.   *(2:464)*

74. (A) The aorta spectral waveform is a triphasic high resistant waveform characteristic of peripheral arteries. The waveform has a rapid rise with a sharp systolic peak and a rapid decline to the baseline during diastole. The velocity is normally in the range of 70–140 cm/s. The aorta is used as a standard by which other abdominal vessels are compared.   *(12:240; 3:196)*

75. (B) The vast majority of atherosclerotic aneurysms are below the level of the renal arteries or infrarenal. The simplest and least expensive test to diagnose and measure the aortic aneurysm is ultrasound. It provides reliable measurement within 3–4 mm of the actual size. The anterior posterior diameter being the best plane to obtain the measurements.   *(3:197; 5:215)*

76. (C) Classically the superior mesenteric changes after eating (postprandial). After ingestion of a meal, the SMA blood flow is significantly increased with a broad systolic peak. There is also increased continuous flow in diastole.   *(3:210; 5:240)*

77. (B) A transverse plane slightly superior to the superior mesenteric artery will demonstrate the celiac artery arising from the aorta with its axis and respective branches; the common hepatic artery, and the splenic artery which are seen as a seagull appearance. The third branch the gastric artery is usually not seen by real-time imaging.   *(2:379; 3:104)*

78. (A) Appendicitis is an inflammatory process and associated with increased vascularity. The vascular supply to the appendix arises from the appendicular artery via the ileocolic and superior mesenteric artery. In cases of acute appendicitis, the color flow Doppler will often show a ring of color around the inflamed appendix.   *(3:222)*

79. (A) The blood supply to the appendix is via the superior mesenteric, ileocolic, and appendicular artery.   *(3:223)*

80. **(D)** Acute tubular necrosis has all of the sonographic characteristics of rejection but can be differentiated from rejection using Doppler and the resistive index. The RI will remain normal with acute tubular necrosis, but it will be abnormal with rejection. *(3:361)*

81. **(C)** Transplantation is the preferred treatment for irreversible end stage renal disease. However, there is a limited availability of donor organs, thus limiting the number of transplants. *(3:357; 9:1015)*

82. **(C)** Characteristics of any high-grade stenosis is narrowing of the vessel with a color jet of mosaic colors caused by turbulence and scattering; followed by poststenotic turbulence and a damping of the vessel. The spectral waveform in the area of the high-grade stenosis will have a dramatically increased peak systolic flow, with filling of the spectral window. Laminar flow is associated with normal flow profiles, and the absence of color would signify an occlusion. *(3:184–187)*

83. **(A)** The term aliasing refers to high velocity waveforms that exceed the Nyquist limit (1/2 of the pulse repetition rate, PRF). It is frequently noted with vessels that have a high-grade stenosis. *(3:15)*

84. **(B)** An orthotopic transplant is where the graft is placed in a normal position. A heterotopic transplantation is where the donor organ is placed in an ectopic location. The most common liver transplant is the orthotopic cadaveric transplant (OLTX). *(3:373)*

85. **(D)** Hepatic artery thrombosis and occlusion is of critical importance because it can mean loss of the liver transplant and even death of the patient. This is a primary cause of graft ischemia, hepatic infarction, sepsis, and ultimately graft failure. Angiography confirms the diagnosis. *(3:381–383)*

86. **(D)** Dialysis access can be performed at home via a peritoneal access. It is the easiest and least expensive method; however, the disadvantage is the possibility of developing peritonitis. *(3:400; 5:285)*

87. **(D)** In the normal dialysis access graft, there is a turbulent mosaic pattern throughout the graft and increased color changes at the anastomotic sites caused by increased velocities. If the color pattern becomes monochrome or homogeneous throughout the graft it is an indication that it is malfunctioning. *(3:406)*

88. **(D)** The dialysis access shunt will be located in a superficial position in the arm or forearm. This makes it ideal for imaging with the linear array transducer, which provides excellent detail and resolution. It is also accessible for palpation for determining the type of graft and its patency. *(3:403; 5:285)*

89. **(C)** Several of the perigraft masses seen on the renal transplant examination can mimic each other. For example, a hematoma and an abscess have similar ultrasound characteristics. Also, the fluid-filled perigraft masses, such as a lymphocele or urinoma, have similar characteristics. To provide a definitive diagnosis, an aspiration or biopsy is required. *(8:171)*

90. **(A)** Thrombosis of the arteriovenous access shunt is the most common cause of access failure and is more frequent in synthetic arteriovenous shunt grafts. *(3:414)*

91. **(B)** Occlusion of the AV shunt will show absence of color filling in the shunt with patency in the adjacent feeding vessels. There are usually echoes filling the shunt with no Doppler signal. *(3:415–417)*

92. **(A)** The functioning AV graft access will be superficially located with two parallel echogenic lines representing the walls of the graft and a sonolucent center. *(3:403)*

93. **(D)** A pseudoaneurysm or false aneurysm results from an injury to the wall of the artery. It is an extraluminal collection of blood that maintains communication with the injured artery via the "neck" whereby blood flows in and out of the pseudoaneurysm with the cardiac cycle. Thus, the forward and reverse flow pattern in the neck. *(3:421)*

94. **(A)** Ultrasound guided compression repair is a safe and effective noninvasive technique for obliteration of the pseudoaneurysm. *(3:424; 14:307–311)*

95. **(D)** The distal pedal pulse is continuously monitored to ensure distal peripheral flow during compression. *(3:424)*

96. **(A)** In cases of acute arterial occlusion, the blood flow is usually instantly interrupted by an emboli, trauma, or thrombi. This will be accompanied by severe pain often associated with numbness. Surgery or interventional procedures are immediately required to restore the blood supply. In cases of acute occlusion, there has not been time for the formation of collateral vessels that can supply the required blood flow. When arterial occlusion occurs over a long time span collateral vessels have time to form, and they provide blood flow patterns to circumvent the occluded vessels. This, in turn, eases the symptoms until the demand for blood exceeds the collateral capacity, as seen with exercise. Then, the symptoms will return, this is what we term claudication pain. *(6:898)*

97. **(D)** Although all the factors listed in the answers are contributors to arterial disease, the etiology for the majority of arterial diseases is atherosclerosis. Atherosclerosis is defined by the World Health

Organization as "a combination of changes in the intima and media. These changes include focal accumulation of lipids, hemorrhage, fibrous tissue, and calcium deposits." *(5:4)*

98. **(C)** Rupture of the aortic aneurysm the most threatening outcome. More recent data indicate that rupture risk escalates when the aneurysm exceeds 5 cm in size. *(5:211–213)*

99. **(D)** A stethoscope reveals bruits when there is significant occlusive disease or stenosis of the aorta or its branches. *(5:23; 5:238)*

100. **(D)** The most common correctable cause of hypertension is renal arterial disease. All of the answers listed are potential causes of renal hypertension; however, as stated, the most common correctable cause is renal arterial disease. *(2:458)*

101. **(D)** The common hepatic artery arises from the right branch of the celiac artery. It then gives off the gastroduodenal artery and the right gastric artery and becomes the proper hepatic artery and enters the liver at the porta hepatis. It further divides into the right and left hepatic arteries. *(2:380,387)*

102. **(A)** The definition of avascular is "not supplied with blood vessels." *(7:144)*

103. **(C)** Brescia–Cimino is the most common autologous arteriovenous fistula access for dialysis. It is has a unique longevity and resistance to infection and hyperplasia. *(3:400; 4:19; 6:413–414)*

104. **(B)** Fusiform aneurysym, a spindle-shaped lesion contiguous with the arterial lumen. There is also thrombus present on the anterior wall. *(3:197)*

105. **(C)** Gray scale ultrasound clearly demonstrates hypoechogenicity with enlargement of the renal pyramids and the thinning of the renal sinus characteristic of rejection. *(8:169–170)*

106. **(D)** Color flow Doppler of the splenic hilum demonstrates the dilated splenic vein with multiple varices. *(3:147)*

107. **(B)** Doppler waveform of the portal vein in a patient with portal hypertension has the classical continuous waveform without respiratory changes. *(3:149)*

108. Fig. 6–40. Transverse real-time image of the abdomen shows the following vessels:

    (1) abdominal aorta
    (2) right renal artery
    (3) splenic vein
    (4) inferior vena cava   *(8:17, 18, 116, 117)*

109. **(A)** Fig. 6–41. Angiogram of the celiac axis demonstrating three primary branches: hepatic, splenic, and gastric. *(3:204–206)*

110. **(B)** The left gastric artery branch of the celiac is usually not seen on the ultrasound examination. *(3:204)*

111. **(C)** Fig. 6–42. SMA stenosis. Color flow Doppler image shows a mosaic color pattern at the site of stenosis caused by extreme turbulence. There is also narrowing and calcification in the walls. The spectral waveform demonstrates aliasing with a velocity of over 450 cm/s. Peak systolic velocity of more than 275 cm/s may indicate a greater than 70% stenosis of the SMA. *(3:210)*

112. **(B)** The superior mesenteric artery (SMA) is best seen in the longitudinal axis just below the origin of the celiac axis. In the longitudinal plane, the origin of the SMA as well as the longest segment can be viewed. Spectral waveforms are also obtained in the longitudinal plane to ensure accuracy. *(3:204)*

113. **(B)** Fig. 6–43. The inferior vena cava is seen with the hepatic vein emptying into the vessel. Also note the changing diameter size and the fact that it runs in a parallel straight plane. In contrast, the aorta remains constant in the size throughout the length of the vessel and slightly ascends to the anterior surface. *(3:213)*

114. **(B)** Fig. 6–44. Contrast venography shows occlusion of the inferior vena cava (arrow) with patency of the common iliac vein (CI) and collateral vessels arising from the internal iliac (II). *(3:213–217)*

115. **(D)** Cystic artery, which arises from the hepatic artery. (See vascular anatomy in the study guide.) *(3:218)*

116. **(C)** Fig. 6–45. Arteriovenous fistula. The color flow image shows a disorganized flow pattern with a multitude of colors in a mosaic pattern. The turbulence extends throughout the adjacent vessels. The spectral analysis shows extreme turbulence and irregular amplitudes with a mixture of arterial and venous signals. *(3:366)*

117. **(C)** Fig. 6–46. Hepatic artery stenosis in a liver transplant. The angiogram shows the redundant kink with the arrow depicting the stenotic zone. The spectral analysis shows the high velocity exceeding 460 cm/s and the high resistant turbulent waveform with spectral broadening. *(3:378, 379)*

118. **(D)** Fig. 6–47. Loop graft of the forearm seen on digital subtraction. Note forearm bones in the background to identify forearm. *(3:401)*

119. **(C)** Fig. 6–48. Angiography with embolism. In Fig. 6–28A, the mycotic aneurysm is seen arising from the gluteal artery. In Fig. 6–28B, the embolization coils are seen postembolization with obliteration of the mycotic aneurysm. *(3:425–427)*

120. Fig. 6–49. Digital subtraction arteriogram of the kidney identifies the following: *(3:179)*

(1) main renal artery
(2) segmental renal artery
(3) interlobar renal artery
(4) arcuate renal artery

121. **(D)** Power Doppler is an excellent mode for demonstrating the perfusion of the kidney. It has the ability to show all of the vessels simultaneously and the patency. However, it does not provide velocity or show the direction of flow. *(3:18, 19)*

122. **(C)** Fig. 6–50. Spectral analysis of the renal artery demonstrates the low resistance with continuous forward flow in diastole. The resistive index is 0.67, which is normal. Upper limit of the RI is 0.7. *(3:177, 178)*

123. **(B)** Distal to the renal artery stenosis, the waveform will present with tardus-parvus. There will be a prolonged systolic acceleration (Tardus) and diminished amplitude with rounding of the systolic peak (parvus). *(3:186)*

124. **(D)** Fig. 6–51. Enlarged gray scale scan depicts the transplanted kidney in a longitudinal plane. There is an area of renal infarct (arrow) in the upper pole seen as an area of hypoechogenicity. Power Doppler is excellent for demonstrating areas of infarction as areas of perfusion deficits. *(3:365)*

125. **(D)** Fig. 6–52. The color scan classically depicts a pseudoaneurysm at the iliac and common femoral junction, which relates to injury secondary to the heart catheterization. There is some turbulence in the native vessel that extends into the pseudoaneurysm at the location of the neck. The neck is not well seen; however, Doppler waveforms would identify the neck with the forward and reverse flow, which would confirm the diagnosis. *(3:421–425)*

126. **(C)** Fig. 6–53. Transverse scan at the level of the xiphoid demonstrates the hepatic veins (left, middle, and right). *(8:18)*

127. **(C)** Fig. 6–54. Transverse scan at the level of the xiphoid demonstrates the superior vena cava filled with thrombus that extends into the hepatic veins. *(3:215)*

128. **(F)** Vascular imaging utilizes a linear array for peripheral vessels with sector scanning transducers such as the phased array and the curved linear array for abdominal vessels. *(15:13; 2:2)*

129. **(D)** Continuous wave transducers are used for Doppler signals only. There is no imaging, and they pick up all signals in the field, there is no discrimination of the vessels. The transducer sends and receives 100% of the time with two crystals. One crystal receives, one crystal sends. Continuous wave can be heard audibly or the waveform can be depicted graphically. *(2:27; 3:14)*

130. **(D)** Hue is a component of the color display. It is the perceived color and is dependent on the frequency shift that is determined by the velocity and the angle of insonation. Luminance is the term used to describe the brightness of the hue and its saturation. *(3:17)*

131. **(A)** To correct for aliasing use a lower frequency, decrease the depth of the sample volume, or adjust the baseline. *(3:15, 35, 38; 2:38)*

132. **(A)** Low wall filters are used for venous imaging to ensure depiction of the low venous flow. The sampling rate (pulse repetition rate) may be decreased and the color sensitivity increased. In addition, power angio may be used because it is more sensitive for low perfusion echoes. The high wall filters are used for arterial studies to eliminate the motion of the vessel walls. *(3:17, 18)*

133. **(A)** The orthotopic cadaver transplant is the most common liver transplant. *(3:373)*

134. **(D)** The abdominal aorta is considered aneurysmal if the diameter (outer wall to outer wall) measures more than 3 cm. *(3:199)*

135. **(A)** Fig. 6–55. Spectral analysis shows a normal hepatic venous flow pattern. A multiphasic waveform with variation in velocity. It is influenced by pressure in the right atrium, compliance of the liver parenchyma, and respiration. *(3:154, 155)*

136. **(B)** Fig. 6–56. Color Doppler scan depicts the TIPS which is filled with echoes and a very minimal flow which is characteristic of pre-occlusive states. *(3:169–171)*

137. **(B)** The splenic vein lies posterior to the body of the pancreas. *(1:819)*

138. **(E)** The renal transplant vascular examination includes the iliac artery, anastomosis with the renal artery, the intrarenal arteries (main renal, segmental, interlobar, interlobular, and arcuate), renal and iliac veins, and usually a perfusion study with power Doppler. The IVC is not included in the examination. *(3:355)*

139. **(D)** Renal arteries are best viewed from the anterior approach using supine, decubitus positions and the transverse and longitudinal planes. *(2:456–457)*

140. **(B)** The cystic artery of the gallbladder is not routinely seen on color flow Doppler examination. In cases of cholecystitis or infectious processes, the vascularity is increased and may be visualized with color Doppler. *(3:217–221)*

141. **(D)** Harmonic imaging depends on the inherent properties of the microbubbles to resonate specific frequencies after they have encountered the ultrasound beam. The signal-to-noise ratio is improved because, in theory, only the echoes arriving back to the transducer from the contrast agent are displayed. *(2:87)*

142. **(D)** The clinical signs and symptoms depend on the degree of venous obstruction associated with portal hypertension. The symptoms include: severe abdominal pain, nausea, vomiting, and rapid enlargement of the abdomen caused by ascites. Because of the elevated venous pressures and congestion of the collateral pathways, secondary signs occur and include: bleeding esophageal varices, hypersplenism, or encephalopathy. *(6:1278–1279)*

143. **(E)** All of the answers are characteristic of aneurysms except the membrane separating the true and false lumen, which is characteristic of a aortic dissection. *(3:197, 203)*

144. **(A)** Because of inflammation and infection of the appendix with appendicitis, it becomes edematous which presents a hypoechoic appearance on the ultrasound examination. On color flow Doppler, the vascular flow will be increased. Appendicitis should be considered if the wall of the appendix is more than 3-mm thick or if the AP diameter of the non-compressible appendix is greater than 7 mm. *(3:222; 16:55–59)*

145. **(A)** Collateral is defined as secondary or accessory or a small side branch, as in a blood vessel. One of the best examples would be venous occlusion with collateral flow. For example, if the common femoral vein is occluded, the blood flow will be rerouted through the collaterals. The collateral can be a secondary vein from the deep or superficial femoral or it can be the greater saphenous vein, which may become the primary vessel to circumvent blood around the occluded common femoral vein. *(7:287)*

146. **(D)** The sonographer should have a good rapport with the surgeon to understand the surgical procedures and before ultrasound examination, to know precisely how the transplant was performed. This should allow them to be familiar with which vessels are anastomosed and any irregularities that may have occurred. If this is not done, the examiner may spend excessive time trying to locate the vessels and their anastomotic sites or have a variant that they do not understand. *(3:369)*

147. **(C)** Subclavian-axillary venous thrombosis is usually associated with central venous catheters. This can be appreciated when monitoring the in-dwelling temporary catheter placed in the subclavian for dialysis access. The majority of the catheters will develop thrombus with possible extension into the jugular vein. Acute diffuse upper limb swelling and discomfort or pain are the usual symptoms. *(5:267)*

148. **(D)** In cases of a ruptured aortic aneurysm, it is imperative the patient be transported to surgery as soon as possible. Any delay will result in deterioration and death of the bleeding patient. *(5:219)*

149. **(F)** Early aortic graft complications include: hemorrhage, thrombosis, colonic ischemia, graft infection, and sexual dysfunction. Late graft complications include: thrombosis, infection, and anastomotic aneurysms. *(5:224)*

150. **(F)** Aneurysmal disease can involve any artery; however, peripheral artery aneurysms occur more frequently in the abdominal aorta, the iliac, femoral, and popliteal arteries. Aortic aneurysms usually form and slowly expand over several years. *(6:212)*

REFERENCES

1. Williams PL, Warwick R, Dyson M, et al. eds. *Gray's Anatomy.* 37th ed. New York: Churchill Livingston; 1989.
2. Zwiebel WL. *Introduction to Vascular Ultrasonography.* 4th ed. Philadelphia: WB Saunders; 2000.
3. Krebs CA, Giyanani VL, Eisenberg RL: *Ultrasound Atlas of Vascular Diseases.* Stamford, CT: Appleton & Lange; 1999.
4. Neumyer MM, King SL, Primozich JF, et al. *Advanced Technology Laboratories Teaching Manual.* Washington, DC: Bothell; 1997.
5. Hallett JW, Brewster DC, Darling RC. *Handbook of Patient Care in Vascular Surgery.* 3rd ed. Boston: Little, Brown & Co; 1995.
6. Schwartz SI, Shires GT, Spencer FC, et al. eds. *Principles of Surgery,* 4th ed. New York: McGraw-Hill; 1984.

7. Bia FJ, Brady JP, Brady LW, et al. Consultants. *Dorland's Illustrated Medical Dictionary.* 26th ed. Philadelphia: WB Saunders; 1974.

8. Krebs CA, Giyanani VL, Eisenberg RL. *Ultrasound Atlas of Disease Processes.* Norwalk, CT: Appleton & Lange; 1993.

9. Cotran RS, Kumar V, Robbins SL. *Robbins Pathologic Basis of Disease.* 4th ed. Philadelphia: WB Saunders; 1989.

10. Mallek R, Mostbeck GH, Reinhard MW, et al. Duplex Doppler sonography of celiac trunk and superior mesenteric artery: comparison with intra-arterial angiography. *J. Ultrasound Med.* 1993;12:337–342.

11. Foshager MC, Ferral H, Nazarian GK, et al. Development of stenosis in transjugular intrahepatic postosystemic hunts. *Radiology.* 1994;192:231–234.

12. Hennerici M, Neuerburg-Heusler D. *Vascular Diagnosis with Ultrasound.* New York: Thieme; 1998.

13. Nichols BT, Rittgers SE, Norris CS, Barnes RW. Noninvasive detection of renal artery stenosis. *Bruit.* 1984; 8:26–29.

14. Corley BD, Roberts AC, Fellmeth DD, et al. Post angiographic femoral artery pseudoaneurysms. Further experience with ultrasound guided compression repair. *Radiology.* 1995;194:307–311.

15. Krebs CA, Odwin CS, Fleischer AC. *Appleton & Lange's Review for the Ultrasonography Examination.* 3rd ed. New York: McGraw-Hill; 2001.

16. Jeffrey RB, Jain KA, Nghiem HV. Sonographic diagnosis of acute appendicitis interpretive pitfalls. *AJR.* 1994;162:55–59.

CHAPTER 7

ENDORECTAL PROSTATE SONOGRAPHY

Dunstan Abraham

Study Guide

The prostate is a heterogeneous, oval-shaped organ that surrounds the proximal urethra. In the adult, the normal gland measures approximately 3.8 cm (cephalocaudal) by 3 cm (anteroposterior) by 4 cm (transverse).[1] It normally weighs about 20 g, but it can be slightly larger in men older than 40. The prostate is composed of glandular and fibromuscular tissue and is located in the retroperitoneum between the floor of the urinary bladder and the urogenital diaphragm. The base of the prostate, its superior margin, abuts the inferior aspect of the urinary bladder. The gland is bounded anteriorly by prostatic fat and fascia, laterally by the obturator internus and levator ani muscles, and posteriorly by areolar tissue and Denonvilliers' fascia, which separates it from the rectum.

The **seminal vesicles** are two sac-like lateral structures that outpouch from the vas deferens and are situated on the posterior–superior aspect of the prostate between the bladder and the rectum. The seminal vesicles join the vas deferens to form the **ejaculatory ducts,** which then enter the base of the prostate to join the urethra at the verumontanum. The **verumontanum** is a midpoint region between the prostatic base and apex and surrounds the urethra. The size and fluid content of the seminal vesicles are variable.

The **prostatic urethra** courses through the substance of the gland and is divided into a proximal and a distal segment. The proximal segment extends from the neck of the bladder to the base of the verumontanum; the distal segment begins at this point and extends to the apex of the gland.

NORMAL SECTIONAL ANATOMY

The earlier anatomic descriptions of the prostate divided the gland into five major lobes (**anterior, posterior, middle,** and **two lateral**) or two zones (**outer** and **inner**). More recent histological studies, however, have divided the prostate into three glandular zones: the **transitional, central,** and **peripheral zones.** There is also a nonglandular region called the **anterior fibromuscular stroma**[2] (Fig. 7–1A, B).

Transitional Zone

The transitional zone represents about 5% of the glandular prostate and is located in the central region on both sides of the proximal urethra.[2] The ducts of the transitional zone run parallel to the urethra and end in the proximal urethra at the level of the verumontanum.

Central Zone

The central zone constitutes approximately 25% of the prostatic glandular tissue and is located at the base of the gland.[2] It is wedge-like in shape, is oriented horizontally, and surrounds the ejaculatory ducts throughout their course. The zone narrows to an apex at the verumontanum. Ducts of the vas deferens and seminal vesicles come together to form the ejaculatory ducts, which pass through the central zone and join the urethra at the verumontanum.

Peripheral Zone

The peripheral zone constitutes about 70% of the glandular tissue.[2] This zone consists of the posterior, lateral, and apical parts of the prostate and also extends anteriorly. The ducts of the peripheral zone enter the urethra at, and distal to, the verumontanum.

Anterior Fibromuscular Stroma

The anterior fibromuscular stroma is a thick nonglandular sheath of tissue that covers the entire anterior surface of the prostate. This tissue is composed of smooth muscle and fibrous tissue.

NORMAL SONOGRAPHIC ANATOMY

Sonographically, the prostate is a homogeneous gland with low-level echoes. The periurethral glandular tissue that

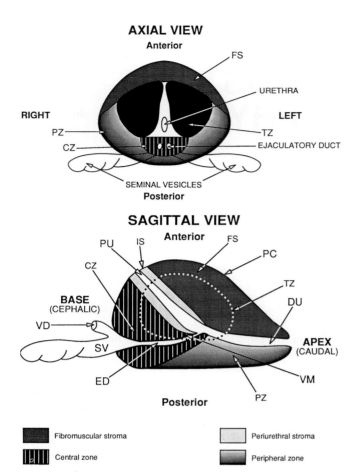

AXIAL VIEW

Figure 7–1. (A) An axial view of normal prostate anatomy: CZ is the central zone, FS is the fibromuscular stroma, TZ is the transition zone, and PZ is the peripheral zone. **(B)** Sagittal view of the normal prostate anatomy: SV is the seminal vesicle, ED is the ejaculatory duct, DU is the distal urethra, PC is the prostatic capsule, VD is the vas deferens, VM is the verumontanum, PU is the proximal urethra, CZ is the central zone, FS is the fibromuscular stroma, TZ is the transition zone, PS is the periurethral stroma, and PZ is the peripheral zone. (*Modified with permission from McNeal JE. Regional morphology and pathology of the prostate. Am J. Clin Pathol. 1968; 49:347–357 and Dakin R., et al. Transrectal ultrasound of the prostate: Technique and sonographic findings. JDMS. 1989; 5:2.)*

surrounds the proximal urethra is homogeneous and isoechoic. The central zone is normally more echogenic than the peripheral zone because it has a greater amount of **corpora amylacea** (calcified deposits) in the central zone. The fibromuscular capsule, located anteriorly, is smooth, hyperechoic, and sharply defined.

The seminal vesicles are visualized as symmetrically paired structures that are slightly less echoic than the prostate. The vas deferens can be depicted as tubular hypoechoic structures joining the seminal vesicles medially. On transverse imaging, they are round or oval and are located between the seminal vesicles. The ejaculatory duct, when empty, can be seen as a hyperechoic line joining the ure-

thra. The empty urethra is identified by its echogenic walls coursing through the prostate. When filled with fluid, the urethra is recognized more easily.

On longitudinal sections, the anterior space between the prostate and the seminal vesicles (**prostate–seminal vesicle angle**) is variable but is the same bilaterally. Similarly, the posterior space between the prostate and the seminal vesicle (or nipple) is symmetrical on both sides.[1]

INDICATIONS FOR SONOGRAPHY

Patients can be referred for endorectal prostate sonography for various reasons such as the following.[3]

- An abnormal digital rectal examination, as indicated by a palpable prostatic nodule or prostate with an asymmetrical size or shape
- Biopsy guidance of sonographically detected abnormal areas
- Clinical evidence of prostate cancer such as an elevated level of prostatic-specific antigen or radiographically detected bone metastasis
- Monitoring of a patient's response to therapy
- Inflammation leading to the formation of a prostatic abscess
- Infertility caused by the absence of the seminal vesicles or a bilateral obstruction of the ejaculatory ducts
- Difficulties in voiding caused by an obstruction of the prostatic urethra

EQUIPMENT AND EXAMINATION TECHNIQUES

Technical innovations have led to the availability of several types of endorectal imaging systems. The original systems were **radial (axial) scanners** that produced transverse-oriented slices of the prostate. Later, **linear array scanners** that imaged the gland in longitudinal sections were introduced. Today, **biplanar endorectal probes** that can produce both longitudinal and transverse sections of the gland are available, thus eliminating the need for two separate probes. The frequency of endorectal probes ranges from 5.0 to 8 MHz. A guide that is attached directly to the probe allows one to biopsy suspicious prostatic lesions safely and accurately.

Preparation of the patient for endorectal sonography begins with a self-administered enema 1 hour before the examination. This not only eliminates fecal material from the rectum that might adversely affect the quality of the image, but also reduces the risk of contamination of the prostate. If biopsy is to be performed, prophylactic antibiotics must be given before the procedure and continued for 24–48 hours afterward.[4]

The patient can be examined in the lateral decubitus, lithotomy, or knee-chest position. The probe is previously sterilized and covered with a condom before insertion. A digital rectal examination is performed to exclude any obstructing lesions or rectal fissures. Axial scanning begins at the level of the seminal vesicles. The probe is then gradually withdrawn to image the gland sequentially down to the level of the apex.

Sagittal imaging begins in the midline and shows the gland from base to apex with portions of the seminal vesicles. The probe is then rotated clockwise and counterclockwise to demonstrate the right and left sides of the gland.

PATHOLOGY

Prostatic Carcinoma

Prostatic carcinoma is the second leading cause of death among American men. In 1995, 244,000 new cases were diagnosed and 44,000 lives were lost to this disease.[5] Although the etiology of prostatic cancer remains unclear, the factors implicated in its causation include age, genetic or racial makeup, hormonal influences, effects of benign prostatic hyperplasia, dietary fat, and infectious agents.[5] Anatomic studies have determined that 70% of prostate cancers originate *de novo* in the peripheral zone, 20% originate in the transitional zone, and 10% originate in the central zone.[1] Clinical symptoms include back pain and an obstruction of urinary outflow that may mimic benign prostatic hypertrophy.

The sonographic characteristics of prostatic carcinoma are variable. Small cancers originating in the peripheral zone are anechoic to hypoechoic. As the tumor enlarges and extends into the central glandular region, it becomes more isoechoic to hyperechoic. The tumor also may spread outward beyond the prostatic capsule and disrupt this normally well-defined echogenic structure.[6] However, the most commonly encountered finding is a hypoechoic peripheral zone lesion. Several entities may have ultrasound characteristics that are similar to those of intraprostatic malignancy. These include hyperplastic nodules, infarcts, focal inflammation, cystic atrophy, blood vessels, and muscle tissue.[7] Invasion of the tumor into the seminal vesicles can be seen as solid material within this normally fluid-filled structure. Invasion may make the size, shape, and echogenicity of the seminal vesicles asymmetrical in appearance.

Obliteration of the nipple or the prostate–seminal vesicle angle is another diagnostic criterion for invasion by the tumor.[1] However, because the nipple is not imaged consistently, the criterion is of limited usefulness. Staging of prostatic cancer with ultrasound is also feasible, but is limited by problems of resolution.

Benign Prostatic Hyperplasia and Hypertrophy

Benign prostatic hyperplasia affects 80–90% of adult men.[1] Its etiology is believed to be related to hormonal factors. The clinical symptoms of the disease may include decreased flow of urine, difficulty in initiating and terminating urination, nocturia, and urinary retention. Benign prostatic hyperplasia originates in the transitional zone and in periurethral glandular tissue.

The sonographic characteristics of hyperplasia nodules are variable. They can be hypoechoic, hyperechoic, or of mixed echogenicity. Enlargement of the central gland by benign prostatic hyperplasia causes lateral displacement of the peripheral zone. The prostatic calculi that are often encountered with benign prostatic hyperplasia are believed to be the result of stasis of prostatic secretions.

Benign prostatic hyperplasia causes the number of cells in the prostate to increase; whereas, **benign prostatic hypertrophy** refers to an increase in the size of existing cells. Hyperplasia and hypertrophy often develop concurrently and result in the enlargement of the prostate gland.

Prostatitis

Inflammation of the prostate can be the result of acute or chronic bacterial infections or of unknown nonbacterial factors. Clinical symptoms of prostatitis may include fever, pelvic and low back pain, urinary frequency and urgency, and dysuria. Although prostatitis usually involves the peripheral zone in its initial stages, it can originate in any area of the gland.

In acute prostatitis, the main sonographic characteristics are (1) a hypoechoic rim surrounding the gland, (2) an echo-free halo surrounding the periurethral zone, and (3) diffuse, low-level echogenic areas within the gland. In chronic prostatitis, diffuse inhomogeneous echogenicity and fluid-filled areas within the prostate is demonstrated, although this is a nonspecific finding.[1] Calculi also may be present.

A prostatic abscess may develop secondary to prostatitis. Endorectal sonography may show hypoechoic areas corresponding to liquefaction within the abscess.

Prostatic Cysts

Prostatic cysts are frequently congenital.[1] Sonographically, these cysts are anechoic, have sharp walls, and demonstrate good sound transmission.

REFERENCES

1. Rifkin M. *Ultrasound of the Prostate.* New York: Raven Press; 1988.
2. Lee F, Torp-Pedersen ST, Siders DB, et al. Transrectal ultrasound in the diagnosis and staging of prostatic carcinoma. *Radiology.* 1989; 170:609.
3. Rifkin M. Prostate cancer ultrasound: Screening tool or hype? *Diagn Imaging.* 1988; 302–305.
4. Brawer M, Chetner M. Ultrasonography of the prostate and biopsy. In: Walsh P, Retik A, Vaughan E, et al. eds. *Campbell's Urology.* 7th ed. Philadelphia: WB Saunders; 1998.
5. Pienta K. Etiology, Epidemiology and Prevention of Carcinoma of the Prostate. In: Walsh P, Retik A, Vaughan, et al. eds. *Campbell's Urology.* 7th ed. Philadelphia: WB Saunders; 1998.
6. Lee F, Littrup PJ, Kumasaka GH, et al. The use of transrectal ultrasound in diagnosis, guided biopsy, staging and screening of prostate cancer. *Radiographics.* 1987; 7:627.
7. Waterhouse RL, Resnick MI. The use of transrectal prostatic ultrasonography in the evaluation of patients with prostatic carcinoma. *J Urol.* 1989; 141:233.

Questions

1. The fibromuscular stroma

   (A) covers the anterior surface of the prostate
   (B) is the major site of benign prostatic hypertrophy
   (C) is a nonglandular region
   (D) A and C

2. Which is not an indication for endorectal prostate sonography?

   (A) a palpable prostate mass
   (B) biopsy guidance of a palpable prostate nodule
   (C) an elevated prostatic–specific antigen
   (D) differentiation of a benign from a malignant nodule

3. Patients having endorectal prostate sonography are commonly examined in which of the following positions?

   (A) the lithotomy position
   (B) the erect position
   (C) the Trendelenburg position
   (D) Fowler's position

4. All of the following statements about the transitional zone are true *except*

   (A) It is located centrally around the urethra.
   (B) It represents about 5% of the gland.
   (C) It is the primary site of benign prostatic hyperplasia.
   (D) It is the primary site of adenocarcinoma.

5. Which one of the following statements is false?

   (A) The central zone constitutes approximately 25% of the glandular tissue.
   (B) The central zone is located at the apex of the prostate.
   (C) The vas deferens join the seminal vesicles in the central zone.
   (D) The central zone surrounds the ejaculatory ducts.

6. The peripheral zone accounts for which percentage of the prostatic glandular tissue?

   (A) 50%
   (B) 10%
   (C) 70%
   (D) 1%

7. Which of the following statements about the prostate is false?

   (A) Its apex is located superiorly.
   (B) Its base abuts the urinary bladder.
   (C) Its has three zones.
   (D) The urethra runs through the gland.

8. Which of the following is a function of the prostate?

   (A) hormonal secretions
   (B) testosterone production
   (C) secretion of alkaline fluid
   (D) spermatozoa production

9. The prostate is bounded anteriorly by

   (A) the obturator muscle
   (B) the levator ani muscle
   (C) fat and fascia
   (D) the obturator and levator ani muscles

10. The seminal vesicles join which of the following to form the ejaculatory duct?

    (A) the Denonvilliers' duct
    (B) the vas deferens
    (C) the verumontanum
    (D) the urethra

11. The ejaculatory duct joins the _____ at the verumontanum

    (A) vas deferens
    (B) efferent ducts
    (C) epididymis
    (D) urethra

12. The seminal vesicles are located on which surface of the prostate?

(A) the anterior–inferior surface
(B) the posterior–inferior surface
(C) the posterior–superior surface
(D) the inferior–lateral

13. Which of the following statements about prostatic cancer is not true?

(A) It originates mainly in the central zone.
(B) It is anechoic to hypoechoic in the early stage.
(C) Its associated factors include benign prostatic hyperplasia and hormonal influence.
(D) Clinical presentation may include urinary obstruction.

14. All of the following are true of benign prostatic hyperplasia *except*

(A) It involves the periurethral tissue.
(B) It affects 80–90% of adult men.
(C) It is sonographically variable.
(D) The incidence decreases with age.

15. Sonographic features of acute prostatitis may include all of the following *except*

(A) a hypoechoic "rim" around the prostate
(B) calcification in the peripheral zone
(C) diffuse low-level echoes within the gland
(D) acute edema of the fibromuscular stroma

16. Approximately what percentage of men are affected by benign prostatic hyperplasia?

(A) 20%
(B) 40%
(C) 50%
(D) 90%

17. Benign prostatic hyperplasia originates in which of the following areas of the prostate?

(A) the fibromuscular stroma
(B) the peripheral zone
(C) the ejaculatory ducts
(D) the transitional zone

18. Corpora amylacea are

(A) part of the anterior fibromuscular capsule
(B) calcified deposits in the prostate
(C) hypoechoic on endorectal ultrasound
(D) never seen on endorectal ultrasound

19. Tumor invasion does not commonly affect which of the following characteristics of the seminal vesicles?

(A) their size
(B) their shape
(C) their echogenicity
(D) Doppler waveform

20. Obliteration of the nipple and the prostate–seminal vesicle angle may indicate

(A) prostatitis
(B) scarring of tissues
(C) tumor infiltration
(D) the need for a higher-frequency probe

21. Prostatic cysts have all the following characteristics *except*

(A) They occur secondary to obstruction.
(B) They can be congenital.
(C) They are anechoic with good enhancement.
(D) They have a high incidence of malignant transformation.

22. Clinical symptoms of prostatitis may commonly include all of the following *except*

(A) fever
(B) dysuria
(C) perineal pain
(D) bloody urethral discharge

23. In its initial stages, prostatitis generally involves the

(A) peripheral zone of the prostate
(B) anterior capsule of the prostate
(C) ejaculatory duct
(D) seminal vesicles

24. All of the following can typically mimic intraprostatic cancer *except*

(A) focal inflammation
(B) blood vessels
(C) muscle tissue
(D) corpora amylacea

25. Sonographic characteristics of prostatic cancer may commonly include all of the following *except*

(A) a hypoechoic nodule in the peripheral zone
(B) distortion of the capsule
(C) obliteration of the "nipple"
(D) marked compression of the prostatic urethra

26. An endorectal examination of the prostate should begin with

(A) transverse scanning
(B) longitudinal scanning
(C) views of the seminal vesicles
(D) a digital rectal examination

27. Prostate cancer is

(A) echogenic
(B) anechoic
(C) hypoechoic
(D) sonographically variable

28. The verumontanum is

(A) a midpoint region between the base and apex of the prostate
(B) a congenital abnormality of the prostate
(C) part of the peripheral zone
(D) part of the seminal vesicle

29. An echo-free "halo" around the periurethral zone may indicate

(A) tumor invasion
(B) benign prostatic hyperplasia
(C) prostatitis
(D) a technical artifact

30. An elevated prostatic-specific antigen may commonly indicate

(A) prostatic inflammation
(B) prostatic cancer
(C) benign prostatic hyperplasia
(D) obstruction of the prostatic ducts

31. Which of the following narrows to an apex at the verumontanum?

(A) the central zone
(B) the peripheral zone
(C) the transitional zone
(D) the fibromuscular stroma

32. The normal adult prostate weights approximately

(A) 10 g
(B) 20 g
(C) 30 g
(D) 40 g

33. Denonvilliers' fascia

(A) is located posterior to the prostate
(B) separates the prostate from the rectum
(C) covers the entire prostate
(D) is located posterior to and separates the prostate from the rectum

34. The normal adult prostate measures approximately

(A) 5 × 8 × 4 cm
(B) 8.3 × 3 × 6 cm
(C) 3.8 × 3 × 4 cm
(D) 5.8 × 4 × 5 cm

35. In 1995 the approximate number of new cases of prostate cancer diagnosed was

(A) 1000
(B) 10,000
(C) 100,000
(D) 200,000
(E) 400,000

36. Which statement about the seminal vesicles is incorrect?

(A) their absence does not usually affect fertility
(B) they are joined by the vas deferens
(C) they are normally less echoic than the prostate
(D) their size varies

37. All of the following describe the normal prostate capsule *except*

(A) smooth and unbroken
(B) highly echogenic
(C) sharply defined
(D) hypoechoic

38. Fig. 7–2 represents a longitudinal scan taken to the right of midline. The structure indicated by the arrow is

(A) the proximal urethra
(B) a seminal vesicle
(C) the verumontanum
(D) the ejaculatory duct

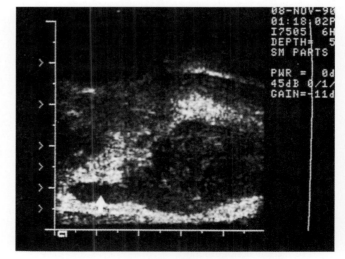

Figure 7–2. Longitudinal scan to the right of midline.

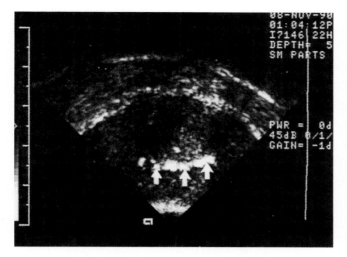

Figure 7–3. Transverse scan of the prostate.

39. Fig. 7–3 represents a transverse scan. The structure indicated by the arrows is

(A) a tumor in the peripheral zone
(B) prostatitis involving the periurethral areas
(C) central gland calcification
(D) distortion of the prostatic capsule

40. Fig. 7–4 represents a longitudinal scan of a 60-year-old patient presenting with urinary frequency. He was referred for an endorectal prostate sonography examination. The area outlined by the markers indicates

(A) obliteration of the "prostate-seminal vesicle angle"
(B) a hypoechoic mass in the central zone
(C) a tumor in the peripheral zone
(D) bulging of the prostatic capsule

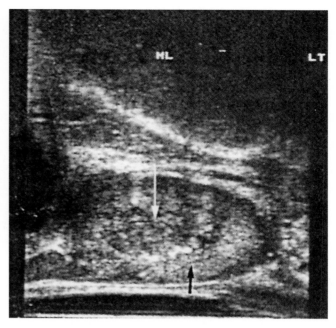

Figure 7–5. Longitudinal scan of the prostate.

41. Fig. 7–5 represents a longitudinal scan. The region indicated by the white arrow is

(A) the fibromuscular stroma
(B) the seminal vesicle
(C) the peripheral zone
(D) the central zone

42. Fig. 7–5 represents a longitudinal scan. The region indicated by the black arrow is

(A) the peripheral zone
(B) the central zone
(C) the prostatic capsule
(D) the vas deferens

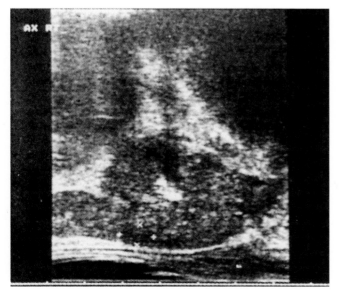

Figure 7–4. Longitudinal scan of the prostate.

43. Fig. 7–6 represents a longitudinal scan taken from a patient presenting with a history of infertility. The findings indicated by the markers probably represent

(A) benign prostatic hypertrophy
(B) a cyst in the ejaculatory duct
(C) extension of a tumor into the nipple region
(D) central gland disease

44. Fig. 7–7 represents a longitudinal scan of a 75-year-old man presenting with voiding difficulties and weight loss. This sonographic finding most likely represents

(A) diffuse cancer
(B) cancer confined to the peripheral zone
(C) benign prostatic hypertrophy
(D) prostatitis

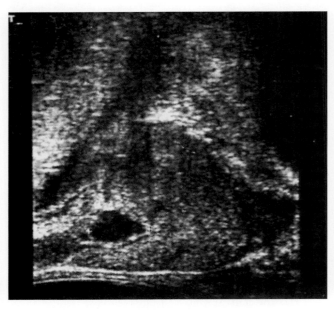

Figure 7–6. Longitudinal scan of the prostate.

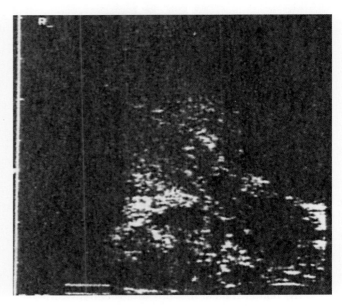

Figure 7–7. Longitudinal scan of the prostate.

Answers and Explanations

At the end of each explained answer there is a number combination in parentheses. The first number identifies the reference source; the second number or set of numbers indicates the page or pages on which the relevant information can be found.

1. **(D)** Both A and C. The fibromuscular stroma is a nonglandular region that covers the anterior surface of the prostate. Therefore, both A and C are correct. *(2:612)*

2. **(D)** Differentiation of a benign from a malignant nodule. Ultrasound cannot make a specific diagnosis of prostatic diseases. Biopsy is required to establish the diagnosis. *(3:303)*

3. **(A)** The lithotomy position. Patients who are having endorectal prostate sonography can be examined in the left lateral decubitus, knee–chest, or lithotomy position. *(1:44)*

4. **(D)** It is the primary site of adenocarcinoma. The transitional zone is located on both sides of the proximal urethra and represents 5% of the gland. It also is the primary site of benign prostatic hyperplasia. *(2:610)*

5. **(B)** The central zone is located at the apex of the prostate. The central zone is a triangular structure located at the base of the prostate with its apex at the verumontanum. *(7:89)*

6. **(C)** 70%. The peripheral zone constitutes more than two-thirds of prostatic glandular tissue. *(2:612)*

7. **(A)** Its apex is located superiorly. The apex of the prostate is located inferiorly. (See Fig. 7–1B in the Study Guide.)

8. **(C)** Secretion of alkaline fluid. The prostate discharges this fluid into the urethra to enhance the motility of sperm. *(6:2)*

9. **(C)** Fat and fascia. The prostate is bounded anteriorly by vessels, fat, lymphatics, nerves, and fascial tissues, collectively termed the anterior prostatic fat and fascia. *(1:5)*

10. **(B)** The vas deferens. The seminal vesicles join the vas deferens to form the ejaculatory duct, which passes through the central zone. *(2:612)*

11. **(D)** Urethra. The ejaculatory duct empties into the urethra at the verumontanum. *(2:612)*

12. **(C)** The posterior-superior surface. *(1:74)*

13. **(A)** It originates mainly in the central zone. Seventy percent of prostatic cancers originate *de novo* in the peripheral zone. *(1:146)*

14. **(D)** The incidence decreases with age. Benign prostatic hyperplasia occurs mostly in the transitional zone, and nodules occasionally develop in the periurethral glandular tissue. It affects 80–90% of men and its incidence increases with age. *(1:191, 196)*

15. **(D)** Acute edema of the fibromuscular stroma. In acute prostatitis, the gland may be surrounded by a hypoechoic rim, have an echo-free halo around the periurethral zone, or have scattered low-level echoes within the gland. *(1:222; 7:218)*

16. **(D)** 90%. It is estimated that 80–90% of adult men will be affected by benign prostatic hyperplasia. *(1:192)*

17. **(D)** The transitional zone (see the explanation for the answer to Question 14).

18. **(B)** Calcified deposits in the prostate. Degenerated epithelial cells of the prostate are shed and become suspended in albuminous fluid. This mass of cells is called corpora amylacea. Calculi are formed by the consolidation of corpora amylacea. *(7:137)*

19. **(D)** Doppler waveform. The diagnostic criteria for neoplasms invading the seminal vesicles include asymmetry in the size, shape, and echogenicity of the vesicles. *(1:239)*

20. **(C)** Tumor infiltration. The tumor will obliterate the "nipple" and "prostate–seminal vesicle angle." *(1:179)*

21. **(D)** They have a high incidence of malignant transformation. Prostatic cysts are frequently congenital

and secondary to obstruction of the seminal vesicle and ejaculatory duct. The differential diagnosis includes a cyst in the mullerian duct and diverticula of the ejaculatory duct.   *(1:235)*

22. **(D)** Bloody urethral discharge. The major symptoms of acute bacterial prostatitis include a high fever, chills, dysuria, perineal pain, urinary frequency and urgency.   *(6:5)*

23. **(A)** Peripheral zone of the prostate. Although prostatitis can originate in any area of the prostate, it initially presents in the peripheral zone.   *(1:14)*

24. **(D)** Corpora amylacea. Hyperplastic nodules, cysts, infarcts, inflammation, blood vessels, and muscle tissue can simulate intraprostatic cancer.   *(4:236)*

25. **(D)** Marked compression of the prostatic urethra. Early prostatic cancers can present as anechoic or hypoechoic lesions in the peripheral zone. They can break through the prostatic capsule causing distortion, or they can invade the seminal vesicles.   *(1:161, 179)*

26. **(D)** A digital rectal examination. This examination should be done before the probe is inserted to exclude obstructing lesions, rectal fissures, or other pathology.   *(9:2508)*

27. **(D)** Sonographically variable. Prostate cancer first appears as anechoic–hypoechoic. It becomes isoechoic to hyperechoic as it spreads to the central gland.   *(5:629)*

28. **(A)** A midpoint region between the base and apex of the prostate (see Fig. 7–1B in the Study Guide).

29. **(C)** Prostatitis. (See the explanation for the answer to Question 15.)   *(Study Guide: 351)*

30. **(B)** Prostatic cancer. An elevated prostatic-specific antigen may indicate prostate cancer.   *(3:304)*

31. **(A)** The central zone. (See Fig. 7–1B in the Study Guide.)

32. **(B)** 20 g. The normal postpubescent prostate weighs approximately that amount.   *(Study Guide: 349)*

33. **(D)** Is located posterior to and separates the prostate from the rectum. Denonvilliers' fascia separates the prostate from the rectum posteriorly.   *(1:5)*

34. **(C)** $3.8 \times 3 \times 4$ cm. This is the average normal size of the prostate.   *(1:5)*

35. **(D)** 200,000. In 1995, 244,000 new cases of prostate cancer were diagnosed, and 44,000 deaths resulted from this disease.   *(8:24)*

36. **(A)** Their absence does not usually affect fertility. In rare cases, infertility can be caused by absence of the seminal vesicles or by an obstruction in the ejaculatory ducts.   *(3:304)*

37. **(D)** Hypoechoic. The normal prostatic capsule is smooth, well defined, and highly echogenic.   *(4:234)*

38. **(B)** A seminal vesicle. The structure demonstrated in Fig. 7–2 is the right seminal vesicle, which joins the vas deferens (not shown) to form the ejaculatory duct.   *(Study Guide: Fig. 7–1B)*

39. **(C)** Central gland calcification. Fig. 7–3 shows bright echoes representing prostatic calcification, which can be solitary or can occur in clusters.   *(Study Guide: 351)*

40. **(C)** A tumor in the peripheral zone. The hypoechoic mass seen on the peripheral zone in Fig. 7–4 is characteristic of prostatic cancer.   *(Study Guide: 351)*

41. **(D)** The central zone. This zone (white arrow) in Fig. 7–5 is clearly demarcated from the peripheral zone (black arrow) by a curved band of echoes.   *(Study Guide: 350)*

42. **(A)** The peripheral zone.   *(Study Guide: 350)*

43. **(B)** A cyst in the ejaculatory duct. The cystic structure shown in Fig. 7–6 is clearly located within the ejaculatory duct.   *(Study Guide: 350)*

44. **(A)** Diffuse cancer. Fig. 7–7 demonstrates diffuse hypoechoic masses throughout the prostate. This inhomogeneous pattern is consistent with diffuse malignancy.   *(Study Guide: 351)*

REFERENCES

1. Rifkin M. *Ultrasound of the Prostate.* New York: Raven Press; 1988.
2. Lee F, Torp-Pedersen ST, Siders DB, et al. Transrectal ultrasound in the diagnosis and staging of prostatic carcinoma. *Radiology.* 1989; 170:609.
3. Rifkin M. Prostate cancer ultrasound: screening tool or hype? *Diagn Imaging.* 1988; 302–305.
4. Waterhouse RL, Resnick MI. The use of transrectal prostatic ultrasonography in the evaluation of patients with prostatic carcinoma. *J Urol.* 1989; 141:233.
5. Lee F, Littrup PJ, Kumasaka GH, et al. The use of transrectal ultrasound in diagnosis, guided biopsy, staging and screening of prostate cancer. *Radiographics.* 1987; 7:627.
6. Paulson D. Diseases of the prostate. *Clin Symposia.* 1989; 41.
7. Resnick M. *Prostatic Ultrasonography.* Philadelphia: BC Decker; 1990.
8. Penta K. Etiology, Epidemiology and Prevention of Carcinoma of the Prostate. In: Walsh P, Retik A, Vaughan, et al. eds. *Campbell's Urology.* 7th ed. Philadelphia: WB Saunders; 1998.
9. Brawer M, Chetner M. Ultrasonography of the prostate and biopsy. In: Walsh P, Retik A, Vaughan E, et al. eds. *Campbell's Urology.* 7th ed. Philadelphia: WB Saunders; 1998.

CHAPTER 8

TRANSVAGINAL SONOGRAPHY

Charles S. Odwin and Arthur C. Fleischer

Study Guide

INTRODUCTION

Transvaginal sonography (TVS) involves the insertion of a specifically designed transducer into the vagina for imaging pelvic structures. Numerous names have been applied to this type of scanning such as endovaginal, endocavity, endosonography and transvaginal. The terms transvaginal and endovaginal are both descriptive of the technical approach to scanning and are not specific for imaging of the vagina. In fact, only a small area of the vagina is imaged; the images are predominantly of the uterus and its adnexa. The terms endosonography and endocavity sonography are general terms used to describe any insertion of the transducer into the body cavity; the vagina, rectum, or esophagus. Any insertion of a medical instrument into a body cavity is classified as an invasive procedure, unlike the term transabdominal or transvesical sonography, in which the transducer is placed on the skin.

PHYSICAL CONCEPTS

The concept of using high-frequency transducers within the vaginal cavity to image the uterus and adnexa derived from the basic concept of ultrasound physics. Placing the transducer in close proximity to the pelvic organs or structures allows the use of higher frequencies, which in turn provides better resolution, both axial and lateral. The close proximity of the transducer also results in reduced attenuation and better focusing. As a result, transvaginal sonography allows for earlier and more definitive diagnosis than is possible with conventional transabdominal techniques.

Transvaginal sonography (TVS) has many clinical obstetric and gynecologic applications because of its ability to delineate the uterus and its adnexa. These include

- evaluation of the endometrium in women with postmenopausal bleeding or dysfunctional bleeding (DUB)
- evaluation of pelvic masses

- diagnosing ectopic pregnancy and other complicated early pregnancy
- evaluation of the cervix
- monitoring the follicles of an infertile patient who is undergoing ovulation induction
- guiding the placement of the needle during follicular inspiration or aspiration of fluid from cul de sac
- evaluating the Fallopian tube
- evaluating blood flow to the gestational sac and uterine artery with Doppler imaging
- achieving additional diagnostic information in conjunction with transabdominal sonography
- detecting the presence of placenta previa
- evaluating the fetal intracranial anatomy and prolapsed of the umbilical cord during the second and third trimester

CONTRAINDICATIONS TO TRANSVAGINAL SONOGRAPHY

- patients who decline the procedure
- infants and children
- virgins
- elderly patients with narrow introitus or atrophic vaginitis who experience pain or discomfort during probe insertion
- unconscious patient (without informed consent)

ADVANTAGES OF TRANSVAGINAL SONOGRAPHY

- higher resolution
- earlier and more definitive diagnosis
- does **not** require a full urinary bladder
- faster medical management
- additional information
- eliminates the discomfort during bladder filling

DISADVANTAGES OF TRANSVAGINAL SONOGRAPHY

- limited field of view
- large masses may not be seen because they are beyond the focal zone of the transducer
- unable to see both ovaries on the same image
- documentation of uterine size may be difficult because of magnification in the near field
- the confined space of the vagina limits the mobility of the transducer; therefore, complete sequential images obtained with transabdominal sonography cannot be achieved with transvaginal sonography
- only the presenting parts of the fetus and cervix can be seen in the second and third trimester pregnancy with the transvaginal approach

PATIENT PREPARATION

The patient should void before the examination begins, and the procedure should be explained to the patient. If a male examiner is to perform the examination, a female chaperone should be present during the entire examination. The chaperone should be a permanent staff of the faculty who is familiar with the procedure. Volunteers and family members are not appropriate chaperones. The name of the chaperone and time of the procedure should be documented. The staff in the room should be introduced to the patient.

TRANSDUCERS

Transducers for transvaginal scanning have a specific size, shape, and frequency. Their diameter ranges from 12 mm to 16 mm; this smaller-than-usual diameter allows easy penetration within the vaginal lumen without patient discomfort. In addition, these transducers are twice as long when compared to transabdominal transducers.

Because the normal length of the vaginal lumen in approximately 7.5–9.5 cm, the transvaginal transducer must be longer than usual so that part of it can be inserted and the other part can serve as a handle for the operator. The normal range of frequency used in transvaginal sonography is 5–10 MHz, with a sector field of view of 90°–115°. The larger the sector fields of view, the larger the portion of the organ or structure that can be visualized.

COLOR DOPPLER

Transvaginal color Doppler is a combination of B-mode image, pulse-wave Doppler, and a color flow display (triplex imaging). The direction of blood flow is indicated by assigning color to the Doppler-shifted echoes that are superimposed on the gray-scale image.

The direction of flow toward and away from the transducer is presented in different colors on the image. For example, red represents flow toward the transducer; whereas, blue represents flow away from the transducer, and a mixture of colors represents turbulent flow. Color Doppler has several advantages. First, because a network of blood vessels occasionally can mimic follicles, color Doppler allows rapid differentiation between vascular structures and follicles. It also allows precise placement of the sample volume for Doppler waveform analysis.

TRANSDUCER PREPARATION

Cross-contamination with reusable medical devices and current methods used in precautionary measures should be addressed. The microorganisms that cause sexually transmitted disease, including the human immunodeficiency virus (HIV), are sometimes present in the vaginal secretions. Although these microorganisms are usually transmitted through sexual contact with an infected partner, they can be transmitted by contaminated reusable instruments. The current methods used to prevent transmission of infection with transvaginal transducers are

1. chemical disinfectants
2. disposable probe cover (condoms, latex gloves, and sheaths)

Both are required to prevent cross-infection from the transducer because, although the probe is covered, a microscopic tear in the cover will expose the transducer to the vaginal membrane and the external cervical os. The transducer should be disinfected before it is returned to the manufacture or technical support staff for maintenance or repair.

The first steps in preparing the transducer for an examination is disinfecting the probe from disease-causing organism bacteria, viruses, and fungi. Several methods of disinfecting agents are available; most are cold chemical disinfectants, which are glutaraldehyde based (e.g., Cidex™, MetriCide™, Wavicide™). The piezoelectric crystal of the transducer is heat sensitive. Therefore, steam autoclaves should not be used because excessive heat could destroy the transducer. The transducer manufacturers normally recommend the type of chemical that is safe for their transducer, specifications, and the time limit for transducer chemical immersion.

Transvaginal transducers are composed of metals, plastic, crystal, bonding materials, and all are not constructed in the same way. Thus, a disinfectant chemical may be safe for some transducers but destructive to others. Sonographers should not attempt to disinfect a transducer until they have carefully reviewed the manufacturer's instruction manual and consulted with the technical support staff regarding any changes that may have occurred since the manual was published. To avoid chemical spills and reduce chemical vapors to health care workers a commercially available immersion station can be used, but must comply with OSHA and JCAHO regulatory requirements.

In addition to disinfectant requirements a probe cover is employed. The probe covers are specially designed sheaths for covering the transducers; they are available in different sizes to fit all types of transducers. These covers are made up of a variety of materials: latex, polyethylene, and polyurethane and are approved by the U.S. Food and Drug Administration (FDA). Probe covers are also available in sterile or nonsterile packs. Patient and health care workers with latex hypersensitivity should use alternate covers and gloves. The used probe cover and gloves should be treated as potentially infectious waste and disposed of accordingly.

POSITION OF THE PATIENT AND THE EXAMINATION TABLE

During the transvaginal examination, the patient is placed in the lithotomy position for insertion of the transducer and for scanning. The probe can be inserted by the patient, the physician, or the sonographer. When the patient does the insertion, the transducer cable should be held so that the patient cannot accidentally drop the transducer.

The ideal table is a gynecologic examination table that allows numerous degrees of pelvic tilt positions and has stirrups for the patient's heels. The table is placed in a slight Fowler's position (also called the reversed Trendelenburg position) (Fig. 8–1). Elevation of the thighs allows the transducer to be moved freely from side to side (horizontal plane). The gynecologic examination table allows free upward and downward movement of the transducer (vertical plane), and the slight Fowler's position of the table allows pooling of the small amount of peritoneal fluid normally found in the region of the cul-de-sac, which allows better delineation of pelvic structures. The Trendelenburg position should not be used because it drains away this fluid. If a gynecologic examination table is unavailable, a flat examination table can be prepared by placing a cushion or inverted bedpan under the patient's pelvis.

SCANNING TECHNIQUES

The commonly used transducer maneuvers for transvaginal sonography are:

a) in and out
b) rotation
c) anterior and posterior angulations
d) right and left angulations

These maneuvers are limited by the size of the vaginal lumen. (Fig. 8–2A) illustrates the in-and-out motion of the transducer used to achieve variation in the depth of the imaging from the cervix to fundus. Imaging from cervix is optimized by gradual withdrawing the probe with up angulations. Fig. 8–2B illustrates the rotating motion of the transducer for obtaining various degrees of semiaxial to semicoronal planes. And (Fig. 8–2C) illustrates the angling motion of the transducer within the vaginal canal to obtain images of the anterior and posterior cul-de-sac. The side-to-side movements are to obtain images of the adnexa (Fig. 8–3 A, B).

Pregnancy Test

Rapid Qualitative Pregnancy Test. This small kit used for detection of hCG (human chorionic gonadotropin) in urine or serum is readily available for immediate hospital or office use and is now available over the counter for private use. Beta hCG is a hormone normally produced by the placenta and present in the serum and urine of a pregnant woman. This rapid kit is an excellent marker on qualitative confirmation of pregnancy while awaiting the result of the more accurate quantitative serum beta hCG. The kit uses a color-coded result in a small result window as the sample contains a detectable amount of hCG in 3 to 5 minutes. A minus (–) result in the result window means not pregnant or below the range of hCG sensitivity. A plus (+) in the result window indicates pregnancy. The first morning urine usually has a higher level of hCG present.

The sensitivity for urine varies from 20 to 25 mIU/mL as early as 7–10 days postconception with an accuracy of

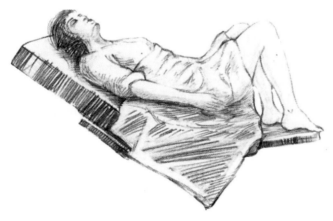

Figure 8–1. Examination table in a slight Fowler's position with a 20° elevation. The patient is in the lithotomy position.

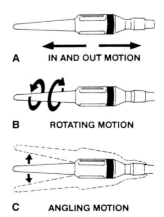

A   IN AND OUT MOTION

B   ROTATING MOTION

C   ANGLING MOTION

Figure 8–2. Scanning techniques: **(A)** in and out; **(B)** rotating motion; **(C)** angling motion. *(Reprinted with permission from Advanced Technology Laboratories, Bothell, Washington.)*

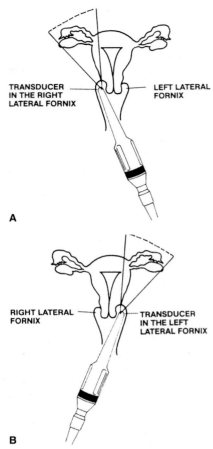

TRANSDUCER
IN THE RIGHT
LATERAL FORNIX

LEFT LATERAL
FORNIX

A

RIGHT LATERAL
FORNIX

TRANSDUCER
IN THE LEFT
LATERAL FORNIX

B

Figure 8–3. (A) Transducer in the right lateral fornix; **(B)** transducer in the left lateral fornix. *(Reprinted with permission from Advanced Technology Laboratories, Bothell, Washington.)*

During the first trimester of pregnancy, the serum beta hCG normally doubles every 48 hours (2 days) or increases at least 66% every 48 hours before 8 weeks of gestation. In the presence of ectopic pregnancy, approximately 80% serum beta hCG have abnormal doubling beta (low doubling time, remain the same, or decrease slightly). However, 10% of ectopic may have a normal doubling in 48 hours, but may eventually drop in titers or plateau.[3] A constant decreasing serial quantitative serum beta hCG in the first trimester is indicative of an abnormal pregnancy, regardless of the pregnancy location.

The serum levels for twins are twice as high as singleton pregnancy, and patients with a benign mole have higher levels than women with a normal pregnancy. Those with invasive mole have higher ratios than those with noninvasive moles, and those with choriocarcinoma have even higher levels than those with invasive moles.[3]

There are various methods of reporting beta hCG. Some laboratories report serum quantitative beta hCG results in terms of International Reference Preparation (1st IRP); whereas, others report the results in terms of Second International Standard (2nd IS). The most current is the Third International Standards (3rd IS). The Third International Standards (3rd IS) is identical to the 1st IRP and 1.8 times those reported for the 2nd IS. Therefore, values in terms of the 3rd IS have been calculated by multiplying the 2nd IS by 1.88 which is the conversion factor.[3]

Serum Beta hCG Correlation With Ultrasound

The level of serum beta hCG to which a gestational sac should be seen on ultrasound is call the discriminatory zone. This concept was developed by Kadar et al., who correlated the ultrasound findings from patients with intrauterine pregnancy with serum beta hCG values using transabdominal scanning. This zone was between 6000 and 6500 mIU/mL of hCG using the First International Reference Preparation (1st IRP).[4] Later, Nyberg et al. reported a modification of the discriminatory zone at 1800 mIU/mL Second International Standard (2nd IS), which is equivalent to 3600 mIU/mL First International Reference Preparation (1st IRP).[5]

The Second International Standard (2nd IS) was released by the World Health Organization (WHO), which is approximately one-half of IRP values.[3] The most current beta hCG levels to which an intrauterine gestational sac can be seen with transvaginal ultrasound is now about 1000 to 1500 mIU/mL, depending on the frequency of the transvaginal probe used.[6] The increased sensitivity in detectable amount of hCG in the urine and serum of pregnant women and the rapid advancement in computers, real-time ultrasound equipment is constantly changing. Therefore, the current level to which a gestational sac should be seen on ultrasound is expected to decrease as the technology advances. If the gestational sac is not seen at this level, the pregnancy may be either abnormal or ectopic. However, a repeated level may be needed to confirm.

99%. A false-negative result can result from a urine sample that is too dilute. Therefore, to avoid a false-negative result, the test should be performed before high volume of fluid ingestion for sonography or high volume of intravenous fluid hydration. The test can also be false-negative if the sensitivity of the detectable hCG levels is below 20 mIU/mL. Fertility drugs containing hCG, such as Pregnyl can alter the result.[1, 2]

Serum Beta hCG Pregnancy Test. This form of pregnancy test is available in qualitative (positive or negative) and quantitative (numerical values).

Human Chorionic Gonadotropin (hCG). hCG is a glycoprotein secreted by the syncytiotrophoblastic cells of the trophoblast.[1] The hCG is composed of two dissimilar subunits, alpha and beta. The antibodies against the beta subunit are used specifically to measure hCG.[1] The quantitative beta hCG is very useful in the diagnosis of ectopic pregnancy, gestational trophoblastic disease or abnormal pregnancy.

The Progesterone Level

Progesterone levels normally increase with gestational age. However, when an ectopic pregnancy is present, the corpus luteum does not secrete as much progesterone as occurs in normal pregnancy. Therefore, the concentration of the serum progesterone is usually lower in ectopic pregnancies. A value of 25 ng/mL or more is, 98% of the time, associated with a normal intrauterine pregnancy; whereas, a value less than 5 ng/mL identifies a nonviable pregnancy, regardless of its location.[7]

The combination use of serum beta hCG, progesterone level, and transvaginal sonography has resulted in great improvement in the diagnosis and management of ectopic pregnancy over the last 15–20 years.

Ectopic Pregnancy

Any pregnancy outside the endometrial cavity is called ectopic pregnancy. The incidence of this type of pregnancy has increased, but the rate of death from ectopic pregnancy has declined. This decrease is the result of earlier diagnosis.[8] Most ectopic pregnancy occurs in the Fallopian tube, approximately 95%. It accounts for approximately 12% of all maternal deaths.[2] It can occur in any anatomic segments of the fallopian tube, but more frequently in the ampullary region. Other less common sites for ectopic implantation are the uterine cervix, ovaries, and abdomen. If the pregnancy is in the abdomen with advanced gestational age, transabdominal scans should be performed first and, if necessary, transvaginal. Abdominal pregnancy is the only form of ectopic that can go to term. The incidence of live birth after abdominal pregnancy is very rare. I have only seen two of these cases go to term in my 22 years of experience, and both were delivered by abdominal surgery. In both cases, the placenta was left in the abdomen after surgery. On occasion, the placenta in an abdominal pregnancy may be adherent to bowel and blood vessels; removal could result in massive hemorrhage. In such cases, the placenta is left in situ and ultimately resorbs.[7, 9]

A coexistent intrauterine pregnancy and ectopic pregnancy known as heterotopic can occur. It was first reported at a rate of 1 in 30,000, then 1 in 16,000 and most currently 1 in 8000. This increase in heterotopic pregnancies may be attributable to increased ovulation induction.[6]

Risk Factors for Ectopic Pregnancy

- salpingitis from chlamydial infection or pelvic inflammatory disease
- previous ectopic pregnancy
- previous operations on the Fallopian tube, bilateral tubal ligation or tuboplasty surgery

Clinical Signs and Symptoms of Unruptured Ectopic Pregnancy

- unilateral pelvic pain, which increases in severity with time
- vaginal spotting or bleeding
- amenorrhea
- adnexal mass
- positive pregnancy test
- nausea and vomiting

Clinical Signs and Symptoms of Ruptured Ectopic Pregnancy

- generalized abdominal pain
- rebound tenderness
- cervical motion tenderness
- bilateral adnexal tenderness
- right shoulder pain
- tachycardia and hypotension
- decreased hematocrit
- syncope
- tachypnea

TRANSVAGINAL ULTRASOUND

Unruptured Ectopic Pregnancy

Ectopic pregnancy should be suspected when there is no intrauterine gestational sac and the serum beta hCG is at a level in which a pregnancy should be seen (values 1500 mIU/mL or greater). The sonographic appearance of ectopic pregnancy primarily depends on if the pregnancy is ruptured, unruptured, its location, and size. The sonographic equipment, the frequency of the transvaginal transducer, as well as the skills of the operator play important roles. Advanced ultrasound equipment in the hands of a skilled operator can, on some occasions depict an ectopic pregnancy before the patient begins to have clinical symptoms. Early depiction of ectopic pregnancy before a tubal rupture occurs is imperative to avoid the potential risk of massive blood loss and tubal damage. However, some patients delay seeking medical treatment when the symptoms start, arriving at the emergency department after rupture.

The sonographic appearance of an unruptured ectopic pregnancy is an adnexal ring-like mass with increased color flow around its periphery ("Ring of Fire"). The center of this adnexal ring is anechoic, and its periphery echogenic, resembling a doughnut. It is imperative for the sonographer to identify and depict the ovary on the side of the adnexal ring. A hemorrhagic corpus luteum cyst could mimic this finding. Rarely, an extrauterine gestational sac is seen with a live embryo.

Fig. 8–4A is a sagittal view demonstrating the uterine cavity free of any intrauterine pregnancy. Fig. 8–4B is of the same patient in a transverse view with an extrauterine gestational sac with an embryo.

Ruptured Ectopic Pregnancy

After an ectopic pregnancy ruptures, blood accumulates in the abdomen and pelvis. It can readily be depicted with both transabdominal and transvaginal sonography. The blood may appear completely anechoic with some areas of echogenic fluid attributable to clotted blood. The patient is scanned in the supine position, allowing the free fluid to accumulate in a gravity-dependent position.

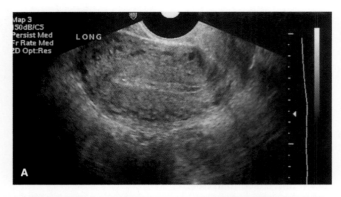

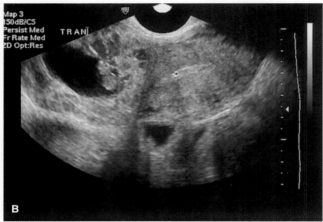

Figure 8–4. (A) Sagittal view of the uterus, free of any intrauterine pregnancy; **(B)** transverse view with a right unruptured ectopic pregnancy.

The regions of Morison's pouch, paracolic gutters, and posterior cul-de-sac are the most common locations for intraperitoneal blood after rupture. A ruptured hemorrhagic corpus luteum cyst could mimic a ruptured ectopic pregnancy both clinically and sonographically. The only type of ectopic pregnancy, which is known to rupture without intraperitoneal collection, is a cervical ectopic pregnancy.

Patients with a large amount of blood in the abdomen may develop right shoulder pain because of diaphragmatic irritation, tachycardia, and hypotension secondary to vascular shock. There is no need to distend the urinary bladder in these cases because the intraperitoneal fluid is a good acoustic medium to view the abdominal and pelvic viscera. The ingestion of fluid to distend the urinary bladder for transabdominal scanning in a patient who is hemodynamically unstable may further delay immediate medical managements and may further interfere with patients who need to be NPO for surgery. Sonographers should have experience in recognizing this emergency and call for assistance immediately.

Treatment

The treatment for ectopic pregnancy depends on whether the pregnancy is ruptured or unruptured, size, location, and the patient's clinical condition. The use of methotrexate, which is a folic acid antagonist that inhibits DNA synthesis in the trophoblastic cells, has been successfully used in treatment of unruptured ectopic pregnancy.[10]

Medical treatment with methotrexate is very useful when the pregnancy is located in the cervix, ovary, or cornua, where surgical treatment carries a significant risk.[7] The purpose of medical treatment is to avoid potential risk of both anesthesia and surgery and spare the fallopian tube from surgical trauma or damage from spontaneous rupture. The success rate is high if the unruptured gestational sac is less than 4 cm and no sonographic evidence of fetal heart activity.[10] This medical treatment is not without failure. There is a possibility of rupture in 3–4% of medically treated cases.[2]

Patients with ruptured ectopic pregnancy usually present with severe pain, accompanied by hypotension and tachycardia. In time, the pain increases in severity and aborts away after rupture. It recurs, as generalized abdominal pain with rebound tenderness secondary to hemoperitoneum. Sonographers must be informed before performing an ultrasound of any patient with a history of diagnosed ectopic pregnancy who is currently undergoing treatment with methotrexate. In a patient in which methotrexate has failed and the patient is hemodynamically unstable, ultrasound scanning may not be helpful because a delay in medical management could result in the patient's going into shock.

Surgical Treatment

Linear salpingostomy is currently the procedure of choice for unruptured ectopic pregnancy. This can be done by laparoscopic techniques or by laparotomy. Laparotomy is indicated when patients are hemodynamically unstable.[7] Sonographers should obtain some past surgical history, if not included on the sonogram request form. Did you have an ectopic pregnancy before? Was your Fallopian tube removed? On which side was the ectopic?

Sonographers should be alert for any abdominal and pelvic surgical scars, which may be a result of previous surgical removal of abdominal/pelvic viscera. Failure to be observant and to obtain patient history pertinent to scanning could result in misdiagnosis.

Salpingostomy: surgical incision of the Fallopian tube for removal of tubal pregnancy. The incision is left open. The Fallopian tube is not removed.

Salpingotomy: surgical incision of the Fallopian tube for removal of tubal pregnancy. The incision is closed by suture. The Fallopian tube is not removed.

Salpingectomy: surgical removal of tubal pregnancy by removing part or all of the Fallopian tube.

ULTRASOUND ANATOMY

Uterus

Visualization of the texture and thickness of the uterus and endometrium is greatly improved with transvaginal sonography. The appearance and thickness of the endometrium will vary, depending on the phase of the patient's menstrual cycle.

Blood supplied to the uterus is from the uterine and ovarian arteries. The uterine artery gives rise to the arcuate arteries, which course within the outer myometrium (Fig. 8–5) of the arcuate venous plexus. Imaging of these vessels can be enhanced with color vaginal sonography. Because of the magnification and the relatively small field of view provided by transvaginal sonography, measurements to indicate the size of the uterus are best obtained with transabdominal sonography.

Endometrial Disorders

Transvaginal sonography (TVS) provides detailed delineation of the thickness and texture of the endometrium. The endometrium should be measured in its thickest anterior/posterior thickness as portrayed in its long axis (bilayer thickness).

Although the image and measurement are used to characterize the endometrium, it must be evaluated completely and characterized by scanning sweeps performed in the long and short axis of the uterus. In women of childbearing age, the endometrium measures between 3–6 mm in the proliferative phase and up to 14–16 mm in the secretory phase.

The texture changes from isoechoic to multilayered in midcycle to echogenic in midsecretory phase. In postmenopausal woman, the endometrium should be less than 6–8 mm in thickness and homogenous in texture. This is true for most women taking hormone replacement therapy. Punctate cyst can be seen in the inner myometrium in women taking Tamoxifen. These are thought to represent reactivated adenomyomas. Polyps typically appear as echogenic endometrial masses that are insinuated between endometrial layers. They are especially seen when saline infusion Sonohysterography is performed.

Sonohysterography uses a flexible catheter that is inserted transcervically. This painless procedure is very accurate in the detection of polyps, submucosal (intracavitary) fibroids, and adhesions. Endometrial carcinoma typically causes asymmetric and irregularity of the endometrium. If there is invasion, the endometrial/myometrial junction is disrupted.

Evaluation of the Cervix

Transvaginal sonography (TVS) provides an objective means to evaluate the uterine cervical length and configuration. The normal cervix is between 2.0 and 2.5 cm in length and shows no funneling or dilation of the endocervical canal. A thin echogenic stripe in the endocervical canal can be seen in most cases and is contiguous with the endometrial canal. Multiple small cysts are sometimes seen in and around the cervical canal and represent nabothian cysts, which are caused by occlusion of the ducts of the cervical secreting glands. These are also known as retention cysts.

Ovaries

The ovaries are normally situated anterior and medial to the internal iliac artery and vein and can be recognized by their ovoid shape, texture, and the presence of Graafian follicles. To image the right ovary, the sonographer moves the transducer handle toward the patient's left thigh so that the tip of the transducer probe is in the right lateral fornix. To image the left ovary, the sonographer moves the handle toward the patient's right thigh so that the tip of the probe is in the left lateral fornix. Although the ovaries can be depicted from almost any parauterine position, they are usually depicted either lateral to the uterus or in the cul de sac. Unlike transabdominal sonography, which allows the simultaneous imaging of both ovaries relatively often, transvaginal sonography can best image only one ovary at a time. In the postmenopausal age group, the ovaries are more difficult to image because of the absence of Graafian follicles and atrophy of the ovaries. In patients who have had a hysterectomy, the ovaries can be difficult to depict because of the air-filled bowel occupying the space left by removal of the uterus.

SONOGRAPHIC PATHOLOGY

Pelvic Mass

Transvaginal sonography is an accurate means of evaluating the ovaries and adnexal structures for the presence or absence of a pelvic mass. Pelvic masses can be characterized as to their location (organ of origin) and internal consistency (cystic, solid, mixed, septated, multiloculated). Such physiologic cysts as the corpus luteum cyst can be characterized as arising from within or around the ovary; whereas, such extra ovarian masses as endometriomas appear outside the ovary.

Cystic masses must be scrutinized with TVS for the intactness of their wall and the presence of any papillary excrescence. Internal structures such as septate or solid areas need to be shown in a minimum of two imaging planes.

Certain pelvic masses have typical features, such as echogenic areas of fluid/fluid layering with dermoid cysts and calcifications within degenerated fibroids. Torsion may occur

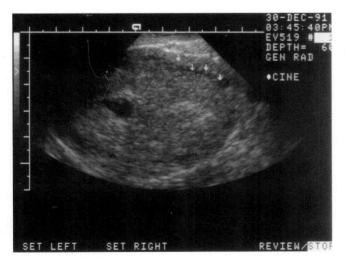

Figure 8–5. Sagittal view of the uterus. Small arrows points to the arcuate venous plexus.

in women with adnexal masses and/or hyperstimulated ovaries. In these patients, the ovaries are enlarged and may contain peripherally located cysts representing follicles. Color Doppler sonography is important in the evaluation of suspected torsion. Refer to Chapter 2 on Color Doppler Sonography (CDS) for further discussion. Malignancy should be suspected in masses containing papillary excrescences.

Early Pregnancy

Documentation of intrauterine pregnancy can be made as early as 4 weeks with transvaginal sonography by the identification of a gestational sac within the uterus. The gestational sac at this time has an anechoic center that represents the chorionic fluid and a highly echogenic ring that represents the developing chorionic villi and decidual tissue. The gestational sac size is about 5 mm when first depicted and increases in size as pregnancy advances with a growth rate of 1 mm per day. The gestational sac is empty and free of an embryo or yolk sac at this early stage. The gestational age at this time can be predicted by measuring the mean sac diameter (MSD).

These measurements are obtained by longitudinal sac diameter, the anteroposterior diameter, and the transverse diameter of the chorionic cavity, excluding the surrounding echogenic ring. All the dimensions are added then divided by 3 to obtain the mean sac diameter (MSD).

At approximately 5 weeks gestational age, the lacunae structures can be seen in a semicircle on one side of the gestational sac in the choriodecidua and represent the beginning of uteroplacental circulation (intervillous spaces).[6] Sonographically, they appear as small rounded hypoechoic structures that measure about 2–3 mm. Transvaginal color Doppler can demonstrate blood flow in these spaces.

Pseudogestational sac is blood or fluid in the uterine cavity mimicking a gestational sac. The differentiation between the gestational sac at 4–5 weeks and the pseudogestational sac are

Gestational sac	Pseudogestational sac
yolk sac	no yolk sac
embryo	no embryo
double decidual sac sign	no double decidual sac sign
highly echogenic ring	thin wall
grows 1 mm per day	no increment in size
lacunar structures with Doppler flow	no lacunar structures

The yolk sac is the first anatomic structure seen within the gestational sac at 5 weeks and measures approximately 5–6 mm. The yolk sac lies in the chorionic cavity (the extraembryonic coelom) between the amnion and chorion. The functions of the yolk sac are

1. form blood cells (hemopoiesis)
2. give rise to sex cell (sperm and egg)
3. supply nutrients from the trophoblast to the embryo

Sonographically, the yolk sac can be depicted between 5 and 10 weeks of gestation. The sac is connected to the midgut by a narrow pedicle called the yolk stalk, the vitelline duct, or the omphalomesenteric duct (Fig. 8–6). The yolk stalk detaches from the midgut by the end of the 6th week, and the dorsal part of the yolk sac is incorporated into the embryo as the primitive gut. As pregnancy advances, the yolk sac shrinks and becomes solid and its stalk becomes relatively longer.[11]

The yolk sac may prevail throughout the pregnancy and be recognized on the fetal surface of the placenta near the attachment of the umbilical cord; this situation is extremely rare and has no significance. In about 2% of adults, the proximal portion of the yolk stalk persists as a diverticulum of the ileum called Meckels diverticulum.[11]

Yolk Sac-Embryo Complex. At approximately 6 weeks of gestation, the crown-rump length of the embryo measures 3–4 mm and abuts the yolk sac. The upper limbs appear first, followed by the lower limb buds at 7 weeks. The heartbeat can be depicted at 6 weeks.

At approximately 8 weeks of gestation, the physiologic herniation of the midgut can be seen sonographically as a hyperechoic bulging of the cord near the point where the cord enters the fetal abdomen. The midgut returns to the abdomen, where it undergoes a second rotation, which is 180° counterclockwise.[11] Thus, the midgut undergoes a total rotation of 270°. If the bowel fails to return to the abdomen during this second stage of rotation, an omphalocele could be the result. Table 8–1 describes the chronological events of early pregnancy.

Nuchal Translucency

Nuchal translucency is thin membrane found along the posterior neck of most fetuses and can be seen at about 10–14 weeks. This translucency disappears by about 15 weeks. The Nuchal translucency measurements are performed as screening test. An increase in nuchal translucency may be a high risk for chromosomal abnormalities or cardiac defects.

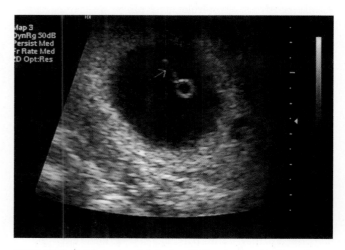

Figure 8–6. Small arrow points to the vitelline duct next to the yolk sac.

TABLE 8–1. CHRONOLOGICAL CHART: TRANSVAGINAL OBSTETRICAL SONOGRAPHY

Length of Gestation	Observations
4 weeks	The gestational sac is first seen at this time. It measures 4–5 mm and is surrounded by decidua with an anechoic center. No embryo or yolk sac is depicted at this time.
5 weeks	The yolk sac is first seen and measures 3–4 mm. The lacunar structures can be seen on one side of the gestational sac, and blood flow from its spaces can be depicted with color Doppler.
6 weeks	The fetal pole can be seen measuring 2–4 mm and abutting the yolk sac (yolk sac/embryo complex). The heartbeats can be seen, and the crown-rump length can be measured.
7 weeks	The limb buds first appear, and the amnion membrane and chorionic cavity can be seen.
8 weeks	Sonolucent brain vesicles and midgut herniation are seen.
9 weeks	The placenta and choroid plexus are seen.
10 weeks	The intraventricular heart septum is seen.
11 weeks	The umbilical cord is visible.
12 weeks	The extraembryonic coelom is obliterated, and the midgut herniation disappears.
13 weeks	The orbital structures are seen.
14 weeks	The four-chamber heart becomes visible.

HYSTEROSONOGRAPHY (HSG) OR SONOHYSTEROGRAPHY (SHG)

The recent developed technique for evaluation of the endometrium using saline infusion into the endometrial lumen during transvaginal sonography, termed sonohysterography (SHG) or hysterosonography (HSG) or saline infusion sonohysterography (SIS), is becoming more frequently used in the gynecologist's office and/or sonographic suites for the evaluation of suspected endometrial and/or certain myometrial disorders.[12] The technique provides a means to detect polypoid endometrial lesions, submucosal fibroids, adhesions, and uterine malformations that affect the lumen and can cause bleeding and/or infertility. Because the CPT code that is used for billing is listed as "hysterosonography," this is the preferred term.

HSG plays an important role in evaluation of the patient with unexplained postmenopausal bleeding and in those patients in whom the endometrium is thickened or indistinct on TVS. Polyps are enigmatic tumors apparently caused by resistance to progesterone-induced apoptosis or exposure to excess endogenous or exogenous estrogen. They typically are associated with intermenstrual bleeding, cramping, and/or infertility. Carcinomas may also be polypoid or arise within polyps.[13] HSG affords clear detection of the polyp and its pedicle. This is in contrast to a thickened endometrium as a result of endometrial hyperplasia and/or carcinoma.

Intraluminal fluid collections are frequently seen on TVS. Although they may be associated with endometrial cancer in some patients, they are more frequently associated with such benign conditions as cervical stenosis.[14] This "natural HSG" can be used to advantage to outline endometrial surfaces. This review provides an overview to the clinical utility, limitations of HSG, and a discussion of the circumstances in which it should be ordered.

TECHNIQUE

With the more extensive use of transvaginal sonography and small flexible catheters, the possibility of improved delineation of the endometrial lumen with intraluminal fluid instillation became possible.[15–18] The technique uses sterile saline as a negative (anechoic) contrast media to outline the endometrial lumen under continuous transvaginal sonographic visualization.[19]

HSG is primarily used for evaluation of endometrial polyps, assessing the presence and extent of submucosal fibroids, detection of uterine synechiae, and in selected cases of uterine malformations that involve the endometrial lumen. The reader is referred to several excellent descriptions of the spectrum of sonographic findings with this technique.[19,20]

Before saline instillation, the standard procedure for transvaginal sonography is followed, including covering the probe with a condom and placement of the transvaginal probe within the vaginal fornix and midvagina to delineate optimally the endometrial interfaces in both long and short axes. The images should be recorded on hard copy film or paper and videotaped for later review.

HSG involves placement of a catheter into the uterine lumen through the endocervical canal. Catheter choices that can be used include insemination catheter, pediatric Foley, pediatric feeding tube, a plastic SHG catheter, or a specially designed flexible catheter with an introducer (Akrad Co, Cranford, NJ). The Akrad catheter is preferred, because it can be introduced easily through the introducer into the cervix without much pain or discomfort (Fig. 8–7). The balloon catheter is recommended when trying to evaluate tubal patency after assessment of uterine lumen patency. Once the cervix is cleansed with a cleansing solution and stabilized with a speculum, the catheter can be advanced into the lumen; and 3–10 cc of sterile saline is injected during sonographic visualization. The slow instillation of saline, allowing reflux out of the cervix, also diminishes the possibility of pain during installation. The endometrium is imaged in both long and short axis, with specific attention to its regularity and thickness (Figs. 8–8, –9, –10). Because the dynamic nature of the examination, videotaping of the procedure is recommended with a few representative frozen images recorded for interpretation.

The procedure is best performed in the early follicular phase. This avoids confusing images arising from mildly

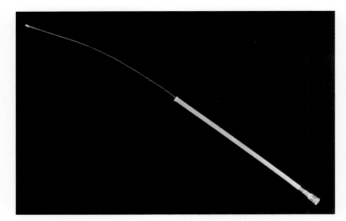

Figure 8–7. Tampa catheter consists of introducer and flexible catheter.

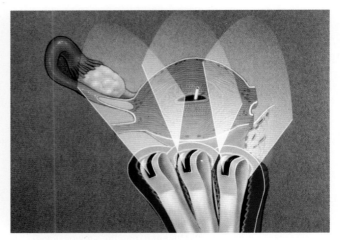

Figure 8–9. Diagram to show transducer sweep in long axis.

irregular interdigitating secretory endometrium or clot that may be encountered in the late secretory portion of the cycle and also decreases the possibility of dislodging an unsuspected early pregnancy. Because most endometrial polyps are echogenic, they can best be seen against the relatively hypoechoic proliferative phase endometrium.[21] Conversely, submucosal fibroids may best be imaged in the secretory phase because they are typically hypoechoic, and their relation to the displaced endometrium may be best delineated during this phase of the cycle.

Contraindications to HSG include hematometra, extensive pelvic inflammatory disease, or significant cervical stenosis. Doxycycline (250 mg p.o. t.i.d.). can be given a few days before HSG if pelvic inflammatory disease is suspected. Rarely an atrophic or stenotic vagina from aging or previous radiation therapy can produce significant discomfort, even with placement of the vaginal speculum.

Typically, the patient does not experience significant discomfort if the catheter is properly placed in the fundus, and only small amounts of fluid are gently infused and

allowed to reflux out of the cervix. Prophylactic antibiotics are usually not needed, but preprocedural, nonsteroidal anti-inflammatories (NSAIDs) are helpful to minimize uterine cramping.

TYPICAL SONOGRAPHIC FINDINGS

The intraluminal surface of the normal endometrium is usually delineated in its entirety after the introduction of intraluminal fluid. On short axis, the normal areas of endometrial invagination in both tubal ostia can be seen. In general, the endometrium measures up to 4 mm in thickness per single layer and should have a relatively regular and homogenous texture. The secretory phase endometrium is mildly irregular and may contain "endometrial wrinkles" a few millimeters in height, representing focal thickenings in the interdigitated endometrial surface. The endometrium is typically similar in thickness and texture, but focal irregularities can be observed in some patients (Figs. 8–11 and 8–12).

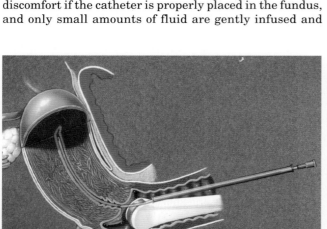

Figure 8–8. Diagram showing catheter in place. The catheter is advanced over the introducer and the tip is best positioned in the fundal portion or the endometrial lumen.

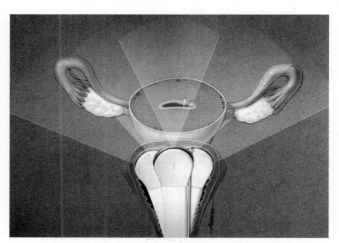

Figure 8–10. Diagram showing transducer sweep in short axis.

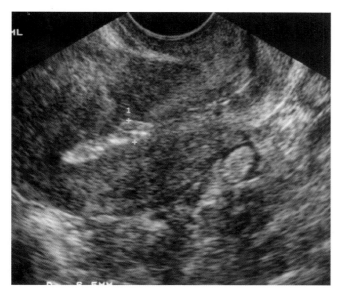

Figure 8–11. Focal endometrial hyperplasia. The TVS shows focal thickening (between cursors) in the corpus.

POLYPS

Endometrial polyps are typically echogenic and project into the endometrial lumen. Larger polyps may contain cystic spaces representing obstructed glands within the polyp (Fig. 8–12). In the nondistended endometrium, they typically displace the median echo, which may represent refluxed cervical mucus, and are best seen just before ovulation. As they enlarge, they can distend the cavity and may be apparent without iatrogenic distension of the endometrial lumen. Some are outlined by trapped intraluminal fluid, mucus, or

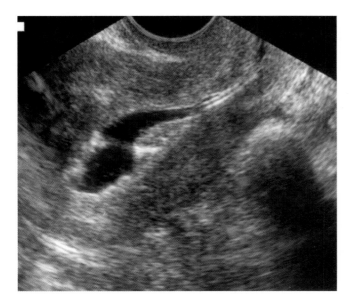

Figure 8–12. Focal endometrial hyperplasia. After saline is instilled, there is focal thickening of the endometrium, which was found to represent hyperplasia.

blood. The vascularity of the pedicle can be demonstrated in some cases with transvaginal color Doppler sonography.

SUBMUCOSAL FIBROIDS

Submucosal fibroids are typically hypoechoic and displace the basalis layer of the endometrium. Amount of extension into the myometrial layers is important to distinguish superficial submucosal fibroids from those that extend into the lumen may be treated with wire loop resections from the lumen; whereas, submucosal and/or intramural fibroids require a transperitoneal approach. If a submucosal fibroid has a thin stalk, it may be removed by wire loop or alligator forceps; whereas, those that extend beyond the endometrial–myometrial interface will not be amenable to wire loop resection.

SYNECHIAE

Synechiae typically occur as the sequelae of intrauterine instrumentation. They may be either echogenic or hypoechoic, depending on their fibrous content. The hypoechoic synechiae are best delineated in the background of the typically echogenic secretory phase endometrium.[22]

OTHER

Certain uterine malformations that affect the lumen, such as bicornuate or septate uteri, may be evaluated using HSG. The presence or absence of a fundal cleft is important in distinguishing bicornuate uteri from septated uteri.

Color Doppler sonography may be helpful to identify the vascular pedicle of a polyp, as well as the vascular rim of certain leiomyomata. HSG is helpful in determining whether a polyp has a wide or narrow pedicle because those with a thin pedicle are more easily removed with a forceps in the office than those with a thick pedicle.

HSG is also particularly helpful in determining whether certain intraluminal cystic areas are within a polyp or the myometrium. Punctate cystic spaces are frequently seen within polyps as a result of glandular obstruction. They may also be seen within the myometrium in women who are on Tamoxifen or a selective estrogen receptor modulator (SERM), possibly a result of reactivation of dormant adenomyosis.[17]

SUMMARY

SHG affords detailed delineation of the endometrial surface. Polyps, submucosal fibroids, and synechiae are readily delineated using this technique.

This study guide provides a description of the major applications of TVS in obstetrics and gynecology. The reader is referred to the references listed at the end of this chapter for further information.

REFERENCES

1. Braunstein GD. *hCG Testing: Volume 1: A Clinical Guide for the Testing of Human Chorionic Gonadotropin.* Abbott Park, IL: Abbott Diagnostics Educational Services; 1993.
2. Speroff L, Glass RH, Kase NG. *Clinical Gynecology Endocrinology and Infertility.* 5th ed. Baltimore: Williams & Wilkins; 1994.
3. Braunstein GD. *hCG Testing: Volume 11: Answers to Frequently Asked Questions about hCG Testing.* Abbott Park, IL: Abbott Diagnostics Educational Services; 1991.
4. Kadar N, DeVore G, Romero R. Discriminatory hCG zone: its use in the sonographic evaluation for ectopic pregnancy. *Obstet Gynecol.* 1981;58:156–161.
5. Nyberg DA, Filly RA, Filho DD, et al. Abdominal pregnancy: early diagnosis by US and serum chorionic gonadotropin levels. *Radiology.* 1986;158:393–396.
6. Timor-Tritsch IE, Rottem S. *Transvaginal Sonography.* 2nd ed. New York: Elsevier; 1991.
7. Mishell DR, Stenchever MA, Droegemueller W, Herbst A. *Comprehensive Gynecology.* 3rd ed. St. Louis, MO: Mosby Year Book, 1997.
8. Lipscomb GH, Stovall TG, Ling FW. Primary Care: nonsurgical treatment of ectopic pregnancy. *N Engl J Med.* 2000;343:1325–1329.
9. Cunningham GF, McDonald PC, Grant NF, et al. *William's Obstetrics.* 19th ed. Norwalk, CT: Appleton & Lange; 1993.
10. Fleischer AC, Kepple DM. *Transvaginal Sonography: A clinical Atlas.* 2nd ed. Philadelphia: J.B. Lippincott Company; 1995.
11. Moore KL, Persaud TVN. *The Developing Human: Clinically Orented Embryology.* 5th ed. Philadelphia: WB Saunders; 1993.
12. Fleischer A. Sonohysterography combined with sonosalpingography: correlation with endoscopic findings in infertility patients. *J Ultrasound Med.* 1997;16:381–384.
13. Salm R. The incidence and significance of early carcinomas in endometrial polyps. *J Pathol.* 1972;108:47–53.
14. Pardo J, Kaplan B, Nitke S, Ovadia J, Segal J, Neri A. Postmenopausal intrauterine fluid collection: correlation between ultrasound and hysteroscopy. *Ultrasound Obstet Gynecol.* 1994;4:224–226.
15. Syrol CH, Sahakian V. Transvaginal sonographic detection of endometrial polyps with fluid contrast augmentation. *Obstet Gynecol.* 1992;79:1041–1043.
16. Parsons A, Lense J. Sonohysterography for endometrial abnormalities: preliminary results. *J Clin Ultrasound.* 1993;21:82.
17. Goldstein S. Unusual ultrasonographic appearance of the uterus in patients receiving Tamoxifen. *Am J Obstet Gynecol.* 1994;170:447–451.
18. Dubinsky T, Parvey H, Gormaz G, Maklad N. Transvaginal hysterosonography in the evaluation of small endometrial masses. *J Ultrasound Med.* 1995;14:1–6.
19. Cullinan J, Fleischer A, Kepple D, Arnold A. Sonohysterography: a technique for endometrial evaluation. *Radiographics.* 1995;15:501–514.
20. Parsons AK, Lense JJ. Sonohysterography, sonosalpingography, and sonohysterosalpinography. In *Sonography in Obstetrics and Gynecology,* Fleischer A, Romero R, Manning R, eds. Stamford, CT: Appleton & Lange; 1995.
21. Cohen Jr, Luxman D, Sagi J, Yovel I, Woman I, David MP. Sonohysterography for distinguishing endometrial thickening from endometrial polyps in postmenopausal bleeding. *Ultrasound Obstet Gynecol.* 1994;4:227–230.
22. Narayan R, Goswamy RK. Transvaginal sonography of the uterine cavity with hysteroscopic correlation in the investigation of infertility. *Ultrasound Obstet Gynecol.* 1993;3:129–133.

Questions

GENERAL INSTRUCTIONS: For each question, select the best answer. Select only one answer for each question unless otherwise specified.

1. The level of serum β-hCG at which the gestational sac can first be depicted with transvaginal or transabdominal sonography is referred to as

   (A) gestational sac levels
   (B) quantitative assay levels
   (C) the discriminatory zone
   (D) serum levels

2. Fusion of the amnion and chorion normally occurs between

   (A) 4 and 6 weeks
   (B) 7 and 8 weeks
   (C) 15 and 16 weeks
   (D) 20 weeks

3. The area outside of the amnion is called

   (A) the extraembryonic coelom
   (B) the amniotic cavity
   (C) the yolk sac
   (D) none of the above

4. At what gestational age should the fetal heart motion be detected on transvaginal sonogram?

   (A) 4 weeks
   (B) 5 weeks
   (C) 6 weeks
   (D) 8 weeks

5. The secondary yolk sac is located

   (A) within the amniotic cavity
   (B) between the amnion and chorion
   (C) within the embryo
   (D) none of the above

6. The position of the patient that enables free movement of the probe in the horizontal plane while performing transvaginal scanning is the

   (A) Trendelenburg position
   (B) lithotomy position
   (C) Sims's position
   (D) prone position

7. The position of the examination table for transvaginal sonography is

   (A) Trendelenburg position
   (B) lithotomy position
   (C) Sims's position
   (D) Fowler's position

8. When a gynecological examination table is not available for performing a transvaginal study, a flat examination table can be used, if a foam cushion is placed under the

   (A) head
   (B) pelvis
   (C) knees
   (D) legs

9. The most important prerequisites for transvaginal sonography is

   (A) emptying of the urinary bladder
   (B) selecting a low-frequency probe
   (C) adequate filling of the urinary bladder
   (D) putting the patient in the Trendelenburg position

10. The anatomic site of ectopic pregnancies with the greatest maternal morbidity is the

    (A) isthmic region of the Fallopian tube
    (B) interstitial region of the Fallopian tube
    (C) ampullary region of the Fallopian tube
    (D) intra-abdominal pregnancy

11. Human fertilization normally occurs in the

    (A) endometrial cavity
    (B) vaginal cavity
    (C) ovaries
    (D) ampullary region of the oviduct

12. Nabothian cyst are located in the

    (A) endometrial cavity
    (B) labia majoria
    (C) cervix
    (D) ovaries

13. The range of transducer frequencies used in transvaginal sonography is

    (A) 2.5–3.5 MHz
    (B) 3.5–5.0 MHz
    (C) 5.0–7.5 MHz
    (D) none of the above

14. Which of the following is not true for transvaginal sonography?

    (A) both ovaries are always seen simultaneously
    (B) an empty bladder is required before scanning
    (C) the ovaries are identified by the presence of follicles
    (D) a large mass can be missed

15. The normal ovary is located in the

    (A) pouch of Douglas
    (B) Waldeyer's Fossa
    (C) broad ligament
    (D) round ligament

16. In the evaluation of a patient with bicornuate uterus, the sonographer should examine the

    (A) liver
    (B) breast
    (C) gallbladder
    (D) kidneys

17. The most appropriate method of disinfecting the transvaginal probes from organisms, including the AIDS virus, is

    (A) diluted household bleach
    (B) ethylene oxide
    (C) glutaraldehyde-based chemical
    (D) an autoclave

18. The normal corpus luteum cyst of pregnancy usually regress at

    (A) 8–10 weeks gestation
    (B) 12–16 weeks gestation
    (C) 20–25 weeks gestation
    (D) 30–36 weeks gestation

19. The most accurate prediction of gestational age is obtained with measurements taken

    (A) 8–10 weeks
    (B) 18–20 weeks
    (C) 20–30 weeks
    (D) 36–40 weeks

20. The first anatomic structure to be apparent within the gestational sac is

    (A) embryo
    (B) placenta
    (C) heartbeat of the embryo
    (D) yolk sac

21. Transvaginal sonography can detect the embryological structures about

    (A) 4 weeks earlier than transabdominal sonography
    (B) 3 weeks earlier than transabdominal sonography
    (C) 1 week earlier than transabdominal sonography
    (D) the same time as transabdominal sonography

22. The diameter of the mature Graafian follicle ranges from

    (A) 3–5 mm
    (B) 10–12 mm
    (C) 17–25 mm
    (D) 26–30 mm

23. Preparation for transvaginal study does not require

    (A) disinfecting of the probe
    (B) emptying of the bladder
    (C) antibiotic therapy before probe insertion
    (D) application of a probe cover

24. Fluid in the posterior cul de sac is uncommon with

    (A) ectopic pregnancy
    (B) pelvic inflammatory disease
    (C) ovulation
    (D) uterine leiomyoma

25. On transvaginal sonography, the embryo is seen within the amniotic cavity and the secondary yolk sac is normally depicted within the

    (A) extraembryonic coelom
    (B) amniotic cavity
    (C) umbilical cord
    (D) trophoblast

26. The crown–rump length (CRL) is obtain by measuring

    (A) limb buds
    (B) yolk sac
    (C) embryo in flexion
    (D) longest axis of the embryo

27. The level of serum quantitative beta human chorionic gonadotropin (hCG) required to depict the gestational sac with transvaginal sonography is approximately

    (A) 6500 mIU/mL IRP
    (B) 3600 mIU/mL 2nd IS
    (C) 1000 to 1500 mIU/mL 3rd IRP
    (D) less than 500 mIU/mL 3rd IRP

28. A fully distended bladder in a patient undergoing transvaginal sonography will

    (A) occupy most of the image and displace organs of interest out of the focal range
    (B) allow better visualization of pelvic organs
    (C) produce low attenuation, resulting in reduced magnification
    (D) increase the focal range, allowing better image enhancement

29. The segment of the Fallopian tube that lies adjacent to the ovary is

    (A) infundibulum
    (B) fimbria
    (C) interstitial
    (D) ampullary

30. The transvaginal probe should be covered with a protective sheath before vaginal insertion. All of the following are recommended for this purpose *except*

    (A) sterile lamb condoms
    (B) latex gloves
    (C) latex condoms
    (D) sterile polyethylene covers

31. Which one of the following lubricants should not be used on latex probe covers?

    (A) coupling gel
    (B) water-based gel
    (C) petroleum jelly
    (D) K-Y jelly

32. Which of the following is not part of the adnexa?

    (A) ovaries
    (B) broad ligaments
    (C) ovarian cyst
    (D) uterus

33. A small cystic space in the posterior cranium of the embryo at approximately 7 to 9 weeks of gestation most likely represents

    (A) rhombencephalon
    (B) Dandy Walker-cyst
    (C) choroid plexus
    (D) mild hydrocephalus

34. The echogenic bulging of the umbilical cord seen with transvaginal sonography near the abdominal insertion at about 8th to 10th week of gestation, most likely represent

    (A) yolk sac
    (B) omphalocele
    (C) gastroschisis
    (D) physiologic herniation of midgut

35. The most common presenting symptoms of ectopic pregnancy is

    (A) bleeding
    (B) cramping
    (C) vaginal discharge
    (D) pain

36. The major limitation of transvaginal sonography is that

    (A) it is limited to the first trimester
    (B) its field of view is limited
    (C) useful only in evaluation intrauterine pregnancy (IUP) and ectopic pregnancy
    (D) not useful in the 2nd and 3rd trimester

37. The use of high-frequency transvaginal transducers results in

    (A) less penetration, more magnification, and better resolution
    (B) more penetration, less magnification, and less resolution
    (C) more penetration, more magnification, and better resolution
    (D) no change

38. Transvaginal sonography is useful for evaluating all of the above *except*

    (A) ectopic pregnancy
    (B) intrauterine growth retardation
    (C) third trimester pregnancy
    (D) placenta previa

39. Transvaginal sonography can depict the fetal heart before a clear sonographic depiction of the embryo can be obtained

    (A) by putting the M-mode curser on the gestational sac
    (B) by putting the M-mode curser on the trophoblast
    (C) by putting the M-mode curser at the periphery of the yolk sac
    (D) by putting the M-mode curser on the amnion

40. All of the following are correct about measuring nuchal translucency *except*

    (A) may be obtained by transabdominal
    (B) obtain after precise calculation of gestational age by crown–rump length (CRL)
    (C) may be obtained by transvaginal
    (D) obtain best when the fetal neck is extended

41. Which of the following is true of focal myometrial contraction?

(A) increased risk of spontaneous abortion
(B) distal acoustic shadow with attenuation of the ultrasound
(C) isoechoic with the adjacent myometrium
(D) distort both the serosal and endometrial contour of the uterus

42. The serum quantitative human chorionic gonadotropin (hCG) normally doubles approximately every

(A) 12 hours
(B) 24 hours
(C) 48 hours
(D) 72 hours

43. Which of the following is not a potential pitfall of first trimester nuchal translucency?

(A) nuchal cord
(B) unfused amnion
(C) neutral position of fetal head
(D) magnification

44. The serum quantitative human chorionic gonadotropin (hCG) normally first detectable, how many days post-conception?

(A) 10
(B) 14
(C) 28
(D) 30

45. Which of the following is not present when imaging the pelvic in post-menopausal patient?

(A) follicles
(B) internal iliac artery and vein
(C) ovaries
(D) color flow of iliac vessels

46. Which of the following can mimic a cornual ectopic pregnancy?

(A) abdominal pregnancy
(B) early intrauterine pregnancy in a bicornuate uterus
(C) cervical pregnancy
(D) corpus luteum cyst

47. The vessel that is located posterolateral to the ovary is

(A) external iliac
(B) infundibulopelvic
(C) common iliac
(D) hypogastric

48. A blighted ovum is

(A) retention of a dead embryo
(B) an ectopic pregnancy
(C) a trophoblastic disease
(D) an anembryonic pregnancy

49. An intrauterine gestational sac can be distinguished from a pseudogestational sac by the presence of

(A) anechoic center
(B) irregular contour
(C) positive pregnancy test
(D) yolk sac

50. Which of the following statements is correct about nuchal translucency?

(A) Nuchal skin fold thickness is measured between 15 and 21 weeks of gestation.
(B) Nuchal translucency measurements are obtained from the outer skull table to the outer skin surface.
(C) Landmarks include the cisterna magna and used to screen Down syndrome.
(D) It is a thin membrane projecting from the posterior aspect of the fetal neck.

For questions 51 through 55, refer to Figs. 8-13 A and B.

51. Figs. 8–13A and B show

(A) the endometrium in long and short axis
(B) the endometrium only in its most fundal area
(C) does not show the endometrium at all
(D) none of the above

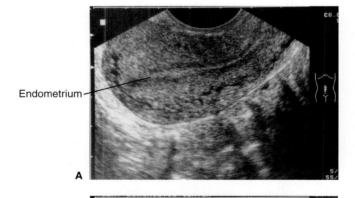

A

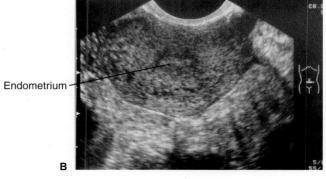

B

Figure 8–13. (A) and **(B)**, Transvaginal sonograms of the uterus.

52. The hypoechoic area adjacent to the endometrium represents

   (A) fluid trapped between the endometrium and the myometrium
   (B) the inner layer of myometrium
   (C) the basal layer of endometrium
   (D) none of the above

53. The arcuate vessels

   (A) are located between the outer and middle (spiral) layers of myometrium
   (B) can not be seen in normal women
   (C) when distended, are a sign of pelvic congestion
   (D) A and C

54. This patient, based on the sonographic appearance of the endometrium, is probably in which phase of her cycle?

   (A) proliferative (follicular)
   (B) secretory (luteal)
   (C) menstrual
   (D) cannot tell

55. The endometrium is best measured

   (A) in single layer thickness
   (B) in bilayer thickness
   (C) in transverse thickness
   (D) cannot be reliably measured

For questions 56 and 57, refer to Fig. 8-14.

56. Based on the sonographic appearance of the endometrium, this patient is probably in which phase of her cycle?

   (A) proliferative (follicular)
   (B) mid cycle (peri-ovulatory)
   (C) secretory (luteal)
   (D) cannot tell

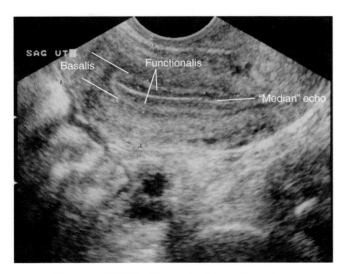

Figure 8–14. TVS of long axis of the endometrium.

57. The central echogenic interface represents

   (A) refluxed mucus
   (B) blood
   (C) sloughed endometrium
   (D) air

For questions 58 and 59, refer to Figs. 8-15 A, B, and C.

58. The figures suggest

   (A) a bicornuate uterus
   (B) a septated uterus
   (C) a uterus didelphys
   (D) none of the above

59. One can distinguish a bicornuate from a septate uterus by

   (A) evaluation of the fundus—because bicornuate uterus has a sharp cleft vs. a septated one which does not
   (B) the lack of agenesis of a kidney
   (C) the presence of two cervices
   (D) none of the above

For questions 60 and 61, refer to Figs. 18–16 A and B.

60. The following findings are shown

   (A) There is asymmetrical thickening at the endometrium suspicious for a polyp.
   (B) The endometrium is normal.
   (C) There are multiple intracavitary fibroids.
   (D) A and C

61. The most likely diagnosis is

   (A) endometrial hyperplasia
   (B) submucosal fibroid
   (C) endometrial carcinoma
   (D) atrophic endometrium

For questions 62 and 63, refer to Figs. 8–17 A and B.

62. The endometrial biopsy could show

   (A) endometrial atrophy
   (B) endometrial cancer
   (C) endometrial hyperplasia
   (D) any of the above

63. To demonstrate the pedicle of this mass, one might

   (A) instill more saline
   (B) reinsert a balloon tipped catheter
   (C) use color Doppler sonography
   (D) any of the above

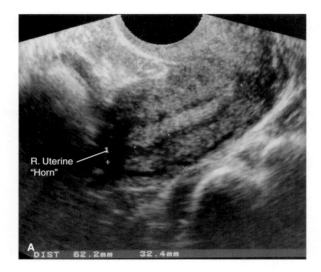

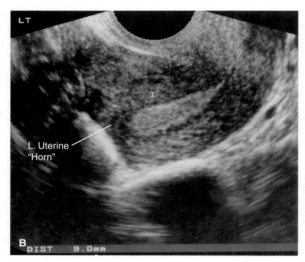

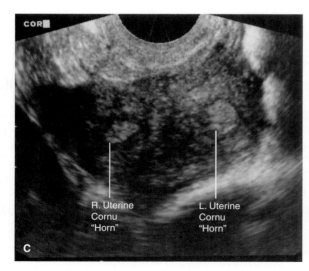

Figure 8–15. Short or coronal axis; **(A)** right, **(B)** coronal, and **(C)** short axis transvaginal sonograms.

64. In Fig. 8–18, the structure marked by the cursors could represent

(A) an endocervical polyp
(B) an organized clot sequestered in a uterine scar
(C) either A or B
(D) neither A nor B

65. In Fig. 8–19, the area marked by the cursors most likely represents

(A) an intramural fibroid
(B) a focal contraction
(C) neither A nor B
(D) either A or B

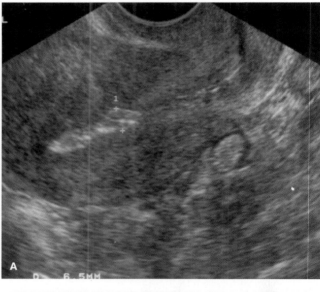

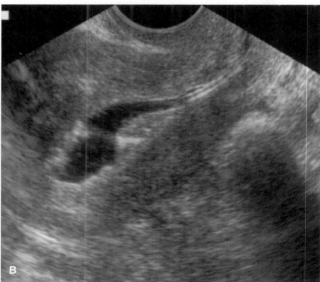

Figure 8–16. TVS **(A)** and sonohysterogram (SHG) **(B)** of a woman presenting with uterine bleeding.

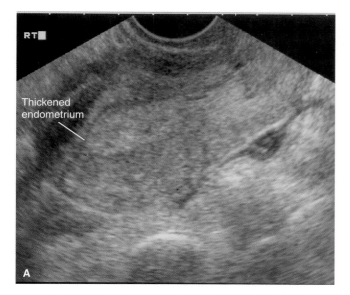

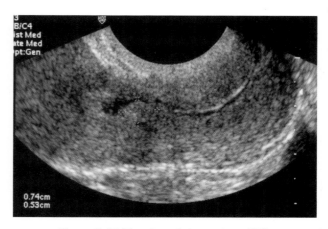

Figure 8–18. The uterus in long axis on TVS.

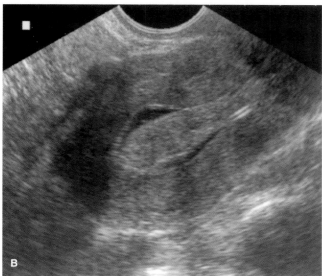

Figure 8–17. (A) and **(B)**, TVS and SHG on a postmenopausal woman with bleeding.

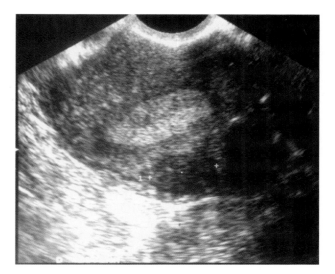

Figure 8–19. Short axis TVS of the uterus in a patient with chronic pelvic pain.

66. In Fig. 8–20, the hypoechoic interface within the cervix most likely represents

(A) cervical fluid
(B) cervical mucus
(C) an artifact
(D) none of the above

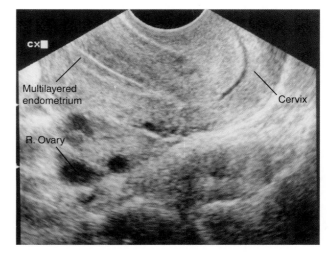

Figure 8–20. The uterus in long axis and the right ovary.

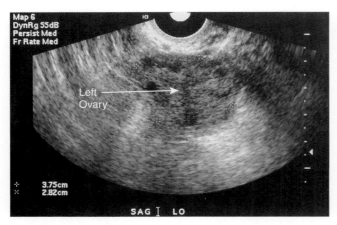

Figure 8–21. TVS of a left ovary of a premenopausal woman.

67. In Fig. 8–21, the left ovary is

(A) normal
(B) polycystic
(C) probably torsed
(D) none of the above

68. For Fig. 8–22, the most likely diagnosis is

(A) hemorrhagic corpus luteum
(B) endometrioma
(C) ovarian carcinoma
(D) cannot tell between A, B, and C

For questions 69 and 70, refer to Fig. 8–23.

69. The abnormal finding is

(A) a papillary excrescence arising from the wall of one of the cystic areas
(B) this is not abnormal, it represents a normal follicle and a corpus luteum
(C) neither A nor B
(D) the presence of cul-de-sac fluid

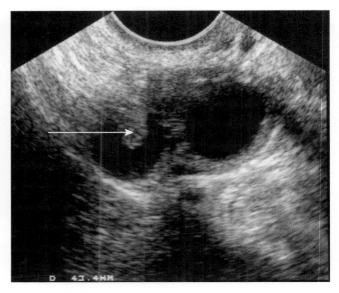

Figure 8–23. TVS of the right ovary in a 26-year-old woman with pelvic pain.

70. The next type of sonographic study should be

(A) transvaginal color Doppler sonography
(B) transabdominal sonography
(C) guided aspiration
(D) none of the above

For questions 71 and 72, refer to Fig. 8–24.

71. The structure measured by the cursors is

(A) the cervix
(B) the left ovary
(C) the right ovary
(D) bowel

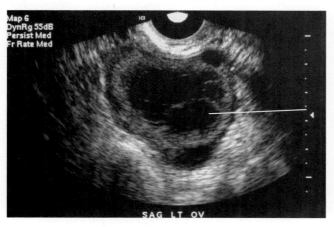

Figure 8–22. TVS of left ovary.

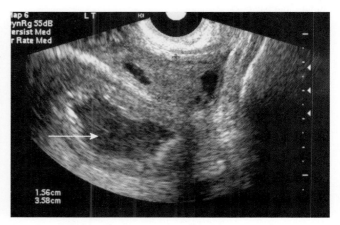

Figure 8–24. TVS of a woman who presented with left adnexal tenderness and fever.

72. Adjacent to the measured structure, the arrow points to

(A) loculated hemorrhagic fluid
(B) a bowel loop containing fluid
(C) the appendix
(D) none of the above

73. In regard to Fig. 8–25, which of the following statements is correct?

(A) This represents a pseudogestational sac of an ectopic pregnancy.
(B) The yolk sac is present within the gestational sac.
(C) The chorionic and decidual layers are intact.
(D) B and C

For questions 74 and 75, refer to Fig. 8–26.

74. Which of the following statements is correct?

(A) There is a nuchal translucency.
(B) There is either a nuchal translucency or cystic hygroma.
(C) This is a normal 9-week fetus.
(D) Karyotyping on this fetus is unnecessary.

75. Karyotyping on this pregnancy should show

(A) normal chromosomes
(B) Turner's syndrome (XO)
(C) Down syndrome
(D) either B or C

76. For Fig. 8–27, the most likely diagnosis is

(A) hydatidiform mole
(B) normal 9 week fetus
(C) neither A nor B
(D) either A or B

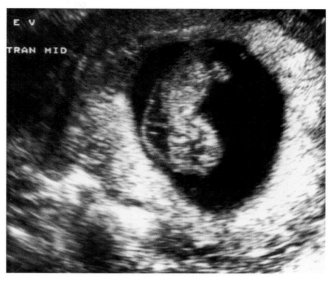

Figure 8–26. TVS of a 9-week fetus.

77. Which of the following statements regarding Fig. 8–28 is correct?

(A) The cervix is shown in long axis.
(B) The cervix is shown in short axis.
(C) There is fluid in the endocervical canal.
(D) There is a clot or polyp in the endocervical canal.
(E) A, C, and D

78. Fig. 8–29 shows

(A) a large polyp in the fundal area
(B) a large submucosal fibroid in the fundal area
(C) either A or B
(D) neither A nor B

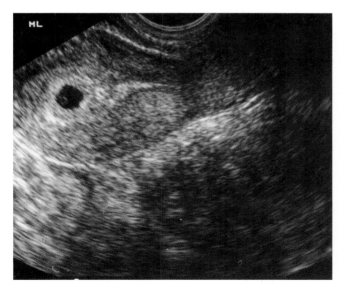

Figure 8–25. TVS of a woman who is 5 weeks pregnant.

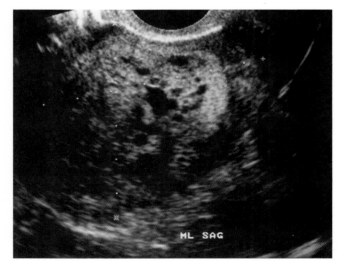

Figure 8–27. TVS of a 9-week pregnancy.

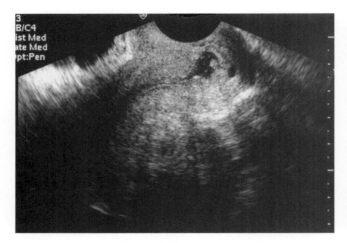

Figure 8–28. TVS of a cervix.

79. The next procedure should be

(A) hysteroscopy
(B) saline infusion sonohysterography
(C) either A or B
(D) neither A nor B

For questions 80 and 81, refer to Figs. 8–30 A and B.

80. Which of the following statements is correct?

(A) The saline infusion sonohysterography (SIS) shows a submucosal fibroid.
(B) The SIS shows a polyp.
(C) The SIS shows a uterine synchae.
(D) A and C

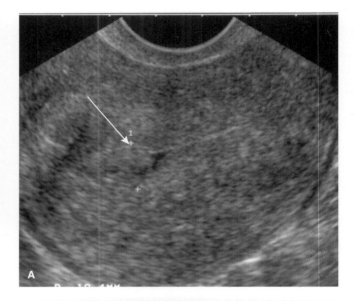

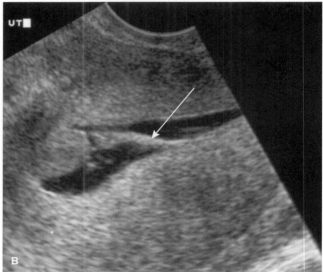

Figures 8–30. The endometrium in long axis before **(A)** and after **(B)** saline infusion sonohysterography.

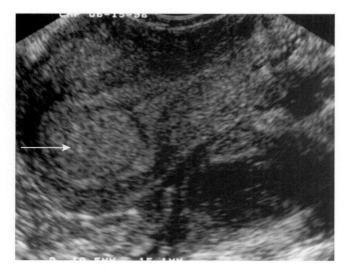

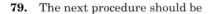

Figure 8–29. TVS of the uterus in long axis.

81. Submucosal fibroids can be distinguished from polyps by

(A) their texture—submucosal fibroids tend to be more echogenic than polyps.
(B) same as A, except polyps tend to be more echogenic than submucosal fibroids
(C) They cannot be distinguished except by histologic examination.
(D) none of the above

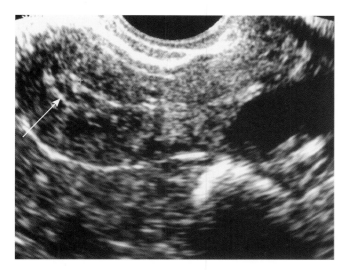

Figure 8–31. The endometrium in long axis (between cursors).

For questions 82 and 83, refer to Fig. 8–31.

82. Which of the following statements is correct?

    (A) The endometrium has a normal texture.
    (B) There are several tiny cysts within the endometrium suggestive of a polyp.
    (C) neither A nor B
    (D) either A or B

83. The next procedure should be

    (A) hysteroscopy
    (B) biopsy
    (C) saline infusion sonohysterography
    (D) none of the above

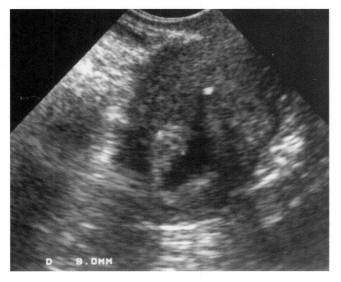

Figure 8–32. Taken during SIS.

For questions 84 and 85, refer to Fig. 8–32.

84. Which of the following statements is correct?

    (A) The endometrium is uniform and normal.
    (B) There is a focal thickening of the endometrium.
    (C) A large polyp is present within the lumen.
    (D) none of the above

85. The next procedure should be

    (A) guided endometrial biopsy
    (B) hysterectomy
    (C) observation
    (D) none of the above

For questions 86 through 89, refer to Figs. 8–33 A and B.

86. Which of the following statements is true?

    (A) This is highly suggestive of a ruptured ectopic pregnancy on the right.
    (B) This is highly suggestive of a normal 6-week intrauterine pregnancy.
    (C) This is highly suggestive of right ovarian torsion.
    (D) none of the above are true

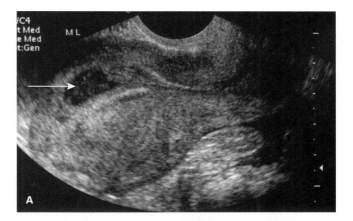

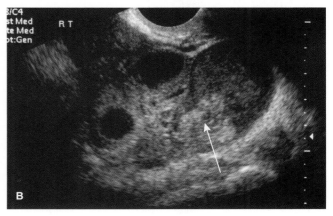

Figures 8–33. Transvaginal sonograms, in **(A)** long-axis uterus and **(B)** short-axis and right adnexal, performed on a woman with positive pregnancy test and pelvic pain.

87. The echogenic material within the uterine lumen suggests

   (A) an intrauterine pregnancy with normal echogenic fluid surrounding the gestational sac
   (B) hemorrhagic fluid within the lumen related to decidual necrosis associated with an ectopic pregnancy
   (C) neither A nor B
   (D) an artifact

88. The TVS of the right adnexa suggests

   (A) an ectopic pregnancy adjacent to a corpus luteum
   (B) hematosalpinx
   (C) both A and B
   (D) neither A nor B

89. The βhCG value that would be expected is

   (A) greater than 1500 mIU/mL
   (B) less than 1500 mIU/mL
   (C) There is no correlation between TVS and βhCG values.
   (D) irrelevant

For questions 90 and 91, refer to Fig. 8–34.

90. Which of the following statements is true?

   (A) The gestational sac does not contain an embryo; therefore, this is a failed intrauterine pregnancy.
   (B) This could represent a "pseudogestational sac" of an ectopic pregnancy.
   (C) One would carefully examine the entire gestational sac for an embryo.
   (D) all of the above

91. At what average dimension of the gestational sac should an embryo first be seen?

   (A) 5–10 mm
   (B) 10–15 mm
   (C) 15–20 mm
   (D) 20–25 mm
   (E) C or D

For questions 92 and 93, refer to Fig. 8–35.

92. Which of the following observations is correct?

   (A) There is a papillary excrescence protruding into the cystic area from the wall.
   (B) There is a fluid/solid tissue interface or clot.
   (C) neither A nor B
   (D) both A and B

93. The next procedure should be

   (A) cyst aspiration
   (B) color Doppler sonography
   (C) CT scan
   (D) none of the above

For questions 94 and 95, refer to Fig. 8–36.

94. Which of the following statements is true?

   (A) There are two cystic areas within the left ovary.
   (B) There is an irregular solid area within the left ovary.
   (C) There is a side lobe artefact overlying the left ovary.
   (D) all of the above

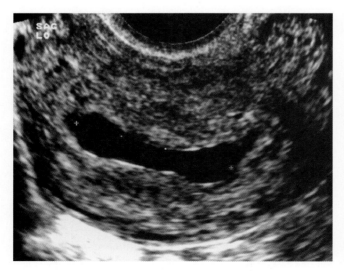

Figure 8–34. Sagittal TVS of a patient who has a positive pregnancy test.

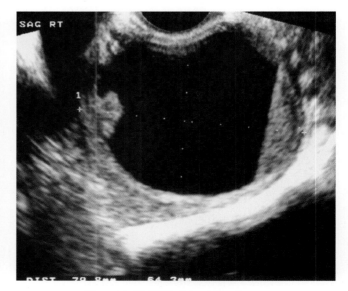

Figure 8–35. TVS of the right adnexa.

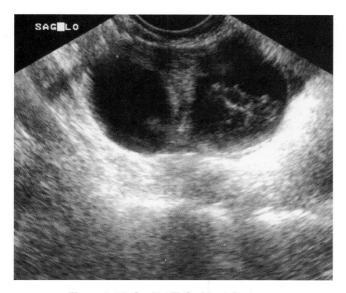

Figure 8–36. Sagittal TVS of the left adnexa.

95. The most likely diagnosis is

(A) ovarian cancer
(B) hemorrhagic cyst
(C) endometrioma
(D) all of the above are possible

96. For Fig. 8–37, the most likely diagnosis is

(A) ovarian cancer
(B) interligamentary fibroid
(C) bowel tumor
(D) endometriosis
(E) cannot tell—all of the above are possible

For questions 97 and 98, refer to Fig. 8–38 A and B.

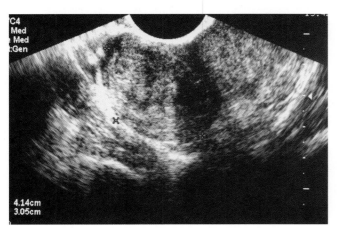

Figure 8–37. TVS of the right adnexa.

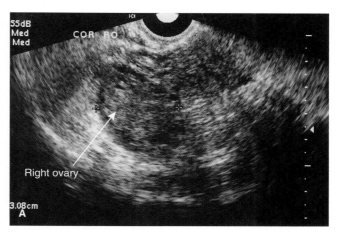

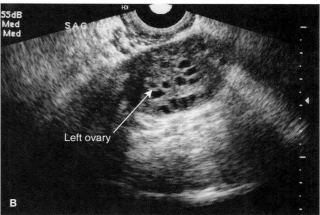

Figures 8–38. TVS of the right **(A)** and left **(B)** ovaries in a woman with amenorrhea.

97. Which of the following statements is correct?

(A) The ovaries appear normal.
(B) The ovaries are rounded but normal.
(C) The ovaries appear to be polycystic.
(D) all of the above

98. The typical TVS finding in polycystic ovaries include

(A) enlarged (over 10 cc), rounded ovaries
(B) as in A, with multiple immature follicles along the periphery
(C) normal ovaries
(D) all of the above

For questions 99 and 100, refer to Fig. 8–39.

99. Which of the following statements is true?

(A) There is a fusiform structure in the right adnexa that contains low level echoes.
(B) There is a bowel loop in the right adnexa.
(C) both A and B
(D) neither A nor B

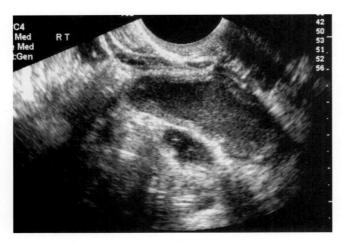

Figure 8–39. TVS of the right adnexa.

100. The most likely diagnosis is

(A) a hydro or pyo-salpinx
(B) rectosigmoid cancer
(C) ovarian carcinoma
(D) cannot tell

For questions 101 and 102, refer to Fig. 8–40.

101. Which of the following statements is true?

(A) There is a corpus luteum in the right ovary.
(B) There is an ectopic gestational sac containing an embryo with heart motion.
(C) neither A nor B
(D) both A and B

102. True statements regarding color Doppler sonography of ectopic pregnancy are (is)

(A) The vascularity of ectopic pregnancies is variable.
(B) Some ectopics may not demonstrate flow in the wall.
(C) both A and B
(D) neither A nor B

103. Which of the following statements is true concerning Fig. 8–41?

(A) There is a highly vascular ectopic.
(B) There is a highly vascular corpus luteum.
(C) neither A nor B
(D) both A and B

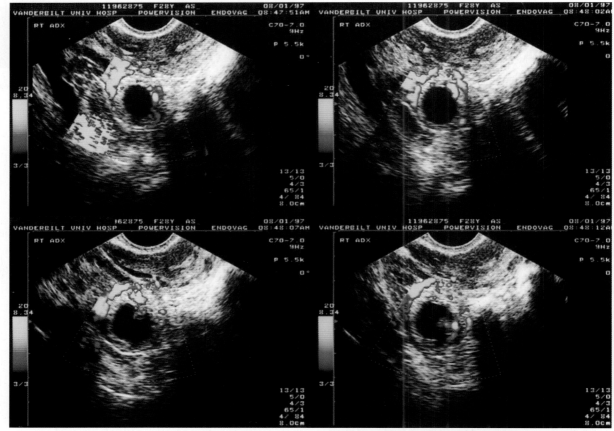

Figure 8–40. Composite of several transvaginal color Doppler sonograms of the right adnexa in a woman with a positive pregnancy test and pelvic pain.

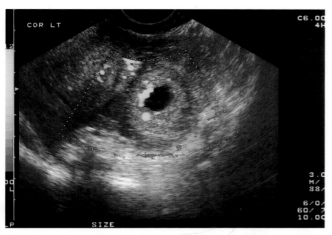

Figure 8–41. Transvaginal color Doppler sonogram of the left adnexa in a woman with a positive pregnancy test.

For questions 104 and 105, refer to Fig. 8–42.

104. Which of the following statements is true?

   (A) There is low impedance flow within the placenta.
   (B) There is high impedance flow within the placenta.
   (C) There is no flow within the placenta.
   (D) none of the above are true

105. Low impedance flow can be seen within

   (A) trophoblastic tissue
   (B) ovarian tumors
   (C) functioning corpus luteum
   (D) all of the above

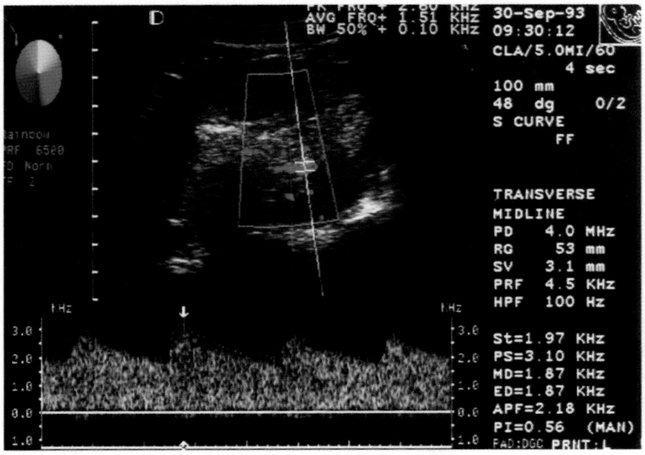

For questions 106 and 107, refer to Fig. 8–43.

106. True statements regarding this mass include

   (A) There is a cystic structure with a highly vascular wall adjacent to a hypovascular smooth walled cyst.
   (B) Both cystic structures are hypervascular.
   (C) Both cystic structures are hypovascular.
   (D) none of the above

107. Differential diagnostic considerations include

   (A) a hemorrhagic corpus luteum
   (B) an ovarian carcinoma
   (C) a normal ovary
   (D) a polycystic ovary
   (E) both A and B

For questions 108 and 109, refer to Fig. 8–44.

108. The most likely diagnosis is

   (A) an ovarian cancer
   (B) a hemorrhagic cyst
   (C) an endometrioma
   (D) none of the above

109. Based on your diagnosis, the following clinical management is appropriate

   (A) Aspirate the mass using transvaginal sonography.
   (B) Repeat the study in 4–6 weeks for signs of spontaneous regression.
   (C) Recommend referral to a gynecologic oncologist.
   (D) Do nothing.

Figure 8–42. Triplex color Doppler sonogram obtained in a woman who was 10 weeks amenorrheic.

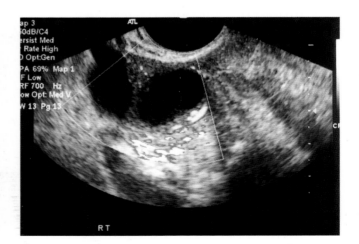

Figure 8–43. Transvaginal color Doppler sonogram of the right ovary in a patient whose mother had ovarian cancer.

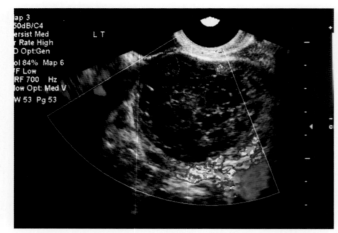

Figure 8–44. Transvaginal color Doppler sonogram of the left adnexa.

For questions 110 and 111, refer to Figs. 8–45 A and B.

110. Which of the following statements is correct?

(A) There are two mature follicles.
(B) There is a cystic area containing a papillary excrescence with a blood vessel.
(C) both A and B
(D) none of the above

111. The most likely diagnosis is

(A) ovarian cancer
(B) two mature follicles
(C) both A and B
(D) neither A nor B

112. Which of the following statements is true concerning Fig. 8–46?

(A) There is a polyp.
(B) There is a polyp with a feeding vessel.
(C) both A and B
(D) the endometrium is normal

For questions 113 and 114, refer to Fig. 8–47.

113. Which of the following statements is correct?

(A) There are two polypoid masses.
(B) There are two polypoid intracavitary masses that have feeding vessels.
(C) There are two large blood clots within the uterine lumen.
(D) The endometrium is normal.

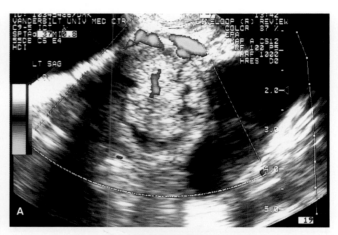

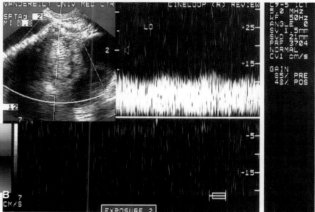

Figures 8–45. (A) and **(B)**, Transvaginal color Doppler sonograms performed for ovulation induction monitoring.

114. The most likely diagnosis is

(A) endometrial carcinoma
(B) submucosal fibroid
(C) polyps
(D) cannot tell between A and C

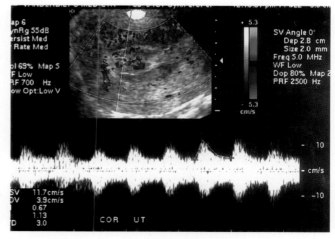

Figure 8–46. Transvaginal color Doppler sonogram of a uterus in a patient with uterine bleeding.

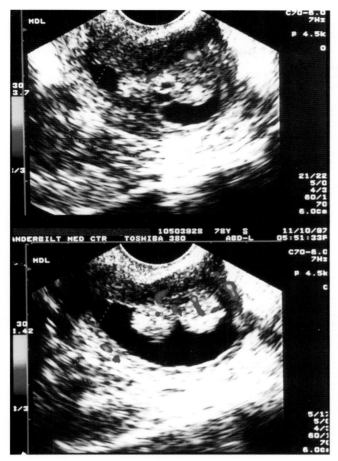

Figure 8–47. Two sagittal TV-CDS of a woman with postmenopausal bleeding.

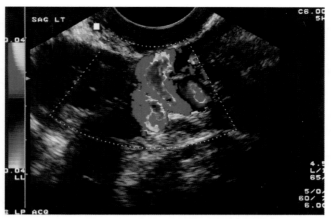

Figure 8–48. Transvaginal CDS of the left adnexa.

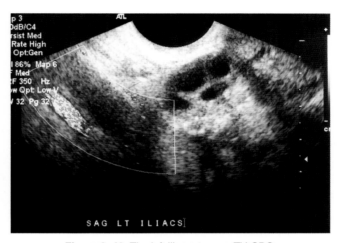

Figure 8–49. The left iliac artery on TV-CDS.

115. The abnormal finding in Fig. 8–48 is

   (A) distended adnexal vessels
   (B) an ectopic pregnancy
   (C) large polyp
   (D) none of the above

116. The abnormal finding in Fig. 8–49 is

   (A) lack of flow within a common iliac vessel
   (B) multiple cysts within the left ovary
   (C) there is nothing abnormal
   (D) both A and B

Answers and Explanations

At the end of each explained answer there is a number combination in parentheses. The first number identifies the reference source; the second number or set of numbers indicates the page or pages on which the relevant information can be found.

1. **(C)** The discriminatory zone. The level of serum β-hCG at which the gestational sac can be depicted with transvaginal or transabdominal sonography is referred to as the "discriminatory" zone of human chorionic gonadotropin. *(1:116–117)*

2. **(C)** The amnion and chorion usually fuse between 15 and 16 weeks. *(1:239)*

3. **(A)** The area outside of the amnion is the chorionic cavity or extraembryonic coelom. *(1:237)*

4. **(C)** 6 weeks. *(1:68)*

5. **(B)** The secondary yolk sac lies between the amnion and chorion. *(1:68)*

6. **(B)** The lithotomy position. The elevated thighs in the lithotomy position allows free movement of the probe from side to side (horizontal plane). *(2:61)*

7. **(D)** Fowler's position. The patient should be lying in the lithotomy position and the examination table in the Fowler's position (reverse Trendelenburg). *(2:61)*

8. **(B)** Pelvis. A thick foam cushion that is 15–20 cm thick can be used to elevate the pelvis, this allows free up-and-down movements of the probe (vertical plane). *(2:61)*

9. **(A)** Emptying of the urinary bladder. This is important because a filled bladder takes up most of the image, displacing adnexal structures out of the image. In addition, it contributes to unnecessary patient discomfort. *(2:62; 1:49)*

10. **(B)** Interstitial region of the Fallopian tube. Ectopic pregnancy in the interstitial segment of the Fallopian tube, also called cornual pregnancy has the most serious potential complications because of its close proximity to major uterine vessels. *(2:115)*

11. **(D)** Human fertilization normally occur in the ampullary segment of the Fallopian tube and implantation occur in the endometrial cavity. *(1:105)*

12. **(C)** Nabothian cyst are located in the cervix. *(2:70)*

13. **(C)** Transvaginal transducers range in frequency from 5 to 7.5 MHz. *(2:8)*

14. **(A)** Transvaginal sonography can best demonstrate only one ovary at a time because of image magnification and the small focal area. *(2:71, 88)*

15. **(B)** Waldeyer's fossa. *(2:71; 1:807)*

16. **(D)** Any women with congenital uterine anomalies should have sonographic evaluation of the kidneys. More than 80% of women with these congenital uterine anomalies have renal abnormalities. *(1:1147; 3:897)*

17. **(C)** Glutaraldehyde-based chemical disinfectants are bactericidal, fungicidal, and virucidal and are effective in inactivating HIV-1 on environmental surfaces. Diluted household bleach is effective in inactivation HIV-1 on environmental surfaces, but it could be destructive to the bonding material and plastic of the transducers. *(4:131)*

18. **(B)** The most common cystic mass that occurs during pregnancy is corpus luteum cyst which usually regress between 12 and 16 weeks gestation. *(1:870)*

19. **(A)** The crown-rump length (CRL) is the most accurate indicators of fetal age and can be measured from 6 to 12 weeks. The most accurate prediction is obtained between 8 and 10 weeks. *(3:153)*

20. **(D)** The first anatomic structure to be apparent within the gestational sac is the yolk sac. *(3:125)*

21. **(C)** Transvaginal sonography can detect the embryological structures about 1 week earlier than transabdominal sonography. *(1:62–68)*

22. (C) The diameter of the mature Graafian follicle ranges from 17 to 25 mm.   *(1:1056)*

23. (C) Preparation for transvaginal study does not require antibiotic therapy before insertion of the vaginal probe. The transvaginal probe should be covered with a protective sheath before vaginal insertion to prevent cross infection.   *(4:13–135)*

24. (D) Fluid in the posterior cul-de-sac is uncommon with uterine fibroids.   *(2:72–73)*

25. (A) The secondary yolk sac lies in the chorionic cavity between the amnion and chorion. The chorionic cavity also known as the extraembryonic coelom.   *(3:109, 118; 2:229)*

26. (D) The crown–rump length (CRL) is obtain by measuring longest axis of the embryo excluding the limb buds and yolk sac.   *(1:145)*

27. (C) The level of serum quantitative beta human chorionic gonadotropin (hCG) required to depict the gestational sac with transvaginal sonography is approximately 1000 to 1500 mIU/ml 3rd IRP.   *(3:913–914; 5:7)*

28. (A) A fully distended bladder in a patient undergoing transvaginal sonography will occupy most of the image and displace organs of interest out of the focal range.   *(2:16)*

29. (B) The segment of the Fallopian tube that lies adjacent to the ovary is the fimbria. The Fallopian has five segments, interstitial (cornual), isthmus, ampullary, infundibulum, and fimbria. The interstitial (cornual) is close to the uterus, and the fimbria is closest to the ovary.   *(3:808)*

30. (A) Lamb condoms, when viewed under the electron microscope, show tiny pores that are larger than the HIV or hepatitis B virus and could permit transmission of viruses.   *(4:130–135)*

31. (C) The type of lubricants recommended for latex condoms are water-based products such as K-Y jelly and ultrasound coupling gel. Petroleum jelly or oil-based products can cause deterioration of the latex that result in fracture.   *(4:130–135)*

32. (D) The uterus is not part of the adnexa.   *(3:801–809)*

33. (A) A small cystic space in the posterior cranium of the embryo at approximately 7–9 weeks of gestation most likely rhombencephalon (hindbrain).   *(1:16)*

34. (D) The echogenic bulging of the umbilical cord seen with transvaginal sonography near the abdominal insertion at about 8th–10th week of gestation, most likely represent physiologic herniation of midgut.   *(2:249)*

35. (D) The most common presenting symptoms of ectopic pregnancy is pain.   *(1:115)*

36. (B) The major limitation of transvaginal sonography is that it has a limited field of view. Transvaginal sonography is useful in evaluation intrauterine pregnancy (IUP), ectopic pregnancy and can be useful in 2nd and 3rd trimester pregnancy.   *(2:7, 221)*

37. (A) The use of high-frequency transvaginal transducers results in less penetration, more magnification, and better resolution.   *(2:29–37)*

38. (B) Transvaginal transducer is limited to the confinement of the vagina, therefore complete segmental obstetrical survey needed to assess intrauterine growth retardation is not possible.   *(2:77–80)*

39. (C) Abutting the yolk sac is the embryological disk, which is too small to be depicted. If the M-mode is placed at the edge of the yolk sac at approximately 5½ to 6 weeks, the heart motion can be depicted, not from the yolk sac, but from the adjacent not-yet-apparent embryo. Transvaginal sonography can depict the fetal heart before a clear sonographic depiction of the embryo can be obtained.   *(3:118–121)*

40. (D) Nuchal translucency may be obtained by either transabdominal or transvaginal sonography. This is performed after precise calculation of gestational age by crown-rump length (CRL). The fetal head should be in a neutral position. An extended fetal neck will result in falsely increased measurements.   *(3:140; 1:91)*

41. (C) Focal myometrial contraction is a physiologic mass, which can be distinguished from uterine myoma. Focal myometrial contraction tends to be isoechoic and resolve spontaneously with time. Uterine myoma has an increased risk of spontaneous abortion, its mass effect tends to distort both the serosal and endometrial contours of the uterus.   *(6:82)*

42. (C) The serum quantitative human chorionic gonadotropin (hCG) normally double approximately every 48 hours.   *(3:914)*

43. (C) The fetal head should be in a neutral position to perform a more precise measurement. Fetal neck flexion or extension may result in poor measurement.   *(3:140; 1:91)*

44. (A) Ten days postconception.   *(1:116)*

45. (A) After menopause the follicles are not present, and the ovaries are atrophic.   *(2:71)*

46. (B) A condition that can be confused with an interstitial (cornual) pregnancy is an early intrauterine pregnancy in a bicornuate uterus.   *(1:128)*

47. (D) The hypogastric artery (internal iliac arteries) is located posterolateral to the ovary.   *(2:151)*

48. (D) A blighted ovum is an empty gestational sac, no embryo, and no yolk sac present, also known as an anembryonic gestational sac.   *(4:126)*

49. (D) An intrauterine gestational sac can be distinguished from a pseudogestational sac, which is associated with an ectopic pregnancy by the presence of a yolk sac. The pregnancy test can be positive with a pseudogestational sac in most cases associated with an ectopic pregnancy.   *(4:118)*

50. (D) Nuchal translucency is best described as a thin membrane projecting from the posterior aspect of the fetal neck. This should not be confused with nuchal fold, which is measured between 15 and 21 weeks.   *(1:90)*

51. (A) These two images show the endometrium in long and short axes.   *(7:28–29)*

52. (B) This is the inner layer of the myometrium. It appears as hypoechoic due to the orientation of the muscle fibers.   *(7:78)*

53. (A) These represent vessels that are circumferentially arranged between the outer and middle layers of myometrium.   *(7:78)*

54. (A) This patient is in the proliferative phase, when the endometrium is relatively thin.   *(7:78)*

55. (B) The endometrium is best measured as a bilayer thickness. When there is intraluminal fluid, each layer can be measured separately and the bilayer thickness expressed as the sum of the two single layer thicknesses.   *(7:78)*

56. (B) This is the multilayered appearance of a midcycle (peri-ovulatory endometrium). The outer echogenic layer represents the basalis layer, the inner relatively hypoechoic layer is the fundus layer, and the central echogenic interface is created by refluxed mucus.   *(7:78)*

57. (A) The central echogenic interface arises from refluxed mucus.   *(7:78)*

58. (B) The fundus lacks a definite cleft and therefore suggests that this is a septated uterus.   *(7:78)*

59. (A) Both bicornuate and septae uteri are associated with unilateral renal agenesis.   *(7:78)*

60. (A) There is focal thickening of the endometrium.   *(7:79)*

61. (A) On SHG, there is focal thickening of the endometrium. Because there is no apparent stalk, this most likely is a focal area of hyperplasia rather than a polyp.   *(7:79)*

62. (D) This patient has a polypoid mass that could represent endometrial cancer or hyperplasia. If the nonguided endometrial biopsy missed sampling the lesion, endometrial atrophy could be found in the nonaffected endometrium.   *(7:79)*

63. (D) Any of the maneuvers or additional exams would be helpful in order to demonstrate the pedicle better.   *(7:79)*

64. (C) The mass could represent either a polyp arising from the endocervical canal or a clot in the sequestered C-section scar defect.   *(7:79)*

65. (A) This is an intramural fibroid.   *(7:78)*

66. (B) Cervical mucus is watery in midcycle.   *(7:25)*

67. (A) This is a normal left ovary.   *(7:25)*

68. (A) This is a hemorrhagic corpus luteum cyst containing typical thin interfaces arising from fibrin strands.   *(7:37)*

69. (A) There is a papillary excrescence projecting into the cystic area of a multiloculated cystic mass. This was found to be a borderline ovarian carcinoma.   *(7:37)*

70. (A) Transvaginal color Doppler sonography could demonstrate whether or not the area in question was vascular. Masses with vascularized solid areas are suspicious for cancer.   *(7:79)*

71. (B) This is the left ovary.   *(7:25)*

72. (B) Adjacent to the left ovary is a bowel loop which contains fluid.   *(7:25)*

73. (D) This is a normal 5-week intrauterine pregnancy showing an intact choriodecidua and containing a yolk sac.   *(7:230)*

74. (B) There is either a nuchal translucency or cystic hygroma.   *(7:337)*

75. (D) There is a nuchal membrane or cystic hygroma which could be associated with either Down syndrome or Turner's syndrome.   *(1:90)*

76. (A) This is the typical appearance of a hydatidiform mole.   *(7:276)*

77. (E) All of the above are true except for the cervix, which is seen in short axis. The long-axis image of the cervix shows it to contain fluid within the endo-cervical canal and a possible polyp or clot. *(7:25)*

78. **(A)** This is a large polyp. *(7:79)*

79. **(C)** The gynecologist could choose to go directly to hysteroscopy. Some would prefer to delineate the pedicle or the polyp before hysteroscopy, though. *(7:111)*

80. **(C)** SIS shows a submucosal fibroid extending from the inner layer of myometrium and a synchae that extends from the endometrium to the fibroid. *(7:111)*

81. **(B)** Polyps tend to be more echogenic than fibroids, but the most important distinguishing feature is that polyps tend to have a pedicle arising from the endometrium; whereas, submucosal fibroids extend from the myometrium. *(7:111)*

82. **(B)** There are several punctate cysts in the endometrium. This is suggestive of a polyp. The cysts represent dilated glandular elements in the polyp. *(7:111)*

83. **(C)** To delineate the abnormality and determine its location (endometrial vs. myometrial), SIS should be performed. *(7:111)*

84. **(B)** There is focal thickening in the endometrium which on re-biopsy revealed endometrial hyperplasia. *(7:79)*

85. **(A)** Once a focal thickening is seen on SIS, guided endometrial biopsy should be performed. *(7:79)*

86. **(A)** These TVSs are highly indicative of a ruptured ectopic pregnancy in the right tube. There is intra-luminal hemorrhage between thickened and irregular endometrium. *(7:276)*

87. **(B)** This represents hemorrhagic fluid within decidualized endometrium of an ectopic pregnancy. This has been referred to as a "pseudogestational sac." *(7:276)*

88. **(A)** As is seen in most patients with an ectopic, the corpus luteum is on the same side as the ectopic. *(7:276)*

89. **(B)** The βhCG value is likely to be less than 1500 mIU/mL. *(7:276)*

90. **(D)** All statements are true. Even though there is no apparent embryo, it is incumbent upon the sonographer to scan the entire gestational sac carefully for the presence of an embryo. *(7:276)*

91. **(C)** At 10 mm, the yolk sac should be seen; whereas, between 10 and 15 mm, an embryo should be detectable. *(7:229)*

92. **(D)** This mass has both a papillary excrescence and a serous fluid/hemorrhagic fluid layer. *(7:132)*

93. **(B)** Color Doppler sonography could be used to ascertain if there was flow within the papillary area. *(7:364)*

94. **(D)** There are two cystic areas within this mass. One has solid components and septate. *(7:132)*

95. **(D)** All are possible. A follow-up scan in 4–6 weeks may be helpful to show if there is spontaneous regression of a physiologic cyst. *(7:132)*

96. **(E)** All are possible. Clinically, the most likely possibility is an interligamentary fibroid, but the other could have a similar sonographic appearance. *(7:133)*

97. **(C)** These ovaries are rounded and enlarged. The left one contains numerous immature follicles suggestive of polycystic ovaries. *(7:131)*

98. **(D)** Polycystic ovaries are typically enlarged and rounded and contain multiple immature follicles. Occasionally, however, some women may have polycystic ovary disease without enlarged ovaries. *(7:131)*

99. **(C)** There is a fusiform mass in the right adnexa adjacent to a bowel loop. *(7:191)*

100. **(A)** This is a pyosalpinx. The echoes inside the mass arise from pus and cellular debris. *(7:191)*

101. **(B)** These scans demonstrate an ectopic pregnancy. There is increased flow around the choriodecidual implanted in the tubal musculature and detectible flow arising from the embryo's heart. *(1:196)*

102. **(C)** Both statements are correct. The vascularity of an ectopic pregnancy varies from hypo- to hyper-vascular. *(1:196)*

103. **(A)** This is an ectopic with marked vascularity around its rim. This can also be seen in functioning corpus luteum. *(1:196)*

104. **(A)** This is low impedance flow typical of trophoblastic tissue. *(1:173)*

105. **(D)** All of the above can contain vessels with low impedance flow. *(1:173; 1:196)*

106. **(A)** There is a bilobed cystic structure which contains a hypervascular wall in one of the cystic areas.   *(1:59)*

107. **(E)** This could represent either a hemorrhagic corpus luteum or an ovarian carcinoma. Polycystic ovaries tend to have multiple immature follicles and normal ovaries typically will contain no more than one corpus luteum.   *(1:62)*

108. **(B)** This most likely represents a hemorrhagic cyst containing areas of formed clot and fibrin strands. It is unlikely to be an ovarian carcinoma because there is no internal flow. Endometriomas tend to have a "ground glass" appearance.   *(1:62)*

109. **(B)** A follow-up scan in 4–6 weeks would be helpful to assess whether or not the mass represents a physiologic cyst.   *(1:62)*

110. **(C)** There are two mature follicles and a papillary excrescence within this ovary.   *(1:62)*

111. **(C)** This was an ovarian cancer adjacent to two mature follicles.   *(1:62)*

112. **(C)** This represents a polyp with a feeding vessel.   *(1:124)*

113. **(B)** This sonogram shows two polypoid masses that are vascular surrounded by intraluminal fluid.   *(1:124)*

114. **(A)** Because of the vascularity and irregular shape of the polyps, carcinoma should be suspected.   *(1:124)*

115. **(A)** The adnexal vessels are distended. This can be seen in "pelvic congestion."   *(1:35)*

116. **(A)** There is thrombosis within the left common iliac vein.   *(1:35)*

REFERENCES

1. Fleischer AC, Manning AF, Jeanty PP, et al. *Sonography in Obstetrics & Gynecology; Principles and Practice.* 6th ed. New York: McGraw-Hill; 2001.
2. Timor-Tritsch IE, Rottem S. *Transvaginal Sonography.* 2nd ed. New York: Elsevier; 1991.
3. Callen PW. *Ultrasonography in Obstetrics and Gynecology.* 4th ed. Philadelphia: WB Saunders; 2000.
4. Odwin C, Fleischer AC, Kepple DM, et al. Probe covers and disinfectants for transducers. *J Diag Med Sonogr.* 1990; 6:130–135.
5. Braunstein GD. *hCG Testing: Volume 11: Answers to Frequently asked Questions About hCG Testing.* Abbott Park, IL: Abbott Diagnostics Educational Services; 1991.
6. Callen PW. *Ultrasonography in Obstetrics and Gynecology.* 3rd ed. Philadelphia: WB Saunders; 1994.
7. Fleischer A, Kepple D. *Transvaginal Sonography: A Clinical Atlas.* Philadelphia: Lippincott; 1995.

CHAPTER 9

OBSTETRICAL AND GYNECOLOGIC SONOGRAPHY

Jayne C. Moser

Study Guide

HISTORICAL PERSPECTIVES AND INTRODUCTORY REMARKS

The introduction of OB/GYN ultrasound began in the late 1950s.[1] Early obstetrical scanning could only answer a few simple questions: (1) fetal viability, (2) fetal number, (3) location of placenta, and (4) gestational age.[2] Early ultrasound examinations were performed on articulated arm (static) B scanners.[3] The articulated arm was passed over the abdomen in successive sweeps, forming a picture. This form of ultrasound allowed for a large field of view and was very helpful for large masses, free fluid, and position of fetus. It was, however, difficult with moving objects because the image was not instantaneous, as with real-time scanning.

Gray scale, real-time imaging became available during the 1970s. It allowed for an instantaneous image to appear on the screen while scanning. This aided in evaluating the moving fetus. The gray scale image also allowed for a better differentiation and resolution of organs and tissue interfaces.[4] The image, however, does have a limited field of view. This can make imaging large structures, such as masses and fluid collections, difficult. With the improvement of computers, real-time ultrasound machines are constantly improving resolution and differentiation of organs and tissues.

Intracavitary, or transvaginal probes have become a very important adjunct to OB/GYN sonography. Because of the close proximity to the organs of interest, less of the sound beam is attenuated when compared to transabdominal scanning. Therefore, a higher frequency may be used resulting in enhanced near-field resolution. Transvaginal scanning (TVS) is limited in its range of motion and depth of view. For gynecologic applications, the pelvic anatomy that can be visualized with sonography can be viewed transvaginally, unless the organ of interest contains a large mass. In obstetrics, TVS can be used to delineate early fetal anatomy (<14 weeks), fetal anatomy in lower uterine segment in obese patients, cervix, placental previa, ectopic pregnancy, and early intrauterine pregnancies.[5]

Doppler and color Doppler sonography were introduced in the 1980s. Doppler imaging can determine the velocity and direction of blood flow in relation to the ultrasound probe. Color Doppler imaging (CDI) applies the color-coded pulsed Doppler information within the B-mode sonographic image. Color is assigned to a direction of flow, with different colors representing flow toward or away from the transducer. For gynecologic disorders, both color Doppler and pulsed Doppler sampling are used to assess blood flow within the pelvic vessels and pelvic masses. In obstetrics, Doppler and color Doppler sonography can be used for the numerous fetal and maternal vessels, as well as obstetrical abnormalities. Because it is low intensity, there are no untoward bioeffects, although it is prudent to limit exposure to the developing fetus. The greatest intensity is used for continuous wave (CW) applications; whereas, color Doppler applications uses only small amounts of energy.[6] Doppler and color Doppler sonography do have limitations. The vessel cannot be sampled at an angle between 60 and 90°, in order for the computer to assess the velocity correctly. With pulsed Doppler, as used with B imaging, a new pulse cannot be sent before the last echo has arrived at the transducer. This limits the absolute maximum velocity that can be detected in high-velocity vessels.[2]

Color Doppler energy (CDE), or color Doppler power, is another method of analyzing blood flow by detecting the energy, or amplitude of Doppler signals generated from moving blood. With power or amplitude mode, intensities are related to the number of blood elements flowing within a vessel. Because the information is obtained differently from CDS, CDE is not angle dependent, not affected by aliasing, and is able to display lower velocities of blood flow. CDE cannot, however, determine velocity or direction of flow. CDE is more sensitive to low-flow vessels than CDS, but is prone to motion artifact.[6]

There are many specialized areas of OB/GYN. Ultrasound has become a vital component to many of these areas. Maternal–fetal medicine, also known as high-risk OB, involves a multidisciplinary team consisting of the perinatologist, genetic counselor, sonographer, and nurse. This team, under the direction of the perinatologist, evaluates pregnancies at risk for genetic, medical, or congenital abnormalities. Ultrasound is used to assess the fetal anatomy, maternal uterine and ovarian anatomy, and give visualization for such invasive procedures as amniocentesis or CVS. The fetal anatomic review is very detailed and focuses on areas not always included in the standard OB ultrasound guidelines set by the AIUM, ACR, or ACOG. The area of focus varies depending on the patients history.

Infertility testing has become a field of its own with multiple methods of assisting couples in reproduction. Many reproductive endocrinologists use sonography as an adjunct to the pelvic exam during the patients initial evaluation. All infertility sonograms are done transvaginally. Sonography is used for follicular monitoring, needle aspiration of oocytes, visualization for catheter insertion, and reinsertion of embryo into the uterus.[2]

Three-dimensional (3-D) sonography research continues in OB/GYN, and its use in the clinical field is increasing. The ultrasound machine stores sequential images, and 3-D reconstructions are produced. These reconstructions are described as surface rendering and volume imaging. Surface rendering allows for the evaluation of the fetal face, limbs, and digits. Surface rendering requires a fluid interface. Volumetric reconstructions are used to show entire organs.[5]

Contrast agents are another investigational area of gynecologic sonography. Contrast agents and/or saline are used to enhance visualization of the endometrial cavity and fallopian tubes. Some IV injected contrast agents have been shown to enhance color and spectral Doppler signals of small blood vessels.

The remaining portion of this chapter deals primarily with OB/GYN, allowing for fetal echocardiography, Doppler, and transvaginal imaging to be discussed in other chapters.

INSTRUMENTATION AND TECHNIQUES

Before starting an ultrasound examination, a thorough review of the patient's history is needed. The patient's referral diagnosis and clinical symptoms should be kept in mind as the history is reviewed. Often, the history will give clues as to the current abnormality. It is important to review the patient's reproductive history as well. Gravida (G) refers to the pregnancies. Primigravida is a first time pregnancy; multigravida is many pregnancies. Nulligravida is a patient that has never been pregnant. Parity (P) is the number of pregnancies carried to term. Typically, parity is displayed as a four digit series. The first number being the term births, the second number being preterm births, the third number being abortions, (spontaneous and elective) as well as complications of pregnancy <20

weeks resulting in abortion, and the fourth number being the number of living children.[7]

In addition to the medical history, lab tests should also be reviewed. For gynecologic sonograms, all blood work should be reviewed. An elevated white blood count could help diagnose an infectious mass, for example. Other tests might include pap smears, biopsies, and ovarian cancer screening tests (CA125). For the obstetric patient, there are many lab tests that may be available at different stages in the pregnancy. Blood type should always be noted, as well as any antibody titers. In early pregnancy, hCG (human chorionic gonadotropin) titers will help with the diagnosis of a threatened abortion. Both gestational sac growth and hCG production relate to trophoblastic function. Any discrepancy between the two can suggest an abnormality in development. Markedly increased hCG is strongly correlated to molar pregnancies. In the second trimester, all pregnant women may elect to have MSAFP3 testing, or maternal serum AFP3. The three refers to the markers tested, including AFP. These are unconjugated estriol and hCG. Assessment of MSAFP3 values is also related to such maternal factors as age, weight, diabetic status, multiple gestation, and race. The test reassigns a risk value for Down syndrome and neural tube defects.

Proper documentation is pertinent to any medical examination. The images should be labeled with patient identification and the anatomy shown on the image. If any abnormalities are identified, the images should also be labeled according to location so that others reviewing the images can locate the abnormality. All exams should be documented in some form of hard copy, such as x-ray film, optic disk, thermal paper, video, or polaroids. In addition, a written report of the exam should be included with the hard copy. This report may contain varied information, but should include any measurements, reason for exam, ultrasound findings, and the doctor's impression. For billing and coding purposes, all reports must contain a diagnosis derived from the exam or referral diagnosis that supports the billing code.

Based on AIUM guidelines, on completion of the exam, all transabdominal probes should have excess gel wiped off with a clean towel and cleaned with a disinfectant cleaner. Commercially available moist towelettes work well and are easy to use. Transvaginal probes should have the cover removed and excess gel wiped off with a paper towel. The transducer should then be cleaned with soap and water and the probe immersed in disinfecting solution for at least 10 minutes. The manufacturers produce cleaning guidelines according to each company's specific guidelines, and these should be compared to the AIUM guidelines.[8]

GYNECOLOGY

The female pelvic organs are divided into four sections: (1) urinary bladder and urethra, (2) cervix, uterus and fallopian tubes, (3) ovaries, and (4) sigmoid colon and rectum (Fig. 9–1).[5]

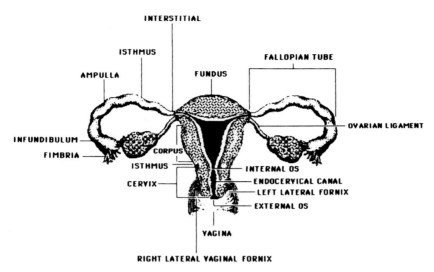

Figure 9–1. Diagram of the female reproductive organs (coronal view).

Uterus

The uterus is situated medially in the pelvis posterior to the bladder and anterior to the rectum. The uterus can be divided into four different regions: (1) cervix, (2) isthmus, (3) corpus, and (4) fundus.[5] The cervix is the most inferior portion of the uterus and invaginates into the vagina. The isthmus is superior to the cervix and begins at the internal os of the cervix. The corpus or body of the uterus is the largest section of the uterus. The fundus is the uppermost portion of the uterus and is located superiorly to where the fallopian tubes arise from the uterus.

The uterus is comprised of three layers of tissue. The outer layer, or peritoneum, is the serosal layer. It is separated from middle (myometrial) layer by the arcuate vessels and is sonographically hypoechoic when compared to the myometrial layer. The largest layer, the muscular portion of the uterus is called the myometrium. It is of midlevel reflectivity. The inner layer, where the two walls of the uterus meet, is called the endometrium. This layer varies in thickness and echogenicity with the menstrual cycle, and is described later in the chapter.[2] The uterus has three primary functions: (1) menstruation, (2) pregnancy, and (3) labor.[7]

Ovaries

The ovaries are ellipsoid in shape, measuring approximately 3 cm in long axis and 2 cm in AP and transverse dimensions.[9] The ovaries are located adjacent to the uterus in the ovarian fossa (also known as the fossa of Waldeyer). The ovarian fossa is bound laterally by the internal iliac artery and the ureter. The medial boundary is the uterus.[2] Appearance of the ovaries are discussed later in the chapter.

Fallopian Tubes

The Fallopian tubes originate at the lateral aspect of the uterus, known as the cornua. Fallopian tubes vary in length from 7 to 12 cm. The Fallopian tube is divided into four subdivisions: (1) interstitial, (2) isthmus, (3) ampulla, and (4) infundibulum.[2] The interstitial portion of the tube sonographically appears as a fine echogenic line extending from the endometrial canal and traveling through the myometrium to cornua of the uterus.[5] The isthmus is the narrowest portion of the tube and is located adjacent to the intersitial segment at the uterine cornua. The tube continues laterally and widens to form the ampulla. The infundibulum is the most lateral portion of the tube and opens to the peritoneum at the fimbria.[2] The purpose of the Fallopian tube is to aid in fertilization and to transport the ova from the ovary to the uterus.

Ligaments

The uterus is loosely suspended in the center of the pelvic cavity with the point of axis being the cervix. The upper portion of the uterus is supported by a series of ligaments. The cardinal ligaments or transverse cervical ligaments originate from the cervix and uterine corpus and insert on a broad portion of the lateral pelvic wall and sacrum. At the distal portion, this ligament is called the uterosacral ligament. This ligament anchors the cervix and is responsible for the uterine orientation.[5]

The round ligament originates from the uterine cornua and passes through the pelvis from anterior to posterior.[5] This ligament is responsible for the anterior tilt of the uterus and aids in stabilizing the fundus of the uterus.

There are two ligaments that are not true ligaments, but folds of peritoneum. The first is the suspensory ligament. It arises from the pelvic side wall and contains ovarian vessels. It aids in supporting both the Fallopian tube and ovary within the broad ligament.[2] The broad ligament is also a double fold of peritoneum. It fans over the adnexa and divides the anterior and posterior portions of the pelvis.[5] It does very little to actually support the uterus.

Muscles

A series of different muscle bundles pass through the female pelvis. Some of these muscles are easily visualized by sonography and can often be confused for adnexal structures. The most commonly visualized muscle is the iliopsoas muscle. On sagittal views, it appears as a long hypoechoic stripe with echogenic linear lines. On transverse images, however, it appears ovoid and is visualized lateral to the uterus.[2] This can often be confused for an ovary until the sagittal view is obtained. The pelvic muscles can be identified sonographically by their appearance. The muscles appear hypoechoic and exhibit linear internal echoes. The borders of the muscles are echogenic representing the fascia.[5]

Bladder and Ureters

The bladder is a thick-walled distendable muscle that lies anterior to the uterus. It is fixed in position inferiorly at the symphysis pubis. This lower region is described as the trigone, defined by the orifices of the two ureters and urethra. The bladder is thicker and more rigid here than at any other location.[5] The ureter originates at the renal pelvis and descends anterior to the internal iliac artery and posterior to the ovary. The ureter travels from posterior to anterior and closely follows the uterine artery in its inferior portion. It then passes anteriomedially to enter the trigone of the bladder.[2]

There are three peritoneal spaces important to pelvic sonography. The peritoneal space posterior to the uterus is the posterior cul-de-sac, also known as the pouch of Douglas. This is the most dependent portion of the peritoneal lining, thus allowing any free fluid within the peritoneum to accumulate here. The peritoneal space anterior to the uterus is the anterior cul-de-sac or vesicouterine pouch. The third peritoneal space is anterior to the bladder and is termed the prevesical or retropubic space.[2]

Blood Supply

The uterine and ovarian arteries are branches of the internal iliac (hypogastric) artery. The uterine artery travels superiorly from the cervix, running lateral to the uterus in the broad ligament. At the junction of the uterus and fallopian tubes, the uterine artery joins with the ovarian artery. The uterine artery branches are called arcuate arteries and supply the outer portion of the myometrium. These vessels are easily identified on ultrasound. The arcuate arteries branch into the radial arteries, which supply the inner layers of the myometrium and endometrium. They then branch into the straight and spiral arteries, which supply the endometrium. The venous channels of the pelvis follow a course similar to the arteries.[2,5]

GYNECOLOGIC PHYSIOLOGY

Uterus

The uterine size varies and is dependent on the patient's age and gestational status. Before puberty and after menopause, the uterus is small in size. During reproductive years, an increase in gravida usually results in a increase in uterine size.[7] A prepubertal uterus is 2–4.4 cm in length, with the corpus (or body of uterus) half the length of the cervix. In an adult nulliparous woman, the uterine length is 6–8.5 cm, width 3–5 cm, and AP dimension 2–4 cm. The corpus and cervix are equal in length. An adult multiparous uterus is 8–10.5 cm × 4–6 cm × 3–5 cm in length, width and AP dimensions with the corpus twice the length of the cervix. In postmenopausal women, the uterus atrophies, regardless of the gravida status premenopausally. The uterine measurements of a postmenopausal woman are 3.5–7.5 × 2–4 × 1.7–3.3 cm, measuring length, width, and AP dimensions respectively.[2]

The uterus can vary slightly in position depending on the distention of the bladder. The following descriptions refer to uterine position with an empty bladder. Ninety percent of the time, the uterus tilts forward in anteverted position, meaning the uterus forms a 90° angle with the cervix. The uterus, however, may be in any of the following positions:

- anteverted: The uterus tilts forward with a 90° angle to cervix.
- anteflexed: The uterine corpus is flexed anteriorly on the cervix, forming a sharp angle at the cervix.
- retroverted: The uterus tilts backwards without a sharp angle between the corpus and cervix.
- retroflexed: The uterine corpus is flexed posteriorly on the cervix, forming a sharp angle at the cervix.
- medianus: midline position
- detroversion: right lateral deviation
- levoversion: left lateral deviation[6]

Congenital abnormalities of the uterus result from improper fusion of the mullerian or paramesonephric ducts. As the ducts fuse, the septum that separates them breaks down, resulting in a single uterine cavity. The lack of septal fusion describes the different anomalies of the uterus, as shown in Fig. 9–2. Because of the close development of the corpus and cervix of the uterus, a uterine malformation

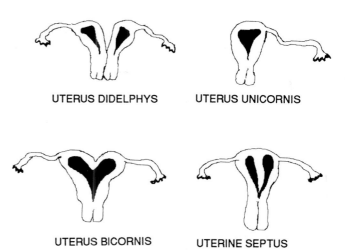

UTERUS DIDELPHYS   UTERUS UNICORNIS

UTERUS BICORNIS   UTERINE SEPTUS

Figure 9–2. Diagram of developmental anomalies of the uterus.

may also affect the cervix and play a part in its function during pregnancy. The uterus develops in synchronicity with the urinary system. When congenital uterine abnormalities are present, the urinary system should be closely evaluated.[2]

The endometrial lining is the innermost layer of the uterus. It is greatly influenced by hormones and is responsible for accepting the embryo for implantation. The endometrium is often described as a "double layer," because of the cyclic inner lining called the Stratum functionale or and the outer, deeper Stratum basale. Sonographic measurements of the endometrium should be done in a sagittal plane of view, measuring from basal layer to basal layer. During the proliferative phase (day 5–9 postmenstruation), the endometrium appears as a thin echogenic line measuring 4–8 mm. During the late proliferative, or periovulatory, phase (day 10–14), the functional zone thickens and sonographically appears hypoechoic to the basal layer. Measurement of the endometrium should include both anterior and posterior basal layers. At this stage, the endometrium has a multilayered appearance, with the outer echogenic layer representing the basal layer and the inner hypoechoic layer arising from the functionalis. Overall measurement of the endometrium at this stage is 6–10 mm. The secretory phase (day 15–28) shows an increased echogenicity of the functional zone as it becomes equal in echogenicity with the basal layer. The increased echogenicity is attributable to the edema of the functional zone, awaiting implantation of an embryo. The overall measurement is 7–14 mm. The appearances and measurements of the endometrium may be greatly affected by oral contraceptives, norplant, postmenopausal changes, and hormone replacement therapy.[2]

Ovaries

Sonographically, the appearance of the ovaries varies with patient age, stage in menstrual cycle, pregnancy status, and body habitus. In reproductive years, the ovaries may be identified by follicles surrounding the outer edge of the ovaries. Follicular cysts are small (<3–5 mm), smooth, thin walled, and anechoic with good sound through transmission. Follicles will increase in size through the cycle with multiple follicles visible at day 5–7. At day 8–12, one or more dominant follicle (>10 mm) will begin to emerge. The dominant follicle reaches a mean diameter of 20 mm with a hypoechoic rim. After the ova is released, bleeding may occur in the follicle, causing it to appear echoic. The follicular cyst becomes a corpus luteal cyst with thick walls and appears anechoic to hypoechoic. The corpus luteal cyst will retain fluid for 4–5 days and measure approximately 2–3 cm. The corpus luteal cyst has a rich blood supply. Color flow doppler will reveal a ring of color around the periphery of the cyst. If no pregnancy occurs, the corpus luteal cyst will gradually atrophy. If pregnancy occurs, the corpus luteal cyst will remain and gradually regress by 14 weeks.[2] The ovarian, follicular, and corpus luteal cysts are all functional cysts

of the ovary.[5] In postmenopausal women, it is more difficult to identify the ovaries because of the absence of follicles and atrophy of the ovaries.[10]

GYNECOLOGIC PATHOLOGY

Uterine Pathology

Uterine pathology may present itself clinically in many different ways. The majority of uterine pathology, both benign and malignant, presents with abnormal uterine bleeding. Other symptoms may include painful menses and increased uterine size on pelvic exam.

The most common uterine tumors are fibroids (also known as leioma, leiomyoma, myoma, and fibromyoma). They are present in 25% of the female population, with a higher percentage in the African American population and becoming more prevalent with advancing female age. Fibroids are thought to be estrogen stimulated so they tend to increase in size during pregnancy and decrease in size after menopause. Often, they are found on pelvic examination without patient symptoms. When symptoms do occur, it can include abnormal bleeding, abdominal pressure, increased urinary frequency, and increased abdominal girth. The malignant form of the leiomyoma, a leiomyosarcoma, although rare, is believed to arise from a preexisting fibroid.[5] On sonogram, it appears similar to the leiomyoma and can be extremely difficult to diagnose preoperatively. Rapid accelerated growth may be the only clinical indication of a possible malignant process.[11]

Adenomyosis is defined as an invasion of endometrial tissue into the myometrium greater than 2 mm. It occurs more often in multiparous women. Symptoms may include menorrhagia, dysmenorrhea, and pelvic tenderness.[12] Sonographically, the uterus is large with small cysts visible in the inner myometrium. Often the myometrium of the uterus will appear inhomogenous, similar to a fibroid, but distinct borders cannot be identified.[5]

In postmenopausal women, the endometrial lining atrophies. Any uterine bleeding during this stage is considered abnormal.[11] A common cause of vaginal bleeding in postmenopausal women is endometrial hyperplasia.[5] It is a increase in endometrial tissue that sonographically appears as a thickened, echogenic, and irregular endometrium. Sonographic differentials may include polyps or endometrial cancer, although both of these entities have a slightly different appearance. Definitive diagnosis is made by an endometrial biopsy.

An endometrial polyp is a focal growth of endometrial tissue. Polyps may occur in the perimenopausal years and may cause metrorrhagia, menorrhagia or both.[5] Sonographically, polyps appear as a focal area of increased echogenicity within the endometrial lining. The ideal time to visualize polyps is day 10–14 of the menstrual cycle, during the proliferative phase. It may still be difficult to distinguish polyps from focal endometrial hyperplasia and endometrial cancer. CDS can help identify the feeding vessel within an endometrial polyp. This may be helpful when the endometrial texture is irregular suggestive of, but not diagnostic of, a polyp.[6] A sonohysterogram, a procedure, where sterile saline is instilled into the endometrial cavity, can outline the polyp for a definitive diagnosis.

Endometrial cancer is more commonly diagnosed in women 60–70 years old, but can occur at earlier ages. Symptoms may include metrorrhagia, menorrhagia, or both. Clinically, these symptoms are similar to endometrial hyperplasia and polyps. In woman not on hormone replacement therapy (HRT), the endometrial lining is usually increased greater than 5–6 mm on sonogram. An endometrial lining of greater than 8 mm is generally considered abnormal in postmenopausal patients on HRT.[2] The endometrial lining appears echogenic and may have irregular contours of the endometrium as the cancer invades into the myometrium. The diagnosis is made by biopsy.[2]

Hematocolpos is an accumulation of blood within the vagina. This condition can be caused by an imperforate hymen or transverse vaginal septum. On ultrasound, the endometrial cavity and vagina will be distended with hypoechoic echoes and possible fluid/fluid levels, representing blood.

Hematometra is an accumulation of blood within the uterine cavity secondary to atrophy of the endocervical canal or cervical stenosis (Table 9–1).

TABLE 9–1. TERMINOLOGY

Menorrhagia—prolonged bleeding occurring at the time of a menstrual period, either in duration or volume
Metrorrhagia—uterine bleeding occurring at irregular intervals
Metromenorrhagia—excessive and prolonged bleeding occurring at irregular, frequent intervals

Ovaries

Benign cystic masses of the ovaries tend to be smooth walled, well-defined, and anechoic with increased posterior acoustic enhancement. Thick irregular walls, thick septations (>3 mm), or echogenic papillary projections protruding into the cyst increase the possibility of malignancy.[2] The role of CDS in distinguishing benign from malignant ovarian masses is somewhat controversial. The actual resistance index (RI) seen in malignancies overlap that seen in some benign ovarian lesions. However, CDS can help establish to the presence of vascularity in papillary excrescence or in irregular areas in the wall of a mass, both of which are suggestive of malignancy.[6]

Malignant ovarian disease has a peak incidence between the ages of 55–59 years old. Other risk factors include family history (maternal or sibling), number of years of ovulation, and environmental (Tables 9–2, –3, –4).[2]

OBSTETRICS

Pregnancy Test

The pregnancy hormone, human chorionic gonadotropin (hCG), is reported in three common standards: the Inter-

TABLE 9–2. CYSTIC OVARIAN TUMORS

Mass	Clinical Findings	Sonographic Findings
Corpus luteum cyst	Associated with pregnancy	Unilocular May contain low-level internal echoes. May appear as multiseptated cystic mass. Normally regress >14th week of pregnancy.
Theca lutein cyst	Represents an exaggerated response to increased hCG Can be associated with ovarian hyperstimulation, molar pregnancy, chorioadenoma destruens, and choriocarcinoma	Bilateral enlarged ovaries Multiple small multiocular cysts
Polycystic ovaries (Stein–Leventhal syndrome)	A build-up of immature follicles with a thick outer covering preventing ovulation. Associated with hirsutism, increased testosterone levels, irregular cycles	Bilaterally enlarged ovaries Multiple small cysts, appearing as "string of pearls"
Ovarian remnant syndrome	Residual ovarian tissue after oophorectomy	Can produced cysts, neoplasms. May cause symptoms. Common with endometriosis and adhesions.
Ovarian torsion	May be caused by large cyst or tumor causing rotation of the ovary.	In early phase, will have an enlarged ovary with intraovarian venous flow, but absent intraovarian arterial flow. In late stages, it will appear as a cystic or complex mass with thick walls and absent blood flow.

Source: References 2–6.

TABLE 9–3. OVARIAN SOLID TUMORS

Mass	Clinical Findings	Sonographic Findings
Dysgerminoma	Uncommon malignant germ cell tumor. Occurs in 2nd–3rd decade of life. One of most common neoplasms in pregnancy. Historically similar to Seminoma.	Predominately solid with hypoechoic internal echoes. Can grow rapidly.
Fibroma	Occurs in 5th–6th decade. Part of stromal family along with the other differentials: thecoma, granulosa cell, androblastoma.	Hypoechoic to echogenic with mixed heterogeneous pattern.
Thecoma	84% occur postmenopausally.	Similar sonographic features as fibroma. Unilocular
Granulosa cell	95% occur postmenopausally.	Similar sonographic features as fibroma. Small tumors are solid. Large tumors are complex.
Androblastoma (Seroli–Leydig cell)	Occurs in 2nd–3rd decade. May cause elevated testosterone and hirsutism.	Similar sonographic features as fibroma.
Transitional cell (Brenner)	Occurs from 4th–8th decade. Most are benign. Symptoms: abnormal uterine bleeding.	Small, hypoechoic tumors. Larger tumors are at greater risk for malignancy.

Source: References 2–6.

national Reference Preparation (IRP), the Second International Standard (2nd IS), and the Third International Standard (3rd IS). The 2nd IS is approximately half the value of the IRP. The first detectable level of hCG is approximately 10 days after conception and considered to be positive at 30 mIU/mL IRP.[7] At a mean level of 1710 IRP, a 4.6 week gestational sac should be visualized by TVS with a mean sac diameter (MSD) of 3 mm.[13] The earliest GA to be able to detect a gestational sac by TAS varies on patient habitus and uterine orientation but is generally considered to be 6 weeks.[2]

The level of hCG above which virtually all normal intrauterine pregnancies can be visualized by ultrasound is called the discriminatory zone. A normal rise of hCG (an average of 66% every 48 hours or double every 72 hours) is indicative of an intrauterine pregnancy; a falling hCG level is indicative of a nonviable intrauterine pregnancy or an ectopic pregnancy.[7] By TVS, a mean sac diameter greater than or equal to 16 mm (34,100 IRP) should visualize a fetal pole. By TAS, a mean sac diameter greater than or equal to 25 mm (82,370 IRP) should visualize a fetal pole (Fig. 9–3).[5]

Duration

The duration of a pregnancy can be calculated from the first day of the last normal menstrual period and is referred to as menstrual age. The average duration of a pregnancy is approximately 280 days, 40 weeks, 9 calendar months, or 10 lunar months.[14] The expected date of delivery can be estimated by Nagele's rule, which is based on a 28-day menstrual cycle:

- Identify the date when the last menstrual period began.
- Add 7 days.
- Subtract 3 months.
- Add 1 year.

The gestational age may be calculated by last menstrual period as described above, with the assumption that conception occurred on day 12. Gestational age may also be calculated by sac size, or most accurately, CRL in the first trimester.[7]

In a clinical setting, many obstetricians will consider 38–40 weeks term, and 40–42 weeks postdates. The pregnancy is divided into three equal segments:

- First Trimester: 0–13 weeks
- Second Trimester: 13–28 weeks
- Third Trimester: 28–42 weeks

Embryological Development

Clinically, the enlargement of the uterus can be followed by examining the fundal height. The fundal height is measured in centimeters from the symphysis pubis to the top of the fundus. The height of the uterus (in cm) should correspond to the gestational age (in weeks). The chronological development of the embryo and fetus during a pregnancy is described in (Table 9–5). The first trimester finding are imaged with TVS.

Basic fetal cardiac evaluation has become an intricate component of obstetrical sonography. Fetal cardiac circulation is shown in Fig. 9–4. Note the three shunts present in fetal circulation that are not present after birth: (1) foramen ovale—between the left and right atria; (2) ductus arteriosus—between the pulmonary trunk and transverse aortic arch; and (3) ductus venosus—between the umbilical vein and inferior vena cava.[15]

The basic cardiac evaluation should include the four chamber view and views showing the outflow tracts origin and relationship to each other. The IVC should also be visualized and a fetal heart rate recorded. Sixty-five percent of cardiac abnormalities can be detected from the four chamber view. Eighty-five percent of defects can be detected if the great vessels views are included (Fig. 9–5).[5]

TABLE 9–4. COMPLEX OVARIAN TUMORS

Mass	Clinical Findings	Sonographic Findings
Endometriosis	Ectopic endometrial tissue that may bleed during menses. Cysts are called endometriomas or chocolate cysts because of blood in the cysts. Symptoms: pain during menses and infertility.	Single or multiple cystic adnexal masses with thick walls and low-level internal echoes. Small echogenic lesions posterior to the uterus.
Benign cystic teratoma (dermoid)	Most common benign germ cell tumor Composed of all three germ cell layers. Varies in composition with fat, bone, hair skin, teeth. More common in reproductive years.	Fluid–fluid levels Distal acoustic shadow Calcifications Tip of the iceberg sign (no through sound transmission)
Serous cystadenoma	Benign. Usually unilateral. Accounts for 25% of benign ovarian tumors. Occurs in 4th–5th decade.	Large cystic mass with thin-walled internal septations
Serous cystadeno-carcinoma	Accounts for 50% of malignant ovarian tumors in 4th–6th decade.	Large, multiocular with papillary projections. Ascites is common.
Mucinous cystadenoma	Largest ovarian tumor. Accounts for 25% of benign ovarian tumors. Occurs in 3rd–5th decade.	Large cystic mass with thick-walled septations. May have debris layering due to thick internal components.
Mucinous cystadeno-carcinoma	Malignant. Account for 5–10% of malignant ovarian tumors	Papillary projections are not as common as with serous cystadenocarcinoma. Associated with ascites.
Endometroid tumor	80% are malignant. Occurs in 5th–6th decade. Arises from endometriosis	Cystic mass with papillary projections. Can occasionally be solid.
Clear cell tumor	Invasive carcinoma occurring in 5th–6th decade.	Complex, predominately cystic mass.
Tubo-ovarian abscess	Infectious process within the tubes and ovaries	Fluid-fluid levels with hydrosalpinx. May be seen as complex or cystic mass with low-level echoes, irregular borders and internal septations.

Source: References 2–6.

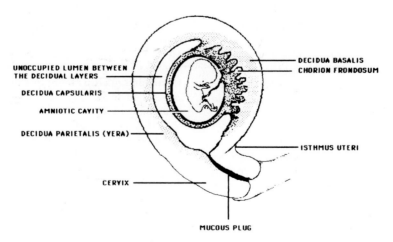

Figure 9–3. Diagram of early pregnancy.

TABLE 9–5. EMBRYOLOGICAL DEVELOPMENT

Gestational Age	Description MSD—mean sac diameter	Developments
4 weeks	avg. MSD 2–3 mm	Small gestational sac surrounded by echogenic rim of tissue
5 weeks	CRL 2–4 mm	"double decidual" sign (two echogenic lines surrounding portion of sac). Yolk sac is visible by end of 5th week. Small CRL visible adjacent to yolk sac.
6 weeks	CRL 4–9 mm	CRL 4–5 mm with cardiac activity > 100 bpm. CRL increases 1 mm/day. CRL changes from flat embryo to c-shaped. All major internal and external structures beginning to form
7–8 weeks	CRL 9–16 mm	Limb buds evolving into upper/lower extremities, fetal trunk elongates. Herniation of midgut into UC begins, base of cord <7 mm. Heart rate >137 bpm
9 weeks	CRL 23–31 mm	Rhombencephalon visible as cystic structure in posterior cranium
11 weeks	CRL 41 mm	Bowel returns to abdomen. Cranium visualized with prominent choroid plexus. Fetal head large, comprising of half of CRL. Good fetal movement is present. All extremities are visualized Anterior abdomen/thorax visualized. Can evaluate nuchal translucency (11–14 weeks). Yolk sac begins to disappear.
12 weeks	CRL 53–67 mm	End of first trimester. Fusion of amnion/chorion begins. Can identify twins, encephaloceles, holoprosencephaly, ectopia cordis, conjoined twins.
13–16 weeks	Multiple parameters	The femur length (FL), abdominal circumference (AC), head circumference (HC) and BPD can be measured. The HC>AC. Can identify cranium, abdominal wall, spine, and extremities.
16–20 weeks	Multiple parameters	Can fully evaluate fetal anatomy. Cardiac anatomy can usually be evaluated after 18 weeks.

Source: References 2–6.

Gestational Age and Growth

Estimated fetal weight is calculated using the parameters listed in Table 9–6. The fetal weight may then be plotted on a normal growth curve to assess the size of the fetus. Macrosomia describes a fetus that weighs more than 4000 g. Large for gestational age (LGA), is a clinical term and refers to the fundal height of the uterus. LGA has many

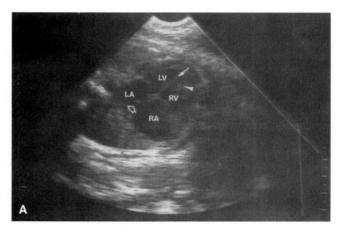

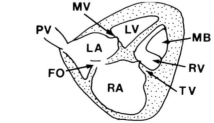

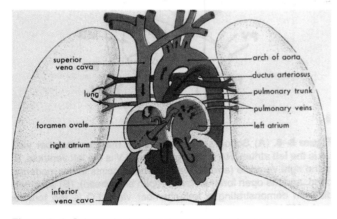

Figure 9–4. Schematic drawing demonstrating fetal cardiac circulation system. *(Reproduced with permission from Moore KL, The Developing Human: Clinically Oriented Embryology, 4th ed, Philadelphia: WB Saunders, 1988, p. 326.)*

Figure 9–5. (A) Sonogram demonstrating the four-chamber view. **(B)** Schematic diagram demonstrating the four-chamber view. *(Reproduced with permission from Cyr DR, et al. A systematic approach to fetal echocardiography using real time/two dimensional sonography. J Ultrasound Med. 1986; 5:343–350)*

TABLE 9–6. GESTATIONAL AGE AND RANGE OF ERROR

Gestational Age	Measurements	Range of Error
First trimester	CRL	± 3-5 days, most accurate
14–20 weeks	BPD, HC, AC, FL	± 10 days
20–30 weeks	BPD, HC, AC, FL	± 14 days
30–40 weeks	BPD, HC, AC, FL	± 21 days

With multiple measurements, the more parameters used, the more accurate the estimated due date. At least two parameters must be used.
Source: Reference 2.

causes, such as a large fetus (>90th percentile), excessive amniotic fluid, fibroids, twins, or a molar pregnancy. Macrosomia is often a manifestation of insulin-dependent diabetes mellitus (IDDM). It is associated with increased muscle mass and fat, leading to an increased AC and thickened shoulders. As well as a large fetus, there is often increased amniotic fluid volume (AFV) and a decreased HC/AC ratio because of the large AC. A macrosomic fetus is at risk for shoulder dystocia, humeral/clavicle fractures, meconium aspiration, prolonged labor, and asphyxial injury. Macrosomia carries an increased perinatal mortality, thus making its diagnosis by ultrasound important.[2]

IUGR or intrauterine growth restriction is defined by ultrasound as a weight <10th percentile. Other measurement findings with IUGR are and increased HC/AC and FL/AC ratios, oligohydramnios (a decrease in amniotic fluid) and advanced placental grade. Symmetrical IUGR refers to overall growth restriction; whereas, asymmetrical IUGR refers to the abdomen measuring smaller than normal for the gestational age and increasing the HC/AC and FL/AC ratios. In asymmetrical IUGR, blood is shunted to the brain in a brain-sparing effort and taken away from the bowel. Early onset IUGR with oligohydramnios is suggestive of a chromosomal abnormality or infection. Other causes of IUGR may be related to placental insufficiency. Maternal conditions that can be associated with IUGR include hypertension, vascular disease, autoimmune disease, and poor nutrition. Pulsed Doppler sonography may aid in assessing fetal well-being in addition to serial scans, AFV assessment, biophysical profile (BPP), and nonstress testing. When there is good umbilical cord blood flow, the waveform (systolic/diastolic ratio) demonstrates continuous diastolic flow.[6] An increased systolic/diastolic ratio of the umbilical artery suggests an increased resistance in the placenta leading to a decrease in blood velocity and volume.[2] The compromised fetus may demonstrate pulsatile or reversed flow in the umbilical vein, another sign of increased resistance to forward blood flow from the placenta to the fetus and a sign of cardiac compromise. CDS may be used to sample the middle cerebral artery and the ductus venosus. Doppler interrogation of these sites is crucial in identifying the fetus that is at high risk of severe compromise. In the severely compromised fetus, the increased flow to the brain is evidenced by increased diastolic flow in the middle cerebral artery. In addition, flow may be shunted away from the liver resulting in ductus venosus flow.[6]

CDS can be used to assess flow in the maternal uterine artery as it branches from the internal iliac artery. Sampling at this point typically reveals a waveform with a diastolic notch. This notch should not be present after 26 weeks, and when it is, it may indicate faulty placentation and a tendency to have pregnancy-induced hypertension (PIH) and/or IUGR.[6]

Biophysical Profile

Real-time sonography is vital to determine fetal condition, as evidenced by physiologic activities seen in fetal "breathing" and body movements. The compromised fetus may exhibit decreased or absent body movement and "breathing." Hypoxia affects certain neurologic autonomic centers in reversed order to their maturation. For example, the central nervous center for body movement and "tone" develops early in fetal maturation followed by centers for cardiac rate variation and "breathing." However, one of the first abnormalities to develop in the hypoxic fetus is lack of fetal heart rate acceleration followed by decreased fetal breathing and body motion.

The standard nonstress test (NST) evaluates changes in heart rate when the fetus moves. A negative (reactive) NST has high negative predictive value but false positives arise and are distressing for the new mothers and her physician.

The biophysical profile incorporates the NST, AF, fetal breathing, and body movements (both gross and tone). Each component is given a score of 2 if present, 0 if absent, with 10 being the highest score. Some biophysical profiles do not include the NST, with 8 being the highest score.

The Doppler techniques mentioned above may also be included in assessing fetal well-being. Thus, there are several sonographic techniques to monitor fetal well-being.[6]

Fetal Demise

Fetal demise is defined as death of the developing fetus after 20 weeks of gestation. The clinical and sonographic signs for fetal demise are numerous. The sonographic signs can be divided into specific and nonspecific. The specific signs are: (1) the failure to find the fetal heart tones on Doppler examination, (2) no fetal cardiac motion on M-mode, and (3) no movements or fetal heart pulsation seen on real-time sonography. The nonspecific signs are:

- overlapping of the fetal sutures (Spalding's sign)
- hydramnios or oligohydramnios
- flattened (oblong) fetal head
- absence of the falx cerebri

- distorted fetal anatomy
- decrease in the biparietal diameter when measurements are repeated from 1 week to the next
- decrease in the size of the uterus
- edematous soft tissue around the head (the "halo" sign or Druel's sign)
- fragmentation of the fetal skin
- diffuse edema of the entire fetus (anasarca)
- separation of the amnion from the chorion after 20 weeks
- gas in the fetal circulatory system (Robert's sign)
- hydropic swelling of the placenta

The clinical and laboratory findings of fetal demise are the failure of the uterus to grow, two negative pregnancy tests (serum beta hCG), no fetal movement, no heart sounds on auscultation, and red or brown amniotic fluid[7] (Fig. 9–6).

Amniotic Fluid

Amniotic fluid (AF) has many functions. It protects the fetus, allows for growth, controls temperature, allows for respiration, allows for normal GI and musculoskeletal development, and prevents infection. In the first trimester and early second trimester, AF is made by the placenta. After 16 weeks, the primary sources of AF are the fetal kidneys and lungs. Fluid is reaccumulated in the body through fetal swallowing. Amniotic fluid volume (AFV) normally increases until 33 weeks gestation. There it peaks and then begins to decline for the remainder of the pregnancy.[5] An exact volume of AFV cannot be obtained with ultrasound; however, the amniotic fluid index (AFI) is an indirect means of quantifying the amount of AF. The maternal abdomen is divided into four quadrants. In each quadrant, an AP measurement of AF is taken that does not contain body parts or umbilical cord. The four quadrant values are totaled with the sum representing the AFI. The AFI can be compared to a normal AFI curve to assess AFV. Another means of measuring AF is the single pocket measurement. The largest pocket of AF that does not contain body parts or umbilical cord is measured in an AP dimension. If a 1-cm pocket of AF cannot be measured, the diagnosis of oligohydramnios can be made.[5] The single pocket measurement is less reliable than the AFI, but it can be useful in such situations as multiple gestations and pre- and postdecompression amniocentesis.

Oligohydramnios is the decrease of AFV below the 2.5th percentile. It may be caused by a renal abnormality or obstruction, placental insufficiency, premature rupture of membranes, or post dates. Oligohydramnios with placental insufficiency is caused by a decreased blood flow to the uterus, which in turn, causes decreased renal perfusion.[2] A lack of AFV can contribute to pulmonary hypoplasia and extremity contractures.

Polyhydramnios is the excessive accumulation of AFV, measuring >95th percentile. Sixty percent of polyhydramnios are idiopathic, 20% are structural, and 20% are maternal (IDDM).[2]

Placenta and Umbilical Cord

The *placenta* is responsible for the maternal/fetal exchange of nutrients, oxygen, and waste. The placenta can attach anywhere in the uterus. The fetal side consists of a fused layer of amnion and chorion, with underlying vessels being located in the chorionic villi. The maternal component consists of cotyledons, composed of maternal sinusoids and chorionic villous structures. Oxygenated maternal blood enters the intervillous spaces that bathe the chorionic villi. Gases and nutrients are exchanged across the walls of the villi, with waste crossing from inside the villi to the intervillous space for the maternal vessels to transport away from the placenta. Maternal blood flow increases in pregnancy to accommodate the increased demand of the placenta. The placenta is a low resistive organ that allows a decrease in resistance to the fetus as the fetus grows.[5] This results in progressively increasing blood flow as the pregnancy advances. Placental insufficiency is related to increased resistance in the vascular bed and results in decreased blood flow to the fetus. Placental insufficiency may be indirectly monitored by umbilical cord pulsed Doppler. The ratio of systolic flow to diastolic flow will show the amount of resistance in the placental bed. A lower ratio is less resistive, a higher ratio is more resistive. Normal ratios vary with gestational age and tables are available listing the normal ranges.

Placenta previa is the condition in which the placenta crosses the internal os of the cervix. Placenta previa is the primary cause of third trimester bleeding, although bleeding may occur from previa at anytime in pregnancy.[2] Placenta previa may be further subcategorized into: (1) complete—placenta totally covers the internal os; (2) partial—placenta is over the edge but does not cross the internal os; (3) marginal—placenta touches the edge of the internal os; and (4) low lying—the placenta is within 2 cm of the internal os. Placentas may have a succenturiate or accessory lobe that is connected to the main lobe of the placenta by blood vessels within a

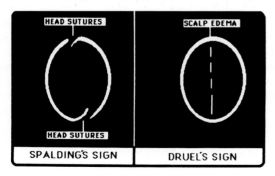

Figure 9–6. Spalding's sign/Druel's sign.

membrane. If these vessels cross the internal os it is considered a vasa previa.[5]

Placental abruption is the premature separation of the placenta from the uterine wall after 20 weeks gestation. Symptoms may include bleeding and abdominal pain. Although the diagnosis is usually made clinically, sonographic findings are a retroplacental, hypoechoic area composed mainly of veins >2 cm, and large periplacental hematomas. Hematoma appearances vary with acute being hyperechoic, becoming isoechoic, and finally becoming hypoechoic to anechoic. Placental abruption is one of the leading causes of perinatal mortality and accounts for 15–20% of all perinatal deaths.[2] It can be associated with maternal vascular disease, hypertension, abdominal trauma, cocaine abuse, cigarette smoking, AMA, and unexplained increased MSAFP.[5]

Placenta accreta is the abnormal adherence of placental tissue to the uterus. It may be further divided into: (1) placenta accreta vera—placental attachment to the myometrium without invasion; (2) placenta increta—invasion of the placenta into the myometrium; and (3) placenta percreta—invasion of the placenta through the uterus and often invasion into the bladder or rectum. Risk factors include uterine scarring from cesarean sections and advanced maternal age. Implantation sites at risk are uterine scars, submucous fibroid, lower uterine segment, rudimentary horn, and uterine cornua. With placenta accreta, the normal hypoechoic 1–2 cm myometrial band is absent or thinned (<2 mm) with loss of placental/myometrial interface.[2] There may be large hypoechoic to anechoic spaces in the placenta, termed "Swiss cheese appearance." Placental vascularity is also increased.[9]

Chorioangioma is the most common benign tumor of the placenta. It is a vascular malformation arising from the chorionic tissue that appears as a well-defined, hypoechoic mass near the chorionic surface and often near the cord insertion site.[2] Color and pulsed Doppler will confirm the increased vascularity of this lesion.

The umbilical cord consists of two arteries and one vein. The vein enters the fetus and drains into the ductus venosum and left portal vein in the liver. The umbilical vein carries oxygenated blood. The umbilical arteries, carrying deoxygenated blood, are seen coursing laterally around the bladder as they leave the fetal body. The vessels in the cord are surrounded by Wharten's jelly for protection. The umbilical cord normally inserts into the central portion of the uterus. It can, however, insert eccentrically or near the membranes. It can also be a velamentous insertion when it inserts into the membranes and courses through the membrane to the placenta.[5] Both of these insertions can play a part in placental insufficiency and fetal growth. Occasionally, only one artery will be present resulting in a two vessel umbilical cord. It may be associated with other abnormalities and could possibly effect fetal growth, although not common. CDS can help identify absence of the umbilical artery, as well as nuchal cord and cord knots.[6]

OBSTETRICAL ANOMALIES

First Trimester Abnormalities
Hydatidiform Mole. This is a component of gestational trophoblastic disease (abnormal proliferation of the trophoblastic elements) that may be partial or complete.

Complete—Sonographic findings are an enlarged uterine cavity filled with complex echoes often resembling placental tissue with multiple cysts. It is associated with a markedly increased β-hCG and may have bilateral theca luteal cysts 18–30% of the time.[11] If not treated, this can progress into malignant choriocarcinoma.[5]

Partial—The combination of a fetus and a localized area of placenta with molar degeneration. Ninety percent of partial moles are triploidy. On ultrasound, a partial mole presents as an enlarged placenta, >4 cm in AP dimension at 18–22 weeks gestation, with focal multicystic, anechoic spaces replacing the normal homogeneous appearance of placenta.[5]

Ectopic Pregnancy. This is implantation of pregnancy anywhere outside the endometrial lumen. The most common site of implantation is the ampullary region of the fallopian tube, followed by the other regions of the fallopian tube, the ovaries, the cervix, and finally the abdomen. Symptoms include vaginal bleeding and abdominal pain. HCG will be positive but values will not rise as fast as an intrauterine pregnancy. Sonographic finding may show an intrauterine pseudosac that has a single decidual layer. The most common ultrasound appearance is an extrauterine and extraovarian complex adnexal mass with free fluid. In some instances, an embryo with fetal heart motion can be visualized.[5] CDS can be used during instillation of saline to determine tubal pregnancy. The patent tube will demonstrate flow within the tube and fluid will be seen egressing from the fibriated end of the tube to collect in the fluid pocket around the ovary.[6]

Blighted Ovum (Anembryonic Demise). This is a large (>2 cm) sac without an appropriately sized embryo that is irregular in shape with a thin choriodecidua.

Missed (Incomplete) Abortion. This is an embryo without fetal heart motion retained in the uterus before 20 weeks. Fetal demise after 20 weeks is called an intrauterine fetal demise (IUFD). In early pregnancy, CDS can identify the presence of retained products of conception by establishing the presence of flow within abnormal tissue within the uterus.[6]

Other first trimester anomalies that may be identified are cranial abnormalities, large spinal defects, abdominal wall defects, severe short limb syndromes.

Fetal Head, Neck, and Spine
Neural Tube Defect. This is a spectrum of malformations of the neural tube including: (1) anencephaly, (2) spina bifida, and (3) cephalocele.

Anencephaly. This is the most severe form of neural tube defect. It is characterized by absence of the upper portion of the cranial vault and underlying cerebral hemispheres. It may be diagnosed as early as 12 weeks by TVS and is associated with a markedly increased MSAFP, polyhydramnios, other spinal defects, and protruding eyes.[2]

Spina Bifida. This is a defect in the lateral processes of the vertebrae allowing the spinal canal to be exposed, which in turn disrupts the muscle and skin covering. Herniation can be limited to meninges (meningocele) or involve the neural tissue as well (myelomeningocele). The most common sites of spina bifida are lumbar, lumbosacral, and thoracolumbar. Cranial finding associated with spina bifida are: (1) banana sign, consistently present with a defect (99%), and (2) lemon sign. The banana sign is the displacement of the cerebrum inferiorly into the upper cervical canal. On the transverse cerebellar view, the cerebellum resembles a banana instead of its characteristic view. The lemon sign, frontal bossing with narrowing of the parietal bones, gives the sonographic impression of a "lemon"-shaped head in the axial scanning plane at the level of the thalamus. Spina bifida is often associated with increased MSAFP, ventriculomegaly, and clubfeet.[2,5,16]

Cephalocele. This is a protrusion of the cranial contents through a bony defect in the skull. An encephalocele contains brain tissue. The majority are occipital (75%).[5] They often cause blockage of CSF and ventriculomegaly results. Very large defects may be associated with microcephaly. Both types have a poor prognosis.[2]

Ventriculomegaly. This is enlargement of the lateral ventricles, >10 mm in the posterior horn. In the absence of a spinal defect, pronounced ventriculomegaly (>15 mm) is most commonly associated with an obstruction of the ventricular system. In order of occurrence, these obstructions are aqueductal stenosis, communicating hydrocephalus, and Dandy–Walker malformation. Congenital hydrocephaly is an X-linked abnormality with only males affected and females being carriers. If there is a strong family history, DNA testing is available.[2] Ventriculomegaly is often associated with other abnormalities.

Dandy–Walker Malformation. This consists of a splaying of the cerebellar vermis, communication with a dilated fourth ventricle, increased cysterna magna (>10 mm), and ventriculomegaly. It can be associated with chromosomal abnormalities and is frequently associated with such other cranial midline defects as agenesis of the corpus callosum. It is often associated with other system abnormalities as well.[2]

Holoprosencephaly. This is a group of midline defects resulting from incomplete cleavage of the prosencephalon. The three major varieties are (1) alobar—single rudimentary ventricle, absent cerebral falx, fused thalamus, absent 3rd ventricle. Facial findings may range from cyclopia to severe hypotelorism. A medial cleft lip/palate is common. A proboscis may replace the nose or the nose may be very flattened; (2) semilobar—the cerebral hemispheres are partially separated posteriorly, with partial separation of the lateral ventricles. Both alobar and semilobar holoprosencephaly are associated with microcephaly; (3) lobar—almost complete separation of cerebellum and ventricles except for the fused anterior horns of the lateral ventricles. Other sonographic findings are absent cavum septum pellicudum. Facial findings are less severe than those found with alobar or semilobar holoprosencephaly.[4]

Cystic Hygroma. This most often occurs at the posterior neck. A hygroma is a sac filled with lymphatic fluid caused by an obstruction of the lymphatic system. It may be multiloculated or contain a midline septum and is often associated with Turner syndrome or Down syndrome.[5]

Choroid Plexus Cyst. This is a cyst in the choroid plexus of the lateral ventricles. With other sonographic findings, it may be associated with trisomy 18 or 21. Alone, many investigators consider this a normal anatomic variant.[2]

Iniencephaly. This is a defect in the occiput involving the foramen magnum characterized by marked retroflexion of the fetal head and frequently shortened spine. This is a rare finding and has a strong association with other abnormalities.[2]

Agenesis of the Corpus Callosum. This cannot be diagnosed until after 18 weeks gestation. Findings to aid in diagnosis include: (1) "teardrop" ventricles—enlargement of the posterior horn of the lateral ventricle without enlargement of the anterior horn. The anterior horns are more laterally positioned in the cerebral cortex; (2) enlargement and upward displacement of the third ventricle. ACC has a strong association with other abnormalities.[2]

Hydranencephaly. A severe destructive process, believed to result from occlusion of the internal carotid arteries. The cerebral cortex is replaced by fluid, causing macrocephaly. The thalamus, brain stem, and cerebellum are spared.[2]

Vein of Galen Aneurysm. This is an arteriovenous (AV) malformation in vein of Galen located posterior to the third ventricle in the midline. Color and pulsed Doppler will demonstrate high-velocity arterial and venous blood flow. Associated with congestive heart failure and hydrops.[2]

Cleft Lip/Palate. Isolated cleft lip and/or palate is the most common congenital facial anomaly. Lateral cleft lip is commonly isolated. Medial cleft lip is associated with chromosomal abnormalities.[2]

Heart

Atrial/Ventricular Septal Defect. This is a congenital malformation of the septum that appears as an opening between the chambers. It is the most common cardiac defect, accounting for 26% of defects.[4]

Atrioventricular (AV) Canal Defect. This is also known as AV septal defect, or endocardial cushion defect. A complete defect has a single ventricle, a single atrium, and a single AV valve. This appearance may vary with partial defects of the atrial or ventricular septums. This is the most common cardiac defect in trisomy 21.[4]

Hypoplastic Left Heart Syndrome. This is hypoplasia of the left ventricle, atrium, mitral valve, and aortic outflow. The right side of the heart will be enlarged.[5] The appearance may vary with different degrees of severity.

Coarctation of the Aorta. This is a narrowed segment of aorta along the aortic arch. It is difficult to see the narrowing but may present as a milder form of hypoplastic left heart syndrome later in pregnancy. Pulsed Doppler studies may also show a decrease in blood flow in the proximal portion of the aorta.[4]

Tetralogy of Fallot. This presents with the following defects: (1) VSD, (2) overriding aorta, (3) pulmonary stenosis or atresia, and (4) right ventricular hypertrophy. It has a strong association with chromosomal abnormalities.[4]

Ebstein Anomaly. This is the inferior displacement of the tricuspid valve. The right atrium is enlarged, and the valve, which is commonly abnormal, may appear thick and irregular in motion. Tricuspid valve regurgitation is often appreciated.[4]

Double Outlet Right Ventricle. The pulmonary artery and aorta both originate from the right ventricle, giving the appearance of the great vessels running parallel. Often a VSD is present.[4]

Transposition of the Great Vessels. The aorta arises from the right ventricle, and the pulmonary artery arises from the left ventricle. The great vessels appear parallel on ultrasound. The pulmonary bifurcation and brachiocephalic vessels must be identified to correctly diagnose this entity. ASD and VSD are often present.[4,5]

Truncus Arteriosus. This is a single large ventricular outflow tract overriding a VSD. Right ventricular outflow tract will not be visualized, and pulmonary artery branches as well as aortic branches will be seen arising from the truncus.[4]

Rhabdomyoma. This is the most common intracardiac tumor. It can be multiple and appears as an echogenic mass located anywhere within the cardiac system. It is not visualized <22 wks and has a strong association with tuberous sclerosis.[4]

Supraventricular Tachycardia (SVT). The fetal heart beat is >200 bpm. Both SVT and atrial flutter can lead to cardiac failure because of increased cardiac output.[4]

Thorax

Congenital Diaphragmatic Hernia (CDH). This is a congenital defect in the diaphragm allowing abdominal contents to herniate into the thorax. It may be left sided (75–90%), right sided (10%), or bilateral (<5%). Sonographically, (1) the fetal heart may be deviated, (2) stomach or bowel may be visualized in the thorax, (3) the area adjacent to the heart may appear inhomogenous, consistent with liver, and (4) polyhydramnios may be present. The intrathoracic abdominal contents can cause pulmonary hypoplasia, a significant factor in the high perinatal mortality (50–80%) of this disorder. If the liver is intrathoracic, CDH has a poorer prognosis (43% survival) versus an intrabdominal liver (80% survival). Associated anomalies (15–45%) and chromosomal abnormalities (5–15%) will also affect perinatal survival.[2]

Congenital Cystic Adenomatoid Malformation (CCAM). This is the most frequently identified mass in the fetal chest. It is typically unilateral and has 3 types: (1) type I, macrocystic—multiple large cysts measuring 2–10 cm, (2) type II—multiple medium sized cysts <2 cm, and (3) type III, microcystic—sonographically appearing as a solid, homogenous echogenic lung mass. Many CCAMs spontaneously regress in size during the third trimester. Prognosis is dependent on size, degree of mediastinal shift, and presence or absence of hydrops and polyhydramnios. Type I and II typically have a better prognosis.[2]

Pulmonary Sequestration. This is a solid, nonfunctioning mass of lung tissue that lacks communication with the tracheobronchial tree. It has its own blood supply commonly arising directly from the aorta and is fed by a single vessel. The majority are visualized as a well circumscribed mass in the left lower lung base. It may cause mediastinal shift and hydrops. Ten percent can be found below the diaphragm and should be considered with any suprarenal mass in the left abdomen. Fifty percent to seventy-five percent of sequestrations regress spontaneously.[2]

Pleural Effusion. This is a fluid accumulation in the pleural lining of the thorax. Most commonly part of the hydrops complex.[2]

Gastrointestinal

Esophageal Atresia. This is an incomplete formation of the esophagus. There are five types of atresia, with 90% of those having a TE fistula that communicates with the fetal stomach. Sonographically, the exam may be normal (because of fistula) or there may be a small to absent stomach bubble and polyhydramnios. Even with a stomach bubble visualized, this must be considered with unexplained polyhydramnios. This has a strong association with other anomalies and chromosomal abnormalities.[2]

Duodenal Atresia. This is a partial to complete obstruction caused by the failure of recanalization of the duodenum. It is the most common perinatal intestinal obstruction. The stomach and duodenum fill proximal to the site of the obstruction creating the classic "double bubble" sign. Fifty percent are associated with other findings including growth restriction, polyhydramnios, GI, and cardiac anomalies. Duodenal atresia has a strong association with trisomy 21.[2]

Gastroschisis. This is an anterior abdominal wall defect, most commonly to the right side of the umbilicus, that allows herniation of abdominal contents into the amniotic cavity. The most common finding is free-floating bowel in the amniotic fluid, but stomach and bladder may also herniate into the amniotic fluid. Exposure to AF and compression at an abdominal wall can lead to dilation and edema of the bowel. Overall, this has a good prognosis and does not have a strong association with chromosomal defects or other anomalies. It is associated with an elevated MSAFP.[2]

Omphalocele. This is a midline defect in the anterior abdominal wall with herniation of abdominal contents into the base of the umbilical cord. The mass is covered by a membrane and may not always have an elevated MSAFP, or may not elevate the MSAFP as significantly as gastroschisis. The umbilical cord can be seen inserting into the abdominal mass. Omphaloceles commonly contain liver, but may contain other abdominal organs such as bowel. They have a strong association with other anomalies (50–80%), particularly cardiac, as well as chromosomal abnormalities (40–60%). If the omphalocele is small and contains only small bowel, the risk of aneuploidy increases.[2]

Pentalogy of Cantrell. This is an anomaly that is sonographically distinctive because of an omphalocele and ectopia cordis. The other components are defects in the lower sternum, diaphragm, and intracardiac anomalies. There are many other associated craniofacial abnormalities, and it often is associated with chromosomal abnormalities.[2]

Beckwith–Wiedemann Syndrome. This is a group of disorders including omphalocele, macroglossia, organomegaly, hypoglycemia, and hemihypertrophy.[2]

Cloacal Exstrophy. This is an association of anomalies including omphalocele, herniated, fluid filled structure inferior to omphalocele in place of urinary bladder, imperforate anus, and neural tube defect. This defect has a marked increased MSAFP.[2]

Meconium Ileus. This is the third most common cause of neonatal bowel obstruction. Sonographic findings include echogenic small bowel, dilated fluid-filled loops of bowel, and echogenic dilated bowel. It has a strong association with cystic fibrosis. If the internal diameter of the small bowel is >7 mm, it is suggestive of obstruction.[2]

Meconium Peritonitis. This is a reaction to bowel perforation. Meconium causes a peritoneal reaction that forms a membrane which seals the perforation and may be seen as thick-walled cyst. Other findings are ascites and meconium calcifications.[2]

Limb–Body Wall Complex (LBWC). This is a complex set of abnormalities caused by failure of the anterior abdominal wall to close. Findings include complete body wall defects, absence of umbilical cord, severe scoliosis, and lower limb abnormalities. Abnormalities are widespread and appearance may be a mass of tissue with few distinctive features.[2]

Amniotic Band Syndrome. This describes a widespread spectrum of defects thought to be caused by amniotic bands that break away from the amnion on one end and disrupt fetal parts and development in the first trimester.[2]

Hydrops. There are two types: (1) Non-immune—accumulation of fluid in body cavities (pleural, pericardial, and peritoneal) and soft tissue. There are many causes for this entity, but major causes are cardiac failure, anemia, arteriovenous shunts, mediastinal compression, metabolic diseases, fetal infections, fetal tumors, congenital fetal defects, chromosomal and placental anomalies; (2) immune—sonographic findings the same. These are caused by maternal antibodies destroying fetal red blood cells, which ultimately leads to congestive heart failure.[2]

Ascites. This is free fluid within the abdominal cavity. It may be part of the hydrops complex or isolated because of bowel perforation or bladder perforation.

Situs Inversus Totalis. This is complete thoracic and abdominal organ reversal. Partial situs involves the abdominal organs only. Often associated with polysplenia and congenital heart defects.[2]

Abdominal Cyst. The differential for an isolated abdominal cyst not related to the GI or GU tract include ovarian cyst, mesenteric cyst, omental cyst, or urachal cyst as the most common listings.

Genitourinary
Ureteropelvic Junction (UPJ) Obstruction. This is an obstruction at the junction of the renal pelvis and ureter.

It is the most common cause of hydronephrosis. A complete obstruction will lead to massive hydronephrosis eventually causing dysplasia.

Ureterovesical Junction (UVJ) Obstruction. This is an obstruction at the junction of the ureter and bladder. Sonographic findings include mild hydronephrosis and hydroureter. Often associated with duplicated renal anomalies including the ureter. The abnormal ureter commonly has a stenotic opening into the bladder and forms an ureterocele, which appears as a cystic structure within or adjacent to the bladder.

Posterior Urethral Valve Bladder Outlet Obstruction (PUV). This is an obstruction of the posterior urethral valves. Overwhelming found in males, the bladder is massively dilated with hydroureters and hydronephrosis. The massive hydronephrosis may lead to atrophy of the kidneys. Anhydramnios is present with complete obstruction. On ultrasound, the bladder has the characteristic "keyhole" appearance as urine fills the proximal urethera. The abdominal wall becomes overly distended, which results in prune belly syndrome (abnormal development of abdominal musculature leading to a lax abdominal wall in newborns). The lack of amniotic fluid causes Potter facies (flattened facies, low set ears) and flexion contractures of the extremities. Pulmonary hypoplasia, caused by anhydramnios, is the primary cause of neonatal death in this syndrome.

Renal Agenesis. Diagnosis is made by the following findings: anhydramnios to severe oligohydramnios, nonvisualized bladder, and absent kidneys without evidence of renal blood flow. The adrenal glands appear flattened and elongated, which may aid in the diagnosis.

Multicystic Dysplastic Kidney (MCDK). This is an obstruction in the first trimester that leads to atretic kidneys and formation of randomly positioned and varying sized cysts in the parenchyma of the kidney. The parenchyma is usually increased in echogenicity as well.

Autosomal Dominant Polycystic Kidney Disease. There must be one affected parent for this disorder to occur. Findings are not always seen in pregnancy and if so, typically do not appear until third trimester. Kidneys may appear enlarged and echogenic with multiple large cysts.

Autosomal Recessive Polycystic Kidney Disease. This is also known as infantile polycystic kidney disease. Multiple microscopic cysts give the appearance of very large, echogenic kidneys with decreased AFV after 20 weeks. Findings may be normal <20 weeks.

Congenital Mesoblastic Nephroma. This is a rare renal tumor that sonographically appears as a large, solid, well-circumscribed, highly vascular mass. The increased vascularity can cause cardiac overload and polyhydramnios.

Neuroblastoma. This malignant tumor is commonly found in the adrenal gland. Sonographically, it appears as echogenic, heterogenous, suprarenal mass.[2]

Skeletal

Limb shortening may be described as: (1) rhizomelic—shortening of the proximal limb, (2) mesomelic—shortening of the forearm bones or lower leg bones, (3) micromelia—shortening of all portions of the limbs, both severe and mild. There are many types of short limb syndromes, and the more common lethal and nonlethal varieties are discussed in this review.

Short limb syndromes are considered lethal if the thoracic circumference is <5th percentile for the gestational age, suggesting pulmonary hypoplasia. Other findings are: (1) severe micromelia, <4 SD of mean, and (2) identification of such specific features as severe fractures.

Lethal

Thanatophoric Dysplasia. This is the most common skeletal dysplasia and is uniformly lethal.

Findings are:

- cranium—macrocrania, hydrocephaly, frontal bossing, cloverleaf shaped skull, depressed nasal bridge
- thorax—severely hypoplastic giving the "bell-shaped" appearance, short ribs
- bones—severe rhizomelia with bowing ("telephone receiver"); hypomineralization; spinal column appears narrow; polyhydramnios

Achondrogenesis—Type I, Most Severe. This exhibits severe micromelia, protruding abdomen, poor skull, and vertebral ossification. Type II, accounts for 80%.

- cranium—macrocrania
- thorax—shortened trunk
- bones—severe micromelia with bowing and decreased mineralization

Osteogenesis Imperfecta Type II—Lethal. OI type II is subcategorized into three types, but all three are discussed in general terms for this text.

- thorax—bell shaped, with small thorax; ribs have multiple fractures, may appear thin and flared
- bones—micromelia; may see fractures or bones may appear thickened, irregular, and bowed because of fractures folding on themselves
- decreased fetal movement and polyhydramnios common

Nonlethal

Heterozygous Achondroplasia. This is the most common form of genetic skeletal dysplasia. It may not always be identified <27 weeks.

- cranium—increased HC, frontal bossing, depressed nasal bridge
- bones—mild to moderate rhizomelic shortening, "trident" hand

Osteogenesis Imperfecta—Type I, III, IV.

- Type I—may not identify <24 weeks; mild micromelia and bowing; may see isolated fractures

- Type III—will show lagging long bone growth early with mild to moderate shortening and bowing
- Type IV—similar to type I

Asphyxiating Thoracic Dysplasia (Jeune Thoracic Dystrophy).
- thorax—may appear bell shaped
- bones—mild to moderate micromelia (rhizomelic) with possible bowing, possible polydactyly polyhydramnios.[2]

Multiple Gestations

Multiple pregnancies account for 1.5% of all pregnancies. Dizygotic, or fraternal twins, occur when two separate ova are fertilized. Monozygotic or identical twins, occur when a single ovum divides. Seventy-five percent of twins are dizygotic, and 25% are monozygotic. The frequency of monozygotic twinning is constant and occurs in 1:250 births. Dizygotic twinning varies widely and is dependent on race, maternal age, parity (increased risk with increased parity), maternal family history, and infertility medication.[2]

It is very important to determine the number of chorionic and amniotic sacs in twin pregnancies. The best and most accurate time to assess this is in the first trimester. All dizygotic twins are dichorionic, diamniotic. Monozygotic twins, on the other hand, may have a variety of presentations depending on the day the zygote divides.[2]

Day of division	Appearance
<4 days	Dichorionic/diamniotic, same gender, occurs 24% of time
4–8 days	Monochorionic, diamniotic, occurs 75% of time
8–12 days	Monochorionic, monoamniotic, 1%
>13 days	Conjoined, monochorionic, monoamniotic

Sonography cannot distinguish between dizygotic and monozygotic twins unless they are different genders. There are sonographic clues to aid in the identification of chorionicity and amniocity.

First trimester sonographic findings are:

Dichorionic—sacs will be divided by a thick echogenic rim, counting the sacs determines the chorionicity

Monochorionic—will appear similar to a single gestation with a thick echogenic gestational sac surrounding both fetuses.

Diamniotic—each sac will have its own yolk sac (>8 wks). The amniotic sac is very thin and can be difficult to identify in the first trimester.[2]

Second trimester—Dichorionic findings:

1) different gender
2) two separate placentas
3) twin peak sign—triangular projection of chorion into dividing membrane appears as a "peak" on ultrasound; strong predictor <28 weeks

4) thickness of membrane—thick membrane, >1 mm, is suggestive of dichorionicity. This finding is more accurate <26 weeks, but is still a weak predictor.[2]

Twin pregnancies carry a 4–6 times higher perinatal mortality, and a two times higher morbidity rate for a variety of reasons. The most common complication of twins is preterm labor. Other complications are growth restriction, anomalies (2–3 times more than a singleton), and such maternal conditions as hypertension and pre-eclampsia.[5]

Twin Abnormalities

Twin-to-Twin Transfusion Syndrome (TTTS).
This condition can occur with monochorionic twins. Arteriovenous communications within the placenta can result in TTTS. One fetus will have blood shunted away and is labeled the donor, while the other fetus will receive the shunted blood and is labeled the recipient. This syndrome presents with a series of sonographic findings related to the shunting of blood. The donor twin is commonly growth restricted with a discordance between the twins >20%. There is often oligohydramnios with the donor and polyhydramnios with the recipient. The donor fetus will appear "stuck" in their sac. This appearance is characteristic of TTTS. The donor will become hypovolemic and anemic. Umbilical cord Dopplers often show an increased systolic/diastolic ratio, demonstrating the increased resistance in the umbilical cord. The recipient will become larger, hypervolemic, and plethoric. Hydrops may occur as the fetus enters into congestive heart failure. The ventricular walls of the heart may thicken, and the contractility of the heart may be decreased as the heart failure becomes worse. As the blood flow increases to the recipient, the S/D ratio decreases, and the overall blood velocity is high. Both fetuses are at a significantly increased risk for intrauterine and perinatal mortality.[2]

Monoamniotic Twins.
This entity carries a 50% mortality risk because of cord entanglement that obstructs blood flow to the fetus. Sonographically, color Doppler may be helpful to look for a mass of cord with areas of increased velocity, suggesting stenotic flow.

Conjoined Twins.
This is rare. Most conjoined twins are born premature, and 40% are stillborn. The most common presentation is fusion of the anterior wall. They may share organs, and those organs can often have abnormalities. Polyhydramnios is present 50% of the time. The most common types are: thoracoomphalopagus (conjoined chest and abdomen), thoracopagus (conjoined chest), and omphalopagus (conjoined abdomen). They account for 56% of the types of conjoined twins.[2,5]

Acardiac Twin.
This is rare. All cases have an arterial-to-arterial shunt and a venous-to-venous shunt allowing for perfusion of the acardiac twin.[2] The acardiac twin either has a rudimentary heart or is completely acardiac. It has a poorly underdeveloped upper body with a small or absent cranium and brain. If it does develop, there are often significant abnormalities. The lungs and abdominal organs

may also be abnormal or absent. The lower extremities are slightly more developed.[4] The normal, or pump twin is at a great risk for congestive heart failure, which will present on ultrasound as polyhydramnios and fetal hydrops. Chromosomes have been reported to be abnormal in up to 50% of the cases. Doppler can verify the reversed flow in the umbilical cord of the acardiac twin.[2]

Chromosomal Abnormalities and Testing

Trisomy 21. This is the most common chromosome disorder. Trisomy 21 occurs when there are three copies of chromosome 21. The Down syndrome frequency increases with advanced maternal age. At this time, the only definitive test to determine Down syndrome is amniocentesis. Noninvasive testing includes blood tests and ultrasound.[4]

First trimester screening combines biochemistry markers, maternal age (MA), and fetal nuchal translucency (NT). Nuchal translucency is a measurement made at the back of the fetal neck on the CRL image. It is applicable from 11–14 weeks. The nuchal translucency increases with gestational age and normal tables are available for comparison; however, any measurement <3 mm is normal. Screening for Down syndrome by maternal age and NT has been shown to identify 80% of fetuses with Down syndrome (with a 5% false-positive rate). Other chromosomal defects (Trisomy 18, 13, triploidy, and Turner syndrome), cardiac defects, skeletal dysplasias, and genetic syndromes can also present with increased NT.[17]

For the NT to be accurate, very strict rules should be followed. The fetus is measured in the sagittal plane, the same used for the CRL. Careful consideration should be taken to bisect the fetus exactly in the midline, evidenced by the umbilical cord insertion. The image should be magnified so that the fetus occupies at least three-fourths of the image. The imager should be able to distinguish between the fetal skin and the amnion, both appearing as a thin membrane. This is accomplished by waiting for the fetus to spontaneously move away from the amnion. The first caliper should be placed so that the horizontal bar of the caliper is on the outside edge of the inner membrane in the nuchal region. The second caliper should be placed so that the horizontal bar is on the inside edge of the fetal skin. The placement of the caliper is very important for the predictability and accuracy of the nuchal translucency. Great care should be taken to achieve the correct image and caliper placement (Fig. 9–7).[17]

First trimester biochemistry includes the analysis of hCG and PAPP-A (pregnancy associated plasma protein A).[4] The higher the hCG and the lower the PAPP-A, the higher the trisomy 21 risk. The detection rate of trisomy 21, combining MA, NT, and biochemistry is 90%, with a 5% false-positive rate.[17]

Second trimester ultrasound markers can be divided into major and minor findings. Major findings warrant offering invasive testing alone; whereas, minor markers require two or more findings to warrant offering invasive testing. Major sonographic markers include: increased nuchal skin fold (>6 mm), cardiac defect, diaphragmatic

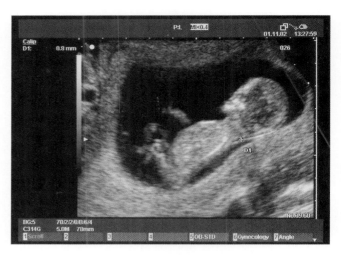

Figure 9–7. Nuchal translucency image.

hernia, omphalocele, facial cleft, and atresia (esophageal or duodenal).[4] Minor markers include abnormal ratio of observed/expected femur and humeral lengths, hypoplasia of midphalanx of 5th digit, echogenic foci of the heart, pyelectasis, echogenic bowel, sandal gap toe, choroid plexus cysts, small ears and, most recently, nasal bone.[4,17]

Second trimester biochemistry or maternal serum AFP 3 (MSAFP3), consists of hCG, AFP, and estriol. A risk of trisomy 21 is calculated based on these values. The risk increases with a higher hCG, lower AFP, and lower estriol. Combining the ultrasound with the biochemistry markers will detect approximately 60% of trisomy 21 fetuses.[17]

Trisomy 18. In this disorder there are three copies of chromosome 18. Ninety-five percent are an intrauterine demise or stillborn.[2] It is commonly, but not always, associated with multiple defects. Sonographically, these major findings may be seen with trisomy 18; growth restriction, increased nuchal translucency, NTD, strawberry-shaped head, choroid plexus cysts, ACC, enlarged cysterna magnum, decreased extremity lengths, cardiac defects, diaphragmatic hernia, esophageal atresia, omphalocele, and renal agenesis. Minor ultrasound findings include clenched hands, echogenic bowel, rockerbottom feet, micrognathia, and single umbilical artery.[4,17] MSAFP3 shows all three markers decreased.[2]

Trisomy 13. In this disorder there is an extra copy of chromosome 13. It may be associated with multiple abnormalities; however, the most common sonographic findings are holoprosencephaly (including the facial spectrums), cardiac defects, postaxial polydactyly, echogenic or polycystic kidneys, omphalocele, and microcephaly.[4,17]

Triploidy. In this disorder there are three complete sets of chromosomes. If paternally derived, the typical finding is a large placenta with multiple cystic areas (partial mole). If maternally derived, multiple findings include severe IUGR with an abnormally large head and small abdomen, hypertelorism, micrognathia, ventriculomegaly, cardiac defects, NTD, holoprosencephaly, Dandy–Walker malformation, cystic hygroma, renal anomalies, clubbed feet, single umbilical artery, and oligohydramnios.[4,17]

Sex Chromosome Abnormalities. The main sex chromosome abnormalities are Turner syndrome, 47, XXX; 47, XXY; and 47, XYY.[17] Sonographically, Turner syndrome findings are cystic hygroma, lymphangiectasia, cardiac defects, renal abnormalities, and hydrops.[4] The other sex chromosome abnormalities do not typically have prenatal sonographic findings.

Invasive Testing

Amniocentesis. This is an invasive procedure in which a needle is inserted into the amniotic cavity and amniotic fluid is withdrawn. The amniotic fluid is typically assessed for karyotype, levels of AF bilirubin associated with Rh disease, amniotic fluid AFP, acetylcholinesterase for spinal defects, infection, fetal lung maturity, and specific DNA studies. Our institution quotes a 1:300 risk of miscarriage with amniocentesis based on the national average. The standard amniocentesis is offered after 14 weeks.

Fluorescence in Situ Hybridization (FISH). This is currently an adjunct to amniocentesis. It is considered experimental at this time, so all findings from this test must be confirmed by amniocentesis results. "Tags" or markers that attach to certain chromosomes (currently testing 13, 18, 21, X and Y) fluorescence. This allows the geneticist to count the chromosomes for extra or deleted chromosomes. Results are available in 24–48 hours.[4]

Early amniocentesis is performed the same as amniocentesis but during the 11- to 14-week gestation. It has been associated with many problems. The loss rate is higher, 1:100, and is technically more difficult to perform because of the lack of fusion of the amnion and chorion. The unfused membranes are difficult to penetrate and often cause the need for multiple sticks, which in turn, increases the loss risk. Early amniocentesis has also been associated with talipes equinovarus.[17]

Chorionic Villi Sampling (CVS). This is a procedure in which a catheter is inserted into the placenta and chorionic villi is aspirated for karyotyping. This procedure may be done transabdominally or transvaginally, depending on placental location. CVS is performed between 10 and 12 weeks and results are obtained in 3–8 days versus 10–14 days for amniocentesis. CVS does not test for amniotic fluid AFP and cannot rule out spinal defects. Although the loss rate is 1:100. Although the loss rate is slightly higher than amniocentesis, the CVS loss rate is comparable to early amniocentesis. CVS performed <10 weeks has an association with severe limb defects and is not typically performed at that time.[2,17]

Percutaneous Umbilical Blood Sampling (PUBS). This is similar to an amniocentesis except that the needle is advanced through the amniotic fluid to the cord insertion site into the placenta. The needle is then inserted into the base of the umbilical cord. CDS can aid in locating the umbilical cord insertion into the placenta.[6] This procedure has a higher loss rate, 1–2%, and is technically more difficult to perform. It allows for rapid karyotyping (48–72 hours). PUBS most common application is with Rh isoimmunization testing. The fetal blood is tested for the amount of bilirubin pigment and allows the perinatalogist to perform a blood transfusion if necessary.[4]

REFERENCES

1. Ballinger PW. *Radiographic Positions and Radiologic Procedures.* 6th ed. St. Louis, MO: Mosby; 1986.
2. Callen PW. *Ultrasounography in Obstetrics and Gynecology.* 4th ed. Philadelphia: WB Saunders; 2000.
3. Fleischer AC, James, AE. *Diagnostic Sonography: Principles and Clinical Applications.* Philadelphia: WB Saunders; 1989.
4. Bianchi DW, Crombleholme TM, D'Alton, ME. *Fetalogy: Diagnosis and Management of the Fetal Patient.* New York: McGraw-Hill; 2000.
5. Berman MC, Cohen HL. *Obstetrics and Gynecology,* 2nd ed. Philadelphia: Lippincott; 1997.
6. Fleischer A, Emerson D. *Color Doppler Sonographics in Obstetrics and Gynecology.* New York: Churchill Livingston; 1993.
7. Odwin CS, Dubinsky T, Fleischer AC. *Appleton & Lange's Review for the Ultrasonography Examination.* 2nd ed. New York: Appleton & Lange; 1993.
8. AIUM guidelines for intracavitary probe cleaning.
9. Guy G, Peisner S, Timor-Tritsch I. Ultrasonographic evaluation of uteroplacental blood flow patterns of abnormally located and adherent placentas. *Am J Obstet Gynecol.* 1990; 163:723.
10. Timor-Tritsch. *Transvaginal Sonography.* 2nd ed. New York: Elesevier; 1987.
11. Fleischer A, Manning F, Jeanty P, Romero R. *Sonography in Obstetrics and Gynecology: Principles and Practice.* 5th ed. Stamford, CT: Appleton & Lange; 1996.
12. Lyons EA. *Abnormal Premenopausal Vaginal Bleeding: Gynecological Causes.* Lecture and paper, SDMS 17th annual conference, 2000.
13. Nyberg DA. *Menstrual Age with Average Gestational Sac Size, Crown-Rump Length, and hCG levels.* Proceeding from SRU, Oct. 1992.
14. Cunningham FG, MacDonald P, Gant N, Leveno L, Gilstrap L. *Williams Obstetrics.* 19th ed. Norwalk, CT: Appleton & Lange; 1993.
15. Tortora GJ, Anagnostakos NP. *Principles of Anatomy and Physiology.* 5th ed. New York: Harper and Row; 1987.
16. Watson W, Cheschier N, Katz V. The role of ultrasound in the evaluation of patients with elevated MSAFP: A review. *Obstet Gynecol.* 1991; 78:123.
17. Noble P. *Course booklet for certification in the 11–14 week scan.* London: Fetal Medicine Foundation; 1999.

Questions

GENERAL INSTRUCTIONS: For each question, select the best answer. Select only one answer for each question unless otherwise specified.

1. The sonographic finding in Fig. 9–8 is

   (A) normal fetal face
   (B) cleft lip
   (C) anencephaly
   (D) hypertelorism

2. Fig. 9–9 demonstrates

   (A) anencephaly
   (B) encephalocele
   (C) cystic hygroma
   (D) craniosynostosis

3. The sonographic finding in Fig. 9–10 include

   (A) equinovarus
   (B) normal foot posture
   (C) an association with spina bifida
   (D) A and C
   (E) all of the above

4. Fig. 9–11 demonstrates

   (A) cystic hygroma
   (B) spina bifida
   (C) encephalocele
   (D) nonimmune hydrops

5. Fig. 9–11 is a sonographic marker for

   (A) Turner syndrome
   (B) Down syndrome
   (C) trisomy 18
   (D) fetal infection

6. The most likely diagnosis for Fig. 9–12 includes

   (A) strawberry skull
   (B) Down syndrome
   (C) "lemon"-shaped skull
   (D) spina bifida
   (E) A and D
   (F) C and D

7. The sonographic finding in Fig. 9–13 is

   (A) fetal abdominal ascites
   (B) meconium peritonitis
   (C) posterior urethral valve obstruction
   (D) nonimmune hydrops

8. Fig. 9–14 demonstrates

   (A) nonimmune hydrops
   (B) cystic hygroma
   (C) increased nuchal sonolucency
   (D) normal findings

9. Fig. 9–15 is an example of

   (A) sonographic artifact
   (B) severe ventriculomegaly
   (C) holoprosencephaly
   (D) none of the above

10. Sonographic findings with Trisomy 18 include all of the following *except*

    (A) IUGR
    (B) clenched hands
    (C) holoprosencephaly
    (D) cystic hygroma

11. Paternally derived triploidy has the following sonographic markers

    (A) complete mole
    (B) severe asymmetrical IUGR
    (C) large placenta with multiple cystic areas
    (D) oligohydramnios
    (E) A and D
    (F) B and D

12. Maternally derived triploidy has the following sonographic markers

    (A) complete mole
    (B) severe assymetrical IUGR
    (C) large placenta with multiple cystic areas
    (D) oligohydramnios
    (E) A and D
    (F) B and D

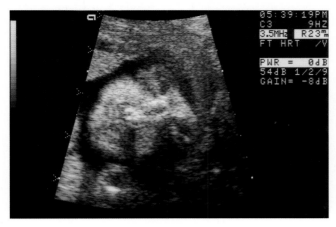

Figure 9–8

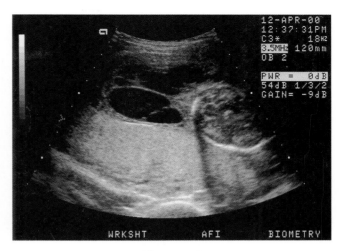

Figure 9–11

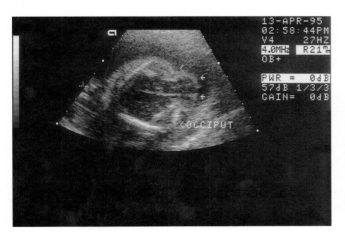

Figure 9–9

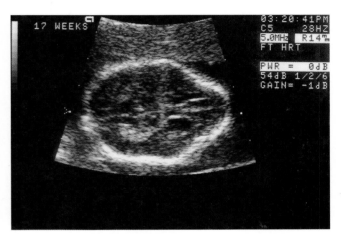

Figure 9–12

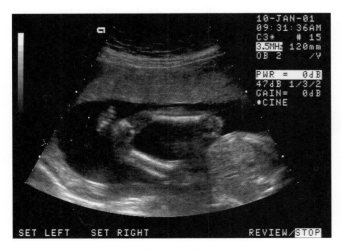

Figure 9–10

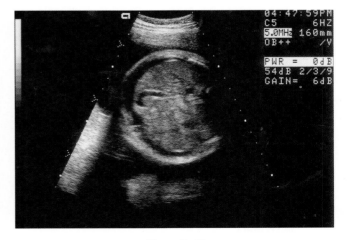

Figure 9–13

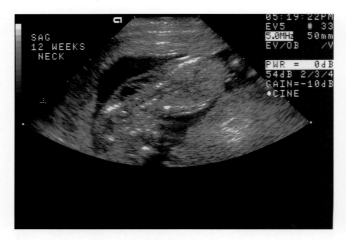

Figure 9–14

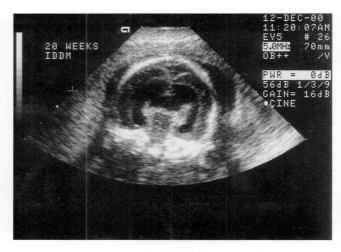

Figure 9–15

Questions 13 through 18: Match the procedures in Column A to the correct description in Column B:

COLUMN A

13. CVS
14. Early amniocentesis
15. FISH
16. Amniocentesis
17. PUBS

COLUMN B

(A) Amniotic fluid is withdrawn from the gestational sac. Performed after 14 weeks with a low loss rate.
(B) Performed 10–12 weeks. Cannot rule out spina bifida.
(C) Performed 11–14 weeks. Increased loss rate and associated with talipes equinovarus
(D) "Tags" chromosomes 13,18,21, X and Y for quick preliminary results
(E) Technically difficult procedure that tests fetal blood

18. The most common twin zygocity is

(A) conjoined twins
(B) monochorionic/diamniotic
(C) dichorionic/diamniotic
(D) monochorionic/monoamniotic

19. The "twin peak" sign is

(A) also known as the beta sign
(B) a triangular projection of chorion into the dividing membrane
(C) a sonographic predictor for dizygotic twins
(D) B and C
(E) all of the above

20. Which of the following statements about conjoined twins is *not* true?

(A) 60% are born alive
(B) 56% of conjoined twins are fused on the ventral wall
(C) polyhydramnios is commonly present
(D) the largest risk of fetal demise is because of cord entanglement

21. The uterine position in Fig. 9–16 would best be described as

(A) retroverted
(B) retroflexed
(C) anteverted
(D) anteflexed

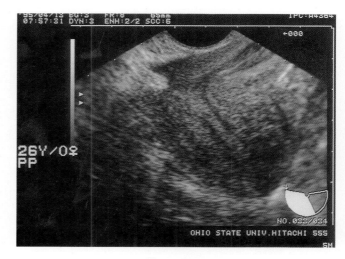

Figure 9–16

Questions 22 through 25. Match the terms in Column A with the definitions in Column B.

COLUMN A

22. rhizomelia
23. mesomelia
24. micromelia
25. acromelia

COLUMN B

(A) shortening of the hand and foot bones
(B) shortening of the proximal limb
(C) shortening of the middle portion of the limb (forearms and lower leg bones)
(D) shortening of all portions of a limb

26. The most common short limb syndrome is

(A) achondrogenesis
(B) thanatophoric dysplasia
(C) osteogenesis imperfecta
(D) jeune thoracic dystrophy

27. What sonographic findings would be identified in a fetus with heterozygous achondroplasia?

(A) hydrocephaly
(B) frontal bossing
(C) "bell shaped" thorax
(D) "trident hand"
(E) A and C
(F) B and D
(G) all of the above

28. Fig. 9–17 is a transverse plane of view through the fundus of the uterus. The two echogenic lines represent

(A) the interstitial portion of the Fallopian tube
(B) two endometrial linings of a duplicated uterus

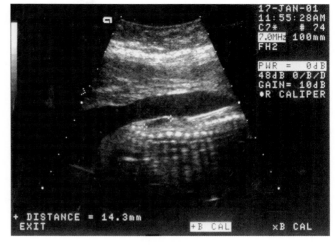

Figure 9–18

(C) single endometrial lining
(D) arcuate vessels

29. Fig. 9–18 demonstrates what fetal anomaly?

(A) sacral agenesis
(B) meningocele
(C) myelomeningocele
(D) sacrococcygeal teratoma

30. Fig. 9–19 is a sonographic example of

(A) placenta accreta
(B) placental abruption
(C) marginal placenta previa
(D) placenta vasa previa

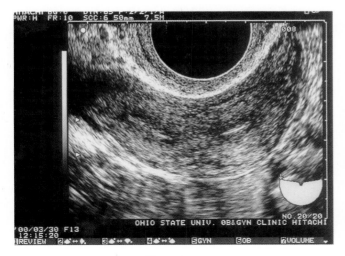

Figure 9–17

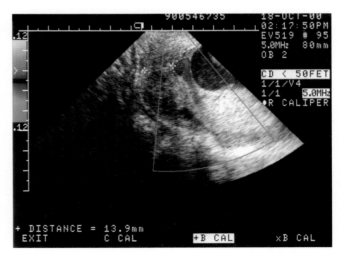

Figure 9–19

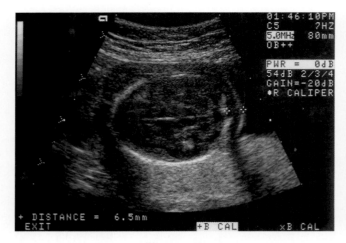

Figure 9–20

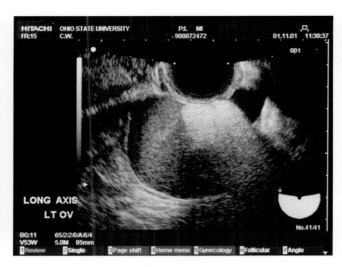

Figure 9–22

31. Fig. 9–20 is a transverse plane of view in the fetal nuchal region. The sonographic finding is

(A) cystic hygroma
(B) increased nuchal skin fold
(C) fetal edema
(D) none of the above

32. Fig. 9–21 is a longitudinal plane of view through the midline of the uterus. The echogenic foci represents

(A) endometrial polyp
(B) IUD
(C) endometrial hyperplasia
(D) endometrial cancer

33. Fig. 9–22 demonstrates what ovarian abnormality?

(A) hemorrhagic corpus luteal cyst
(B) tubo-ovarian abscess

(C) benign cystic teratoma
(D) ovarian torsion

34. Fig. 9–23 demonstrates what ovarian abnormality?

(A) ectopic pregnancy
(B) corpus luteal cyst
(C) polycystic ovarian disease
(D) ovarian neoplasm

35. Fig. 9–24 is an image of a fetus at 8 weeks gestational age. The cystic structure within the fetus is

(A) rhombencephalon
(B) cystic hygroma
(C) increased nuchal translucency
(D) all of the above

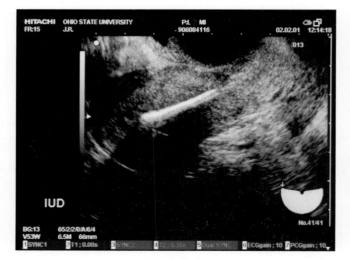

Figure 9–21

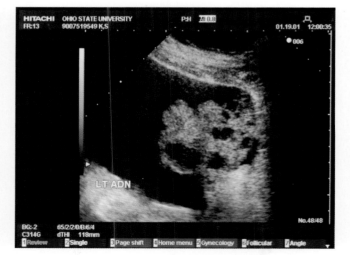

Figure 9–23

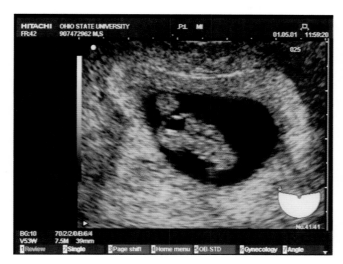

Figure 9–24

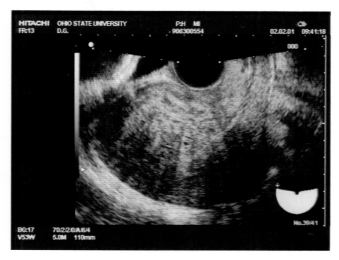

Figure 9–26

36. The cardiac abnormality demonstrated in Fig. 9–25 is a

   (A) hypoplastic left heart
   (B) hypoplastic right heart
   (C) Ebstein's anomaly
   (D) left ventricular aneurysm

37. Fig. 9–26 is a longitudinal uterine image. The patient is G4P4 with complaints of menorrhagia and uterine tenderness. The most likely diagnosis would be

   (A) normal uterus
   (B) intramuscular fibroid
   (C) endometrial hyperplasia
   (D) adenomyosis

38. The differential diagnosis for the ovarian image in Fig. 9–27 is

   (A) mucinous cystadenoma
   (B) dermoid
   (C) hemorrhagic corpus luteal cyst
   (D) tuboovarian abscess
   (E) A and C
   (F) all of the above

39. The abnormality in Fig. 9–28 is

   (A) abdominal ascites
   (B) hydrops fetalis
   (C) anasarca
   (D) prune-belly syndrome

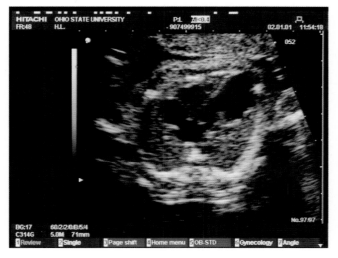

Figure 9–25

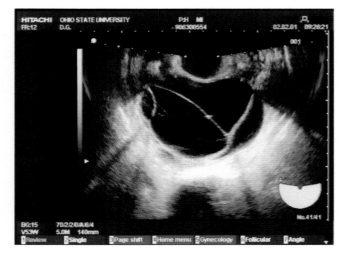

Figure 9–27

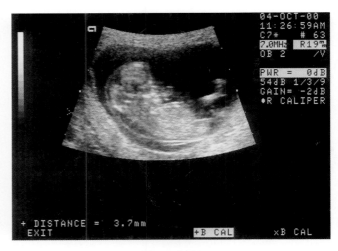

Figure 9–28

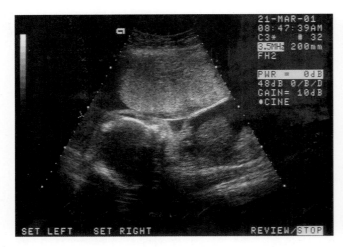

Figure 9–30

40. Fig. 9–29 demonstrates what sonographic abnormality

    (A) hemivertebrae
    (B) rachischisis
    (C) sacral agenesis
    (D) none of the above

41. The sonographic image in Fig. 9–30 is consistent with what findings

    (A) 60% positive predictive value for trisomy 21
    (B) increased nuchal translucency
    (C) 80% positive predictive value for trisomy 21
    (D) A and B
    (E) A and C

42. The findings in Fig. 9–30 are associated with

    (A) cardiac defects
    (B) skeletal dysplasia

    (C) Down syndrome
    (D) A and C
    (E) all of the above

43. Fig. 9–31 demonstrates what fetal bladder abnormality?

    (A) ureterocele
    (B) posterior urethral valve obstruction
    (C) cloacal exstrophy
    (D) normal full bladder

44. Fig. 9–32 is a sonographic image of what cardiac defect?

    (A) ventricular septal defect
    (B) overriding aorta
    (C) tetralogy of Fallot
    (D) A and C
    (E) all of the above

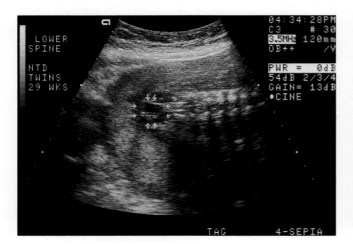

Figure 9–29

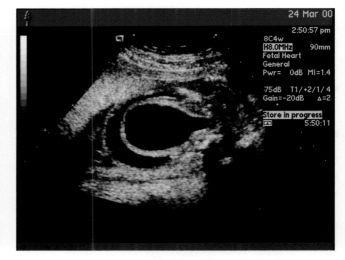

Figure 9–31

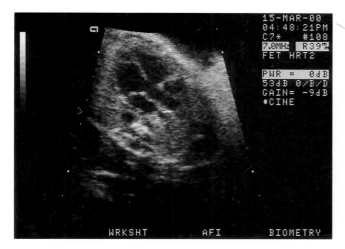

Figure 9–32

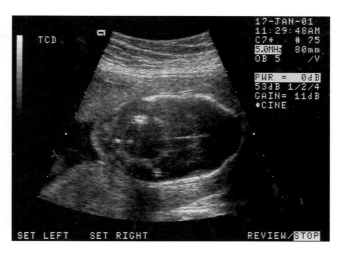

Figure 9–34

45. Fig. 9–33 is a sonographic image of

(A) normal fetal thorax and heart
(B) congenital cystic adenomatoid malformation of the lung, type III
(C) pulmonary sequestration
(D) congenital left diaphragmatic hernia

46. Fig. 9–34 demonstrates what sonographic finding?

(A) Dandy–Walker malformation
(B) normal cerebellum
(C) arachnoid cyst
(D) Arnold–Chiari malformation

47. Fig. 9–35 is a sonographic example of

(A) gastroschisis
(B) omphalocele
(C) normal first trimester physiological umbilical cord herniation
(D) duodenal atresia

48. Fig. 9–36 demonstrates what sonographic finding?

(A) normal kidneys
(B) dysplastic kidneys
(C) infantile polycystic kidney disease
(D) enlarged kidneys

49. Fig. 9–37 demonstrates what fetal abnormality?

(A) micrognathia
(B) macroglossia
(C) frontal bossing
(D) normal fetal profile

50. What is the most likely diagnosis if Figs. 9–35, –36, and –37 are found in the same fetus?

(A) trisomy 18
(B) trisomy 13
(C) Beckwith–Wiedemann syndrome
(D) Finnish nephrosis

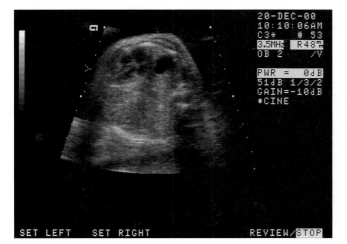

Figure 9–33

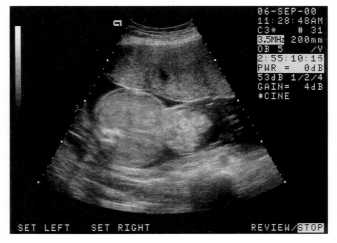

Figure 9–35

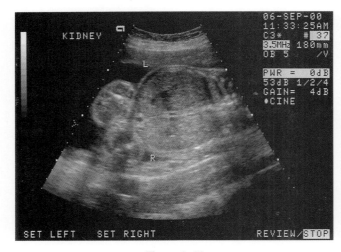

Figure 9–36

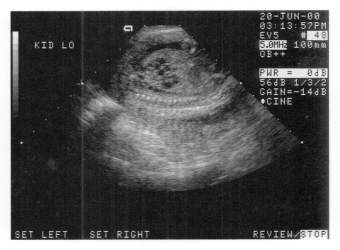

Figure 9–38

51. Fig. 9–38 is a sonographic example of

(A) multicystic dysplastic kidney disease
(B) infantile polycystic kidney disease
(C) UPJ obstruction
(D) A and B
(E) A and C

52. What is the most common congenital facial anomaly?

(A) proboscis
(B) hypotelorism
(C) isolated cleft lip/palate
(D) low set ears

53. 3-D surface rendering is used to

(A) obtain volume measurements
(B) obtain technically difficult images
(C) image fetal spine
(D) image fetal face

54. The earliest age at which a gestational sac may be visualized by transvaginal sonography is

(A) 4 weeks
(B) 6 weeks
(C) 8 weeks
(D) 10 weeks

55. The optimal time for imaging cardiac structures is

(A) 14–18 weeks
(B) 18–24 weeks
(C) 24–28 weeks
(D) 28–32 weeks

56. 3D volumetric reconstructions are used to show all of the following except

(A) fetal face
(B) fetal limbs
(C) organs
(D) digits

57. By 12 weeks gestational age, the sonographer can identify what abnormalities?

(A) conjoined twins
(B) anencephaly
(C) duodenal atresia
(D) A and B
(E) all of the above

58. An unexplained increased MSAFP3 can cause what third trimester complications?

(A) premature rupture of membranes
(B) placental abruption
(C) preterm labor
(D) A and B
(E) all of the above

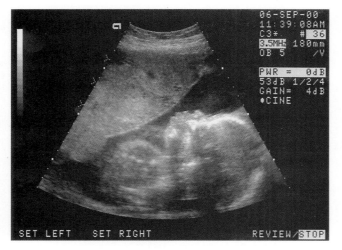

Figure 9–37

59. A markedly increased MSAFP would be associated with

(A) amniotic sheets
(B) cloacal exstrophy
(C) congenital diaphragmatic hernia
(D) Smith–Lemli–Opitz syndrome

60. If the triple marker screen shows a decreased AFP, a decreased estriol, and a decreased hCG, the fetus is at risk for

(A) trisomy 21
(B) Smith–Lemli–Opitz syndrome
(C) trisomy 18
(D) trisomy 13

61. Which is not a direct sonographic finding of posterior urethral valve obstruction?

(A) "keyhole" bladder
(B) anhydramnios
(C) hydronephrosis
(D) pulmonary hypoplasia

62. What cranial finding can cause congestive heart failure and hydrops?

(A) vein of Galen aneurysm
(B) periventricular leukomalacia
(C) Dandy–Walker malformation
(D) iniencephaly

63. What is the name of the cardiac abnormality with one outflow tract giving rise to both the pulmonary and aortic branches and associated with a ventricular septal defect?

(A) truncus arteriosis
(B) double outlet right ventricle
(C) tetralogy of Fallot
(D) transposition of the great vessels

64. The cardiac abnormality consisting of a VSD, an overriding aorta, a small or atretic pulmonary trunk, and right ventricular hypertrophy describes

(A) double outlet right ventricle
(B) hypoplastic left heart syndrome
(C) transposition of the great vessels
(D) tetralogy of Fallot

65. Which of the following describes congenital cystic adenomatoid malformation?

(A) may spontaneously regress
(B) poor survival rate
(C) divided into two subsets, solid and cystic
(D) none of the above

66. Which of the following statements regarding congenital diaphragmatic hernia are true?

(A) more commonly right sided than left sided
(B) carries a poor prognosis

(C) may be associated with chromosomal abnormalities
(D) all of the above
(E) A and C
(F) B and C

67. Esophageal atresia is

(A) diagnosed by ultrasound 90% of the time
(B) associated with oligohydramnios
(C) is a component of the VACTERL complex
(D) can be diagnosed in the first trimester

68. An increased MSAFP is associated with all of the following *except*

(A) trisomy 21
(B) neural tube defect
(C) maternal preeclampsia
(D) gastroschisis

69. The uterine ligament responsible for uterine orientation is

(A) transversal ligament
(B) broad ligament
(C) uterosacral ligament
(D) round ligament

70. Which two ligaments are not true ligaments?

(A) uterosacral and broad ligament
(B) suspensory and broad ligament
(C) uterosacral and round ligament
(D) cardinal and suspensory ligament

71. The most commonly visualized pelvic muscle often mistaken for an ovary is

(A) piriformis muscle
(B) levator ani muscle
(C) coccygeus muscle
(D) iliopsoas muscle

72. The most dependent portion of the peritoneum is called

(A) pouch of Douglas
(B) vesicouterine pouch
(C) retropubic space
(D) none of the above

73. The three peritoneal spaces in the pelvic cavity are: (PCDS—posterior cul-de-sac, ACDS—anterior cul-de-sac)

(A) PCDS, ACDS, and vesicouterine
(B) PCDS, pouch of Douglas, ACDS
(C) PCDS, ACDS, and prevesical
(D) PCDS, ACDS, and interstitial

74. AIUM guidelines for cleaning a transvaginal probe are

(A) clean with soap and water
(B) immerse in disinfecting solution
(C) clean with moist towelette
(D) A and B
(E) A and C
(F) all of the above

75. An invasive mole is also known as

(A) hydatidiform mole
(B) triploid molar pregnancy
(C) endometrioma
(D) chorioadenoma destruens

76. Which of the following is true regarding a hydatidiform mole and coexistent fetus?

(A) consistent with maternally derived trisomy 13
(B) consistent with paternally derived trisomy 13
(C) can progress to choriocarcinoma
(D) A and C
(E) B and C

77. In what portion of the fallopian tube does fertilization usually occur?

(A) interstitial
(B) isthmus
(C) ampulla
(D) infundibulum

78. The sonographic appearance of an ectopic gestation includes all of the following *except*

(A) increased endometrial lining
(B) irregular adnexal mass or ovarian mass with ring of color flow Doppler
(C) fluid in the cul-de-sac
(D) absence of sac within the uterus

79. Rank the following ectopic pregnancy implantation sites from the most common to the least common.

(1) ampullary
(2) ovarian
(3) isthmus
(4) cervical
(A) 1,2,3,4
(B) 4,2,3,1
(C) 1,3,2,4
(D) 3,1,4,2

80. Fetal demise is the detection of an absent heart beat after 16 weeks.

(A) True
(B) False

81. Which of the following is not true of dysgerminoma?

(A) It is a solid malignant germ cell tumor of the ovary.

(B) It is a counterpart of seminoma of the testis.
(C) It is a relatively uncommon tumor accounting for about 2% of all ovarian cancers.
(D) 90% are unilateral.
(E) It is a solid benign tumor.

82. Which of the following is not true of dermoid tumors?

(A) may cast an acoustic shadow
(B) encountered more in women over 40 years
(C) also called benign cystic teratoma
(D) most common benign germ cell tumor in the female
(E) unilateral in about 80% of cases
(F) The tumor has elements such as hair, tooth, bone, endoderm, ectoderm, mesoderm, and thyroid glandular tissue.
(G) may be echogenic because of fat content and sonographically produce "tip of the iceberg" effect

83. The normal adult ovaries measure

(A) $3 \times 2 \times 2$ cm
(B) $2 \times 2 \times 4$ cm
(C) $3 \times 3 \times 2$ cm
(D) $3 \times 2 \times 1$ cm

84. The first definitive sonographic sign of an intrauterine pregnancy is

(A) gestational sac
(B) yolk sac
(C) fetal pole
(D) double decidua sign

85. What percentage of cardiac defects can be detected from the four-chamber view?

(A) 50
(B) 65
(C) 80
(D) 85

86. What percentage of cardiac defects can be detected from the four-chamber view and outflow tracts?

(A) 50
(B) 65
(C) 80
(D) 85

87. A simple cyst may exhibit all of the following *except*

(A) anechoic interior
(B) posterior enhancement
(C) thin walled
(D) distal acoustic shadows

88. The cyst commonly associated with hydatidiform mole is

(A) follicular
(B) paraovarian

(C) theca lutein
(D) corpus luteal

89. The most accurate method for establishing EDC is

(A) first trimester ultrasound
(B) second trimester ultrasound
(C) LMP
(D) Nagele's rule

90. The accuracy of gestational age in the first trimester is

(A) 3–5 days
(B) ± 10 days
(C) ± 14 days
(D) ± 21 days

91. The accuracy of gestational age from 13–20 weeks is

(A) 3–5 days
(B) ± 10 days
(C) ± 14 days
(D) ± 21 days

92. The accuracy of gestational age from 20–30 weeks is

(A) 3–5 days
(B) ± 10 days
(C) ± 14 days
(D) ± 21 days

93. The accuracy of gestational age in the third trimester is

(A) 3–4 days
(B) ± 10 days
(C) ± 14 days
(D) ± 21 days

94. The normal rise of hCG in a viable pregnancy should

(A) double in 24 hours
(B) double in 48 hours
(C) double in 72 hours
(D) double in 1 week

95. Conditions associated with a poorly rising or decreasing hCG include all of the following except

(A) twin pregnancy
(B) ectopic pregnancy
(C) anembryonic demise
(D) incorrect dates

96. An ovarian mass identified on sonogram is complex, predominately hypoechoic with septations. The patient complains of severe pain during menses. The most likely diagnosis is

(A) corpus luteal cyst
(B) granulosa cell
(C) thecoma
(D) endometrioma

97. If a patient's LMP is 6/15/2001, by Nagele's rule, the EDC should be

(A) 2/22/2002
(B) 2/30/2002
(C) 3/22/2002
(D) 3/30/2002

98. The differential diagnosis for a thick-walled ovarian cyst with blood flow surrounding the periphery is

(A) follicular cyst
(B) oocyte
(C) corpus luteal cyst
(D) all of the above

99. The following are true characteristics of a mucinous cystadenoma *except*

(A) the largest abdominal tumor
(B) thick septations
(C) benign
(D) may have debris layering within cyst

100. Another name for polycystic ovarian syndrome is

(A) Stein–Leventhal syndrome
(B) Seroli–Leydig cell
(C) Brenner's tumor
(D) Chocolate cyst

101. The etiology of hydatidiform mole is

(A) trophoblastic changes in a blighted ovum
(B) hydatid swelling of the retained placenta in a missed abortion
(C) fertilization of an ovum without any active chromosomal material
(D) A and B

102. All of the following characteristics of color Doppler energy are false *except*

(A) CDE can determine the direction of blood flow
(B) CDE can determine the velocity of blood flow
(C) the different colors represent flow toward or away from the transducer
(D) CDE is based on the amplitude of the soundwave

103. The term trophoblast denotes

(A) the extra-embryonic peripheral cells of the blastocyst
(B) a rigid state of the flagellate microorganism
(C) the gestation sac
(D) the characteristics of a disease

104. The mean diameter of a dominant follicular cyst at the time of ovulation is

(A) 10 mm
(B) 15 mm
(C) 20 mm
(D) 25 mm

105. The most common uterine tumor is

(A) leiomyoma
(B) adenomyosis
(C) leiomyosarcoma
(D) endometrial hyperplasia

106. A complex adnexal mass is identified in a patient with tenderness and elevated temperature. The most likely diagnosis is

(A) tubo-ovarian abscess
(B) corpus luteal cyst
(C) serous cystadenoma
(D) Brenner's tumor

107. The endometrium can appear echogenic (1) in the secretory phase, (2) in patients with pelvic inflammatory disease, (3) after dilation and curettage, (4) in patients with endometritis, (5) after removal of an intrauterine contraceptive device

(A) 1 and 3 only
(B) 4 only
(C) 1,2,3, and 5
(D) all of the above

108. The endometrial lining in postmenopausal women *not* on hormone replacement therapy should be less than

(A) 10 mm
(B) 8 mm
(C) 6 mm
(D) 2 mm

109. The endometrial lining in postmenopausal women on hormone replacement therapy should be less than

(A) 10 mm
(B) 8 mm
(C) 6 mm
(D) 2 mm

110. The best time to visualize a polyp is during what stage of the menstrual cycle?

(A) menstruation phase
(B) follicular phase
(C) proliferative phase
(D) secretory phase

111. The date of the last menstrual period indicates

(A) the date when fertilization occurred
(B) the date when menstrual bleeding ended
(C) the date when ovulation occurred
(D) the date when menstrual bleeding began

112. Which of the following diagnoses does not mimic the sonographic characteristic of hydatidiform mole?

(A) endometriosis
(B) hematoma
(C) uterine leiomyoma
(D) anembryonic demise

113. What percentage of patients diagnosed with hydatidiform mole will usually follow a benign course?

(A) 20%
(B) 10%
(C) 50%
(D) 80%

114. The uterus can be divided into regions. List them from inferior to superior.

(A) cervix, isthmus, corpus, fundus
(B) serosal, myometrial, endometrial
(C) fundus, isthmus, corpus, cervix
(D) cervix, corpus, isthmus, fundus

115. The uterine layers are

(A) cervix, isthmus, corpus, fundus
(B) serosal, myometrial, endometrial
(C) fundus, isthmus, corpus, cervix
(D) peritoneum, serosal, and myometrial

Match the following:

116. prepubertal uterus

117. adult nulliparous woman

118. adult multiparous woman

(A) corpus twice the length of cervix
(B) corpus and cervix equal in length
(C) corpus half the length of the cervix

119. The normal size of a multiparous uterus is

(A) 5 × 4 × 3 cm
(B) 7 × 5 × 4 cm
(C) 10 × 6 × 5 cm
(D) 6 × 4 × 3 cm

120. In postmenopausal women, the uterus will not atrophy as much in multigravid women as nulligravid women

(A) true
(B) false

121. Congenital abnormalities of the uterus result from improper fusion of the

(A) mesonephric ducts
(B) paramesonephric ducts
(C) Gartner's duct
(D) Wolffian ducts

122. During the early proliferative phase, the endometrium appears

    (A) thin, echogenic line, 4–8 mm
    (B) thin, hypoechoic line, 4–8 mm
    (C) thickened and hypoechoic medially with an echogenic basal layer
    (D) thickened and echogenic throughout

123. During the periovulatory phase, the endometrium appears

    (A) thin, echogenic line, 4–8 mm
    (B) thin, hypoechoic line, 4–8 mm
    (C) thickened and hypoechoic medially with an echogenic basal layer
    (D) thickened and echogenic throughout

124. During the secretory phase, the endometrium appears

    (A) thin, echogenic line, 4–8 mm
    (B) thin, hypoechoic line, 4–8 mm
    (C) thickened and hypoechoic medially with an echogenic basal layer
    (D) thickened and echogenic throughout

125. Women with endometriosis may have

    (A) dyspareunia
    (B) metromennorhagia
    (C) dysmenorrhea
    (D) all of the above

126. Endometriosis is

    (A) ectopic endometrial tissue
    (B) benign invasion of endometrial tissue into the myometrium
    (C) endomyosarcoma with chocolate tissue
    (D) inflammation of the endometrium

127. The most common location for a dermoid cyst is

    (A) posterior cul-de-sac
    (B) right adnexa
    (C) left adnexa
    (D) superior to the uterine fundus

128. Macrosomia is

    (A) fetus weighing >4,000 g
    (B) fetus >90% for gestational age
    (C) fetus with a shoulder thickness >10mm
    (D) LGA fetus

129. LGA is a term referring to

    (A) a fetus weighing >4,000 g
    (B) fetus >90%
    (C) a clinical assessment of an increased fundal height
    (D) polyhydramnios

130. A macrosomic fetus is at risk for

    (A) shoulder dystocia
    (B) increased perinatal morality
    (C) prolonged labor
    (D) all of the above

131. Macrosomia may be associated with

    (A) IDDM
    (B) GDM
    (C) HTN
    (D) Rh isoimmunization
    (E) A and B

132. An increased fundal height may be caused by

    (A) macrosomic fetus
    (B) polyhydramnios
    (C) twins
    (D) all of the above

133. IUGR is

    (A) EFW <10%
    (B) decreased AFV
    (C) increased umbilical cord dopplers
    (D) abnormal growth ratios

134. An increased HC/AC is a suggestion of

    (A) late onset of IUGR
    (B) brain sparing effort
    (C) placental insufficiency
    (D) all of the above

135. Causes of IUGR include

    (A) fetal infection
    (B) chromosomal abnormality
    (C) placental insufficiency
    (D) all of the above

136. IUGR can be caused by all *except*

    (A) diabetes
    (B) maternal hypertension
    (C) chromosomal abnormalities
    (D) spina bifida

137. Doppler testing of vessels that may aid in the diagnosis of IUGR are

    (A) umbilical cord
    (B) straight sinus
    (C) celiac axis
    (D) jugular vein
    (E) A and C
    (F) all of the above

138. Doppler sampling of the maternal uterine artery <26 weeks shows a diastolic notch. This notch is indicative of

(A) IUGR
(B) maternal HTN
(C) normal
(D) A and B

Questions 139–156. Match the structures in Fig. 9–39 with the list of terms in Column B.

COLUMN A   COLUMN B

139. _____   (A) uterine cervix
140. _____   (B) fimbria
141. _____   (C) uterine fundus
142. _____   (D) right lateral vaginal fornix
143. _____   (E) left lateral vaginal fornix
144. _____   (F) interstitial portion of the fallopian tube
145. _____   (G) vagina
146. _____   (H) isthmus uteri
147. _____   (I) external os of the cervix
148. _____   (J) ovary
149. _____   (K) ovarian ligament
150. _____   (L) uterine corpus
151. _____   (M) fallopian tube
152. _____   (N) infundibulum
153. _____   (O) internal os of cervix
154. _____   (P) isthmus tubae
155. _____   (Q) ampulla
156. _____   (R) endocervical canal

Rank the following in order of their neurologic development, earliest to latest.

COLUMN A   COLUMN B

157. _____   (A) body motion
158. _____   (B) fetal tone
159. _____   (C) breathing
160. _____   (D) fetal heart rate acceleration

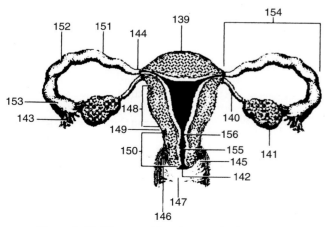

Figure 9–39. Diagram of female reproductive organs.

161. Placental grading is an important component of BPP.

(A) true
(B) false

162. The components of BPP are

(A) fetal breathing, Doppler, NST, gross body movement, and AFV
(B) placental grade, NST, gross body movement, and AFV
(C) NST, Doppler, gross body movement, AFV, and fetal flexion/extension
(D) AFV, gross body movement, fetal flexion/extension, fetal breathing, and NST

163. Fetal breathing must last how long to be counted in the BPP?

(A) 20 seconds
(B) 30 seconds
(C) 1 minute
(D) 2 minutes

164. In a normal fetus, if the middle cerebral artery is sampled, one would expect to find

(A) an increased S/D ratio
(B) a decreased S/D ratio
(C) retrograde flow
(D) absent flow

165. The only purpose of amniotic fluid is to allow the fetal lungs to develop and to allow for fetal movement.

(A) true
(B) false

166. The amniotic fluid production is performed primarily by the fetus after what gestational age in pregnancy?

(A) 8 weeks
(B) 10 weeks
(C) 16 weeks
(D) 25 weeks

167. When does the amniotic fluid volume peak in pregnancy?

(A) 20 weeks
(B) 24 weeks
(C) 33 weeks
(D) 38 weeks

168. An exact volume of amniotic fluid can be determined by measuring the four quadrants of the maternal abdomen.

(A) true
(B) false

169. In the single pocket method, when is the diagnosis of oligohydramnios made?

(A) a single pocket of 2 mm cannot be measured
(B) a single pocket of 1 cm cannot be measured
(C) a single pocket of 2 cm cannot be measured
(D) a single pocket of 4 cm cannot be measured

170. In the amniotic fluid index method of measuring four quadrants, the diagnosis of oligohydramnios is made

(A) when the amniotic volume is less than 300 mL
(B) when the amniotic volume is less than 200 mL
(C) when the amniotic fluid index is less than the 10th percentile
(D) when the amniotic fluid index is less than the 2.5th percentile

171. The nonspecific signs of fetal death are which of the following: (1) echoes in the amniotic fluid, (2) the absence of the falx cerebri, (3) a decrease in the biparietal diameter (BPD) measurements, (4) a double contour of the fetal head (sonographic halo sign).

(A) 3 and 4
(B) 4 only
(C) all of the above
(D) none of the above

172. How long after fetal death can scalp edema be seen?

(A) 2–3 days
(B) 5–10 days
(C) 10–20 days
(D) 20–30 days

173. The term decidua denotes the transformed endometrium of pregnancy. The different regions of the decidua are divided into

(A) two regions called decidua basalis and chorionic villi
(B) one region called decidual reaction
(C) three regions called decidua basalis, decidua parietalis, and decidua capsularis
(D) three regions called endoderm, mesoderm, and ectoderm

174. Cystic masses in the vagina could include all of the following except

(A) Gartner's duct cyst
(B) Nabothian cyst
(C) hematocolpos
(D) vaginal agenesis

175. The functions of the secondary yolk sac are which of the following

(A) nutrients for the embryo
(B) hematopoiesis
(C) contributing to the development of the reproductive system
(D) all of the above

176. In about 2% of adults, the yolk sac persists as a diverticulum of the ileum. This is known as

(A) Michael's diverticulum
(B) Meckel's diverticulum
(C) Turner's diverticulum
(D) Smith's diverticulum

177. The location of the yolk sac is

(A) inside the umbilical cord
(B) inside the amniotic cavity
(C) in the chorionic cavity between the amnion and the chorion
(D) outside the chorionic cavity between the chorion and the endometrial wall

178. On transvaginal sonography, when is the yolk sac visible?

(A) 4 weeks
(B) 5.5 weeks
(C) 6 weeks
(D) 7 weeks

Questions 179–182: Arrange in sequence in Column A the embryologic stages following fertilization listed in Column B.

COLUMN A	COLUMN B
179. _____	(A) morula
180. _____	(B) cleavage
181. _____	(C) zygote
182. _____	(D) blastocyst

183. All of the following are complications of oligohydramnios *except*

(A) clubfeet
(B) hand posturing
(C) urethral stenosis
(D) pulmonary hypoplasia

184. The umbilical cord S/D ratio normally

(A) increases throughout the pregnancy
(B) decreases throughout the pregnancy
(C) remains the same throughout pregnancy
(D) is controlled by the fetal cerebellum

185. Placental insufficiency is indirectly monitored by

(A) an increasing umbilical cord S/D ratio
(B) a decreasing umbilical cord S/D ratio
(C) Doppler of placental intervillous spaces
(D) Doppler of maternal arcuate arteries

186. The terminology vasa previa describes

(A) placenta near the internal os
(B) placenta touching the internal os
(C) placenta crossing the internal os
(D) placenta vessels crossing the internal os

187. The primary cause of third trimester bleeding is

(A) placenta previa
(B) preterm labor
(C) cervical bleeding
(D) abruption

188. An ectopic pregnancy will usually be on the same side as the corpus luteal cyst.

(A) true
(B) false

189. Which of the following statements *is not true* concerning the yolk sac?

(A) The yolk sac should be included in measurements of CRL.
(B) The yolk sac shrinks as pregnancy advances.
(C) The yolk sac plays a role in blood development and transfer of nutrients.
(D) The yolk sac is attached to the body stalk and is located between the amnion and chorion.

190. The vessels of the normal umbilical cord consist of

(A) two arteries, one vein
(B) two veins, one artery
(C) one artery, one iliac vein, and the iliac artery
(D) one artery, one vein

191. The term "neural tube defect" refers to

(A) spinal defect
(B) open tube defect
(C) anencephaly
(D) cephalocele
(E) all of the above

192. Myelomeningocele refers to the herniation of

(A) meninges
(B) meninges and neural tissue
(C) meninges at the lumbar level
(D) meninges and neural tissue below L5

193. The most accurate way to diagnosis a spinal defect is

(A) in the longitudinal plane of the spine
(B) in the coronal plane of the spine
(C) in the sagittal plane of the spine
(D) the "lemon and banana" signs of the fetal cranium

194. The "lemon" sign of the fetal cranium in diagnosing spina bifida refers to

(A) the narrowing of the vertebral process at the area of the defect
(B) the overall appearance of the fetal spine in the presence of a defect
(C) the appearance of the cerebellum in the presence of a spinal defect
(D) the appearance of the fetal skull in the presence of a spinal defect

195. The "banana" sign of the fetal cranium in diagnosing spina bifida refers to

(A) the narrowing of the vertebral process at the area of the defect
(B) the overall appearance of the fetal spine in the presence of a defect
(C) the appearance of the cerebellum in the presence of a spinal defect
(D) the appearance of the fetal skull in the presence of a spinal defect

196. The "banana" sign is present with spinal defects

(A) 50% of the time
(B) 75% of the time
(C) 85% of the time
(D) 99% of the time

197. Which of the following is true about the "lemon" sign and neural tube defects?

(A) The "lemon" sign is not as accurate as the "banana" sign.
(B) The "lemon" sign may be present in the normal fetus in the third trimester.
(C) The "lemon" sign can be artificially produced at the level of the ventricles.
(D) The "lemon" sign is a predictor for spina bifida.
(E) all of the above

198. The diagnosis of placenta previa is most accurately made

(A) transabdominally with a full maternal bladder
(B) transabdominally with an empty maternal bladder
(C) transrectally
(D) transvaginally

199. The definition of "low lying placenta" in the third trimester is

(A) placental edge >3 cm from internal os
(B) placental edge <2 cm from internal os
(C) placental edge <3 cm from internal os
(D) placental edge in lower uterine segment

200. The rotation of the heart in the fetal chest should be

(A) 45° with apex pointed to the right
(B) 45° with apex pointed to the left

(C) 60° with apex pointed to the right

(D) the heart should not be rotated in fetal chest

201. The fetal heart is horizontal in the chest because of

(A) large spleen
(B) flat diaphragm
(C) large liver
(D) large thorax

202. The majority of cephaloceles are parietal.

(A) true
(B) false

203. What percentage of cephaloceles are occipital?

(A) 50
(B) 60
(C) 75
(D) 99

204. The diagnosis of ventriculomegaly may be made when the ventricle measures

(A) greater than 10 mm in the posterior horn
(B) greater than 15 mm in the posterior horn
(C) when the third ventricle may be visualized
(D) when the choroid does not touch the medial wall of the lateral ventricle

205. The most common type of obstruction causing ventriculomegaly is

(A) Dandy–Walker malformation
(B) communicating hydrocephalus
(C) aqueductal stenosis
(D) congenital hydrocephaly

206. Congenital hydrocephalus is

(A) genetically linked affecting both male and females
(B) able to be detected in both male and females by DNA testing
(C) expressed in males only
(D) A and C
(E) B and C
(F) all of the above

207. Mild ventriculomegaly is described as

(A) posterior horn measuring >15 mm
(B) posterior horn measuring >5 mm
(C) choroid is separated from the medial wall of the ventricle >5 mm
(D) visualization of the third ventricle

208. Mild ventriculomegaly may be associated with

(A) agenesis of the corpus callosum
(B) trisomy 21
(C) normal
(D) all of the above

209. Other findings associated with a spinal defect are

(A) clubfeet
(B) ventriculomegaly
(C) single umbilical artery
(D) A and B
(E) all of the above

210. The severity of impairment in a child with hydrocephaly may be predicted by the severity of their fetal hydrocephaly.

(A) true
(B) false

211. In the case of spina bifida, the fetal sonogram is able to accurately predict the child's impairment.

(A) true
(B) false

212. The cysterna magna is considered increased when

(A) the measurement is >5 mm
(B) the cerebellum may be seen outlined by fluid
(C) the cerebellar vermis is splayed
(D) the measurement is >10 mm

213. Findings on ultrasound include an increased cysterna magna, agenesis of the cerebellar vermis with communication to the fourth ventricle and ventriculomegaly. The most likely diagnosis would be

(A) Dandy–Walker malformation
(B) Dandy–Walker malformation variant
(C) arachnoid cyst
(D) communicating hydrocephaly

214. Findings on ultrasound include hydrocephaly, an enlarged cysterna magna, and an intact cerebellar vermis elevated by a cyst in the posterior fossa. The most likely diagnosis would be

(A) Dandy–Walker malformation
(B) Dandy–Walker malformation variant
(C) arachnoid cyst
(D) communicating hydrocephaly

215. Other findings associated with Dandy–Walker malformation include

(A) holoprosencephaly
(B) facial clefting
(C) cardiac defects
(D) all of the above

216. Associated findings occur with Dandy–Walker malformation

(A) rarely
(B) 10–25% of the time
(C) 50–70% of the time
(D) always

217. Complications associated with Dandy–Walker malformation include

(A) chromosomal abnormalities
(B) subnormal intelligence after birth
(C) increased neonatal death
(D) A and B only
(E) all of the above

218. The most common cause of hypotelorism is

(A) Dandy–Walker malformation
(B) Arnold–Chiari type II
(C) Goldenhar syndrome
(D) holoprosencephaly

219. Cyclopia, hypotelorism, proboscis, cebocephaly, and cleft lip/palate are

(A) abnormal intracranial findings
(B) abnormal facial findings
(C) associated with hydrocephaly
(D) all of the above

220. The most common chromosomal abnormality associated with holoprosencephaly is

(A) trisomy 21
(B) trisomy 18
(C) trisomy 13
(D) Turner syndrome

221. The most common cause of hypertelorism is

(A) anterior cephalocele
(B) holoprosencephaly
(C) hydranencephaly
(D) craniosynostosis

222. Teratomas in pregnancy are located in

(A) the sacrococcygeal region
(B) intracranial
(C) cervical
(D) all of the above

223. Maternal Grave's disease and Hashimoto thyroiditis may cause what finding in the fetus?

(A) fetal ascites
(B) fetal goiter
(C) oligohydramnios
(D) there is no effect on the fetus

224. The most common cause of macroglossia is

(A) micrognathia
(B) trisomy 18
(C) Beckwith–Wiedemann syndrome
(D) obstruction of the fetal airway

225. Macroglossia may cause polyhydramnios.

(A) true
(B) false

226. Macroglossia is present how often in Beckwith–Wiedemann syndrome?

(A) 15% of the time
(B) 25% of the time
(C) 50% of the time
(D) 97% of the time

227. The most common type of isolated cleft lip/palate is

(A) unilateral cleft lip
(B) unilateral cleft lip and palate
(C) bilateral cleft lip
(D) bilateral cleft lip and palate

228. The most common associated anatomic abnormalities of cleft lip are

(A) genitourinary
(B) gastrointestinal
(C) cardiac
(D) there are no associated abnormalities

229. A medial cleft lip has a strong association with what abnormality?

(A) hydrocephaly
(B) Turner syndrome
(C) holoprosencephaly
(D) hydranencephaly

230. Micrognathia may be associated with which of the following syndromes?

(A) Pierre Robin syndrome
(B) trisomy 18
(C) campomelic dysplasia
(D) all of the above

231. In the presence of micrognathia, polyhydramnios is present how often?

(A) 15% of the time
(B) 25% of the time
(C) 50% of the time
(D) 70% of the time

232. If a fetal nose is not visualized, one should look for

(A) cebocephaly
(B) cyclopia
(C) proboscis
(D) all of the above

233. All cases of alobar holoprosencephaly will demonstrate facial anomalies.

(A) true
(B) false

234. Agenesis of the corpus callosum cannot be diagnosed by ultrasound before

(A) 10 weeks
(B) 14 weeks
(C) 18 weeks
(D) 28 weeks

235. In 90% of cases with agenesis of the corpus callosum, what other sonographic finding is present?

(A) polyhydramnios
(B) omphalocele
(C) polydactyly
(D) teardrop ventricles

236. Absent cerebral cortex is found in what cranial abnormality?

(A) holoprosencephaly
(B) hydrocephaly
(C) hydranencephaly
(D) agenesis of the corpus callosum

237. Microcephaly is defined as

(A) HC <–2SD of mean
(B) HC <–3SD of mean
(C) 2 week lag in HC
(D) A and B
(E) all of the above

238. A fetus presents with an anechoic midline lesion in the brain, fetal hydrops, and congestive heart failure. The most likely diagnosis for the lesion is

(A) agenesis of the corpus callosum
(B) dilation of the third ventricle
(C) arachnoid cyst
(D) AV malformation

239. Choroid plexus cysts, when found with other associated abnormalities, have a strong association with

(A) Noonan's syndrome
(B) trisomy 18
(C) trisomy 13
(D) X-linked hydrocephaly

240. The risk of aneuploidy is increased in cases where the choroid plexus cysts are multiple, bilateral, and/or large.

(A) true
(B) false

241. The nuchal skin fold in the second trimester should be measured at what level?

(A) the level of the BPD
(B) the same image as the OOD
(C) the level of the TCD in the axial plane
(D) the level of the ventricles

242. When measuring the lateral ventricle, the anterior portion of the ventricle should always be measured.

(A) true
(B) false

243. The TCD may be measured in either the axial or coronal view.

(A) true
(B) false

244. If the cephalic index is >85, it is an indication for what condition?

(A) brachycephaly
(B) dolicocephaly
(C) microcephaly
(D) macrocephaly

245. If the cephalic index is <75, it is an indication for what condition?

(A) brachycephaly
(B) dolicocephaly
(C) microcephaly
(D) macrocephaly

246. Dolicocephaly will demonstrate

(A) a large BPD and shorter OFD for gestational age
(B) a small BPD and longer OFD for gestational age
(C) an HC <3SD of mean for GA
(D) an HC >2SD of mean for GA

247. Brachycephaly will demonstrate

(A) a large BPD and shorter OFD for gestational age
(B) a small BPD and longer OFD for gestational age
(C) an HC <3SD of mean for GA
(D) an HC >2SD of mean for GA

248. Dolicocephaly is often associated with what conditions?

(A) breech fetus
(B) oligohydramnios
(C) LGA fetus
(D) A and B
(E) A and C
(F) all of the above

249. Brachycephaly is associated with what conditions?

(A) trisomy 21
(B) normal variant
(C) myelomeningocele
(D) A and B
(E) A and C
(F) all of the above

Questions 250–252: The ratio of head circumference to body circumference normally changes as pregnancy progresses. Match the weeks of gestation in Column A with the head and body ratio in Column B.

COLUMN A   COLUMN B

250. 12–24 _____   (A) abdomen larger than
251. 32–36 _____   head
252. 36–40 _____   (B) head and body are equal
                        (C) head larger than
                            abdomen

253. If performing a BPD measurement and the midline echo is continuous and unbroken, this would indicate that the scanning plane is

   (A) normal
   (B) too high
   (C) through the fetal neck
   (D) correct

254. The fluid within a cystic hygroma is

   (A) serous fluid
   (B) amniotic fluid
   (C) ascites
   (D) lymphatic fluid

255. Cystic hygromas are caused by

   (A) obstruction of the lymph system at the level of the jugular veins
   (B) obstruction of the lymph system at the level of the iliac veins
   (C) obstruction of the venous system at the level of the jugular veins
   (D) carotid artery obstruction

256. Cystic hygromas differ from cervical masses because

   (A) a cystic hygroma is hypoechoic with internal septations
   (B) a cystic hygroma is a cystic mass separated by a midline septum
   (C) a cystic hygroma appears as two completely separate sacs
   (D) cystic hygromas may not be differentiated from other cervical masses

257. Eighty percent of cystic hygromas occur in what region?

   (A) the axilla
   (B) the mediastinum
   (C) the cervical region
   (D) none of the above

258. Cystic hygromas are associated with

   (A) Potter's syndrome
   (B) Beckwith–Weidemann syndrome
   (C) elevated levels of AFP
   (D) Turner syndrome
   (E) C and D
   (F) B and D
   (G) all of the above

259. Cystic hygromas are always associated with a chromosomal abnormality.

   (A) true
   (B) false

Questions 260–268: Match the structures in Fig. 9–40 with the list of terms in Column B.

COLUMN A   COLUMN B

260. _____   (A) isthmus uteri
261. _____   (B) chorion frondosum
262. _____   (C) decidua parietalis (vera)
263. _____   (D) decidua capsularis
264. _____   (E) cervix
265. _____   (F) amniotic cavity
266. _____   (G) decidua basalis
267. _____   (H) unoccupied lumen between the
268. _____   decidual layers
                 (I) mucous plug

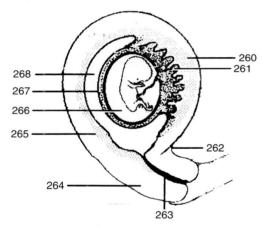

Figure 9–40. Diagram of early pregnancy.

Questions 269–278: Match the structures in Fig. 9–41 with the list of terms in Column B.

COLUMN A   COLUMN B

269. _____   (A) placenta
270. _____   (B) inferior vena cava
271. _____   (C) portal sinus
272. _____   (D) umbilical vein
273. _____   (E) aorta
274. _____   (F) left hepatic vein
275. _____   (G) right hepatic vein

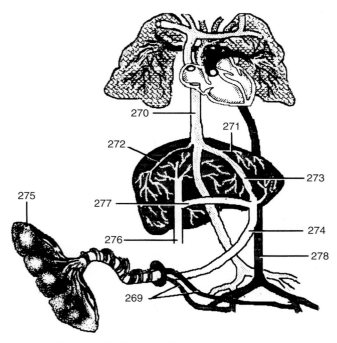

270

271

272

273

275

277

276

274

278

269

Figure 9–41. Diagram of fetal circulatory system.

276. _____
277. _____
278. _____

(H) ductus venosus
(I) portal vein
(J) umbilical arteries

279. The fetal shunt between the left and right atria is

(A) ductus venosum
(B) ductus arteriosis
(C) foramen ovale
(D) pulmonary ductus

280. The fetal shunt connecting the transverse aortic trunk and the main pulmonary trunk is

(A) ductus venosum
(B) ductus arteriosis
(C) foramen ovale
(D) pulmonary ductus

281. Hydranencephaly is thought to result from

(A) chromosomal abnormalities
(B) a vascular accident of the jugular veins
(C) a vascular accident of the internal carotid arteries
(D) none of the above

282. The differential diagnosis for hydranencephaly may be

(A) semilobar holoprosencephaly
(B) alobar holoprosencephaly
(C) severe hydrocephaly

(D) A and C
(E) B and C
(F) all of the above

283. Hemivertebrae may be identified on sonogram

(A) as a narrowing of the individual vertebrae in the coronal plane of view
(B) as a narrowing of the individual vertebrae in the sagittal plane of view
(C) as a narrowing of the individual vertebrae in the axial plane of view
(D) all of the above

284. The downward displacement of the cerebellar vermis, the fourth ventricle, and medulla oblongata through the foramen magna is termed

(A) "lemon" sign
(B) Dandy–Walker malformation
(C) arachnoid cyst
(D) Arnold–Chiari malformation

285. Large encephaloceles may be associated with

(A) hydranencephaly
(B) hypotelorism
(C) microcephaly
(D) all of the above

286. A patient presents for an anatomy scan. The fetal head shows a single ventricle, single choroid, two cerebellar hemispheres, and fused thalamus. The abnormality is most likely

(A) semilobar holoprosencephaly
(B) alobar holoprosencephaly
(C) hydranencephaly
(D) hydrocephaly

287. A patient presents for an anatomy scan. The fetal head shows a single large cystic cavity with a rim of cerebral cortex. A fused thalamus is also identified. The most likely diagnosis is

(A) alobar holoprosencephaly
(B) semilobar holoprosencephaly
(C) hydranencephaly
(D) hydrocephaly

288. A patient presents for an anatomy scan. The fetal head shows the cranium filled with anechoic fluid, and no cerebral cortex is identified. The brain stem is identified. The most likely diagnosis is

(A) semilobar holoprosencephaly
(B) alobar holoprosencephaly
(C) hydranencephaly
(D) hydrocephaly

289. How early can anencephaly be detected on ultrasound?

(A) 10 weeks
(B) 14 weeks
(C) 16 weeks
(D) 20 weeks

290. Acrania is described as

(A) abnormal brain tissue with absent calvarium
(B) the first stage of anencephaly before prolonged exposure to amniotic fluid
(C) normal brain tissue with abnormal facies
(D) A and B
(E) all of the above

For questions 291–295, which numbers in the term "parity G7P3214" correspond to the following?

291. The number of living children _____

292. The number of preterm infants _____

293. The number of pregnancies total _____

294. The number of abortions _____

295. The number of full term pregnancies _____

296. A patient has had six pregnancies: three full term, one preterm delivery of twins, one spontaneous abortion, one fetal loss at 22 wks. This would be listed as

(A) G6P3215
(B) G6P3124
(C) G7P5411
(D) G7P2135

297. Spina bifida occulta may be diagnosed on ultrasound by the lemon and banana sign.

(A) true
(B) false

298. An increased MSAFP3 may be associated with

(A) anencephaly
(B) spina bifida occulta
(C) skin covered spina bifida
(D) A and C

299. A gestational sac is identified within the uterus. The CRL measures 3 mm. What is the approximate age of the embryo?

(A) <4 weeks
(B) 5 weeks
(C) 6 weeks
(D) 8 weeks

300. CRL is the appropriate dating measurement until what gestational age?

(A) 8 weeks
(B) 10 weeks

(C) 13 weeks
(D) 15 weeks

301. In a fetus without abnormalities in the second and early third trimester, the best parameters to use for EFW are

(A) CRL
(B) FL/AC
(C) BPD, HC, AC, FL
(D) BPD/FL

302. When measuring the femur, the calipers should be placed at

(A) the outermost edge of the bone
(B) include epiphyseal plate
(C) the diaphysis of the shaft of the femur
(D) the edges of the entire bone, including the head and neck of the femur

303. Polyhydramnios is most commonly associated with what finding?

(A) insulin-dependent diabetes mellitus
(B) duodenal atresia
(C) idiopathic
(D) micrognathia

304. Polyhydramnios may be associated with which of the following?

(A) osteogenesis imperfecta
(B) cleft lip
(C) maternal diabetes
(D) twin–twin transfusion
(E) A and B
(F) all of the above

305. At what gestational age should the amnion and chorion be fused?

(A) 8 weeks
(B) 10 weeks
(C) 16 weeks
(D) 20 weeks

306. The placenta is responsible for all of the following *except*

(A) exchange of nutrients
(B) hematopoiesis
(C) oxygen exchange
(D) barrier to some medications

307. Placental abruption is primarily diagnosed by ultrasound.

(A) true
(B) false

308. Placental abruption is

(A) the premature separation of placenta before 20 weeks
(B) the premature separation of placenta after 20 weeks
(C) the premature separation of placenta at any gestational age
(D) the same as a retrochorionic clot

309. Sonographic signs of placental abruption include

(A) retroplacental veins >2 cm
(B) echogenic periplacental hematomas
(C) hypoechoic periplacental hematomas
(D) A and C
(E) all of the above

310. Placental abruption is associated with

(A) drug abuse
(B) fibroids
(C) maternal vascular disease
(D) A and C
(E) all of the above

311. Risks for placenta accreta include

(A) maternal hypertension
(B) isoimmunization
(C) previous cesarean section
(D) infertility

312. "Swiss cheese" appearance retroplacentally is associated with what abnormality?

(A) placenta previa
(B) placental abruption
(C) placenta accreta
(D) placental chorioangioma

313. Placenta percreta refers to

(A) invasion of placental tissue through the uterus into bladder
(B) invasion of placental tissue into myometrium
(C) invasion of placenta up to the serosal layer
(D) placental attachment to the myometrium without invasion

314. Name the placental vascular malformation that appears as a hypoechoic mass near the cord insertion.

(A) fetal vascular anastomosis
(B) placental lake
(C) placental aneurysm
(D) chorioangioma

315. The fetal umbilical vein carries deoxygenated blood.

(A) true
(B) false

316. The vessels in the umbilical cord are protected by.

(A) Wharten's jelly
(B) amniotic fluid
(C) serosal fluid
(D) myometrium

317. A cyst in the umbilical cord is called?

(A) allantoic cyst
(B) yolk sac cyst
(C) Meckel's cyst
(D) ectodermal cyst

318. The umbilical cord inserting in the membranes and coursing to the placenta is termed

(A) normal cord insertion
(B) succenturiate cord insertion
(C) eccentric cord insertion
(D) velamentous cord insertion

319. The umbilical cord inserting into the edge of the placenta is called?

(A) normal cord insertion
(B) marginal cord insertion
(C) eccentric cord insertion
(D) velamentous cord insertion

320. The most common cardiac defect is

(A) hypoplastic left heart syndrome
(B) atrial/ventricular septal defect
(C) tetralogy of Fallot
(D) none of the above

321. The left side of the heart is responsible for perfusing

(A) cranial aspects of the fetus
(B) systemic aspects of the fetus
(C) placenta
(D) none of the above

322. The right side of the heart is responsible for perfusing

(A) cranial aspects of the fetus
(B) systemic aspects of the fetus
(C) placenta
(D) none of the above

323. The heart should occupy what percentage of the fetal thorax?

(A) 25%
(B) 30%
(C) 60%
(D) 75%

324. If the axis of the heart is pointed to the right, the sonographer should look for

(A) an interrupted IVC
(B) other heart abnormalities
(C) abdominal organ orientation
(D) all of the above

325. The most common cardiac defect associated with trisomy 21 is

(A) atrial/ventricular septal defect
(B) hypoplastic left heart syndrome
(C) AV canal defect
(D) transposition of the great vessels

326. From the four-chamber view, the transducer is tilted toward the fetal left shoulder. This will obtain what cardiac view?

(A) five-chamber view
(B) short axis view
(C) long axis view
(D) aortic arch

327. What anatomy should be evaluated in the four-chamber view?

(A) junction of the AV valves with the atrial and ventricular septum intact
(B) equally sized ventricular chambers
(C) contractility of the heart
(D) A and B
(E) all of the above

328. All ventricular septal defects can be detected in the four-chamber view.

(A) true
(B) false

329. Hypoplastic left heart syndrome is easily apparent at 18 weeks.

(A) true
(B) false

330. Which of the following heart abnormalities are difficult or unable to be identified on fetal echocardiography?

(A) coarctation of the aorta
(B) Ebstein's anomaly
(C) double outlet right ventricle
(D) none of the above

331. The majority of congenital diaphragmatic hernias are

(A) left sided
(B) right sided
(C) bilateral
(D) midline

332. On sonogram, the fetal heart is deviated to the right with apex pointed to the left. The sonographer should consider what possible abnormalities?

(A) congenital diaphragmatic hernia
(B) congenital cystic adenomatoid malformation
(C) teratoma
(D) A and B
(E) all of the above

333. In the identification of congenital diaphragmatic hernia, the sonographer should also assess

(A) the location of the fetal liver
(B) fetal kidneys
(C) fetal bladder
(D) all of the above

334. The significant perinatal mortality of fetuses with congenital diaphragmatic hernia is caused by

(A) chromosomal abnormalities
(B) oligohydramnios
(C) associated cardiac defects
(D) pulmonary hypoplasia

335. Congenital diaphragmatic hernia has a poorer prognosis if

(A) it is a left-sided defect
(B) the stomach is located on the left and anterior
(C) if bowel is identified in the chest
(D) if liver is identified in the chest

336. The most frequently identified chest mass is

(A) right-sided diaphragmatic hernia
(B) left-sided diaphragmatic hernia
(C) congenital cystic adenomatoid malformation
(D) pulmonary sequestration

337. Congenital cystic adenomatoid malformation is divided into three types. Type I is

(A) microcystic
(B) medium-sized cysts
(C) macrocystic
(D) mixed-size cysts

338. Type II congenital cystic adenomatoid malformation is

(A) microcystic
(B) medium-sized cysts
(C) macrocystic
(D) mixed-size cysts

339. Type III congenital cystic adenomatoid malformation is

(A) microcystic
(B) medium-sized cysts
(C) macrocystic
(D) mixed-size cysts

340. Pulmonary sequestrations may be found in the fetal abdomen.

(A) true
(B) false

341. The majority of pulmonary sequestrations are found

(A) inferior to the diaphragm
(B) in the lower left lung base
(C) in the lower right lung base
(D) in the upper left pulmonary lobe

342. Esophageal atresia is routinely diagnosed by ultrasound because of an absent or small stomach bubble.

(A) true
(B) false

343. What percentage of esophageal atresias have a tracheoesophageal fistula?

(A) 25%
(B) 50%
(C) 75%
(D) 90%

344. Eighty percent of fetuses with esophageal atresia have what associated condition in the third trimester?

(A) intrauterine growth retardation
(B) macrosomia
(C) polyhydramnios
(D) decreased abdominal circumference

345. Esophageal atresia has a strong association with what chromosomal abnormality?

(A) trisomy 21
(B) trisomy 18
(C) trisomy 13
(D) translocation

346. The "double bubble" sign refers to

(A) two-vessel umbilical cord
(B) duodenal atresia
(C) ureterocele
(D) hypotelorism

347. Fifty percent of fetuses with duodenal atresia also have which of the following abnormalities?

(A) spinal defects
(B) cardiac defects
(C) macrosomia
(D) A and B
(E) all of the above

348. Duodenal atresia has a strong association with what chromosomal abnormality?

(A) trisomy 21
(B) trisomy 18

(C) trisomy 13
(D) unbalanced translocation

349. The physiological herniation of bowel into the umbilical cord is complete by what gestational age?

(A) 8 weeks
(B) 9 weeks
(C) 11 weeks
(D) 13 weeks

350. Gastroschisis has more associated defects and chromosomal abnormalities than omphaloceles.

(A) true
(B) false

351. MSAFP is elevated more with omphaloceles than with gastroschisis.

(A) true
(B) false

352. Which of the following about gastroschisis is true?

(A) more common with advanced maternal age
(B) often associated with other abnormalities
(C) has a very good prognosis with 80–90% survival rate
(D) has an autosomal recessive inheritance

353. Sonographic signs of bowel perforation include all of the following *except*

(A) thickened bowel loops
(B) abdominal calcifications
(C) meconium cysts
(D) oligohydramnios

354. Intrauterine complications of gastroschisis include all of the following *except*

(A) IUGR
(B) edematous bowel wall
(C) intestinal obstruction
(D) dilated fetal stomach
(E) none of the above

355. Gastroschisis is a break in the abdominal wall at the level of the umbilical cord. Where does this typically occur?

(A) right side of the umbilical cord
(B) left side of the umbilical cord
(C) at the umbilical cord insertion with cord attaching to the gastroschisis
(D) medially and inferior to the umbilical cord

356. Physiological herniation <12 weeks may also include bowel and liver.

(A) true
(B) false

357. Large omphaloceles have a worse prognosis than small omphaloceles.

(A) true
(B) false

358. A midline defect in the anterior abdominal wall with herniation of abdominal contents into the base of the umbilical cord is called

(A) gastroschisis
(B) omphalocele
(C) cloacal exstrophy
(D) pentalogy of Cantrell

359. Omphaloceles are associated with all of the following except

(A) advanced maternal age
(B) chromosomal abnormalities
(C) maternal smoking
(D) cardiac abnormalities

360. The terminology for a midline defect of the chest with the heart herniated to the outside of the chest is

(A) rachyschisis
(B) ectopia cordis
(C) cloacal extrophy
(D) limb–body wall complex

361. An omphalocele and ectopia cordis are identified on sonogram. What condition should be included in the differential?

(A) pentalogy of Cantrell
(B) trisomy 18
(C) Beckwith-Wiedemann syndrome
(D) A and B
(E) all of the above

362. Beckwith–Wiedemann syndrome is a group of which of the following disorders?

(A) omphalocele
(B) shortening of limbs unilaterally
(C) macroglossia
(D) polyhydramnios
(E) A and C
(F) all of the above

363. If the bladder is herniated through the ventral wall and a spinal defect is identified, what condition should be considered?

(A) bladder exstrophy
(B) cloacal exstrophy
(C) pentalogy of Cantrell
(D) limb–body wall complex

364. A condition in which no umbilical cord may be identified, along with ventral wall defects, and scoliosis is most likely

(A) cloacal exstrophy
(B) amniotic synechia
(C) limb-body wall complex
(D) complete ventral wall defect

365. Amniotic bands differ from amniotic sheets because

(A) amniotic bands are attached to the uterus at both ends
(B) amniotic sheets often cause disruption in the first trimester
(C) amniotic bands can cause amputation or limb deformities
(D) there is no difference between amniotic bands and sheets

366. Rh isoimmunization results from which of the following combinations?

(A) mother Rh– and father Rh–
(B) mother Rh+ and father Rh–
(C) mother Rh+ and fetus Rh–
(D) mother Rh– and fetus Rh+

367. The Rh immune globulin is effective against the anti-D antibody; therefore, immune hydrops no longer exists in anyone able to receive rhogam.

(A) true
(B) false

368. The hemolytic process of destruction of fetal red blood cells by the maternal antibodies is termed

(A) hypercoagulation
(B) erythroblastosis fetalis
(C) thrombocytopenia
(D) nonimmune hydrops

369. Immune and nonimmune hydrops may be differentiated by their sonographic appearances.

(A) true
(B) false

370. Signs of congestive heart failure in the fetus are

(A) serous effusions
(B) enlarged fetal liver
(C) fetal ascites
(D) all of the above

371. How is the diagnosis of fetal hydrops made by sonography?

(A) two fetal sites of fluid accumulation
(B) fetal ascites and one site of accumulated fluid
(C) one site of fluid accumulation and oligohydramnios
(D) A and B
(E) A and C
(F) all of the above

372. In cases of fetal distress in diabetic mothers, the fetal heart may

(A) have thickened ventricular walls
(B) have decreased contractility
(C) have increased cardiac output
(D) A and B
(E) all of the above

373. The main causes for nonimmune hydrops include

(A) fetal abnormalities
(B) parvovirus
(C) anti-Kell antibodies
(D) A and B
(E) A and C
(F) all of the above

374. A quick way to check for organ orientation is to assure that the heart and stomach are on the same side of the fetus.

(A) true
(B) false

375. Partial situs inversus is associated with more significant abnormalities than complete situs inversus.

(A) true
(B) false

376. In cases of partial situs inversus, the sonographer should consider

(A) cardiac defects
(B) polysplenia
(C) asplenia
(D) interrupted IVC
(E) B and C
(F) all of the above

377. On a sonogram, the fetus has unilateral hydronephrosis, nonvisualized ureters, normal bladder, and normal AFV. This most likely represents

(A) unilateral UVJ obstruction
(B) unilateral UPJ obstruction
(C) PUV
(D) none of the above

378. A UVJ obstruction is associated with what other findings?

(A) ureterocele
(B) unilateral hydronephrosis
(C) pelvic kidney
(D) A and C

379. A hydroureter will appear differently than dilated bowel on sonogram because

(A) ureters are predominately lateral structures in the fetal abdomen
(B) ureters will appear predominately anechoic

(C) bowel will appear predominately anechoic
(D) dilated large bowel mainly found in the midline of the fetus

380. The trigone refers to is

(A) the point at which the ureter enters the kidney
(B) the region where the urethra exits the body
(C) the region of the bladder containing the orifices of the ureters and urethra
(D) the region of the bladder containing the orifice of the urethra

381. Posterior urethral valve obstruction is found only in males.

(A) true
(B) false

382. Complete posterior urethral valve obstruction has all of the following ultrasound characteristics *except*

(A) hydramnios
(B) hydronephrosis
(C) hydroureter
(D) "keyhole" bladder
(E) lax abdominal wall

383. Potter's facies refers to

(A) flattened facial features caused by the lack of amniotic fluid in PUV syndrome
(B) abnormal development of the abdominal muscles caused by the overdistended bladder in PUV syndrome
(C) the appearance of the fetal bladder in PUV syndrome
(D) other name for urinary ascites

384. The primary cause of death in posterior urethral valve outlet syndrome is

(A) renal failure
(B) sepsis
(C) cardiac overload
(D) pulmonary hypoplasia

385. Sonographic features of renal agenesis include all *except*

(A) inability to demonstrate blood flow in renal arteries
(B) elongated adrenal glands in the renal fossa
(C) low amniotic fluid
(D) unable to visualize fetal bladder

386. How often does the fetal bladder fill?

(A) every 10 minutes
(B) every 30 minutes
(C) every hour
(D) every 2 hours

387. During organogenesis, the kidneys migrate from

(A) the thorax, moving inferiorly to the renal fossa
(B) the anterior midgut to the posterior renal fossa
(C) the pelvis, moving superiorly to the renal fossa
(D) the kidneys do not migrate

388. In the early stages of organogenesis, how many kidneys form?

(A) 2
(B) 3
(C) 4
(D) 6

389. What other organ system has a strong correlation with renal abnormalities?

(A) cardiac
(B) uterine
(C) ovarian
(D) muscular

390. All of the following about multicystic dysplastic kidney disease is true *except*

(A) caused by a first trimester obstruction
(B) caused by a second trimester obstruction
(C) multiple, varying sized cysts in the parenchyma
(D) echogenic parenchyma

391. In the case of unilateral, multicystic, dysplastic kidney disease, the contralateral kidney will often

(A) enlarge
(B) become obstructed
(C) have decreased function
(D) remain the same

392. If one parent has autosomal dominant polycystic kidney disease, the risk for the fetus having the same disease is

(A) 25%
(B) 50%
(C) 75%
(D) 100%

393. A 26-week fetus presents with large echogenic kidneys that contain some small cysts. The amniotic fluid volume is normal. Differential diagnosis includes

(A) autosomal recessive polycystic kidney disease
(B) autosomal dominant polycystic kidney disease
(C) Meckel's syndrome
(D) A and C
(E) all of the above

394. The kidneys should occupy how much of the fetal abdomen in an axial plane of view?

(A) ¼
(B) ⅓
(C) ½
(D) ⅔

395. Anechoic cysts that surround the periphery of the kidney in a "string of pearls" appearance most likely represent

(A) multicystic dysplastic kidney disease
(B) autosomal dominant polycystic kidney disease
(C) normal renal pyramids
(D) early-stage obstructed renal pyramids

396. The fetus begins to produce urine at what gestational age?

(A) 10 weeks
(B) 13 weeks
(C) 17 weeks
(D) 20 weeks

397. It is possible for the fetal bladder to rupture in utero.

(A) true
(B) false

398. In the second trimester, the normal renal pelvis size is

(A) less than 20 mm
(B) less than 15 mm
(C) less than 8 mm
(D) less than 6 mm

Match the renal grading system in Column A to the description in Column B.

COLUMN A	COLUMN B
399. Grade 0 _____	(A) renal pelvis and calices dilated
400. Grade I _____	(B) no dilation
401. Grade II _____	(C) renal pelvic dilation with or without infundibula visible
402. Grade III _____	(D) renal pelvis and calices dilated with parenchymal thinning
403. Grade IV _____	(E) renal pelvic dilation with calices visible

404. A rare renal tumor that is large, solid, and highly vascular is

(A) neuroblastoma
(B) renal teratoma
(C) congenital mesoblastic nephroma
(D) none of the above

405. A malignant adrenal gland tumor that appears as an echogenic, heterogenous mass is

 (A) neuroblastoma
 (B) teratoma
 (C) Wilm's tumor
 (D) none of the above

406. A congenital mesoblastic nephroma is also known as a

 (A) neuroblastoma
 (B) teratoma
 (C) Wilm's tumor
 (D) William's tumor

Questions 407–410: Match the type of developmental anomalies of the uterus shown in Fig. 9–42 with the terms in Column B.

COLUMN A   COLUMN B

407. _____   (A) bicornuate
408. _____   (B) septate
409. _____   (C) unicornis
410. _____   (D) didelphic

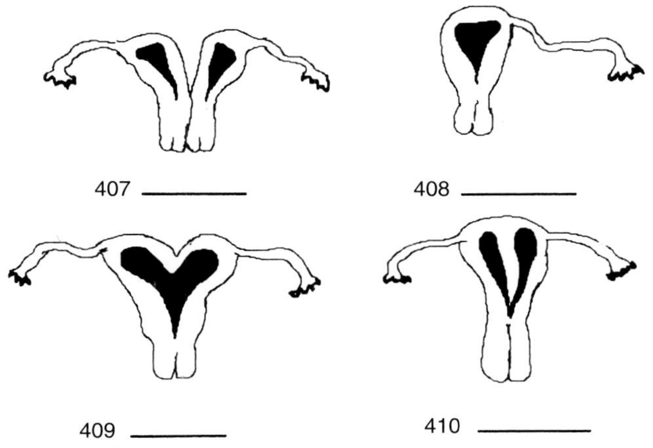

407 _____   408 _____

409 _____   410 _____

Figure 9–42. Diagram showing developmental anomalies of the uterus.

411. The degree to which the head shapes may affect biparietal diameter (BPD) can be estimated by which of the following formulas?

 (A) HC = BPD2 + OFD
 (B) V = 7(pi/6(bpd/OFD)
 (C) CI = BPD/OFD × 100
 (D) BPD = BPD × OFD/1.256

412. The most common cause for ovarian torsion is

 (A) ovarian tumors
 (B) hyperstimulation of the ovary
 (C) adhesions
 (D) hypervascularity to the ovary

413. Causes for ovarian hyperstimulation may include

 (A) oral contraceptives
 (B) hyperstimulation of the ovaries by infertility medications
 (C) hydatidiform mole
 (D) all of the above

414. Ovaries that have been overstimulated by infertility medication are at risk for

 (A) producing grossly enlarged cysts
 (B) torsion
 (C) endometriosis
 (D) A and B
 (E) all of the above

415. The sonographic characteristics of ovarian torsion are

 (A) enlarged ovaries
 (B) edematous ovarian walls
 (C) decreased intraovarian blood flow
 (D) all of the above

416. Fibroids are estrogen-stimulated tumors.

 (A) true
 (B) false

417. A rapidly growing fibroid in the first trimester of pregnancy is not as worrisome as a rapidly growing fibroid in a postmenopausal woman because

 (A) of the rapid rise of progesterone in the first trimester
 (B) of the decrease of estrogen in postmenopausal women
 (C) rapid fibroid growth is not worrisome
 (D) both cases are cause for concern

418. A rapidly growing fibroid in a postmenopausal woman not on hormone replacement therapy could indicate

 (A) leiomyosarcoma
 (B) fibrous degeneration
 (C) hemorrhagic infiltration
 (D) calcific changes

419. In the first and second trimesters, the fetal lung is

 (A) of greater echogenicity than the fetal liver
 (B) of decreased echogenicity compared to the fetal liver
 (C) isoechoic to the fetal liver
 (D) variable in appearance

420. In the third trimester, the fetal lung is

 (A) of greater echogenicity than the fetal liver
 (B) of decreased echogenicity compared to the fetal liver
 (C) isoechoic to the fetal liver
 (D) variable in appearance

421. The femoral epiphyseal plates are visualized on sonogram after

(A) 13 weeks
(B) 20 weeks
(C) 24 weeks
(D) 32 weeks

422. Postaxial polydactyl is

(A) an extra digit on the ulnar aspect of the fetal hand
(B) an extra digit on the radial aspect of the fetal hand
(C) curvature of the last digit on the ulnar aspect
(D) an extra digit on the fetal foot

423. Preaxial polydactyl is

(A) an extra digit on the ulnar aspect of the fetal hand
(B) an extra digit on the radial aspect of the fetal hand
(C) curvature of the last digit on the ulnar aspect
(D) an extra digit on the fetal foot

424. Concordant growth in twins refers to

(A) <10% difference in EFW between the twins
(B) <20% difference in EFW between the twins
(C) both fetus within normal range on a normal growth curve
(D) fetus remaining at the same EFW percentile from exam to exam

425. Concordant twin growth is more important in dichorionic twins than monochorionic twins.

(A) true
(B) false

426. The formula for determining EFW discordance is?

(A) smallest EFW + largest EFW/smallest EFW
(B) smallest EFW × 2 − largest EFW/largest EFW
(C) largest EFW − smallest EFW/largest EFW × 100
(D) largest EFW × 100 − smallest EFW/largest EFW

427. What is frank breech?

(A) when both feet are prolapsed into the lower uterine segment
(B) when one foot is prolapsed into the vagina
(C) when the fetal head is to the maternal right and the buttocks are to the maternal left
(D) when the buttocks descend first, the thighs and legs are extended upward along the anterior fetal trunk

428. What is complete breech?

(A) when both feet are prolapsed into the lower uterine segment

(B) when both feet are prolapsed into the vagina
(C) when the buttocks descend first, the knees are flexed, baby sitting cross-legged
(D) when the thighs and legs are extended upward along the anterior fetal trunk

429. What is footling breech?

(A) when one or both feet are prolapsed into the lower uterine segment
(B) when one foot is prolapsed into the fundus
(C) when the buttocks descend first, the knees are flexed, fetus sitting cross-legged
(D) when the thighs and legs are extended upward along the anterior fetal trunk

430. A fetal karyotype is 46 XY. This fetus is

(A) affected with Down syndrome
(B) affected with Turner syndrome
(C) a boy
(D) a girl

431. A fetal karyotype is 47X. This fetus is

(A) affected with Down syndrome
(B) affected with Turner syndrome
(C) a boy
(D) a girl

432. In a twin pregnancy with only one placenta, a dividing membrane is the only structure that needs to be identified to determine zygocity.

(A) true
(B) false

433. When labeling twins, fetus A should be

(A) the first fetus identified
(B) the fetus closest to the fundus
(C) the fetus closest to the internal os
(D) any of the above methods is appropriate

434. The fetus is vertex with the spine on the maternal right. The fetal left side should be

(A) anterior
(B) posterior
(C) inferior
(D) superior

435. The fetus is transverse with head on the maternal left. The fetal spine is inferior. The fetal left side should be

(A) anterior
(B) posterior
(C) inferior
(D) superior

436. The fetus is breech with the spine on the maternal left. The fetal left side should be

(A) anterior
(B) posterior
(C) inferior
(D) superior

437. Subchorionic placental lakes are

(A) associated with IUGR
(B) associated with oligohydramnios
(C) also known as subchorionic fibrin deposition
(D) all of the above

438. Early placental maturation may be associated with

(A) hypertension
(B) gestational diabetes mellitus
(C) maternal smoking
(D) A and C
(E) all of the above

439. A thin placenta (<1.5 cm) may be associated with all of the following except

(A) preeclampsia
(B) IUGR
(C) insulin dependent diabetes mellitus
(D) triploidy

440. A thick placenta (>5 cm) may be associated with all of the following except

(A) gestational diabetes mellitus
(B) infection
(C) multiple gestations
(D) hypertension

441. Maternal causes of IUGR may include all of the following except

(A) maternal infection
(B) diabetic mothers with vasculopathy
(C) maternal smoking
(D) gestational diabetes mellitus

442. If an insulin-dependent mother is in good diabetic control in the first trimester, the risk of structural abnormalities is decreased.

(A) true
(B) false

443. Caudal regression syndrome is associated with

(A) insulin-dependent diabetes mellitus
(B) chromosomal abnormalities
(C) Noonan's syndrome
(D) hypertension

444. Ultrasound findings in caudal regression syndrome include all of the following except

(A) agenesis of the sacrum
(B) hypoplasia of the lower extremities

(C) agenesis of the coccyx
(D) exstrophy of the bladder

445. A definitive diagnosis of trisomy 18 can be made by ultrasound if the fetus has multiple structural abnormalities.

(A) true
(B) false

446. Turner syndrome affects males and females

(A) equally
(B) males more than females
(C) females more than males
(D) males only
(E) females only

447. The fetus of an insulin-dependent diabetic mother may suffer from IUGR.

(A) true
(B) false

448. Fetal complications caused by maternal diabetes may include

(A) caudal regression syndrome
(B) cardiac defects
(C) shoulder dystocia
(D) A and B
(E) all of the above

449. Lung maturity amniocentesis is used in what cases?

(A) IUGR fetus with decreasing EFW
(B) insulin-dependent diabetes mellitus
(C) complete PROM
(D) A and B
(E) all of the above

450. Sonographic markers that may be used to assess macrosomia include all of the following *except*

(A) humeral shoulder thickness
(B) cheek-to-cheek diameter
(C) HC/AC ratio
(D) AFV

451. In the case of anhydramnios, how can karyotype be obtained?

(A) PUBS
(B) CVS
(C) cystocentesis
(D) all of the above

452. Amniocentesis may be used to test for

(A) fetal infection
(B) fetal bilirubin
(C) specific short limb syndromes
(D) A and B
(E) all of the above

453. Maternal hypertension may have what effect on pregnancy?

(A) fetal abnormalities
(B) chromosomal abnormalities
(C) IUGR
(D) delayed lung maturation

454. An excessively accelerated calcific placenta in the second trimester is associated with

(A) excessive maternal smoking
(B) chromosomal abnormality
(C) precursor to third trimester IUGR
(D) all of the above

455. The abbreviation BBOW refers to

(A) baby below outer water
(B) brachycephalic baby on way
(C) bulging bag of water
(D) baby below occipital wing

456. The abbreviation PROM refers to

(A) partially ruptured outer membrane
(B) previous rip of mucus plug
(C) partial range of motion
(D) premature rupture of membranes

457. Overdistension of the urinary bladder may cause

(A) anterior placenta to appear previa
(B) closure of an incompetent cervix
(C) distortion or closure of the gestational sac
(D) obscured visualization of the internal iliac vein
(E) A and B only
(F) all of the above

458. Ovulation occurs approximately

(A) always after intercourse
(B) on the 7th day of the menstrual cycle
(C) on the 14th day of the menstrual cycle
(D) on the 2nd day of the menstrual cycle

Questions 459–467: Match the terms in Column A to the correct description in Column B.

COLUMN A

459. Gravida _____
460. Multipara _____
461. Nullipara _____
462. Primipara _____
463. Nulligravida _____
464. Primigravida _____
465. Multigravida _____
466. Para _____
467. Trimester _____

COLUMN B

(A) a woman who has given birth two or more times
(B) one who has never been pregnant
(C) a woman who is pregnant
(D) a woman who has never given birth to a viable infant
(E) pregnant for the first time
(F) one who has been pregnant several times
(G) the number of pregnancies that have continued to viability
(H) a woman who has given birth one time to a viable infant
(I) a 3-month period during gestation

468. Puerperium refers to the period

(A) surrounding conception time
(B) after death
(C) 6–8 weeks before delivery
(D) beginning with the expulsion of the placenta

469. A postpartum gynecologic sonogram may be needed for

(A) assessing maternal hydronephrosis
(B) examining the uterus for retained placenta
(C) checking for maternal bowel obstruction
(D) all of the above

470. It is not possible to get pregnant while lactating.

(A) true
(B) false

471. Which of the following structures is most likely not seen in a postpartum pelvic sonogram?

(A) uterus
(B) endometrial echo
(C) vagina
(D) ovaries

472. A sonogram approximately 1 week after delivery would visualize the uterus

(A) above the umbilicus
(B) 38 cm from the symphysis pubis
(C) 30 cm from the symphysis pubis
(D) below the umbilicus

473. The most common complication during the postpartum period is?

(A) hemorrhage
(B) thromboembolism
(C) infection
(D) A and B
(E) all of the above

474. In a nongravid uterus, a previous cesarean section scar may be visualized on sonogram.

(A) true
(B) false

475. What percentage of fetuses are breech at term?

(A) 25%
(B) 7%
(C) 4%
(D) 1%

476. Term breech fetuses are more likely to have abnormalities than vertex fetuses.

(A) true
(B) false

477. The abbreviation VBAC refers to

(A) vaginal blockage and closure
(B) vaginal blockage after cesarean
(C) vaginal birth after cesarean
(D) none of the above

478. What sonographic findings may help determine mothers that are not VBAC candidates?

(A) decreased cervical length
(B) large amount of maternal abdominal scarring from previous cesarean section
(C) uterine wall <5 mm in the lower uterine segment
(D) sonogram cannot aid in determining VBAC candidates

Questions 479–484: Match the terms in Column A to the correct description in Column B.

COLUMN A   COLUMN B

479. placenta   (A) abnormal adherence of
       previa _____   part or all of the pla-
                                  centa to the uterine
                                  wall
480. placenta
       accreta _____   (B) premature separation
                                  of the placenta after
481. placenta   20 weeks of gestation
       succenturiata _____   (C) accessory lobe of
                                  placenta
482. abruptio   (D) implantation of the pla-
       placentae _____   centa in the lower uter-
                                  ine segment
483. placenta   (E) abnormal adherence of
       increta _____   part or all of the pla-
                                  centa in which the the
                                  chorionic villi invade
484. placenta   the myometrium
       percreta _____   (F) abnormal adherence
                                  of part or all of the
                                  placenta in which chori-
                                  onic villi invade the
                                  uterine wall

485. The chorion frondosum progressively develops to become

(A) fetal component of the placenta
(B) maternal component of the placenta
(C) the amniotic cavity
(D) the yolk sac and stalk

486. The decidua basalis progressively develops to become

(A) fetal component of the placenta
(B) maternal component of the placenta
(C) the amniotic cavity
(D) the yolk sac and stalk

487. The following information about HELLP syndrome is true *except*

(A) abbreviation for hemolysis, elevated liver enzymes, and low platelets
(B) abbreviation for hemivertebrae, elevated liver enzymes, and low lying placenta
(C) treated similar to severe preeclampsia
(D) Doppler may help in assessing HELLP syndrome

488. Infections that may affect the fetus include all of the following *except*

(A) parvovirus
(B) cytomegalovirus
(C) HIV
(D) none of the above

489. Varicella-zoster virus is also known as

(A) 5ths disease
(B) chicken pox
(C) "slapped cheek" disease
(D) herpes simplex

490. The most common intrauterine viral infection is

(A) toxoplasmosis
(B) HIV
(C) parvovirus
(D) cytomegalovirus

491. Ultrasound is not able to differentiate between different infections.

(A) true
(B) false

492. Parvovirus is also described as

(A) 5th's disease
(B) chicken pox
(C) "slapped cheek" disease
(D) A and C
(E) B and C

493. Sampling of the middle cerebral artery is helpful in determining

(A) IUGR and related complications
(B) prediction of fetal anemia
(C) the need for a fetal transfusion
(D) all of the above

494. Ovarian tumors that appear similar to a fibroma include all of the following *except*

(A) androblastoma
(B) endometroid
(C) thecoma
(D) all of the above

495. A 24-year-old patient presents for an ultrasound. The sonogram shows a solid hypoechoic ovarian mass. The differential is most likely

(A) granulosa cell
(B) thecoma
(C) dysgerminoma
(D) fibroma

496. All of the following about stromal tumors is correct *except*

(A) All have a similar sonographic appearance and can't be differentiated from one another.
(B) solid, hypoechoic ovarian tumors
(C) Types include: fibromas, thecomas, Sertoli–Leydig cell tumors.
(D) Types include: fibromas, thecomas, Brenner tumors.

497. Endometrioma may appear similar to

(A) benign cystic teratoma
(B) mucinous cystadenoma
(C) thecoma
(D) serous cystadenoma

498. Hydrosalpinx may be differentiated from a multicystic ovarian mass on sonogram by

(A) following the cystic spaces to ensure that they all communicate
(B) using color Doppler to follow the ovarian artery to the ovary
(C) having the patient roll to lengthen out the fallopian tube
(D) the two cannot be differentiated

499. An anechoic, smooth-walled cyst is identified in a patient who has had a hysterectomy/oophorectomy. The differential diagnosis should include

(A) paraovarian cyst
(B) ovarian cyst
(C) mesonephric cyst
(D) all of the above

500. The hydatid of Morgagni is

(A) a complex ovarian mass
(B) a section of sigmoid colon visible on transvaginal ultrasound
(C) paramesonephric cyst
(D) another name for ovarian remnant syndrome

501. The formula for determining ovarian volume is

(A) $d1 \times d2 \times d3 \times .523$
(B) $d1 + d2 + d3 \times 3.14$
(C) $d1 \times d2 \times d3 \times 3.14$
(D) $d1 \times d2/d1 + d2 + d3$

502. The image in Fig. 9–43 represents

(A) arachnoid cyst
(B) communicating hydrocephaly
(C) "banana" sign
(D) Dandy–Walker malformation

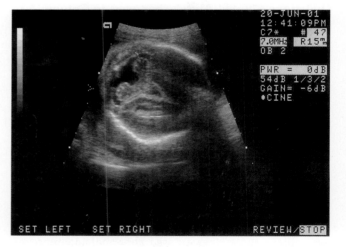

Figure 9–43

Answers and Explanations

At the end of each explained answer there is a number combination in parentheses. The first number identifies the reference source; the second number or set of numbers indicates the page or pages on which the relevant information can be found.

1. **(C)** The fetal calvarium is absent superior to the eyes. This finding is consistent with anencephaly. *(1:19)*

2. **(B)** The image shows a defect in the posterior cranial vault. Because brain tissue is herniated through the defect, this would be an occipital encephalocele. This fetus also demonstrates microcephaly caused by the large defect. *(1:19)*

3. **(D)** Equinovarus, or clubfoot, may be isolated or associated with other defects, most commonly neural tube defects. *(2:363)*

4. **(A)** The image represents a cystic hygroma. The multiple septations differentiate it from hydrops. The intact cranium differentiates it from an encephalocele. Cranial findings associated with spina bifida are found within the calvarium. *(2:992)*

5. **(A)** Seventy-five percent of fetuses with cystic hygromas have a chromosomal abnormality, most commonly Turner syndrome. *(2:56)*

6. **(C)** The image is an example of a "lemon"-shaped skull. It is most commonly associated with spinal defects, but can be present with encephaloceles and in normal fetuses 1–2% of the time. *(2:286)*

7. **(A)** Abdominal ascites outlines the abdominal viscera. Ascites associated with meconium peritonitis may have particles of debris within it, and echogenic foci are often present in the fetal liver. Nonimmune hydrops must have two fluid collections or one fluid collection with anasarca. *(2:470–471)*

8. **(B)** The septation within the cystic mass is characteristic of a cystic hygroma. *(1:20)*

9. **(C)** Alobar holoprosencephaly is characterized by a single ventricle, single choroid, and fused thalamus. *(1:20)*

10. **(D)** Cystic hygroma is associated with Turner syndrome, not trisomy 18. *(3:499–502)*

11. **(C)** Paternally derived triploidy is associated with a relatively well-grown fetus that has a proportionate head size. The placenta is large with multiple cystic spaces resembling a molar pregnancy. This accounts for 90% of triploidy. *(2:850)*

12. **(F)** Maternally derived triploidy is associated with a small placenta. The fetus has severe asymmetric growth restriction and oligohydramnios. *(2:851; 3:506)*

13. **(B)** Chorionic villi sampling can test for karyotype only. AFP is a fetal protein that may be tested for by concentration levels in the amniotic fluid or in maternal serum. *(2:25)*

14. **(C)** Early loss rate is thought to be associated with the unfused chorion and amnion. They are difficult to penetrate and often require multiple sticks. *(1:32)*

15. **(D)** FISH is considered experimental and requires amniocentesis follow-up. Fluorescent chromosomal markers are introduced into the amniotic fluid that "tag" or attach to certain chromosomes. These markers and chromosomes fluorescence allow for early preliminary detection of chromosomal abnormalities. *(1:32)*

16. **(A)** Amniocentesis may be performed after 14 weeks. It has a 0.3% risk of miscarriage. *(1:32)*

17. **(E)** PUBS—percutaneous umbilical blood sampling—is the insertion of a needle into the fetal umbilical cord and the withdrawal of fetal blood. It may be used in cases of anhydramnios, testing for isoimmunization, fetal blood typing, hemophilias, and other disorders. *(2:33)*

18. **(C)** Seventy-five percent of twins are dizygotic. *(1:27)*

19. **(D)** The twin peak is formed when the placental tissue migrates between the chorionic layers. This is 94–100% predictive of dizygotic twins. *(2:182–183)*

20. **(D)** Forty percent of conjoined twins are born stillborn. Fifty-six percent of conjoined twins are thoracoomphalopagus, thoracopagus, and omphalopagus. Polyhydramnios is present 50% of the time. Commonly, there is one umbilical cord that may have an abnormal number of vessels and is shared by the conjoined fetuses. *(1:29)*

21. **(B)** Retroflexion of the uterus is described as the uterine corpus is flexed posteriorly on the cervix, forming a sharp angle at the cervix. *(1:7)*

22. **(B)** Shortening of the humerus and femur. *(2:337)*

23. **(C)** Shortening of the radius/ulna and tibia/fibula. *(2:337)*

24. **(D)** Shortening of the entire limb, but can also refer to shortening of a limb without specific reference. *(2:337)*

25. **(A)** Shortening of the hand and foot bones. *(2:337)*

26. **(B)** The occurrence rate for thanatophoric dysplasia is 1/6000–1/17,000 births. Sonographic findings are polyhydramnios, severe rhizomelia, and micromelia with bowing. The thorax is bell-shaped, and the cranium is cloverleaf-shaped with hydrocephaly and frontal bossing. *(2:343; 1:28)*

27. **(F)** Heterozygous achondroplasia accounts for 80% of achondroplasias. It is the most common form of genetic skeletal dysplasia. It is often not identified before 26–27 weeks. *(1:27)*

28. **(B)** The two lines represent two endometrial linings in a duplicated uterus. The degree of duplication cannot be determined from this image. The interstitial portion of the fallopian tube runs through the cornua, or superior lateral portion of the fundus. *(2:824; 932)*

29. **(B)** A meningocele is a spina bifida with herniation of the meninges only. *(1:19)*

30. **(D)** A vasa previa is an accessory placenta with vessels crossing the internal os. *(1:17)*

31. **(B)** This is an image of an increased nuchal skin fold (>6 mm). Edema would surround the entire cranium. A cystic hygroma would have a midline septation. *(1:30)*

32. **(B)** The thin, well-defined, very bright reflection without any through transmission is characteristic of an IUD. *(3:849)*

33. **(C)** The image represents a benign cystic teratoma. A differential for this mass could be an endometrioma. *(1:Table 9–4)*

34. **(D)** The ovary is large, irregular in contour, and surrounded by ascites. This was a metastatic ovarian neoplasm. *(2:883)*

35. **(A)** The cystic structure represents the rhombencephalon. It is a normal structure seen between 7–9 weeks and contributes to the fourth ventricle, brain stem, and cerebellum. *(2:139)*

36. **(D)** The image represents a left ventricular aneurysm. Notice the normal sized right ventricle and atria, as well as the normally positioned valves. The coexistent normal findings would rule out hypoplasia and Ebstein's anomaly. *(4:377, 395)*

37. **(D)** The uterus is large with a heterogenous appearance and no definite masses. This finding and the patient's symptoms would be consistent with adenomyosis. *(1:9)*

38. **(E)** This mass may be either a hemorrhagic corpus luteal cyst or a mucinous cystadenoma. The patient's history, age, and stage in menstrual cycle may help to further differentiate the mass. *(1:Table 9–4)*

39. **(B)** Hydrops fetalis is an accumulation of fluid in body cavities and soft tissue. This image shows abdominal ascites, pleural effusion and anasarca. *(1:24)*

40. **(D)** The abnormality is spina bifida of the lumbar spine. The differential may include a sacrococcygeal teratoma based on the image alone, however, this fetus had a +lemon/banana sign. *(1:19)*

41. **(E)** The image is an increased nuchal translucency. It has an 80% positive predictive value for trisomy 21. If combined with the first trimester biochemistry, it has a 90% positive predictive value for trisomy 21. *(1:30)*

42. **(E)** An increased nuchal sonolucency is associated with specific chromosomal abnormalities, genetic syndromes, and structural defects. *(1:30)*

43. **(B)** The dilation of the proximal urethra gives the fetal bladder the classic "keyhole" appearance associated with posterior urethral valve obstruction. *(1:25)*

44. **(E)** Tetralogy of Fallot is comprised of a VSD, overriding aorta, pulmonary stenosis, and right ventric-

ular hypertrophy. The hypertrophy is not always present, particularly in the early to mid second trimester. This image shows the VSD and overriding aorta. *(1:21)*

45. (D) The stomach is located posterior to the fetal heart, which is deviated to the right side of the chest. The solid appearance on the left side of the thorax is consistent with the liver. *(1:22)*

46. (D) Arnold–Chiari malformation is also known as the "banana sign." It is characterized by the inferior displacement of the cerebellum and has a strong association with spinal defects. *(2:73)*

47. (B) The image is an example of an omphalocele. Atypically, the bowel is herniated instead of the liver. Notice the membrane around the bowel and the umbilical cord inserting into the membrane. *(1:23)*

48. (D) The image is consistent with enlarged kidneys. Dysplastic kidneys would have multiple cysts. Infantile polycystic kidney disease is associated with large kidneys; however, they are echogenic and oligohydramnios is present. *(2:543)*

49. (B) The tongue can be seen protruding from the mouth, consistent with macroglossia. The chin, forehead, and profile are normal. *(4:225)*

50. (C) Beckwith–Wiedemann syndrome is a group of disorders including omphalocele, macroglossia, organomegaly, and hemihypertrophy. *(1:24)*

51. (A) Multicystic, dysplastic kidneys have multiple cysts of various sizes. The cysts occur randomly and do not follow any pattern, as with dilated renal pyramids. The parenchyma is usually echogenic. *(1:25)*

52. (C) It has a variable prevalence, with Native American being the highest at 3.6/1000 births. *(2:322)*

53. (D) Three-dimensional imaging of the internal organs is termed volume imaging. Three-dimensional images of surface structures, such as the fetal face, is surface rendering. *(1:1020)*

54. (A) A gestational sac can be visualized by transvaginal scanning as early as 4 weeks. *(1:Table 9–5)*

55. (B) Cardiac imaging can be done earlier than 18 weeks, but is dependent on maternal habitus. After 24 weeks, the fetal bones become denser and more calcified and begin to limit the sonographic windows that allow visualization of the cardiac structures. *(2:378–379)*

56. (A) Three-dimensional imaging of surface structures, such as the fetal face, is termed surface rendering. *(1:1020)*

57. (D) Although duodenal atresia has been detected in the first trimester, the classic "double bubble" sign is not usually present until the late second and early third trimesters. *(2:466)*

58. (E) When the increased AFP is unexplained, it is thought to be because of an increased placental transfer of AFP. The placental dysfunction can occur with various placental abnormalities that may cause third trimester complications. *(2:30)*

59. (B) Cloacal exstrophy is characterized by an abdominal wall defect inferior to the umbilical cord insertion with exstrophy of a cloacal sac and a neural tube defect. It is associated with a markedly increased MSAFP. Amniotic sheets and congenital diaphragmatic hernia do not increase MSAFP. Smith–Lemli–Opitz syndrome is associated with a low level of maternal uE3 and normal MSAFP. *(2:29, 503)*

60. (C) If AFP (<0.6 MoM), uE3 (<0.5 MoM), and hCG (<0.3 MoM) are all decreased, the triple screen will show an increased risk for trisomy 18. *(2:29)*

61. (D) Pulmonary hypoplasia can be assumed by the small thoracic circumference and anhydramnios, but underdeveloped fetal lungs are not visible by sonography. *(1:25)*

62. (A) Vein of Galen aneurysm is an AV malformation located posterior to the third ventricle in the midline of the brain. *(1:21)*

63. (A) Truncus arteriosis consists of one outflow tract overriding a VSD. The right ventricular outflow tract is absent. Differential diagnosis includes tetralogy of Fallot with pulmonary atresia. Identifying the pulmonary arteries branching from the main trunk would differentiate the defect. *(4:390)*

64. (D) The most predictive sonographic findings is the overriding aorta and VSD. If the VSD is perimembranous, it will not appear on the four chamber view. The right ventricle may appear larger than the left, but this is not a consistent finding and is dependent of the degree of pulmonary stenosis. Differential diagnosis would include truncus arteriosis. *(4:426)*

65. (A) Congenital cystic adenomatoid malformation (CCAM) is divided into three subsets; macro, medium, and microcystic. Survival rate combines all types and sizes and is 75–80%. Studies have shown that CCAM regresses 55–69% of the time. *(2:439–441)*

66. (F) Congenital diaphragmatic hernia is left sided 75–90% of the time. Prognosis is poor, particularly if the liver is herniated into the chest. Five to fifteen percent of congenital diaphragmatic hernias are associated with chromosomal abnormalities, commonly trisomy 18. *(2:433–438)*

67. (D) Ninety percent of esophageal atresias have a tracheoesophageal fistula. This allows amniotic fluid to reach the stomach, but at a slower rate. The stomach will be visualized, but may be smaller than usual. Polyhydramnios occurs in the mid to late second trimester. The VACTERL complex is: vertebral anomalies, anal atresia, cardiac abnormalities, tracheoesophageal atresia, renal anomalies, and limb anomalies. At least three of the anomalies listed must be present to diagnosis the VACTERL condition.   *(2:103, 460)*

68. (A) Trisomy 21 is associated with a decreased MSAFP and an increased hCG.   *(5:71)*

69. (C) The uterosacral ligament is the distal portion of the cardinal ligament. It anchors the cervix and is responsible for uterine orientation.   *(1:5)*

70. (B) Both the suspensory and broad ligaments are folds of peritoneum.   *(1:5)*

71. (D) The iliopsoas muscle runs laterally to the uterus, near the iliac vessels. In transverse, it is ovoid and hypoechoic and may be mistaken for an ovary. *(2:785)*

72. (A) The most dependent portion is the pouch of Douglas, or the posterior cul-de-sac. It is located posterior to the cervix and anterior to the rectum. *(1:6)*

73. (C) The posterior cul-de-sac (pouch of Douglas) is located posterior to the uterus. The anterior cul-de-sac (vesicouterine pouch) is located anterior to the uterus. The prevesical space (retropubic space) is anterior to the bladder. They form the peritoneal spaces of the pelvic cavity.   *(1:6)*

74. (D) Transvaginal probes need to be cleaned with soap and water as well as soaked in a disinfecting solution. Transabdominal probes may be cleaned with a moist towelette.   *(1:4)*

75. (D) An invasive mole and a hydatidiform mole are excessive trophoblastic proliferation. Unlike the hydatidiform mole, chorioadenoma destruens is malignant and invades into the myometrium.   *(3:734)*

76. (E) Paternally derived trisomy 13 presents with a large placenta sometimes termed a partial mole. Less commonly, a dizygotic pregnancy may occur. One fetus results from normal fertilization of one egg and a complete molar pregnancy results from the fertilization of the other egg. In those cases, it is possible for the hydatidiform mole to advance to choriocarcinoma.   *(3:734)*

77. (C) The ovum enters the fallopian tube at the fimbriated ends. It courses to the ampulla where fertilization occurs 24–36 hours after ovulation.
   (6:211–212)

78. (D) The decidual reaction may resemble an early intrauterine sac. A yolk sac or embryonic pole will confirm an intrauterine pregnancy.   *(6:198)*

79. (C) The occurrence rates for ectopic locations are: ampullary—most common, 75–80%, isthmus—second most common, 10–15%, ovarian—0.5% and cervical—0.1%.   *(2:919)*

80. (B) Fetal demise is defined as an absence of fetal heart tones after 20 weeks.   *(1:14)*

81. (E) Dysgerminoma is a malignant tumor.   *(7:434)*

82. (B) Dermoid cysts are more common in younger women.   *(7:434)*

83. (A) Normal adult ovarian size is $3 \times 2 \times 2$ cm.   *(2:5)*

84. (B) The first finding is a gestational sac, however ectopic pregnancies may also present with a pseudo-sac. A yolk sac is the earliest definitive sonographic sign of an intrauterine pregnancy.   *(6:198)*

85. (B) The detection rate is 65%, but may vary among patients depending on the maternal habitus, fetal position, AFV, ultrasound machine, and expertise of the sonographer and physician.   *(6:325)*

86. (D) The detection rate is 85%, but may vary among patients depending on the maternal habitus, fetal position, AFV, ultrasound machine, and expertise of the sonographer and physician.   *(6:325)*

87. (D) Distal acoustic shadowing is associated with a solid mass.   *(6:124)*

88. (C) Theca lutein cysts are present in 18–37% of hydatidiform moles.   *(3:731)*

89. (A) The CRL is the most accurate because fetal growth is very uniform and is rarely affected by pathological disorders. The choices C and D are based on maternal LMP, which assumes ovulation on day 14.
   (3:138)

90. (A) Fetal growth in the first trimester is very uniform, thus allowing for accurate dating. *(1:Table 9–6)*

91. (B) Fetal growth is starting to show variation and multiple parameters are used to calculate the EDC. Both of these factors allow for an increased range of error.   *(1:Table 9–6)*

92. (C) Fetal growth is showing a moderate amount of variation, which allows for an increasing range of error.   *(1:Table 9–6)*

93. (D) Fetal growth has a large amount of variation in the third trimester and obtaining the images for

EFW can be challenging depending on fetal position and size. This allows for the largest range of error in the pregnancy.   *(1:Table 9–6)*

94. **(B)** The hCG doubles in approximately 48 hours until 6 weeks.   *(6:195)*

95. **(A)** Twin pregnancy is associated with an elevated hCG.   *(6:225)*

96. **(D)** The internal component of an endometrioma is typically blood from bleeding ectopic endometrial tissue during menstruation. Differential diagnosis may include a dermoid tumor; however, most women tend to be asymptomatic with dermoids.   *(1:Table 9–4)*

97. **(C)** Nagele's rule is: (1) identify the LMP, (2) add 7 days, (3) subtract 3 months, and (4) add one year.   *(1:397)*

98. **(C)** A corpus luteal cyst and ectopic pregnancy may mimic each other, and the sonogram should be correlated with clinical findings.   *(3:288, 916)*

99. **(A)** A mucinous cystadenoma is the largest ovarian tumor.   *(2:876)*

100. **(A)** Seroli-Leydig cell tumor is an androblastoma and Brenner's cell tumor is a transitional cell tumor. Chocolate cyst is another name for endometrioma.   *(1:Table 9–9, 3, 4)*

101. **(C)** The etiology of hydatidiform mole is fertilization of an ovum without any active chromosomal material.   *(7:357)*

102. **(D)** Blood flow direction and velocity are characteristics of color Doppler imaging.   *(1:1–2)*

103. **(A)** The extra-embryonic peripheral cells of the blastocyst. The trophoblast forms these cells, which form the wall of the blastocyst.   *(7:357)*

104. **(C)** By approximately day 14 of the menstrual cycle, one or more dominant follicles will reach a mean diameter of 20 mm with a hypoechoic rim.   *(1:8)*

105. **(A)** Leiomyomas are present in 25% of the female population with a higher percentage in African American women and becoming more prevalent in the fourth generation of life.   *(1:9)*

106. **(A)** The majority of tubo-ovarian abscesses are bacterial in origin. Symptoms are similar to other bacterial infections including pain, fever, and increased white blood cell count.   *(6:123)*

107. **(D)** All of the above. Decidual proliferation in ectopic pregnancy and endometrial carcinoma can also cause the endometrium to appear echogenic.   *(7:360)*

108. **(C)** Normal endometrial lining in postmenopausal women not on hormone replacement therapy is <5–6 mm.   *(1:10)*

109. **(B)** Normal endometrial lining in postmenopausal women on hormone replacement therapy is <8 mm.   *(1:10)*

110. **(C)** In the proliferative phase, the lining is thick, but the internal component is hypoechoic. This allows for the echogenic polyp to be seen. In the secretory phase, the entire endometrial lining is echogenic and will mask a polyp.   *(1:10)*

111. **(D)** LMP refers to the first day of the last cycle.   *(1:11)*

112. **(A)** The differential diagnoses that may mimic hydatidiform moles are missed abortions, leiomyomas, and hematomas. Endometriosis is endometrial tissue outside of the endometrial lining.   *(7:424)*

113. **(D)** 80%.   *(7:424)*

114. **(A)** The cervix is the most inferior portion of the uterus and invaginates into the vagina. Moving superiorly, the next section is the isthmus beginning at the internal os. The body, or corpus, of the uterus is the largest section of the uterus. The most superior portion is the fundus.   *(1:4)*

115. **(B)** The outer layer is the serosal, or peritoneal layer. The large muscular middle layer is the myometrium, and the inner layer is the endometrium.   *(1:4–5)*

116. **(C)** The cervix is larger than the body of the uterus in prepuberty.   *(1:7)*

117. **(B)** If the woman has not delivered a child before, the cervix and corpus are equal in size.   *(1:7)*

118. **(A)** After a full term pregnancy, the corpus is twice as long as the cervix.   *(1:7)*

119. **(C)** A nulliparous uterus is $8 \times 5 \times 4$ cm. A postmenopausal uterus is $7 \times 4 \times 3$ cm.   *(1:7)*

120. **(B)** False. The uterus atrophies equally in both multigravid and nulligravid women.   *(1:7)*

121. **(B)** Congenital abnormalities result from improper fusion of the mullerian, or paramesonephric ducts.   *(2:824)*

122. **(A)** The proliferative phase is day 5–9 postmenstruation.   *(1:8)*

123. **(C)** The periovulatory, or late proliferative phase is day 10–14 postmenstruation.   *(1:8)*

124. **(D)** The secretory phase is day 15–28 postmenstruation. The echogenicity is a result of edema of the functional zone of the endometrium.   *(1:8)*

125. **(D)** Symptoms of endometriosis caused by adhesions include dysmenorrhea, low back pain, dyspareunia (painful sexual intercourse), irregular bleeding and infertility.   *(2:868)*

126. **(A)** The most common locations for endometriosis are: ovaries, uterine ligaments, rectovaginal septums, posterior cul-de-sac, and pelvic peritoneum.   *(2:868)*

127. **(D)** Dermoid tumors are most commonly located superior to the uterine fundus.   *(7:436)*

128. **(A)** A fetus greater than the 90th percentile for estimated fetal weight is termed large for gestational age (LGA). A fetus greater than 4000 g is macrosomic.   *(3:544; 2:215)*

129. **(B)** LGA refers to a fetus measuring greater than the 90th percentile for gestational age.   *(3:544; 2:215)*

130. **(D)** All of the above. Identification of a macrosomic fetus can alert the obstetrician to watch for complications of macrosomia during delivery.   *(2:215)*

131. **(E)** Insulin-dependent diabetes mellitus (IDDM) and gestational diabetes mellitus (GDM) may both cause macrosomia. If the IDDM involves vascular disease, the fetus may actually be at risk for intrauterine growth retardation.   *(3:543)*

132. **(D)** Other causes for an increased fundal height include fibroids, incorrect dates, and molar pregnancy.   *(2:215; 6:465)*

133. **(A)** Although the other features, such as oligohydramnios, do often coexist and interact with IUGR, the diagnosis of IUGR is a fetus <10% for gestational age.   *(2:206)*

134. **(B)** An increased HC/AC ratio is the result of redistribution of fetal blood away from the bowel and directed to the fetal head.   *(3:522)*

135. **(D)** All of the above. IUGR may be found in chromosomal abnormalities, infection early in pregnancy, and placental insufficiency.   *(2:207)*

136. **(D)** Spina bifida is not associated with IUGR. Diabetes with vasculopathy, maternal HTN, and chromosomal abnormalities may all be associated with IUGR.   *(6:499)*

137. **(A)** An increase in systolic/diastolic ratio has been shown to have a correlation with placental insufficiency.   *(2:214)*

138. **(C)** The diastolic notch is normal before 26 weeks and is related to trophoblastic invasion.   *(2:685)*

139–156. See Fig. 9–44. Diagram of the fetal reproductive organs (frontal view).

157. **(B)** The central nervous center that regulates fetal tone functions first at 7.5–8.5 weeks.   *(2:663)*

158. **(A)** The central nervous center that regulates body movements starts functioning at 9 weeks.   *(2:663)*

159. **(C)** The central nervous center that regulates fetal breathing starts at 21 weeks.   *(2:663)*

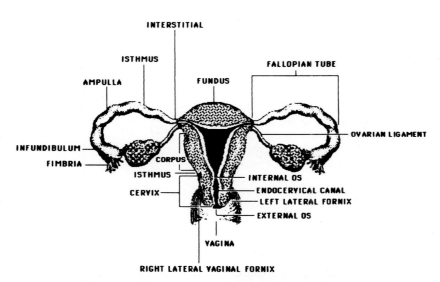

Figure 9–44. Diagram of female reproductive organs, labeled.

160. **(D)** The central nervous center for fetal heart rate reactivity functions by the end of the second trimester or beginning of the third trimester. *(2:663)*

161. **(B)** Components of a BPP include flexion/extension, gross body movement, breathing, amniotic fluid, and NST. *(1:14)*

162. **(D)** If the component (i.e., movement) is present, it is given a score of two. If it is absent, it is given a zero with the total score being 10. *(1:14)*

163. **(B)** Fetal breathing must last at least 30 seconds in a 30-minute time period in order to score a 2 in the BPP. *(2:663)*

164. **(A)** In response to hypoxia, the fetus reroutes blood to the brain in a brain-sparing effort. The middle cerebral artery is normally of higher resistance, but it will decrease to compensate for the increased blood flow and brain-sparing effort. *(2:690–691)*

165. **(B)** Amniotic fluid also controls temperature, protects the fetus, allows growth, and prevents infection. *(5:15)*

166. **(C)** Although the kidneys produce some urine prior to 16 weeks, they do not take over the majority of urine production until after 16 weeks. *(2:517)*

167. **(C)** The maximum amniotic fluid volume peaks at approximately 33 weeks, and then begins to decline. *(1:15)*

168. **(B)** The exact uterine volume cannot be determined by the sonogram. *(1:15)*

169. **(B)** This method is not as accurate as the amniotic fluid index. *(2:642)*

170. **(D)** All four quadrants are added and compared to an expected amniotic fluid volume for that fetus' gestational age. The normal range extends from 2.5% to 97.5%. *(8:1168)*

171. **(C)** All of the above. Nonspecific signs of fetal death are double contour of the fetal head caused by scalp edema, absence of the falx cerebri because of liquefaction of the brain, echoes in the amniotic fluid because of fragmentation of the fetal skin, and a decrease in biparietal diameter measurements because of collapse of the cranial sutures after death. *(7:429)*

172. **(A)** Scalp edema can be seen 2–3 days, or 24–72 hours, after fetal death. *(7:429)*

173. **(C)** The decidua of early intrauterine pregnancy is divided into decidua basalis, decidua parietalis (vera), and decidua capsularis. This marked hypertrophic change in the endometrium occurs no matter where the pregnancy is located. The uterine mucosa responds by a decidual reaction caused by hormonal stimuli. However, when an ectopic pregnancy occurs, the uterine decidua responds by a cast off-decidual cast. This should not be confused with the normal decidua in an early pregnancy. *(7:431)*

174. **(D)** Vaginal agenesis is the absence of a vagina. Gartner's duct cyst, Nabothian cyst, and hematocolpos will appear as a cystic mass in the vagina. *(2:940)*

175. **(D)** All of the above. The functions of the yolk sac are: nutrition-transfer of nutrients to the embryo; hemopoiesis-blood cell development; and development of sex cells that later become spermatogonia or oogonia. *(7:431)*

176. **(B)** The yolk sac reduces in size as pregnancy advances. However, it may persist throughout pregnancy and continue to persist into adulthood. In about 2% of adults, the proximal intra-abdominal part of the yolk sac is presented as a diverticulum of the ilium, called Meckel's diverticulum. *(7:431)*

177. **(C)** The yolk sac is located adjacent to the embryonic plate in early pregnancy and is located within the chorion. *(2:113)*

178. **(B)** The yolk sac may be visible as early as 5 weeks, but is virtually always seen by 5.5 weeks. *(2:118)*

179. **(C)** Zygote. *(7:433)*

180. **(B)** Cleavage. *(7:433)*

181. **(A)** Morula. *(7:433)*

182. **(D)** Blastocyst. *(7:433)*

183. **(C)** Oligohydramnios can cause restrictive deformities such as clubfoot, hand posturing, and scoliosis due to restricted fetal movement. Oligohydramnios may also cause pulmonary hypoplasia. It will not cause urethral stenosis. *(2:649)*

184. **(B)** As the pregnancy advances, the placenta becomes less resistive. This allows for more blood and oxygen to reach the growing fetus. *(2:687)*

185. **(A)** An increasing S/D ratio of the umbilical cord is a sign of vascular resistance within the placenta, which ultimately leads to a decrease in oxygen to the fetus. *(2:268)*

186. **(D)** Vasa previa may also be described as a succenturiate placenta with vessels crossing the internal os. *(2:601)*

187. (A) The incidence of placenta previa at term is 0.5–1%, with 90% of previas bleeding before 38 weeks.   *(9:403)*

188. (A) The ovum is usually found on the side of the corpus luteum from which it was released. It is possible for the ovum to contralaterally implant one-third of the time.   *(2:919)*

189. (A) The yolk sac lies in the chorionic cavity between the amnion and chorionic sac. It measures 5 mm to 1 cm. The yolk sac shrinks as pregnancy advances. It should not be measured in the CRL.   *(7:427)*

190. (A) The umbilical cord normally consists of two arteries and one vein.   *(1:17)*

191. (E) Open tube defect, anencephaly, and cephalocele are part of the neural tube defect spectrum.   *(1:19)*

192. (B) Herniation of meninges alone is termed a meningocele.   *(1:19)*

193. (D) Cranial signs are present 99% of the time with spinal defects. The second most accurate technique would be visualizing the spine in the transverse plane of view, looking for vertebral splaying and a break in the skin line.   *(1:19)*

194. (D) The "lemon" refers to the narrowing of the parietal bones giving the appearance of a lemon-shaped cranium in the axial view.   *(1:19)*

195. (C) The "banana" refers to the displacement of the cerebellum inferiorly into the upper cervical canal. On transverse view, the cerebellum is small and resembles a banana.   *(1:19)*

196. (D) 99% of the time.   *(1:19)*

197. (E) The lemon sign is found in 1–2% of normal fetuses.   *(2:286)*

198. (D) There is no contraindication to scanning a placenta previa transvaginally, and it provides the most accurate diagnosis. Transabdominal scanning may give a false-positive caused by a full maternal bladder compressing the internal os or an inadequate view of the internal os.   *(2:591)*

199. (B) If the placenta is greater than 2 cm from the internal os, a vaginal delivery is considered safe. *(2:591)*

200. (B) The normally positioned heart should be rotated approximately 45° with the apex pointed to the left.   *(2:384)*

201. (C) The horizontal position of the fetal heart is largely due to a large liver size.   *(7:432)*

202. (B) 75% of cephaloceles are occipital.   *(1:19)*

203. (C) 75% of cephaloceles are occipital.   *(1:19)*

204. (A) In the absence of a spinal defect, if the lateral ventricles measure greater than 10 mm, it is commonly associated with an obstruction of the ventricular system.   *(1:19)*

205. (C) The order of occurrence of obstruction from most common to least common is: aqueductal stenosis, communicating hydrocephaly, Dandy–Walker malformation, congenital hydrocephaly.   *(3:701)*

206. (E) Congenital hydrocephaly is an X-linked abnormality, with the expression in males and the females being carriers. It is able to be detected through DNA testing.   *(1:19)*

207. (C) Mild ventriculomegaly may be described as a separation of choroid from the medial ventricular wall >5 mm (but not dangling) or a measurement of the ventricular atrium between 10 and 15 mm.
(3:376; 6:246–247)

208. (D) Agenesis of the corpus callosum has mild ventriculomegaly, but the ventricle is also shaped like a "teardrop" in most cases. Mild ventriculomegaly has been associated with trisomy 21, but may also a normal variant.   *(2:44, 282)*

209. (D) Clubfeet and ventriculomegaly have a strong association with spinal defects.   *(2:619)*

210. (B) The prognosis of hydrocephaly remains unclear from the prenatal imaging.   *(2:283)*

211. (B) The site and extension of the lesion may aid in a very general prognosis, but it is impossible to accurately and clearly predict an individual fetus' prognosis by in utero findings.   *(2:286)*

212. (D) The cysterna magna is enlarged if the measurement is greater than 10 mm.   *(6:245)*

213. (A) A true Dandy–Walker malformation must have agenesis of the cerebellar vermis with communication to the fourth ventricle. A Dandy–Walker malformation variant is described as having some degree of cerebellar vermis agenesis, but not complete agenesis. An arachnoid cyst will push the cerebellum superiorly without splaying the cerebellum.   *(2:292)*

214. (C) An arachnoid cyst will not cause splaying of the cerebellum and the cerebellar vermis will be intact.   *(2:292)*

215. (A) Dandy–Walker malformation is associated with other midline defects including agenesis of the corpus callosum and cephaloceles, as well as holoprosencephaly, clefting and cardiac defects. Dandy–Walker malformation has a 50–70% risk of associated abnormalities. *(2:292)*

216. **(C)** Dandy–Walker malformation may occur as part of the mendelian disorder (abnormalities in multiple different organ systems) and is associated with chromosomal abnormalities. *(2:292)*

217. **(E)** Subnormal intelligence is reported in 40–70% of cases. Morbidity rates are 24%, but are improving with increased anesthesia and surgical techniques. *(2:295)*

218. **(D)** The most common cause of hypotelorism is holoprosencephaly. Hypotelorism is found in many different syndromes and chromosomal abnormalities and is strongly associated with abnormalities of the brain. *(2:309; 4:223)*

219. **(B)** Cyclopia—absent nose with protrusion of tissue at level of eye sockets; hypotelorism—close set orbits; cebocephaly—single nostril nose; and cleft lip/palate are all abnormal facial findings strongly associated with holoprosencephaly. *(2:309–311)*

220. **(C)** Thirty to fifty percent of fetuses with holoprosencephaly have chromosomal abnormalities, the most common being trisomy 13. *(4:119)*

221. **(A)** The most common cause of hypertelorism is a defect that prevents the migration of the eyes to their normal position. An anterior cephalocele is the most common blockage of that migration. *(2:311)*

222. **(D)** Teratomas can occur in many different locations. The most common region is sacrococcygeal accounting for 50% of fetal teratomas. The second most common location is orofacial (including intracranial) and cervical, accounting for 5% of fetal teratomas. *(2:317)*

223. **(B)** Maternal Graves disease and Hashimoto thyroiditis produce antibodies that cross the placenta and may affect fetal thyroid production. *(2:318)*

224. **(C)** Macroglossia is present in 97.5% of Beckwith–Weidemann syndrome. *(2:320)*

225. **(A)** Macroglossia may prevent effective fetal swallowing causing polyhydramnios. *(2:320)*

226. **(D)** Other findings of Beckwith–Wiedemann syndrome include omphalocele, organomegaly, hemihypertrophy, and hypoglycemia. *(1:24)*

227. **(B)** Of the isolated cleft lip and palate cases, 40% are unilateral cleft lip and palate, 29% are unilateral cleft lip, 27% are bilateral cleft lip and palate, and 5% are bilateral cleft lip. *(2:324)*

228. **(C)** The risk of significant abnormalities seems to increase with the severity of the cleft. A wide variety of abnormalities are associated with clefts, but cardiac abnormalities are the most prevalent. *(2:324)*

229. **(C)** Medial cleft lip is associated with a spectrum of midline defects, the most common being holoprosencephaly. *(2:314)*

230. **(D)** Pierre Robin syndrome, trisomy 18, and campomelic dysplasia are all associated with micrognathia and polyhydramnios. Micrognathia commonly causes difficulty swallowing resulting in polyhydramnios. *(2:56, 327, 352)*

231. **(D)** Due to the small mandible and normal sized tongue, normal swallowing is inhibited. *(2:327)*

232. **(C)** If the nose is not visualized, the sonographer should look superiorly on the fetal face for a proboscis. The orbits should also be identified, looking for hypotelorism or cyclopia. *(2:327)*

233. **(B)** It is possible to have a normal face with holoprosencephaly, although the majority of cases will not have facial anomalies. *(6:254–255)*

234. **(C)** Development of the corpus callosum occurs between 12–18 weeks; therefore, visualization is not possible less than 18 weeks. *(2:290)*

235. **(D)** The "teardrop" appearance (enlargement of the atria and occipital horns and lateral displacement of the anterior horns) is present 90% of the time. *(2:290; 6:255)*

236. **(C)** Hydranencephaly exists when the cerebral hemispheres are replaced by fluid. The brain stem is usually spared. Causes are thought to be infection or obstruction of the internal carotid artery. *(2:297)*

237. **(D)** Microcephaly has been described as an HC between –2 and –3 standard deviations (SD) of the mean. *(2:298)*

238. **(D)** A Vein of Galen aneurysm is a type of AV malformation. Agenesis of the corpus callosum, third ventricular dilation, and an arachnoid cyst are cystic midline lesions, but they will not have the high, turbulent blood flow of an AV malformation. *(2:301)*

239. **(B)** Isolated choroid plexus cyst has a small risk for trisomy 18. If other abnormalities are identified along with the choroid plexus cyst, the risk for trisomy 18 increases. *(2:301)*

240. **(B)** The data do not support an increased risk attributable to size or number of choroid plexus cysts. *(2:301)*

241. **(C)** The image should also show the cavum septum pellucidum. The measurement is taken from the outer edge of the cranium to the outer edge of the skin.

(6:245)

242. **(B)** The lateral ventricle should be measured at the widest portion of the atrium from the medial to the lateral wall. It should not exceed 10 mm. *(6:246)*

243. **(B)** The data for transverse cerebellar diameter is based on imaging in the axial plane of view. *(2:163)*

244. **(A)** A cephalic index >85 describes an increased BPD when compared to a shorter OFD. The head has a rounded appearance on ultrasound. *(6:244)*

245. **(B)** Dolicocephaly is a long, narrow head with a small BPD when compared with a longer OFD.

(6:381)

246. **(B)** Dolicocephaly appears as a long, narrow head.

(6:381)

247. **(A)** Brachycephaly appears as a short, rounded head.

(6:381)

248. **(D)** Dolicocephaly is associated with breech fetuses and oligohydramnios. *(2:991)*

249. **(F)** Brachycephaly with a flat occiput is a feature of trisomy 21. Brachycephaly may also be present with a spina bifida due to ventricular enlargement. Most commonly, brachycephaly is a normal variant.

(4:1009)

250. **(C)** The head is larger than the abdomen at 12–24 weeks. *(7:434)*

251. **(B)** At 32–36 weeks, the head and body are about the same size. *(7:434)*

252. **(A)** After 36 weeks, the abdomen is larger than the head. *(7:434)*

253. **(B)** The scanning plane is too high. When performing a biparietal diameter measurement (BPD), the fetal head should be ovoid and the measurement obtained at the level of the thalami and cavum septum pellucidum. *(7:440)*

254. **(D)** The fluid within a cystic hygroma is lymphatic fluid from an obstructed lymph system. *(6:263)*

255. **(A)** A cystic hygroma occurs when the jugular lymph sacs fail to communicate with the venous system. The obstructed lymphatic fluid fills the sacs and forms the cystic hygroma. *(6:263)*

256. **(B)** The midline septum represents the medial walls of the two obstructed lymph sacs. *(6:263)*

257. **(C)** The cervical region. *(7:426)*

258. **(E)** C and D. Cystic hygromas are associated with elevated MSAFP and Turner syndrome. *(7:365)*

259. **(B)** Seventy-five percent of cystic hygromas are associated chromosomal abnormalities. If the cystic hygroma is isolated, the outcome for the fetus is typically good.

(2:56; 4:255)

260–268. See Fig. 9–45.

269–278. See Fig. 9–46.

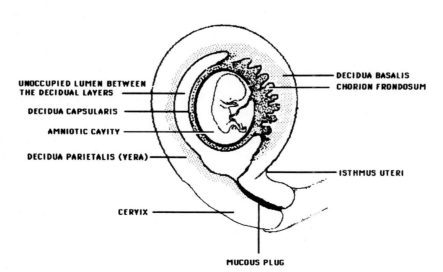

Figure 9–45. Diagram of early pregnancy, labeled.

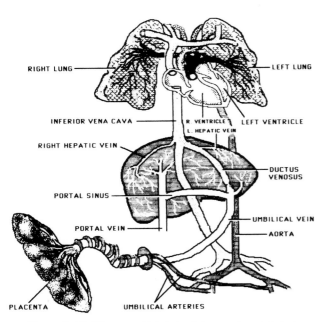

Figure 9–46. Diagram of fetal circulatory system, labeled.

Labels on figure: RIGHT LUNG, LEFT LUNG, INFERIOR VENA CAVA, R VENTRICLE, LEFT VENTRICLE, L. HEPATIC VEIN, RIGHT HEPATIC VEIN, PORTAL SINUS, DUCTUS VENOSUS, PORTAL VEIN, UMBILICAL VEIN, AORTA, PLACENTA, UMBILICAL ARTERIES

279. **(C)** The foramen ovale allows for oxygenated blood to pass from the right atrium to the left atrium. *(6:323)*

280. **(B)** The ductus arteriosis allows for approximately 70% of the blood to bypass the nonfunctioning lungs. *(6:323)*

281. **(C)** It is a destructive process that obliterates the cerebral cortex. The brain stem is usually spared. Other causes include infection and intrauterine strangulation. *(3:385)*

282. **(E)** Alobar holoprosencephaly and severe hydrocephaly may sonographically present similar to hydranencephaly. Lobar holoprosencephaly sonographically presents with a interhemispheric fissure anterior and posterior, thus being excluded in the differential. *(2:299)*

283. **(D)** Hemivertebrae is easiest to view in the sagittal plane of view because the other vertebrae may be used as a reference of normal. It is visible in the other planes of view also, but requires more meticulous scanning. *(3:456)*

284. **(D)** Arnold–Chiari malformation is most commonly associated with myelomeningocele and hydrocephaly. *(2:73)*

285. **(C)** Microcephaly is a result of a large portion of the brain tissue being herniated out of the cranium. *(1:19)*

286. **(A)** Semilobar holoprosencephaly is a single anterior ventricle with partial separation of the posterior cerebellar hemispheres. *(1:20)*

287. **(A)** The most likely diagnosis would be alobar holoprosencephaly. Differential diagnosis would include hydranencephaly and hydrocephaly. Hydranencephaly would not show any cerebral cortex and only brain stem would be spared. Hydrocephaly would show a bi-lobed thalamus with a dilated third ventricle. *(1:20)*

288. **(C)** Hydranencephaly will present with no visible cerebral cortex. The differential includes alobar holoprosencephaly (fused thalamus) and severe hydrocephaly (bi-lobed thalamus with dilated third ventricle). *(1:20)*

289. **(B)** It may be possible to diagnose anencephaly as early as 12 weeks, but it should be definitely diagnosed by 14 weeks. *(1:19)*

290. **(D)** Acrania is theorized to be the first trimester finding of anencephaly. With prolonged exposure to the amniotic fluid, the abnormal brain tissue is eroded, and the second trimester finding of anencephaly is appreciated. *(3:379–380)*

291. **(4)** The last number stands for the number of living children. *(1:3)*

292. **(2)** The number of preterm births is the second number after parity. *(1:3)*

293. **(7)** G refers to the gravida or number of pregnancies. *(1:3)*

294. **(1)** The third number after parity represents the number of abortions (spontaneous and elective). *(1:3)*

295. **(3)** The first number after parity represents the number of full term pregnancies. *(1:3)*

296. **(A)** The number of pregnancies is listed after gravida (G). The first number after parity (P) is the number of full term pregnancies (3), the second number is the number of preterm pregnancies (1 set of twins, single pregnancy and 1 preterm fetal death >20 weeks = 2), the third number is the number of abortions (1), and the final number is the number of living children (5). *(1:3)*

297. **(B)** Spina bifida occulta is a mild form of spina bifida that does cause a break in the skin. Because the spinal cord does not herniate out of the spinal canal, it does not cause a lemon or banana sign. *(3:380)*

298. **(A)** AFP is produced by the fetus. An abnormal concentration occurs whenever there is an abnormal opening in the fetus allowing an increased amount of the protein in the amniotic fluid.   *(2:25)*

299. **(B)** 5 weeks.   *(1:Table 9–5)*

300. **(C)** After 13 weeks, the fetus is larger and it is technically more difficult to obtain the correct view to measure a CRL.   *(1:Table 9–5)*

301. **(C)** Multiple parameters help to increase the accuracy of estimated fetal weight.   *(3:146)*

302. **(B)** Only the shaft of the femur should be measured in femur length, excluding the femoral neck and other epiphyseal calcification centers.   *(7:442)*

303. **(C)** Of the cases with polyhydramnios, 60% are idiopathic, 20% are structural, and 20% are maternal insulin dependent diabetes mellitus.   *(1:16)*

304. **(F)** Polyhydramnios has many causes that may include increased urine production or decreased fetal swallowing.   *(2:348; 651, 1:29)*

305. **(C)** Amnion begins to fuse with the chorion at 12 weeks and is routinely complete by 14–16 weeks.   *(2:124)*

306. **(B)** Hematopoiesis, or red blood cell production, is done by the fetus. The placenta is responsible for the exchange of nutrients, oxygen, and waste. The placenta also acts as a barrier although some medication can cross through the placenta.   *(1:16)*

307. **(B)** The diagnosis is determined by the history and physical findings. Most commonly, the patient presents with vaginal bleeding and abdominal or back pain.   *(9:406)*

308. **(C)** Placental abruption usually occurs in the third trimester, although it is possible at any point in the pregnancy.   *(2:612)*

309. **(D)** The hypoechoic region behind the placenta should measure 1–2 cm in thickness. Any increase in thickness of this area should alert the sonographer to a possible hematoma.   *(2:611)*

310. **(E)** Other risk factors include: abdominal trauma, smoking, sudden decompression of the uterus (i.e. delivery of a twin or PROM), prolonged PROM, uterine anomaly, high pariety, and prior abruption.   *(9:406)*

311. **(C)** Implantation sites at risk for placenta accreta are uterine scars, submucosal fibroids, lower uterine segment, rudimentary horn, and uterine cornua.   *(2:613–614)*

312. **(C)** The "swiss cheese" appearance is referring to large anechoic spaces in and behind the placenta and increased placental vascularity.   *(1:17; 2:615)*

313. **(A)** Placenta accreta may be divided into (1) placenta accreta vera—placental attachment to the myometrium without invasion, (2) placenta increta—invasion of placenta into the myometrium and (3) placenta percreta—invasion of placenta through the uterus and into other organs.   *(1:17)*

314. **(D)** Chorioangioma is a vascular mass arising from chorionic tissue and is similar to a hemangioma.   *(2:612)*

315. **(B)** The umbilical vein carries oxygenated blood.   *(1:17)*

316. **(A)** Wharten's jelly is a mucoid connective tissue that surrounds the umbilical vein and artery.   *(6:440)*

317. **(A)** A true cord cyst is attributable to allantoic duct remnants and is thought to be more common in the first trimester.   *(3:212; 2:621)*

318. **(D)** A velamentous cord insertion is associated with IUGR, particularly in monochorionic twins.   *(2:620)*

319. **(C)** An eccentric cord insertion is considered a normal variant and is of no clinical significance.   *(3:206; 2:620)*

320. **(B)** Atrial and ventricular septal defects are the most common defects accounting for 26% of the cardiac abnormalities.   *(1:21)*

321. **(A)** Generally, the left side of the heart perfuses the fetal cranium.   *(7:449)*

322. **(B)** Generally, the right side of the heart perfuses the systemic circulation of the fetus.   *(7:449)*

323. **(B)** The ratio of the heart circumference to the thoracic circumference should be 30–50%.   *(2:384)*

324. **(D)** This condition is called situs inversus (partial or total), dextrocardia and heterotaxy syndrome. Along with dextrocardia, there may be significant intracardiac anomalies, anomalies of the great vessels, an interrupted IVC, an anomalous venous return system, asplenia or polysplenia, and possible heterotaxy of the abdominal organs depending on whether it is complete or partial.   *(4:385)*

325. **(C)** 50% of trisomy 21 cases have a cardiac defect, the majority being AV canal defects.   *(2:45)*

326. (C) This view allows for visualization of the right ventricular outflow tract, the left ventricular outflow tract and the crossing of the outflow tracts. *(2:385)*

327. (E) Other structures to evaluate include atrial sizes, foramen ovale, coronary vessels, thickness of the ventricular walls, cardiac orientation and size. *(2:385)*

328. (B) Ventricular septal defects can be divided into the muscular and membranous regions. A muscular VSD is within the muscular portion of the septum and may be detected from a four-chamber view. A membranous VSD is just below the aortic valve and is confirmed in the long axis view of the heart. *(4:438)*

329. (B) In most cases, hypoplastic left heart syndrome (HLHS) is easily visualized by 18 weeks. It is possible for HLHS to evolve through the pregnancy due to aortic coarctation. *(7:396)*

330. (A) Coarctation of the aorta is a narrowing of the aorta, usually near the ductus arteriosis. It may be very difficult to image depending on the degree of stenosis. Often diagnosis relies on the ventricular discrepancy indicating that a stenosis is present. *(4:366)*

331. (A) Of the diaphragmatic hernias, 75–90% are left sided, 10% are right and <5% are bilateral. *(2:433)*

332. (E) Whenever the heart is deviated with the correct apex orientation, the sonographer should consider a thoracic mass. *(2:429, 433, 440, 6:290)*

333. (A) It is important to identify the location of the fetal liver. If the liver is intrathoracic, the prognosis for survival is 43%. If the liver is intrabdominal the prognosis is 80% survival. *(1:22)*

334. (D) Although chromosomal abnormalities and associated anomalies are prevalent in congenital diaphragmatic hernia, the significant factor in mortality is pulmonary hypoplasia. *(1:22)*

335. (D) If the liver is intrathoracic, the survival rate is 43%, if the liver is intrabdominal, the survival rate is 80%. *(1:22)*

336. (C) CCAM accounts for 75–80% of congenital lung malformations with over 95% of those being unilateral. *(2:439)*

337. (C) Macrocystic is defined as multiple large cysts measuring 2–10 cm. *(1:22)*

338. (B) Type II cysts are <2 cm, but still visible. *(1:22)*

339. (A) Sonographically, these appear as a solid, homogenous, echogenic lung mass. *(1:22)*

340. (A) Approximately 10–15% of pulmonary sequestrations are found within or below the diaphragm, typically on the left side. *(2:444)*

341. (B) The most common appearance detected prenatally is a well-circumscribed echogenic mass in the left lower lung base. *(2:441)*

342. (B) Ninety percent of esophageal atresias have a TE fistula that communicates with the stomach. Polyhydramnios may not develop until the third trimester, making a second trimester diagnosis difficult. *(1:23)*

343. (D) There are five types of TE fistulas. They comprise 90% of the cases of esophageal atresia. *(2:460)*

344. (C) Regardless of the presence of a TE fistula, 80% of fetuses derive polyhydramnios by the third trimester. *(2:457)*

345. (B) Esophageal atresia is a very strong marker for trisomy 18. *(2:4547)*

346. (B) Amniotic fluid fills the stomach and duodenum proximal to the site of obstruction. The ultrasound appearance resembles a "double bubble." *(2:466)*

347. (D) Thirty-three percent will have spinal defects, 36% will have cardiac defects. *(2:466)*

348. (A) Thirty percent of fetuses with duodenal atresia have trisomy 21. *(2:466)*

349. (C) The bowel begins to herniate at 8 weeks and becomes most visible at 9–10 weeks on ultrasound, because of the rotation of the bowel. The bowel then returns to the abdomen by the end of the 11th week. *(2:139)*

350. (B) Chromosomal and associated defects (nongastrointestinal) with gastroschisis are very rare. *(2:492)*

351. (B) Gastroschisis is a defect in the abdominal wall in which the bowel herniates into the amniotic fluid. This allows the AFP to enter the amniotic fluid directly from the abdominal wall defect, cross the placenta, and enter the maternal blood stream. The mean AFP value for gastroschisis is 7 MoM versus 4.1 MoM for omphaloceles. *(4:474)*

352. (C) Gastroschisis is rarely associated with chromosomal or nongastrointestinal disorders and has an excellent survival rate. *(2:492)*

353. **(D)** When the bowel perforates, meconium enters the peritoneal space. A membrane forms that seals off the intestine at the site of the perforation. The meconium that entered the peritoneum may cause calcium deposits. Other findings are polyhydramnios, ascites with echogenic debris, and bowel dilation.

(2:470–471)

354. **(E)** All of the above. They may all cause a complication in gastroschisis and should be monitored with ultrasound throughout the pregnancy. *(2:497)*

355. **(A)** Although left-sided gastroschisis have been reported, it is typically to the right of the umbilical cord. *(4:473–474)*

356. **(B)** The physiological hernia is the outpouching of the intestines as they rotate around the SMA and then return to the abdomen. *(2:139)*

357. **(B)** The presence of bowel without liver in the smaller omphaloceles has a stronger association to abnormal karyotypes and perinatal mortality. *(4:486)*

358. **(B)** Small omphaloceles may be mistaken for a cord hematoma. If the defect at the base of the cord insertion is >7 mm it is most likely an omphalocele.

(4:484)

359. **(C)** Omphaloceles are not associated with teratogens, such as maternal smoking. *(4:484)*

360. **(B)** Ectopia cordis results from underdevelopment or agenesis of the fetal sternum. It is rarely isolated and is most commonly part of the pentalogy of Cantrell.

(4:467)

361. **(D)** Pentalogy of Cantrell involves defects of the lower sternum, diaphragm, diaphragmatic pericardium, abdominal wall, and intracardiac defects. It is associated with trisomy 13 and trisomy 18.

(2:501; 4:493)

362. **(F)** Beckwith–Wiedemann syndrome is due to a dysfunction of the placenta excreting increased levels of growth hormone. This causes organomegaly, macroglossia, omphalocele, hemi hypertrophy, and cardiac abnormalities. *(2:501)*

363. **(B)** Cloacal exstrophy is believed to arise from irregular development of the cloacal membrane. Neural tube defects are present 50% of the time. *(2:508)*

364. **(C)** Limb–body wall complex (LBWC) is the most severe abdominal wall defect with the entire ventral wall disrupted. If the umbilical cord is visualized at all, it is very short and severe scoliosis is present.

(2:508; 4:453–455, 762)

365. **(C)** Amniotic band syndrome is a rupture of the amnion early in pregnancy. That rupture allows bands of amniotic tissue to float freely in the amniotic fluid. If these bands come in contact with the fetus, they can cause strictures, amputations, and adhesions to the band itself. Amniotic sheets, also known as uterine synechia, are caused by scars or adhesions in the uterus. The amnion and chorion grow around the synechia and form a thick membrane with two layers of amnion and chorion on either side of the membrane. It is attached to the uterus at both ends and does not impede the fetus in any way. *(2:502–504, 511; 4:762–766)*

366. **(D)** If a mother is Rh-, she will produce antibodies against an Rh+ fetus. The mother's antibodies will perceive the fetal blood as foreign and attack the fetal red blood cells resulting in erythroblastosis fetalis. *(9:413)*

367. **(B)** There are many other antibodies in addition to the anti-D antibody that can cause immune hydrops. *(9:413)*

368. **(B)** This condition will cause immune hydrops in the fetus *(9:413)*

369. **(B)** Both immune and nonimmune hydrops present the same sonographically. *(2:551)*

370. **(D)** Other signs of heart failure include pericardial effusions, decreased contractility, increased ventricular thickness, abnormal umbilical cord, and middle cerebral artery Doppler. *(3:276; 2:567; 6:492)*

371. **(D)** Fetal hydrops is defined as two sites of fluid accumulation or one site of fluid accumulation and fetal ascites. *(2:551)*

372. **(D)** The cardiac ventricular walls will thicken and contractility decreases. This causes the cardiac output to decrease. This may lead to acidosis, increased hematocrit, and increased neonatal morbidity.

(3:339)

373. **(D)** The list of causes for nonimmune hydrops fetalis (NIHF) is more than 120 conditions, some of which are rare. Major causes are: cardiac arrhythmias and tumors, abnormal chromosomes, cardiac failure, anemia, AV shunts, mediastinal compression, metabolic disease, fetal infection, fetal tumors, congenital fetal defects, and placental defects. *(1:24)*

374. **(B)** A complete situs inversus will appear with the heart and normally positioned left-sided abdominal organs on the right side. A complete situs inversus has a minimally increased risk of abnormalities and is not as significant as a partial situs inversus.

(6:272)

375. **(A)** Partial situs inversus, divided into asplenia and polysplenia, has a 40% incidence of anomalies. They include complex heart disease, absent gallbladder, interrupted IVC with an azygous venous return, and splenic abnormalities.   *(2:480; 6:274)*

376. **(F)** Partial situs inversus, divided into asplenia and polysplenia, has a 40% incidence of anomalies. They include complex heart disease, absent gallbladder, interrupted IVC with an azygous venous return and splenic abnormalities.   *(2:480; 6:274)*

377. **(B)** A ureteropelvic junction (UPJ) obstruction is an obstruction at the junction of the ureter and renal pelvis. Therefore, the fetal urine is obstructed within the kidney causing hydronephrosis, but not hydroureter. As long as the contralateral kidney is functioning normally, the amniotic fluid should remain normal.   *(1:25)*

378. **(A)** A ureterovesicle junction (UVJ) obstruction is an obstruction at the junction of the ureter and fetal bladder. It is associated with ureter anomalies, such as duplication and abnormal insertion sites. There is often an ureterocele caused by the abnormal insertion of the ureter. Hydroureter and mild hydronephrosis are commonly present.   *(2:527; 1:25)*

379. **(B)** Ureters will typically appear anechoic and tortuous on sonogram. Bowel is typically hypoechoic with peristalsis.   *(6:277)*

380. **(C)** The trigone is located at the inferior portion of the posterior bladder wall.   *(6:44)*

381. **(B)** Although it is overwhelmingly found in males, it may rarely be found in females. In females, it is usually caused by a cloacal malformation or urethral atresia.   *(2:529)*

382. **(A)** Complete PUV obstruction does not allow for any fetal urination, therefore severe oligohydramnios occurs.   *(2:535)*

383. **(A)** Potter's facies also includes low set ears, clubfoot, and hip dislocation.   *(2:536)*

384. **(D)** The primary cause of neonatal death in PUV syndrome is pulmonary hypoplasia, although the other entities are also serious complications.   *(1:25)*

385. **(C)** In cases of renal agenesis, particularly after 16 weeks, anhydramnios is present.   *(2:537)*

386. **(B)** A normal fetal bladder should empty every 30–45 minutes.   *(6:281)*

387. **(C)** Kidneys begin to develop at 7 weeks. Between 7 and 11 weeks, the kidneys migrate cephalically into the renal pelvis.   *(3:433)*

388. **(D)** Three pairs of kidneys form in successive stages: pronephros, mesonephros, and metanephros with metanephros remaining as the functioning kidney.   *(10:687)*

389. **(D)** The urinary system develops closely with the uterine development. Twenty to thirty percent of patients with uterine anomalies also have renal ectopia or agenesis.   *(2:828)*

390. **(B)** Multicystic dysplastic kidney disease is caused by a first trimester obstruction. The kidney is nonfunctioning with ureteral atresia.   *(2:541)*

391. **(A)** In cases of a unilateral nonfunctioning kidney, the contralateral kidney will often enlarge to compensate. The unilateral kidney usually provides enough function to be sufficient for the individual.   *(2:5440)*

392. **(B)** The risk to the fetus in an autosomal dominant disease with one parent affected is 50%.   *(2:542)*

393. **(B)** Autosomal dominant polycystic kidney disease does not typically cause renal disease prenatally therefore the amniotic fluid is normal. The kidneys may appear large and echogenic. Autosomal recessive polycystic kidney disease does affect renal function and is associated with oligohydramnios. Meckel's syndrome is associated with encephaloceles and postaxial polydactyly.   *(2:545)*

394. **(B)** Although kidneys grow throughout gestation, the ratio of kidneys to abdomen remains constant at 0.27–0.30.   *(2:519)*

395. **(C)** Unless the kidney is echogenic or obstructed, the anechoic cysts in the periphery represent normal renal pyramids.   *(3:518, 534)*

396. **(B)** Fetal urine production begins at 12 weeks, but the fetal kidneys do not produce the majority of the fetal urine until 16 weeks.   *(2:517; 6:296)*

397. **(A)** In PUV cases, the fetal bladder may rupture creating urine ascites.   *(2:532)*

398. **(D)** Although this is somewhat debated, many sources quote a number from 4–6 mm as the upper limit of normal in the second trimester.*(3:496, 2:520)*

399. **(B)** Grade 0—no dilation.   *(2:521)*

400. **(C)** Grade I—renal pelvic dilation with or without infundibula visible.   *(2:521)*

401. **(E)** Grade II—renal pelvic dilation with calices visible.   *(2:521)*

402. **(A)** Grade III—renal pelvis and calices dilated.
(2:521)

403. **(D)** Grade IV—renal pelvis and calices dilated with parenchymal thinning. *(2:521)*

404. **(C)** Because of its vascularity, the fetus may experience heart failure and polyhydramnios. On ultrasound, a congenital mesoblastic nephroma will resemble a Wilm's tumor. *(2:548)*

405. **(A)** A neuroblastoma appears as a suprarenal mass and should be considered when a mass is identified superior to the kidney. *(2:549)*

406. **(C)** Nephroblastoma, also known as Wilm's tumor, is a malignant renal tumor that sonographically appears similar to a mesoblastic nephroma.
(4:880–881)

407–410. See Fig. 9–47.

411. **(C)** A change in head shape, such as brachycephaly or dolicocephaly, affects accurate measurement in predicting gestational age. The degree to which fetal head shape affects BPD can be estimated with the formula:

$$CI = BPD/OFD \times 100 \qquad (7:438)$$

412. **(A)** Ovarian tumors account for 50–81% of torsion.
(2:872)

413. **(B)** Risks for ovarian hyperstimulation syndrome include: advanced maternal age, polycystic ovarian disease, oral contraceptives, and obesity. *(2:866)*

414. **(D)** Hyperstimulated ovaries produce large cysts that may torse, as well as cause fullness and nausea to the patient. Rarely, more severe complications can occur because of the shift in fluid resulting in ascites and effusions. *(2:866)*

415. **(D)** Torsed ovaries will appear edematous with a change in blood flow patterns. First is the loss of venous flow, followed by the lack of arterial flow in a complete ovarian torsion. *(3:800; 2:872)*

416. **(A)** Fibroids are estrogen dependent and will increase with pregnancy and decrease postmenopausally. *(2:841)*

417. **(B)** Fibroids are estrogen dependent and commonly increase in pregnancy and decrease postmenopausally. The only sonographic difference between a leiomyoma and a leiomyosarcoma is a rapid increase in growth. *(2:841)*

418. **(A)** On ultrasound, a leiomyoma and a leiomyosarcoma appear the same. Clinically, the only difference is a rapid increase in growth in postmenopausal women. *(2:841)*

419. **(C)** The fetal lung is isoechoic to the fetal liver in the second trimester. *(2:634)*

420. **(A)** Although the lung increases in echogenicity throughout the pregnancy, researchers have not been able to correlate the increase with lung maturity.
(2:634; 6:272)

421. **(D)** Visualization of the femoral epiphyseal plate is seen on fetuses with a gestational age greater than 33 weeks with 95% accuracy. *(2:632)*

422. **(A)** Polydactyly may be isolated or occur as part of a syndrome. The extra digit may have a bone or be soft tissue only. Postaxial refers to the ulnar aspect of the hand. *(2:362)*

423. **(B)** Polydactyly may be isolated or occur as part of a syndrome. The extra digit may have a bone or be soft tissue only. Preaxial refers to the radial aspect of the hand. *(2:362)*

424. **(B)** Discordance in dichorionic/diamniotic twins is more acceptable because of their different genetic makeup, provided that the smaller twin is not less than the 10th percentile in EFW. In monochorionic twins, EFW should be concordant and not differ by more than 20%. *(2:184)*

425. **(B)** Discordance in dichorionic/diamniotic twins is more acceptable because of their different genetic makeup, provided that the smaller twin is

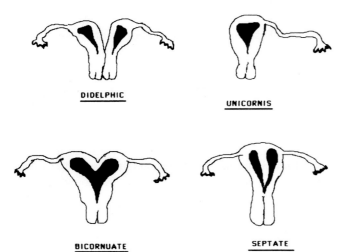

DIDELPHIC

UNICORNIS

BICORNUATE

SEPTATE

Figure 9–47. Diagram showing developmental anomalies of the uterus.

not less than the 10th percentile in EFW. In mono-chorionic twins, EFW should be concordant and not differ by more than 20%.   *(2:184)*

426.   **(C)** Twin fetal discordance is determined by subtracting the largest twin from the smallest twin and dividing by the largest twin. This number is multiplied by 100 to determine the percentage.   *(2:184)*

427.   **(D)** Frank breech is described as the buttocks descending first with the thighs and legs extending upward along the anterior fetal trunk.   *(7:445)*

428.   **(C)** Complete breech is described as the buttocks descending first with the knees flexed, and the fetus sitting cross-legged.   *(7:445)*

429.   **(A)** A footling breech is when one or both feet are prolapsed into the lower uterine segment.   *(7:445)*

430.   **(C)** XY karyotype indicates a male fetus. XX karyotype indicates a female fetus. Down syndrome is labeled 47, +21, and Turner syndrome is labeled 45X.   *(2:20–21)*

431.   **(B)** XY karyotype indicates a male fetus. XX karyotype indicates a female fetus. Down syndrome is labeled 47, +21, and Turner syndrome in labeled 45X.   *(2:20–21)*

432.   **(B)** A membrane may be present with a dichorionic/diamniotic or monochorionic/diamniotic pregnancy. A zygocity indicator would be fetal genders (if different).   *(1:28)*

433.   **(C)** The fetus (regardless of the body part), as well as the sac, closest to the internal os is labeled fetus A.   *(6:467)*

434.   **(A)** The fetus would be lying on its right side, with left side closest to the maternal abdominal wall.   *(7:432)*

435.   **(A)** The fetus would be lying on its right side, with the left side closest to the maternal abdominal wall.   *(7:432)*

436.   **(A)** The fetus would be lying on its right side, with the left side closest to the maternal abdominal wall.   *(7:432)*

437.   **(C)** Placental lakes are areas of fibrin under the chorion, on the fetal side of the placenta. They carry no clinical significance.   *(2:603)*

438.   **(D)** Hypertension and maternal smoking can cause the placenta to undergo early maturation. Smoking can cause an increase in calcifications in the placenta. Unfortunately, placenta maturation has not proved to be a reliable tool in assessing placental function or fetal well-being.   *(2:604)*

439.   **(D)** Triploidy from the paternal component, presents with a large cystic placenta.   *(2:599; 6:421)*

440.   **(D)** Maternal hypertension can cause a restrictive flow in the uterine vessels, which in turn, may decrease the placental perfusion.   *(2:599; 6:421)*

441.   **(D)** Gestational diabetes mellitus is a cause for macrosomia because of the increased maternal blood sugars.   *(2:215)*

442.   **(A)** Studies have shown a 22% rate of congenital abnormalities if hemoglobin (a reflection of blood sugar control) was >8.5% before 14 weeks. A 3% rate of congenital abnormalities was reported if hemoglobin was <8.5%.   *(1:540)*

443.   **(A)** Caudal regression syndrome is associated with insulin-dependent diabetes mellitus in up to 16% of the cases. It is thought to occur with poor glucose control in the first trimester. Findings include sacral agenesis, spinal, and lower limb abnormalities, femoral hypoplasia, GI and GU abnormalities.   *(2:364–366)*

444.   **(D)** Other findings of caudal regression syndrome may include renal, gastrointestinal, facial, and spinal abnormalities.   *(2:365)*

445.   **(B)** The only definitive test for any chromosomal abnormality is karyotyping of fetal cells.   *(2:21)*

446.   **(E)** The phenotype for Turner syndrome is 45X, indicating only one single X, or female, chromosomes.   *(2:21)*

447.   **(A)** If the diabetic mother has significant vascular disease as a component of her diabetes, it may cause intrauterine growth retardation in the fetus.   *(3:543)*

448.   **(E)** Caudal regression syndrome and cardiac defects are first trimester insults and a risk of occurrence increases with increasing blood sugar levels in the first trimester. Shoulder dystocia can occur with delivery of macrosomic fetuses.   *(3:544)*

449.   **(D)** Depending on the fetal gestational age, lung maturity amniocentesis may be performed to assure lung maturation before delivery. In cases of complete PROM, often there is not an adequate sample of amniotic fluid available for maturity testing.   *(2:628)*

450.   **(D)** Although an increased AFV is associated with macrosomia, it is not a direct assessment of macrosomia.   *(3:544)*

451. **(D)** CVS and PUBS may be performed provided the placenta or umbilical cord are accessible. If the fetal bladder is full, as in cases of PUV syndrome, fetal urine may be tested for karyotype.   *(2:32)*

452. **(E)** Amniocentesis can be used to test the level of fetal bilirubin, infection, and for a limited amount of short limb syndromes.   *(2:33, 566)*

453. **(C)** Hypertension can affect the vascular bed of the placenta resulting in intrauterine growth retardation.   *(2:214)*

454. **(A)** Excessive maternal smoking has been linked to accelerated maturation of the placenta. It is not predictive, however, in actual placenta perfusion to the fetus.   *(6:420)*

455. **(C)** BBOW, bulging bag of water, refers to the amniotic membrane bulging into the vagina.   *(13:156)*

456. **(D)** PROM, premature rupture of membranes, is the rupture of membranes before 37 weeks.   *(2:588)*

457. **(E)** All of the above. Overdistension of the urinary bladder can result in serious diagnostic error. Overdistension of the urinary bladder may result in closure of an incompetent cervix due to bladder compression on the cervix; placenta previa caused by bladder compression on the lower uterine segment; closure of the gestational sac caused by bladder compression that causes both sides of the sac walls to meet resulting in a loss of the anechoic center or a change in sac shape (distortion); nonvisualization of the internal iliac vein because of displacement.   *(7:432)*

458. **(C)** Ovulation occurs approximately 14 days after the first day of the last menstrual period.   *(7:432)*

459. **(C)** Gravida is a woman who is pregnant.   *(7:435)*

460. **(A)** Multipara is a woman who has given birth two or more times.   *(7:435)*

461. **(D)** Nullipara is a woman who has never given birth to a viable infant.   *(7:435)*

462. **(H)** Primipara is woman who has given birth one time to a viable infant, regardless of whether the child was living at birth and regardless of whether the birth was single or multiple.   *(7:435)*

463. **(B)** Nulligravida is a woman who has never been pregnant.   *(7:435)*

464. **(E)** Primigravida is a woman who is pregnant for the first time.   *(7:435)*

465. **(F)** Multigravida is a woman who has been pregnant several times.   *(7:435)*

466. **(G)** Para is the number of pregnancies that have continued to viability.   *(7:435)*

467. **(I)** Trimester is a 3-month period during gestation.   *(7:435)*

468. **(D)** The puerperium period begins with the expulsion of the placenta and continues until maternal physiology and anatomy return to a prepregnancy level, approximately 6–8 weeks.   *(6:533)*

469. **(B)** Sonographic assessment of the maternal kidneys and bowel would not be considered a gynecological sonogram.   *(6:533)*

470. **(B)** It is possible to ovulate during lactation. The risk of ovulation in the first 6 months while breast feeding is 1–5%.   *(12:692)*

471. **(D)** The ovaries are least likely to be seen on a postpartum pelvic sonogram. This may be because of extrapelvic position of the ovaries caused by the large uterus.   *(7:438)*

472. **(D)** The uterus has a dramatic decrease in size and returns to a position between the symphysis pubis and umbilicus.   *(6:533)*

473. **(E)** Hemorrhage, thromboembolism, and infection are the most common complications during the postpartum period. Placenta previa is an antepartum complication.   *(7:438)*

474. **(A)** A cesarean section scar will appear at the cervicocorpus junction on the anterior myometrial wall.   *(3:749)*

475. **(C)** 25% of fetuses are breech at 28 weeks, 7% at 32 weeks, and 3–4% at term.   *(9:451)*

476. **(A)** The incidence of abnormalities in a breech fetus is 6.3% versus 2.4% in a vertex fetus.   *(9:451)*

477. **(C)** VBAC is a commonly used abbreviation for vaginal birth after cesarean section.   *(12:370)*

478. **(C)** Although adhesions cannot be seen on ultrasound, occasionally changes related to previous cesarean sections may be appreciated. These changes are found in the lower uterine segment and may include thinning, ballooning, and wedge defects. A thin uterine wall is felt to be at increased risk for uterine rupture.   *(3:749)*

479. **(D)** Placenta previa is the implantation of the placenta in the lower uterine segment.   *(7:438)*

480. (A) Placenta accreta is the abnormal adherence of part or all of the placenta to the uterine wall.
(7:439)

481. (C) Placenta succenturiata is an accessory lobe of placenta.
(7:439)

482. (B) Abruptio placentae is the premature separation of the placenta after 20 weeks of gestation.
(7:439)

483. (E) Placenta increta is the abnormal adherence of part or all of the placenta in which the chorionic villi invade the myometrium.
(7:439)

484. (F) Placenta percreta is the abnormal adherence of part or all of the placenta in which the chorionic villi invade the uterine wall.
(7:439)

485. (A) The fetal component of the placenta.
(7:447)

486. (B) The maternal component of the placenta.
(7:447)

487. (A) Sonographic fetal HELLP findings include IUGR, oligohydramnios, and possible signs of fetal distress (poor BPP, abnormal UC Dopplers for example).
(2:86)

488. (D) Parvovirus, CMV, and HIV are all infections that may be transmitted across the placenta.
(2:566–568)

489. (B) Varicella-zoster is also known as chicken pox.
(3:676)

490. (D) With a maternal CMV infection, the risk of transmission to the fetus is 40–50%, regardless of gestational age.
(2:567)

491. (A) Infections, regardless of the type, present in the fetus with the same spectrum of sonographic findings. These may be IUGR, oligohydramnios, ventriculomegaly, microcephaly, and nonimmune hydrops fetalis.
(2:567)

492. (D) Parvovirus have also be referred to as 5th's disease and "slapped cheek" disease.
(12:1225)

493. (D) In the case of IUGR, the fetus will direct more blood flow to the brain. This will lower the PI and S/D ratio of the middle cerebral artery (MCA). More recently, multiple studies have been conducted showing that the peak velocity of the MCA is a good predictor of fetal anemia. The peak velocity is measured and plotted of a curve to determine whether the fetus is in need of a fetal blood transfusion because of fetal anemia.
(2:689–690, 11:13)

494. (B) Androblastoma, fibroma, thecoma, and granulosa cell are all sex cord-stromal tumors, with fibromas being the most common.
(2:881)

495. (C) Dysgerminoma is one of the most common malignant tumors of pregnancy. Granulosa cell and thecoma tumors typically occur postmenopausally, and fibromas usually occur in the 5–6th decade.
(2:881)

496. (D) Sex cord-stromal tumors are: fibroma, thecoma, granulosa cell, and androblastoma (Seroli–Leydig cell). They appear hypoechoic to echogenic with a mixed heterogeneous pattern and appear similar to each other on ultrasound.
(2:874, 877)

497. (A) An endometrioma may have a variety of appearances, but primarily appears as a cystic to hypoechoic mass with internal echoes or debris layering consistent with blood. Teratomas also have a variety of appearances, but can be hypoechoic with internal echoes and a layering of debris.
(1:Table 9–4)

498. (A) A hydrosalpinx may initially look like a cystic mass with septations. On closer examination, the septations are not complete. The sonographer is able to follow the connection of the cystic spaces. This assumes that the structure is tubular and communicates as with hydrosalpinx.
(2:870)

499. (D) A paraovarian, or mesonephric cyst originates from the mesonephric duct. A paraovarian cyst may form, regardless of uterine or ovarian status. Ovarian tissue does occasionally remain after an oophorectomy, especially if adhesions were present. The remaining ovarian tissue can still function and produce a cyst. It is called ovarian remnant syndrome and should be considered with any cystic mass identified in a postoophorectomy patient.
(2:867–868)

500. (C) Hydatid of Morgagni is the most common paramesonephric cyst. It measures 2–10 mm and appears similar to ovarian cysts.
(2:868)

501. (A)
(2:861)

502. (D) The image is a Dandy–Walker malformation. The cerebellum is splayed, and the vermis is absent. There is communication with the fourth ventricle.
(1:20)

REFERENCES

1. Krebs C. *Appleton & Lange's Review for the Ultrasonography Examination.* 3rd ed. New York: Appleton & Lange; 2001.

2. Callen PW. *Ultrasonography in Obstetrics and Gynecology.* 4th ed. Philadelphia: WB Saunders; 2000.

3. Fleischer A, Manning F, Jeanty P, Romero R. *Sonography in Obstetrics and Gynecology: Principles and Practice.* 5th ed. Stamford, CT: Appleton & Lange; 1996.

4. Bianchi DW, Cromblelholme TM, D'Alton ME. *Fetalogy: Diagnosis and Management of the Fetal Patient.* New York: McGraw-Hill; 2000.

5. Nyberg D, Mahony B, Pretorius D. *Diagnostic Ultrasound of Fetal Anomalies.* St. Louis, MO: Mosby-Year Book; 1990.

6. Berman MC, Cohen HL. *Obstetrics and Gynecology.* 2nd ed. Philadelphia: Lippincott; 1997.

7. Odwin CS, Dubinsky T, Fleischer AC. *Appleton & Lange's Review for the Ultrasonography Examination.* 2nd ed. Norwalk, CT: Appleton & Lange; 1993.

8. Moore TR, Cayle JE. The amniotic fluid index in normal human pregnancy. *Am J Obstet Gynecol.* 1990;162: 1168–1173.

9. Zuspan F, Quilligan E, Blumenfeld M. *Handbook of Obstetrics, Gynecology, and Primary Care.* St. Louis, MO: Mosby-Year Book; 1998.

10. Tortaora GJ, Anagnostakos NP: *Principles of Anatomy and Physiology.* 5th ed. New York: Harper and Row; 1987.

11. Mari G, et. al. *Proceedings SMFM.* Miami Beach, FL, January 2000.

12. Gabbe S, Niebyl J, Simpson JL. *Obstetrics: Normal and Problem Pregnancies.* New York: Churchill Livingstone; 1996.

13. Thomas C. *Taber's Cyclopedic Medical Dictionary.* Philadelphia: F.A. Davis; 1982.

CHAPTER 10

FETAL ECHOCARDIOGRAPHY

Julia A. Drose and Teresa M. Bieker

Study Guide

INTRODUCTION

Congenital heart disease is a leading cause of infant mortality, with a reported incidence of approximately 1 in 100 live births.[1] However, these numbers are based on live born infants, and therefore, probably underestimate the true incidence in the fetus.[2] Early fetal loss and stillbirths are often the result of complex cardiac defects or chromosomal defects, which have an associated heart defect. For this reason, the incidence of congenital heart disease in the fetus has been reported to be as much as five times that found in live born children[1] (Table 10–1).

In utero diagnosis of congenital heart disease allows a variety of treatment options to be considered, including delivery at an appropriate facility, termination, and in some cases, in utero therapy.[3] Conversely, a normal fetal echocardiogram in the setting of an increased risk factor provides reassurance for both the patient and physician.

INSTRUMENTATION AND TECHNIQUE

The AIUM Technical Bulletin on the performance of a basic fetal cardiac ultrasound recommends that a four-chamber view and both the right and left ventricular outflow tracts, be obtained on all obstetrical ultrasound exams.[4] Evaluation of a four-chamber view alone may substantially decrease the detection rate of major cardiac malformations.

When risk factors increase the likelihood of congenital heart disease, a formal fetal echocardiogram should be performed.

Various reports advocate evaluation of the fetal heart at different gestational ages;[5] however, the AIUM Technical Bulletin recommends that fetal echocardiographic exams be performed between 18 and 22 weeks gestation.[4] During this period, optimum image quality and, therefore, diagnostic accuracy is achieved. It should be borne in mind that even at 18 weeks gestation, the fetal heart is a very small structure. Before this age, many cardiac structures may be too small to evaluate accurately, even with endovaginal scan-

ning.[6] In addition, cardiac lesions such as coarctation of the aorta and hypoplastic left heart syndrome may be progressive lesions.[7] Therefore, scanning the fetus too early in gestation may result in a false-negative diagnosis.

Later in gestation, the echocardiographic exam may be hindered by increased attenuation from the fetal skull, ribs, spine, and limbs, as well as decreased amniotic fluid as pregnancy progresses.[6]

Equipment

Fetal echocardiography requires the use of high-resolution ultrasound equipment.[8] Preferred transducer frequencies usually range from 5 MHz to 7 MHz, depending on gestational age, maternal body habitus, and the amount of amniotic fluid present. Equipment utilized for fetal echocardiography should have M-mode, and pulsed Doppler capabilities to provide physiologic assessment, as well as color Doppler capabilities to assess spatial and directional information. All of these modalities are vital to performing a complete and accurate examination.

Indications

A family history of congenital heart disease is the most common indication to perform a fetal echocardiogram. Recurrence risk for fetuses varies depending on the type of lesion and their relationship to the affected relative.

The risk of congenital heart disease for a fetus with an affected sibling is approximately 2%–4%.[9–10] If two or more siblings are affected, this risk increases to approximately 10% (Table 10–2). When the mother of the fetus has a congenital heart abnormality, the recurrence risk is also approximately 10–12%.[10] An affected father carries a lower risk (Table 10–3).[9–10]

Exposure to known cardiac teratogens also increases the risk of having a fetus with a cardiac defect.[11] The list of substances considered teratogenic is extensive.[12] Specific occurrence risk varies with length and type of exposure as well as the specific substance involved.

Chromosomal abnormalities have been reported to occur in 13% of live born infants with a congenital heart defect.[13,14]

TABLE 10-1. FREQUENCY OF CONGENITAL HEART LESIONS AMONG AFFECTED ABORTUSES AND STILLBORN INFANTS

Defect	Frequency (%)
Ventricular septal defect	35.7
Coarctation of the aorta	8.9
Atrial septal defect	8.2
Atrioventricular septal defect	6.7
Tetralogy of Fallot	6.2
Single ventricle	4.8
Truncus arteriosus	4.8
Hypoplastic left heart	4.6
Complete transposition of the great arteries	4.3
Double outlet right ventricle	2.4
Hypoplastic right heart	1.7
Single atrium	1.2
Pulmonic stenosis	0.7
Aortic stenosis	0.5
Miscellaneous	10.6

(Modified from: Hoffman JIE. Incidence of congenital heart disease: II. Prenatal incidence. *Pediatr Cardiol.* 1995; 16:155–165.)

The incidence of abnormal karyotype in the fetus with a congenital heart abnormality is approximately 35%.[2,15]

The specific type and occurrence risk of a congenital heart defect varies depending on the chromosomal abnormality. Trisomy 21 is associated with a 40–50% occurrence of congenital heart disease,[13] whereas, in trisomy 13 and trisomy 18, the association is almost 100%.[16] As with teratogenic agents, the list of abnormal karyotypes and syndromes associated with cardiac defects is extensive.[12]

Several maternal conditions may also carry an inherent risk to the fetus. Congenital heart disease is increased fivefold among infants of diabetic mothers,[17] whereas phenylketonuria has a reported risk of 12–16%.[18]

TABLE 10-2. RECURRENCE RISK IN SIBLINGS FOR ANY CONGENITAL HEART DEFECT

| Defect | Suggested Risk % ||
	If One Sibling Affected	If Two Siblings Affected
Aortic stenosis	2	6
Atrial septal defect	2.5	8
Atrioventricular canal	3	10
Coarctation of the aorta	2	6
Ebstein anomaly	1	3
Endocardial fibroelastosis	4	12
Hypoplastic left heart	2	6
Pulmonary atresia	1	3
Pulmonary stenosis	2	6
Tetralogy of Fallot	2.5	8
Transposition	1.5	5
Tricuspid atresia	1	3
Truncus arteriosus	1	3
Ventricular septal defect	3	10

(Adapted from Nora JJ, Fraser FC, Bear J, et al. *Medical Genetics: Principles and Practice.* 4th ed. Philadelphia: Lea & Febiger; 1994:371.)

TABLE 10-3. SUGGESTED OFFSPRING RECURRENCE RISK FOR CONGENITAL HEART DEFECTS GIVEN ONE AFFECTED PARENT (%)

| Defect | Suggested Risk % ||
	Father Affected	Mother Affected
Aortic stenosis	3	13–18
Atrial septal defect	1.5	4–4.5
Atrioventricular canal	1	14
Coarctation of the aorta	2	4
Pulmonary stenosis	2	4–6.5
Tetralogy of Fallot	1.5	2.5
Ventricular septal defect	2	6–10

(Adapted from Nora JJ, Fraser FC, Bear J, et al. *Medical Genetics: Principles and Practice.* 4th ed. Philadelphia: Lea & Febiger; 1994:371.)

Complete heart block in the fetus is associated with maternal collagen vascular disease (systemic lupus erythematosus). In these patients, circulating antinuclear antibodies of the SSA or SSB types damage the developing conduction tissue.[19]

Maternal infections such as human parvovirus and cytomegalovirus also have a reported association with cardiac defects in the fetus.[20]

Another indication for performing a fetal echocardiogram is the presence of extracardiac anomalies in a fetus.[21] The overall incidence of extracardiac malformations in children identified as having a congenital heart abnormality ranges from 25–45% (Table 10–4).[21] Cardiac abnor-

TABLE 10-4. INCIDENCE (%) OF ASSOCIATED CONGENITAL HEART DEFECTS OCCURRING WITH EXTRACARDIAC MALFORMATIONS IN INFANTS

System or Lesion	Frequency of CHD (%)
Central nervous system	
Hydrocephalus	4.5–14.8
Dandy–Walker malformation	2.5–4.3
Agenesis of the corpus callosum	14.9
Meckel–Gruber syndrome	13.8
Gastrointestinal	
Tracheoesophageal fistula	14.7–39.2
Duodenal atresia	17.1
Jejunal atresia	5.2
Anorectal anomalies	22
Imperforate anus	11.7
Ventral wall	
Omphalocele	19.5–32
Gastroschesis	0–7.7
Diaphragmatic hernia	9.6–22.9
Genitourinary	
Renal agenesis (bilateral)	42.8
Renal agenesis (unilateral)	16.9
Horseshoe kidney	38.8
Renal dysplasia	5.4
Ureteral obstruction	2.1

(Modified from: Copel JA, Pilu G, Kleinman CS. Congenital heart disease and extracardiac anomalies: associations and indications for fetal echocardiography. *Am J Obstet Gynecol.* 1986; 154:1121–1132.)

malities such as atrioventricular septal defects are associated with extracardiac defects in more than 50% of cases, while atrial septal defects, ventricular septal defects, tetralogy of Fallot, and cardiac malpositions are associated with extracardiac malformations in about 30% of cases.[21]

A suspected structural or rhythm abnormality seen in the fetal heart on a routine obstetrical examination should also warrant a formal fetal echocardiogram to rule out an underlying structural abnormality or, in some cases, to implement in utero therapy.

Nonimmune hydrops fetalis is also an indication for fetal echocardiography. In some cases, it may reflect structural heart disease, while in others, it is the result of a dysrhythmia.[19] Finally, massive polyhydramnios is a recognized indication for fetal echocardiography.[19] An increase in amniotic fluid may be the result of congestive heart failure, but it is more likely related to associated defects in the fetus, such as those that cause difficulty in swallowing or compression of the esophagus. Although there are several predisposing indications to perform a fetal echocardiogram, up to 90% of congenital heart disease occurs in unselected "normal" obstetric patients.[1] Therefore, routine obstetric scanning should identify the majority of fetuses with cardiac lesions that will need a formal fetal echocardiogram.

Position

A fetal echocardiographic exam should always begin by determining fetal position. Unlike a pediatric or adult patient, the fetus cannot be placed in a standard position, nor can the heart be evaluated consistently from routine angles. Although the fetus may move throughout the exam, establishing basic position will allow the examiner to identify various cardiac structures more quickly.[6] Once fetal position is determined, the location and orientation of the heart should be established. In a cross-sectional transverse view of the fetal chest, the correct orientation for the fetal heart is with the apex pointing to the left and the bulk of the heart occupying the left chest. The normal angle of the fetal heart, relative to midline is 45 ± 20°.[22] The left atrium should be located closest to the fetal spine and the right ventricle nearest to the anterior chest wall. This normal orientation is termed levocardia.

The normal fetal heart should occupy approximately one-third of the fetal thorax.[23] Fetal cardiac size can be calculated by measuring the diameter or the circumference of the heart and comparing it to the diameter or circumference of the fetal chest, respectively. When calculating this ratio, both measurements must be obtained from the same image.

Scanning Technique

The first view to obtain when beginning a fetal echocardiographic examination, is the four-chamber view.[12] There are two different four-chamber views. The apical four-chamber view and the subcostal four-chamber view. The apical four-chamber view is obtained in a transverse view of the fetal chest, with the transducer imaging the fetal heart from either the anterior or posterior aspect.

In the apical four-chamber view, the interventricular and interatrial septae are perpendicular to the transducer (Fig. 10–1). From this projection, all four cardiac chambers can be visualized. In addition, color and/or pulsed Doppler interrogation of the mitral and tricuspid valves can be performed. Doppler should be performed on the atrial side of the valves to assess for valvular insufficiency; whereas, Doppler distal to the valves should be done to evaluate for stenosis or atresia. The two superior pulmonary veins should also be identified entering the left atrium from this projection. The two inferior pulmonary veins are usually not visualized on a fetal echocardiogram.

The apical four-chamber view is not optimal for evaluating the interventricular septum. In this view, the angle of incidence of the sound beam is parallel to the interventricular septum, and may result in an artifactual dropout of echoes at the level of the membranous portion, simulating a "pseudo" septal defect (Fig. 10–2).[24]

By sliding the transducer cephalad from an apical four-chamber view, the aorta and pulmonary artery should be visualized side by side (Fig. 10–3). This confirms that both are present and normally of equal size.

The subcostal four-chamber view is obtained by imaging the fetal chest in a transverse projection from the anterior chest wall and angling the transducer slightly cephalad (Fig. 10–4). This view also allows identification and comparison of both atria and ventricles. It is ideal for obtaining M-mode measurements of the ventricles and interventricular septum by placing an M-mode cursor perpendicular to the septum at the level of the atrioventricular valves (Fig. 10–5).

Atrial measurements can be obtained by moving the M-mode cursor through both atria. The subcostal four-chamber view is also preferable for evaluating a fetal dysrhythmia by placing the M-mode cursor through an atrial wall and a ventricular wall simultaneously (Fig. 10–6). This allows visualization of the timing of dysrhythmic events and may aid in making a definitive diagnosis.

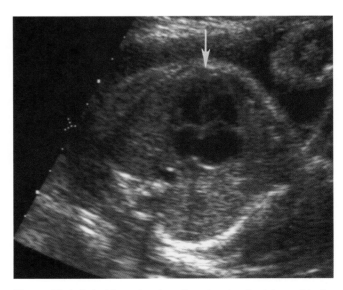

Figure 10–1. Apical four-chamber view showing the interventricular and interatrial septae perpendicular to the transducer. Arrow = apex of heart.

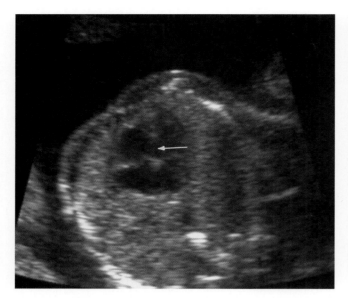

Figure 10–2. Apical four-chamber view showing a "pseudo" interventricular septal defect (arrow), caused by the septum being parallel to the sound beam.

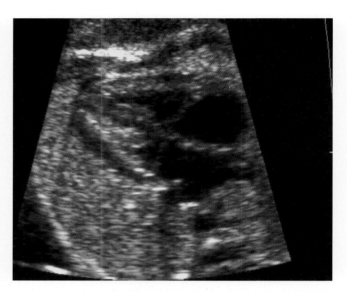

Figure 10–4. Subcostal four-chamber view with the interventricular and interatrial septae perpendicular to the sound beam.

Either pulsed Doppler or color Doppler can be used to evaluate the foramen ovale in this projection. Documentation of flow from the right atrium to the left atrium by either modality rules out restriction of the foraminal flap (Fig. 10–7). It is also valuable in assessing altered flow direction secondary to a structural defect. A spectral Doppler tracing will display normal foraminal flow as being twice the fetal heart rate.

The interventricular septum is best evaluated in the subcostal four-chamber view. Color Doppler is the best means of achieving this because it allows a large area to be evaluated simultaneously (Fig. 10–8). Pulsed Doppler may

not detect flow across a septal defect if the sample volume is not precisely located.

Larger ventricular septal defects may be detected with gray scale imaging alone; however, many remain undetected by any means. Even when a ventricular septal defect is present, the pressures in the fetal heart are such that no flow may be appreciated across the interventricular septum.

Obtaining a subcostal four-chamber view is critical in performing a complete fetal echocardiogram. By angling the transducer systematically toward the fetal right shoulder from this view, most of the remaining fetal heart views are obtained.

A slight angulation from the subcostal four-chamber view toward the fetal right shoulder will result in visualization of a long-axis view of the proximal aorta. In this

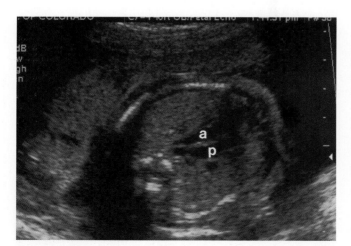

Figure 10–3. The aorta (a) and pulmonary artery (p) can be seen as two parallel structures by angling the transducer cephalad from the apical four-chamber view. This view allows you to confirm that both great vessels are present and are of similar size.

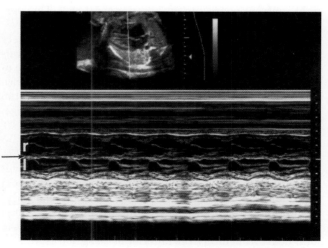

Figure 10–5. M-mode tracing of the right (r) and left (l) ventricles at the level of the atrioventricular valves. Arrow = IVS.

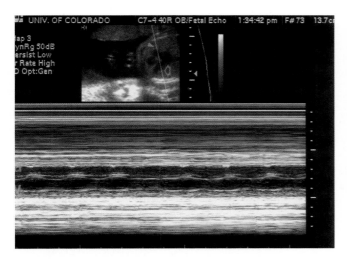

Figure 10–6. M-mode tracing through the right atrial (a, arrowhead) and left ventricular (v, open arrow) wall simultaneously to assess the response of each in the setting of a dysrhythmia.

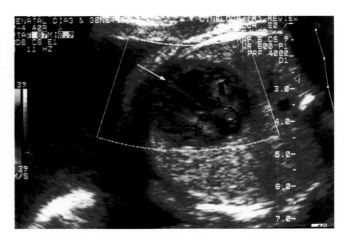

Figure 10–8. Color Doppler image showing no flow crossing the intact interventricular septum (arrow).

view, continuity of the anterior wall of the aorta with the interventricular septum and the posterior wall with the anterior leaflet of the mitral valve can by determined (Fig. 10–9). The aortic valve can be interrogated with pulsed Doppler in this view, both proximally looking for aortic insufficiency, and distally to detect stenosis or atresia.

The long-axis view of the aorta also provides another means of evaluating a dysrhythmia. By utilizing a wide sample gate and placing the pulsed Doppler cursor between the mitral and aortic valves, both left ventricular inflow and outflow can be evaluated simultaneously (Fig. 10–10). The inflow through the mitral valve will reflect rhythm disturbances occurring in the atria; whereas, the left ventricular outflow through the aorta reflects the ventricular response. Being able to visualize both events simultaneously may help in differentiating the type of dysrhythmia present.

The right ventricular outflow tract is visualized next by rotating the transducer further in the direction of the fetal right shoulder. In the normal fetus, this view demonstrates the pulmonary artery coursing cephalad, leftward, and posteriorly from the right ventricle (Fig. 10–11). The course of the pulmonary artery should cross the aorta in the normal fetus. In other words, by angling the transducer from the long-axis view of the aorta to the long-axis view of the pulmonary, the great vessels should "criss-cross" directions if they are correctly oriented. Color and/or pulsed Doppler are again used in this projection to evaluate the valve proximally for pulmonic insufficiency and distally for pulmonic stenosis or atresia.

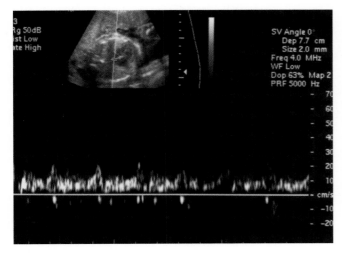

Figure 10–7. Pulsed Doppler tracing of the foramen ovale documenting flow from the right atrium into the left atrium.

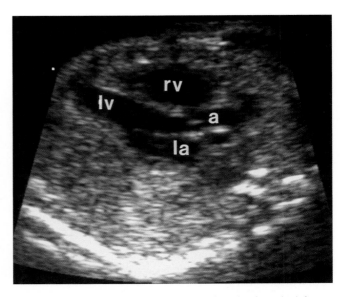

Figure 10–9. Long-axis view of the aorta (a) arising from the left ventricle (lv). Continuity can be appreciated between the anterior wall of the aorta and the interventricular septum, and the posterior wall of the aorta with the anterior leaflet of the mitral valve. rv = right ventricle, la = left atrium.

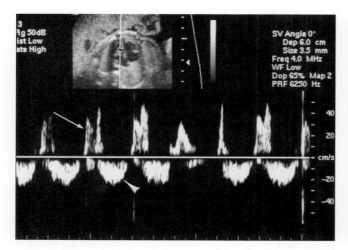

Figure 10–10. Pulsed Doppler tracing showing the mitral valve inflow (arrow) simultaneously with the aortic valve (arrowhead) outflow.

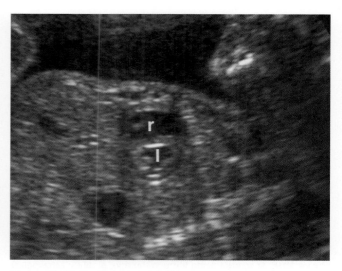

Figure 10–12. Sagittal view of the fetus, showing a short-axis view of the right (r) and left (l) ventricles.

A further rightward rotation of the transducer will result in a sagittal view of the fetal thorax and thus a short-axis view through the ventricles (Fig. 10–12). The echogenic moderator band should be apparent near the apex to help in identifying the right ventricle.

The short-axis view of the ventricles is useful for obtaining measurements of the ventricular free walls and interventricular septum, as well as chamber size. Color Doppler should be used in this view to again evaluate the interventricular septum for defects. With the color Doppler activated, the ventricles should be scanned from the apex to the level of the atrioventricular valves. If color is seen crossing the septum, pulsed Doppler can be used to confirm a septal defect.

From the short-axis view of the ventricles, a short-axis view of the great vessels can be obtained by angling the transducer slightly toward the fetal left shoulder (Fig. 10–13). In this view, the aorta appears as a circular structure with the pulmonary artery draping over it. The aortic, pulmonic, and tricuspid valves are usually well visualized in this projection. The main pulmonary artery can often be seen bifurcating into the ductus arteriosus and the right pulmonary artery. This view provides a reasonable angle

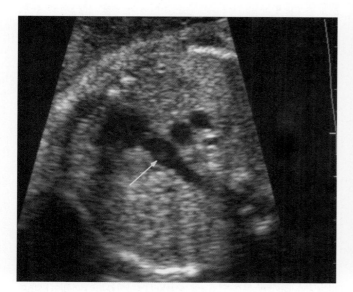

Figure 10–11. Continuous angulation of the transducer toward the fetal right shoulder from the long-axis view of the aorta, results in a long-axis view of the pulmonary artery (arrow) arising from the right ventricle.

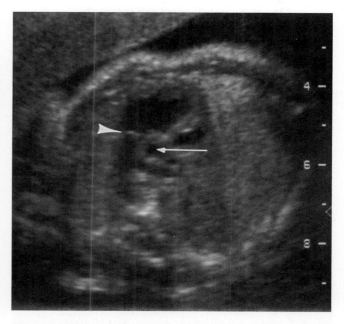

Figure 10–13. Angulation toward the fetus's left shoulder from the short-axis view of the ventricles (Fig. 10–12), results in a short-axis view of the great vessels. The pulmonary artery (arrowhead) can be seen normally draping over the aorta (arrow).

from which the pulmonary and tricuspid valves can be interrogated with pulsed Doppler for insufficiency or stenosis or atresia.

Simultaneous M-mode through the aorta, and left atrium (which will be below the aorta in this projection) is another useful method for evaluating fetal dysrhythmias (Fig. 10–14). The atrial contraction will be depicted in atrial wall movement, while the ventricular response is reflected in the motion of the aortic valve.

In the normal heart, the short-axis view of the great vessels confirms the perpendicular relationship of the aorta to the pulmonary artery, thereby excluding such defects as complete or *d*-transposition of the great arteries or truncus arteriosus.

The aortic arch view is obtained from a sagittal plane of the fetal torso, with the transducer angled from the left shoulder to the right hemithorax. The aortic arch can be differentiated from the flatter, broader, more caudally located ductal arch by identifying the three brachiocephalic vessels arising from its superior aspect (Fig. 10–15). The aortic arch has been described as having a rounded "candy cane" appearance.[23]

Pulsed Doppler should be used to evaluate the arch from the aortic valve to the descending aorta, looking for areas of increased or decreased velocities. Of particular importance is the section of the arch between the origin of the left subclavian artery and the insertion of the ductus arteriosus, as this is where most in utero coarctations occur. It should be borne in mind, however, that diagnosis of coarctation of the aorta is extremely difficult, and a coarctation may be present even in the setting of a normal appearing aortic arch, with normal velocities. When evaluating the aortic arch, it is also important to remember to confirm a left-sided location of the descending aorta.

The ductal arch view is obtained by returning to a more anteroposterior axis of the thorax. It is often helpful to image the short-axis view of the great vessels and then angle

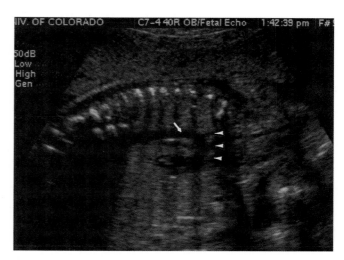

Figure 10–15. Sagittal view of the aortic arch (arrow) with the three brachiocephalic vessels (arrowheads) arising from it.

the transducer slightly until the pulmonary artery/ductus arteriosus confluence connects with the descending aorta (Fig. 10–16). The ductal arch has a flatter appearance than the aortic arch. It is often referred to as having a "hockey stick" appearance.[23] The ductal arch comprises the pulmonary artery, ductus arteriosus, and the descending aorta.

The final view that should be obtained is the right atrial inflow view, allowing visualization of the inferior and superior vena cavae. This is achieved by sliding the transducer rightward from the aortic arch, while remaining in a sagittal plane of the fetus (Fig. 10–17).

Pulsed Doppler

Pulsed Doppler substantially enhances the ability to detect cardiac malformations in utero. It is an effective means of quantitating flow velocity in the cardiac vessels and across the heart valves, as well as determining flow direction. It is also a useful adjunct in differentiating dysrhythmias.[19]

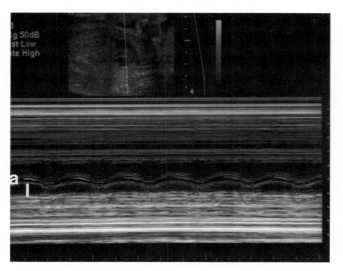

Figure 10–14. Simultaneous M-mode through the aorta (a) and the left atrium (l) is a useful means of assessing a dysrhythmia.

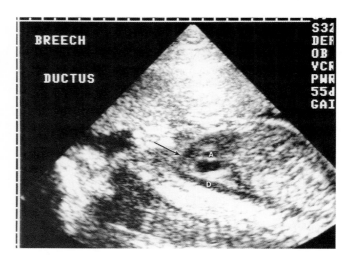

Figure 10–16. Sagittal view of the ductal arch (arrow) with a flatter appearance than the aortic arch. A = aorta, D = descending aorta.

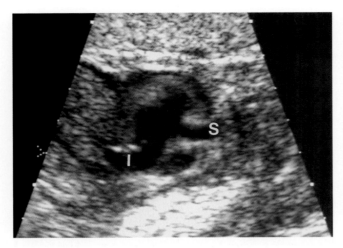

Figure 10–17. Right atrial inflow view showing the inferior vena cava (I) and the superior vena cava (S) entering the right atrium.

In a standard fetal echocardiogram, pulsed Doppler should be used to evaluate all four cardiac valves, both proximal and distal to the valve. Pulsed Doppler interrogation of the foramen ovale should be done to document the presence of flow into the left atrium. The ductus arteriosus and aortic arch should also be interrogated to document the presence and normality of flow. In addition, pulsed Doppler of the pulmonary veins can be used to confirm their presence and course into the left atrium.

Technical factors to consider include attempting to place the Doppler cursor in the area of interest at an angle as close to 0° as possible by using transducer angulation and the angle correction capabilities of the equipment used. The sample gate should be set small enough so that interference from wall noise and transmitted flow from adjoining vessels or valves can be minimized. Wall filter should be set to eliminate unnecessary noise without losing essential low flow information, and velocity scale should be set to record maximum velocities accurately.

Color Doppler

Color Doppler also plays an essential role in fetal echocardiography by providing a more efficient and expedient means of assessing normal and abnormal flow patterns in the fetal heart. Color Doppler supplies information on the presence or absence of flow, flow direction, and flow patterns. By superimposing color over the gray-scale image, morphologic and hemodynamic information can be assessed simultaneously.

Color Doppler allows visualization of flow in entire structures, such as the aortic arch, thus making it much more time efficient than pulsed Doppler. This efficiency is also prudent when imaging a fetus because color Doppler imaging produces lower peak intensities than pulsed Doppler.

Color Doppler can simplify the investigation of valvular stenosis or insufficiency, again, by sampling a large area and identifying areas of turbulence or flow reversal. In some cases, color may aid in visualizing such cardiac structures as the outflow tracts, which may be difficult to see with gray-scale imaging alone. Also, it may occasionally lead to detection of an abnormality not obvious on the gray-scale image, such as valvular stenosis, small VSDs, and flow reversal within the aortic and ductal arches.

Equipment used for fetal echocardiography should have specific fetal cardiac capabilities utilizing higher pulse repetition frequencies, which allow color imaging at a frame rate fast enough to evaluate the rapid fetal heart rate. Using a narrow color field or reducing the image depth, when possible, may be necessary to maintain an adequate frame rate.

It is important to remember that color Doppler will only provide mean velocity information; therefore, pulsed Doppler is a necessary adjunct to color Doppler to provide quantitative information regarding peak velocities.

Power Doppler

Power Doppler, in general, may hold several advantages over color Doppler, such as increased sensitivity, lack of aliasing, and direction independence. In the fetal heart, however, flow direction and maximum velocities are essential in making an accurate diagnosis. Therefore, power Doppler may not be useful except for establishing the presence of blood flow.

M-Mode

Although M-mode echocardiography is not routinely necessary in fetal echocardiographic examinations, it is essential to differentiate some dysrhythmias.[25] By placing the M-mode cursor through both an atrial and ventricular wall or structure simultaneously, the response of both structures can be visualized, aiding in identifying the type of dysrhythmia. M-mode can also be used to acquire measurements of chamber size and wall thickness; however, it is not absolutely necessary because these measurements can also be obtained from two-dimensional (2-D) images.

M-mode is also helpful in evaluating contractility in heart abnormalities, which may affect wall motion, such as cardiomyopathies, and is a quick and accurate method of measuring fetal heart rate.

ANATOMY AND PHYSIOLOGY

Several important structural and physiologic differences exist between the fetal and adult cardiovascular systems.[12] Unlike the adult, fetal oxygen and carbon dioxide exchange takes place in the placenta. For oxygenated blood to reach the systemic circulation and deoxygenated blood to return to the placenta for oxygenation, the fetal cardiovascular system contains several shunts not present in the adult.

In utero, oxygenated blood travels from the placenta to the fetus via the umbilical vein. After entering the fetus, the majority of this blood travels through the ductus venosus, bypassing the liver, and entering the inferior vena cava. The remainder of this oxygenated blood enters the liver and mixes with the portal circulation.

After entering the inferior vena cava, this oxygenated blood mixes with deoxygenated blood returning from the lower extremities of the fetus. It then enters the right atrium. As it enters the right atrium, the majority of blood is shunted across the foramen ovale into the left atrium. A smaller amount of blood mixes with the desaturated blood returning from the fetal head and upper extremities. This blood travels into the right atrium and into the pulmonary artery. Resistance to blood flow is high in utero; therefore, the majority of the blood that enters the pulmonary artery passes directly into the descending aorta via the ductus arteriosus.

The blood that was shunted through the foramen ovale into the left atrium, mixes with a small amount of desaturated blood returned from the lungs by way of the pulmonary veins. This blood then enters the left ventricle and then the aorta. As this blood travels through the aortic arch, a majority passes through the head and neck vessels to supply the fetal head and upper extremities. The remainder continues down the descending aorta, mixes with blood from the ductus arteriosus, and flows out of the fetus by way of the umbilical arteries to the placenta.

The three shunts present in utero, the ductus venosus, the foramen ovale, and the ductus arteriosus, all normally close after birth. The ductus arteriosus closes almost immediately after birth. This results in increased pressure within the left atrium, which combined with decreased pressure in the right atrium causes the foramen ovale to close. Complete fusion of the foramen ovale is usually complete by 1 year of age. The umbilical arteries also close immediately after birth. This leads to closure of the ductus venosus.

CONGENITAL CARDIAC ABNORMALITIES

Ventricular Septal Defect

The pooled reported frequency of congenital heart lesions among affected abortuses and stillborn infants, shows that ventricular septal defect (VSD) is the most common type of heart defect found (Table 10–1).[12]

In children, VSDs account for 20–57% of cases of congenital heart defects.[2] Unfortunately, it is also one the most commonly missed defects in utero. The sonographic diagnosis of a VSD is based on identifying an interruption in the ventricular septum. This area of dropout may be bordered by a hyperechoic specular reflector, representing the blunted edge of the intact portion of the septum (Fig. 10–18). The subcostal four-chamber view is often the most useful view in detecting a VSD.

VSDs vary in size and may be singular or multiple. Obviously, smaller defects are more difficult to recognize in utero. In addition, spontaneous closure of a VSD may occur during later gestation. Therefore, a defect that was present earlier in pregnancy may not be present when re-evaluated.

Pulsed and/or color Doppler are useful in making the diagnosis of a VSD. In fact, some small defects that are virtually unseen by 2-D alone, may be visualized with the utilization of color. However, it should be borne in mind that because of the almost equal pressures of the right and left ventricles in utero, flow across a small VSD may not be appreciated by either color or pulsed Doppler.

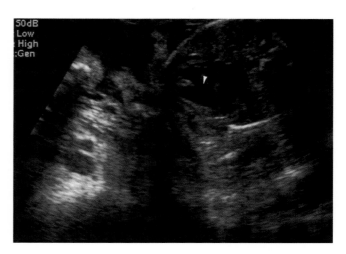

Figure 10–18. Subcostal, four-chamber view showing an anechoic area (arrowhead) in the membranous portion of the interventricular septum representing a VSD.

Atrial Septal Defect

Atrial septal defects (ASD) account for approximately 6.7% of congenital heart disease in live born infants.[26] Overall, ASDs are twice as common in females as in males. It is difficult to make the diagnosis of ASD in utero because of the normal atrial shunt, the foramen ovale, which allows blood flow from the right atrium to the left atrium in the fetus. Most in utero ASDs are best visualized in the subcostal, four-chamber view (Fig. 10–19).

An ostium secundum ASD would appear as a larger than expected area of dropout in the vicinity of the foramen ovale. As ostium primum ASD would result in the absence of the lower portion of the atrial septum, just above the

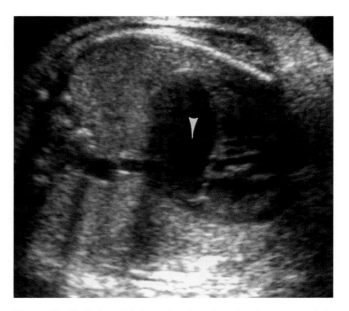

Figure 10–19. Subcostal, four-chamber view showing an anechoic area (arrowhead) in the interatrial septum representing an ASD.

atrioventricular valves. As with VSDs, color Doppler may be a useful adjunct in making the diagnosis.

Atrioventricular Septal Defect

Atrioventricular septal defect (AVSD) refers to a constellation of cardiac malformations that include abnormal development of the interatrial septum, the interventricular septum, and the atrioventricular (mitral and tricuspid) valves. It is also referred to as an atrioventricular canal defect or endocardial cushion defect. Approximately 30% of AVSDs in the fetus are associated with polysplenia.[3] Of these, most are accompanied by complete heart block. Chromosomal abnormalities, especially Down syndrome, are associated in up to 78% of cases.[3] When an AVSD is present without complete heart block, it is more likely to be associated with abnormal chromosomes.

A complete AVSD can usually be appreciated from either a subcostal or apical four-chamber view (Fig. 10–20). The endocardial cushion is absent, creating a wide opening within the center of the heart. The continuity between the interatrial and interventricular septa and the atrioventricular valves is lost. Instead of identifying separate mitral and tricuspid valves, one single, multileaflet valve is seen.

A partial form of AVSD occurs less frequently. With this, two atrioventricular valves are present; however, their leaflet formation is always abnormal. This may be difficult to appreciate by ultrasound, with the presence of an atrial and a ventricular septal defect being the only clue that an abnormality is present. In a partial AVSD, the apical four-chamber view is useful in demonstrating the abnormal

insertion level of the atrioventricular valves. In the normal heart, the tricuspid valve has a more apical insertion than the mitral valve. When a partial AVSD is present, the two atrioventricular valves appear to insert at the same level.[5]

Additional echocardiographic views of the heart, such as a short-axis view and long-axis views of the aorta and pulmonary artery, may be useful in defining the extent of the AVSD, as well as identifying associated cardiac malformations.

Hypoplastic Left Heart Syndrome

Hypoplastic left heart syndrome (HLHS) refers to a group of structural abnormalities affecting the left side of the heart. Its hallmark is a small left ventricle, which can be accompanied by aortic atresia, a hypoplastic ascending aorta, an atretic or hypoplastic mitral valve, and a small left atrium (Fig. 10–21).[4] HLHS results from decreased blood flow into or out of the left ventricle. This lack of blood flow results in the underdevelopment of the left ventricle.[6] Sonographically, a very small left ventricle is usually seen. This is apparent in either four-chamber view as well as a short-axis view of the ventricles.

When a small left ventricle is identified, accompanying abnormalities of the mitral and/or aortic valves must be determined. With valve atresia or hypoplasia, the valve orifice will appear smaller than normal for gestational age. Color and pulsed Doppler will demonstrate a lack of blood flow through the valve. The aorta itself will also appear small or atretic. In some cases, the walls of the aorta will appear more hyperechoic than expected. Blood flow through the ascending aorta may be absent or may be reversed. Reversal of flow represents blood flowing through the ductus arteriosis and then retrograde through the ascending aorta.

HLHS has a very poor prognosis, carrying a 25% mortality rate within the first week of life. All untreated infants die within the first 6 weeks. Treatment of this lesion usu-

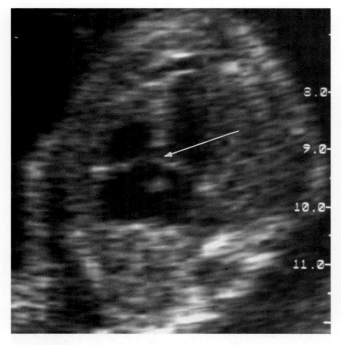

Figure 10–20. Apical four-chamber view in a fetus with an AVSD. A singular atrioventricular valve (arrow) can be seen closing within a ventricular and atrial septal defect.

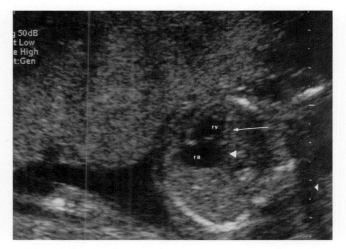

Figure 10–21. Apical four-chamber view in a fetus with hypoplastic left heart syndrome. The left ventricle (arrow) and left atrium (arrowhead) are nearly obliterated; whereas, the right ventricle (rv) and right atrium(ra) are enlarged.

ally involves surgical repair via a two-stage Norwood procedure or heart transplantation.[8]

Hypoplastic Right Heart

Hypoplastic right heart is the result of either pulmonary atresia with intact ventricular septum or tricuspid atresia.[12] As with HLHS, it occurs when normal blood flow into or out of the ventricle is compromised. Sonographic findings include a small right ventricle accompanied by a small or atretic and pulmonary artery and valve. Either an apical or subcostal four-chamber view is most useful in assessing this abnormality (Fig. 10–22). Color and pulsed Doppler will confirm the absence of blood flow across the pulmonary valve.

In tricuspid atresia, flow will be absent or substantially decreased across the tricuspid valve. The pulmonic valve is usually stenotic, so an increased velocity may be appreciated distal to the valve. If severe stenosis is present, no flow may be detectable, making differentiation from pulmonary atresia difficult. Color Doppler is essential for evaluating the interventricular septum for defects. As stated previously, this should be done in a subcostal four-chamber view.

Both tricuspid atresia and pulmonary atresia with intact ventricular septum are associated with a large left atrium and a dilated, often hypertrophied, left ventricle. The aortic root may be dilated with either entity. This left-sided enlargement is a result of the vast quantity of blood being forced across the foramen ovale because it is unable to enter the right ventricle.[8] Retrograde blood flow within the ductus arteriosis is also possible because of the increased flow through the aorta and the accompanying decreased or absent flow through the pulmonary artery.

Univentricular Heart

Univentricular heart is defined as the presence of two atrioventricular valves or a common atrioventricular valve emptying into a single ventricle. From either four-chamber view, only three chambers are present, two atria and one large ventricle (Fig. 10–23).

If two atrioventricular valves are identified, but one appears atretic, the most likely diagnosis is tricuspid or mitral atresia, which is usually considered a defect separate from a univentricular heart. The aorta and pulmonary artery are almost always transposed in the setting of a univentricular heart. Pulmonary atresia or stenosis is also common. Univentricular heart has been associated with asplenia or polysplenia in 13% of cases.[9]

Coarctation of the Aorta

When the diagnosis of coarctation of the aorta is made in utero or in early infancy, it is easily correctable, but if left undetected, the effects can be devastating. Coarctation is a narrowing of the aortic lumen, which results in an obstruction to blood flow. In 98% of cases, this narrowing occurs between the origin of the left subclavian artery and the ductus arteriosus.[10] The severity of a coarctation can range from a slight narrowing of the distal end of the arch to severe hypoplasia of the entire arch.

Intuitively, the in utero diagnosis of a coarctation seems straightforward. It is in fact, extremely difficult. Subtle changes associated with coarctation, such as a narrowing of the aortic arch, may not be appreciated, even when the arch is well visualized (Fig. 10–24). This may be caused by the physiological shunts present in the fetal heart, allowing for the severity of the narrowing not to present until after birth.

These shunts may also explain why Doppler velocities may not be affected in the presence of a coarctation. Interestingly, one of the most reliable signs of a coarctation in utero to be reported is a right ventricular dimension greater

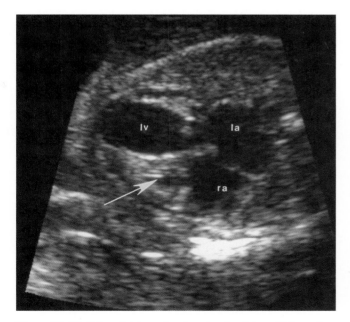

Figure 10–22. Subcostal, four-chamber view in a fetus with hypoplastic right heart syndrome. The right ventricle (arrow) is nearly obliterated; whereas, the right atrium (ra), left atrium (la) and left ventricle (lv) are enlarged.

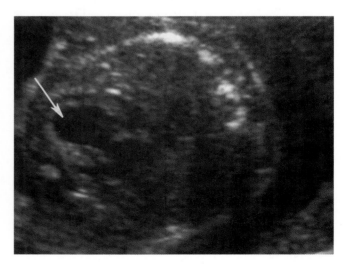

Figure 10–23. Subcostal, four-chamber view showing the single ventricle (arrow) present in a univentricular heart.

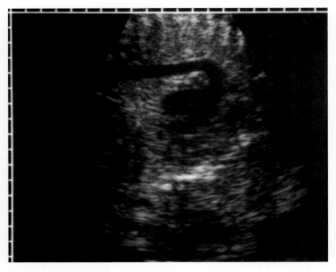

Figure 10–24. Sagittal view of the aortic arch showing a normal appearing arch in the setting of a coarctation of the aorta.

than that expected for a gestational age (Fig. 10–25). Pulmonary artery size may also be increased.[11]

This finding may be subtle, therefore, measurements of the ventricles and great vessels should always be performed in the fetus at risk for coarctation, such as those with Turner syndrome (XO) or a prior family history of left heart anomalies. It is also important to remember that coarctation of

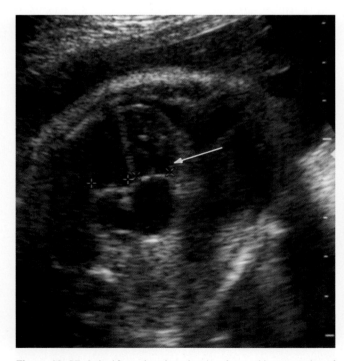

Figure 10–25. Apical four-chamber view in a fetus with coarctation of the aorta. The only clue in this case was a right ventricle (arrow) that was slightly larger than expected for gestational age.

the aorta is often a progressive lesion, with the distal arch becoming more hypoplastic as pregnancy advances. Reversal of blood flow through the foramen ovale is often, but not always, present with a coarctation.

Ebstein Anomaly

Ebstein anomaly is defined as the inferior displacement of the tricuspid valve leaflets from their normal location. Ebstein anomaly is an uncommon cardiac lesion, with a reported incidence of 1 in 20,000 live births.[13] It has often been associated with maternal lithium use; however, more recent data have shown this association to be substantially less than previously reported.[14]

The sonographic diagnosis of Ebstein anomaly is usually straightforward. Apical displacement of the tricuspid valve leaflets is readily apparent from either four-chamber view (Fig. 10–26). This results in "atrialization" of the right ventricle, which, along with the tricuspid insufficiency that is almost always present, causes an often massively enlarged right atrium. This is turn, causes the axis of the heart to be severely levocardic, giving the heart a very horizontal position within the fetal chest. Pulmonary atresia or stenosis, as well as dysrhythmias are not uncommon with Ebstein anomaly. Ebstein anomaly frequently causes in utero cardiac dysfunction, resulting in cardiomegaly and hydrops fetalis.

Tetralogy of Fallot

Tetralogy of Fallot consists of four classic structural defects: a ventricular septal defect, aortic override of the VSD, pulmonary stenosis, and right ventricular hypertrophy.[12] Because of the normal shunts present in the fetus, the right ventricular hypertrophy may not occur in utero. To diagnose this malformation in utero, an aortic root overriding the interventricular septum must be identified (Fig. 10–27).

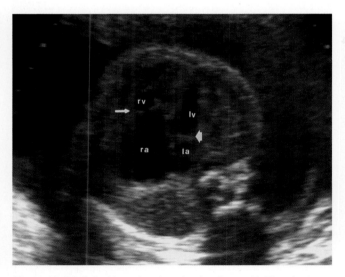

Figure 10–26. Apical four-chamber view in a fetus with Ebstein anomaly. The tricuspid valve (arrow) is displaced apically, causing atrialization of the right atrium (ra) and a small right ventricle (rv). La = left atrium, lv = left ventricle.

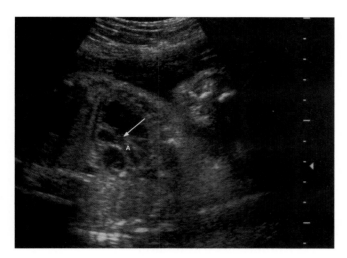

Figure 10–27. Apical view of heart in a fetus with tetralogy of Fallot showing the aorta (A) overriding a ventricular septal defect (arrow).

It is often not possible to make this diagnosis solely from a four-chamber view, either apical or subcostal. The VSD may be seen on the four-chamber view; however, color Doppler should be used to confirm that the defect is real and not artifactual. A slight angulation of the transducer toward the fetus' right shoulder from a subcostal four-chamber view, or cephalad from an apical four-chamber view should allow the overriding aorta to be appreciated. Dilation of the aortic root is usually present in later gestation.[15]

Once an overriding aorta has been observed, the diagnosis of tetralogy of Fallot relies on the evaluation of the right ventricular outflow tract. This is usually best accomplished in either a long-axis view of the pulmonary artery or a short-axis view of the great vessels. The pulmonary artery will appear small, often so much so that it cannot be identified. Pulsed Doppler interrogation of the pulmonic valve may show a greatly increased velocity, indicative of stenosis, or absence of flow in the setting of severe stenosis or atresia. Retrograde flow through the ductus arteriosus may also be present. Making an accurate diagnosis of tetralogy of Fallot relies on identifying the pulmonary artery. If a pulmonary artery cannot be visualized, the differential diagnosis would include pulmonary atresia with a VSD. If there is no main pulmonary artery arising from the right ventricle, but smaller pulmonary artery branches are seen arising from the overriding aorta, the diagnosis is truncus arteriosus.

When the diagnosis of tetralogy of Fallot is established, the laterality of the aortic arch should be determined because approximately 25% of cases are associated with a right-sided aortic arch.[16]

Truncus Arteriosus

Truncus arteriosus is rare. It is an embryological failure that results in a single great vessel arising from the heart.[12] The systemic, pulmonary, and coronary circulations are all supplied by this single great vessel. Sonographically, truncus arteriosus appears very similar to tetralogy of Fallot. A VSD is present, and the singular great vessel overrides the defect, similar to the aorta in tetralogy of Fallot (Fig. 10–28). The difference is that the pulmonary artery arises from this great vessel, not the right ventricle. Depending on the type of truncal defect present, the number and position of the pulmonary arteries on the great vessel will vary.[17]

The in utero diagnosis of truncus arteriosus may be challenging. The definitive diagnosis can be made only if the origin of the pulmonary artery can be identified arising from the large, single great vessel. Because of the inherent technical factors associated with fetal echocardiography, this may be difficult.

As with tetralogy of Fallot, identification of the overriding great vessel is usually accomplished with slight angulation from either the apical or subcostal four-chamber view. Several views, including long- and short-axis views of the right outflow tract must be obtained to confirm the absence of a pulmonary artery. Evaluation of the aortic arch is also important. A right-sided arch has been reported in 15–30% of cases. Interruption of the aortic arch as also been associated with truncus arteriosus.[17]

Complete Transposition of the Great Arteries

Eighty percent of fetuses with transposition of the great arteries have complete or *d*-transposition.[18] In this setting, the connections between the atria and ventricles are normal, meaning that the right atrium connects through the tricuspid valve to the right ventricle, and the left atrium connects through the mitral valve to the left ventricle. However, the aorta arises from the right ventricle, and the pulmonary artery arises from the left ventricle. This results in two parallel circulations that will only allow mixing of venous and arterial blood through the ductus arteriosus, interatrial, or interventricular connections.

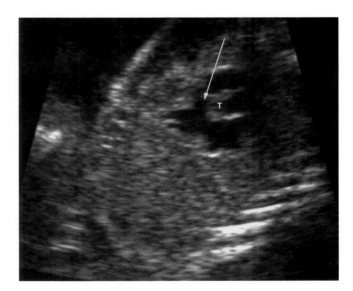

Figure 10–28. Subcostal view of the heart in a fetus with truncus arteriosus showing a single truncal vessel (T) overriding a ventricular septal defect (arrow).

The four-chamber views are often normal in the presence of complete transposition. The diagnosis is made by identifying the aorta arising from the right ventricle and connecting to the aortic arch and descending aorta, and identifying the pulmonary artery arising from the left ventricle and then branching into the left and right pulmonary arteries. From a long-axis view of the great vessels, the aorta and pulmonary artery will appear to run in a parallel fashion. The short-axis view, at the level of the great vessels, is also useful in making this diagnosis. In this view, both the pulmonary artery and aorta appear as circular structures adjacent to each other, instead of their normal relationship of the pulmonary artery draping over the aorta. A ventricular septal defect is present in 20% of cases, so color Doppler should be used to assess the interventricular septum thoroughly.[19]

Congenitally Corrected Transposition of the Great Arteries

Congenitally corrected or *l*-transposition of the great arteries comprises the remaining 20% of transposition cases.[18] In corrected transposition, the great vessels arise from the correct sides; however, the left and right ventricles and the left and right atrioventricular valves are transposed. In other words, the right atrium is connected to the left ventricle, and the left atrium is connected to the right ventricle. The aorta then arises from the left-sided right ventricle, and the pulmonary artery arises from the right-sided left ventricle. Blood circulation in this abnormality is in series, as it is in the normal heart; therefore, surgical correction is not required unless associated cardiac anomalies are present.

Sonographic identification of this abnormality can be subtle. Correct identification of the cardiac chambers is crucial in making this diagnosis. In the normal heart, the tricuspid valve insertion is slightly more apical than the mitral valve. The right ventricle also has a prominent moderator band near the apex that is usually seen on fetal echocardiography. If these findings appear to be left sided, the diagnosis of corrected transposition can be entertained. As with complete transposition, the great vessels exit the heart in a more parallel relationship than seen in the normal heart. This may be appreciated on a short-axis view of the great vessels, but is far more subtle than in complete transposition. It is not uncommon to miss the diagnosis of corrected transposition in utero, particularly when no other cardiac defects are present.

VSDs have been reported in about 50% of patients with corrected transposition. Pulmonic stenosis and abnormalities of the mitral and tricuspid valves are also common.[18]

Double Outlet Right Ventricle

Double outlet right ventricle (DORV) is a condition in which more than 50% of both the aortic root and the main pulmonary artery arise from the right ventricle. A VSD is almost always present.[20]

This, again, is one of many cardiac defects easily missed when only a four-chamber view is obtained. The long-axis views of the aorta and pulmonary artery are most useful in identifying both great vessels as arising from the right ventricle (Fig. 10–29). In DORV, the most common relationship of the great vessels is side by side, with the aorta right and lateral to the pulmonary artery. When this occurs, the normal perpendicular course of the great vessels is lost. As with transposition of the great arteries, they will appear parallel to each other. Differentiating DORV from transposition relies on identifying both great vessels as arising from the right ventricle. This can be challenging in utero. As with all congenital cardiac abnormalities, the surgical intervention depends heavily on the presence or absence of other cardiac anomalies. Therefore, a thorough interrogation of the fetal heart must be undertaken.

Double outlet left ventricle, in which both the aortic root and the main pulmonary artery arise from the left ventricle has also been reported, but it is exceedingly rare.[21]

Total Anomalous Pulmonary Venous Connection

Total anomalous pulmonary venous connection (TAPVC) is an anomaly in which all of the pulmonary veins drain either directly into the right atrium or into channels that terminate in the right atrium.[22] In the normal heart, venous return is to the left atrium. TAPVC is rare and as with many other congenital cardiac anomalies, is a difficult diagnosis to make in the fetus.

The diagnosis relies on the inability to identify any pulmonary veins entering the left atrium and the identification of all four pulmonary veins entering the right atrium or abnormally converging and entering the superior vena cava, inferior vena cava, portal vein, or ductus venosus.

If any pulmonary veins are seen entering the left atrium or if all pulmonary veins are not seen entering an ectopic structure, the diagnosis of TAPVC is excluded. Partial anomalous pulmonary venous connection may be present in this setting, but cannot be definitively ascertained in utero.

The pulmonary veins are best identified in either a subcostal or apical four-chamber view. Usually only the

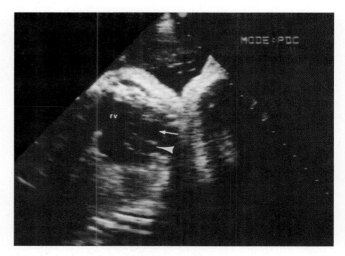

Figure 10–29. Double outlet right ventricle in a fetus. The aorta (arrowhead) and the pulmonary artery (arrow) are both arising from the right ventricle (rv).

two superior veins are identified in utero (Fig. 10–30), adding to the difficulty of making this diagnosis. Enlargement of the right ventricle and pulmonary artery may be secondary signs of TAPVC.[22]

When enlargement of these structures are present, and the normal pulmonary veins cannot be identified as they drain into the left atrium, the possibility of TAPVC should be entertained. Using color Doppler to identify an abnormal convergence of veins posterior to the right atrium may also be useful.

Cardiac Axis and Position

As stated previously, determining cardiac axis and position is one of the first steps in performing a fetal echocardiogram. Abnormal cardiac axis or position may be an important clue that a structural defect is present.[12]

Normal cardiac axis is termed levocardia, meaning the apex of the heart points to the left side of the fetal chest (Fig. 10–31). Even if a heart is levocardic, if its axis is greater than 45° ± 20° to the left, an abnormality may be present. Cardiac anomalies that result in severe levocardia are usually those that cause an enlarged right atrium, such as Ebstein anomaly (Fig. 10–35). It is thought that this enlargement causes the heart to shift and lie more horizontally. The terms dextrocardia or dextroversion refer to the apex of the heart pointing abnormally to the right (Fig. 10–32). Isolated dextrocardia is associated with a structural cardiac abnormality in 95% of cases.[12] Dextrocardia associated with abdominal situs abnormalities carries a lower risk. Dextroposition is present when the apex of the heart points normally to the left side of the fetal chest, but the heart itself is positioned in the right chest (Fig. 10–33).

When dextroposition is present, two possibilities should be considered. Either the heart is being displaced to the right by a left-sided thoracic defect, such as a diaphrag-

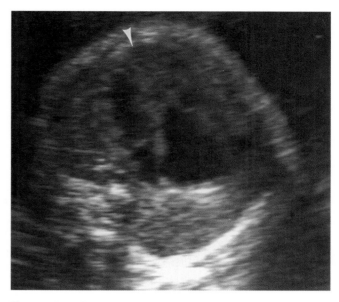

Figure 10–31. Severe levocardia in a fetus with Ebstein anomaly. The apex of the heart (arrowhead) is angled too far to the left chest.

matic hernia or a cystic adenomatoid malformation, or the heart is filling a potential space in the right thorax. This may be indicative of an absent or hypoplastic right lung.

Whenever a fetal echocardiogram is performed, special attention should be paid to identifying cardiac axis and position. Any deviation from normal may be indicative of an underlying intra or extracardiac defect.

Dysrhythmias

The normal fetal heart rate is regular and between 100 and 180 beats per minute. A dysrhythmia if present if the fetal

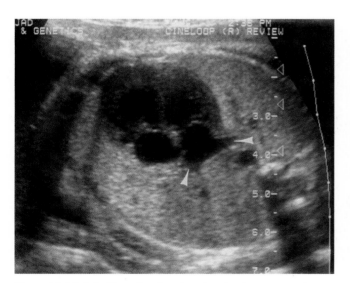

Figure 10–30. Apical four-chamber view showing the two normal superior pulmonary veins appropriately entering the left atrium.

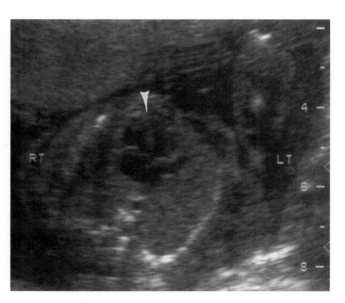

Figure 10–32. Dextrocardia of the fetal heart. The apex of the heart (arrowhead) is pointing incorrectly to the right chest.

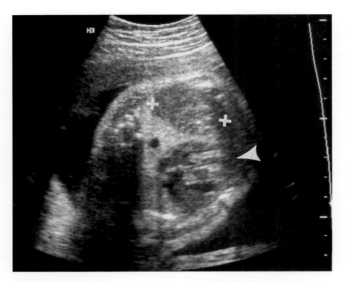

Figure 10–33. Dextroposition of the fetal heart. The apex of the heart (arrowhead) is pointing correctly to the left chest; however, the entire heart is being displaced into the right chest by the mass in the left chest (calipers).

heart rate is noted to be abnormally fast, slow, or irregular. Dysrhythmias are detected in approximately 1% of fetuses.[26]

Most dysrhythmias are benign; however, in a small number of cases, they may be life threatening. M-mode is the most useful method of assessing the type of dysrhythmia present. As stated previously, the M-mode cursor should be placed simultaneously through a structure in the fetal heart that represents an atrial beat (atria wall or atrioventricular valve) and the ventricular response (ventricle wall or semilunar valve).

Premature atrial contractions (PACs) are the most common dysrhythmia encountered in the fetus (Fig. 10–34).[12] They have been associated with a redundant foraminal flap,

as well as maternal use of caffeine, cigarettes, or alcohol.[27] Rarely, PACs may evolve into a sustained tachycardia; however, most resolve around the time of delivery and seldom present a problem in the newborn. Tachycardias are the second most common dysrhythmia seen in the fetal population. Tachycardias are classified as:

- Supraventricular tachycardia—heart rate of 180–280 bpm, with atrial-ventricular concordance (Fig. 10–35)
- Atrial flutter—atrial heart rate of 280–400 bpm, with variable ventricular response (Fig. 10–36)
- Atrial fibrillation—atrial heart rate of >400 bpm, with variable ventricular response

Sustained SVT can result in fetal hydrops or death and represents a fetal medical emergency.[28] SVT is associated with structural heart disease in 5–10% of cases.[29]

The treatment of SVT in utero is difficult. Immediate medical therapy should be implemented if there are signs of fetal compromise. Digoxin has been the initial drug of choice when treating fetal SVT; however, several other medications are available and may be used in place of or in combination with digoxin.

Bradycardia may also be encountered in the fetus. Transient bradycardia is often encountered during the course of an ultrasound examination secondary to pressure from the transducer. The bradycardia is resolved when the transducer is removed. This entity should not be confused with pathologic bradycardias that result in a sustained slow heart rate.

Ninety-six percent of fetuses with sustained bradycardia will have second- or third-degree heart block.[12] Second-degree heart block is commonly referred to as a 2:1 or 3:1, etc., heart block, referring to the fact that the ven-

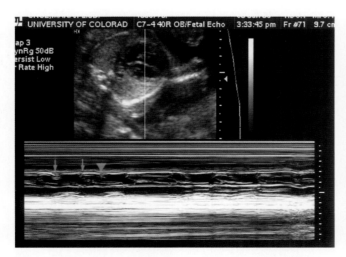

Figure 10–34. M-mode tracing of premature atrial contractions in a fetus. Normally spaced atrial beats (arrows) can be seen followed by a premature beat (arrowhead).

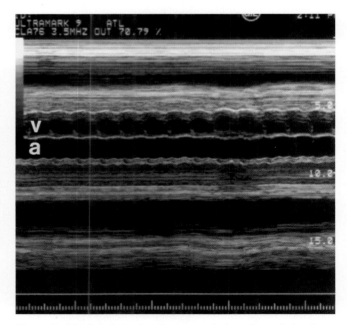

Figure 10–35. M-mode tracing of supraventricular tachycardia in a fetus. Both the ventricular (v) and atrial (a) rates were 240 beats per minute.

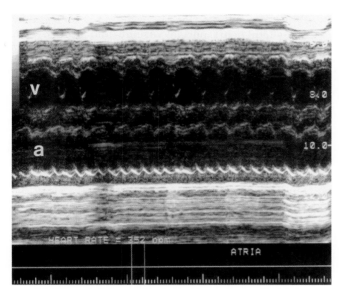

Figure 10–36. M-mode tracing of a fetal heart with atrial flutter. The atrial (a) rate was 352 beats per minute, while the ventricular (v) rate was 180 beats per minute.

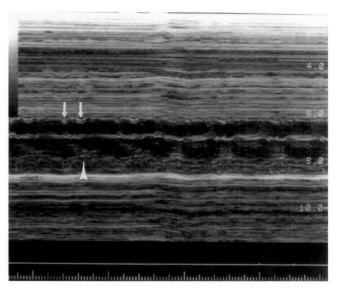

Figure 10–37. M-mode tracing of a fetal heart with a 2:1 heart block. The atrial rate is 120 beats per minute, whereas the ventricular rate is 60 beats per minute.

tricular rate will be a submultiple of the atrial rate. In other words, two atrial contractions will occur for every one ventricular contraction, or three atrial contractions will occur for every one ventricular contraction, and so on (Fig. 10–37).

Third degree or complete heart block is present when there is complete dissociation between the atrial and ventricular rates, with the atrial rate being faster. Approximately 50% of fetuses with complete heart block have significant structural heart disease, specifically, atrioventricular septal defects, corrected transposition of the great arteries, cardiac tumors, or a cardiomyopathy.[12] Complete heart block associated with an atrioventricular septal defect is highly suggestive of polysplenia syndrome.[30] In fetuses with complete heart block without structural defects, there is a high association with maternal connective tissue diseases such as lupus.[31]

Second- and third-degree heart block are difficult to treat in utero. Increasing fetal heart rate through the maternal administration of sympathomimetic agents and placement of an in utero pacemaker have been attempted, but with dismal results.[32] Administration of maternal steroids has also been reported.[33]

The prognosis for fetuses with complete heart block and structural heart disease is poor. In fetuses without structural heart disease, outcome is dependent on the atrial and ventricular rate and the presence of fetal hydrops.

REFERENCES

1. Hoffman JIE. Incidence of congenital heart disease: II. Prenatal incidence. *Pediatr Cardiol.* 1995; 16:155–165.
2. Allan LD, Crawford DC, Anderson RH, et al. Spectrum of congenital heart disease detected echocardiographically in prenatal life. *Br Heart J.* 1985; 54:523–526.
3. Allan LD. Fetal cardiology. *Ultrasound Obstet Gynecol.* 1994; 4:441–444.
4. AIUM Technical Bulletin: Performance of the fetal cardiac ultrasound examination. American Institute of Ultrasound in Medicine. *J Ultrasound Med.* 1998; 17:601–607.
5. Dolkart LA, Reimers FT. Transvaginal fetal echocardiography in early pregnancy: Normative data. *Am J Obstet Gynecol.* 1991; 165:688–691.
6. DeVore GR, Medearis AL, Bear MB. Fetal echocardiography: Factors that influence imaging of the fetal heart during the second trimester of pregnancy. *J Ultrasound Med.* 1993; 12:659–663.
7. Allan LD. Diagnosis of fetal cardiac abnormality. *Br J Hosp Med.* 1988; 40:290–293.
8. Fyfe DA, Kline CH. Fetal echocardiographic diagnosis of congenital heart disease. *Pediatr Clin North Am.* 1990; 37:45–67.
9. Nora JJ, Fraser FC. Cardiovascular Disease. In: *Medical Genetics: Principles and Practice.* 3rd ed. Philadelphia: Lea & Febiger; 1989: 321–337.
10. Nora JJ, Nora AH. Maternal transmission of congenital heart diseases: new recurrence risk figures and the question of cytoplasmic inheritance and vulnerability to teratogens. *Am J Cardiol.* 1987; 59:459–463.
11. Reed KL. Introduction to fetal echocardiography. *Ob Gyn Clin N Am.* 1991; 18:811–822.
12. Drose JA. *Fetal Echocardiography.* Philadelphia: WB Saunders; 1998: 1–300.
13. Berg KA, Boughman JA, Astemboroski JA, et al. Implications for prenatal cytogenetic analysis from Baltimore–Washington study of liveborn infants with confirmed congenital heart defects (CHD). *Am J Hum Genet.* 1986; 39:A50.

14. Berg KA, Clark EB, Astemboroski JA, et al. Prenatal detection of cardiovascular malformations by echocardiography: an indication for cytogenetic evaluation. *Am J Obstet Gynecol.* 1988; 159:477–481.

15. Stewart PA, Wladimiroff JW, Reuss A, et al. Fetal echocardiography: A review of six years experience. *Fetal Ther.* 1987; 2:222–231.

16. Nicolaides K, Shawwa L, Brizot M, et al. Ultrasonographically detectable markers of fetal chromosomal defects. *Ultrasound Obstet Gynecol.* 1993; 3:56–59.

17. Rowland TW, Hubbel JP, Nadas AS. Congenital heart disease in infants of diabetic mothers. *J. Pediatr.* 1973; 83:815–820.

18. Levy HL, Waisbren SE. Effects of untreated maternal phenylketonuria and hyperphenylalaninemia on the fetus. *N Engl J Med.* 1983; 309:1269–1274.

19. Nyberg DA, Emerson DS. Cardiac malformations. In: Nyberg DA, Mahony BS, Pretorius DH, eds. *Diagnostic Ultrasound of Fetal Anomalies: Text and Atlas.* Chicago: Yearbook Medical Publishers, Inc.; 1990: 300–341.

20. Drose JA, Dennis MA, Thickman D. Infection in utero: Ultrasound findings in 19 cases. *Radiology.* 1991; 178:369–374.

21. Coper JA, Pilu G, Kleinman CS. Congenital heart disease and extracardiac anomalies: Associations and indications for fetal echocardiography. *Am J Obstet Gynecol.* 1986; 154:1121–1132.

22. Comstock CH. Normal fetal heart axis and position. *Obstet Gynecol.* 1987; 70:255–257.

23. DeVore GR. The prenatal diagnosis of congenital heart disease-A practical approach for the fetal sonographer. *J Clin Ultrasound.* 1985; 13:229–245.

24. Brown DL, DiSalvo DN, Frates MC, et al. Sonography of the fetal heart: normal variants and pitfalls. *AJR.* 1993; 160:1251–1255.

25. Allan LD, Joseph MC, Boyd EG, et al. M-mode echocardiography in the developing human fetus. *Br Heart J.* 1982; 47:573–583.

26. Southhall DP, Richard J, Hardwick RA, et al. Prospective study of fetal heart rate and rhythm patterns. *Arch Dis Child.* 1980; 55:506–511.

27. Steward PA, Wladimiroff JW. Fetal atrial arrhythmias associated with redundancy/aneurysm of the foramen ovale. *J Clin Ultrasound.* 1988; 16:643–650.

28. Allan LD. Cardiac ultrasound of the fetus. *Arch Dis Child.* 1984; 59:603–605.

29. Beall MH, Paul RH. Artifacts, blocks, and arrhythmias confusing nonclassical heart rate tracings. *Clin Obstet Gynecol.* 1986; 29:83–85.

30. Machado MV, Crawford DC, Anderson RH, et al. Atrioventricular septal defect in prenatal life. *Br Heart J.* 1988; 59:352–355.

31. McCue CM, Mantakas ME, Tingelstad JB, et al. Congenital heart block in newborns of mothers with connective tissue disease. *Circulation.* 1977; 56:82–85.

32. Carpenter RJ, Strasburger JF, Farson A, et al. Fetal ventricular pacing for hydrops secondary to complete atrioventricular block. *J Am Coll Cardiol.* 1986; 8:1434–1440.

33. Kaaja R, Julkunen HA, Ammala P, et al. Congenital heart block: successful prophylactic treatment with intravenous gamma globulin and corticosteroid therapy. *Am J Obstet Gynecol.* 1991; 165:1333–1335.

Questions

1. The first step in beginning a fetal echocardiogram is to determine

   (A) fetal heart rate
   (B) fetal position
   (C) gestational age
   (D) amount of amniotic fluid present

2. The most important view when performing a fetal echocardiogram is

   (A) apical four-chamber view
   (B) subcostal four-chamber view
   (C) long-axis view of the aorta
   (D) long-axis view of the pulmonary artery

3. Pulsed Doppler should be used to interrogate all valves proximally for

   (A) stenosis
   (B) atresia
   (C) contractility
   (D) insufficiency

4. In addition to a four-chamber view, all routine obstetrical ultrasound exams should include

   (A) views of the aorta and pulmonary artery
   (B) views of the mitral and tricuspid valves
   (C) views of the anterior and posterior pulmonary veins
   (D) views of the aortic and ductal arches

5. To assess a fetal dysrhythmia, the M-mode cursor should be placed simultaneously through which structures?

   (A) the mitral and tricuspid valves
   (B) the right and left ventricles
   (C) an atrial and ventricular wall
   (D) the foraminal flap

6. The normal direction of blood flow through the foramen ovale is from

   (A) the right atrium to the left atrium
   (B) the left atrium to the right atrium
   (C) the right ventricle to the left ventricle
   (D) the left ventricle to the right atrium

7. All of the following are indications for performing a fetal echocardiogram, *except*

   (A) mother with lupus
   (B) mother with diabetes
   (C) mother with cytomegalovirus
   (D) mother with influenza

8. Which of the following chromosomal abnormalities carries the highest risk of an associated congenital heart defect?

   (A) trisomy 21
   (B) trisomy 18
   (C) Turner syndrome
   (D) DiGeorge syndrome

9. Equipment used for fetal echocardiography should be equipped with all of the following modalities, *except*

   (A) pulsed Doppler
   (B) color Doppler
   (C) power Doppler
   (D) M-mode

10. Congenital cardiac abnormalities occur in approximately how many live births

    (A) 1/400
    (B) 1/300
    (C) 1/200
    (D) 1/100

11. The most common type of congenital heart disease found in abortuses and stillbirths is

    (A) ASD
    (B) VSD
    (C) AVSD
    (D) coarctation of the aorta

12. The most appropriate view to interrogate the interventricular septum is

(A) apical four-chamber
(B) subcostal four-chamber
(C) short-axis of the great vessels
(D) long-axis of the aorta

13. A fetal echocardiogram should be performed at approximately

(A) 10–12 weeks
(B) 15–16 weeks
(C) 18–22 weeks
(D) 24–28 weeks

14. The apex of the normal heart points

(A) toward the left
(B) toward the right
(C) superior
(D) posterior

15. The angle of the normal fetal heart compared to midline is approximately

(A) 20°
(B) 45°
(C) 70°
(D) 90°

16. The normal position of the heart is termed

(A) levocardia
(B) dextrocardia
(C) mesocardia
(D) mesoposition

17. The normal fetal heart occupies

(A) ¼ of the chest
(B) ⅔ of the chest
(C) ⅓ of the chest
(D) ½ of the chest

18. The apical four-chamber view is obtained when the septae of the heart are directed

(A) toward the fetus's right
(B) parallel the transducer
(C) toward the fetus's left
(D) perpendicular to the transducer

19. The apical four-chamber view is *not* the ideal view to visualize

(A) all four chambers
(B) the mitral and tricuspid valves
(C) chamber size
(D) the interventricular septum

20. The sonographer has obtained a subcostal four-chamber view. The transducer is then angled toward the fetus's right shoulder. What view will be visualized first?

(A) cross-section view of the ventricles
(B) short-axis view of the aorta with the pulmonary artery crossing over
(C) right ventricular outflow track
(D) long-axis view of the aorta

21. The orientation of the great vessels is correct if they

(A) run parallel to each other
(B) criss-cross
(C) join to form one vessel
(D) originate from the right ventricle

22. The moderator band can be identified in the

(A) left ventricle
(B) left atrium
(C) right ventricle
(D) right atrium

23. Which of the following views is *not* used to identify interventricular septal defects?

(A) subcostal four-chamber view
(B) long axis of the proximal aorta
(C) short-axis view of the ventricles
(D) short-axis view of the great vessels

24. While demonstrating a short-axis view of the great vessels, the main pulmonary artery is often seen bifurcating into the

(A) ductus arteriosus and the right pulmonary artery
(B) right and left pulmonary arteries
(C) ductus arteriosus and the left pulmonary artery
(D) ductus arteriosus and the aorta

25. Which of the following does *not* describe the appearance of the aortic arch?

(A) brachiocephalic vessels are visualized
(B) has an appearance of a candy cane
(C) is superior to the ductal arch
(D) has an appearance of a hockey stick

26. The portion of the aortic arch just distal to where the ductus arteriosus inserts is important to evaluate with pulsed Doppler because this is where

(A) aortic valve insufficiency is identified
(B) aortic coarctations occur
(C) aortic stenosis occurs
(D) pulmonary valve insufficiency is identified

27. The ductal arch is comprised of all of the following *except* the

(A) descending aorta
(B) pulmonary artery
(C) ascending aorta
(D) ductus arteriosus

28. A fetus is *most* likely to develop a congenital heart defect if

(A) one sibling has a heart defect
(B) the father of the fetus has a heart defect
(C) the mother of the fetus has a heart defect
(D) the paternal grandmother has a heart defect

29. Which of the following is *not* an indication for a fetal echocardiography exam?

(A) nonimmune hydrops
(B) polyhydramnios
(C) suspicion of abnormal chromosomes
(D) suboptimal heart views on a 12-week ultrasound

30. Which of the following is *not* an advantage of using color Doppler during a fetal echocardiography exam?

(A) identifying areas of turbulence
(B) indicating direction of flow
(C) indicating peak velocity
(D) identifying small VSDs

31. In which of the following situations is M-mode *not* helpful?

(A) measuring chamber size
(B) measuring wall thickness
(C) documenting dysrhythmias
(D) documenting direction of flow

32. As blood enters the fetus, much of the blood bypasses the liver by traveling through the

(A) foramen ovale
(B) ductus venosus
(C) ductus arteriosis
(D) ligamentum venosum

33. Pulsed Doppler of the pulmonary veins is useful in determining flow

(A) into the left atrium
(B) out of the left atrium
(C) into the right atrium
(D) out of the right atrium

34. When performing pulsed Doppler on the fetal heart, the Doppler angle should be

(A) as close to 90° as possible
(B) as close to 60° as possible
(C) as close to 30° as possible
(D) as close to 0° as possible

35. The sample gate for the pulsed Doppler cursor is set

(A) small; so that many vessels can be interrogated at once
(B) large; so that many vessels can be interrogated at once
(C) large; to ensure the vessel of interest is obtained
(D) small; to avoid interference while obtaining the vessel of interest

36. Oxygenated blood flows from the placenta to the fetus by way of the

(A) umbilical vein
(B) umbilical artery
(C) ductus venosum
(D) fetal shunts

37. The blood that enters the right atrium is

(A) deoxygenated blood
(B) oxygenated blood
(C) oxygenated and deoxygenated blood
(D) maternal blood

38. Which of the following is *not* a shunt present in the fetus?

(A) ductus venosum
(B) foramen ovale
(C) ductus arteriosus
(D) umbilical vein

39. The least useful modality in diagnosing a VSD is

(A) 2-D imaging
(B) color Doppler
(C) pulsed Doppler
(D) M-mode

40. An atrioventricular septal defect (AVSD) includes abnormal development of all of the following *except*

(A) aortic arch
(B) interatrial septum
(C) interventricular septum
(D) atrioventricular valves

41. In hypoplastic left heart syndrome (HLHS), the left ventricle becomes hypoplastic because of

(A) decreased blood flow into or out of the left ventricle
(B) increased blood flow into or out of the left ventricle
(C) decreased blood flow due to a closed foramen ovale
(D) a large VSD

42. In a fetus with HLHS, abnormalities may be seen in which of the following valves?

(A) aortic and pulmonary
(B) mitral and tricuspid
(C) tricuspid and pulmonary
(D) mitral and aortic

43. With HLHS, blood flow through the ascending aorta is usually

(A) absent or reversed
(B) high velocity
(C) normal
(D) low velocity

44. AVSDs are commonly associated with

(A) asplenia
(B) oligohydramnios
(C) polysplenia
(D) polyhydramnios

45. Which of the following chromosomal abnormalities is most commonly associated with an AVSD?

(A) trisomy 13
(B) trisomy 18
(C) trisomy 21
(D) Turner syndrome

46. Which of the following heart anomalies has the best prognosis?

(A) Ebstein anomaly
(B) isolated VSD
(C) truncus arteriosus
(D) undetected coarctation of the aorta

47. Which of the following heart anomalies usually has the poorest prognosis?

(A) hypoplastic left heart syndrome
(B) hypoplastic right heart syndrome
(C) mild aortic stenosis
(D) isolated ASD

48. Which of the following structures could be small with hypoplastic right heart syndrome?

(A) aortic valve
(B) pulmonary valve
(C) aorta
(D) pulmonary veins

49. When a valve is stenotic, which of the following is seen?

(A) decreased velocity proximal to the valve
(B) decreased velocity distal to the valve
(C) increased velocity proximal to the valve
(D) increased velocity distal to the valve

50. Which of the following is *not* visualized with HRHS?

(A) retrograde flow through the foramen ovale
(B) large left-sided heart
(C) increased flow through the pulmonary artery
(D) dilated aortic root

51. Which condition is almost always present with an univentricular heart?

(A) transposition of the great vessels
(B) coarctation of the aorta
(C) hypoplastic left heart syndrome
(D) Ebstein anomaly

52. Which of the following is *not* associated with an univentricular heart?

(A) two normal atrioventricular valves
(B) pulmonary stenosis
(C) asplenia
(D) polysplenia

53. Coarctation of the aorta is

(A) absence of the aorta
(B) an aneurysm of the aorta
(C) narrowing the aortic lumen
(D) enlargement of the aortic lumen

54. The majority of coarctations of the aorta occur between the

(A) thoracic and abdominal aorta
(B) aortic valve and the ductus arteriosus
(C) right subclavian artery and the ductus arteriosus
(D) left subclavian artery and the ductus arteriosus

55. All of the following are signs of coarctation of the aorta *except*

(A) enlarged right ventricle
(B) enlarged left ventricle
(C) increased velocities in the aorta
(D) narrowing of the aorta

56. Coarctation of the aorta is most common in which genetic condition?

(A) Turner syndrome
(B) trisomy 13
(C) trisomy 18
(D) trisomy 21

57. Ebstein anomaly is

(A) inferior displacement of the mitral valve
(B) superior displacement of the mitral valve
(C) inferior displacement of the tricuspid valve
(D) superior displacement of the tricuspid valve

58. Ebstein anomaly has been associated with maternal use of

(A) lithium
(B) alcohol
(C) codeine
(D) tobacco

59. Which of the following defects is *not* seen in a newborn with tetralogy of Fallot?

(A) VSD
(B) overriding aorta
(C) pulmonary stenosis
(D) aortic stenosis

60. A tetralogy of Fallot defect that may not be present in utero is

(A) large VSD
(B) ASD
(C) right ventricular hypertrophy
(D) overriding aorta

61. Which of the following defects is present with truncus arteriosus?

(A) coarctation of the aorta
(B) hypoplastic right heart
(C) ASD
(D) VSD

62. An accurate description of truncus arteriosus would be

(A) a single vessel arising from the heart; the pulmonary arteries arise from this great vessel
(B) a single vessel arising from the heart; the aorta arises from this great vessel
(C) two vessels arise from the heart; running parallel
(D) two vessels arise from the heart and criss-cross

63. A right-sided aortic arch may be seen in all of the following *except*

(A) truncus arteriosus
(B) congenitally corrected transposition of the great vessels
(C) tetralogy of Fallot
(D) situs inversus above the diaphragm

64. Truncus arteriosus can be mistaken for which other anomaly?

(A) transposition of the great vessels
(B) tetralogy of Fallot
(C) Ebstein anomaly
(D) univentricular heart

65. Which view cannot be obtained with complete transposition of the great vessels?

(A) apical four chamber
(B) subcostal four chamber

(C) short-axis view of the great vessels
(D) aortic arch

66. With complete transposition of the great vessels

(A) the atria, ventricles, and valves are in the appropriate location; the aorta arises from the right ventricle, the pulmonary artery from the left ventricle
(B) the atria, ventricles, and valves are in the appropriate location; the aorta arises from the left ventricle, the pulmonary artery from the right ventricle
(C) the atria, ventricles, and valves are reversed; the aorta arises from the right ventricle, the pulmonary artery from the left ventricle
(D) the atria, ventricles, and valves are reversed; the aorta arises from the left ventricle, the pulmonary artery from the right ventricle

67. To identify congenitally corrected transposition of the great vessels, the moderator band can be seen in the

(A) right-sided left ventricle
(B) left-sided left ventricle
(C) right-sided right ventricle
(D) left-sided right ventricle

68. With congenitally corrected transposition of the great vessels

(A) the atria, ventricles, and valves are in the appropriate location; the aorta arises from the left ventricle, the pulmonary artery from the right ventricle
(B) the atria, ventricles, and valves are in the appropriate location; the aorta arises from the right ventricle, the pulmonary artery from the left ventricle
(C) the right atrium and left ventricle are connected, the left atrium and right ventricle are connected; the aorta arises from the right-sided left ventricle; the pulmonary artery from the left-sided right ventricle
(D) the right atrium and left ventricle are connected, the left atrium and right ventricle are connected; the aorta arises from the left-sided right ventricle; the pulmonary artery from the right-sided left ventricle

69. The best view to identify double outlet right ventricle is

(A) long-axis views of the aorta and pulmonary artery
(B) apical four-chamber view
(C) subcostal four-chamber view
(D) long-axis view of the pulmonary artery

70. With double outlet right ventricle, the great vessels run

(A) right to left
(B) left to right
(C) parallel
(D) perpendicular

71. With total anomalous pulmonary venous connection, the pulmonary veins drain into the

(A) right ventricle
(B) left ventricle
(C) right atrium
(D) left atrium

72. Which of the following anomalies is most likely to be identified in utero, if only a four-chamber heart view is obtained?

(A) double outlet right ventricle
(B) truncus arteriosus
(C) transposition of the great vessels
(D) hypoplastic left heart syndrome
(E) tetralogy of Fallot

73. Severe levocardia can be defined as

(A) heart is pointed toward the left at a 45° angle
(B) heart is pointed toward the left at an angle greater than 65°
(C) heart is pointed toward the right at a 45° angle
(D) heart is pointed toward the right at an angle greater than 65°

74. When the apex of the heart is pointed toward the right side, it is termed

(A) levocardia
(B) levoposition
(C) dextrocardia
(D) dextroposition

75. The heart can be displaced to the right side of the chest due to all of the following *except*

(A) tricuspid insufficiency
(B) diaphragmatic hernia

(C) cystic adenomatoid malformation
(D) hypoplastic right lung

76. The most common type of dysrhythmia is

(A) supraventricular tachycardia
(B) tachycardia
(C) atrial flutter
(D) premature atrial contractions

77. If supraventricular tachycardia is sustained, it can lead to

(A) hypoplastic right heart
(B) hypoplastic left heart
(C) oligohydramnios
(D) hydrops

78. Pressure from the transducer may cause which transient dysrhythmia?

(A) premature atrial contractions
(B) atrial flutter
(C) bradycardia
(D) tachycardia

79. A second-degree heart block of 3:1 can be described as

(A) two atrial contractions for every one ventricular contraction
(B) three atrial contractions for every one ventricular contraction
(C) two ventricular contractions for every one atrial contraction
(D) three ventricular contractions for every one atrial contraction

80. All of the following can be associated with complete heart block *except*

(A) digoxin use
(B) ASD
(C) cardiac tumors
(D) polysplenia

Answers and Explanations

At the end of each explained answer there is a number combination in parentheses. The first number identifies the reference source; the second number or set of numbers indicates the page or pages on which the relevant information can be found.

1. **(B)** A fetal echocardiogram should always begin by determining fetal position. Once fetal position is determined, situs (position of the heart and stomach) and cardiac structures can be accurately identified. *(Study Guide: 469)*

2. **(B)** In the subcostal four-chamber view, all four chambers can be identified along with the interventricular and interatrial septae. Subcostal four-chamber is the best view to evaluate for ASDs and VSDs, because the septae are perpendicular to the transducer. The long-axis views are important in determining appropriate position of the outflow tracks. *(Study Guide: 470)*

3. **(D)** When valves are insufficient, complete closure of the valve does not occur. Blood, therefore, flows back and can be detected with pulsed Doppler proximal to the valve. *(Study Guide: 474)*

4. **(A)** A four-chamber heart view does *not* exclude all anomalies. To increase the chance of identifying abnormalities, outflow tracks must be obtained. Long-axis views of the aorta and pulmonary should be seen "criss-crossing." *(Study Guide: 467)*

5. **(C)** Dysrhythmias involve both the atria and ventricle. An atrial beat and a ventricular response can be evaluated if the M-mode cursor is placed through both the atria and ventricle. *(Study Guide: 469)*

6. **(A)** Blood flows from the right atrium into the left atrium. The foraminal flap opens into the left atrium. *(Study Guide: 474)*

7. **(D)** Complete heart block is associated with mothers who have Lupus. Diabetic mothers are more likely to have babies with congenital heart disease, double-outlet right ventricle, cardiomyopathies, and truncus arteriosus. Cytomegalovirus is associated with dilated cardiomyopathy. *(Study Guide: 467)*

8. **(B)** Trisomies 13 and 18 are associated with heart defects almost 100% of the time. Trisomy 21 has a 40–50% defect rate. *(Study Guide: 468)*

9. **(C)** Pulsed and color Doppler and M-mode are essential tools for a fetal echocardiogram. Even though power Doppler can have higher sensitivity, it has increased flash artifact and cannot determine direction of flow. *(Study Guide: 467)*

10. **(D)** Congenital heart defects occur in 1/100 live births. *(Study Guide: 467)*

11. **(B)** VSDs are the most common heart defect, occurring in approximately 20–57% of heart defect cases. *(Study Guide: 475)*

12. **(B)** In the subcostal four-chamber view, the septa are perpendicular to the transducer; therefore, it is more likely a defect will be identified. In the apical four-chamber view, the chambers are identified, but the septae is parallel to the transducer. In this position, a pseudodefect is often seen. *(Study Guide: 470)*

13. **(C)** A fetal echocardiogram should be performed between 18 and 22 weeks. Before this time, the heart is too small to visualize accurately. After 22 weeks, artifact from bony structures and decreased fluid volume makes evaluation difficult. *(Study Guide: 467)*

14. **(A)** The apex of the heart points toward the left. This is termed levocardia. Dextrocardia is when the apex points toward the right. *(Study Guide: 469)*

15. **(B)** The heart sits in the chest at an angle approximately 45°. The angle, however, can vary 20° in either direction. (i.e., 25°–65°). *(Study Guide: 469)*

16. **(A)** Levocardia is the normal orientation of the fetal heart. Dextrocardia occurs when the heart is in the right chest and the apex points toward the right. When the heart is situated in the midline and the apex points midline, this is termed mesocardia. Dextroposition is when the heart is in the right chest but the apex points toward the left. Mesoposition is not a term used to describe fetal heart position. *(Study Guide: 469)*

17. (C) The normal fetal heart occupies one-third of the fetal chest. *(Study Guide: 469)*

18. (B) The apical four-chamber view is obtained with a transverse view of the chest. The heart (apex) is directed toward or away from the transducer. In other words, the interventricular and interatrial septa run parallel to the beam of the transducer. *(Study Guide: 469)*

19. (D) An apical four-chamber view of the heart allows visualization of all four chambers, the size of the chambers, and the mitral and tricuspid valves. The ventricular septum is not well visualized because the septum is parallel to the transducer. *(Study Guide: 469)*

20. (D) Once a subcostal four-chamber view is obtained, the transducer can be rotated toward the fetus's right shoulder. The first view seen will be a long-axis view of the aorta (left ventricular outflow track). If rotation continues, the long axis of the pulmonary artery will be visualized (right ventricular outflow track). A short-axis view of the ventricles will be seen next. The short-axis view of the aorta with the pulmonary artery crossing over completes the rotation. *(Study Guide: 470)*

21. (B) The great vessels should be documented criss-crossing. If the great vessels run parallel, this could indicate transposition of the great vessels. Truncus arteriosus is when one vessel arises from the ventricle. When both vessels arise from the right ventricle, this is termed double outlet right ventricle. *(Study Guide: 471)*

22. (C) The moderator band is located in the right ventricle. This can be helpful in determining situs, especially with congenitally corrected transposition of the great arteries. *(Study Guide: 480)*

23. (D) The subcostal four-chamber view, long-axis view of the aorta, and the short-axis view of the ventricles are all useful in determining pathology of the ventricular septum. The short-axis view of the great vessels does not demonstrate the ventricular septum. It is, however, beneficial in determining correct orientation of the great vessels. *(Study Guide: 470)*

24. (A) In the fetus, the main pulmonary artery bifurcates into the ductus arteriosus and the right pulmonary artery. *(Study Guide: 472)*

25. (D) The aortic arch does not have the appearance of a hockey stick. The ductal arch is flat and broader, much like a hockey stick. *(Study Guide: 473)*

26. (B) The majority of coarctations occur just distal to where the ductus arteriosus inserts into the aorta. Aortic valve insufficiency is obtained proximal to the aortic valve. Aortic stenosis occurs at the level of the aortic valve. Pulmonary valve insufficiency would be identified in the right ventricle, proximal to the pulmonary valve. *(Study Guide: 477)*

27. (C) The ductal arch has a hockey stick appearance. The pulmonary artery, ductus arteriosus, and the descending aorta comprise the ductal arch. *(Study Guide: 473)*

28. (C) The most common indication for a fetal echocardiogram is family history. The risk for a reoccurring heart defect is highest when the mother has a defect (10–12%). The percentages are lower with other family members. *(Study Guide: 467)*

29. (D) Suboptimal heart views on a 15-week ultrasound are not an indication for a fetal echocardiogram. At 15 weeks, the fetal heart is small and structures are difficult to visualize. If the heart is suboptimal on an 18- to 20-week ultrasound, a fetal echocardiogram should be performed. *(Study Guide: 467)*

30. (C) Peak velocities can only be obtained with pulsed Doppler. Color Doppler, however, can help in determining areas of increased velocity or turbulence. *(Study Guide: 474)*

31. (D) M-mode is not useful in determining direction of flow. Color or pulsed Doppler can be used to determine direction. *(Study Guide: 474)*

32. (B) In the fetus, oxygenated blood travels from the umbilical veins through the ductus venosus, bypassing the liver. This blood then enters the IVC. The blood that enters the liver mixes with the portal system. Once the fetus is born, the ductus venosus closes and becomes the ligamentum venosum of the liver. *(Study Guide: 474)*

33. (A) The pulmonary veins enter the left atrium. Pulsed Doppler is helpful in determining appropriate direction and location of the pulmonary veins. *(Study Guide: 474)*

34. (D) The Doppler angle should be as close to zero as possible. With a 90° angle, a Doppler signal cannot be obtained. *(Study Guide: 474)*

35. (D) The Doppler gate should be small to avoid interference of other structures and vessels. *(Study Guide: 474)*

36. (A) Blood flows from the placenta to the fetus by way of the umbilical vein. The umbilical arteries return blood back to the placenta. The ductus venosum is a shunt that allows blood to bypass the liver. *(Study Guide: 474)*

37. (C) Oxygenated blood flows from the placenta through the umbilical vein. Most of this blood bypasses the liver via the ductus venosum and enters the IVC. Deoxygenated blood from the lower extremities travels up the IVC and mixes with the oxygenated blood. This oxygenated and deoxygenated blood then enters the right atrium. *(Study Guide: 475)*

38. **(D)** The umbilical vein is not considered a shunt. It carries blood from the placenta to the fetus. The ductus venosus allows blood to bypass the liver. It closes shortly after birth and becomes the ligamentum venosum in the liver. The foramen ovale shunts blood from the right atrium to the left atrium. The ductus arteriosus is a shunt between the pulmonary artery and the descending aorta. It also closes shortly after birth and becomes the ligamentum arteriosum. Closure of the ductus arteriosus causes a pressure change in the heart. After birth the pressure is higher in the left side of the heart, causing the foramen ovale to close. *(Study Guide: 475)*

39. **(D)** M-mode is not very useful in identifying a VSD in the fetus. It is useful in determining heart rate and rhythm, chamber size, and wall thickness. *(Study Guide: 474)*

40. **(A)** An AVSD is an abnormal development of the interatrial septum, interventricular septum, and the atrioventricular valves (tricuspid and mitral valves). *(Study Guide: 476)*

41. **(A)** With HLHS, there is a decreased in the blood flow coming in or out of the ventricle. The decrease in flow results in underdevelopment of the ventricle. *(Study Guide: 476)*

42. **(D)** Because HLHS affects the left heart, the mitral and aortic valves can be abnormal. *(Study Guide: 476)*

43. **(A)** With HLHS, the flow through the ascending aorta may be absent or reversed. This is caused by the blood flowing back through the ductus arteriosis into the ascending aorta. *(Study Guide: 476)*

44. **(C)** AVSDs are associated with polysplenia approximately 30% of the time. *(Study Guide: 476)*

45. **(C)** Approximately 78% of AVSDs are associated with Down syndrome (trisomy 21). *(Study Guide: 476)*

46. **(B)** An isolated VSD has the best prognosis. With Ebstein anomaly, the displacement of the tricuspid valve can lead to an enlarged right atrium, pulmonary atresia or stenosis, and cardiomegaly. Truncus arteriosus has a poor prognosis when left untreated. When treated, there is still mixing of oxygened and deoxygenated blood. If a coarctation of the aorta is untreated it is fatal. *(Study Guide: 475)*

47. **(A)** Hypoplastic left heart syndrome has the poorest prognosis. If left untreated, it is uniformly fatal. The poor prognosis is because of the small left heart, hypoplastic mitral valve, and ascending aorta. Hypoplastic right heart syndrome, however, has a better prognosis with a survival rate of approximately 25%. A *mild* aortic stenosis and an isolated ASD are treatable and have a good prognosis. *(Study Guide: 476)*

48. **(B)** With hypoplastic right heart syndrome, the pulmonary artery and valve can be small or atretic. The aorta and pulmonary veins are not affected with HRHS. *(Study Guide: 477)*

49. **(D)** When a valve is stenotic, the velocity will be increased distal to the valve. The sample gate can be placed proximal to the valve to determine valvular regurgitation. *(Study Guide: 474)*

50. **(C)** With the decrease of size and flow through the right side of the heart, there is decreased flow through the pulmonary artery. *(Study Guide: 477)*

51. **(A)** A univentricular heart has two atria and one ventricle. Often, when a univentricular heart is present, there is transposition of the great vessels coming off of this one ventricle. *(Study Guide: 477)*

52. **(A)** With univentricular heart, two atrioventricular valves may be seen. One, however, is usually atretic, indicating tricuspid or mitral atresia. This atresia is not related to the univentricular heart, but is considered a separate pathology. Pulmonary stenosis, asplenia, and polysplenia are all associated with univentricular heart. *(Study Guide: 477)*

53. **(C)** Coarctation is a narrowing of the aorta. Coarctation is often difficult to visualize in utero. *(Study Guide: 477)*

54. **(D)** Approximately 98% of coarctations occur between the left subclavian artery and the ductus arteriosus. *(Study Guide: 477)*

55. **(B)** Coarctation of the aorta is often difficult to visualize in utero. A narrowing of the aorta or increased velocities in the aorta can help to confirm the diagnosis. A large right ventricle may be a secondary sign of a coarctation. *(Study Guide: 477)*

56. **(A)** Coarctation of the aorta is most commonly seen with Turner syndrome. *(Study Guide: 477)*

57. **(C)** Ebstein anomaly is a right-sided heart anomaly. The tricuspid valve is displaced inferiorly. *(Study Guide: 478)*

58. **(A)** Maternal use of lithium has been associated with Ebstein anomaly. *(Study Guide: 478)*

59. **(D)** The four criteria for tetralogy of Fallot are a VSD, overriding aorta, pulmonary stenosis, and right ventricular hypertrophy. *(Study Guide: 478)*

60. **(C)** Right ventricular hypertrophy may not be seen in utero because of the presence of fetal shunts. An ASD is not a defect associated with tetralogy of Fallot. *(Study Guide: 478)*

61. **(D)** VSDs are present with truncus arteriosus. The single vessel overrides this defect. *(Study Guide: 479)*

62. (A) With truncus arteriosus, a single vessel arises from the heart. The pulmonary arteries then branch off this single vessel.   *(Study Guide: 479)*

63. (B) Congenitally corrected transposition of the great vessels occurs when ventricles are switched. The aorta arises from the left-sided right ventricle and follows the normal course toward the left side. With truncus arteriosus, a right-sided aortic arch is seen in approximately 15–30% of cases. Tetralogy of Fallot has a right side aortic arch in 25% of cases. With situs inversus of the chest, all anatomy above the diaphragm would be flipped.   *(Study Guide: 478–480)*

64. (B) Truncus arteriosus and tetralogy of Fallot appear similar sonographically. Both pathologies have a single vessel overriding a VSD. Truncus arteriosus, however, occurs when the pulmonary arteries arise from this single vessel; where with tetralogy of Fallot, the pulmonary artery arises from the right ventricle. A univentricular heart's vessels are often transposed.   *(Study Guide: 478–479)*

65. (C) With complete transposition of the great vessels, the great arteries arise from the heart parallel; therefore, a normal short-axis view of the great vessels cannot be obtained. A normal four-chamber heart can be obtained. This stresses the point of why outflow tracks should always be obtained.   *(Study Guide: 479)*

66. (A) With complete transposition of the great vessels, the atria, ventricles, and valves are in the appropriate location. The aorta arises from the right ventricle, and the pulmonary artery arises from the left ventricle. This differs from congenitally corrected transposition of the great vessels. With congenitally corrected transposition, the right atrium and left ventricle are connected, and the left atrium and right ventricle are connected. The aorta arises from the left-sided right ventricle, and the pulmonary artery arises from the right-sided left ventricle. Identification of the moderator band in the right ventricle is helpful in the diagnosis of congenitally corrected transposition of the great vessels.   *(Study Guide: 479)*

67. (D) The moderator band will always be located in the right ventricle. In congenitally corrected transposition of the great vessels, the right ventricle is located on the left side of the chest.   *(Study Guide: 480)*

68. (D) With congenitally corrected transposition, the right atrium and left ventricle are connected, and the left atrium and right ventricle are connected. The aorta arises from the left-sided right ventricle, and the pulmonary artery arises from the right-sided left ventricle. Identification of the moderator band in the right ventricle is helpful in the diagnosis of congenitally corrected transposition of the great vessels. With complete transposition of the great vessels, the atria, ventricles and valves are in the appropriate location.

The aorta arises from the right ventricle, and the pulmonary artery arises from the left ventricle.   *(Study Guide: 480)*

69. (A) When the long-axis views of the aorta and pulmonary artery are obtained, both great arteries would be visualized arising from the right ventricle. Four-chamber views of the heart will not demonstrate double outlet right ventricle.   *(Study Guide: 480)*

70. (C) Double outlet right ventricle occurs when both great arteries arise from the right ventricle running parallel.   *(Study Guide: 480)*

71. (C) The pulmonary veins normally drain into the left atrium. When total anomalous pulmonary venous connection is present, all four pulmonary veins will drain into the right atrium, or other venous structures.   *(Study Guide: 480)*

72. (D) Of the choices listed, hypoplastic left heart would be the most likely diagnosed in utero when only a four-chamber heart view is visualized. All of the other pathologies listed can be diagnosed with careful interrogation of the outflow tracks.   *(Study Guide: 476)*

73. (B) Severe levocardia is defined as the heart's apex pointing toward the left at an angle greater than the normal 45° ± 20°. Severe levocardia is commonly seen with Ebstein Anomaly, or other cardiac lesions that cause right-sided enlargement.   *(Study Guide: 481)*

74. (C) Dextrocardia is when the heart is in the right chest, and the apex of the heart is pointed toward the right. Levocardia is the normal position of the heart. Severe levocardia is defined as the heart's apex pointing toward the left at an angle greater than the normal 45° ± 20°. Dextroposition is when the heart's apex points toward the left, but the heart is in the right chest.   *(Study Guide: 481)*

75. (A) A diaphragmatic hernia and cystic adenomatoid malformation can push the heart into the right chest. Hypoplastic right lung causes a potential space on the right side that the heart can move into. Tricuspid insufficiency will not cause abnormal cardiac axis or position.   *(Study Guide: 481)*

76. (D) The most common dysrhythmia is premature atrial contractions. PACs can be caused by maternal use of caffeine, cigarettes or alcohol, or by a redundant foraminal flap. The majority of PACs resolve by delivery.   *(Study Guide: 482)*

77. (D) Supraventricular tachycardia occurs when the fetal heart rate is 180–280 bpm, and there is also atrial–ventricular concordance. If SVT remains throughout pregnancy, fetal hydrops or death can occur.   *(Study Guide: 482)*

78. (C) Transducer pressure can lead to bradycardia. When pressure is released, normal rate returns.   *(Study Guide: 482)*

79. **(B)** A second-degree heart block of 3:1 occurs when there are three atrial contractions for every one ventricular contraction.   *(Study Guide: 482)*

80. **(A)** ASDs, cardiac tumors, and polysplenia are all associated with complete heart block. Digoxin is a drug used to treat fetal supraventricular tachycardia.   *(Study Guide: 482)*

CHAPTER 11

VASCULAR SONOGRAPHY— CEREBROVASCULAR

Carol A. Krebs, Sandra L. Hughes, Karen K. Rawls, and Thomas G. Hoffman

Study Guide

INTRODUCTION

Stroke is the third leading cause of death in the United States with more than 500,000 strokes annually.[1] It is the leading cause of disability in the adult population and often leaves the patient crippled and unable to maintain a normal lifestyle.[2] Thus, stroke has become a national issue, and there have been important advances in the diagnosis and treatment of stroke patients. The emphasis has been placed on early diagnosis and treatment in the hopes of preventing long-term disability. In some geographic areas, there are stroke centers or specialized stroke treatment units that provide rapid evaluation of the stroke patient using computerized axial tomography (CT) perfusion imaging to rule out other diagnoses and to determine if the stroke is ischemic or hemorrhagic. A newer technique, magnetic resonance imaging (MRI) diffusion imaging can diagnosis stroke immediately, and MRI perfusion imaging shows where the blood is flowing. The goal is to define hyperacute cerebral ischemia (deficiency of blood caused by constriction or obstruction of a blood vessel)[3] with differentiation of reversible from irreversible ischemic damage and to identify those patients who qualify for thrombolytic therapy. The impact of a stroke is governed by multiple factors: the size of the stroke, the area of the brain involved, and whether the stroke is ischemic or hemorrhagic. In ischemic stroke, such drugs as tissue plasminogen activator (t-PA) are administered within 3 hours after onset. They can often dissolve the clot, restore the blood flow, and reverse the stroke effects.[4] However, thrombolytic therapy cannot be used with massive strokes or when hemorrhaging is involved.

Stroke is defined as a sudden and often severe impairment of the blood flow to the brain. There are three basic types of stroke.

Thrombotic strokes are the result of a clot blocking the blood flow in the artery of the brain, and approximately 60% of all strokes fall into this category.

Embolic stroke occurs when a piece of clot or embolus breaks loose, and the bloodstream carries it to the brain and blocks the artery. This occurs in approximately 20% of all strokes.

Hemorrhagic stroke occurs when a blood vessel in the brain breaks and spills blood into the brain and surrounding areas. High blood pressure is often associated with this type of stroke, and it occurs in 20% of strokes.

Symptoms

Internal Carotid Artery Symptoms. Internal carotid artery disease affects the cerebral hemispheres and is associated with the following symptoms.

- Paralysis on the contralateral side. For example, if the stroke occurs on the right side of the brain, the left side of the body will be affected.
- Speech deficit with involvement of the dominant hemisphere
- Hemianopsia (blindness in one half of the field of vision, can be bilateral or unilateral) from occlusion of the middle cerebral artery
- Decreased level of consciousness
- Amaurosis fugax (fleeting eye blindness) on the side of the diseased artery, which is caused by an embolus in the ophthalmic artery or one of its branches

Vertebrobasilar Artery Disease Symptoms. It often affects the posterior areas of the brain, including the occipital lobes, brain stem, and cerebellum and has the following symptoms.

- Vertebrobasilar artery disease is often bilateral and involves either arms or legs.
- Tinnitus (noise in the ears)[3]
- Dizziness
- Vertigo (loss of equilibrium)
- Diplopia (two images)[3]
- Dysarthria (imperfect articulation of speech)[3]
- Dysphagia (difficulty swallowing)
- Ataxia (muscular uncoordination)
- Vomiting
- Headache
- One of the most common symptoms is the drop attack where the patient falls to the ground with no warning. However, they recover quickly with only residual dizziness or mild ataxia.[2]

The classic stroke as a result of unilateral carotid disease presents with ipsilateral blindness and contralateral hemiplegia (paralysis of one side of the body).[3] Of less severity are the fleeting focal neurologic defects, such as transient monoplegia, transient hemiplegia, or transient ipsilateral blindness. These are sudden and abrupt episodes and are gone in minutes to hours after the onset and are termed *transient ischemic attacks* (TIA).[2] There are various terms used to describe the neurologic events and conditions that are associated with stroke and they include.

- *Transient Ischemic Attack (TIA).* A TIA is an acute neurologic event in which there are neurologic deficits, but the symptoms completely resolve in less than 24 hours.
- *Reversible Ischemic Neurologic Deficit (RIND).* A RIND lasts longer than 24 hours, but resolves completely within a week.
- *Completed Stroke.* In a completed stroke, neurologic defects last longer than 24 hours and do not resolve; symptoms may be severe, and cell death occurs in the brain tissue.
- *Stroke in Evolution.* Stroke in evolution is where the neurologic defects become progressively worse over time. The duration can be up to 2 weeks.
- *Acute Brain Death.* Brain death may be caused by a lack of blood supply (ischemia) or the effect of the blood outside of normal vessels (hemorrhage). There are generally two basic types of strokes, ischemic stroke (80%) and hemorrhagic stroke (20%).[5]

Some of the more common causes of ischemic stroke include:[2,6,7]

- Atherosclerosis (cause in the majority of patients)
- Embolus from the heart
- Hypertensive arteriolar sclerosis
- Dissection
- Prethrombotic states
- Vasospasm: subarachnoid hemorrhage, idiopathic
- Fibromuscular hyperplasia

- Obliterative arteritis of the great vessels
- Blunt or penetrating trauma

TECHNIQUE AND INSTRUMENTATION

Equipment, understanding their design and use, and manipulation for specific vascular examinations are vital in the performance of high-quality examinations. There have been numerous changes over the last 20 years in instrumentation, and subsequently, our performance of vascular examinations. There can be no doubt that color flow Doppler units that combine realtime two-dimensional (2D) imaging, spectral analysis with calculations, and color flow Doppler is the method of choice in ultrasound cerebrovascular examinations. They have come of age, and we are now seeing further new innovative techniques. These include power Doppler, and the use of contrast media with intracerebral, as well as extracerebral examinations. In some vascular laboratories, we continue to see such supplementary examinations as periorbital, ocular plethysmography, and small operative units that do spectral tracings in the surgical suites and bedside.

CW or continuous wave Doppler was explained in the arterial principles and instrumentation, and is an indirect evaluation of the cerebrovascular system. It is frequently used in the transcranial evaluation for portable bedside examinations or in the surgical suite during operative procedures. It is also used in the indirect testing methods described below.

Ocular Pneumoplethysmography (OPG)

OPG is based on pressure measurements of the ophthalmic artery to detect hemodynamically significant lesions (greater than 50%). A significant stenosis will cause an arterial pressure decrease. When there are ophthalmic artery pressure differences of 5 mmHg or more between the right and left sides, a hemodynamically significant lesion should be considered present. The examination is performed by anesthetizing the eye, placing eyecups on the sclera, and applying a vacuum (300–500 mmHg). When the vacuum is released, tracings are made of the returning pulsations of both eyes. This examination can be used in the assessment of collateral circulation that occurs secondary to critical stenosis or occlusion.

Periorbital Doppler

This method of testing examines the direction of blood flow in the ophthalmic artery branches (supraorbital, frontal, and nasal arteries). These arteries serve as collateral pathways with internal carotid artery disease.

Determining the direction of flow in the periorbital arteries requires a directional Doppler velocity detector. The frontal and supraorbital arteries are examined separately. Flow in each artery is assessed in its normal state and with compression of the superficial temporal, facial, and infraorbital arteries. In the normal state, the periorbital arterial flow is toward the face. Compression of the external carotid artery branches can cause no change or can increase the periorbital arterial flow. With internal carotid artery critical stenosis or occlusion, flow in the periorbital arteries can be reversed; or rather, flowing backward into the orbit. Compression of the external carotid artery branches will decrease or obliterate the Doppler signal.

Duplex and Color Flow Doppler

Color flow Doppler is achieved by estimating and displaying the mean velocity relative to the ultrasound beam direction and the reflectors. Echo signals from moving reflectors are generally displayed so color hue, saturation, or brightness indicates relative velocity.[7]

Initially, a high-resolution gray-scale image is obtained of the cerebrovascular vessels using a 7.5 MHz or 10 MHz linear array transducer. A linear array with multiple elements (64–256) with electronic focusing and beam steering is the most common transducer for carotid imaging. Occasionally, a 10 MHz may be employed for extremely superficial vessels or very small necks and a lower frequency is routinely used for transcranial structures. In gray-scale imaging, the beam is always perpendicular to the vessel for the best delineation of the structures. However, Doppler information is obtained with the beam parallel to the vessel.[8] This is best achieved by using a 45–60° angle. When the Doppler angle exceeds 60–70°, the accuracy declines to the point where there is no velocity change detected at a Doppler angle of 90°.[9] Angle correction is mandatory when using velocity to represent the Doppler shift. The Doppler shift may be recorded in frequency or velocity; however, velocity allows for a universal standard for comparison.[9] Color flow Doppler provides a rapid localization of vessels and easily demonstrates turbulent or disturbed flow associated with disease processes. It is also superior for demonstrating occluded vessels and stenotic zones. Spectral analysis provides the quantification, and it is obtained by placing a sample volume with a narrow gate (minimum usually 1.5 mm) at a specific depth (Fig. 11–1). Spectral analysis determines the presence, direction, and characteristics of the blood flow.

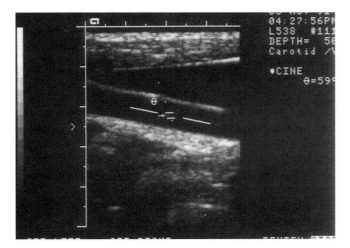

Figure 11–1. The sample volume (arrowhead) is seen as two parallel lines. The axial dimension (gate width) is determined by the operator.

The sample volume can be moved along an electronic cursor, which is steered on the real-time image. The ability to range gate allows the selection of depth from which the Doppler information is obtained. In actuality, a real-time delay is used to decipher information from the sample volume area. The frequency spectrum is displayed in graph form that shows relative amplitude of each frequency in the Doppler signal. It is usually analyzed by the interpreter for peak velocity, peak end diastolic velocity, and systolic/diastolic ratios between the ICA and CCA.[9] One of the artifacts with pulsed Doppler is aliasing, which occurs when the frequencies exceed the Nyquist limit (pulse repetition frequency/2) and is seen as a wraparound or folding over of the waveform. This may be overcome by a change in the probe position, decreasing the depth, increasing the PRF, increasing the Doppler angle, or lowering the frequency.[8]

Power Doppler

There are various terminologies for power Doppler used by different manufacturers, such as: ultrasound angiography, color power angiography, and color Doppler energy. Power Doppler is extremely sensitive in low-flow states and often supplemental in the color flow Doppler evaluation.[10] Power Doppler provides a perfusion-type display of blood flow in the vascular beds of tissues and can often display longer segments of the vessels. It encodes the power in the Doppler signal in color by using the amplitude information from the color Doppler signal and raising the noise floor. It does not rely on frequency shift information, is not dependent on beam angle, and is free from the aliasing artifact. The disadvantage of power Doppler is the failure to provide information about speed or direction of flow. It insonates all vessels in its path, and excessive motion can seriously degrade the image. In most units, there are additional motion suppression mechanisms.[5] Power Doppler is especially beneficial in defining occlusive states where there is no flow or low flow states, both intra and extracerebral.

ANATOMY

The blood supply to the brain is supplied by the cerebrovascular vessels (Fig. 11–2). They are further described as extracranial (extracerebral), which means outside of the cranium, or intracranial (intracerebral), which means inside of the cranium. These cerebrovascular vessels arise from the aortic arch and course cephalad (Fig. 11–3).

Brachiocephalic Trunk (Innominatae) Artery

This arises from the aortic arch and courses to the right and branches into the right common carotid artery superiorly and the right subclavian artery laterally. The subclavian artery continues descending into the right extremity to become the axillary and the brachial.

Subclavian Artery

This arises from the brachiocephalic on the right and from the aortic arch on the left. It is a direct continuation and is named according to location. Subclavian artery from the

The right common carotid artery arises from the brachio-cephalic and the left common carotid artery arises directly from the aortic arch. It bifurcates into the internal carotid artery and the external carotid artery. The location of the bifurcation is variable but is usually at the level of the thyroid cartilage.

Internal Carotid Artery (ICA)

This artery carries blood to the cerebral hemispheres of the brain. It supplies the eye and accessory organs, forehead, and part of the nose. It is divided into four sections; cervical, petrous, cavernous, and intracranial. There are no branches of the internal carotid artery in the cervical section. Small branches arise from the petrous and cavernous portions. The ophthalmic artery is the first major branch coursing from the cavernous portion. The intracranial portion feeds the middle cerebral artery, the anterior cerebral artery, and the posterior communicating artery. Branches of the ICA include:

Petrous branches
- Caroticotympanic
- Pterygoid

Cavernous branches
- Cavernous
- Hypophyseal
- Semilunar
- Anterior Meningeal
- Ophthalmic. This artery courses anteriorly from the cavernous portion of the internal carotid artery. It supplies blood to the eye. The three distal branches are the supraorbital, frontal, and nasal arteries. These arteries can become sources of collateral circulation with the distal branches of the external carotid artery in the event of internal carotid artery occlusive disease.

Cerebral branches
- Anterior cerebral
- Middle cerebral
- Posterior communicating
- Choroidal

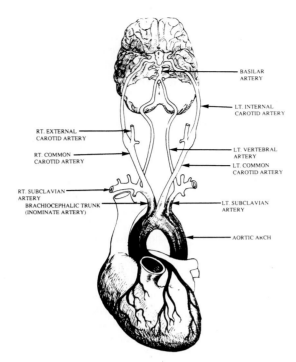

Figure 11–2. Blood supply to the brain.

arch to the border of the first rib, axillary artery from the first rib to the teres major muscle, and brachial artery from the teres major to the bifurcation at the elbow. Branches of the subclavian include:

- Vertebral
- Internal thoracic
- Thyrocervical trunk
- Costocervical trunk
- Dorsal scapular

Common Carotid Artery (CCA)

This artery is the main branch of the carotid system, which is the main blood supply for the cerebrovascular circulation.

External Carotid Artery (ECA)

This artery carries blood to the face and scalp. Unlike the internal carotid artery, it can be identified by its numerous branches in the cervical region. The superior thyroid artery is the first branch. The location of the superficial temporal artery is important for performing a tapping maneuver for positive identification of the external carotid artery during Doppler examination. Branches of the ECA include:

- Superior thyroid
- Ascending pharyngeal
- Lingual
- Internal and external maxillary
- Occipital
- Posterior auricular
- Superficial temporal

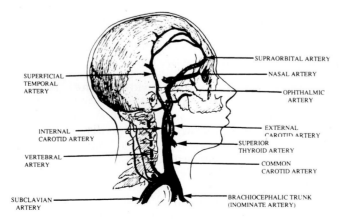

Figure 11–3. Cerebrovascular anatomy.

Vertebral Artery

The vertebral artery arises from the superoposterior aspect of the subclavian and is the first branch of the subclavian. It courses superiorly to enter the foramina of the transverse processes of the sixth cervical vertebra. It enters the skull at the foramen magnum. The two vertebral arteries unite to form a single basilar artery at the junction of the medulla and pons. Branches of the vertebral artery include:

Cervical Branches
- Muscular
- Spinal

Cranial Branches
- Meningeal
- Posterior and Anterior Spinal
- Posterior inferior cerebellar
- Medullary

Basilar Artery

This is an intracranial vessel arising from the unison of the vertebral arteries. Branches of the basilar artery include:

- Pontine
- Internal auditory (labyrinthine)
- Anterior Cerebellar
- Superior Cerebellar

Circle of Willis

The circle of Willis is an anastomosis found at the base of the brain formed by a network of arteries that arise from the internal carotid arteries and the vertebral artery (Fig. 11–4). The arteries can vary in caliber, be maldeveloped, absent or have anomalies, and in some instances, the circle may not be intact. The internal carotid artery, which courses superiorly into the base of the brain, branches into the anterior cerebral artery, middle cerebral artery, and the anterior and posterior communicating arteries. The vertebral arteries converge to form a single basilar artery, which bifurcates to form the posterior cerebral arteries. Communicating arteries form an important network of collateral circulation in the circle of Willis. The anterior communicating artery connects the two anterior cerebral arteries. The posterior communicating arteries connect the posterior cerebral arteries with the anterior circulation (middle, cerebral, and anterior cerebral arteries). Three predominant arterial trunks arise from the circle of Willis and supply the cerebral hemisphere. The anterior portions are supplied by the two anterior cerebrals, the anterolateral portions by the middle cerebrals, and the posterior portion by the posterior cerebral. Each of these trunks give rise to numerous vessels that supply the brain. The circle of Willis is an important collateral pathway for circulation. Collateral pathways are often complex and can make it difficult to interpret the cerebrovascular examination. Transcranial Doppler examinations have proved valuable in identification of these collateral pathways. Some of the more common pathways include:[5]

- Right to left anastomoses that provides redistribution of blood flow between the sides of the body and occurs

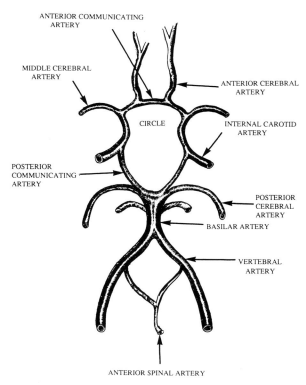

Figure 11–4. Circle of Willis.

via the anterior communicating arteries (AcoA) and the basilar artery (BA)
- Carotid to vertebral anastomoses via the posterior communicating arteries (PcoA)
- ICA to ECA ipsilateral anastomoses involving the supraorbital and supratrochlear arteries
- Subclavian to carotid and subclavian to vertebral anastomoses, which involve the deep cervical artery, spinal branches of the vertebral artery, and ascending cervical artery
- Cortical anastomoses can provide collateral flow between the anterior cerebral artery (ACA), middle cerebral artery (MCA), and posterior cerebral artery (PCA) territories.

NORMAL SONOGRAPHIC CAROTID EXAMINATION

Indications for Carotid Examination[5,7]
- Asymptomatic cervical bruit
- Nonspecific neurologic symptoms (dizziness, numbness, transient loss of vision)
- Classic transient ischemic attack (TIA)
- Amaurosis fugax (transient monocular blindness)
- Ischemic oculopathy
- Retinal artery or vein occlusion
- Carotid endarterectomy follow-up
- Pre-op major surgeries

- Follow-up patients with mild asymptomatic carotid stenosis
- Baseline data on symptomatic patients
- Hollenhorst plaques (cholesterol embolus in a retinal arteriole noted on a routine retinoscopy)
- Pulsating mass in the carotid regions

The normal extracranial carotid examination includes interrogation of the following vessels:

- Right brachiocephalic artery
- Bilateral subclavian arteries
- Bilateral vertebral arteries
- Bilateral common carotid arteries
- Bilateral common carotid bulb and bifurcation
- Bilateral internal carotid artery
- Bilateral external carotid artery

Each vessel is imaged with representative view obtained. Spectral analysis is performed in midstream of the vessel with peak systolic velocity recorded. Any required routine calculations are performed. If there is disease present or any narrowing seen, close up characterization of the area is obtained with views in the longitudinal and transverse planes. A percentage stenosis is calculated for any narrowed segment and should be in agreement with the peak systolic velocity recordings. If not, these parameters should be rechecked to ensure accuracy. Spectral analysis is obtained in the pre- and poststenotic zones. It is also helpful to walk the sample volume cursor through the vessel with the sample volume gate open to obtain the maximum velocity ranges. Color flow Doppler will also denote the highest velocity ranges, with mosaic color changes, and color turbulence in the poststenotic zones.

The extracranial vessels normally have laminar flow because blood flows through an artery in concentric layers, with the fastest flow in the central portion of the lumen. Blood flow becomes slower as each layer becomes closer to the arterial wall. In theory, the layer next to the arterial wall will display little or no flow. At the bulb of the common carotid artery, there will be a boundary layer separation, which is a reversal of flow toward the outer edge with some turbulence in the mainstream of the vessel. On real-time images, the vessels are seen as tubular anechoic structures, and color Doppler shows color filling of the patent vessel lumen. Power Doppler may be used for better delineation of the walls and to define any area that has poor filling. The spectral analysis is narrow in systolic and somewhat wider in early and late diastole. There is usually a blank zone between the spectral line and zero velocity baselines, which represents the spectral window. There are distinct differences in the ICA and ECA spectral waveforms.

The internal carotid artery is a low-resistance waveform supplying the low-resistance circulation of the brain and has a flow similar to other low-resistance arteries, such as the renal artery and vertebral arteries. The most common feature of a low resistance arterial waveform is the large quantity of forward flow, which continues throughout diastole (Fig. 11–5).

The external carotid artery is a high-resistance waveform that supplies the high-resistance vasculature of the

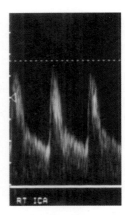

Figure 11–5. Internal carotid artery waveform with characteristic continuous flow in diastole.

facial musculature. It presents as a highly pulsatile signal resembling a peripheral artery[9] (Fig. 11–6). In cases where the ICA is occluded or has a high-grade stenosis, the waveform characteristic may change because the blood is being diverted to the ECA it will take on an ICA characteristic. In some instances, it may be difficult to define the vessels and necessary to verify the specific vessel. The ECA may be further identified by seeing the first branch because the ICA has no cervical branches. A "wobble" maneuver can also be performed by tapping the superficial temporal while imaging the vessel. If the ECA has a wobble motion in the waveform during the maneuver, it confirms that it is the ECA.

The common carotid artery is a mixture of the ICA and ECA waveforms but more often resembles the ICA waveform (Fig. 11–7). Approximately 80% of blood flowing from the CCA goes through the ICA and 20% goes through the ECA.[9]

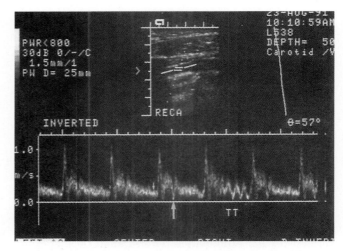

Figure 11–6. External carotid artery waveform with resistive flow pattern. Note the return of flow to the baseline (large arrow) in early diastole and the close proximity to the baseline in end diastole (small arrow). Positive identification of the external can be made by tapping the superficial temporal artery and noting the transmitted pulsations along the diastolic portion of the waveform (TT).

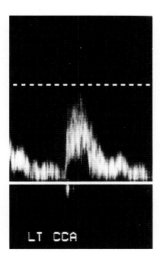

Figure 11–7. Common carotid artery with a combination of ICA and ECA characteristics.

The vertebral arteries are seen arising as the first branch of the subclavian and ascending through the transverse processes up to the transverse foramina. The origin of the vertebral artery is carefully evaluated in the transverse plane at the level of the subclavian artery. In some cases, plaque, stenosis, or even absence of the vertebral artery may be noted. In a longitudinal plane at the level of the common carotid artery, the transducer is angled laterally until the vertebral is be seen passing through the transverse processes. The spectral waveform analysis will depict a low-resistance waveform pattern similar to that of the common carotid artery (Fig. 11–8).

Percentage Stenosis

The basic principles of hemodynamics in the section on Arterial Principles and Instrumentation should be reviewed to aid in the understanding of arterial occlusive and aneurysm disease.

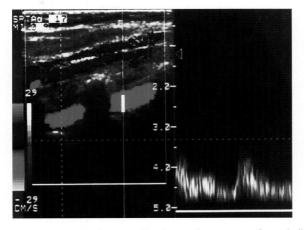

Figure 11–8. Vertebral artery with a low-resistance waveform similar to the common carotid artery.

Symptoms of arterial disease usually become evident when a critical arterial stenosis is reached. *Critical stenosis* is defined as a stenosis that causes a significant reduction in flow and pressure.[4] The blood flow and pressure are not significantly affected until 75% of the cross-sectional area of the vessel is obliterated. This is equal of a 50% reduction in lumen diameter. A hemodynamically significant stenosis is one that exceeds 50–60% diameter reduction (75% area reduction) (Fig. 11–9, Fig. 11–10). It is at this point when flow velocities begin to increase (both systolic and end diastolic), and flow volume begins to decrease. Therefore, stenotic lesions in the fourth and fifth category are considered hemodynamically significant. When a hemodynamically significant lesion is present, certain flow characteristics are evident at the prestenotic, stenotic, and poststenotic sample sites.

Prestenotic Site. Located proximal to a hemodynamically significant stenosis (Fig. 11–11).

Peak systolic velocities are within normal limits

A resistive flow pattern may be noted in diastole

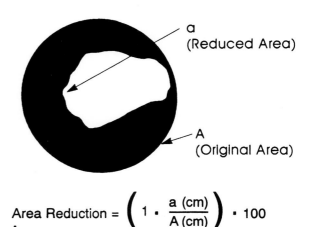

$$\text{Area Reduction} = \left(1 \cdot \frac{a\ (cm)}{A\ (cm)}\right) \cdot 100$$

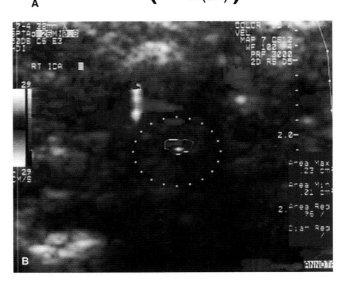

Figure 11–9. Cross-sectional area reduction.

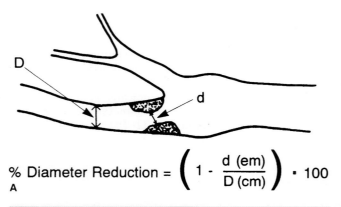

$$\text{\% Diameter Reduction} = \left(1 - \frac{d\ (em)}{D\ (cm)}\right) \cdot 100$$

A

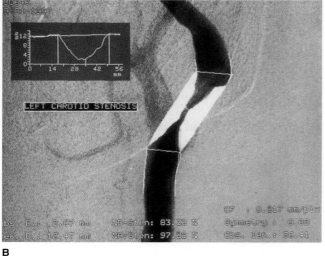

B

Figure 11–10. Lumen diameter reduction.

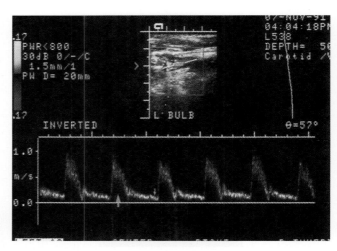

Figure 11–11. Waveform proximal to a stenosis with a decreased diastolic portion caused by distal resistance (arrow). Note the laminar flow pattern with a clear spectral window (large arrow).

consists of both forward and reverse components as blood flow changes The turbulence usually occurs in the poststenotic zone because of the kinetic energy dissipating by the turbulent eddies. These is also indication that the atherosclerotic lesions form near areas of blood flow separation and low shear stress. The layer of blood adjacent to the arterial wall is slower moving than the mainstream laminar flow and is termed the boundary layer. The flow in the center of the artery is rapid and laminar, but the areas of boundary layer separation have slower more disturbed currents. These areas of boundary layer separation and low shear force generally occur at the outer wall of arterial bifurcations where atheroma formation is more frequently seen.[1]

Interpretation of the cerebrovascular examination includes evaluation of the spectral analysis and its characteristics as defined in the following section.

Stenotic Site (Fig. 11–12)
Peak systolic velocities increase
End-diastolic velocities increase
Spectral broadening

Poststenotic Site (Fig. 11–13)
Peak systolic velocities decrease
End–diastolic velocities decrease
Turbulent flow is noted (flow reversal as well as forward flow)

Other factors also affect the critical stenosis but to a lesser degree. These include the length of the stenosis, blood viscosity, and peripheral resistance.[1] It has been noted that a series of subcritical stenoses can have an additive effect and be equal to a single critical stenosis. Turbulence is the most important cause of blood flow changes and pressure drop across a stenosis. Turbulent flow is seen when blood flow looses its laminar characteristics as it travels past areas of atheromatous deposits.

The degree of turbulent flow depends upon the degree of disease; as the stenotic area becomes increasingly narrow, the degree of turbulence increases. Turbulent flow

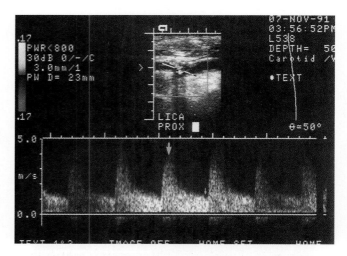

Figure 11–12. ICA stenosis with a dramatic increase in the peak systolic velocity (large arrow) and the end diastolic velocity (small arrow). Also filling in of the spectral window.

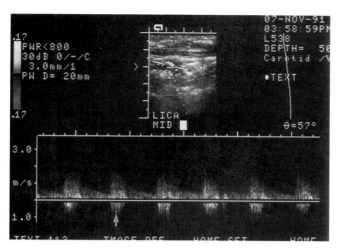

Figure 11–13. Poststenotic zone distal to a stenosis. The peak systolic velocities and end diastolic velocities are decreased with turbulent and reversed flow.

Spectral Doppler Waveform in Progressive Disease States of the Internal Carotid Artery (Fig. 11–14)

Normal
- Narrow range of velocities in systole and diastole
- Clear spectral window
- Peak systolic velocities do not exceed 125 cm/s

Mild disease (0–15% diameter reduction)
- Range of velocities in diastole mildly increases
- Spectral window may still remain clear
- Peak systolic velocities do not exceed 125 cm/s

Moderate disease (16–49% diameter reduction)
- Spectral broadening (range of velocities increases)
- Spectral window filling
- Peak systolic velocities do not exceed 125 cm/s

Severe disease (50–79% diameter reduction)
- Marked spectral broadening with spectral window filling
- Peak systolic velocities exceed 125 cm/s
- End diastolic velocity increases but does not exceed 100 cm/s

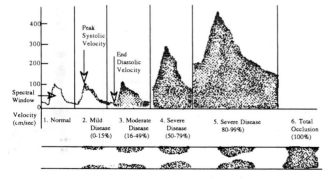

Figure 11–14. Spectral Doppler waveform in progressive disease states in the internal carotid artery.

Severe disease (80–99% diameter reduction)
- Marked spectral broadening with spectral window filling
- Peak systolic velocities exceed 125 cm/s and may be in the 300–400 cm/s range
- End diastolic velocity exceeds 140 cm/s

Total occlusion
- Absence of spectral information because of no flow in the occluded state

DISEASE AND PATHOLOGY

The etiology of most arterial diseases is atherosclerosis. It has been defined by the World Health Organization as a combination of changes in the intima and media, which include: focal accumulation of lipids, hemorrhage, fibrous tissue, and calcium deposits.[1]

Atheroma Formation
Atheroma formation is a complicated process whereby plaque is initially formed in the intimal layer of tissue and evolves into an accumulation of fibrotic materials, hemorrhagic products, and calcifications. Atheroma formation begins with the infiltration of lipid materials into the endothelial layer of the intima of the artery. On real, time 2-D, the intima echo is bright with a uniform, narrow width. Lipid infiltration is depicted as an irregular thickening that varies throughout the length of the lumen. The simple lipid (fatty) plaque can evolve into a more complex structure. Hemorrhage may occur within the plaque as the endothelial layer becomes eroded, and the surface of the intima becomes irregular. Ulceration of the plaque can lead to the release of platelet aggregates into the circulation. These become microemboli, and neurologic symptoms may occur as small vessels become occluded. Irregular plaque surfaces can lead to thrombus formation. Thrombus can narrow the arterial lumen and, eventually, cause a total occlusion. It can also break free from the plaque site and become a large embolus, causing neurologic symptoms. Arterial bifurcations are common sites for plaque formation. The most common site in the extracerebral vascular circulation is the bifurcation of the common carotid artery into the internal and external carotid arteries.

Inherent risk factors include:[1,5]

- Advanced age
- Hypertension
- History of transient ischemic attacks
- Cigarette smoking
- Heart disorders
- Associated embolism
- Family history of cerebrovascular accident
- Use of oral contraceptives
- Diabetes
- Physical inactivity
- Obesity
- Hypercholesterolemia
- Hyperlipidemia

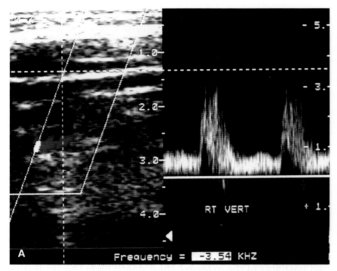

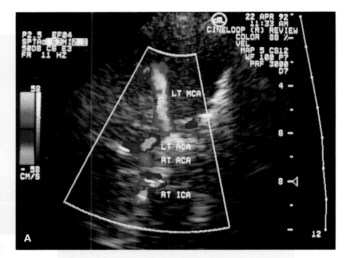

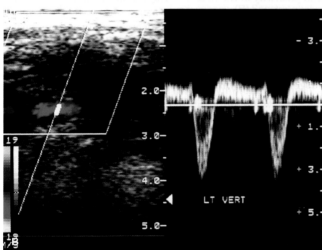

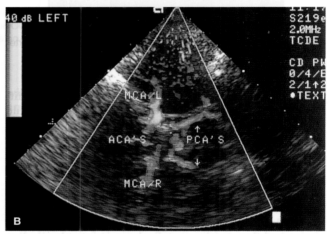

Figure 11–32. (A) Transcranial vessels illustrated with color Doppler imaging. **(B)** Transcranial vessels illustrated with color Doppler power energy mode.

Figure 11–31. Subclavian steal. **(A)** Right vertebral has a normal waveform with increased flow. **(B)** Left vertebral is reversed indicating subclavian steal.

Primary TCD parameters are vital for identification of specific intracranial arteries especially using the blind method without imaging. These parameters include:

- Insonation depth
- Direction of blood flow at the specific depth
- Mean flow velocity
- Probe position
- Direction of ultrasound beam

Cerebral blood flow can be altered by multiple physiological changes. The examiner must understand these changes so as not to mistake them for pathological changes.

- Heart rate increase will increase velocities, and conversely, a decrease in heart rate will decrease the velocities.

- Increased intracranial pressure will decrease the diastole flow.
- Decreased hematocrit will lower velocities.
- Increasing age will lower velocities.
- Children and young adults will have higher velocities.

The primary anatomy involved in the transcranial Doppler examination is the vasculature of the circle of Willis as seen in Fig. 11–4 includes the following arteries:

MCA—Middle cerebral artery (M1, M2 segments)
ICA—Internal carotid artery
PCA—Posterior cerebral artery (P1, P2 segments)
VA—Vertebral artery
BA—Basilar artery
CS—Carotid siphon (C1, C2, C3, C4 segments)
ACoA—Anterior communicating artery (A1, A2 segments)
PCoa—Posterior communicating artery
Oa—Ophthalmic artery

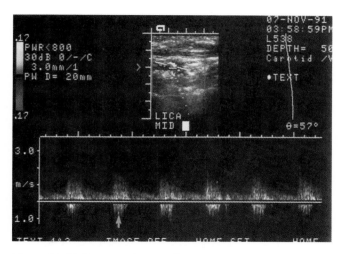

Figure 11–13. Poststenotic zone distal to a stenosis. The peak systolic velocities and end diastolic velocities are decreased with turbulent and reversed flow.

Spectral Doppler Waveform in Progressive Disease States of the Internal Carotid Artery (Fig. 11–14)

Normal
- Narrow range of velocities in systole and diastole
- Clear spectral window
- Peak systolic velocities do not exceed 125 cm/s

Mild disease (0–15% diameter reduction)
- Range of velocities in diastole mildly increases
- Spectral window may still remain clear
- Peak systolic velocities do not exceed 125 cm/s

Moderate disease (16–49% diameter reduction)
- Spectral broadening (range of velocities increases)
- Spectral window filling
- Peak systolic velocities do not exceed 125 cm/s

Severe disease (50–79% diameter reduction)
- Marked spectral broadening with spectral window filling
- Peak systolic velocities exceed 125 cm/s
- End diastolic velocity increases but does not exceed 100 cm/s

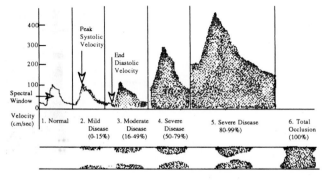

Figure 11–14. Spectral Doppler waveform in progressive disease states in the internal carotid artery.

Severe disease (80–99% diameter reduction)
- Marked spectral broadening with spectral window filling
- Peak systolic velocities exceed 125 cm/s and may be in the 300–400 cm/s range
- End diastolic velocity exceeds 140 cm/s

Total occlusion
- Absence of spectral information because of no flow in the occluded state

DISEASE AND PATHOLOGY

The etiology of most arterial diseases is atherosclerosis. It has been defined by the World Health Organization as a combination of changes in the intima and media, which include: focal accumulation of lipids, hemorrhage, fibrous tissue, and calcium deposits.[1]

Atheroma Formation
Atheroma formation is a complicated process whereby plaque is initially formed in the intimal layer of tissue and evolves into an accumulation of fibrotic materials, hemorrhagic products, and calcifications. Atheroma formation begins with the infiltration of lipid materials into the endothelial layer of the intima of the artery. On real, time 2-D, the intima echo is bright with a uniform, narrow width. Lipid infiltration is depicted as an irregular thickening that varies throughout the length of the lumen. The simple lipid (fatty) plaque can evolve into a more complex structure. Hemorrhage may occur within the plaque as the endothelial layer becomes eroded, and the surface of the intima becomes irregular. Ulceration of the plaque can lead to the release of platelet aggregates into the circulation. These become microemboli, and neurologic symptoms may occur as small vessels become occluded. Irregular plaque surfaces can lead to thrombus formation. Thrombus can narrow the arterial lumen and, eventually, cause a total occlusion. It can also break free from the plaque site and become a large embolus, causing neurologic symptoms. Arterial bifurcations are common sites for plaque formation. The most common site in the extracerebral vascular circulation is the bifurcation of the common carotid artery into the internal and external carotid arteries.

Inherent risk factors include:[1,5]

- Advanced age
- Hypertension
- History of transient ischemic attacks
- Cigarette smoking
- Heart disorders
- Associated embolism
- Family history of cerebrovascular accident
- Use of oral contraceptives
- Diabetes
- Physical inactivity
- Obesity
- Hypercholesterolemia
- Hyperlipidemia

Plaque. Plaque should be documented, characterized, and evaluated for surface contours. Acoustical shadowing may be present and, on occasion, so dense that the spectral analysis cannot be obtained. Alternate positioning or changes in frequency may help to overcome this problem.

Characteristics of Plaque

Fatty Streaks (Fig. 11–15). These are the earliest lesions and are primarily lipid.[1]

Soft Plaque (Fig. 11–16, 17). It may be technically difficult to visualize soft plaque because of the low-level echoes it contains and, in some instances, may be anechoic. Careful scanning techniques must be utilized to optimize visualization and characterize the plaque.

Dense Fibrous Plaque. (Fig. 11–18). It is easy to identify a dense plaque because it is echogenic on the 2-D images. They usually occur later in life and are primarily located at arterial bifurcations. These plaques have a lipid core surrounded by a capsule of elastin and collagenous tissue.[1]

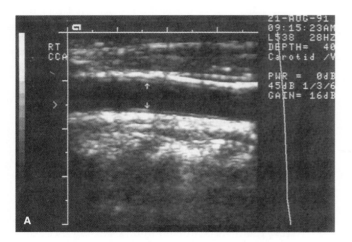

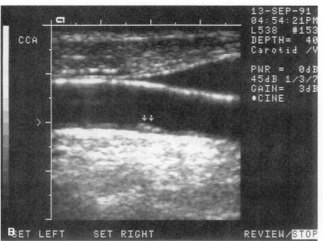

Figure 11–15. (A) Normal intimal echo in the carotid artery (arrows). **(B)** Abnormally thickened intimal echo consistent with lipid (fatty infiltration (arrows).

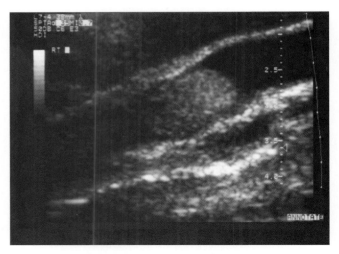

Figure 11–16. Soft plaque with low level echoes.

Calcified Plaque (Fig. 11–19). Calcified plaque is identified by the bright echo appearance and posterior acoustic shadowing on the 2D image.

Complicated Lesions. These lesions usually begin with the fibrous plaque, but calcifications may also be present. Necrosis of the plaque often leads to ulceration where thrombi may occur. Ulcerated plaque can be a nidus for emboli and is often associated with intraplaque hemorrhage. Neither ultrasound nor angiography is highly accurate for defining ulceration. Findings, on ultrasound, which suggest ulceration are: continuous contours showing a focal depression, well-defined break in plaque surface, and anechoic plaque area within a plaque extending to the surface.[9] Intramural hemorrhage may also be seen with or without ulceration. The vessel lumen can become narrowed because of the atherosclerotic process, or the wall may degenerate and dilate, forming an aneurysm.[1] This type of lesion will be heterogeneous on the ultrasound image.

Surface Characteristics of Plaque
Smooth Borders (Fig. 11–20). Plaque may have a smooth surface with no irregularities.

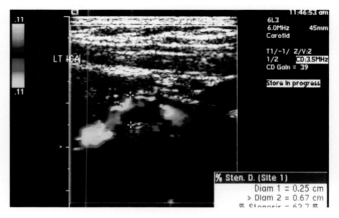

Figure 11–17. Soft plaque that is anechoic.

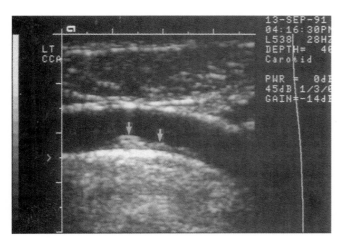

Figure 11–18. Dense plaque (arrows).

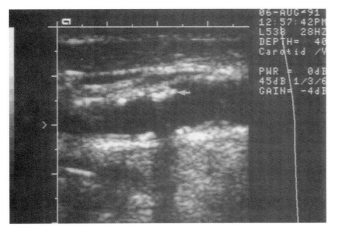

Figure 11–19. Calcified plaque (arrow) with posterior acoustic shadowing.

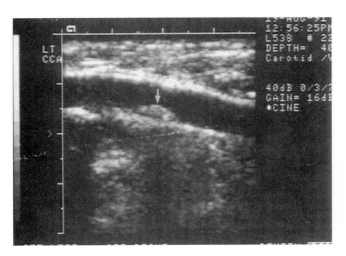

Figure 11–20. Smooth-bordered plaque (arrow).

Irregular Borders (Fig. 11–21). Plaque may have irregularities, with pitted surfaces, and the presence of ulcers.

Internal Echo Characteristics

Homogeneous Echo Content (Fig. 11–22). In a homogeneous plaque, all the echoes within the plaque are uniform. The borders are usually smooth. On the 2-D images, the plaque may range from mildly echogenic to very echogenic.

Heterogeneous Plaque (Fig. 11–23). In a heterogeneous plaque, a complex echo pattern is noted. Echo-poor areas may be caused by intraplaque hemorrhage. Calcifications may be noted. Irregular surfaces, ulcer formation, and thrombus formation may occur.

Carotid Fibromuscular Dysplasia (FMD). This is a noninflammatory process with hypertrophy of the muscular and fibrous arterial walls separated by abnormal areas of fragmentation.[9] It is usually a benign condition and appears as a series of thin vascular webs interposed between smooth rounded areas of focal dilatation.[5] However it has been associated with TIA's and can lead to dissection or aneurysm. It sonographically appears as a low-level homogeneous thickening of the arterial wall. There may be no narrowing of the vessel since there is often focal dilatation; therefore the spectral analysis will be normal unless there is a narrowing present. These lesions may not be seen on the angiogram if there is no impingement or narrowing of the internal lumen.

Carotid Endarterectomy. This is the most common operation for extracranial cerebrovascular disease. The goals of endarterectomy are to remove stenotic or ulcerated plaque and to close the surgery without stenosis or thrombosis occurring. In some instances, synthetic or venous patches or grafts may be required (Fig. 11–24). There have been three randomized clinical trials that document the supe-

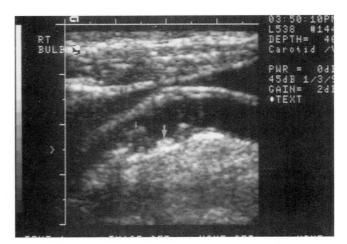

Figure 11–21. Irregular-bordered plaque with echogenic (large arrow) and echo-poor (small arrow) regions.

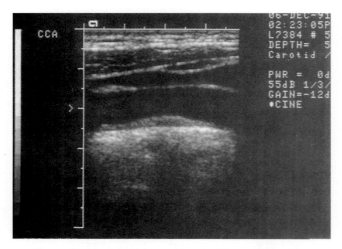

Figure 11–22. Homogeneous plaque with smooth borders.

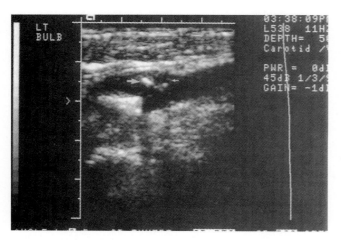

Figure 11–23. Heterogeneous plaque with echo-poor (small arrow) and echogenic areas (large arrow). The echo-poor area may be caused by hemorrhage within the plaque.

riority of carotid endarterectomy over anticoagulation in preventing neurologic events in symptomatic patients with high-grade (>70%) carotid stenosis. (North American Symptomatic Carotid Endarterectomy Trial (Nascet), European Carotid Surgery Trial, and Veterans Affairs Symptomatic Carotid Endarterectomy Trial).[1] CW Doppler is frequently used in the operating suite or recovery room to verify patency of the carotid artery. Color flow Doppler is used as a post-surgical follow-up to demonstrate patency and to evaluate for any stenosis, residual plaque, occlusion, or flaps. There normally will be absence of the intimal lining in the area of the endarterectomy, with mild increased velocity that will persist for several months. Turbulence will be seen at the anastomotic sites, but there should be no narrowing or stenosis present. Stenosis will produce a greatly elevated velocity appropriate to the degree of narrowing. Both the ICA and ECA should be identified to rule out occlusion or stenosis (Fig. 11–25).

Tortuosity, Coils, and Kinks. Tortuosity is very common and usually presents as an S or C shape elongation or curving of the artery (Fig. 11–26). Tortuosity is more common than kinking or coiling and gradually occurs in patients who are hypertensive or in advanced age. There will be multiple color changes with mildly increased velocity and turbulence as the vessel curves and bends. Prominence of the vessels at the base of the neck are frequently seen with long-standing hypertension. They often present as a pulsatile mass that must be differentiated from an aneurysm.[5] Kinks are usually a sharp angulation that usually occur 2–4 cm above the carotid bifurcation and exhibit increased velocities in the kinked segment. Coiling is an exaggerated and redundant S-shaped curve or a complete circle in the long axis of the artery. This is most likely a congenital anomaly that accentuates with aging.[5]

Color flow Doppler and power Doppler are helpful in demonstrating tortuous vessels and to determine their true

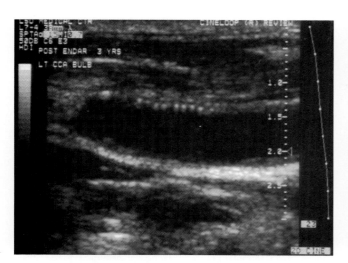

Figure 11–24. Endarterectomy with patching.

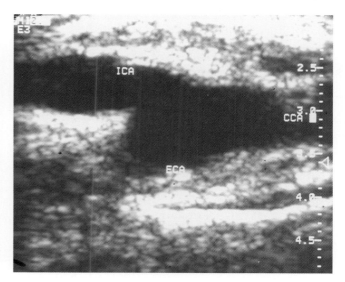

Figure 11–25. Endarterectomy with occlusion of the ECA.

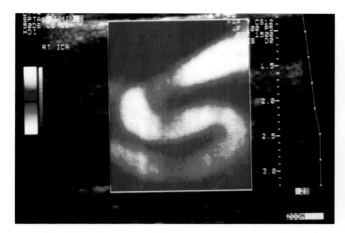

Figure 11–26. Power angio demonstrating tortuosity of the ICA.

course. There will be a slight increase in the Doppler shift in the tortuous segments and in the bend of the kinks. This is a normal finding, and as a rule, there is no stenosis present.

Stenosis. Carotid artery stenosis (50% decrease in diameter or 70% cross section) reduces the blood flow and continues to decrease gradually until the critical level (70% diameter, 90% cross section) is reached. Low levels of stenosis will demonstrate no flow abnormalities. As the degree of stenosis increases, mild turbulence will be noted in the form of spectral broadening. When a stenosis increases beyond hemodynamic significance, the velocity of blood through the stenosis must increase to maintain flow volume. This produces a jet of high velocity through the stenosis and a variable amount of turbulence at or just distal to the stenosis. Flow velocities increase dramatically in the stenotic area, followed by a poststenotic turbulence. More distally, the flow will assume a more normal pattern. Velocities increase in systole as well as diastole.[11] Peak systolic velocity has proved to be an accurate determination of stenotic lesions by Doppler. End-diastolic velocity ratios have also proved to be useful in distinguishing between degrees of high-grade stenosis[9] (Fig. 11–27).

Aneurysms, Pseudoaneurysms. These are relatively uncommon lesions in the extracranial vessels but the most frequent causes include: atherosclerosis, trauma, infection, and previous carotid surgery. A true aneurysm results from a weakness of the media and produces dilatation of all three layers of the arterial wall; as opposed to the pseudoaneurysm or false aneurysm which do not have a true arterial wall and are usually the result of a vascular injury caused by trauma or previous surgery. These lesions appear as a pulsating anechoic mass with an internal swirling slow motion of the blood. Color flow Doppler shows the change in colors as the blood swirls around, and the spectral waveform will have a classical positive and negative direction. The pseudoaneurysm often has a neck or tract from the native artery to the pseudoaneurysm. The spectral analysis will show a pulsatile positive and negative flow during pulses of the cardiac cycle.

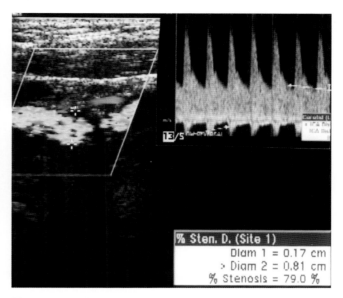

Figure 11–27. ICA stenosis demonstrated with color flow as a severe narrowing. Spectral waveform has elevated systolic and diastolic velocities and filling of the spectral window.

Occlusion. This is diagnosed when there is no flow in the vessel. However, in some instances, it may be difficult to define a high-grade stenosis because it approaches occlusion with only a trickle of blood flow present. As a stenosis approaches the point of occlusion, there may be a drop in flow volumes and a decrease in velocities so great that it may be indistinguishable from a total occlusion. Color flow is unique in defining a trickle flow when set to display low flow states. It is of utmost importance to define an occlusion clearly versus a high-grade stenosis or trickle flow because a total occlusion is inoperable; whereas, a trickle flow can be surgically restored (Fig. 11–28, A–D). In total occlusion of the ICA, color flow or spectral analysis detects no flow. The CCA velocity waveforms resemble the ECA with a high resistance pattern, and the ECA waveform may become more of a low-resistance flow pattern mimicking the ICA.

Dissection. Dissection occurs as a result of a break in the intima followed by hemorrhage into the media. The vessel becomes enlarged, with a reduced size of the true lumen and the addition of a false lumen. Real-time imaging demonstrates an echogenic membrane within the vessel lumen moving in the bloodstream (Fig. 11–29 A, B).

This should be seen in both a longitudinal and a transverse plane so as not to be confused with image artifacts. Color Doppler can demonstrate the true lumen with color flow as well as the false lumen with a reversal of flow or no flow. The spectral analysis will show increased velocity in the true lumen caused by the narrowing and reversal of flow in the false lumen. Spikes in the Doppler signal represent the motion of the moving membrane.

Carotid Body Tumor. This is a paraganglioma that is a benign well-encapsulated mass that occurs at the carotid

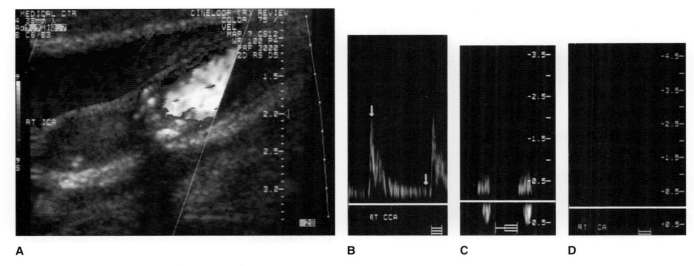

Figure 11–28. (A) ICA occlusion is see on color flow Doppler as an abrupt end to the blood flow with the remainder of the ICA filled with echoes. **(B)** Spectral analysis of the CCA demonstrates increased pulsatility. **(C)** Reversal of flow is seen at the entrance to the ICA. **(D)** There is no Doppler signal in the ICA indicating no flow.

bifurcation. As a rule, they are slow growing tumors but highly vascular in nature. The initial symptom is usually a palpable mass in the neck. Ultrasound shows a well-encapsulated solid tumor with variable echogenicity located between the internal and external carotid arteries. Color flow Doppler or power Doppler demonstrates the extreme vascularity of the tumor.

Vertebral Artery Pathology

The vertebral arteries are best seen on the longitudinal views with the probe angled laterally from the CCA. They will be seen segmentally between the transverse processes and continue to the foramina magnum to enter the base of the skull and then join to form the basilar artery.[8]

Stenosis. The majority of vertebral stenoses occur at the origin of the vertebral artery. They can often be difficult to visualize because of their location in the thorax. Care should be taken to demonstrate the narrowing of the vessel with associated mosaic color patterns and increased velocities. Just distal to the stenosis will be a poststenotic turbulence, and the waveform may become damped. In some instances, plaque may be shown (Fig. 11–30).

Occlusion. Vertebral artery occlusion may be difficult to determine, especially because the vertebral artery can be

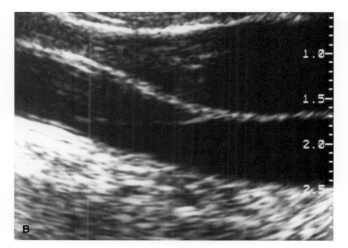

Figure 11–29. (A) Transverse CCA with thin moving membrane that is characteristic of dissection. **(B)** Longitudinal scan of the CCA demonstrates the membrane.

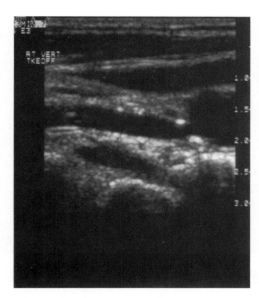

Figure 11–30. Vertebral plaque and stenosis at the origin of the vertebral artery.

congenitally absent or the origin of the vertebral artery difficult to visualize. However, the same guidelines would apply as with any occluded vessel. An occluded artery would present as a tubular structure filled with debris with absence of color flow and Doppler signals.

Subclavian Steal. This is a condition where there is stenosis or occlusion of the subclavian proximal to the vertebral artery. This condition occurs as the proximal obstruction of the subclavian artery decreases the pressure and causes a reversal of flow in the vertebral artery via the basilar artery and contralateral vertebral artery, hence the term "steal."[2] The bilateral blood pressure will show a difference of greater that 10 mmHg with the lower value on the side of obstruction. The steal may be incomplete or complete. The incomplete steal causes a decrease in systolic blood flow velocity, and if more severe, an alternating blood flow pattern will be seen in the vertebral artery on the side of the subclavian lesion. Complete steal demonstrates a reversal of flow. (Fig. 11–31, A, B). Exercise of the upper extremity on the side of the subclavian steal will enhance the Doppler findings and clinical symptoms.[12] The ischemic arm steals blood from the basilar circulation via retrograde vertebral artery flow during arm exercise producing symptoms of vertebrobasilar insufficiency.[13] This condition can be easily identified with color flow Doppler and spectral analysis. There will be a reversal of color as well as a reversed spectrum. In some instances, there may be a partial steal, with blood flow in a positive and negative pattern.[14–16]

Transcranial Doppler (TCD). Transcranial Doppler is a noninvasive technique that measures blood flow in the major intracranial brain vessels. It is now possible for ultrasound to evaluate and record intracranial blood flow velocity directly. Applications include:

- Evaluating and monitoring vasospasm
- Assessing intracranial collateral flow in patients with extracranial occlusive disease
- Identification and localization of intracranial stenosis
- Identification of arteriovenous malformations (ATM) and aneurysms
- Evaluation of brain death
- Evaluation of revascularization
- Evaluation of vertebrobasilar symptoms
- Intraoperative and postoperative monitoring
- Evaluation and monitoring of sickle cell patients to determine, predict impending stroke conditions

There are two types of TCD; one is the classic or nonimaging method, and the other is the newer color flow Doppler imaging method. The nonimaging method assesses the blood flow with a knowledge of the anatomical location and pathway of the arteries, their depth from the skull surface, and the direction of flow as related to the transducer position. These units produce spectral analysis waveforms with capabilities of mapping flow and calculating a pulsatility index (PI) and resistive index (RI) and in some units, provide visual mapping. These small, portable units can go to surgery, recovery room, and bedside and are ideal for monitoring. They are also equipped with stable probe fixation, which allows for simultaneous examination of both sides of the intracranial cerebrovascular system for comparison. The other type of TCD is the color flow Doppler imaging unit, which provides 2-D or real-time imaging, color flow, and Doppler spectral analysis. Color flow Doppler has the ability to image the vessel to provide anatomical data with depth location and direction of flow (Fig. 11–32). Color flow Doppler imaging can visualize the vascular segments and selectively examine the vessel by using a gated sample volume. These techniques use a low-frequency transducer, such as 2–2.5 MHz and specific windows for placement of the probe to penetrate the skull and image the underlying vessels.

Positions for the examination include: transtemporal, suboccipital, submandibular, and transorbital (Fig. 11–33, A, B, C).

Transtemporal window allows insonation of the middle cerebral artery (M1–M2 segments), anterior cerebral artery, the posterior cerebral artery (P1 and P2 segments), and the C1 segment of the carotid siphon.

Suboccipital window allows insonation of the vertebral arteries and basilar artery.

Submandibular window allows insonation of the retromandibular ICA (distal).

Transorbital window allows insonation of the anterior circulation through the orbit. The vessels identified include the ophthalmic artery and the carotid siphon (C2, C3, and C4). However, this approach may not be approved by the FDA on all instruments.

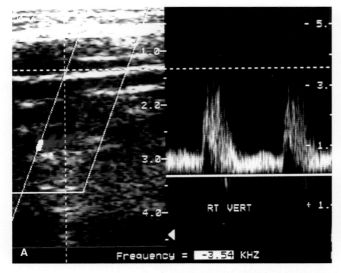

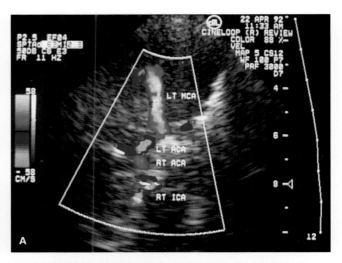

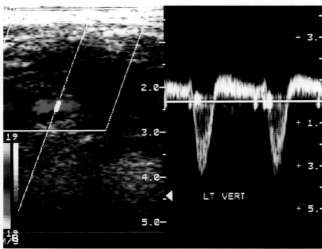

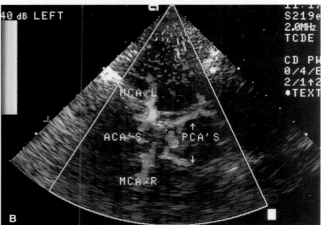

Figure 11–32. (A) Transcranial vessels illustrated with color Doppler imaging. **(B)** Transcranial vessels illustrated with color Doppler power energy mode.

Figure 11–31. Subclavian steal. **(A)** Right vertebral has a normal waveform with increased flow. **(B)** Left vertebral is reversed indicating subclavian steal.

Primary TCD parameters are vital for identification of specific intracranial arteries especially using the blind method without imaging. These parameters include:

- Insonation depth
- Direction of blood flow at the specific depth
- Mean flow velocity
- Probe position
- Direction of ultrasound beam

Cerebral blood flow can be altered by multiple physiological changes. The examiner must understand these changes so as not to mistake them for pathological changes.

- Heart rate increase will increase velocities, and conversely, a decrease in heart rate will decrease the velocities.

- Increased intracranial pressure will decrease the diastole flow.
- Decreased hematocrit will lower velocities.
- Increasing age will lower velocities.
- Children and young adults will have higher velocities.

The primary anatomy involved in the transcranial Doppler examination is the vasculature of the circle of Willis as seen in Fig. 11–4 includes the following arteries:

MCA—Middle cerebral artery (M1, M2 segments)
ICA—Internal carotid artery
PCA—Posterior cerebral artery (P1, P2 segments)
VA—Vertebral artery
BA—Basilar artery
CS—Carotid siphon (C1, C2, C3, C4 segments)
ACoA—Anterior communicating artery (A1, A2 segments)
PCoa—Posterior communicating artery
Oa—Ophthalmic artery

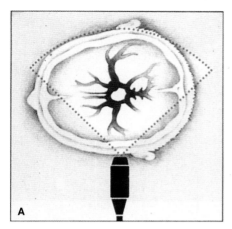 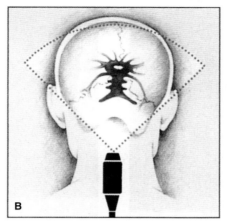 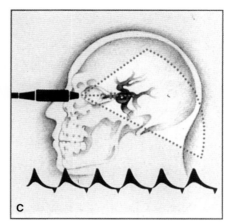

Figure 11–33. Transcranial positions for performing the Transcranial Doppler examination. **(A)** Transtemporal. **(B)** Transoccipital. **(C)** Transorbital.

NORMAL VALUES FOR THE TCD EXAMINATION INDEXES (FIG. 11–34)

The common index used is the pulsatility index (PI). A pulsatility index is normal between 0.8 and 1.2. Increased pulsatility index greater than 1.2 may indicate elevated intracranial pressure, vasospasm, hypercapnia, or systemic hemodynamic changes (aortic insufficiency).[12] A damped index less than 0.8 is usually seen in post stenotic vessel sites, in vessels supplied by collateral circulation and local vessel enlargement.

DISEASE AND PATHOLOGY

Carotid Artery Occlusion or High Grade Stenosis

When there is an occlusion or a high-grade stenosis of the ipsilateral extracranial carotid artery, the middle cerebral artery (MCA) velocity is reduced or absent. The ophthalmic artery will have decreased flow or may have reversed flow direction. There may be increased velocities in other arteries, which become part of the collateral pathway[5] (Fig. 11–35 A, B).

Subclavian Steal

Subclavian steal can be detected in the intracranial vertebral arteries and the basilar artery. There may be an abnormal oscillating or reversed flow in the ipsilateral vertebral artery or biphasic flow in the basilar artery. However, in most instances, basilar artery flow is not critically affected, unless there is a high-grade stenosis of the vertebral artery supplying the steal. The velocities and PI will be decreased.[5]

Occlusion

MCA is the more common occlusion of the intracranial vessels and is often seen in acute strokes. It results in absence of flow in the vessel with reduced flow in the proximal vascular segments. The MCA should be evaluated in all of its segments to determine patency or absence of flow. It should also be remembered that the adjacent vessels can be seen, and patency can be demonstrated to prove the adequacy of the transcranial sonographic window being used.[12] Collateral flow patterns may be seen with increased velocity or reversed flow[5] (Fig. 11–36 A, B).

Intracranial Vessel Stenosis

Stenosis of the intracranial vessels will exhibit the same characteristics as other vessels. There will be a focal increase in the mean blood flow velocity at the site of the vessel narrowing. Color flow Doppler will show a multiple color pattern. This compared with the demonstration of normal flow in the contralateral vessel of the same location aids in the diagnosis of stenosis. Secondary findings include: abnormal flow immediately downstream from the site of stenosis with deceased velocities and pulsatility and decreased velocity and increased pulsatility proximal to the stenosis.[5]

	Systolic	Mean	Diastolic	Age
MCA	94.5 ± 13.6	58.4 ± 8.4	45.6 ± 6.6	<40
	91.0 ± 16.9	57.7 ± 11.5	44.3 ± 9.5	40–60
	78.1 ± 15.0	44.7 ± 11.1	31.9 ± 9.1	>60
ACA	76.4 ± 16.9	47.3 ± 13.6	36.0 ± 9.0	<40
	86.4 ± 20.1	53.1 ± 10.5	41.1 ± 7.4	40–60
	73.3 ± 20.3	45.3 ± 13.5	34.2 ± 8.8	>60
PCA	53.2 ± 11.3	34.2 ± 7.8	25.9 ± 6.5	<40
	60.1 ± 20.6	36.6 ± 9.8	28.7 ± 7.5	40–60
	51.0 ± 11.9	29.9 ± 9.3	22.0 ± 6.9	>60
Vertebral/basilar	56.3 ± 7.8	34.9 ± 7.8	27.0 ± 5.9	<40
	59.5 ± 17.0	36.4 ± 11.7	29.2 ± 8.4	40–60
	50.9 ± 18.7	30.5 ± 12.9	21.2 ± 9.2	>60

Figure 11–34. Normal velocities of the circle of Willis arteries.

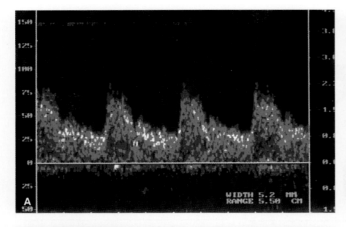

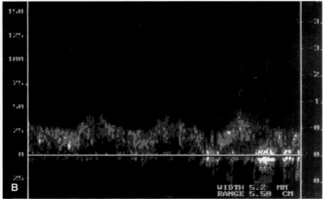

Figure 11–35. (A) Normal spectral analysis of the normal middle cerebral artery (MCA). (B) Abnormal spectral analysis of the middle cerebral artery with proximal carotid artery high-grade stenosis.

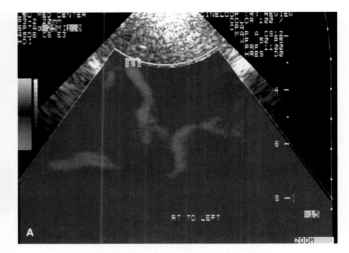

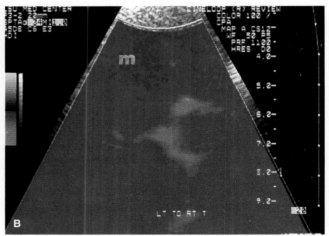

Figure 11–36. (A) Normal middle cerebral artery. (B) Occlusion of the middle cerebral artery.

Arteriovenous Malformation (AVM)

AVM is usually seen in the third decade of life and is caused by persistent connections between arterial and venous sides of the embryonic vascular plexus. The arteriovenous malformation nidus, feeding arteries, and draining veins demonstrate unusual hemodynamics; increased blood flow velocity and vessel diameter, decreased arterial pressure, increased venous pressure, and diminished or absent autoregulation. A characteristic transcranial Doppler appearance of accelerated flood flow with a damped waveform can be seen. The AVM can also have an associated induced subarachnoid hemorrhage with vasospasm. The AVM will appear on color flow imaging as a conglomeration of vessels in a focal area. The feeding arteries will present with a marked elevation of velocity and a reduced PI. There will be bidirectional flow, and the adjacent arteries will have decreased flow velocities. TCD can be used to monitor the effects of surgical or drug therapies.[12]

Embolus

An embolus passing through the intracranial vessels will show a bright brief blip passing through the Doppler beam. These are termed "HITS" or high-intensity transient signals. They are usually less than 0.1 s, unidirectional, and occur at random in the cardiac cycle. They can be heard as whips or clicks, depending on their density and velocity.[5]

Vasospasm

Vasospasm is commonly seen following subarachnoid hemorrhage because of the rupture of an intracranial aneurysm or other pathologic conditions. Vasospasms usually occur within the first few days after subarachnoid hemorrhage and gradually increase for a week, thus, peaking between 11 and 17 days. Criteria for the diagnosis of vasospasm should include a relative increases in blood flow velocity of greater than 50% determined in serial studies. However, is has been stated by most authors that some degree of vasospasm is present with a velocity of 120 cm/s, and that velocities greater than 200 cm/s correlate with a risk of infarction.[12] The PI will also be increased. TCD is used to monitor during such surgical procedures as neuroradiological interventional procedures, carotid endarterectomy, or cardiopulmonary bypass.[5]

Brain Death

TCD may also be used to confirm cerebral circulatory arrest; however, the diagnosis of brain death must ultimately be made by the attending physician on the basis of clinical findings in addition to the results of the diagnostic studies. The TCD Doppler appearance of brain death is seen in a progression of patterns observed during three stages of increased intracranial pressure. Intracranial pressure increases to a point where blood flow into the peripheral circulation is prevented, a characteristic pattern of to and from blood flow is seen in the middle cerebral artery and other basal intracranial arteries. The transcranial Doppler demonstration of this to and from pattern or complete cessation of intracranial blood flow is suggestive of cerebral circulatory arrest. However, these patterns are not synonymous with brain death in all cases, although; it has also been noted that blood flow velocity in the middle cerebral artery of less than 10 cm/s for longer than 30 minutes is not compatible with survival.[12]

REFERENCES

1. Hallett JW, Brewster DC, Darling RC. *Handbook of Patient Care in Vascular Surgery.* 3rd. ed. Boston: Little, Brown & Co.; 1995.
2. Schwartz SI, Shires GT, Spencer FC, et al. *Principles of Surgery.* 4th ed. New York: McGraw-Hill, 1984: 941–948.
3. *Dorlands Illustrated Medical Dictionary.* 26th ed. Philadelphia: WB Saunders; 1974.
4. Staff. Better stroke care. *Adv Radiol Sci Professionals.* 1999; 12:38–41.
5. Krebs CA, Giyanani VL, Eisenberg RI. *Ultrasound Atlas of Vascular Diseases.* Stamford, CT: Appleton & Lange; 1999.
6. Scoutt LLM, Sawin ML, Taylor JW. Doppler US. Part II. Clinical applications. *Radiology* 1990; 174:309–319.
7. Zwiebel WJ. *Introduction to Vascular Ultrasonography.* 4th ed. Philadelphia: WB Saunders; 2000.
8. Bluth EI: The carotid and vertebrals: technique, anatomy and hemodynamics. Proceedings of the Color Doppler Ultrasonography Course, American Institute of Ultrasound in Medicine, Feb. 23, 24, 1991: 29–32.
9. Carroll BA: Color Doppler ultrasound of the carotids and vertebrals: detection and analysis of atherosclerotic plaque. Proceedings of the Color Doppler Ultrasonography Course, American Institute of Ultrasound in Medicine, Feb. 23, 24, 1991: 35–43.
10. Erickson SJ, Mewissen MW, Foley WD, et al: Color Doppler evaluation of arterial stenoses and occlusions involving the neck and thoracic inlet *Radiographics.* 1989; 9.
11. Robinson ML. Duplex sonography of the carotid arteries. *Semin Roentgenol.* 1992; 27:17–27.
12. Lupetin AR, Davis DA, Beckman DO, et al: Transcranial Doppler sonography, part 2. *Radiographics,* 1995; 15:193–209.
13. Polak, JF: *Peripheral Vascular Sonography. A Practical Guide.* Baltimore: Williams & Wilkins; 1992.
14. Foley WD: *Color Doppler Flow Imaging.* Boston: Andover Medical Publishers, Inc.; 1991.
15. Taylor KJW, Burns PN, Wells PNT, eds. *Clinical Applications of Doppler Ultrasound.* New York: Raven Press; 1988.
16. Gerlocl AJ, Giyanani VL, Krebs CA. *Applications of Noninvasive Vascular Techniques.* Philadelphia: WB Saunders; 1988.

Questions

GENERAL INSTRUCTIONS: For each question, select the best answer. Select only one answer for each question unless otherwise specified.

1. Stroke is ranked in the United States as the following cause of death annually

   (A) 1st with 800,000 deaths
   (B) 2nd with 600,500 deaths
   (C) 3rd with 500,000 deaths
   (D) none of the above

2. The emphasis of stroke as a national issue is based on

   (A) defining the stroke as ischemic or hemorrhagic
   (B) preventing long-term disability
   (C) deciding which treatment is to be used
   (D) early diagnosis and treatment to prevent long-term disability

3. The newest technique for early determination of a stroke as hemorrhagic or ischemic is which of the following imaging modalities?

   (A) ultrasound of the carotid arteries
   (B) computerized axial tomography (CT)
   (C) magnetic resonance imaging (MRI) diffusion imaging
   (D) digital subtraction arteriography (DSA)

4. Stroke is defined as

   (A) sudden increase of blood flow to the brain causing syncope
   (B) total blockage of the internal carotid artery
   (C) sudden and often severe impairment of blood flow to the brain
   (D) none of the above

Match the following terms with the correct definition.

5. Transient ischemic attack (TIA) _____

6. Stroke in evolution (SIE) _____

7. Reversible ischemic neurologic deficit (RIND) _____

8. Completed stroke _____

9. Acute brain death _____

   (A) neurologic symptoms that last longer than 24 hours, but completely resolve
   (B) this is caused by either lack of blood supply or effect of blood outside of normal vessels
   (C) ischemic neurologic symptoms that last less than 24 hours and completely resolve
   (D) stable neurologic deficit that had sudden onset and persists longer than 3 weeks
   (E) ischemic neurologic symptoms that actively worsen during a period of observation

10. Which is currently the major cause of vascular disease?

    (A) hypertension
    (B) intracerebral hemorrhage
    (C) smoking more than one pack of cigarettes per day
    (D) atherosclerosis

11. Internal carotid artery symptoms include all of the following *except*

    (A) paralysis on the contralateral side
    (B) decreased level of consciousness
    (C) amaurosis fugax
    (D) ataxia

12. A neurologic symptom related to atherosclerotic disease in the posterior circulation (vertebrobasilar disease) is

    (A) amaurosis fugax
    (B) contralateral extremity weakness
    (C) orthostatic hypotension
    (D) vertigo

13. Continuous wave or CW Doppler is used in all of the following *except*

    (A) periorbital Doppler
    (B) extracranial arteries
    (C) ocular pneumoplethysmography
    (D) transcranial Doppler

14. Ocular pneumoplethysmography (OPG) can be used to detect

    (A) hemodynamically significant lesions (greater than 50%)
    (B) in the assessment of collateral circulation
    (C) both (A) and (B)
    (D) none of the above

15. Color Doppler units provide which of the following information?

    (A) real-time imaging
    (B) Doppler waveform analysis
    (C) color depiction of the flow characteristics
    (D) all of the above
    (E) B and C

16. The optimal transducer for high-resolution gray-scale image is obtained by which frequency transducer?

    (A) 2.5 MHz linear array
    (B) 5 MHz curved array
    (C) 5 MHz linear array
    (D) 7.5 MHz linear array

17. Doppler information in the extracranial arterial system is best achieved using which of the following angles?

    (A) 60–70° angle to the artery
    (B) 0° angle to the artery
    (C) 45–60° angle to the artery
    (D) 20–35° angle to the artery

18. The most utilized of the Doppler criteria for estimation of percentage diameter stenosis is

    (A) end diastolic velocity
    (B) peak diastolic velocity divided by end diastolic velocity
    (C) peak systolic velocity
    (D) none of the above

19. What is mandatory when using velocity to represent the Doppler shift?

    (A) angle correction
    (B) high-frequency linear array transducer
    (C) electronic steering of transducer
    (D) both B and C

20. One of the artifacts with pulsed Doppler in a hemodynamically significant stenosis is

    (A) spectral broadening
    (B) turbulence
    (C) aliasing
    (D) both A and B

21. Aliasing occurs when high frequencies exceed the Nyquist limit and may be corrected by

    (A) increasing the transducer frequency and increasing the sample volume
    (B) positioning the sample volume deeper by transducer manipulation
    (C) change in probe position, decreasing the depth, increasing the PRF, increasing the Doppler angle or lowering the frequency
    (D) none of the above

22. Two advantages of power Doppler

    (A) extremely sensitive to high flow state of intracranial arteries
    (B) more sensitive frequency shift information
    (C) beneficial in defining occlusive vessels
    (D) is not dependent on beam angle and free from aliasing artifact
    (E) both A and B
    (F) both C and D

Match the following three layers of an artery wall with the correct definition.

23. Media _____   (A) elastic inner layer
24. Adventitia _____   (B) layer of muscle and elastic
25. Intima _____   tissue
                         (C) outer loose filmy layer

26. Variable plaque morphology may be termed

    (A) soft (homogeneous low-level gray echoes)
    (B) dense (highly echogenic)
    (C) calcified (increased echogenicity with acoustic shadowing)
    (D) ulcerated (irregular margins or craters)
    (E) all of the above

27. The cerebrovascular vessels arise from which of the following?

    (A) vertebral artery
    (B) costocervical trunk
    (C) internal thoracic
    (D) aortic arch

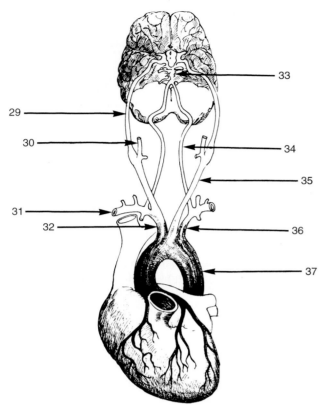

Figure 11–37. Blood supply to the brain.

28. Branches of the subclavian artery include

    (A) vertebral
    (B) internal thoracic
    (C) thyrocervical and costocervical trunk
    (D) dorsal scapular
    (E) all of the above

Match the following to Fig. 11–37.

29. _____	(A)	basilar artery
30. _____	(B)	right external carotid artery
31. _____	(C)	left subclavian artery
32. _____	(D)	right common carotid artery
33. _____	(E)	left vertebral artery
34. _____	(F)	right subclavian artery
35. _____	(G)	left common carotid artery
36. _____	(H)	aortic arch
37. _____	(I)	brachiocephalic trunk
	(J)	right internal carotid artery

38. The main branch of the carotid system is which of the following?

    (A) internal carotid artery
    (B) vertebral artery
    (C) common carotid artery
    (D) external carotid artery

Match the following extracranial arteries with the correct spectral analysis description.

39. internal carotid artery _____

40. external carotid artery _____

41. common carotid artery _____

42. carotid bulb _____

    (A) exhibits a complicated turbulent flow pattern
    (B) demonstrates a rapid increase in velocity during systole with a clear window and a continuous antegrade flow during diastole
    (C) combination of the pattern of internal and external carotid arteries
    (D) demonstrates a brisk systolic upstroke, sharp peak, abrupt downstroke

Match the following extracranial waveforms with the proper normal waveform.

43. external carotid artery _____
44. internal carotid artery _____
45. common carotid artery _____

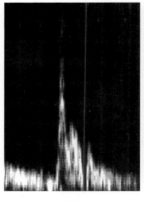
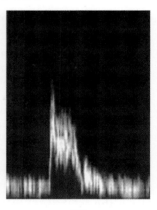

(A)   (B)

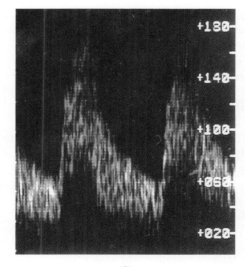

(C)

46. Which of the following radiographic modalities is the method of choice for opacifying the entire cerebral arterial system?

(A) carotid duplex examination with transcranial Doppler
(B) computerized axial tomography with contrast
(C) magnetic resonance imaging with contrast
(D) digital subtraction angiography

Match the transverse scans of the extracranial carotid arteries in the proper order according to examination protocol.

47. _____
48. _____
49. _____
50. _____
51. _____

(A) origin of the vertebral artery
(B) carotid bifurcation with internal and external carotid arteries
(C) common carotid artery
(D) carotid bulb
(E) brachiocephalic artery and bifurcation of the subclavian and carotid arteries

Match the following longitudinal scans of the extracranial carotid arteries in the proper order according to examination protocol.

52. _____
53. _____
54. _____
55. _____
56. _____

(A) vertebral artery from origin and as far distal as possible
(B) carotid bifurcation (carotid bulb and proximal portion of internal and external carotid arteries)
(C) external carotid artery as far distal as possible
(D) common carotid artery (from clavicle to mandible)
(E) internal carotid artery as far distal as possible

Match the following gray-scale image to the normal extracranial carotid arteries.

57. _____ external carotid artery.   a.
58. _____ internal carotid artery.   b.
59. _____ common carotid artery.   c.
60. _____ bulb   d.

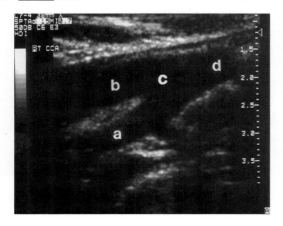

61. Normal flow in the normal carotid artery is

(A) laminar
(B) turbulent
(C) helical
(D) parabolic

62. The first major branch of the internal carotid artery with clinical significance is the

(A) middle cerebral artery
(B) anterior cerebral artery
(C) ophthalmic artery
(D) posterior communicating artery

63. The internal carotid artery supplies blood to

(A) cerebral hemispheres of the brain only
(B) cerebral hemispheres of the brain, eyes and accessory organs, forehead, and part of the nose
(C) posterior portion of the brain and face
(D) none of the above

64. The external carotid artery supplies blood to

(A) cerebellum
(B) scalp, face, and most of the neck
(C) face, eyes, and temporal portion of the brain
(D) all of the above

65. Which of the following maneuvers will identify that the Doppler signal is coming from the external carotid artery?

(A) swallowing
(B) compression of the mandibular artery
(C) temporal tapping
(D) none of the above

66. Which common carotid artery arises directly from the aortic arch?

(A) right branch of the common carotid
(B) left branch of the common carotid

67. Nonatheromatous causes of turbulent flow in the carotid arteries may include

(A) sudden increase in the diameter of the vessel
(B) kinking of the internal carotid artery
(C) tortuosity of the internal carotid artery
(D) all of the above
(E) none of the above

68. An increased resistivity index in the common carotid artery may indicate

(A) stenotic disease proximal to the sample site
(B) stenotic disease distal to the sample site
(C) disease at the sample site
(D) sample volume site placed too close to the arterial wall

69. Factors affecting the Doppler shift frequency include

    (A) Doppler angle
    (B) transducer
    (C) velocity of the red blood cells
    (D) B and C
    (E) A, B, and C

70. The most common site for atherosclerotic plaque formation is

    (A) distal internal carotid artery
    (B) distal common carotid artery
    (C) carotid bifurcation
    (D) vertebral artery origin

71. Which branch of the internal carotid artery is in the cervical section of the neck?

    (A) caroticotympanic
    (B) cavernous
    (C) posterior communicating
    (D) none of the above

72. The gradual decrease in blood flow due to vascular narrowing does not produce symptoms until it reaches the point of "critical arterial stenosis." Which of the following diameter reductions constitutes a critical stenosis?

    (A) 20% diameter reduction
    (B) 30–45% diameter reduction
    (C) 50% diameter reduction
    (D) 25–30% diameter reduction

Identify the following plaque morphology with the appropriate image.

73. soft _____
74. dense _____
75. calcified _____
76. ulcerated _____
77. intraplaque hemorrhage _____

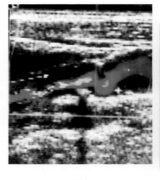
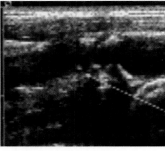

(A)   (B)

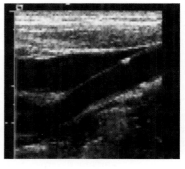

(C)

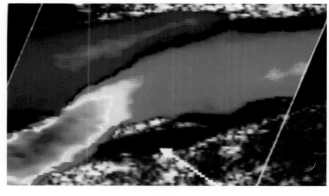

(D)

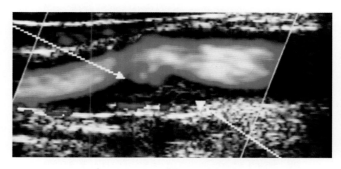

(E)

Match the following with the appropriate image:

78. critical stenosis _____
79. occlusion of ICA _____

80. reversal of flow in bulb proximal to ICA occlusion _____
81. moderate stenosis by diameter reduction _____
82. mild stenosis by diameter reduction _____

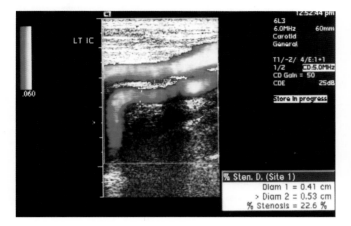

(A)

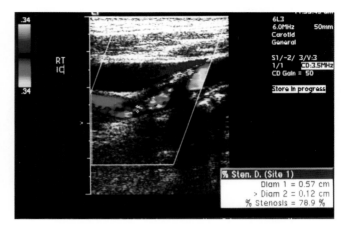

(B)

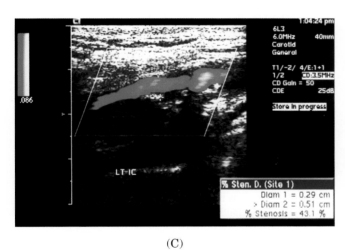

(C)

(D)

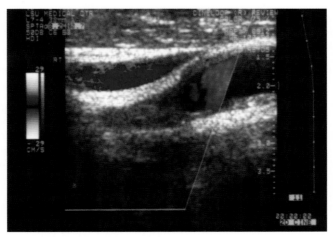

(E)

83. Distal to a critical stenosis, the spectral analysis depicts which of the following characteristics?

   (A) peak systole velocities decrease
   (B) end diastole velocities decrease
   (C) turbulent flow is present in the spectral analysis
   (D) all of the above

84. Carotid body tumors are

   (A) rare neoplasms
   (B) composed of paraganglionic tissue
   (C) occur only at the carotid bifurcation
   (D) A and B
   (E) all of the above

85. Which of the following variations of the extracranial carotid artery is associated with the symptom of ischemia?

   (A) coiling of the internal carotid artery
   (B) kinking of the internal carotid artery
   (C) tortuosity of the internal carotid artery
   (D) all of the above

86. According to the North American Symptomatic Carotid Endarterectomy Trial (NASCET) which is the most common treatment to risk reduction for stroke?

   (A) identifying and operating on appropriately severe common carotid bifurcation lesion
   (B) treating all patients with aspirin therapy and perform carotid Doppler exam once a year
   (C) once the stenosis reaches a moderate level perform the endarterectomy before symptoms occur
   (D) none of the above

Match the following vessels to Fig. 11–38.

87. _____	(A)	superficial temporal artery
88. _____	(B)	supraorbital artery
89. _____	(C)	subclavian artery
90. _____	(D)	internal carotid artery
91. _____	(E)	ophthalmic artery
92. _____	(F)	common carotid artery
93. _____	(G)	external carotid artery
94. _____	(H)	superior thyroid artery
95. _____	(I)	brachiocephalic trunk
96. _____	(J)	vertebral artery

97. Which of the following is not a branch of the subclavian?

   (A) vertebral
   (B) internal thoracic
   (C) thyrocervical trunk
   (D) costocervical trunk
   (E) hypophyseal

98. The extracranial posterior circulation of composed of

   (A) paired vertebral arteries in the back of the neck
   (B) basilar artery
   (C) brachiocephalic
   (D) B and C

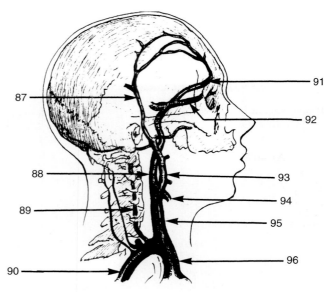

Figure 11–38. Cerebrovascular anatomy. (*Reproduced with permission from Zwiebel, WJ: Introduction to Vascular Ultrasonography, 2nd ed. Philadelphia: WB Saunders, 1986.*)

99. Subclavian steal causes which of the following symptoms?

   (A) ataxia
   (B) limb paralysis
   (C) vertigo
   (D) syncope
   (E) all of the above
   (F) C and D

100. The hallmark sign of the subclavian steal is

   (A) difference of blood pressure (10–20 mm Hg) between the two arms
   (B) decreased peripheral pulse in the affected upper extremity
   (C) difference of blood pressure (20–30 mm Hg) between the two arms
   (D) all of the above
   (E) A and B
   (F) B and C

101. Doppler waveform characteristics of subclavian steal include

   (A) deceleration, reversed, or alternating flow in the contralateral vertebral artery
   (B) decreased velocities/frequencies at the site of subclavian stenosis
   (C) diminished waveform distal to the stenosis or occlusion
   (D) all of the above
   (E) A and C

102. The normal vertebral artery spectral analysis will depict

(A) high-resistant flow similar to external carotid artery
(B) monophasic flow
(C) low-resistance waveform pattern similar to the internal carotid artery
(D) none of the above

103. Normally the vertebrobasilar system provides the following percentage of blood flow to intracranial system

(A) 40%
(B) 10%–20%
(C) 20%–30%
(D) none of the above

104. The vertebral artery can be visualized

(A) medial to the jugular
(B) transverse just lateral to common carotid artery
(C) longitudinal plane at the level of common carotid with the transducer angled laterally until the vertebral is seen passing through the transverse processes
(D) A and C
(E) B and C

105. Subclavian steal syndrome is asymptomatic

(A) when exercising contralateral side
(B) when exercising ipsilateral side
(C) at rest
(D) none of the above

Match the following arteries in Fig. 11–39.

106. _____   (A) anterior cerebral artery
107. _____   (B) posterior communicating artery

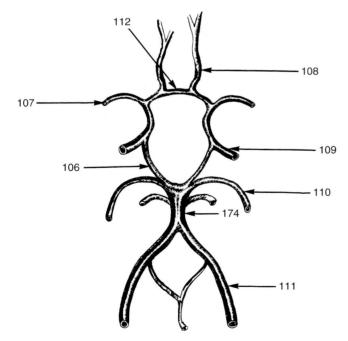

Figure 11–39. Circle of Willis.

108. _____   (C) anterior communicating artery
109. _____   (D) middle cerebral artery
110. _____   (E) basilar artery
111. _____   (F) internal carotid artery
112. _____   (G) vertebral artery
113. _____   (H) posterior cerebral artery

114. The transcranial Doppler examination requires

(A) high-frequency continuous wave transducer
(B) high-frequency linear array
(C) low-frequency (2 MHz) transducer
(D) appropriate computerized software for calculations
(E) C and D

115. The suboccipital window examines

(A) vertebral arteries
(B) posterior communicating arteries
(C) basilar artery
(D) A and C
(E) A and B

116. Transcranial Doppler is described as follows

(A) invasive technique that measures and visualizes the major intracranial vessels
(B) displays intracerebral hemorrhages
(C) noninvasive technique to measure the velocity of blood flow in the major intracranial brain vessels by using Doppler
(D) B and C

117. Transcranial imaging has the advantage of

(A) observation of narrowing of the vessel lumen
(B) visual assessment of the transcranial vessels for localization
(C) observation of vessel tortuosity
(D) calculation of the vessel lumen
(E) all of the above
(F) B and D

118. The following artery is the largest branch of the cerebral ICA

(A) ophthalmic artery
(B) middle cerebral artery
(C) anterior cerebral artery
(D) all of the above

119. The middle cerebral artery (MCA) supplies

(A) occipital lobe
(B) frontal lobe
(C) temporal lobe
(D) parietal lobe
(E) A, B, and C
(F) B, C, and D

120. The middle cerebral artery is divided into which of the following segments

(A) M1
(B) M2

(C) M3

(D) A-1

(E) A, B, and C

121. The posterior communicating artery anastomoses with

(A) anterior cerebral artery

(B) posterior cerebral artery

(C) posterior cerebral artery and middle cerebral artery

(D) A and C

122. The ophthalmic artery forms extensive anastomoses with the following artery

(A) anterior communicating artery

(B) anterior cerebral artery

(C) middle cerebral artery

(D) external carotid artery

123. The anterior cerebral artery and its branches supplies which of the following?

(A) frontal and parietal lobes

(B) corpus callosum

(C) septum pellucidum

(D) basil ganglia

(E) anterior limb of the internal capsule

(F) all of the above

(G) A, B, and C

124. The vertebral arteries unite to form the

(A) posterior communicating artery

(B) posterior cerebral artery

(C) basilar artery

(D) A and C

125. The various parts of the brainstem are supplied by which of the following arteries

(A) middle cerebral artery

(B) posterior communicating artery

(C) basilar artery

(D) all of the above

126. The basilar artery gives rise to all but which of the following

(A) anterior inferior cerebellar artery

(B) posterior communicating artery

(C) superior cerebellar artery

(D) posterior cerebral arteries

127. The anastomotic arteries that is formed by the major cerebral arteries is the

(A) middle cerebral and anterior communicating artery

(B) vertebral arteries and basilar

(C) anterior cerebral and anterior communicating arteries

(D) circle of Willis

(E) A and C

Match the following collateral pathway systems that supply blood by existing anastomoses in the brain.

128. right-to-left anastomoses provide redistribution of blood flow between the sides of of the body and occur via _____

129. carotid-to-vertebral anastomoses via _____

130. subclavian-to-carotid and subclavian-to-vertebral anastomoses _____

131. ICA-to-ECA ipsolateral anastomoses _____

132. optical anastomoses can provide collateral flow between _____

(A) involve the deep cervical artery, spinal branches of the vertebral arteries, and the ascending cervical artery

(B) superorbital and supratrochlear arteries

(C) anterior communicating (AcoA) and basilar artery (BA)

(D) posterior communicating arteries (PcoAs)

(E) anterior cerebral artery (ACA), middle cerebral artery (MCA), and posterior communicating artery (PCA)

133. Pulsitility index represents the degree of

(A) pliability of the artery

(B) stenosis of the artery

(C) peripheral resistance

(D) all of the above

134. A pulsitility index of greater than 1.2 may indicate

(A) increased intracranial pressure

(B) vasospasm

(C) hypercapnia

(D) aortic insufficiency

(E) all of the above

135. Transtemporal window allows insonation of the

(A) middle cerebral artery (M1–M2 segments)

(B) anterior cerebral artery

(C) posterior cerebral artery and C1 segment of the carotid siphon

(D) distal ICA

(E) A, B, and C

136. Suboccipital window allows insonation of

(A) carotid siphon (C2, C3, and C4)

(B) vertebral arteries

(C) basilar artery

(D) B and C

(E) A, B, and C

137. Submandibular window allows insonation of the

(A) ophthalmic artery

(B) carotid siphon

(C) retromandibular ICA (distal)

(D) A and B

138. Transorbital window allows insonation of

(A) ophthalmic artery
(B) carotid siphon (C2, C3, and C4)
(C) anterior communicating artery
(D) A and B
(E) all of the above

Match the following acoustic windows with the proper name.

139. transorbital window _____
140. transtemporal window _____
141. transoccipital window _____

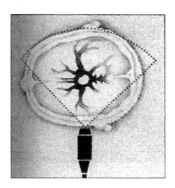

(A)

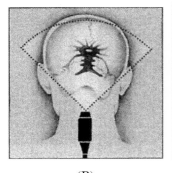 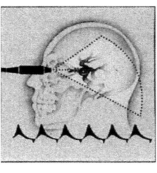

(B)   (C)

142. Each TCD examination includes all of the following except

(A) color Doppler imaging
(B) spectral waveform analysis with notation of depth, speed, and direction of flow
(C) mean velocity
(D) measurements of all arteries in the circle of Willis

Match the direction of flow for the following vessels.

143. carotid siphon _____
144. ICA bifurcation _____
145. M1 segment of MCA _____
146. vertebral artery _____
147. basilar artery _____
148. ACA _____
149. PCA, P1 segment _____
150. PCA, P2 segment _____
151. ophthalmic artery _____

(A) bidirectional
(B) away from the probe
(C) toward the probe
(D) any

152. With the occlusion or a critical stenosis of the ipsilateral extracranial carotid artery

(A) middle cerebral artery velocity is decreased or absent
(B) middle cerebral artery end diastole is increased
(C) ophthalmic artery will decrease in flow or may have reverse flow
(D) A and C
(E) A and B

153. Subclavian steal can be detected in which of the following intracranial vessels?

(A) cervical vertebrals
(B) intracranial vertebral arteries
(C) basilar artery
(D) all of the above
(E) B and C

154. Intracranial vessel stenosis will exhibit which of the following characteristics?

(A) focal increase in the mean blood flow velocity distal to the stenosis
(B) focal increase in the mean blood flow velocity at the site of the vessel stenosis
(C) color flow Doppler will show multiple color patterns
(D) all of the above
(E) A and C
(F) B and C

155. Which of the intracranial vessels is the most common to occlude and seen with acute stroke?

(A) basilar artery
(B) anterior cerebral artery (ACA)
(C) ophthalmic artery
(D) middle cerebral artery (MCA)

156. Transcranial color Doppler can be used to examine which of the following conditions?

(A) brain death
(B) vasospasms
(C) arteriovenous malformations
(D) embolus
(E) all of the above

Answers and Explanations

At the end of each explained answer there is a number combination in parentheses. The first number identifies the reference source; the second number or set of numbers indicates the page or pages on which the relevant information can be found.

1. **(C)** Stroke is ranked in the United States as the 3rd leading cause of death annually.
(Study Guide:497)

2. **(D)** The emphasis of stroke as a national issue is on early diagnosis and treatment to prevent long-term disability. *(4:38–41)*

3. **(C)** The newest technique for early determination of a stroke a hemorrhagic or ischemic is magnetic resonance imaging (MRI) diffusion imaging. *(4:38–41)*

4. **(C)** Stroke is defined as sudden and often severe impairment of blood flow to the brain.
(Study Guide:497)

5. **(C)** Transient ischemic attack is an acute neurologic symptoms that last less than 24 hours and completely resolve. *(5:59)*

6. **(E)** Stroke in evolution is ischemic symptoms that actively worsens during a period of observation.
(5:59)

7. **(A)** Reversible ischemic neurologic deficit is a neurologic symptoms that last longer than 24 hours and completely resolves. *(5:59)*

8. **(D)** Completed stroke is a stable neurologic deficit that had sudden onset and persists longer than 3 weeks.
(5:59)

9. **(B)** Acute brain death is caused by either lack of blood supply or effect of blood outside of normal vessels.
(5:59)

10. **(D)** Atherosclerosis is the major cause of vascular disease. *(5:58)*

11. **(D)** Ataxia is a symptom of vertebrobasilar insufficiency not internal carotid artery symptoms.
(2:941–948)

12. **(D)** Vertigo is a neurologic symptom of vertebrobasilar disease. *(5:106)*

13. **(C)** Ocular pneumoplethysmography is used with pressure cups over the ocular globe. *(13:84–85)*

14. **(C)** Ocular pneumoplethysmography is used to detect hemodynamically significant lesions (greater than 50%) and in the assessment of collateral flow.
(13:84–85)

15. **(D)** All of the above. Color Doppler units provide real-time imaging, Doppler waveform analysis, and color depiction of the flow characteristics. *(5:16)*

16. **(D)** 7.5 MHz linear array is the optimal transducer for high-resolution gray-scale imaging of the carotid arteries. *(8:29–32)*

17. **(C)** 45–60° angle to the artery gives the best Doppler information. *(5:5)*

18. **(C)** Peak systolic velocity is the most utilized of the Doppler criteria for estimation of percentage diameter reduction. *(14:36)*

19. **(A)** Angle correction is mandatory when using velocity to represent Doppler shift. *(5:5)*

20. **(C)** Aliasing is an artifact that occurs with pulsed Doppler in a hemodynamically significant stenosis.
(5:15)

21. **(C)** Change in probe position, decreasing the depth, increasing the PRF, increasing the Doppler angle, or lowering the frequency can correct aliasing. *(5:15)*

22. **(F)** Both C and D. Two advantages of power Doppler is in defining occlusive vessels and it is not dependent on beam angle and free from aliasing artifact.
(5:19)

23. (B) The arterial layer of muscle and elastic tissue is the media.   *(5:23:Fig. 3–3)*

24. (C) The outer loose filmy layer of the artery wall is the adventitia.   *(5:23:Fig. 3–3)*

25. (A) The elastic inner layer of the artery wall is the intima.   *(5:23:Fig. 3–3)*

26. (E) All of the above. Variable plaque morphology may be termed as soft, dense, calcified, and ulcerated.   *(5:28–29)*

27. (D) Aortic arch is the vessel from which the cerebrovascular vessels arise.   *(5:57)*

28. (E) All of the above: The vertebral, internal thoracic, thyrocervical, costocervical, and dorsal scapular all arise from the subclavian artery.   *(5:57)*

29. (J) right internal carotid artery   *(Study Guide, Fig. 11–2)*

30. (B) right external carotid artery   *(Study Guide, Fig. 11–2)*

31. (F) right subclavian artery   *(Study Guide, Fig. 11–2)*

32. (I) brachiocephalic trunk   *(Study Guide, Fig. 11–2)*

33. (A) basilar artery   *(Study Guide, Fig. 11–2)*

34. (E) left vertebral artery   *(Study Guide, Fig. 11–2)*

35. (G) left common carotid artery   *(Study Guide, Fig. 11–2)*

36. (C) left subclavian artery   *(Study Guide, Fig. 11–2)*

37. (H) aortic arch   *(Study Guide, Fig. 11–2)*

38. (C) The common carotid artery is the main branch of the carotid system.   *(5:57)*

39. (B) The internal carotid artery demonstrates a rapid increase in velocity during systole with a clear window and continuous antegrade flow during diastole. *(5:60)*

40. (D) The external carotid artery has a brisk systolic upstroke, sharper peak, abrupt downstroke because it supplies a high-resistance system.   *(5:60)*

41. (C) Common carotid artery combines the pattern of the internal and external carotid artery.   *(5:60)*

42. (A) Carotid bulb exhibits a complicated turbulent flow pattern.   *(5:60)*

43. (B) external carotid artery   *(5:60–61:Fig. 5–14)*

44. (C) common carotid artery   *(5:60–61:Fig. 5–12)*

45. (A) internal carotid artery   *(5:60–61:Fig. 5–13)*

46. (D) digital subtraction angiography is the radiographic modality that is the method of choice for opacifying the entire cerebral arterial system.   *(5:62)*

The following are the transverse scans of the extracranial carotid arteries in the proper order according to the examination protocol:

47. (E) brachiocephalic artery and bifurcation of the subclavian and carotid arteries   *(5:53)*

48. (C) common carotid artery   *(5:53)*

49. (D) carotid bulb   *(5:53)*

50. (B) carotid bifurcation with internal and external arteries   *(5:53)*

51. (A) origin of the vertebral artery   *(5:53)*

The following longitudinal scan of the extracranial arteries in the proper order according to examination protocol:

52. (D) Common carotid artery from clavicle to mandible.   *(5:53)*

53. (B) Carotid bifurcation (carotid bulb and proximal portion of internal and external carotid arteries.   *(5:53)*

54. (E) Internal carotid artery as far distal as possible.   *(5:53)*

55. (C) External carotid artery as far distal as possible.   *(5:53)*

56. (A) Vertebral artery from origin as far distal as possible.   *(5:53)*

57. (A) External carotid artery   *(5:54:Fig. 5–4)*

58. (B) Internal carotid artery.   *(5:54:Fig. 5–4)*

59. (D) Common carotid artery   *(5:54:Fig. 5–4)*

60. (C) Carotid bulb   *(5:54:Fig. 5–4)*

61. (A) Laminar flow is the normal flow pattern in the carotid artery.   *(5:60)*

62. (C) Ophthalmic artery is the first major branch of the internal carotid artery with clinical significance.   *(5:120)*

63. (B) Cerebral hemispheres of the brain, eyes and accessory organs, forehead, and part of the nose are

supplied by blood from the internal carotid artery.
(5:58)

64. **(B)** Scalp, face, and most of the neck are supplied by blood from the external carotid artery.   (5:57)

65. **(C)** Temporal tapping is the maneuver to identify that the Doppler signal is coming from the external carotid artery.   (9:35–43)

66. **(B)** The left branch of the common carotid artery arises directly from the aortic arch.
(Study Guide, Fig. 11–2)

67. **(D)** All have the above. Turbulent flow does not necessarily have to be caused by atheromatous plaque. Sudden increase in the diameter of the blood vessel can cause turbulence. This can be seen in the carotid bulb region where the boundary layer separates from the arterial wall with an inherent reversal of flow. Tortuous arteries also can cause turbulence as blood flow is forced to change direction. Carotid kinks can cause turbulence as the arterial lumen is narrowed.
(16:18–19)

68. **(B)** An increase resistivity index in the common carotid artery can indicate stenotic or occlusive disease distal to the sample site. Total occlusion of the internal carotid artery can cause a decrease in diastolic flow in the common carotid artery because of increased resistance to flow.   (16:88)

69. **(E)** Doppler shift frequencies are affected by Doppler angle, transducer frequency, and the velocity of the red blood cells.   (16:5–7)

70. **(C)** Carotid bifurcation is the most common site for atherosclerotic plaque formation.   (5:59)

71. **(D)** None of the above. The internal carotid artery does not have a branch in the cervical section.   (5:58)

72. **(C)** 50% diameter reduction constitutes the beginning of a critical arterial stenosis where symptoms manifest.   (5:68)

Identification of the plaque morphology:

73. **(E)** Soft   (5:64–65)

74. **(C)** Dense   (5:64–65)

75. **(A)** Calcified   (5:64–65)

76. **(B)** Ulcerated   (5:64–65)

77. **(D)** Intraplaque hemorrhage   (5:64–65)

78. **(B)** Critical stenosis   (5:73:Fig. 5–49)

79. **(D)** Occlusion of ICA   (5:73:Fig. 5–49)

80. **(E)** Reversal of flow in bulb proximal to ICA occlusion   (5:73:Fig. 5–49)

81. **(C)** Moderate stenosis by diameter reduction
(5:73:Fig. 5–49)

82. **(A)** Mild stenosis by diameter reduction
(5:73:Fig. 5–49)

83. **(D)** All of the above, Distal to a critical stenosis, the spectral analysis depicts peak systole velocities decrease, end diastole velocities decrease, and turbulent flow is seen in the spectral analysis.   (5:67–73)

84. **(D)** Carotid body tumors are composed of paraganglionic tissue and are rare neoplasms.   (5:97)

85. **(B)** Kinking of the internal carotid artery is associated with the symptom of ischemia.   (5:91)

86. **(A)** Identifying and operating on appropriately severe common carotid bifurcation lesions is the most common treatment to risk reduction for stroke according to NASCET.   (5:93–94)

87. **(A)** The superficial temporal artery.
(Study Guide, Fig. 11–3)

88. **(D)** The internal carotid artery.
(Study Guide, Fig. 11–3)

89. **(J)** The vertebral artery.   (Study Guide, Fig. 11–3)

90. **(C)** The subclavian artery.   (Study Guide, Fig. 11–3)

91. **(B)** The supraorbital artery.   (Study Guide, Fig. 11–3)

92. **(E)** The ophthalmic artery.   (Study Guide, Fig. 11–3)

93. **(G)** The external carotid artery.
(Study Guide, Fig. 11–3)

94. **(H)** The superior thyroid artery.
(Study Guide, Fig. 11–3)

95. **(F)** The common carotid artery.
(Study Guide, Fig. 11–3)

96. **(I)** The brachiocephalic trunk. (Study Guide, Fig. 11–3)

97. **(E)** The hypophyseal is not a branch of the subclavian.   (5:4)

98. **(A)** The extracranial posterior circulation is composed of paired vertebral arteries in the back of the neck.   (5:105)

99. **(E)** The subclavian steal causes ataxia, limb paralysis, vertigo, and syncope as symptoms.   (5:116)

100. **(E)** The hallmark sign of the subclavian steal is the difference of blood pressure (10–20 mmHg) between the two arms and decreased peripheral pulse in the affected upper extremity. *(5:116)*

101. **(E)** The Doppler waveform characteristics of subclavian steal include deceleration, reversed, or alternating flow in the contralateral vertebral artery and diminished waveform distal to the stenosis or occlusion. *(5:116)*

102. **(C)** The normal vertebral artery spectral analysis will depict low-resistance waveform pattern similar to the internal carotid artery. *(5:107)*

103. **(B)** Normally the vertebrobasilar system provides a 10%–20% percentage of blood flow to the intracranial system. *(5:106)*

104. **(C)** The vertebral artery can be visualized by the longitudinal plane at the level of common carotid with the transducer angled laterally until the vertebral is seen passing through the transverse processes. *(5:105)*

105. **(C)** The subclavian steal syndrome is asymptomatic at rest. *(5:116)*

106. **(B)** The posterior communicating artery. *(Study Guide, Fig. 11–4)*

107. **(D)** The middle cerebral artery. *(Study Guide, Fig. 11–4)*

108. **(A)** The anterior cerebral artery. *(Study Guide, Fig. 11–4)*

109. **(F)** The internal carotid artery. *(Study Guide, Fig. 11–4)*

110. **(H)** The posterior cerebral artery. *(Study Guide, Fig. 11–4)*

111. **(G)** The vertebral artery. *(Study Guide, Fig. 11–4)*

112. **(C)** The anterior communicating artery. *(Study Guide, Fig. 11–4)*

113. **(E)** The basilar artery. *(Study Guide, Fig. 11–4)*

114. **(E)** The transcranial Doppler examination requires low-frequency (2 MHz) and the appropriate software for spectral analysis calculations and computations. *(5:117)*

115. **(D)** The suboccipital window examines vertebral arteries and basilar artery. *(5:117)*

116. **(C)** The transcranial Doppler is described as a noninvasive technique to measure the velocity of blood flow in the major intracranial brain vessels by using pulsed-waved Doppler. *(5:118)*

117. **(E)** Transcranial imaging has the advantage of observation of the narrowing of the vessel lumen, visual assessment of the transcranial vessels for localization, observation of vessel tortuosity, and calculation of the vessel lumen. *(5:120)*

118. **(B)** The middle cerebral artery is the largest branch of the cerebral ICA. *(5:120)*

119. **(F)** The middle cerebral artery (MCA) supplies frontal lobe, temporal lobe, and parietal lobe. *(5:120)*

120. **(E)** The middle cerebral artery is divided into M1, M2, and M3 segments. *(5:121)*

121. **(B)** The posterior communicating artery anastomoses with the posterior cerebral artery. *(5:121)*

122. **(D)** The ophthalmic artery forms extensive anastomoses with the external carotid artery. *(5:120)*

123. **(F)** The anterior cerebral artery and its branches supply the frontal and parietal lobes, the corpus callosum, the septum pellucidum, the basil ganglia, and the anterior limb of the internal capsule. *(5:120)*

124. **(C)** The vertebral arteries unite with the basilar artery. *(5:121)*

125. **(C)** The basilar artery supplies the various parts of the brainstem. *(5:121)*

126. **(B)** The basilar artery does not give rise to the posterior communicating artery. *(5:121)*

127. **(D)** The anastomotic arteries that is formed by the major cerebral arteries is the circle of Willis. *(5:121)*

Collateral pathway systems that supply blood by existing anastomoses in the brain:

128. **(C)** Right-to-left anastomoses provide redistribution of blood flow between the sides of the body and occur via anterior communicating (AcoA) and basilar artery (BA). *(5:122)*

129. **(D)** Carotid-to-vertebral anastomoses via posterior communicating arteries (PcoAs). *(5:122)*

130. **(A)** Subclavian-to-carotid and subclavian-to-vertebral anastomoses involve the deep cervical artery, spinal branches of the vertebral arteries, and the ascending cervical artery. *(5:122)*

131. (B) ICA-to-ECA ipsolateral anastomoses super-orbital and supratrochlear arteries.   *(5:122)*

132. (E) Optical anastomoses can provide collateral flow between anterior cerebral artery (ACA), middle cerebral artery (MCA), and posterior communicating artery (PCA).   *(5:122)*

133. (C) Pulsitility index represents the degree of peripheral resistance.   *(5:122)*

134. (E) A pulsitility index of greater than 1.2 may indicate an increased intracranial pressure, vasospasm, hypercapnia, and aortic insufficiency.   *(5:123)*

135. (E) Transtemporal window allows insonation of the middle cerebral artery (M1-M2 segments), anterior cerebral artery, and posterior cerebral artery and C1 segment of the carotid siphon.   *(5:117)*

136. (D) Suboccipital window allows insonation of vertebral arteries and basilar artery.   *(5:117)*

137. (C) Submandibular window allows insonation of the retromandibular ICA (distal).   *(5:117)*

138. (D) Transorbital window allows insonation of ophthalmic artery and carotid siphon (C2, C3, and C4).   *(5:117)*

139. (C) Transorbital window.   *(5:117)*

140. (A) Transtemporal window.   *(5:117)*

141. (B) Transoccipital window.   *(5:117)*

142. (D) Each TCD examination does not include measurements of all arteries in the circle of Willis.   *(5:117)*

143. (D) The carotid siphon can flow in any direction.   *(5:119:Table 5–1)*

144. (A) ICA bifurcation flow is bi-directional.   *(5:119:Table 5–1)*

145. (C) M1 segment of MCA flow is toward the probe.   *(5:119:Table 5–1)*

146. (B) Vertebral artery flow is away from the probe.   *(5:119:Table 5–1)*

147. (B) Basilar artery flow is away from the probe.   *(5:119:Table 5–1)*

148. (B) ACA flow is away from the probe.   *(5:119:Table 5–1)*

149. (C) PCA, P1 segment flows toward the probe.   *(5:119:Table 5–1)*

150. (B) PCA, P2 segment flow is away from the probe.   *(5:119:Table 5–1)*

151. (C) Ophthalmic artery flow is toward the probe.   *(5:119:Table 5–1)*

152. (D) With the occlusion or a critical stenosis of the ipsilateral extracranial carotid artery the middle cerebral artery velocity is decreased or absent, and ophthalmic artery will decrease in flow or may have reverse flow.   *(5:125)*

153. (E) Subclavian steal can be detected in intracranial vessels of the intracranial vertebral arteries and basilar artery.   *(5:125)*

154. (F) Intracranial vessel stenosis will exhibit characteristics of focal increase in the mean blood flow velocity at the site of the stenosis and color flow Doppler will show multiple color patterns.   *(5:127)*

155. (D) The middle cerebral artery (MCA) is the most common intracranial vessel to occlude and seen with acute stroke.   *(5:127)*

156. (E) Transcranial color Doppler can be used to examine conditions of brain death, vasospasms, arteriovenous malformations, and embolus.   *(5:129–132)*

REFERENCES

References appear on page 515.

CHAPTER 12

VASCULAR SONOGRAPHY— PERIPHERAL VEINS

Carol A. Krebs, Sandra L. Hughes, Karen K. Rawls, and Thomas G. Hoffman

Study Guide

INTRODUCTION

Diseases of the venous system are not new. One of the oldest depictions of varicose veins can be seen in the leg of an Athenian warrior in an ancient frieze in Greece. Epidemiologic studies suggest that approximately 50% of the adult population in the United States have some form of chronic venous disorder. Acute venous problems are often asymptomatic but carry a sequel that can either be fatal or cause chronic debilitation. Although we are very familiar with the risk factors for acute and chronic venous diseases, there is still very little scientific knowledge about the pathophysiology of these entities.

The true incidence of acute deep vein thrombosis is difficult to determine. Randomized clinical trials on different prophylactic regimens in which serial testing of patients was performed from the time of hospital admission probably provides the most accurate prevalence data. These studies reported a 20% incidence of deep vein thrombosis (DVT) in general medical and surgical patients over 40 years old and a 60–80% incidence in patients with long bone fracture or undergoing total joint replacements.[1-5] An even more significant finding was that 50% of these patients were asymptomatic. Acute DVT that remains confined to the extremity is relatively benign in the short term. However, the primary clinical concern in DVT is the complication of pulmonary embolism (PE), which is fatal in 1% of patients with diagnosed DVT. Although the clinical course of the majority of patients with acute DVT is uneventful, the thrombotic process causes permanent damage to the deep venous system. Scarring of the vein wall and residual thrombus leads to *postphlebitic syndrome*. Symptoms of this condition appear between 18 months and 10 years after the thrombotic event. Eighty percent of patients who develop acute DVT will have some symptoms of postphlebitic syndrome within 10 years. It has been postulated that early intervention and treatment may halt the progression of thrombus and reduce the incidence of embolism. Earlier diagnosis and treatment may also prevent later disability associated with chronic venous disease.

INSTRUMENTATION AND TECHNIQUES

Over the last few years, a resurgence of interest in the venous system has occurred, and new technologies have been applied to increase our knowledge of the venous system. Advances in diagnostic techniques have far outpaced our knowledge of the disease itself. Until the last few years, ascending contrast venography was the standard method used. Today, noninvasive laboratory techniques have all but replaced venography to confirm the diagnosis of deep vein thrombosis. Early noninvasive vascular techniques for evaluating the veins included; electrical, strain gauge, and plethysmography. Photoplethysmography was used to determine venous incompetency and discriminate between superficial and deep vein thrombosis and is still in use in some laboratories.

Doppler ultrasound examination is a subjective test where the examiner compares the audible Doppler velocity signals of the extremity using limb compression maneuvers. It is performed with the patient in the supine position with the legs exposed and externally rotated. In a normal venous Doppler examination, the venous signal is heard when the transducer is placed over the vein located next to the accompanying artery. This characteristic is referred to as spontaneity. The only location where a spontaneous venous signal may normally not be heard is the posterior tibial vein at the ankle. In this location, the blood flow rate may be below the sensitivity of the Doppler velocity detector. Most commercially available Doppler velocity detectors cannot detect movement below 6 cm/s. The audible signal is evaluated to determine if it is phasic (waxes and wanes with respiration), continuous, or pulsatile. A normal venous signal is phasic. A continuous venous signal indicates either internal obstruction of flow or external compression of the vein proximal to the position of the transducer. Compression of the vein by the transducer also can cause a continuous venous signal. The normal response to distal augmentation is a rapid increase in the pitch (frequency) of the signal followed by a slow decay and than a return to the normal phasicity. If the Doppler velocity signal increases rapidly and then abruptly stops or no response is heard with augmentation, the vein is considered to be obstructed proximal to or at the location of the transducer.

Valvular competence of the vein is evaluated by manually compressing the extremity above the transducer. If the valves are competent between the transducer and the location of the manual compression, there will be no audible venous signal during the compression. On release of the compression, the signal will resume in a manner similar to the response of the distal augmentation. If a signal is heard during proximal compression, the valves between the area of compression and the transducer are incompetent.

Venous Doppler examination is started at the posterior tibial vein and proceeds to the popliteal, superficial, and common femoral veins, respectively. The venous Doppler evaluation is highly accurate in the detection of hemodynamically significant obstruction of the popliteal, superficial femoral, and common femoral veins. However, because of the extreme compliance and redundancy of the venous system, it cannot reliably detect partial obstructions that do not cause changes in the venous flow pattern. This procedure also cannot accurately detect thrombosis confined to the calf veins. In addition, according to the physiologic nature of this examination, it cannot differentiate acute from chronic or intrinsic from extrinsic causes of obstruction.

Venous imaging and Color flow Doppler is now considered the method of choice for evaluating the venous system and to screen for thrombus. Over the last few years ultrasonic venous imaging has been shown to image accurately the entire venous system and detect venous thrombosis with an accuracy similar to contrast venography.[6–10] More recently, it has been used to assess valve function, locate and map the sites of venous reflux, and differentiate between acute and chronic venous obstruction.[11–14] Ultrasonic venous imaging can be performed using any commercial high-resolution system that has "small parts" capabilities. The ideal transducer frequency is 7.15 MHz, with an imaging field depth of 6–7 cm. Linear-array transducers with their rectangular shape and wide footprint are ideally suited for extremity imaging. The patient population and the clinical indications for the examination influence the sequence and extent of the venous evaluation. B-Mode real-time imaging and color flow Doppler:

- provide anatomic and physiologic information
- reliably assess venous flow patterns
- determine extent of vascular incompetence
- identify sites of venous obstruction

Color flow Doppler is unique because of its ability to demonstrate patency quickly with color flow through the vessel lumen. It demonstrates occlusion or partial occlusions with associated thrombus and, in some cases, determines whether the thrombus is acute or chronic. Collateral flow patterns can be documented circumventing any occluded segment, and follow-up studies can evaluate the regression or progression of disease.

Normal veins have a thin, echogenically homogeneous wall with elliptical valve sinuses that contain long thin valve leaflets. Perforating and small tributary veins are rarely visualized in the normal venous system. Venous flow characteristics may be assessed by direct observation of moving luminal echoes created by the ultrasonic reflection of red blood cell aggregates.[15] In veins containing acute thrombus, a hypoechoic or anechoic mass is seen with the luminal echoes flowing around it (Fig. 12–1). The visualization of an anechoic mass usually indicates a very recent thrombotic process. When the vein is externally compressed with the transducer, the vein walls will not compress, and the echogenicity of the luminal mass will increase because of the density change caused by the compression maneuver. If the mass does not change in echogenicity, it is an older stable thrombus and is not considered to be part of the acute disease process. It is not unusual, however, to visualize acute thrombus on either side of an older obstruction.

Chronic venous disease is characterized by hyperechoic heterogeneous protrusions from the vein wall that may partially or totally occlude the vein (Fig. 12–2). Any vein not visualized in its normal anatomic position is classified as chronically obstructed. However, it is rare to find the entire length of the vein totally obstructed.[16] Veins that at one time contained thrombus that has resolved by the normal lytic process have hyperechoic thick walls and are classified as recanalized. Incompetent collateral and perforating veins leading to intramuscular or superficial varicosities are frequently observed. Valve sinuses are rarely distinguishable but, when present, have absent or short, thickened, nonfunctional valve leaflets that are frequently misaligned.

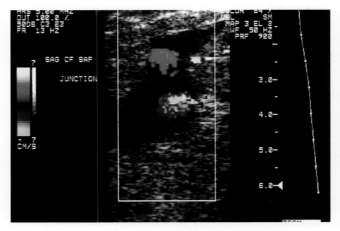

Figure 12–1. Color flow Doppler scan of the common femoral saphenous junction containing anechoic thrombus.

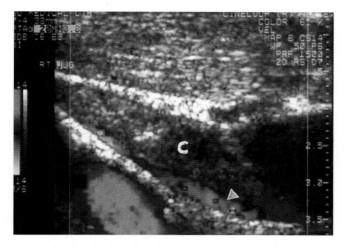

Figure 12–2. Color flow Doppler scan of the jugular vein with aged thrombus and partial flow (arrowhead).

Photoplethysmography techniques assess reflux and differentiate between superficial and deep vein incompetency. These techniques provide indirect information about location and extent of venous insufficiency. These methods are less time consuming than the color flow Doppler for screening the bilateral lower extremities and can be a great value when there are a large number of patients. Photoplethysmography involves a photoelectric cell placed above the medial malleolus. This photocell actually has an infrared light emitting diode and a photodetector that is attached to an amplifier and a strip chart recorder in the direct current (DC) mode. The patient is placed in a sitting position with the legs hanging in a dependent, nonweight-bearing position. Either the patient dorsiflexes the foot to contract the calf muscles or the calf is squeezed to empty the veins. The leg is allowed to relax and the refilling time of the veins is recorded. The normal venous refilling time is 20 seconds or greater. Less than 20 seconds indicates venous incompetency[17] (Fig. 12–3). Venous incompetency can be confined to the superficial veins or involve the deep veins. It is important to discriminate which systems are involved since the superficial veins can be surgically corrected but the deep veins cannot be surgically corrected. If the initial examination is positive for incompetency the test is repeated with

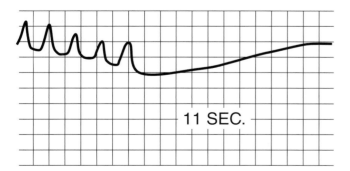

11 SEC.

Figure 12–3. Photoplethysmograph recording of venous incompetency with an 11-second refill time.

a tourniquet placed above the knee to occlude the superficial veins. If the test with the tourniquet is positive it indicates the deep system is also incompetent.

Venography (phlebography) is defined as radiography of the veins after injection of contrast medium. The venogram allows us the opportunity to study the anatomy and function of the veins in vivo and to diagnose venous pathology.[17] Contrast material is injected into the venous system and flows into the deep and superficial venous system because of specific gravity. There are two types of venography *ascending* and *descending* depending on the injection site. Ascending venography will be injected into a peripheral vein and the contrast material carried centripetal by the venous flow. Descending venography will be injected into a proximal vein in the leg and the contrast media carried distally by induced retrograde venous flow.[18]

The normal venogram of the lower extremity demonstrates the deep and superficial system as well as the external and common iliac vein. In some instances, special maneuvers (compression or muscular contraction) may be required to delineate the venous structures fully. The veins are quite variable among different individuals but are usually shown as deep venous trunks that are well defined and easily recognized. The valves are best seen after muscular contraction. The perforators will be defined between the deep venous trunks and the superficial veins.[18]

Venous thrombosis obstructs the draining vein and creates a filling defect on the venogram (Fig. 12–4). The thrombus causes venous flow to be rerouted into the superficial or collateral veins. These collateral veins will become dilated because of the increased pressure/flow and have abnormally high velocities. In the wall of the vein where the thrombus is attached, there will be various degrees of inflammation and edema (phlebitis). In the acute stage, the thrombus may be free-floating, and the complete extension of the thrombus must be seen. After occlusive thrombus, the vein lumen will be irregular and the valves nonfunctioning. With such conditions as incompetent perforating veins or varicose veins, there are no working valves allowing the blood to flow in both a forward or reverse pattern. The veins will appear as irregular tortuous vessels that have rapid filling of contrast medium on the venogram.[18]

ANATOMY

Because of the complex nature of the venous system and its diseases, the vascular laboratory staff must have a thorough knowledge of anatomy, physiology, and pathophysiology. In addition, the technical aspects of diagnostic procedures must be well known to provide the clinician with an accurate appraisal of the pathology. The intent of this chapter is to provide an overview of venous anatomy and physiology as well as ultrasonic diagnostic procedures. This chapter includes the upper and lower extremity venous systems; however, epidemiologic studies have found that 95% of venous disease originates in the lower extremities.

The tripartite structure of the vein wall is composed of an inner *intima*, a *media* and an outer *adventitia*.

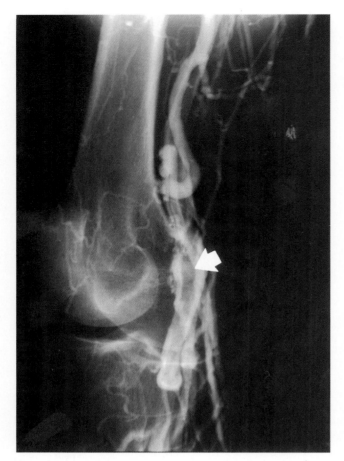

Figure 12–4. Venogram demonstrates the thrombus in the vein as a filling defect (arrow).

Tunica intima. The innermost lining of the vein consists of a thin layer of endothelial cells. Folds of endothelial tissue form the inherent semilunar valves.

Tunica media. The media or middle layer of the vein contains smooth muscle cells with a loose network of collagen and elastin fibrils. It varies in thickness in different veins, for example, the superficial veins have a thicker layer than many deep veins.

Tunica adventitia. The outer layer of the vein consisting of collagen and smooth muscle. Vein wall structure is similar to that of an artery. In veins, the main differences are that the media is very thin with the elastin concen-

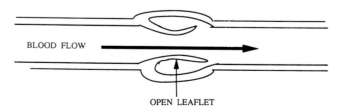

Figure 12–5. Venous valve open.

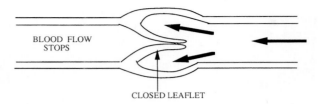

Figure 12–6. Venous valve closed.

tration substantially reduced, and the muscle fibers predominantly oriented longitudinally. The adventitia is the thickest and strongest part of the vein wall.

Venous valves are found in the tunica intima. They are thin, paired structures consisting of endothelial and connective tissue. A normal valve allows blood to flow only in one direction toward the heart. The valve is found in a broadened area of the vein called a valve sinus. Valves open in the deep system when venous blood is forced upward by muscular contractions of the calf (Fig. 12–5). Valves close when pressure on the venous blood is released (Fig. 12–6). Blood pools in the valve sinus when the valve is closed. A functioning valve is said to be competent when it will not allow reversal of blood flow. To ensure flow in a forward direction back to the heart, veins contain one-way valves that are generally bicuspid and consist of smooth muscle cells and loose connective tissue covered by endothelial cells (Fig. 12–7). This connection is associated with a localized area of vein wall dilatation or "sinus" immediately above the valve ring. The number of valves in the venous system varies depending on the distance from the heart. In the calf, valves can be found every 1.5–2 cm. As many as 10–15 valves may be present in each vein. In the thigh, three to five valves are present; whereas, valves are rarely found in the iliac veins and vena cava. Valves are more numerous in the deep calf veins and decrease in number in the popliteal and femoral veins. The location of venous valves are inconsistent within each vein, but they are most commonly found at the orifices of branches or just beyond the joining or confluence of two or more veins. Formation of deep vein thrombosis in the valve sinus may cause injury to the valve. Valve leaflets may become frozen in the open position, and venous blood will flow retrograde when pressure on the venous system is released. This is referred to as an incompetent valve. Valves in the deep veins prevent reversal of flow in the deep system. Valves in the communicating veins prevent flow from the deep to superficial veins. Those in the superficial veins prevent flow from the deep to superficial system as well as retrograde flow in the superficial system. They are located throughout the greater and lesser saphenous veins. For a comparison of veins and arteries see (Table 12–1).

LOWER EXTREMITY VEINS

Deep Venous System

In the lower extremity, there are four components to the venous system. These are the *deep, superficial, intramuscu-*

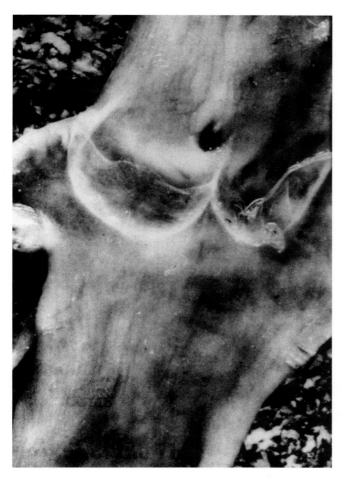

Figure 12–7. Venous valve leaflets. *(Reprinted with permission from Gottlob R. Venous Valves. New York: Springer; 1986:27.)*

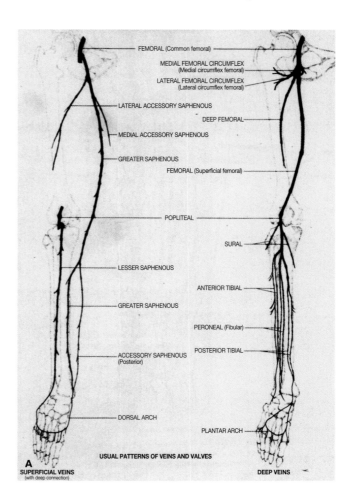

lar, perforating, or *communicating* veins (Fig. 12–8 A, B). The deep veins are the primary channels that transport the blood from the extremity to the heart. They are located beneath the muscle close to the bones from which their names are derived. These veins run in close association with the corresponding arteries (Fig. 12–9 A, B). These primary veins include:

- external iliac
- common femoral (CFU)
- superficial femoral (SFV)
- profunda or deep femoral (PFV)
- popliteal (POP)
- posterior tibial (PTV)

TABLE 12–1. COMPARISON OF VEINS AND ARTERIES

Veins	Arteries
Thin walls	Thick walls
Walls collapse easily	Rigid walls
Valves	No valves
Nonpulsatile	Pulsatile

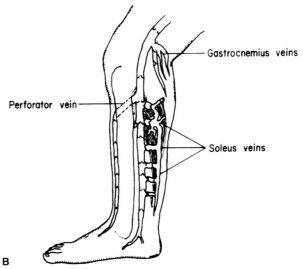

Figure 12–8. (A) Superficial and deep veins of the lower extremity. *(Reprinted with permission from DeWeese JA, Rogoff SM, Tobin CE. Radiographic Anatomy of Major Veins of Lower Limb (chart). Rochester, NY: Eastman Kodak Company.)* **(B)** Anatomical drawing of the gastrocnemius, soleus, and perforating veins of the lower extremity.

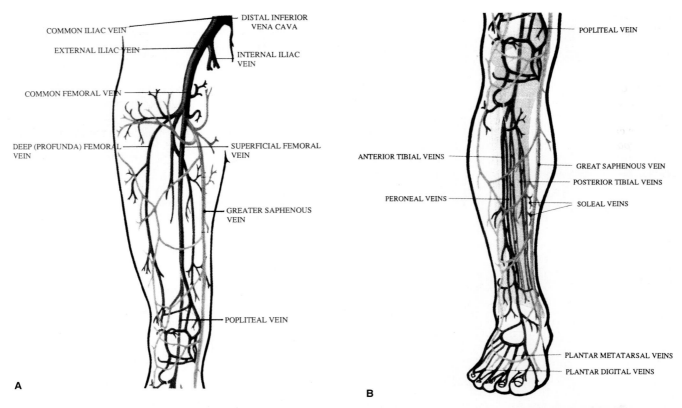

Figure 12–9. (A) Veins of the thigh. **(B)** Veins of the leg. *(Reprinted with permission from Abbott Laboratories. North Chicago, Il. Medical illustration by Scott Thorn Barrows, AMI.)*

- peroneal
- anterior tibial (ATV).

The three deep veins of the calf, (PTV, peroneal, and ATV), are classified as venae comitantes because they are intimately associated to the artery of the same name and are duplicated throughout their course. The deep veins of the calf are paired vessels that accompany the arteries. Each set of veins runs within a specific muscofascial compartment of the leg. The posterior tibial veins are formed by the union of the superficial and deep plantar veins behind the medial malleolus. These veins course proximally lying on the tibialis posterior muscle, which separates them from the interosseous membrane. The posterior tibial veins lie in the posterior crural compartment and are covered superficially by the soleus and gastrocnemius. They drain the flexors of the calf and soleus muscle and tributaries of the greater saphenous system and enter these veins through a series of perforating veins. In the upper third of the calf, posterior tibial veins unite to form a single vessel that ascends for 1–3 cm before anastomosing with the peroneal trunk to form the tibioperoneal confluence. This ascends another few centimeters, where it is joined by the anterior tibial vein and forms the popliteal vein.

The popliteal vein lies deep in the popliteal fossa and lies medial to the popliteal artery. It crosses from the medial to the lateral aspect of the artery as it courses upward into the adductor (*Hunter's*) canal. It is joined by the termination of the lesser saphenous vein (*saphenopopliteal confluence*) 1–5 cm above the popliteal fossa. The *gastrocnemius* veins usually enter the popliteal veins at the same level as the lesser saphenous. The medial gastrocnemius vein anastomoses to the popliteal vein just inferior to the lesser saphenous. However, it may quite commonly anastomose with the lesser saphenous more directly and enter the popliteal as a single trunk. The lateral gastrocnemius vein almost always joins to the popliteal vein separately.

The peroneal veins lie directly beneath and medial to the fibula. In the distal third of the lower leg, the peroneal veins are small and run deep to the *flexor hallucis longus* (tendons) in close proximity to the interosseous membrane. Near the top of the lower third of the leg, a lateral perforating vein that drains the soleus muscle joins the peroneal vein. At this point, the peroneal veins dramatically increase and double in size. In the middle third of the lower leg, the peroneal veins emerge from under the flexor hallucis muscle in the deep posterior compartment. The peroneal veins unite to form a single trunk in the upper third of the leg and continue their ascension to join the posterior tibial vein at the tibioperoneal confluence. The anterior tibial veins are a continuation of the *dorsalis pedis* veins coursing with the anterior tibial artery. They lie on the interosseous membrane between the tibia and fibula in the anterior compartment and are beneath the extensor muscles. In the upper third of the leg, these veins unite to form a single trunk. At this point, the anterior tibial vein travels posteriorly and medially close to the fibular head to join with the tibioperoneal to constitute the *popliteal vein*. The *superficial femoral vein* is a continuation of the popliteal vein and begins at the adductor canal. It lies lateral to the artery. As it ascends into *Scarpa's triangle*, it crosses behind the artery to assume a more medial position. Five to ten cm below the inguinal ligament, the profunda femoral vein unites with it posteriorly

to form the common femoral vein that ascends medial to the artery. The common femoral vein passes underneath the inguinal ligament to become the external iliac Fig. 12–10, A–D illustrate the veins in cross section from the pelvis to the knee.

Superficial Venous System

The superficial venous system primarily consists of the *greater and lesser* saphenous veins along with their multitude of branches. These veins drain the skin and subcutaneous tissue and run beneath the superficial fascia above the muscle fascia (Fig. 12–11). Perforating, or communicating veins as they are often called, connect the superficial to the deep veins and transport blood into the deep systems where more efficient flow is present. Intramuscular

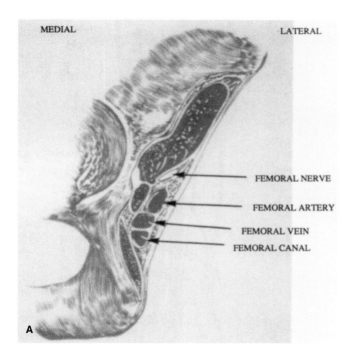

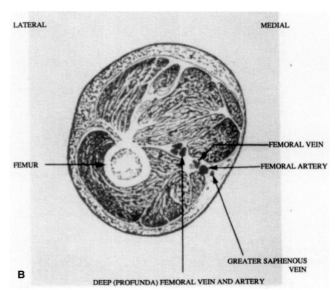

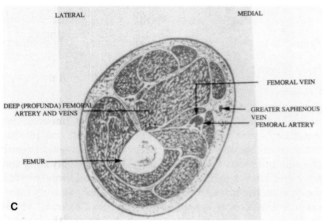

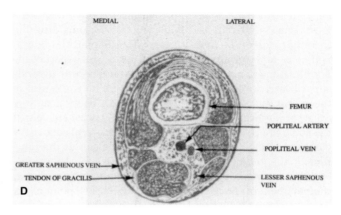

Figure 12–10. (A) Lateral surface of the right pelvic girdle. **(B)** Cross section of the proximal thigh. **(C)** Cross section of the midthigh. **(D)** Cross section of the popliteal space. *(Reprinted with permission from Gray H, Clemente CD. Anatomy of the Human Body. Philadelphia: Lea & Febiger; 1985.)*

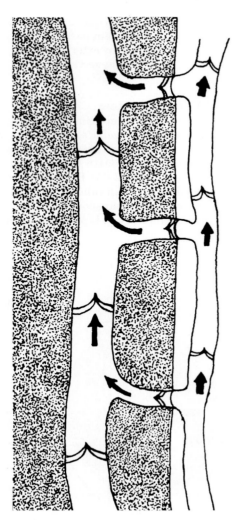

Figure 12–11. Venous flow pattern. Superficial to deep veins via the perforators.

veins drain the muscles of the lower extremity into the deep venous system. These are often paired.

The lesser saphenous vein is formed by the union of the lateral marginal vein and numerous small veins draining the outer side of the foot. It arises from behind the lateral malleolus and continues upward on the lateral aspect of the Achilles tendon in its lower third. From there it ascends superficially to the gastrocnemius muscle up the center of the calf to the popliteal fossa (Fig. 12–12). There is a large constant perforating vein draining into the peroneal vein at the point where the saphenous crosses the lateral edge of the gastrocnemius fascia. In the middle of the calf at the junction of the tendinous and muscular part of the gastrocnemius muscle, the lesser saphenous enters the intrafascial compartment of the gastrocnemius muscle. The point of the lesser saphenous entry into the popliteal space is variable; usually it is 1.5 cm above the skin crease behind the knee.

The greater saphenous vein is formed by the union of veins from the inner part of the foot and the *medial mar-*

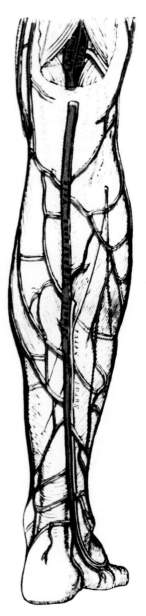

Figure 12–12. Lesser saphenous vein and tributaries. *(Reprinted with permission from Gray H. In: Goss CM, ed. Anatomy of the Human Body. Philadelphia: Lea & Febiger; 1973: 718.)*

ginal vein. The greater saphenous vein is the longest vein in the body. At the ankle, it lies in the groove between the anterior border of the medial malleolus and the tendon of the tibialis anterior. It ascends obliquely posteriorly over the subcutaneous medial surface of the lower fourth of the tibia and along the medial border of the tibial to the medial condyle at the knee. Around the knee, the greater saphenous receives three large tributaries: a calf branch, which drains the posterior calf and connects with the lesser saphenous; an anterior branch, which arises from the dorsum of the foot and ascends on the anterior surface of the leg; and a posterior arch branch, which is formed by a series of small venous arches connecting the medial calf perforators that ascend the medial aspect of the leg. The greater saphenous vein then courses over the posteromedial aspect of the knee joint and behind the medial condyle of the femur. Above the knee, it ascends the anteromedial aspect of the thigh into the fossa ovalis, where it joins the common femoral vein (Fig. 12–13). Just distal to its termination, it receives the posteromedial branch that runs up the posterior aspect of the thigh under the deep fascia, which later in its ascension pierces the deep fascia to become subcutaneous and medial. The greater saphenous vein at this level also unites with an anterolateral branch that courses diagonally upward from the lateral side of the leg, knee, and thigh. The branches of

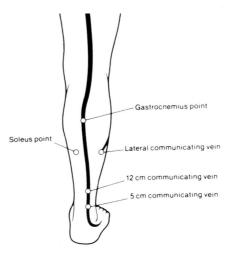

Figure 12–14. Common posterior perforators associated with the lesser saphenous, including the gastrocnemius point. *(Reprinted with permission from Brose NL, Burnand KG, Thomas ML. Disease of the Veins: Pathology, Diagnosis and Treatment. Kent, England: Edward Arnold Division of Hodder & Stoughtton; 1988: 46.)*

the saphenous vein near its termination are highly variable in number and location.

The muscular veins of the calf include a series of large venous sinuses in the soleus muscles, which are reported to be devoid of valves. They are drained by a series of short but compliant veins into the posterior tibial and peroneal veins, as previously described. During rest, they assume a tortuous appearance that may be mistaken for deep varicosities; however, this is necessary to accommodate the wide range of movement when the soleus muscle contracts. The gastrocnemius muscles contain several parallel veins in each head that contain many valves and are accompanied by an artery and nerve. The paired gastrocnemius veins emerge from the inner (ventral) surface of the heads to form a singular trunk in each head. These veins join the popliteal vein at or above the level of the knee joint. Distally, the gastrocnemius veins are united in the posterior midline of the midcalf, where they are joined by a midcalf perforator that communicates with the lesser saphenous vein. This perforator is often referred to as the *gastrocnemius point* (Fig. 12–14).

The *calf muscle pump* consists of calf muscle contractions that cause compression of the venous sinuses and deep veins of the calf. This forces blood upward into the more proximal deep venous system (Fig. 12–15). The major reservoirs of this pump are the *soleus* and *gastrocnemius sinusoids*. Pressures in excess of 100 mm Hg occur when the muscles contract.[19] Venous valves prevent reversal of blood flow.

UPPER EXTREMITY VEINS

Upper extremity veins include a superficial and deep venous system with a large capacity for the formation of collaterals (Fig. 12–16). Although deep vein thrombosis is more

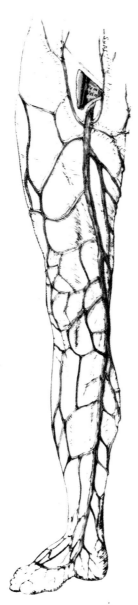

Figure 12–13. Greater saphenous vein and branches. *(Reprinted with permission from Gray H. In: Goss CM, ed. Anatomy of the Human Body. Philadelphia: Lea & Febiger; 1973: 717.)*

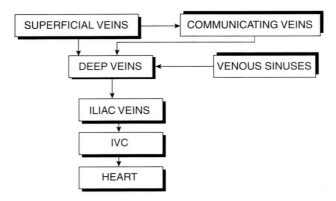

Figure 12–15. Venous flow pattern in the lower extremity.

prevalent in the lower extremities, there are cases that involve the upper extremities such as the presence of indwelling catheters or the dialysis patient with an upper extremity AV shunt.

Superficial Venous System

The superficial venous system begins in the dorsum of the hand. The digital veins drain the digits into the dorsal venous arch. Arising from the arch are the two main superficial veins of the upper extremity. The *cephalic* and *basilic* veins. The cephalic vein originates from the radial side of the dorsal venous arch and ascends along the lateral aspect of the arm. It runs between the deltoid and the pectoralis major muscles, perforates the costocoracoid membranes, and enters the axillary vein just below the clavicle. The cephalic vein communicates with the basilic vein through the medial cubital vein in the cubital fossa at the elbow.[17] The basilic vein is the second major superficial vein in the upper extremity that arises from the medial side of the dorsal venous arch. The vein runs along the ulnar aspect of the forearm and arm. It penetrates the deep fascia of the arm and unites with the brachial vein to form the axillary vein. There are numerous valves in the cephalic and basilic veins.[16]

Deep Venous System

The veins of the deep venous system are often paired and usually accompany the artery from which they are named. The digital veins drain into the superficial and deep palmar venous arches, which correspond with the superficial and deep palmar arterial arches. The *radial* and *ulnar* veins arising from the arch join at the elbow to form the brachial vein. The *brachial* vein ascends along the brachial artery to join the basilic vein to form the *axillary* vein at the lower border of the teres major muscle. The axillary vein begins at the lower border of the teres major muscle and is joined

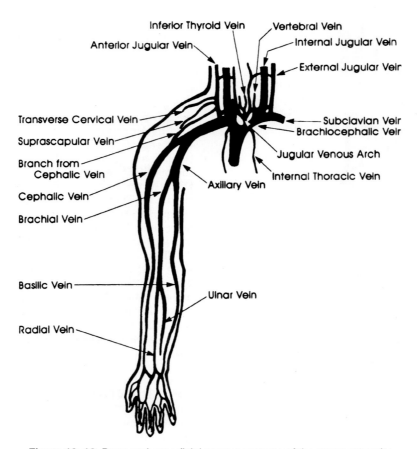

Figure 12–16. Deep and superficial venous systems of the upper extremity.

by the cephalic vein before its termination into the *subclavian* vein at the outer border of the first rib. The subclavian vein is a continuation of the axillary vein and joint the *internal jugular* vein near the medial end of the clavicle to form the *innominate* vein. The subclavian artery lies behind and superior to the subclavian vein, which is usually located anterior to the anterior scalenus muscle and the phrenic nerve. The innominate or brachiocephalic vein is formed by the subclavian and the internal jugular veins. The left innominate vein is longer than the right innominate vein, and the two join to form the superior vena cava.

PHYSIOLOGY

Veins are thin-walled vessels that collapse when empty. This feature of the venous system allows it to contain large volumes of blood with little change in venous pressure. As the vein begins to fill with blood, it changes from a collapsed state to an elliptical shape. The pressure within the vein is directly proportional to the force that is exerted on the vein wall by the column of blood within it. The vein during this shape transition is very compliant; therefore, the pressure change is minimal. As the volume of blood increases, the shape of the vein becomes oval and finally circular. During this transition, the venous pressure increases only slightly until the circular state is reached. At this point, increased blood volume will result in large increases in pressure until the maximum expansion of the vessel has been reached.

The ability of the venous system to adjust shape and size makes it ideally suited for the storage of blood. In fact 75–80% of the blood volume is contained within the venous system. When a person is resting in the supine position, the blood volume is equally distributed. The venous pressure of a normal individual at the ankle is 7–10 mm Hg. When an erect position is assumed, approximately 500 mL of blood volume is redistributed to the lower extremities. This redistribution causes an increased venous pressure in the extremities and is referred to as the hydrostatic *gradient*. The change in pressure caused by positional change can be calculated by multiplying the density of blood by the distance from the right atrium to a specific location in the extremity (e.g., the ankle). The pressure (e.g., in the ankle) is to be determined times gravity. Pressure increased because of gravity effects both the venous and arterial systems (Fig. 12–17). However, because of a lower initial pressure within the venous system, the effect of this change is more dramatic.

In the supine person, the venous pressure at the ankle is approximately 10 mm Hg, whereas, the pressure in the right atrium is ±2 mm Hg. This pressure differential encourages flow toward the heart. Venous flow also is aided by the pressure differential created by movement of the diaphragm during respiration. During inspiration, the intra-abdominal venous pressure increases, preventing flow from the lower extremities but allowing inflow from the upper portions of the body. During exhalation, the building volume of blood in the lower extremities rushes into empty intrathoracic vessels. The phasic flow pattern created by the activity of respiration is characterized by sharp increases in flow followed by a complete cessation. Flow patterns in the venous system

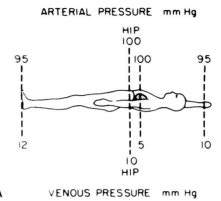

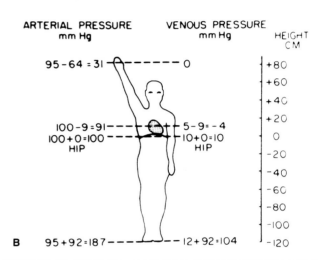

Figure 12–17. Graph showing changes in venous pressure caused by changes in body position. *(Reprinted with permission from Strandness DE. Sumner DS. Hemodynamics for Surgeons. New York: Grune & Stratton; 1975: 123.)*

can be altered by changing the breathing pattern. For example, if you take a deep breath and hold it, venous flow will stop. Respiratory changes have a profound effect on the vein diameter. These changes can be seen with deep inspiration or a valsalva maneuver. A totally occluded vein will have no diameter changes with respiration (Fig. 12–18). Blood flow also can be augmented by manual compression of an area. When a person stands upright, the venous return is not adequate. To augment, venous blood flow from the periphery muscular contractions helps propel blood toward the heart.

In the lower extremity, the predominant peripheral pumps are the muscles of the calf and, to a lesser extent, contraction of the foot and thigh muscles. Venous return is enhanced by the network of valves. The venous valves open and close in response to a pressure differential. A functioning valve is said to be competent when it will not allow reversal of blood flow. When venous pressure is higher than the valve, it closes to prevent reverse flow (*venous reflux*). When the muscles of the leg contract, the venous pressure is higher, and blood from the deep veins of the calf is expelled into the thigh, and the calf veins collapse. Because some

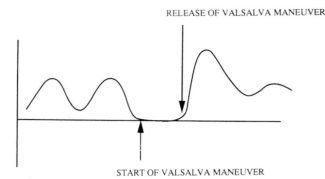

Figure 12–18. Normal venous response to a Valsalva maneuver.

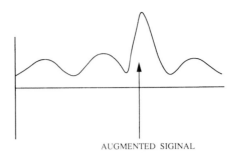

Figure 12–20. Venous augmentation pattern.

blood in the calf is forced downward by the collapse of the vein, the pressure increases distally and closes the inferior valves. During muscle relaxation, blood from the superficial system and the foot rush into empty veins. Venous pressure in the thigh is now higher than in the calf, which closes the valves above the knee. The combination of competent valves and muscle pumps provides an efficient mechanism that propels blood from the lower extremities. If either the valves or the muscle pump do not function, then the efficiency of the venous return is compromised and ambulatory *venous hypertension* in the leg occurs. Valves in the deep system prevent reversal of flow in the deep system. Valves in the communicating (perforating) veins prevent flow from the deep to superficial veins. Those in the superficial veins prevent flow from the deep to superficial system as well as retrograde flow in the superficial in the superficial system.

VENOUS CHARACTERISTICS

Normal veins exhibit certain characteristics which include the following:

- *Spontaneous flow,* which consists of a phasic signal that, is automatically elicited in all major veins. The venous sounds are low surges of blood intermittently flowing.
- *Phasic flow* occurs with respiration and is controlled by intra-abdominal pressure. In the supine position, the greatest flow is during expiration. A decrease or cessation in flow will be noted during inspiration (Fig. 12–19).

- *Distal squeezing or compression* demonstrates augmentation in the normal vein. The venous flow will be enhanced, which indicates patency of the venous channels from the site of compression (Fig. 12–20).
- *Nonpulsatility.* Normally the veins are not pulsatile. Variations in the diameter of veins are caused by respiration, rather than the cardiac cycle. Exceptions to this general rule include cardiac disease, extreme bradycardia, and overtranfusion, which can cause pulsatility (Fig. 12–21).
- *Compressibility.* The normal veins are thin walled and easily compressible. This is one of the most important criteria for venous examinations. When external compression is applied with a transducer, a normal vein will collapse until opposing walls touch. A partially occluded vein will only partially collapse and a total occluded vein will not compress at all (Fig. 12–22).

Demonstration of the absence of vein compression indicates the presence of venous thrombi.

Competency of valves can be demonstrated using the Valsalva maneuver (forcibly exhaling against a closed glottis). The venous flow should stop until the maneuver is discontinued. There should be no reversal of venous flow. Release of the maneuver will show a brief compensatory increase venous flow velocity. Valve competency can also be determined by using a compression maneuver proximal to the site being examined (Fig. 12–23). A change in the phasic pattern may be noted, but no reversal of venous flow should be demonstrated. Normally when the vein is compressed, there will be only one venous sound as it surges through the vein with the compression. In cases of venous incompetency, there will be two sounds, a forward and a reverse sound as the blood travels in two directions. This can be demonstrated with the spectral waveform analysis or with color flow Doppler changing colors with one compression (Figs. 12–24, 25).

DISEASE AND PATHOLOGY

The more common venous diseases include: varicose veins, superficial and deep venous thrombosis, pulmonary embolism, and postphlebitic syndrome.[19]

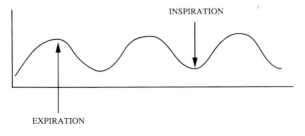

Figure 12–19. Venous phasic flow pattern.

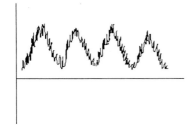

Figure 12–21. Pulsatile venous flow pattern.

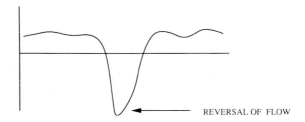

REVERSAL OF FLOW

Figure 12–23. Proximal compression with reversal of flow.

Deep Vein Thrombosis

Deep vein thrombosis (DVT) of the lower extremity is a major cause for pulmonary embolus.[20] A combination of primary contributing factors for DVT formation is known as *Virchow's triad* (blood stasis, hypercoagulability and damage to the endothelial layer of the vein. Researchers in the 20th century determined that some mechanical and medical conditions placed individual patients at a higher risk of developing acute DVT during their course of hospitalization. These risk factors include: age, patient immobility, major abdominal, pelvic, or orthopedic surgery, malignancy, pregnancy and postpartum state, trauma to lower limbs, heart failure, use of oral contraceptives, obesity, and previous DVT. The risk factor with the highest predictive value is a previous history of venous disease. It has been associated with an 80–100% incidence of recurrent thrombosis.[1,6] The initial clinical evaluation of the venous system involves a careful medical history with emphasis on the risk factors. Clinical findings in acute deep vein thrombosis are highly variable and can be asymptomatic. It has also been demonstrated that an equal number of patients with signs and symptoms suggestive of deep vein thrombosis have normal venous systems. Because DVT most commonly occurs in the calf veins, most symptoms begin at that level. Pain, consisting of a dull posterior calf ache that increases over several hours or days and is exacerbated by ambulating, is most common. This may be localized over the area of thrombosis. The physical findings include tenderness over the affected area, unilateral leg swelling, edema, and, if the proximal veins are involved, the calf may become erythematous and hot, mimicking a bacterial cellulitis.

Thrombus formation has been described from accumulated data as the following sequence. The platelets begin to accumulate in the area of intimal injury or from stasis or possible instability of the platelet/plasma relationship. The congregated platelets disintegrate slowly and fibrin deposits are noted. These fibrin deposits incorporate leuko-

cytes and this mixed cellular mass occlude the lumen of the vein (Fig. 12–26).[21] Propagating from the mass toward the heart is a thrombus tail. The tail may completely fill the vein and adhere to the wall or it may be a thin membrane moving in the venous stream (Fig. 12–27). When major obstruction of the iliofemoral system occurs, massive swelling of the entire lower extremity associated with a white or deeply cyanotic limb may occur and is termed *phlegmasia cerulea dolens*. The signs of iliofemoral thrombosis represent the few clinical features that reliably identify acute DVT. Unfortunately, the overall diagnostic accuracy of physical examination is only about 50%, and thus, the diagnosis must be confirmed with objective testing. Historically, ascending contrast venography was considered the "gold standard." It is highly accurate but invasive and results in patient discomfort.[22] With the advent of Doppler and ultrasound technology, especially color flow Doppler over the last 20 years, noninvasive testing has replaced contrast venography for the diagnosis of deep venous thrombosis in most instances.[23] Color flow Doppler combined with duplex imaging allows us to visualize the entire deep venous system reliably and to diagnose acute and chronic thrombosis with an accuracy similar to contrast venography.[6-8]

In the acute stage, the thrombus may be anechoic (not visible on ultrasound), (Figs. 12–28, 29) isoechoic (echogenic filling of vein but less echogenic than vein walls), or hyperechoic (vein filled with bright echoes. The diameter of

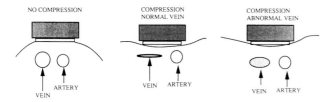

Figure 12–22. Venous compression.

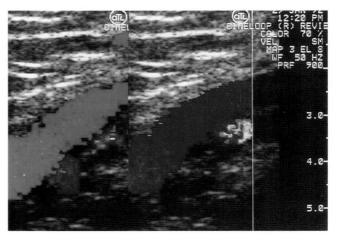

Figure 12–24. Color flow Doppler demonstrates reflux in the popliteal vein.

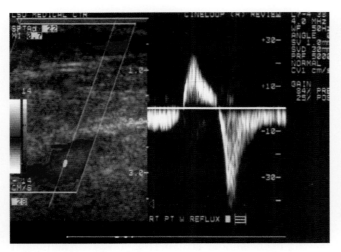

Figure 12–25. Spectral analysis demonstrates reflux in the posterior tibial vein.

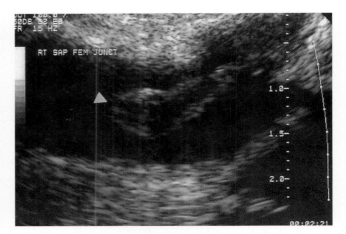

Figure 12–27. Real-time image of a free-floating clot (arrowhead).

the vein increases because of the inflammatory nature of the acute stage, and the obstruction may be partial or complete. The vein may partially compress, but the vein walls do not touch completely. There may be a "free floating clot" within the vein lumen attached to the valve and moving freely within the vein. If the lumen of the vein is occluded or partially occluded, the Doppler signals are not sponta-

neous or phasic and do not augment well. With total occlusion of the vein, there will be no signal. In partial occlusion, there will be an increased high-pitched signal in the patent portion of the lumen and damped or absence of the signal in the occluded portion (Fig. 12–30). Reflux will often be present because of the inability of the valves to function. As the thrombus ages, it becomes more echogenic (usually brighter than vein walls), adheres to the vein wall (nonmobile), and becomes rigid (difficult to compress). The diameter of the vein decreases as the inflammatory stage declines, and recanalization (return of venous flow) of the obstructed vein occurs. The vein wall becomes thickened, and there are usually collateral veins present.[24]

Lower Extremity Pathology that may clinically be indistinguishable from deep vein thrombosis:

- cellulitis of the calf with painful swelling
- baker's cyst causing swelling and pain in the popliteal fossa and calf
- lymphedema causing swelling of the lower extremity
- swelling caused by external compression of pelvic or thigh veins

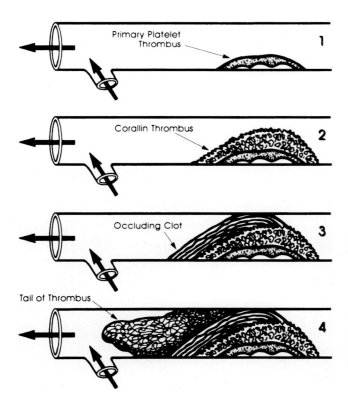

Figure 12–26. Pathology diagram of thrombus; Aschoff's classic description.

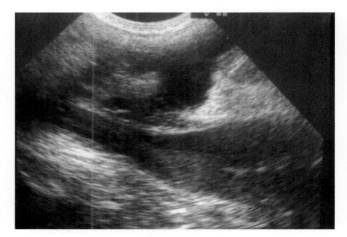

Figure 12–28. Thrombus in the acute stage containing low level echoes.

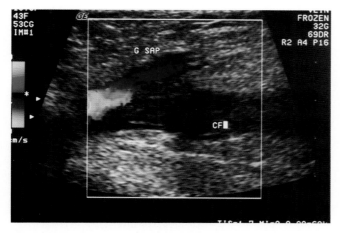

Figure 12–29. Thrombus in the acute stage that is primarily anechoic with some scattered low-level echoes.

- muscle pain
- plantaris tear

Chronic Venous Disease

The primary cause of chronic deep vein abnormalities is acute thrombosis. Following the initial event, thrombi variably lyse, but persistent obstruction and valvular damage occur. The chronic venous hypertension that ensues causes a "blowout" of the perforating veins and results in "secondary" varices. Over a period of time, the chronic venous disease causes chronic leg pain, swelling, edema, hyperpigmentation, stasis dermatitis, and ankle ulceration. This is the well-known post-thrombotic syndrome. Diagnosis of chronic venous disease is more straightforward because varicose veins, leg swelling, and distal leg skin changes resulting from chronic venous obstruction and valvular reflux are often obvious. These clinical manifestations result from chronic venous hypertension caused by anatomic derangements in the superficial, perforating, and deep vein. Doppler can demonstrate retrograde blood flow with proximal compression of the vein.

Treatment of venous thrombosis includes the following:

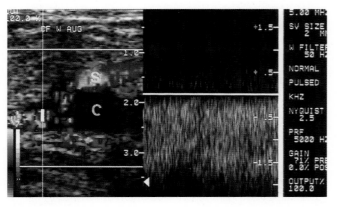

Figure 12–30. Partial occlusion of the vein with flow circumventing the obstruction. The venous sound is high pitched and continuous.

Anticoagulants. The propagation of thrombus may be prevented with such anticoagulants as heparin or one of the couman derivatives. Heparin is usually the initial treatment for a short term with a hospital stay and is followed by coumadin administered on an outpatient basis. Coumadin is usually the prophylactic therapy or long term therapy.[9]

Greenfield Filter. Vena cava filtering prevents pulmonary embolus in approximately 90% of the patients. Recurrent pulmonary embolism after adequate anticoagulation or when anticoagulation is contraindicated is generally considered an indication for a vena cava filter. Current preference is the Greenfield (birdnest) filter. It is placed percutaneously via the jugular or femoral vein into the inferior vena cava.[19] This prevents the upward extension of clot to the lung (pulmonary embolism) (Fig. 12–31 A, B).[25–28]

Superficial Thrombophlebitis occurs when there is thrombus formation in the greater or lesser saphenous veins with an inflammatory reaction. This condition is usually diagnosed clinically because the painful cords (thrombosed veins) may be palpated below the skin surface. This condition should be carefully evaluated because it may extend or progress into the deep venous system (Fig. 12–32).

Varicose Veins

Varicose veins are the most common form of venous disease and affect approximately 15% of the population.[15] Contrary to popular belief, they are equally prevalent in men and women and are usually associated with low morbidity and mortality rates. Epidemiologic data indicate that the greatest risk factor for the development of varicose veins is genetic predisposition. This familial pattern is sex linked to the male. There is usually progressive, functional failure of the valves rather than absence of valves.[15] Primary varicose veins are dilated tortuous superficial veins, often related to the saphenous system and its branches (Figs. 12–33, 34). Perforating veins carry blood from the superficial venous system to the deep venous system.[29] Reflux is prevented by subfascial valves. Occasionally, primary incompetence of perforating veins occurs; particularly in patients whose occupations require prolonged standing. In addition, chronic superficial venous reflux in the saphenous vein may cause secondary dilatation and damage to the perforating veins with resulting valvular incompetence. The exact etiology of primary varicose veins remains controversial. However, they are most likely caused by such mechanical factors as pregnancy and prolonged standing. Secondary varicose veins occur following acute deep vein thrombosis. Chronic deep vein obstruction and reflux lead to ambulatory venous hypertension and incompetence of normal valves. Commonly, the saphenous veins and their branches become dilated as venous outflow channels are created through destruction of perforating vein valves and reflux into the saphenous system. In the past, the presence of incompetent perforating veins was thought to be indicative of previous deep vein thrombosis. However, a multitude of investigators have reported that incompetent perforating veins occur without any evidence of a previous thrombotic process.

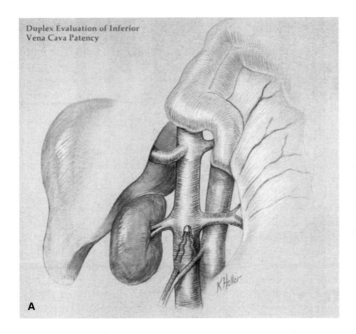

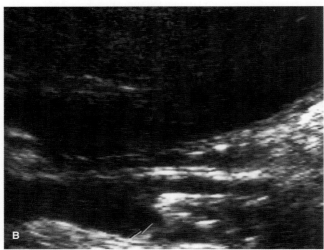

Figure 12–31. (**A**) Schematic of the inferior vena cava filter. *(Reproduced with permission from the Journal of Vascular Technology.)* (**B**) Real-time image shows the echogenic Greenfield filter in the inferior vena cava.

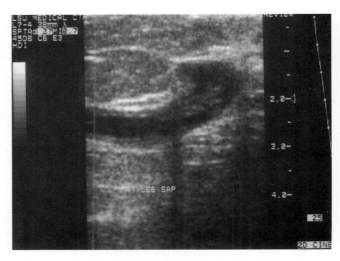

Figure 12–32. Distended lesser saphenous vein with thrombus.

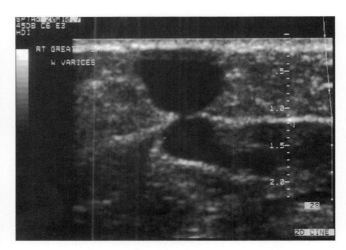

Figure 12–33. Real-time image of the superficial varices.

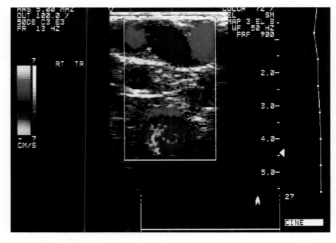

Figure 12–34. Color flow Doppler of superficial varices.

There are several methods of treatment for varicose veins. These include:

nonoperative treatment with the use of support stockings, feet elevation, and walking to improve the musculo-venous pump of the calf.[19]

surgical stripping and ligation may be performed on varicose veins of the great and small saphenous veins.[19]

sclerotherapy by injection of a sclerosing agent into the varicose vein to damage its endothelium and cause an aseptic thrombosis, which organizes and closes the vein.[19]

REFERENCES

1. Borow M, Goldson H. Postoperative venous thrombosis—Evaluation of five methods of treatment. *Am J Surg.* 1981; 141: 245–251.

2. Caprini JA, Chucker JL, Zuckerman L, et al. Thrombosis prophylaxis using external compression. *Surg Gynecol Obstet.* 1983; 156:599–602.

3. Hartman JT, Pugh JL, Smith RD, et al. Cyslic sequential compression of the lower limb in prevention of deep venous thrombosis. *J Bone Joint Surg.* 1982; 64-A:1059–1062.

4. Hills NH, Pflug JJ, Jeyasingh K, et al. Prevention of deep vein thrombosis by intermittent pneumatic compression of calf. *Br Med J.* 1972; 1:131–135.

5. Oster G, Tuden RL, Colditz GA. Prevention of venous thromboembolism after general surgery: cost-effectiveness analysis of alternative approaches of prophylaxis. *Am J Med.* 1987; 82:889–899.

6. Raghavendra BN, Rosen R. Deep venous thrombosis detection of high resolution real time ultrasonography. *Radiology.* 1984; 152:789–793.

7. Hannan LJ, Stedke KJ, Cranley JJ, et al. Venous imaging of the lower extremities: our first 2,500 cases. *Bruit.* 1986; 10:29–31.

8. Semrow CM, Friedell ML, Buchbinder D, et al. The efficacy of ultrasonic venography in the detection of calf vein thrombosis. *J Vasc Technol.* 1988; 12:240–244.

9. Flanagan LD, Sullivan ED, Cranley JJ. Venous imaging of the extremities using real-time B-mode ultrasound. In: Bergan JJ, Yao JST, eds. *Surgery of the Veins.* Orlando, FL: Grune & Stratton; 1984:89–98.

10. Langsfield M, Hershey FB, Thorpe, et al. Duplex B-mode imaging for the diagnosis of deep venous thrombosis. *Arch Surg.* 1987; 122:587–591.

11. Rollins DL, Semrow CM, Friedell ML, et al: The use of ultrasonic venography in the evaluation of venous valve function. *Am J Surg.* 1987; 154:189–191.

12. Rollins DL, Semrow CM, Buchbinder D, et al. Diagnosis of recurrent deep venous thrombosis using B-mode ultrasonic imaging. *Phlebology.* 1986; 1:181–188.

13. Szendro G, Nicolaides AN, Zukowski AJ, et al: Duplex scanning in the assessment of deep venous incompetence. *J Vasc Surg.* 1986; 4:237–242.

14. Semrow CM, Laborde A, Buchbinder D, et al. Preoperative mapping of varicosities and perforating veins: a preliminary report. *J Vasc Technol.* 1990; 14(2):72–74.

15. Semrow CM, Friedell ML, Buchbinder D, et al. Characterization of lower extreme venous disease using real-time B-mode ultrasonic imaging. *J Vasc Technol.* 1987; 11:187–191.

16. Rollins DL, Semrow CM, Friedell ML, et al. Origin of deep vein thrombi in an ambulatory population. *Am J Surg.* 1988; 156:122–125.

17. Gerlock AJ, Giyanani VL, Krebs CA. *Applications of Noninvasive Vascular Techniques.* Philadelphia: WB Saunders; 1988.

18. Abrams HI: *Angiography.* 2nd ed. Vol. II. Boston: Little Brown; 1971: 1251–1271.

19. Hallett JW, Brewster DC, Darling RC. *Handbook of Patient Care in Vascular Surgery.* 3rd ed. Boston: Little Brown; 1995: 257–280.

20. Janssen HF, Schachner J, Hubbard J, et al. The risk of deep venous thrombosis: a computerized epidemiologic approach. *Surgery.* 1987; 1010:205–212.

21. Filip DJ, Eckstein JD, Veltkemp JJ. Heredity antithrombin three deficiency and the thrombo embolic diseases. *Med J Hematol.* 1978; 1:343–349.

22. Haeger K. Problems of acute deep vein thrombosis. *Angiology.* 1969; 20:219–223.

23. Yao JS, Horres JP, Rubo N, et al. Diagnosis of deep venous thrombosis by Doppler ultrasound and impedance plethysmography. In Kwaan HL, Bowie EJC, et al. *Thrombosis.* Philadelphia: WB Saunders; 1982: 224–235.

24. Zwiebel WJ: *Introduction to Vascular Ultrasonography.* 4th ed. Philadelphia: WB Saunders Co.; 2000.

25. Schwarts SI, ed. *Principles of Surgery,* 4th ed. New York: McGraw-Hill; 1984.

26. Krebs CA, Giyanani VL, Eisenberg RL. *Ultrasound Atlas of Disease Process.* Norwalk, CT: Appleton & Lange; 1993.

27. Krebs CA, Giyanani VL, Eisenberg RL. *Ultrasound Atlas of Vascular Diseases.* Stanford, CT: Appleton & Lange; 1999.

28. Talbot SR, Oliver MA. *Techniques of Venous Imaging.* Pasadena, CA: Appleton Davies, Inc.: 1992.

29. Thibodeau GA, Patton KT. *Anatomy & Physiology.* St Louis: Mosby; 1999.

Questions

1. All deep veins of the lower leg are usually paired, communicate with the superficial vein system, and contain at least how many valves?

    (A) 10
    (B) 7
    (C) 15
    (D) 5

2. Within 15 minutes of standing still, what percentage of the body's total volume of blood may be pooled to the lower extremity veins?

    (A) 20–30
    (B) 10–15
    (C) 30–40
    (D) 15–20

3. The longest vein in the body is the

    (A) cephalic vein
    (B) superficial femoral vein
    (C) greater saphenous vein
    (D) inferior vena cava vein (IVC)

4. The popliteal vein is formed from the posterior tibial and anterior tibial veins at the knee, then extends upward through what to become the superficial femoral vein?

    (A) profunda hiatus
    (B) adductor (Hunter's) canal
    (C) Scarpa's triangle
    (D) flexor hallucis longus

5. Which vein is not part of the superficial venous system?

    (A) greater saphenous vein
    (B) superficial femoral vein
    (C) lesser saphenous vein
    (D) basilic vein

6. Normal veins exhibit all the characteristics below except

    (A) spontaneous flow
    (B) phasic flow
    (C) pulsatility
    (D) compressibility

7. What percentage of blood in the body can be found within the venous system?

    (A) 60–65
    (B) 50–65
    (C) 70–75
    (D) 75–80

8. Veins differ from arteries in all the ways listed below except

    (A) veins have thicker walls with very little muscles.
    (B) veins are distensible
    (C) veins are collapsible
    (D) veins can be divided into deep and superficial systems

9. The primary clinical concern in deep vein thrombosis (DVT) is the complication of

    (A) claudication
    (B) pulmonary embolism (PE)
    (C) valve competency
    (D) loss of extremity

10. Duplex scanning on the deep venous system of the lower extremities is usually performed with

    (A) the patient placed in the supine position with the leg straight
    (B) the patient placed in the supine position with the leg externally rotated
    (C) the patient placed in the supine position with the leg internally rotated
    (D) the patient placed in the prone position with leg internally rotated

11. Venous Doppler evaluation of the lower extremities is highly accurate in the detection of

(A) differentiating intrinsic from extrinsic causes of obstruction

(B) partial obstructions that do not cause changes in the venous flow pattern

(C) detect thrombosis confined to the calf veins

(D) detecting hemodynamically significant obstruction of the popliteal, superficial, femoral, and common femoral veins.

12. When testing for venous incompetency using photo-plethysmography, the normally refilling time is

(A) 15 seconds or greater
(B) 25 seconds or greater
(C) 10 seconds or greater
(D) 20 seconds or greater

13. The vein wall is very thin and is comprised of three layers: the outermost layer is called

(A) tunica media
(B) tunica intima
(C) tunica adventitia
(D) tunica endothelium

14. The only location where a spontaneous venous signal may normally not be heard in the lower extremity veins is the

(A) external iliac vein
(B) posterior tibia vein
(C) profunda or deep femoral vein
(D) peroneal vein

15. A normal venous signal is described as being

(A) continuous
(B) phasic
(C) pulsatile
(D) oscillating

16. The development of extensive iliofemoral thrombosis occurring and producing a clinical pattern of tight leg edema, severe pain, and cyanotic mottled skin; is commonly referred to as

(A) Raynaud's phenomenon
(B) claudication
(C) Byrum trace syndrome
(D) phlegmasia cerulea dolens

17. Deep vein thrombosis often destroys the venous valves sometimes resulting in postphlebitic syndrome, which leads to everything *except*

(A) thin vessel walls
(B) chronic induration
(C) stasis dermatitis
(D) ulcers (in later years)

18. Varicose veins are the most common form of venous disease. These veins also

(A) affect approximately 45% of the human population
(B) are equally prevalent in both men and women
(C) are not of genetic predisposition
(D) are usually caused by absence of valves

19. In the acute stage, fresh venous thrombus

(A) is usually echogenic
(B) vein is usually compressible
(C) is usually anechoic
(D) collateral veins usually start to appear adjacent to the vessel

20. Respiration plays a major role on the venous flow patterns. During inspiration, the intra-abdominal venous pressure increases

(A) blood flows smoothly throughout the body, at the moment of exhalation the valves close, then quickly reopen again
(B) decreasing blood flow from the lower extremities while increasing the flow from the upper part of the body
(C) increasing blood flow from the lower extremities while decreasing the flow from the upper part of the body
(D) respiration does not play a big role in the venous flow pattern

21. Photoplethysmography assess reflux involving the placement of a photoelectric cell to measure the subcutaneous blood flow. The photoelectric cell is constructed of

(A) a small electric wire that is designed to deliver small shocks to the leg along with a crystal to receive the returning sound waves
(B) an infrared light emitting diode and a photo detector
(C) a small crystal to send and receive sound waves that are recorded on photo paper
(D) a small camera that records the subcutaneous blood flow on photo paper

22. When performing a Doppler ultrasound examination of the venous system, the normal response to a distal augmentation is

(A) a rapid increase in frequency followed by a abrupt cessation of the signal, and then a normal return to phasicity
(B) a rapid increase in frequency followed by a slow decay, and then a normal return to phasicity
(C) a slow increase in frequency followed by a abrupt cessation of the signal, and then a normal return to phasicity
(D) no response is heard with augmentation

23. The pressure within a vein is

(A) indirectly proportional to the cardiac output
(B) equal to the arterial pressure
(C) directly proportional to the force that is exerted on the vein wall by the blood volume within it
(D) directly proportional to the rate of respiration and the pulmonary status

24. Varicose veins with incompetent superficial vein valves and competent deep vein valves are termed primary varicose veins. Varicose veins with incompetent valves in both the superficial and deep veins are termed secondary varicose veins. Patients with primary varicose veins do

(A) improve after excision and ligation of the varicosities
(B) have a chronic venous problem that is rarely cured or significantly improved by surgical intervention
(C) both primary and secondary varicose veins are treatable with the same results
(D) both primary and secondary varicose veins are rarely cured or significantly improved

25. Chronic venous insufficiency can be evaluated by all the following test *except*

(A) photoplethysmography
(B) descending contrast venography
(C) ascending contrast venography
(D) CAT scan

26. The greater saphenous vein enters the common femoral vein in the groin region just below the inguinal ligament at the

(A) foramen ovale
(B) foramen Penn
(C) foramen Adcock
(D) foramen fascial

27. "Virchow's triad" places the risk factors for venous thrombosis into three categories. All of the following are correct *except*

(A) changes or injury to the vessel wall
(B) hypercoagulability of blood
(C) immobility of extremity
(D) stasis or slowing of blood flow

28. Calf pain on passive dorsiflexion of the foot is the nonspecific sign suggesting the diagnosis of deep vein thrombosis known as

(A) Sullivan's sign
(B) Rich–Durbin's sign
(C) Madison's sign
(D) Homans sign

29. Which vessels distal landmark is the area between the medial malleolus and the Achilles tendon, near the skin surface?

(A) anterior tibial veins
(B) posterior tibial veins
(C) lesser saphenous vein
(D) greater saphenous vein

30. Venous valves are semilunar and are attached to the vein walls by a circular ring of collagen and elastin fibers. Which layer of the vein wall are they attached to?

(A) tunica adventitia
(B) tunica intima
(C) tunica media
(D) tunica lateral

31. One of the ways angiography plays a role in the treatment of deep vein thrombosis is the placement of a filter (e.g., Greenfield), to prevent extension of clot to the lung (pulmonary embolism). This filter is normally placed in the

(A) right internal jugular
(B) inferior vena cava
(C) superior vena cava
(D) external iliac of thrombosed leg

32. Which vein arises medial to the lateral malleolus of the ankle, then in the lower two thirds of the leg follows the medial surface of the fibula, finally in the upper third it turns to join the posterior tibial vein?

(A) peroneal vein
(B) anterior tibial vein
(C) posterior tibial vein
(D) lesser saphenous vein

33. Using ultrasound duplex scanning to look at the venous system, a partial obstruction will present as

(A) partial fixed lumen that is very easy to compress, with complete closure
(B) partial fixed lumen that is very hard to compress, with limited closure
(C) complete fixed lumen that is very easy to compress, with complete closure
(D) complete fixed lumen that is very hard to compress, with limited closure

34. When scanning the subclavian vein toward the shoulder, what branch does it give off just before becoming the axillary vein?

(A) costocoracoid vein
(B) basilic vein
(C) cubital vein
(D) cephalic vein

35. After the "deep vein muscular pump" activates (contracts) the leg muscles and valves, everything listed below happens *except*

(A) blood is forced out of the deep veins up the leg
(B) once the blood is pumped into the thigh, the valves close at the popliteal vein to hold it there
(C) the perforating (communicating veins) will open to fill the superficial veins
(D) blood flows from the superficial system into the deep system

36. When testing for incompetency using photoplethysmography (PPG), if the venous refill time is less than 20 seconds this indicates valvular incompetency. Next, the study is repeated, but a tourniquet has been placed just below the knee, the refill time has now become 20 seconds or more. This indicates that

(A) superficial venous system incompetency
(B) deep venous system incompetency
(C) both superficial and deep venous systems are incompetent
(D) the person had a large leg, the tourniquet helped to obtain an accurate study

37. Saphenous vein mapping allows for preoperative planning. When ultrasound indicates certain inadequacy, these vessels are normally no longer explored surgically. All of the following would be a problem for the surgeon *except*

(A) absent
(B) sclerotic
(C) too dilated
(D) too narrow

38. Care should be taken when measurements are made during venous mapping, because the veins are easily compressed. If a vein measures 2.5 mm in the cross-section plane, what should it be able to dilate to under arterial pressure?

(A) 3.5 mm
(B) 2.5 mm
(C) 4.0 mm
(D) 7.7 mm

39. The two major muscle plexus veins are the soleus and gastrocnemius in the lower legs. The gastrocnemius plexus drains the blood from the gastrocnemius muscle and empties into the

(A) posterior tibial vein
(B) anterior tibial veins
(C) popliteal vein
(D) peroneal vein

40. Which vessel arises from the medial end of the dorsal venous arch at the foot and ascends in the ankle in front of the medial malleolus of the tibia, and after ascending up the calf it crosses behind the medial condyle of the femur at the knee?

(A) lesser saphenous vein
(B) posterior tibial vein
(C) greater saphenous vein
(D) anterior tibial vein

41. Which vein arises from the medial side of the dorsal venous arch, runs along the ulnar aspect of the forearm and upper arm, finally penetrating the deep fascia to unite with the brachial vein to form the axillary vein?

(A) basalic vein
(B) cephalic vein
(C) median cubital vein
(D) radial vein

42. The innominate or brachiocephalic vein lies anterior and lateral to the innominate artery, and receives all the veins below except

(A) brachiocostal vein
(B) vertebral vein
(C) internal mammary vein
(D) inferior thyroid

43. Thrombosis of the axillary and subclavian veins is an uncommon primary disorder, occurring in fewer than 2% of cases of acute thrombophlebitis of deep vein of the extremities. The low frequency of this disorder may be attributable to everything listed below *except*

(A) rapid emptying of blood from the arm
(B) fewer veins
(C) a shorter course of blood flow
(D) increased quantity of clot-resolving enzymes

44. The dynamic venous pressure normally measures about 15–20 mm Hg in the venules. What does it normally measure in the right atrium?

(A) 15–20 mm Hg
(B) 100 mm Hg
(C) 0 mm Hg
(D) 50 mm Hg

45. As venous thrombus ages, it becomes everything listed below *except*

(A) echogenic
(B) the vein distends
(C) the vein doesn't compress
(D) anechoic

46. To ensure sonographic visualization of low-frequency venous flow

(A) a high wall filter setting is used
(B) a low wall filter setting is used
(C) the same setting is used for arterial and venous flow
(D) a medium wall filter setting is used

47. Compression of the venous system by external pressure often compromises the flow of the vessel. Which of the following cannot compromise the flow?

    (A) Baker's cyst
    (B) lymph nodes
    (C) varicose veins
    (D) hematomas

48. Normal veins characteristics do not include the following

    (A) phasicity
    (B) spontaneity
    (C) compressibility
    (D) augmentation
    (E) continuous signal without respiratory movements

49. The cephalic vein communicates with the basilic vein in the cubital fossa at the elbow through the

    (A) lateral cubital vein
    (B) median cubital vein
    (C) inter cubital vein
    (D) inferior cubital vein

50. There are no valves present in which of these veins?

    (A) innominate veins
    (B) axillary vein
    (C) external jugular vein
    (D) internal jugular vein

51. The perforating veins of the lower extremities do everything listed below *except*

    (A) connect the superficial veins to the deep veins
    (B) penetrate the deep fascia
    (C) allow blood to flow from the superficial to the deep veins
    (D) connect the anterior arch of the greater saphenous vein with the deep veins

52. The superficial veins of the lower extremities can be demonstrated sonographically within 1–2 cm of the skin surface, they lie

    (A) within the subcutaneous fat
    (B) within the connective tissue sheath
    (C) just below the subcutaneous fat
    (D) just above the deep fascia

53. The greater saphenous veins of the lower extremities have two primary tributaries veins in the legs, the first one joining at the knee (posterior arch and anterior veins of the legs) and the second one at the foramen ovale, includes all veins listed below *except*

    (A) superficial external pudendal veins
    (B) superficial epigastric veins
    (C) deep external pudendal veins
    (D) superficial iliac circumflex

54. There are multiple techniques for providing hemodialysis access, including peritoneal access, dialysis catheters, synthetic arteriovenous shunt grafts, and autologous arteriovenous fistulas. The most common type of autologous arteriovenous fistulas is the Brescia–Cimino which is created surgically between the

    (A) distal ulnar artery and basilic vein
    (B) cephalic vein and the radial artery
    (C) proximal radial artery and transpose basilic vein
    (D) brachial artery and cephalic vein

55. Deep vein thrombosis of the upper extremity is becoming more frequent because of

    (A) Increased number of patients having radiation therapy and complications
    (B) Increased incidence of trauma patients with complications
    (C) Increased incidence of thoracic outlet syndrome
    (D) Increased use of central venous catheters

56. The normal route of venous flow in the lower extremity is

    (A) superficial veins to perforator veins to the deep veins
    (B) deep veins to the perforator veins to the superficial veins
    (C) deep veins to superficial veins to perforator veins
    (D) superficial veins to the deep veins to perforator veins

57. In the lower extremity what provides the energy required to circulate blood during strenuous exercise?

    (A) soleus sinusoids
    (B) gastrocnemius sinusoids
    (C) musculovenous pump
    (D) venous pressure changes

58. Blood is propelled from one point to another by an energy gradient and is slowed by resistance. The total fluid energy at any one point in the venous system is the sum of the hydrostatic pressure, gravitational potential energy, kinetic energy, and dynamic pressure produced by the left ventricle contraction and surrounding skeletal muscle according to

    (A) Bernouilli's principle
    (B) Poiseuille's law
    (C) Reynolds law
    (D) Rawls principle

59. Which vein is a continuation of the dorsalis pedis and lies between the tibia and fibula on top of the interosseous membrane?

    (A) popliteal vein
    (B) anterior tibial vein
    (C) lesser saphenous vein
    (D) peroneal vein

60. A large series of veins drain into what sinuses to form the main collecting chambers of the calf muscle pump?

    (A) gastrocnemial sinuses
    (B) medial calf sinuses
    (C) peroneal sinuses
    (D) soleal sinuses

61. What arises from the dorsal venous system that is formed by the digital and metacarpal veins?

    (A) the venous arch
    (B) radial and ulnar veins
    (C) innominate vein
    (D) cephalic and basilic veins

62. Which veins make up the superficial venous system in the upper extremity?

    (A) axillary vein
    (B) subclavian vein
    (C) brachial vein
    (D) cephalic vein
    (E) basilic vein
    (F) A, B, and C
    (G) D and E
    (H) all of the above

63. The right testicular vein drains directly into the inferior vena cava (IVC), what route does the left testicular vein take?

    (A) left internal iliac
    (B) left renal vein
    (C) inferior vena cava
    (D) right testicular vein

64. Thrombosis is the most frequent etiology of hemodialysis graft failure; many factors contribute to this development. Of the answers listed below, which one is the least likely to lead to thrombosis?

    (A) deposition of platelets and fibrin
    (B) high flow and turbulence
    (C) pulmonary embolism
    (D) shear stresses

65. Sclerotherapy is

    (A) surgical removal of the superficial veins
    (B) use of support stockings and appropriate exercise
    (C) injection of superficial veins with agent to induce thrombosis
    (D) injection of deep and superficial veins with agent to induce thrombosis

66. There are several causes of chronic venous insufficiency that result in venous stasis. Which one listed below is incorrect?

    (A) varicose veins
    (B) surgery
    (C) post-thrombotic syndrome
    (D) chronic recurrent thrombosis

67. Lower extremity venous examination for patency includes

    (A) compression and augmentation at each landmark site
    (B) proximal compression at each landmark site
    (C) spectral analysis at each landmark site
    (D) color flow Doppler at each landmark site

68. Pathologic conditions can mimic deep vein thrombosis but can be easily demonstrated by ultrasound. Which one of the answer listed below is *not* a pathologic condition?

    (A) enlarged lymph nodes
    (B) hematomas
    (C) cast on broken bone, causing swelling
    (D) popliteal (Baker's) cyst

69. Ultrasound cannot accurately detect thrombosis in which lower extremity veins?

    (A) calf veins
    (B) superficial veins
    (C) deep veins
    (D) perforating veins

70. To determine reflux in the vein, manual compression is performed

    (A) proximal to the transducer and vein in question
    (B) distal to the transducer and vein in question
    (C) at the level of the transducer and vein in question
    (D) in 5-minute intervals at the level of the transducer

71. Which one of the following is not used to augment veins?

    (A) distal compression of the vein
    (B) coughing
    (C) Valsalva
    (D) compression of the vein with the transducer probe

72. The condition for chronic venous insufficiency of the extremity that continues to deteriorate with progressive leg pain described as an aching or bursting sensation with prolonged walking is called

    (A) Young syndrome
    (B) venous claudication
    (C) Ryan syndrome
    (D) arterial claudication

73. The veins serve as the passageway of blood flow to the heart, pulmonary veins carry

(A) deoxygenated blood from the heart back to the lungs
(B) blood from the portal system to the heart
(C) oxygenated blood from the lungs to the heart
(D) blood from the inferior vena cava (IVC) to the heart

74. Varicocele is an abnormal venous dilation of the pampiniform plexus. All the facts listed below are true *except*

(A) is more common on the right side
(B) occurs in about 15–20% of the male population
(C) has a higher incidence (20–40) among men presenting with infertility
(D) is associated with decreased sperm motility, oligospermia, and abnormal sperm morphology

75. The venogram shows the clot in the vein as

(A) echogenic mass within the vein
(B) filling defect within the vein
(C) heterogeneous mass within the vein
(D) dilated vein with a spongy appearing mass in the lumen

76. Following an episode of deep vein thrombosis (of the lower extremity), the venous valves have probably become irreversibly incompetent. This results in continual high venous pressure which causes everything listed below *except*

(A) chronic edema
(B) dilated incompetent perforators
(C) development of varices
(D) calf is cold to the touch

77. Acute thrombus is soft and may be easily compressed to a certain extent; chronic thrombus

(A) is not compressible to any extent
(B) may be easily compressed to a certain extent
(C) will easily compress completely
(D) with some difficulty (pressure) will compress completely

78. Duplex imaging is able to give the sonographer high-resolution images along with Doppler techniques. When scanning one of the extremities venous systems, the frequencies of choice would be

(A) 7.5 or 10 MHz for imaging with 3.5 or 4.5 MHz for detecting Doppler blood flow
(B) 5 or 7.5 MHz for imaging with 3.5 or 5 MHz for detecting Doppler blood flow
(C) 5 or 7.5 MHz for imaging with 2 or 3.5 MHz for detecting Doppler blood flow
(D) 7.5 or 10 MHz for imaging with 4.5 or 5 MHz for detecting Doppler blood flow

79. Collateralization caused by obstruction may be confusing for the examiner and may be mistaken for a patent vessel. They exhibit all the characteristics below except

(A) continuous in nature
(B) pulsatile in nature
(C) abnormally located
(D) difficult to compress

80. The high-pitched continuous signal that will not augment, below an obstructed vein, is called

(A) trickster effect
(B) windstorm effect
(C) rainstorm effect
(D) snowstorm effect

81. The soleus plexus veins in the posterior calf drain the soleus muscle and empty into the

(A) lesser saphenous vein
(B) peroneal vein
(C) posterior tibial vein
(D) greater saphenous vein

82. Venous stasis leads to chronic venous insufficiency, which is characterized clinically by everything, listed below *except*

(A) no leg pain
(B) varicose veins
(C) chronic swelling of the leg
(D) cutaneous hyperpigmentation

83. Primary varicose veins normally affect the superficial system. Their exact cause is unknown. Listed below are what is believed to be a few of the contributing factors. Which one is incorrect?

(A) abnormal wall weakness
(B) increased distending force
(C) large arteriovenous fistulas
(D) multiple arteriovenous fistulas

84. Although venography is the "gold standard" for the diagnosis of venous disease offering the opportunity to study both the anatomy and the function of the veins in vivo, ascending venography cannot

(A) assess the function of the proximal valves in the lower extremity
(B) determine the location of incompetent perforator
(C) localize recanalized channels indicating previous thrombophlebitis
(D) determine the absence or presence of varicosities

85. Varicose veins with competent deep vein valves and incompetent superficial veins are termed

(A) secondary varicose veins
(B) primary varicose veins

(C) first varicose veins
(D) thigh varicose veins

86. Which vein(s) arise(s) from and drain the plantar venous arch and superficial venous net of the foot?

   (A) anterior tibial veins
   (B) posterior tibial veins
   (C) greater saphenous vein
   (D) lesser saphenous vein

87. Which vein receives both the superficial and deep venous systems of the upper extremity?

   (A) innominate vein
   (B) cephalic vein
   (C) brachial vein
   (D) subclavian vein

88. The walls of the veins are somewhere between one-third to one-tenth as thick as the arteries, depending on their location. The axillary veins consist of 5% smooth muscle; whereas, the feet contain

   (A) 60–80% smooth muscle
   (B) 35–50% smooth muscle
   (C) 25–45% smooth muscle
   (D) 75–85% smooth muscle

89. Each toe has two dorsal digital and two plantar veins that unite to form the dorsal metatarsal veins that join to form the

   (A) dorsal metatarsal venous arch
   (B) superficial dorsal venous arch
   (C) deep dorsal venous arch
   (D) planter–dorsal venous arch

90. The communicating veins or "perforators" are located throughout the leg, in most legs there are

   (A) more than 50 of these veins
   (B) more than 1000 of these veins
   (C) more than 100 of these veins
   (D) more than 500 of these veins

91. The only point in the body (in any position ex: upright) where the arteriovenous pressure gradient remains the constant (83 mm Hg) is the hydrostatic indifferent point (HIP), which is located

   (A) at the external jugular
   (B) at the hip
   (C) at the aorta bifurcation
   (D) just below the diaphragm

92. After thrombus fills the vein and adheres to the wall of the vessel, it will then contract, and recanalization will begin. This general takes

   (A) about 10 days after formation
   (B) about 3 days after formation

(C) about 5 days after formation
(D) about 12 days after formation

93. There are a number of variables that are associated with an increase in the likelihood of developing deep vein thrombus, one that decreases the chances is

   (A) obesity
   (B) the use of oral contraception
   (C) over 60 age group
   (D) smoking

94. Deep vein thrombus can originate anywhere in the venous system, but studies have shown the single most common site to be

   (A) soleal sinusoids
   (B) posterior tibial vein
   (C) ilio-femoral veins
   (D) saphenous–femoral junction

95. The veins in the sole of the foot form the planter cutaneous arch, which drains into the medial and lateral marginal veins, which in turn empty into

   (A) greater and lesser saphenous veins
   (B) anterior and posterior tibial veins
   (C) anterior tibial vein and lesser saphenous vein
   (D) greater saphenous vein

96. What type of venography offers the ability of assessing valvular functions?

   (A) posterior venography
   (B) descending venograph
   (C) ascending venograph
   (D) visceral venograph

97. Several abdominal organs do not pour their blood directly into the inferior vena cava; they send their blood to the liver by means of the hepatic portal vein. Which one of the organs listed below does not go through the portal vein?

   (A) spleen
   (B) gallbladder
   (C) renal
   (D) pancreas

98. The venous valves are found in the

   (A) tunica intima
   (B) tunica media
   (C) tunica adventitia
   (D) A and C

99. The right ovarian vein drains directly into the inferior vena cava. The left ovarian vein drains into

   (A) the right ovarian vein
   (B) the left internal iliac vein
   (C) the inferior vena cava
   (D) the left renal vein

100. A functioning valve is competent if

(A) it simultaneously opens and closes
(B) it allows both forward and reverse venous flow
(C) it will not allow reversal of venous blood flow
(D) it stays open continuously allowing continuous venous flow

Questions 101 through 108: Match the structures in Fig. 12–35 with the terms in Column B.

COLUMN A

101. _____
102. _____
103. _____
104. _____
105. _____
106. _____
107. _____
108. _____

COLUMN B

(A) popliteal vein
(B) greater saphenous vein
(C) superficial femoral vein
(D) distal inferior vena cava
(E) internal iliac vein
(F) deep femoral vein (profunda)
(G) external iliac vein
(H) common femoral vein

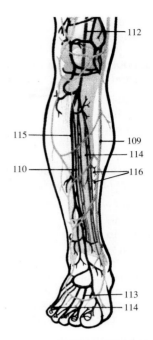

Figure 12–36. Veins of the leg. *(Reprinted with permission from Abbott Laboratories, North Chicago, IL. Medical illustration by Scott Thorn Barrows, AMI.)*

Questions 109 through 116: Match the structures in Fig. 12–36 with the terms in Column B.

COLUMN A

109. _____
110. _____
111. _____
112. _____
113. _____
114. _____
115. _____
116. _____

COLUMN B

(A) anterior tibial veins
(B) plantar digital veins
(C) soleal veins
(D) posterior tibial veins
(E) plantar metatarsal veins
(F) peroneal veins
(G) popliteal vein
(H) greater saphenous vein

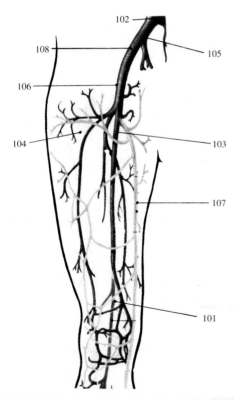

Figure 12–35. Veins of the thigh. *(Reprinted with permission from Abbott Laboratories, North Chicago, IL. Medical illustration by Scott Thorn Barrows, AMI.)*

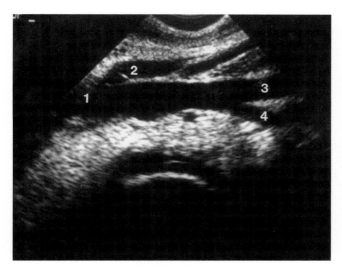

Figure 12–37.

Questions 117 through 120: Match the structures in Fig. 12–37 with the numbers in Column B.

COLUMN A	COLUMN B
117. common femoral vein _____	4
118. deep femoral vein _____	1
119. greater saphenous vein _____	3
120. superficial femoral vein _____	2

121. Fig. 12–38 shows a transverse view of the groin area, that demonstrates

   (A) normal right common femoral vein—with compression
   (B) thrombosed right common femoral vein—no compression
   (C) normal left common femoral vein—with compression
   (D) thrombosed left common femoral vein—no compression

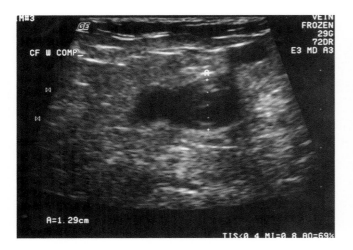

Figure 12–38.

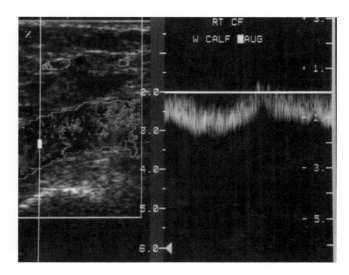

Figure 12–39.

122. The Doppler signal in Fig. 12–39 represents the common femoral vein with augmentation of the calf, this demonstrates

   (A) normal phasic flow
   (B) good augmentation of the calf—veins clear from calf to thigh
   (C) no augmentation of the calf—thromboses in calf
   (D) reflux

123. Fig. 12–40 shows the hepatic veins, along with the middle hepatic veins waveform, which demonstrates

   (A) normal multiphasic waveform, with variation in the velocity and direction of blood flow
   (B) normal triphasic waveform, no variation in the direction of blood flow, with variation in the velocity
   (C) abnormal multiphasic waveform, no variation in the direction of blood flow, with variation in the velocity
   (D) abnormal triphasic waveform, no variation in direction of blood flow or in the velocity

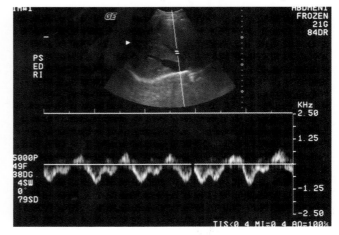

Figure 12–40.

124. Posterior to the neck of the pancreas, what two veins join to form the portal vein?

(A) splenic vein and hepatic vein
(B) hepatic vein and superior mesenteric vein
(C) hepatic vein and celiac vein
(D) splenic vein and superior mesenteric vein

Questions 125 through 138: Match the letter in Column B as seen in Fig. 12–41 with the veins in Column A.

COLUMN A	COLUMN B
125. Ulna _____	(A)
126. Left subclavian _____	(B)
127. Vertebral _____	(C)
128. Cephalic _____	(D)
129. External jugular _____	(E)
130. Axillary _____	(F)
131. Basilic _____	(G)
132. Radial _____	(H)
133. Internal jugular _____	(I)
134. Brachiocephalic _____	(J)
135. Brachial _____	(K)
136. Inferior thyroid _____	(L)
137. Right subclavian _____	(M)
138. Internal thoracic _____	(N)

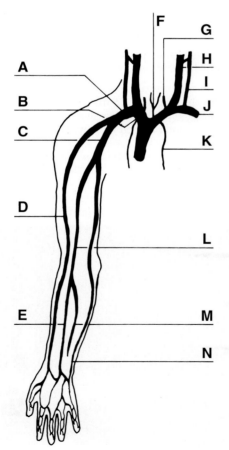

Figure 12–41.

139. What percentage of patients with deep vein thrombosis will be likely to develop venous insufficiency in 5–10 years?

(A) 50%
(B) 60%
(C) 70%
(D) 80%

140. A pathological condition, which can mimic a deep vein thrombosis, is

(A) aortic aneurysm
(B) Baker's cyst
(C) phlegmasia cerulea dolens
(D) decreased skin temperature

141. Fig. 12–42 demonstrates a normal thin-walled vein with

(A) a closed valve
(B) a opened valve
(C) the early stages of a thrombosis
(D) an artifact

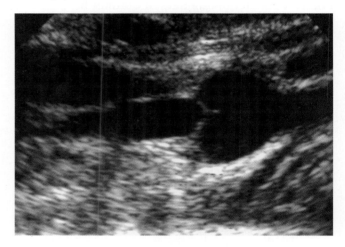

Figure 12–42.

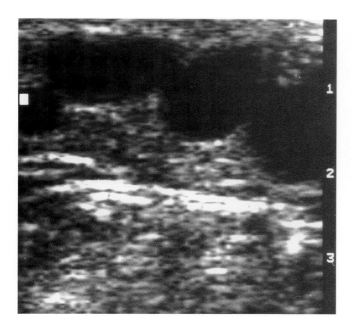

Figure 12–43.

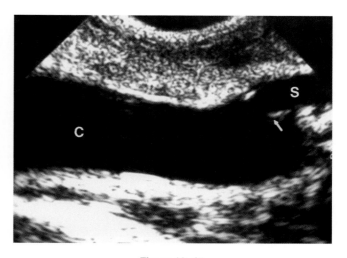

Figure 12–45.

142. The gray scale image in Fig. 12–43 of the subcutaneous region, demonstrates what?

(A) dilated greater saphenous vein
(B) bulbous lesser saphenous
(C) Baker's cyst
(D) varices

143. The spectral analysis in Fig. 12–44 shows venous flow with

(A) normal respiratory movements
(B) augmentation
(C) collateral flow pattern
(D) vein pulsatility

144. Fig. 12–45 is a gray-scale image of the common femoral vein (C) at the saphenous–femoral junction. The arrow is pointing to

(A) plaque at the saphenous–femoral junction
(B) an artifact
(C) open valves at the saphenous–femoral junction
(D) early stages of thrombosis at the saphenous–femoral junction

145. The spectral analysis of the portal vein in Fig. 12–46 shows normal respiratory movements and

(A) blood flow away from the liver
(B) flow that is bidirectional
(C) pulsatility
(D) blood flow toward the liver

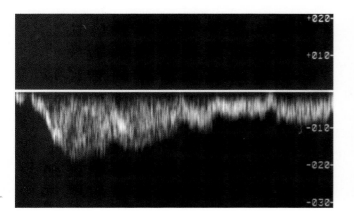

Figure 12–44.

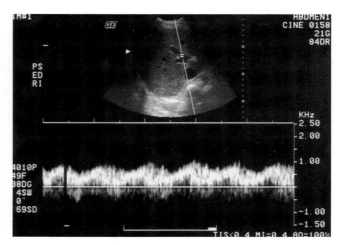

Figure 12–46.

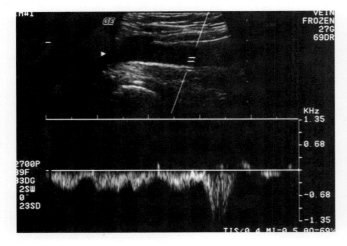

Figure 12–47.

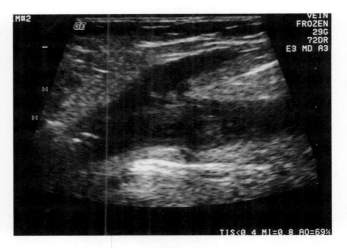

Figure 12–49.

146. The image in Fig. 12–47 is of the common femoral vein with a Doppler waveform demonstrating

   (A) normal distal augmentation
   (B) augmentation demonstrating venous insufficiency
   (C) normal phasic wave form
   (D) augmentation demonstrating proximal thrombus

147. The spectral analysis of the middle hepatic vein in Fig. 12–48 shows the characteristics of

   (A) a woman in her third trimester of pregnancy
   (B) congestive heart failure
   (C) during expiration
   (D) during inspiration

148. The picture in Fig. 12–49 is of the common femoral and greater saphenous vein. This photograph demonstrates

   (A) a normal common femoral and greater saphenous vein

   (B) thrombus in the greater saphenous vein, normal common femoral vein
   (C) thrombosis in the common femoral vein, normal greater saphenous vein
   (D) thrombosis in both the common femoral vein and greater saphenous vein

149. Fig. 12–50 shows the orientation of the iliac vein with an area anterior and superior to its origin. This area is

   (A) Baker's cyst
   (B) lymph node
   (C) button cyst
   (D) honey node

150. After an episode of deep vein thrombosis, the venous valves are destroyed and become incompetent. This is termed

   (A) thrombophlebitis
   (B) Raynaud's phenomenon
   (C) postphlebitic syndrome
   (D) phlegmasia cerulea dolens

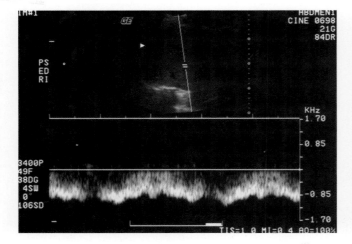

Figure 12–48.

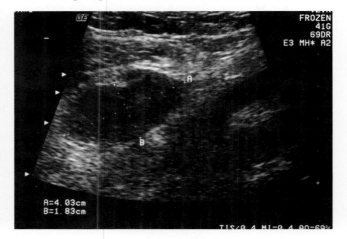

Figure 12–50.

Answers and Explanations

At the end of each explained answer there is a number combination in parentheses. The first number identifies the reference source; the second number or set of numbers indicates the page or pages on which the relevant information can be found.

1. **(A)** All deep veins of the lower leg contain at least 10 valves. As many as 10–15 may be present in each vein. They are usually paired and communicate with the superficial system. *(Study Guide)*

2. **(D)** The venous anatomy of the lower extremity is capable of containing a large volume of blood. As much as 15 to 20% of the body's total blood volume may be pooled in the lower extremity veins within 15 minutes of standing absolutely still. This accounts for the well-known example of soldiers fainting after standing at attention for extended periods of time. *(Study Guide)*

3. **(C)** The longest vein in the body is the greater saphenous located in the both lower extremities. The superficial femoral vein is also located in the lower extremities. The inferior vena cava (IVC) is located in the abdomen; whereas, the cephalic vein is found in both upper extremities. *(Study Guide)*

4. **(B)** The popliteal vein extends upward through the adductor (Hunter's) canal to become the superficial femoral vein. The flexor hallucis longus are tendons in close proximity to the interosseous membrane in the distal third of the lower leg. The superficial femoral vein ascends into Scarpa's triangle, then crosses behind the artery to assume a more medial position. *(Study Guide)*

5. **(B)** The superficial femoral vein located in the lower extremities, is part of the deep venous system. The greater and lesser saphenous veins are also in the lower extremities. The basilic vein is found in the upper extremity. *(Study Guide)*

6. **(C)** Normally the veins are not pulsatile. Exceptions include cardiac disease, extreme bradycardia and overtransfusion, which can cause pulsatility. Varia-

tions in the diameter of veins are caused by respiration, rather than the cardiac cycle. *(Study Guide)*

7. **(D)** Seventy-five to 80% of the blood volume is contained within the venous system. The ability of the veins to adjust shape and size makes it ideally suited for the storage of blood. *(Study Guide)*

8. **(A)** Veins have thinner walls with very little muscle, resulting in their being both distensible and collapsible. They can also be divided into deep and superficial systems, unlike arteries. *(Study Guide)*

9. **(B)** The primary clinical concern in DVT is the complication of pulmonary embolism. Claudication is an arterial disease. Valvular incompetence frequently results from a DVT. *(Study Guide)*

10. **(B)** Duplex scanning of the deep vein system of the lower extremities is usually performed with the patient supine and the leg externally rotated. It is important that the leg also be relaxed for ease of blood flow. The popliteal vein can be visualized with the patient in a prone position. *(Study Guide)*

11. **(D)** The venous Doppler evaluation is highly accurate in the detection of hemodynamically significant obstruction of the popliteal, superficial femoral, and common femoral veins. It cannot reliably detect partial obstructions that do not cause changes in the venous flow pattern. In addition, it cannot accurately detect thrombosis confined to the calf veins or differentiate acute from chronic or intrinsic from extrinsic causes of obstruction. *(Study Guide)*

12. **(D)** The normal venous refilling time is 20 seconds or greater. Less than 20 seconds indicates venous incompetency. *(Study Guide)*

13. **(C)** The tunica adventitia, the outer layer is the strongest part of the vein wall. It is composed of collagen fibers. Tunica media is the middle layer. Tunica intima is the inner layer that contains the venous valves. *(Study Guide)*

14. (B) A spontaneous venous signal may not be heard at the posterior tibial vein at the ankle. In this location, the blood flow rate may be below the sensitivity of the Doppler velocity detectors. Most Doppler velocity detectors cannot detect movement below 6 cm/s. *(Study Guide)*

15. (B) A normal venous signal is phasic and spontaneous. A continuous venous signal indicates either internal obstruction of flow or external compression of the vein proximal to the position of the transducer. *(Study Guide)*

16. (D) Phlegmasia cerulea dolens produces a clinical pattern of tight leg edema, severe pain, and cyanotic mottled skin when extensive iliofemoral thrombosis occurs. Raynaud's syndrome is a functional vasospastic disorder affecting the small arteries and arterioles of the extremities. *(Study Guide)*

17. (A) In patients that have had previous episodes of deep vein thrombosis the vessel walls are thickened not thinned. Postphlebitic syndrome often leads to chronic induration, stasis dermatitis, and ulcers in later year. Symptoms of this condition appear between 18 months and 10 years after the thrombotic event. *(Study Guide)*

18. (B) Varicose veins are equally prevalent in men and women. They also affect approximately 15% of the population, are genetic predisposition and are usually caused by functional failure of the valves rather than absence of them. *(Study Guide)*

19. (C) In acute stages, fresh venous thrombus is usually anechoic. The vein will not compress. Collateral veins can appear as the recanalization begins. *(Study Guide)*

20. (B) Respiration causes the diaphragm to descend. This increases intra-abdominal pressure, decreasing blood flow from the lower extremities while increasing the flow from the upper part of the body. *(Study Guide)*

21. (B) Photoplethysmography's photoelectric cell actually has an infrared light emitting diode and a photodetector that is attached to an amplifier and a strip chart recorder. It is used to assess reflux and differentiate between superficial and deep vein incompetency. *(Study Guide)*

22. (B) The normal response to distal augmentation is a rapid increase in the pitch (frequency) of the signal followed by a slow decay and then a return to the normal phasicity. If the Doppler velocity signal increases rapidly and then abruptly stops or no response is heard, the vein is considered to be obstructed proximal to or at the location of the transducer. *(Study Guide)*

23. (C) The transmural pressures are governed by the pressure–volume relationship. The difference in pressure between the intraluminal pressure trying to expand the vein and the outside tissue pressure trying to collapse the vein is called transmural pressure. If this pressure is increased, the volume of blood within the vein increases due to the flexibility of the vein wall. *(Study Guide)*

24. (A) Patients with primary varicose veins improve after excision and ligation of the varicosities. Those with secondary varicose veins have a chronic venous problem and that is rarely cured or significantly improved by surgical intervention on the superficial varicosities alone. *(Study Guide)*

25. (D) CT scan cannot evaluate chronic venous insufficiency. Photoplethysmography, Doppler, ultrasound, descending contrast venography, ascending contrast venography, and ambulatory venous pressure can evaluate chronic venous insufficiency. *(Study Guide)*

26. (A) The greater saphenous vein ascends along the medial aspect of the leg then enters the common femoral vein at the foramen ovale, just below the inguinal ligament. It is located within subcutaneous tissue receiving numerous superficial tributaries before entering through the fascial defect. The superficial femoral vein joins the deep femoral vein in the groin to become the common femoral vein. *(Study Guide)*

27. (C) Immobility of extremity is not one of the categories of "Virchow's triad." Rudolf Virchow was the German pathologist who introduced the theory between 1845 and 1856. There are many risk factors that may increase a patient's chances of developing thrombosis, but all factors should fit into one of the three categories. *(Study Guide)*

28. (D) Homans sign of calf pain on passive dorsiflexion of the foot suggests the diagnosis of deep vein thrombosis. Calf hematomas may also produce the symptoms of pain with dorsiflexion. *(Study Guide)*

29. (B) The posterior tibial veins distal landmark is the area between the medial malleolus and the Achilles tendon. After identifying the vessels, they can be followed up the medial surface of the calf. The veins are paired, one vein on either side of the posterior tibial artery. *(Study Guide)*

30. (B) The tunica intima (inner layer) is the thin layer of endothelial cells that contains the venous valves. The valves consist of two leaflets that maintain the blood flow in one direction, toward the heart. *(Study Guide)*

31. (B) The filter is placed in the inferior vena cava (via the jugular or femoral approach) to prevent the upward extension of clot to the lung. The Greenfield filter consists of a small cone-shaped filter that is placed usually below the levels of the renal veins in the IVC. *(Study Guide)*

32. (A) The peroneal vein arises medial to the lateral malleolus of the ankle. While in the lower two thirds of the leg it follows the medial surface of the fibula, and then in the upper third, it turns medially to join the posterior tibial vein. *(Study Guide)*

33. (B) Partial venous obstruction will present as a partially fixed lumen that is very hard to compress, with limited closure. Deep vein thrombosis in a totally occluded vessel will present as an echogenic filled lumen that does not compress and has no Doppler venous sounds. *(Study Guide)*

34. (D) As soon as the subclavian vein gives off the cephalic vein branch it changes its name to the axillary vein. This happens at the outer border of the first rib. Usually, only one valve is found in the axillary vein. *(Study Guide)*

35. (C) Blood flows from the superficial system to the deep system by way of the perforating (communicating) veins. After the deep veins empty, the superficial veins fill with blood, causing their pressure to increase. This activates the communicating veins to open so that blood can flow into the deep system. *(Study Guide)*

36. (A) If the venous refilling time becomes normal (20 seconds or more) after the placement of a tourniquet, superficial venous system incompetency is indicated. If there is no change in the venous refill time, that it remains abnormal, the deep venous system is considered incompetent. *(Study Guide)*

37. (C) When ultrasound identifies veins that are absent, sclerotic or too narrow they are normally not explored surgically. This helps in preoperative planning and decreases operating time. *(Study Guide)*

38. (C) The vein should be able to dilate to 4 mm under arterial pressure if it measured 2.5 by ultrasound. All measurements should be taken carefully because of pressure of the transducer and taken in the cross section plane. *(Study Guide)*

39. (C) The gastrocnemius plexus empties into the popliteal vein. The soleus plexus veins empty into the posterior tibial vein. *(Study Guide)*

40. (C) The greater saphenous vein arises from the medial end of the dorsal venous arch at the foot; next it ascends in the ankle just in front of the medial malleolus of the tibia. After that, it spirals around the medial aspect of the leg posteriorly to cross behind the medial condyle of the femur at the knee. *(Study Guide)*

41. (A) The basilic vein arises from the inner side of the dorsal venous arch, then runs along the ulnar aspect of the forearm and upper arm until it penetrates the deep fascia of the arm and unites with the brachial vein to form the axillary vein. It is the second major superficial vein in the upper extremity. *(Study Guide)*

42. (A) The innominate veins receive the vertebral vein, the internal mammary vein, the inferior thyroid vein, and sometimes the superior intercostals vein. The innominate veins are formed by the subclavian and internal jugular veins, and then unite to form the superior vena cava. *(Study Guide)*

43. (B) The low frequency of this disorder may be caused by rapid emptying of blood from the arm, a shorter course of blood flow, and increased quantity of clot resolving enzymes. Thrombophlebitis usually occurs in males between 20 to 40 years of age and generally affects the right arm. *(Study Guide)*

44. (C) The right atrium pressure is normally 0 mm Hg and is termed central venous pressure. When it measures 0 mm Hg, the blood flows from the systemic veins into the right atrium. *(Study Guide)*

45. (D) As the thrombus tends to age it become more echogenic, the vein distends, and does not compress. Various patterns of collateral veins can appear. Thrombus is anechoic in its acute stage. *(Study Guide)*

46. (B) Low wall filters are used to demonstrate the low-frequency venous flow. The high wall filters are used with arterial flow. *(Study Guide)*

47. (C) Varicose veins can not compromise the flow of a vessel by external compression. Baker's cyst, tumors, or hematomas often produce external compression that can compromise the flow. *(Study Guide)*

48. (E) Vein characteristics include phasicity, spontaneity, compressibility, and augmentation. They do not have a continuous sound without respiratory motion, this is characteristic of collateral venous flow. *(Study Guide)*

49. (B) The cephalic vein communicates with the basilic vein through the median cubital vein in the cubital fossa at the elbow. Unlike the veins in the deep system, these veins do not accompany the major arteries in the forearm. *(Study Guide)*

50. (A) There are no valves in the innominate veins. Valves are present in the external and internal jugular veins, axillary veins, and the subclavian vein. *(Study Guide)*

51. (D) The perforating veins connect the posterior arch of the greater saphenous vein with the deep veins.

They also connect the superficial veins to the deep veins, penetrate the deep fascia, and allow blood to flow from the superficial to the deep system.

(Study Guide)

52. **(A)** The superficial veins of the lower extremities lie within 1 to 2 cm of the skin surface within the subcutaneous fat. The system consists of dorsal venous arch, marginal veins, and lesser and greater saphenous veins. *(Study Guide)*

53. **(A)** The greater saphenous vein's second primary tributary is at the foramen ovale and consist of the superficial epigastric, superficial iliac circumflex, and the deep external pudendal veins. The greater saphenous can serve as a collateral pathway to bypass obstruction in the deep system. *(Study Guide)*

54. **(B)** The Brescia–Cimino fistula is created surgically between the cephalic vein and the radial artery at the wrist. It has a 3-year patency rate of 80–90%, and is the most durable dialysis access. It requires 3 to 6 weeks to mature. *(Study Guide)*

55. **(D)** Deep vein thrombosis is occurring more frequently due to the increased use of central venous catheters. *(Study Guide)*

56. **(A)** The veins of the lower extremity flow from the superficial veins through the perforators(communicating veins) to the deep veins. Valves maintain the flow in one direction. Flow in the opposite directions is abnormal. *(Study Guide)*

57. **(B)** The musculovenous pump mechanism. When the leg muscles contract around the intramuscular and surrounding veins the blood is propelled toward the heart. The main reservoir of the pump mechanism is the soleus and gastrocnemius sinusoids.

(Study Guide)

58. **(A)** According to Bernouilli's principle, the blood is propelled from one point to another by energy gradient and is slowed by resistance, that the energy within the moving fluid is determined by the pressure, gravitational energy, and kinetic energy. Poiseuille's law states the effect of the radius of the vessel and the viscosity of the blood and is a variation of Ohm's law. *(Study Guide)*

59. **(B)** The anterior tibial vein is a continuation of the dorsalis pedis and lies between the tibial and fibula, located in the anterior compartment just on top of the interosseous membrane. In the upper part of the calf they join the popliteal vein. *(Study Guide)*

60. **(D)** The soleus muscle is drained by a large series of veins located within the soleal sinuses, which form the main collecting chamber of the calf muscle pump. These veins then empty into larger valved veins that send blood from the distal to the proximal portion of the muscle, and finally into the posterior tibial and peroneal veins. *(Study Guide)*

61. **(D)** The cephalic and basilic veins arise from the dorsal venous system that is formed by the digital and metacarpal veins. The cephalic vein begins along the radial aspect of the hand, while the basilic vein arises along the ulnar side. *(Study Guide)*

62. **(H)** The cephalic and basilic veins and their tributaries constitute the superficial venous system of the upper extremity. The axillary, subclavian, and brachial veins are part of the upper extremity deep venous system. *(Study Guide)*

63. **(B)** The left testicular vein drains into the left renal vein, while the right drains directly into the inferior vena cava. The pampiniform plexus provides venous drainage from the testes and the scrotum.

(Study Guide)

64. **(C)** Pulmonary embolism will not lead to thrombosis causing hemodialysis graft failure. High flow, turbulence, and shear stresses can lead to intimal hyperplastic reaction and accelerate atherosclerosis in the venous limbs of the dialysis fistulas. The deposit of platelets and fibrin can also lead to fibrosis.

(Study Guide)

65. **(C)** Sclerotherapy is the injection of a sclerosing agent into the superficial veins to damage the endothelium and cause thrombosis which organizes and closes the veins. *(Study Guide)*

66. **(B)** Some of the causes of chronic venous insufficiency are varicose veins, chronic recurrent thrombosis, and post-thrombotic syndrome. Venous stasis, the result of the failure of the venous pump mechanism reflects chronic venous insufficiency.

(Study Guide)

67. **(A)** Venous sonographic examination of the lower extremity include compression and augmentation at each landmark site, this documents patency of the vessels. Proximal compression is used for reflux studies to document venous incompetency.

(Study Guide)

68. **(C)** A cast placed on a broken bone that causes swelling is not a pathologic condition that can mimic deep vein thrombosis. Those that can are popliteal aneurysm, superficial thrombophlebitis, popliteal (Baker's) cyst, enlarged lymph nodes, cellulites, hematomas, pseudoaneurysm, and post-phlebitic syndrome.

(Study Guide)

69. **(A)** Ultrasound cannot accurately detect thrombosis confined to the calf veins. It has been well documented that the diagnostic results of calf vein ultrasound are poor when visualization is inadequate.

(Study Guide)

70. (A) To determine and verify reflux with Doppler techniques, manual compression is performed proximal to the transducer and the vein in question. This maneuver forces the blood backward against the valve to check competency. If it is competent, there will be no backward flow, if it is incompetent, the flow will be forced backward and then forward. Distal compression maneuvers are used to augment the veins and demonstrate patency.   *(Study Guide)*

71. (D) Compression of the vein with the transducer probe is a maneuver used to confirm patency and rule out the presence of clot. It is not the maneuver used for augmentation. Distal compression, valsalva, or cough maneuvers are the methods for augmenting the veins.   *(Study Guide)*

72. (B) Chronic venous insufficiency of the extremity that continues to deteriorate with progressive leg pain described as aching or bursting sensation with prolonged walking is called venous claudication. Other symptoms include swelling, hyperpigmentation, and stasis dermatitis.   *(Study Guide)*

73. (C) Pulmonary veins serve as the passageway that carry oxygenated blood from the lungs to the heart. The portal vein returns venous blood from the intestinal tract and spleen, while the systemic veins return the venous blood from the rest of the body.   *(Study Guide)*

74. (A) Varicocele is more common on the left side (85–95%) than the right. It also occurs in about 15–20% of the male population and has a higher incidence among men presenting with infertility. Varicocele is also associated with decreased sperm motility, oligospermia, and abnormal sperm morphology, which is an increased number of immature and tapered sperms.   *(Study Guide)*

75. (B) Venous thrombus or clot obstructs the draining vein and creates a filling defect on the venogram.   *(Study Guide)*

76. (D) Incompetent valves lead to only a minimal drop in venous pressure with exercise resulting in chronic edema, the development of varices, and dilated incompetent perforators. Arterial problems result in the lower extremities being cold to the touch.   *(Study Guide)*

77. (A) Chronic thrombus is not compressible to any extent. Acute thrombus is soft, and may be compressed to a certain extent.   *(Study Guide)*

78. (D) When scanning one of the extremities venous systems, the frequency of choice would be 7.5 or 10 MHz for imagining with 4.5 or 5 MHz for detecting Doppler blood flow. The 10 MHz would provide excellent resolution, while the 7.5 would be required for deeper structures.   *(Study Guide)*

79. (B) Collateral vessels can be very confusing, they usually are continuous in nature, difficult to compress, and abnormally located close to the obstructed vessel. They can easily be mistaken for a patent vessel.   *(Study Guide)*

80. (B) The "windstorm effect" is the high-pitched continuous signal that will not augment below an obstructed vein. It is associated with collateral flow and reflects the extent of venous hypertension that exists.   *(Study Guide)*

81. (C) The soleus plexus veins drain the soleus muscle and empty into the posterior tibial vein. The gastrocnemius plexus veins grain the gastrocnemius muscle and empty into the popliteal. Deep vein thrombosis occurs frequently in the soleus plexus veins.   *(Study Guide)*

82. (A) Venous stasis is characterized by chronic swelling of the leg, malleolar ulceration, cutaneous hyperpigmentation, varicose veins, and leg pain. Venous stasis leads to chronic venous insufficiency.   *(Study Guide)*

83. (C) Small not large arteriovenous fistulas have been suggested as a possible contributing factor to primary varicose veins. Other factors are abnormal wall weakness, increased distending force, and multiple arteriovenous fistulas. Primary varicose veins are associated with venous valvular incompetency.   *(Study Guide)*

84. (A) Ascending venography cannot assess the function of the proximal valves in the lower extremity. Only descending venography can offer that capability. Ascending venograph can offer the location of incompetent perforators; localize recanalized channels indicating previous thrombophlebitis and the absence or presence of varicosities.   *(Study Guide)*

85. (B) Varicose veins with competent deep vein valves and incompetent superficial veins are termed primary varicose veins. Veins with both incompetent superficial and deep vein valves are termed secondary varicose veins.   *(Study Guide)*

86. (B) The posterior tibial veins arise from and drain the plantar venous arch and superficial venous net of the foot. They also receive the peroneal veins farther up the calf.   *(Study Guide)*

87. (D) The subclavian vein receives both the superficial and deep venous system of the upper extremity. An occlusion of this vein blocks both these major systems. Acute pain, swelling, and edema of the entire upper extremity can occur.   *(Study Guide)*

88. (A) The feet contain 60–80% smooth muscle. Veins consist largely of smooth muscle and have relative little elastin.   *(Study Guide)*

89. **(B)** The dorsal digital and plantar veins unite to form the dorsal metatarsal veins that join to form the superficial dorsal venous arch. The plantar cutaneous arch eventually drains into the greater and lesser saphenous veins.   *(Study Guide)*

90. **(C)** Normally, there are more than 100 communicating veins located throughout most limbs. They are mainly less than 2 mm in diameter and are usually described in groups.   *(Study Guide)*

91. **(D)** The hydrostatic indifferent point (HIP) is just below the diaphragm. It is the only point that remains constant.   *(Study Guide)*

92. **(C)** Generally about 5 days after the thrombus fills the vein, it will start to contract. The next step is recanalization. Valves within the thrombus are usually destroyed.   *(Study Guide)*

93. **(D)** Smokers have shown a decrease in deep vein thrombus (DVT), compared to nonsmokers. The over 60-age group, use of oral contraception, and obesity increase the chances of developing a DVT.
    (Study Guide)

94. **(A)** The soleal sinusoids are the most common site to develop a DVT according to recent studies. DVTs can originate any place with the venous system.
    (Study Guide)

95. **(A)** The planter cutaneous arch empties into the greater and lesser saphenous veins. The superficial dorsal venous arch also ends up at the greater and lesser saphenous veins.   *(Study Guide)*

96. **(B)** The descending venography offers the ability of assessing valvular functions. It directly visualizes the venous valves.   *(Study Guide)*

97. **(C)** The renal system does not go through the portal vein. The spleen, stomach, pancreas, gallbladder, and intestines do send their blood to the liver by way of the portal vein.   *(Study Guide)*

98. **(A)** The inherent semilunar venous valves are found in the tunica intima; the intermost lining of the vein.
    (Study Guide)

99. **(D)** The left ovarian vein drains into the left renal vein. The right empties directly into the inferior vena cava.   *(Study Guide)*

100. **(C)** Valves are competent if they do not allow reversal of flow. The valves ensure flow in the forward direction toward the heart.   *(Study Guide)*

101. **(A)** Popliteal vein   *(Study Guide)*

102. **(D)** Distal inferior vena cava   *(Study Guide)*

103. **(C)** Superficial femoral vein   *(Study Guide)*

104. **(F)** Profunda (deep) femoral vein   *(Study Guide)*

105. **(E)** Internal iliac vein   *(Study Guide)*

106. **(H)** Common femoral vein   *(Study Guide)*

107. **(B)** Greater saphenous vein   *(Study Guide)*

108. **(G)** External iliac vein   *(Study Guide)*

109. **(H)** Greater saphenous vein   *(Study Guide)*

110. **(F)** Peroneal veins   *(Study Guide)*

111. **(B)** Plantar digital veins   *(Study Guide)*

112. **(G)** Popliteal vein   *(Study Guide)*

113. **(E)** Plantar metatarsal veins   *(Study Guide)*

114. **(D)** Posterior tibial veins   *(Study Guide)*

115. **(A)** Anterior tibial veins   *(Study Guide)*

116. **(C)** Soleal vein   *(Study Guide)*

117. **(1)** Common femoral vein   *(Study Guide)*

118. **(4)** Deep femoral vein   *(Study Guide)*

119. **(2)** Greater saphenous vein   *(Study Guide)*

120. **(3)** Superficial femoral vein   *(Study Guide)*

121. **(B)** Fig. 12–38 demonstrates a transverse view of the right groin. The right common femoral vein has a chronic thrombosis that is not compressing. Brightly echogenic thrombus is a sign of a clot that has started the aging process.   *(Study Guide)*

122. **(C)** The flow pattern of the common femoral vein can appear normal, when there is a thrombosed area in the calf. Augmentation maneuvers of the calf usually do not produce any response or a minimal response.
    (Study Guide)

123. **(A)** The spectral waveform from the hepatic veins is multiphasic, with variation in the velocity and direction of blood flow. It is influenced by respiration, pressure in the right atrium, and compliance of the hepatic parenchyma.   *(Study Guide)*

124. **(D)** The splenic vein and the superior mesenteric vein join posterior to the neck of the pancreas to form the portal vein. The main portal vein courses toward the right, superiorly, and anteriorly.   *(Study Guide)*

125. **(M)** Ulna vein   *(Study Guide)*

126. **(J)** Left subclavian vein   *(Study Guide)*

127. (G) Vertebral vein   *(Study Guide)*

128. (D) Cephalic vein   *(Study Guide)*

129. (H) Internal jugular vein   *(Study Guide)*

130. (C) Axillary vein   *(Study Guide)*

131. (N) Basilic vein   *(Study Guide)*

132. (E) Radial vein   *(Study Guide)*

133. (H) Internal jugular vein   *(Study Guide)*

134. (B) Brachiocephalic vein   *(Study Guide)*

135. (L) Brachial vein   *(Study Guide)*

136. (F) Inferior thyroid vein   *(Study Guide)*

137. (A) Right subclavian vein   *(Study Guide)*

138. (K) Internal thoracic vein   *(Study Guide)*

139. (D) About 80% of patients with deep vein thrombosis will be likely to develop venous insufficiency in the next 5–10 years. The incidence of serious venous problems is increasing in the United States according to recent studies.   *(Study Guide)*

140. (B) Baker's cyst is a pathological condition that can mimic a deep vein thrombosis. It can also be easily demonstrated by ultrasound, along with the patency of the deep veins.   *(Study Guide)*

141. (A) Fig. 12–42 demonstrates a normal thin-walled vein with a closed valve. This valve contains leaflets that are attached by convex edges to the venous wall. The concave margins of the valves are positioned in the direction of blood flow; they lie flat against the wall as long as the blood is flowing toward the heart. When the blood flow reverses, the valves close.   *(Study Guide)*

142. (D) The gray-scale image in Fig. 12–43 of the subcutaneous region, demonstrates irregular varices. They appear as tortuous, dilated vessels.   *(Study Guide)*

143. (A) The spectral analysis in Fig. 12–44 shows venous flow with normal respiratory movements. It is phasic with respiration and controlled by intra-abdominal pressure.   *(Study Guide)*

144. (C) Fig. 12–45 is a gray-scale image of the common femoral vein at the saphenous–femoral junction, with an arrow pointing to open valves at the junction. The margins of the valves are positioned in the direction of blood flow, and lie flat against the wall as long as the flow is going toward the heart. The valves close when the flow reverses.   *(Study Guide)*

145. (D) The spectral analysis of the portal vein in Fig. 12–46 show normal respiratory movements and blood flow toward the liver. This is called hepatopetal flow.   *(Study Guide)*

146. (A) The image in Fig. 12–47 is of the common femoral vein with a Doppler waveform demonstrating normal augmentation distal to the transducer. Squeezing the distal portion of the extremity forces the flow of the blood to increase at a rapid speed.   *(Study Guide)*

147. (A) The spectral analysis of the middle hepatic vein in Fig. 12–48 shows the characteristics of a woman in her third trimester of pregnancy. Hepatic venous waveforms change from their normal pulsatile nature to become completely flat, with increasing gestation.   *(Study Guide)*

148. (C) The picture in Fig. 12–49 is one of the common femoral and greater saphenous vein. This photograph demonstrates thrombosis in the common femoral vein. There is normal flow in the greater saphenous vein, which can serve as a collateral pathway to bypass obstruction in the deep venous system.   *(Study Guide)*

149. (B) Fig. 12–50 demonstrates the iliac vein with a lymph node anterior and superior to its origin. Compression of the venous system by external pressure from lymph nodes, Baker's cyst, tumors, or hematomas may compress the vessel along with compromising the flow but can easily be demonstrated with ultrasound.   *(Study Guide)*

150. (C) Deep vein thrombosis results in the postphlebitic syndrome and venous incompetency. The venous valves are destroyed with deep vein thrombosis leading to venous incompetency. In later years, there will be chronic induration, stasis, dermatitis, and ulceration associated with venous incompetency.   *(Study Guide)*

CHAPTER 13

VASCULAR SONOGRAPHY— PERIPHERAL ARTERIAL

Carol A. Krebs, Sandra L. Hughes, Karen K. Rawls, and Thomas G. Hoffman

Study Guide
Part I: Principles and Instrumentation

INTRODUCTION

All ultrasound specialties begin with physics, basic principles, and instrumentation. The basic theory is necessary to understand the technology and to perform clinical applications effectively. Vascular ultrasound has technical principles as well as hemodynamic principles that must be understood to evaluate the vascular system and make a clinical evaluation.

Physical Principles

Probably the most important vascular concept in vascular examinations is the Doppler effect and the Doppler equation. The Doppler effect was introduced by Christian Doppler in 1842 and states, that a change in frequency of the sound wave is relative to the motion between the source and the receiver[1] (Fig. 13–1). The equation defines the parameters, which include:

- *The difference in the transmitted frequency and the received frequency is the Doppler shift*
- *Flow toward the receiver or probe has higher frequency*
- *Flow away from the receiver has a lower frequency*
- *The Doppler shift frequency (f) increases with increased transmitted frequency (F)*
- *There is a direct proportional relationship between the blood flow velocity and frequency*
- *The Doppler shift can be measured in frequency or velocity.* Most clinicians prefer velocity primarily because the results of different units can be compared for research, applications, and setting up normal and abnormal values. Using this method requires angle correction for each vessel interrogated. Frequency may be used to measure the Doppler shift, and the advantage is no angle correction is required. However, before comparing with other units or using normal or abnormal values from another unit, the

carrier Doppler frequency must be known and must be the same.
- *The cosine angle is the angle of the transducer and ultrasound beam relative to the vessel/blood flow.*

The maximum frequency shift occurs when flow is at zero or 180°. However, this is not usually attainable in clinical practice so it is recommended that a 40–60° angle be maintained for accuracy in Doppler examinations. There will be no frequency shift at a 90° angle.

INSTRUMENTATION

Continuous Wave Doppler (CW)

CW is one of the oldest and simplest methods to demonstrate patency and evaluate blood flow. CW operates with a single frequency and does not have aliasing, which is associated with pulsed systems. The CW transducer transmits a continuous sound wave and receives continuous sound waves at the same time. This is done by having two piezoelectric crystals in one probe, one sending and one receiving. Conversely, all imaging systems have pulsed sound waves; whereas, CW has continuous soundwaves. This increases the biological factor because of the continuous emission of sound waves. CW Doppler can be heard audibly, recorded by a chart strip recording, or recorded on film. It is usually a simple analog waveform without the distribution of frequencies that are displayed in the spectral analysis. The primary disadvantage of the CW Doppler is the fact that there is no discrimination between the vessels in the path of the beam. Because there is no associated imaging, it can be difficult and time consuming to localize and interrogate specific vessels.

Plethysmography

Plethysmography is generally a measurement of volume changes in the extremities for measuring blood flow. It has

$$Fs = \frac{2VFo\ Cos\ 0}{C}$$

Fs = frequency shift
V = velocity of the source
Fo = transmitted frequency
Cos = angle of incidence to blood flow
C = speed of sound in tissue

Figure 13–1. Doppler equation.

been used in the past for venous flow studies, venous reflux studies, and arterial studies. There are several types of plethysmography, which include:

Air plethysmography uses air flow to measure volume changes in a limb. Often performed using pneumatic cuffs inflated to a low pressure and measuring the relative changes in pressure. These instruments provide a good arterial pulse contour waveform.

Strain gauge plethysmography or mercury strain gauge plethysmography uses small silicone tubes filled with mercury or a liquid metal alloy.[2] These tubes are placed around the limb to measure the volume changes in the limb as it is maneuvered (squeezing or exercising). This can be used to obtain a volume pulse recording and has been used extensively in venous disease to document the filling and refilling time of the veins.

Impedance plethysmography is based on the principle that the resistive impedance of a body segment is inversely proportional to its total fluid content. Thus the changes in blood volume of a limb are reflected by the change in electrical impedance.[3] This technique was used extensively in venous testing for deep vein thrombosis but has gener-

ally been replaced with the duplex and color flow Doppler systems.

Photoplethysmography is a small photocell placed on the extremity, which contains an infrared light (light-emitting diode and a phototransistor). This photocell identifies subcutaneous flow and produces a pulse contour that can be recorded.[2] This technique is frequently used in vascular examinations to detect blood flow when it becomes difficult with conventional techniques. For example, in diabetics where toe pressure must be obtained, the photocell is placed on the toe to obtain a Doppler signal and take a pressure recording.

Spectral Analysis

Spectral analysis is the method of choice for displaying the Doppler signals. It is a mathematical computation of the reflected pulse and is computed using the Fast Fourier Transform (FFT) method. This technique displays all of the Doppler frequencies with individual amplitudes for each frequency displayed in a horizontal plane and the time displayed in the parallel plane. In essence, it is a frequency spectrum of the cardiac cycle. The spectral analysis demonstrates the presence, direction, and the characteristics of the blood flow (Fig. 13–2). In the vascular examination, the spectral waveform analysis has the capabilities of showing the degree of stenosis, site of occlusion, type of vessel, flow disturbances and turbulence, peripheral resistance, and relative flow velocity.[1]

The normal arterial waveform demonstrates a sharp systolic peak that is the Doppler shift with a quick reversal caused by early diastole and a continuous forward flow, which represents the late diastolic flow. The waveform has a spectral window that is normally clear or void of echoes and a narrow bandwidth representing the frequency spectrum. Peripheral arteries are generally very pulsatile due

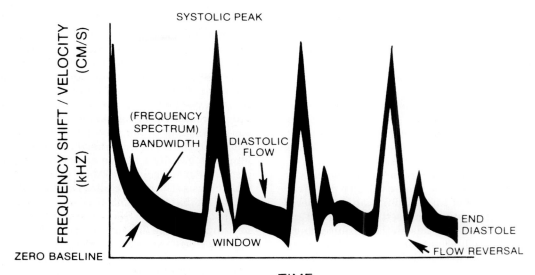

Figure 13–2. Spectral analysis.

to the resistance.[1] The Doppler Spectral waveform is used to define flow characteristics and to evaluate arterial disease that affects those characteristics (Fig. 13–3). The specific waveform parameters are outlined below.

Pulsed Wave Doppler Spectral Display[3,4]

- *Normal*
    Triphasic waveform
    Clear, crisp spectral window
    Quick upstroke to systolic peak
- *Mild disease (less than 20% diameter reduction)*
    Triphasic waveform
    Minimal spectral broadening with minimal filling of the spectral window
    Quick upstroke to systolic peak
- *Moderate disease (less than 50% diameter reduction)*
    Peak systolic velocity at least 30% greater than the proximal segment waveform
    Biphasic waveform
    Spectral window filling, spectral broadening
- *Severe disease (diameter reduction greater than 50%)*
    Peak systolic velocity increases by 100% or greater over the proximal segment waveform
    Severe disease may have monophasic pattern with increased diastolic flow
    Severe spectral broadening
- *Occluded artery*
    Absence of spectral information
- *Flow distal to an occluded site (because of collateral channels)*
    Decreased systolic flow
    Sluggish upstroke to peak systole
    Spectral broadening
    Monophasic

Duplex Scanning and Color Flow Doppler

Duplex units are pulsed ultrasound units that allow monitoring the blood velocity at various depths through the sample volume. Sample volume is the localized area along the Doppler beam path where the signal is accepted for processing. Inherent in these units is aliasing that is defined as frequencies that exceed the Nyquist limit. To explain, the audio Doppler output signal has a frequency that is lower than one half the pulse repetition frequency (PRF) of the pulsed Doppler. This is the Nyquist frequency. Therefore, the Nyquist limit is one half the pulse repetition frequency (PRF/2) Aliasing occurs in frequencies that exceed the Nyquist limit and will appear with the exceeding frequency reversing in direction or a "folding over of the waveform" (Fig. 13–4). The duplex units combine real-time imaging with Doppler waveform analysis and were the precursor for the color flow Doppler units. Primarily, all vascular ultrasound imaging units now have color flow Doppler incorporated. These are the state of the art for vascular imaging. The color flow Doppler units combine B-mode real-time imaging with Doppler, waveform analysis, and color Doppler imaging. The Doppler waveform analysis is imperative for quantitative data and includes: Doppler shift measurements of frequency and velocity, characteristics of the waveform, and direction of flow. Color flow Doppler also demonstrates motion, the direction of flow, and velocity ranges. However, the actual measurements and calculations come from the Doppler spectral analysis. Duplex and color flow Doppler units include measurement and calculation software that allows automated calculations. These include the pulsatility index (Fig. 13–5), the resistive index (Fig. 13–6), percent diameter reduction (Fig. 13–7), percent area reduction (Fig. 13–8) and volume flow (Fig. 13–9).[5]

The majority of color flow Doppler units acquire color information by the asynchronous imaging where grayscale and Doppler information are obtained separately.

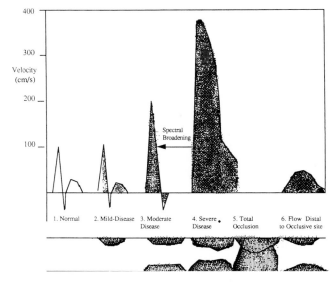

Figure 13–3. Spectral Doppler waveform in progressive disease states.

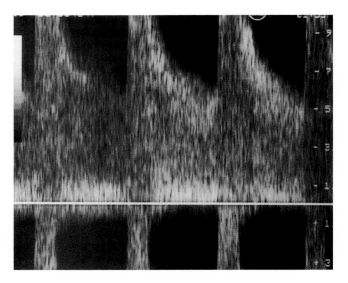

Figure 13–4. Aliasing with wraparound of the waveform.

$$PI = \frac{A\ (cm/s) - B\ (cm/s)}{TA\ (cm/s)}$$

A = Velocity in cm/s at peak systole on the spectral waveforce trace.
B = Velocity in cm/s at the minimum point of diastole on the spectral waveform trace.
TA = (Time-averaged peak velocity)
Velocity time integral of the spectral waveforce trace. (Can be calculated for frequency using kHz in place of cm/sec)

Figure 13–5. Pulsatility index.

$$RI = \frac{A\ (cm/s) - B\ (cm/s)}{A\ (cm/s)}$$

A = Velocity in cm/s at peak systole on the spectral waveforce trace.
B = Velocity in cm/s at the minimum point of diastole on the spectral waveform trace. (Can be calculated with frequency using kHz in place of cm/s)

Figure 13–6. Resistive index.

$$\%\ Diameter\ Reduction = \left(1 - \frac{d(cm)}{D(cm)}\right) \times 100$$

d = reduced diameter of vessel in cm.
D = original diameter of vessel in cm.

Figure 13–7. Percent diameter reduction.

$$\%\ Area\ Reduction = \left(1 - \frac{a(cm^2)}{A(cm^2)}\right) \times 100$$

a = reduced area of vessel in cm.
A = original area of vessel in cm.

Figure 13–8. Percent area reduction.

$$Volume\ (mm/min) = A(cm^2).\{TA\ mean\}\ (cm/s) \times 60\ s$$

A = measured area of vessel.
TA Mean (time-averaged mean velocity) = average of the intensity-weighted mean velocity

Figure 13–9. Volume flow.

Color Doppler requires powerful computer processing, fast beam forming capabilities with excellent signal detection and processing. Therefore, linear array or phased array transducers are utilized because they have a large number of elements. The processing of the color Doppler informa-tion is usually by the autocorrelation method that compares two or more samples and subtracts the stationary echoes from the data, leaving the Doppler shift echoes. This method is faster and has superior spectral resolution. The color display has three main parameters that include hue, saturation, and luminance. These parameters are used to indicate the sign, magnitude of the mean, and sometimes the magnitude of the variance of the Doppler shift.[1] Color power Doppler is a specialized component of the color flow Doppler units that increases the sensitivity to flow without angle dependence and aliasing. This technique is similar to CW Doppler in that it shows any flow or motion throughout the field, and there is no discrimination of the vessels. It is an excellent technique to demonstrate perfusion of flow in organs or vascular beds. Conventional color Doppler shows flow by encoding in color an estimate of the mean Doppler frequency shift at a particular position; whereas, power Doppler encodes the power in the Doppler signal in color by using the amplitude from the color Doppler signal and rais-ing the sensitivity of the low echoes.[1] However, it must be remembered that power Doppler provides no information as to speed or direction of flow and is extremely sensitive to any motion or blood flow. Most units incorporate a motion suppression mechanism to eliminate artifactual motion.

Radiographic Examinations

Radiology offers a variety of diagnostic imaging examina-tions for the vascular system as well as interventional ther-apeutic treatments. It is extremely important that the sonographer become familiar with the various radiologic procedures and be able to compare the findings with the sonographic examination. In some cases, ultrasound will be the initial examination, and the radiologic procedure will verify the findings. In other cases, ultrasound may be used as follow-up or correlation with the radiologic procedure. If ultrasound is utilized for comparison or for localization and the pathological area has been identified on another radio-logic procedure, it is important to review the procedure to make sure the precise area is identified for comparison. The various radiologic procedures are described and listed below.

Computerized Axial Tomography (CT)

CT units have an x-ray tube, two scintillation detectors, a line printer, teletyper, and a computer and magnetic disc unit that are used to attain a series of detailed visualiza-tions of the tissues of the body at any depth desired. It is painless, noninvasive, and requires no special preparation; however, there is associated radiation. The body is scanned in two planes simultaneously at various angles. The computer calculates tissue absorption, displays a printout of the numerical values, and produces a visualization of the tissues that demonstrates the densities of the various structures. Tumor masses, infarctions, bone displacement, and accumulations of fluid may be detected.[6]

Angiography, Arteriography, and Digital Subtraction Angiography (DSA)

Angiography or ateriography is defined as "the roentgenographic visualization of blood vessels following introduction of contrast material and is used as a diagnostic aid."[7] It is a radiology procedure where a rapid sequence of films is obtained after injection of contrast material through a catheter that is introduced percutaneously through the femoral or axillary artery. The catheter tip is placed into the selective artery or its branches. Early films show the contrast material in the major arteries followed in subsequent the filling of the smaller arteries. Angiography has the ability to demonstrate intrinsic vascular abnormalities such as atherosclerotic plaques, strictures, occlusions, and malformations. In the extremities, it can also assess the degree of collateral circulation and the patency of the distal vessels.[8] It has long been considered the "gold standard" for vascular examinations and is usually done before surgery or interventional techniques. In some instances, it also solves such diagnostic dilemmas as vasospastic disorders versus occlusive disease of the hands, Buerger's disease, ergotism, temporal arteritis, and periarteritis nodosa.[1] However, angiography is invasive, and has some inherent risks with radiation exposure.

Magnetic Resonance Imaging (MRI)

Magnetic resonance imaging shows proton density in the body and obtains dynamic studies of certain physiologic functions. Basically, it induces transitions between energy states by causing certain atoms to absorb and transfer energy. This is done by directing a radiofrequency pulse at a substance placed within a large magnetic field. The various measures of time required for material to return to a baseline energy state (relaxation time) can be translated by a complex computer algorithm to a visual image. Magnetic resonance images can be obtained in the transverse, coronal, or sagittal plane. It can penetrate bone without significant attenuation with the underlying tissue clearly imaged. There is no associated radiation.[8]

Positron Emission Tomography (PET)

Positron emission tomography (PET) is a nuclear medicine imaging modality that uses radiopharmaceuticals to measure differences in metabolic activity between tissues. Fluorine-18-fluoro-2-deoxyglucose (FDG) is the most common radiopharmaceutical used. Once injected, the FDG is absorbed by the malignant tissues at a faster rate than normal cells. Inside the tumor cell, FDG metabolism is arrested quickly, which causes a buildup of the compound. As it decays, photons are released in opposite directions and detected by the PET scanner, which translates the activity into a visual image. The visual image can be displayed and maneuvered into a coronal, sagittal, transaxial plane or by three-dimensional (3-D) surface projections.[8]

Vascular Interventional Procedures

Percutaneous transluminal angioplasty is a radiology procedure where an angiographic balloon catheter is placed directly into a narrowed or stenotic vessel and dilated to enlarge the vessel lumen. Major complications from the procedure are less than those expected from the surgical procedure.

Stents are artificial devices placed inside the vessel, duct, or shunt to prevent recoil or restenosis. The stent is introduced through a catheter that can be preloaded or handloaded into a balloon catheter. Angiograms are performed before placement of stents to determine the diameter of the vessel and exact location for placement.[8]

Transcatheter embolization is used to control bleeding or stop blood flow to a tumor or vascular malformation without requiring a surgical procedure. The angiogram demonstrates the area of bleeding, aneurysm, arteriovenous malformation, or vascular tumors. The embolization agent is introduced via a vascular catheter. Permanent embolization agents include stainless steel coils, polyvinyl alcohol, silicone beads, and detachable balloons. Temporary agents include: gelfoam, or a vasoconstricting drug.[8]

Inferior vena cava (IVC) filters are permanent implants placed to prevent pulmonary embolism in patients with deep vein thrombosis, who are at risk of migrating emboli traveling from the lower extremity veins through the IVC and lodging in the pulmonary arteries. Inferior vena cava filters are placed when anticoagulation treatment is contraindicated because of recent surgery or bleeding. The filter may be placed percutaneously through the jugular vein or the femoral vein.[8]

Transjugular intrahepatic portasystemic shunt (TIPS) is a radiologic procedure where a shunt is created inside the liver parenchyma extending from the hepatic vein to a main branch of the portal vein. The shunt decreases pressure in the portal venous system by allowing blood to be shunted away from the liver into the systemic circulation. Indications for TIPS include: cirrhosis of the liver, ascites, and failed sclerotherapy of bleeding esophageal or gastric varices.[8]

Thrombolytic therapy is performed for the treatment (lysis) of an acute thrombus (blood clot). An angiographic infusion catheter is placed directly into the thrombus, and such thrombolytic agents as urokinase are infused to dissolve the blood clot. The patient is closely monitored for any signs of bleeding during the entire treatment, and usually anticoagulation medications are administered to prevent further blood clot formation.[8]

VASCULAR HEMODYNAMICS

The physiology of circulation is termed hemodynamics. Blood flows as a result of the difference in energy or pressure. The arterial system represents the high energy/pressure, and the veins represent the low energy/pressure.

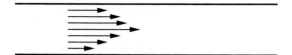

Figure 13–10. Laminar flow profile.

Pressure/energy levels decrease from the arterial to venous ends because of the lost energy as a result of blood viscosity and its inertia. There are layers and particles inherent in the vessels that create resistance and cause a loss of energy. The energy is restored by the pumping action of the heart to maintain the arterial pressure/energy difference required for the blood flow. Blood flow through the arterial system is termed *laminar flow* and is defined as blood movement in concentric layers with the highest velocity in the center of the vessel creating a parabolic flow profile[2] (Fig. 13–10). There are several laws and equations that govern blood flow and influence the results of the Doppler evaluation of the arterial system. *Poiseuille's Law* states that in a cylindric tube model, the mean linear velocity of laminar flow is directly proportional to the energy difference between the ends of the tube and the square of the radius. It is inversely proportional to the length of the tube and viscosity of the fluid. Volume flow is proportional to the fourth power of the vessel radius[2] (Fig. 13–11). Small changes in the radius results in large changes in flow. Laminar flow may be disturbed or turbulent. The factors affecting the development of turbulence are expressed by the Reynolds number (Fig. 13–12).

The development of turbulence depends mainly on the size of the vessel and the velocity of flow. Laminar flow is stable, and the streamline tends to remain intact. Whereas unstable flow has broken discontinuous streamlines that produce eddy currents (circular, backward movements of the fluid) and vortices (radial rotation of the fluid within a body of fluid) (Fig. 13–13). The stability of a fluid can be reasonably predicted by the Reynolds number.[9] Laminar flow tends to be disturbed if the Reynolds number exceeds 2000.[2]

In cases of arterial stenosis specific characteristics are seen. Proximal to the stenosis, blood forms a velocity gradient across the vessel lumen as it moves. The flow velocity increases upon entering the stenosis because of the decreased cross-sectional area. Inside the stenosis, the flow may be increased but remain stable. It maintains its

$$Q = \frac{r^4 (P_1 - P_2)}{8Ln}$$

Q	= Flow
r	= Radius
$P_1 - P_2$	= Pressure Difference between two points
L	= Distance (between two points)
n	= Viscosity

Figure 13–11. Poiseuille's Law.

$$Re = \frac{v \times r}{\dfrac{n}{p}}$$

Re	=	Reynold's Number
v	=	Velocity of Blood (cm/sec)
r	=	Radius (cm)
n	=	Viscosity (poises)
p	=	Density

Figure 13–12. Reynolds Number.

streamlines and organization. Distal moving to the larger opening, there is an unstable flow pattern. At the orifice of the stenosis, there is usually flow separation that produces a stagnant region around the narrowing. In the center of the stenosis, the high-velocity jet flows into the larger opening and creates flow reversals, eddy currents, and vortices. As the flow continues down the vessel, the energy present in the flow turbulence dissipates and stability returns to the flowing blood.[9]

Bernoulli's equation plays a central role in the quantitative applications of Doppler. The equation makes the assumption that the total energy along a streamline is constant. The energy simply changes from one form to another as the conditions of the streamline changes.

Bernoulli's equation states that the moving fluid shifts energy from one form to another, depending on the conditions. The total energy remains constant. If the flow is horizontal, the hydrostatic pressure makes contribution.[10,11]

Bernoulli's Principle:

$$P_1 + pgh_1 + \tfrac{1}{2} pu_1^2 = P_2 + pgh_2 + \tfrac{1}{2} pu_2^2 + \text{heat}$$

where   P = pressure
pgh = gravitational potential energy
$\tfrac{1}{2} pu^2$ = kinetic energy

Sum of velocity and kinetic energy of a fluid flowing through a tube is constant.

The volume of blood flow through tissue in a given period of time (milliliters per minute) is termed the blood flow. The velocity of blood flow (centimeters per second) is

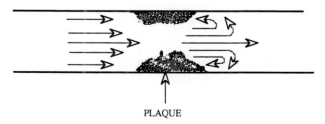

PLAQUE

Figure 13–13. Turbulent flow profile. Forward and reverse flow seen after blood flow passes narrowed segment.

inversely related to the cross-sectional area of the blood vessel. Therefore the blood flows slowest where the cross-sectional area is greatest.[12] Blood pressure (BP) is the pressure exerted by blood on the wall of a blood vessel. Blood pressure is created by the contraction of the ventricles. In the aorta of a resting young adult, BP rises to approximately 120 mm Hg during systole (contraction) and drops to approximately 80 mm Hg during diastole (relaxation). If the carbon monoxide rises, the blood pressure rises. If the total volume of blood in the system decreases, the BP decreases. As blood flows into small arteries, the resistance increases, and pressure begins to fall.[6] The expansion and contraction of arteries after each systole of the left ventricle creates a pressure wave termed the pulse, which is transmitted down the aorta into the peripheral arteries. Normally, the pulse rate is the same as the heart rate. Resting pulse is between 70 and 80 beats per minute. Tachycardia is the term for a rapid resting heart or pulse rate (over 100/min) and brachycardia is the term for a slow resting heart or pulse rate (under 60/min). If pulses are missed, it is irregular.[13]

Blood pressure is usually measured in the left brachial artery using a sphygmomanometer.

Study Guide
Part II: Clinical Applications

INTRODUCTION

Arterial diseases are one of the leading causes of death and disability in the United States.[10] Advances in the accurate diagnosis and treatment of arterial diseases has been rapid with the introduction of new diagnostic methods as well as numerous interventional and surgical techniques. Ultrasound has made a major impact on the diagnosis of arterial disease with the impressive addition of color flow Doppler. Color flow Doppler has enhanced noninvasive testing and, in some instances, become a major diagnostic screening tool.

INSTRUMENTATION AND TECHNIQUES

Patient history and physical examination of the lower extremity is required before the ultrasound examination. The patient history may often establish the diagnoses of lower extremity disease and suggest the underlying causes. Predisposing factors include:

- smoking
- aging
- hypertension
- hyperlipidemia
- diabetes mellitus
- family history of vascular disorders[1]

Pain is the key symptom of ischemia or arterial occlusion.[14] It is important to know the type of pain; whether it is during stress or at rest and how the pain is relieved. Other clinical symptoms include:[1]

- numbness
- tingling
- coldness
- edema
- cyanosis or color changes
- tissue breakdown such as ulceration or necrosis
- absence of pulses

The patient history should include:

- traumatic injuries
- major diseases that affect the peripheral arteries, such as diabetes or hypertension
- previous vascular surgery or interventional procedures
- previous vascular examinations both invasive and noninvasive with their outcomes

Noninvasive vascular examinations identify vascular abnormalities, document the severity of disease, identify the location, and provide a physiological baseline study before treatment as well as an objective assessment of outcome after treatment.[10] The nonimaging vascular systems usually incorporate: continuous wave bidirectional Doppler, plethysmography, pulse volume recording, automated cuff inflation, computerized data storage, and examination computation and printout.

Nonimaging peripheral arterial examination requires segmental pressures with corresponding Doppler waveforms, and ankle brachial index (Fig. 13–14).

If the patient falls into a claudication category (0.6–0.9), exercise with a treadmill with speeds of 1.5 and 2.5 mph, at a 10–12.5% grade for a maximum of 5 minutes is recommended to demonstrate the severity of the disease.[1] Alternate methods of exercise would be hyperemia testing or exercise by walking.

Segmental Pressures

Segmental pressures are an indirect noninvasive test that indicates the level and degree of arterial disease. Preferably four pressure cuffs are placed on the lower extremity (high thigh, above knee, below knee, and above ankle). Three cuffs may be used; however, there will be no differentiation between the common femoral and superficial femoral lesions. A manometer is used to measure pressure with a Doppler probe placed at the posterior tibia artery to record the pressure as each individual cuff is activated. If the posterior tibial is absent or not clearly audible, the dorsalis pedis or anterior tibial may be used. The pressure is taken at the site where the cuff is inflated and deflated, even though the pressure recordings are recorded at the posterior tibial artery. The cuff at each site is inflated until the systolic pressure sound disappears. The cuff is then slowly released until the sound or the Doppler waveform returns. This measurement is recorded. Bilateral brachial pressures are used as the standard and should be within 10 mm Hg of each other. If there is a greater difference in the bilateral brachial measurements, this would indicate upper extremity arterial disease. The highest value of the normal two pressures is used as the standard.[1]

Interpretation:

Normal
   systolic ankle pressure is equal to or greater than brachial systolic pressure (1.0 or greater)

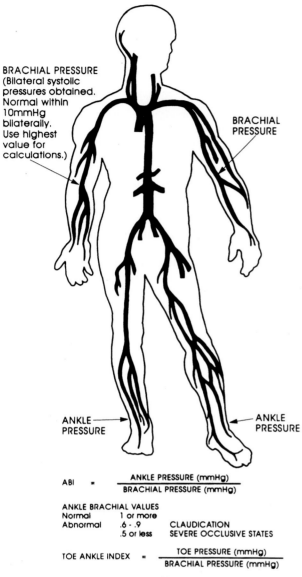

BRACHIAL PRESSURE
(Bilateral systolic
pressures obtained.
Normal within
10mmHg
bilaterally.
Use highest
value for
calculations.)

BRACHIAL
PRESSURE

ANKLE
PRESSURE

ANKLE
PRESSURE

$$ABI = \frac{ANKLE\ PRESSURE\ (mmHg)}{BRACHIAL\ PRESSURE\ (mmHg)}$$

ANKLE BRACHIAL VALUES
Normal   1 or more
Abnormal   .6 - .9   CLAUDICATION
             .5 or less   SEVERE OCCLUSIVE STATES

$$TOE\ ANKLE\ INDEX = \frac{TOE\ PRESSURE\ (mmHg)}{BRACHIAL\ PRESSURE\ (mmHg)}$$

Toe pressure is equal to 60% of the ankle pressure.

Figure 13–14. Ankle brachial index and corresponding values.

Claudication
   0.6–0.9 indicates claudication (requires exercise testing)

Severe occlusive disease
   0.5 or less indicates severe occlusive disease (does not require exercise testing)[1]

• Pressure gradient of more than 20 mm Hg between cuff levels indicates a hemodynamically significant lesion.
• Bilateral pressure gradients should be approximately equal for comparison

Fig. 13–15 is a normal lower extremity segmental arterial examination.

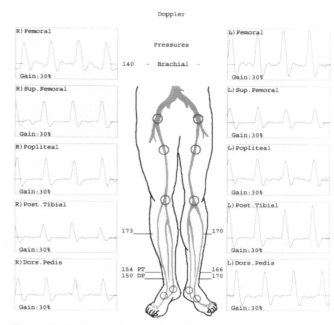

Figure 13–15. Normal lower extremity arterial segmental pressure examination.

Limitations of this examination;

• Severe calcified vessels that are often seen in the diabetic patient may not be compressible so the leg pressure is falsely elevated possibly higher than 300 mm Hg. In these cases toe pressures are required.[10] The normal toe pressure is 60% of the brachial pressure.[1]
• Collateral blood flow may be so well developed that a 20 mm gradient is not seen across a significant occlusive segment.[10]

Recommendations include combining the physical findings, Doppler waveforms, and exercise testing for a more accurate identification of hemodynamic significant disease.

Exercise. Leg exercise normally increases total limb flow, however in cases of significant arterial occlusive disease the ankle pressures drop. This is due to the narrowing and turbulence across a stenosis and the fact that blood flow is diverted into the higher resistance collateral beds of the leg muscles. In other words, the artery and its collateral's are able to supply sufficient blood during the resting state of the extremity but during exercise, when there is an increased need for blood supply, the vessel cannot provide sufficient blood flow due to the diseased state. The normal segmental pressure findings after exercise include the following;

Interpretation After Exercise.

   Normal vessels—no change or an increase

   Single level disease—2–6 minutes to return to the baseline measurement

Multiple levels of disease—12 or more minutes to return to baseline measurement

Severe occlusive disease—30 minutes or longer to return to baseline measurement

Monitoring for 10–15 minutes after exercise is sufficient to determine the severity of the disease[15] (Fig. 13–16).

VASCULAR ANATOMY

The blood vessels are a closed system of tubes that carry oxygenated blood away from the heart to the tissues of the body and then return deoxygenated blood to the heart. The system consists of arteries (large elastic tubes) dividing into medium size muscular arteries and into smaller arteries that branch into arterioles that branch into microscopic vessels termed capillaries.[11] The systemic circulation includes all the arteries and arterioles that carry oxygenated blood from the left ventricle to the systemic capillaries plus the veins and venules that carry deoxygenated blood returning to the right atrium after flowing through the organs and tissue. Subdivisions of the systemic circulation are the coronary, cerebral and the hepatic portal circulation.[11]

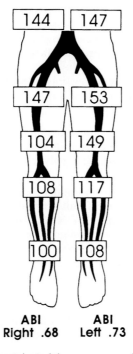

**ABI
Right .68**   **ABI
Left .73**

Figure 13–16. Segmental arterial pressure examination with bilateral lower extremity disease. ABI's indicate claudication requiring exercise testing. Segmental pressure differences indicate disease bilaterally in the iliac, right superficial femoral, and left popliteal artery. Exercise testing produced bilateral calf pain and a drop in pressures which required 4 minutes to return to normal indicating moderate disease.

The composition of large and medium size arteries include:

- *intima (tunica interna)* The intima is the innermost layer which is a monolayer of flattened endothelial cells and a thin underlying matrix of collagen and elastic fibers.
- *media (tunica media)* The media is a thick middle layer of varying amounts of smooth muscle, collagen, and elastic fibers. It has an outer border of external elastic membrane separating it from the adventitia.
- *adventitia (tunica externa)* The adventitia is the outermost layer of an artery composed of collagen and elastin, which provides the strength of the arterial wall.[10]

The composition of the arteries provides two important functional properties: elasticity and contractility. The ventricles of the heart contract and eject blood from the heart, the large arteries expand and accommodate the increased blood flow. The ventricles relax, and the elastic recoil of the arteries forces the blood onward. As the sympathetic stimulation is increased, the smooth muscle of the artery contracts and narrows the vessel lumen, which is termed vasoconstriction. Conversely, as the sympathetic stimulation decreases, the smooth muscle relaxes and the vessel dilates, termed vasodilatation.[11]

All systemic arteries arise from the heart and branch from the aorta, which are termed according to the location. Terminology includes: the ascending aorta, aortic arch, the descending aorta, thoracic aorta, and the abdominal aorta. The lower abdominal aorta bifurcates into the common iliac arteries to supply the pelvis and lower extremities. The arteries of the pelvis include: the common iliac arteries, internal iliac (hypogastric) arteries and external iliacs.

UPPER EXTREMITY ARTERIES[1,9,3]

The majority of the upper extremities are listed below with the corresponding branches given for each (Fig. 13–17). An asterisk (*) denotes the primary vessels routinely evaluated in the arterial examination.

Aortic arch (begins at the aortic annulus, part of the base of the left ventricle)

*Innominate or brachiocephalic (Present only on right side, on the left side the subclavian arises from the aortic arch and is the largest branch of the aorta)

*Subclavian (divided into three parts and arches over the cervical pleura and pulmonary apex)

*Vertebral (first branch of first part of the subclavian)
Cervical branches
Cranial branches

Thyrocervical (second branch of the first part of the subclavian divides almost at once)
Inferior thyroid
Superficial cervical
Suprascapular

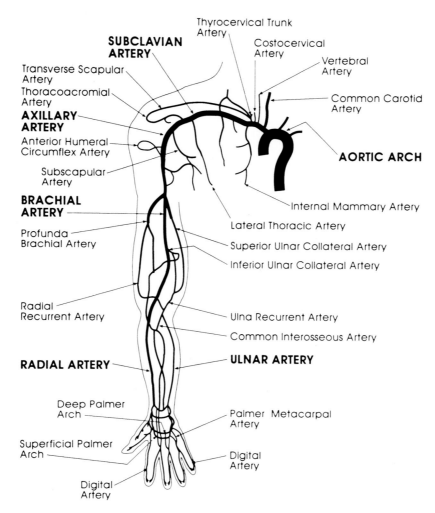

Figure 13–17. Normal upper extremity anatomy.

Internal mammary (arises inferiorly from lower margin of first part of the subclavian below thyrocervical)
Pericardiacophrenic artery
Mediastinal
Pericardial branches
Sternal branches
Anterior intercostal branches
Perforating branches
Musculophrenic
Superior epigastric

Costocervical trunk (arises posteriorly from the second part of the subclavian on the right and from the first portion on the left)
Superior intercostal artery
Deep cervical
Dorsal scapular

*Axillary (direct continuation of the subclavian)
Superior thoracic
Acromiothoracic
Lateral thoracic

Subcapsular
Posterior circumflex
Humeral
Anterior circumflex

*Brachial (is a continuation of the axillary and originates at the lateral border of the teres major and ends in the cubital fossa)
Profunda brachial
Superior ulnar collateral
Inferior ulnar collateral (supratrochlear)
Muscular

*Radial (a continuation of the brachial and the smaller of the two branches of the brachial and begins opposite the neck of the radius and travels along the lateral thumb side of the arm from forearm to wrist)
Radial recurrent artery
Muscular
Palmar carpal branch
Superficial palmar branch
Dorsal carpal branch

First dorsal metacarpal
Princeps pollicis (supplies the thumb)
Palmar digital
Dorsal digital
Radialis indicis (supplies the radial side of index finger)
Deep palmar arch (at the wrist the radial artery gives off
    the posterior carpal arch before it ends in the palm
    of the hand by anastomosing with the deep branch
    of the ulna artery to form the deep palmar arch)
    Palmar metacarpal
    Perforating
    Recurrent

*Ulna (the other terminal branch of the brachial artery)
    Ulnar anterior and posterior recurrent
    Common interosseous
    Anterior and posterior interosseous
    Muscular
        Palmar carpal branch
        Dorsal carpal branch
        Deep plantar branch
    Superficial palmer arch (fed mostly by ulnar artery and
        anastomosis with radial artery branches to form
        the superficial and deep palmar arches)
    Palmar digital
    Digital (arises from convex side of the superficial pal-
        mar arch and is joined by the palmar metacarpal
        branch from the deep palmar arch)

LOWER EXTREMITY ARTERIES[1,15,3]

The abdominal aorta bifurcates into the common iliac artery that divides into the internal and external iliac arteries. The internal iliac divides into the anterior and posterior trunks. The anterior trunk supplies the superior and inferior vesical artery, middle rectal artery, uterine artery, vaginal artery, obturator artery, internal pudendal artery, perineal artery, penile arteries, urethral artery, and inferior gluteal artery.

Listed below are the arteries of the lower extremity. This is an extensive listing of the main vessels as well as the smaller vessels. In disease states, many of these vessels participate in performing collateral flow, and the examiner should be aware of the complex vascular network (Fig. 13–18, 19). An * will signify the primary vessels that are routinely demonstrated on the arterial examination.

*Common femoral artery (a continuation of the external iliac
    and supplies the psoas major muscle, inferior epigastric
    artery, and deep circumflex iliac branches. Proximally,
    it is in the femoral triangle and distally in the adductor
    canal (hunters canal). It passes under the inguinal lig-
    ament and lies lateral to the common femoral vein. It
    bifurcates into the superficial femoral artery and the
    profunda femoral artery.
    Superficial epigastric
    Superficial circumflex iliac
    Superficial external pudendal
    Deep external pudendal
    Muscular branches

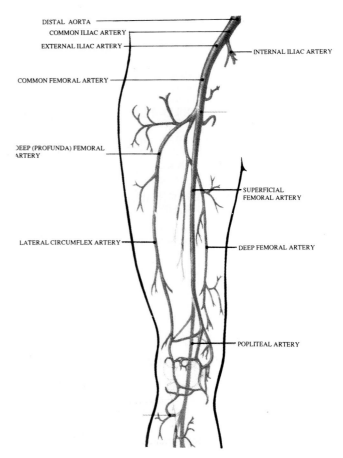

Figure 13–18. Normal arteries of the thigh.

*Superficial femoral artery (the common femoral bifurcates
    into the superficial femoral and the deep femoral. It lies
    anterior to the superficial femoral vein and descends to
    the adductor canal in the distal third of the thigh and
    becomes the popliteal artery.

*Profunda (deep) femoral artery. (courses deep into the thigh
    muscles and is paired with the deep femoral vein)
    Lateral circumflex femoral
    Medial circumflex femoral
    Perforating
    Muscular branches
    Genicular

*Popliteal (continuation of the superficial femoral artery. It
    courses inferiorly from the level of the adductor canal
    to the proximal portion of the calf. It divides into the
    anterior tibial artery and the tibioperoneal trunk.)
    Cutaneous branches
    Superior muscular branches

Sural
    Geniculars

*Anterior tibial (courses anteriorly through the interosseous
    membrane and travels inferiorly to form the dorsalis
    pedis artery in the foot.)

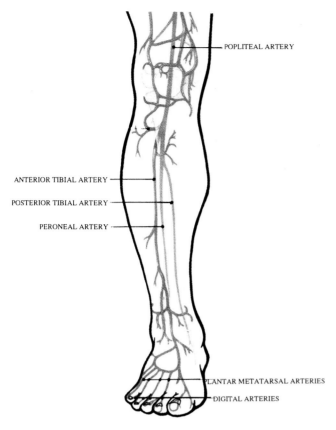

Figure 13–19. Normal arteries of the lower leg.

Posterior tibial recurrent
Anterior tibial recurrent
Muscular branches
Anterior medial malleolar
Anterior lateral malleolar
Dorsalis pedis (continuation of the anterior tibial)
Tarsal
Arcuate
Metatarsal
Deep plantar

Posterior tibial—peroneal trunk
  Tibial (courses medially and posteriorly from the tibio-
    peroneal trunk and ends at the medial aspect of
    the ankle)
  Nutrient
  Muscular
  Posterior medial malleolar
  Communicating
  Medial calcaneal

Peroneal (courses posteriorly and laterally from the tibio-
    peroneal trunk and ends at the lateral aspect of the
    ankle)
  Nutrient
  Muscular branches
  Communicating branches

Medial malleolar branches
Calcanean branches

Plantar Arch
  Perforating
  Plantar metatarsal branches
  Digital

DISEASE AND PATHOLOGY

Sudden arterial occlusion caused by emboli, thrombi, or trauma results in severe pain often associated with numbness of the entire extremity beginning below the occlusion. When the arterial occlusion develops over a longer period of time, ischemia is usually subtle and may not become manifest until the demand for blood exceeds the basic requirement, such as with exercise. Claudication pain is present during the exertion and disappears upon cessation of activity. Chronic arterial disease progresses until the intermittent pain is replaced by continuous pain at rest. Rest pain is worsened by elevation of extremity and is relieved by placing the extremity in a dependent position.[14]

The cause of the majority of arterial diseases today is atherosclerosis. Atherosclerosis refers to changes in the intima and media that includes focal accumulation of lipids, hemorrhage, fibrous tissue, and calcium deposits. The development of atherosclerotic lesions is a complex biochemical and cellular process. However, plaque is generally described as soft, dense, calcified, or complex.[1] Atherosclerosis usually manifests by gradual occlusion of blood flow. Symptoms occur when a critical arterial stenosis is reached. The blood flow and pressure are not significantly diminished until at least 75% of the cross-sectional area of the vessel is obliterated. This figure is equated with a 50% reduction in lumen diameter. The formula for the area of a circle (area = $3.14 \times radius^2$) explains the relationship between vessel diameter and cross-sectional area.[1] A decrease in radius is a major factor in a critical stenosis; however, other factors also influence a critical stenosis. They include: length of the stenosis, blood viscosity and peripheral resistance.[10] Lower extremity disease can be divided into three groups according to the level of involvement. These groups are aortoiliac, femoropopliteal, and tibioperoneal.[14] The most common site for atherosclerotic occlusion in the lower extremities are the distal superficial femoral artery within the adductor canal.[14]

Arterial Stenosis

Arterial stenosis can occur in the upper or lower extremities; however, it is more common in the lower extremities. Stenosis of the upper extremity may be caused by atherosclerosis, systemic diseases (scleroderma, lupus erythematosus) thromboangitis, arteritis, trauma, aneurysm, dialysis access, emboli, electrical injury, burns, and mechanical compression.[1]

Critical stenosis demonstrates a diminished pressure and flow distal to the lesion. However, extensive changes must be present before hemodynamic changes are evident.[2] How severe a stenosis is depends on several factors:[2]

- Length and diameter of the narrowed segment
- Roughness of endothelial surface
- Degree of narrowing or irregularity
- Ratio of cross section of narrowed segment to the normal segment
- Rate of flow
- Arteriovenous pressure gradient
- Peripheral resistance beyond the stenosis

At the site of the stenosis, real-time imaging will show a narrowing of the vessel, and there may be associated calcification or hyperplasia seen. There will be a marked disturbance with irregular travel of particles in various directions at different velocities.[2] This will be seen on the waveform as irregular random amplitudes. Color flow Doppler will demonstrate a mosaic type color pattern in the area of narrowing. There will be a significant increase in the peak systolic velocity with spectral broadening of the waveform.[1] Immediately past the stenosis (poststenotic zone), there will be turbulence, followed by damping of the waveform that results in a monophasic damped waveform.[1] A study by Sachs determined that a velocity of ration of 2.0 (100%) in velocity corresponds to a 70% reduction in diameter of the peripheral artery lumen.[1] (Figs. 13–20 A, B; Figs. 13–21 A, B, and C).

Occlusion of the artery may be acute or chronic. Acute occlusion without warning may be the result of embolism, trauma, or thrombosis and can progress to ischemic necrosis within hours.[1]

- *Thrombus* is the formation of clotted blood within the cardiovascular system.
- *Blood clot* is formed by the interaction of blood vessel walls and blood elements and involves only the coagulation sequence in its formation.
- *Embolus* is a detached mass that is carried by the blood to a site distant from its origin.

Acute occlusion requires prompt diagnosis and treatment to prevent loss of limb. There are five characteristic signs associated with acute arterial occlusion, termed the five Ps:

- Pain
- Paralysis
- Paresthesia
- Pallor
- Absence of pulses.[1]

Chronic occlusion is generally associated with atherosclerosis. Thromboangitis obliterans, or Berger's disease, is an inflammatory obliterative disease of the blood vessels of the extremities, primarily the lower extremities, which causes ischemia and gangrene. Real-time imaging demonstrates occlusion with the arterial lumen filled with echoes. However, if acute thrombus or emboli is present, the lumen may be sonolucent. Color flow Doppler demonstrates the stenotic lesion versus the occluded lesion and defines the patency. In occlusive lesions, the color flow is absent in the lumen of the vessel, and no Doppler signal is

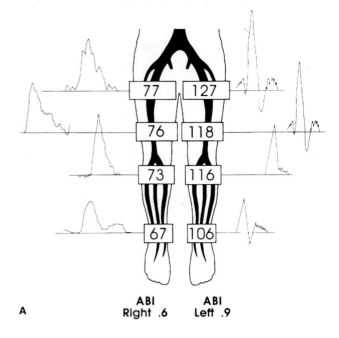

BRACHIAL PRESSURE LEFT 109

77   127
76   118
73   116
67   106

A   ABI Right .6   ABI Left .9

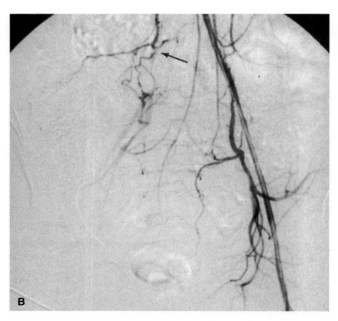

B

Figure 13–20. (A) Segmental artery pressure examination demonstrates 0.6 on the right and 0.9 on the left. The pressures in the left leg were normal. In the right leg, there is an abnormal pressure drop below the brachial pressure. The Doppler waveforms on the right indicate a damped monophasic collateral type waveform of the entire lower extremity, which is consistent with severe occlusive disease of the right iliac artery. **(B)** Angiography shows occlusion of the right iliac artery with collateral flow.

BRACHIAL PRESSURE RIGHT 190

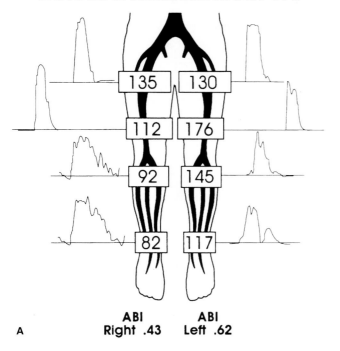

135	130
112	176
92	145
82	117

A   ABI
Right .43   ABI
Left .62

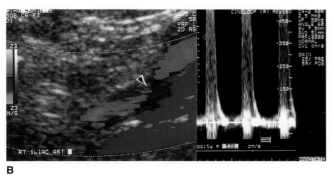

B

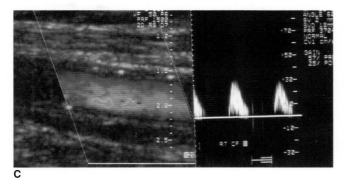

C

Figure 13–21. (A) Segmental artery pressure examination shows 0.4 on the right and 0.6 on the left indicating severe occlusive disease bilaterally. Doppler waveforms show damped monophasic waveforms bilaterally in all of the vessels, indicating bilateral iliac arterial disease. **(B)** Color flow Doppler shows the critical stenosis of the right iliac artery with a high velocity of 538 cm/s. **(C)** Damped monophasic waveform distal to the stenosis.

detected. Doppler waveforms may be damped proximal to the occlusion[1] (Figs. 13–22, 23).

A common stenosis of the upper extremity is subclavian steal. Defined as stenosis or occlusion of the subclavian artery proximal to the vertebral origin. Classically, this entity produces the subclavian steal syndrome. This condition is characterized by a reversal of blood flow within the vertebral artery and is more common on the left side. The retrograde vertebral flow on the side of the lesion is siphoned from the contralateral vertebral artery ultimately stealing blood from the basilar artery. The severity of the steal often determines the patient's symptoms, and they may experience ataxia, limb paralysis, vertigo, diplopia, dysarthria, syncope, or sensory disturbances. The hallmark sign of the subclavian steal is the difference in blood pressure (over 10 mm Hg) between two arms and a decreased peripheral pulse in the affected upper extremity.[1] The Doppler waveforms will demonstrate reversed or alternating flow in the ipsilateral vertebral artery. There will be increased velocities at the site of stenosis in the subclavian artery followed by damping of the waveform distal to the stenosis (Figs. 13–24 B, C, D; Figs. 13–25 A, B).

Thoracic Outlet Syndrome or Thoracic Outlet Compression

This condition occurs as a result of the subclavian arteries lying in close proximity to the clavicle, first rib, and the scalene muscles resulting in intrinsic compression of the vessels by these structures. Because this condition is not vascular in nature, but rather a compression syndrome, special maneuvers are required. These maneuvers include the military position, hyperabduction, and Adson maneuver. The radial artery is used to monitor the waveforms during the maneuver and is usually recorded with photoplethysmography to maintain stability during the maneuver. This test is not definitive, but if a positive is denoted, it indicates further testing. In abnormal examinations, the

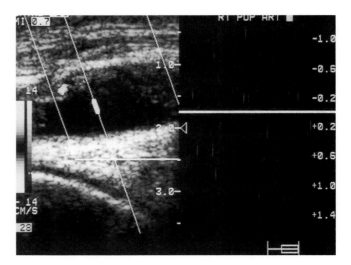

Figure 13–22. Popliteal artery occlusion with no color flow in the vessel and no signal on the Doppler waveform.

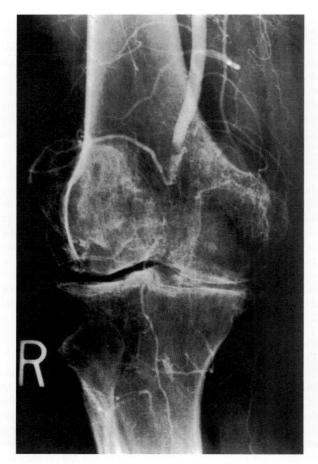

Figure 13–23. Angiography shows occlusion of the popliteal artery.

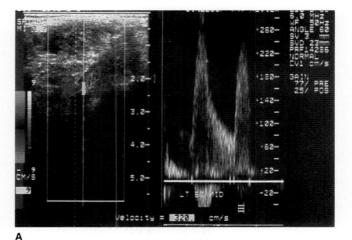

A

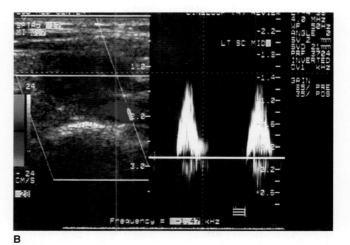

B

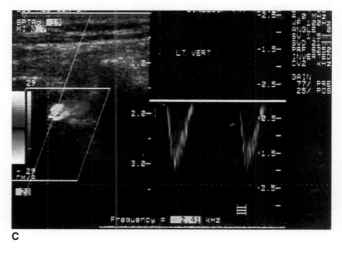

C

Figure 13–24. (A) Subclavian steal with markedly elevated waveform in the subclavian artery proximal to the vertebral origin. **(B)** Subclavian steal with reversed flow in the vertebral artery. **(C)** Subclavian steal with damped monophasic waveform in the distal subclavian artery.

photoplethysmograph recording will be obliterated during maneuvers indicating compression of the proximal arteries (Figs. 13–26 A, B; Figs. 13–27 A, B).

Raynaud's Phenomenon and Raynaud's Disease

Raynaud's disease (syndrome) is a functional vasospastic disorder that affects the small arteries of the extremities, most commonly the upper extremity. Cold and emotional stimuli trigger the response with the fingers turning white, blue, and finally red. With this condition, the arterial examination becomes abnormal when the patient is subjected to cold stimulation indicating vasospasm.

Raynaud's phenomenon is an obstructive arterial disease with an underlying systemic or vascular abnormality. It can be associated with arteriosclerosis, connective tissue disease (scleroderma), thromboangitis obliterans (Buerger's Disease) cryoglobulinemia, multiple myeloma, primary pulmonary hypertension, and rarely, carcinoma.[1,16] With this condition, there is absence of digital waveforms indicating occlusion.[1] Angiography will confirm occlusion of the digital arteries (Figs. 13–28 A, B; Figs. 13–29 A, B).

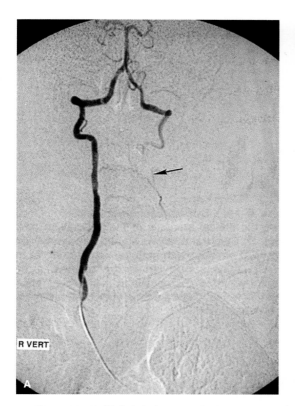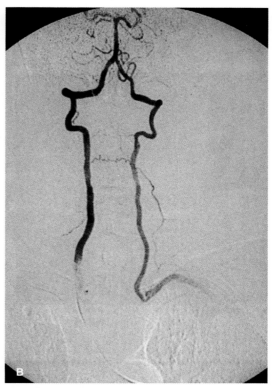

Figure 13–25. (A) Subclavian steal. Angiogram in early film with no flow in the left vertebral (arrow). **(B)** Angiogram in late film shows the delayed filling of the left subclavian artery and the delayed retrograde filling of the vertebral artery.

Aneurysm, Pseudoaneurysm, Mycotic Aneurysm

Aneurysm is an abnormal dilatation of the blood vessel wall. This abnormality is potentially dangerous because of the inherent ability to rupture or hemorrhage. They may be caused by atherosclerosis, hypertension, trauma, infection or a congenital weakness in the vessel wall. An aneurysm may be described as saccular, or fusiform. It can be seen on plain radiographs if there is calcification present in the wall or it displaces other structures. CT, MRI, and ultrasound can provide a more detailed evaluation.

Real-time ultrasound identifies the dilated sac with identification of the external lumen and internal lumen as well as any associated thrombus. Color flow Doppler or spec-

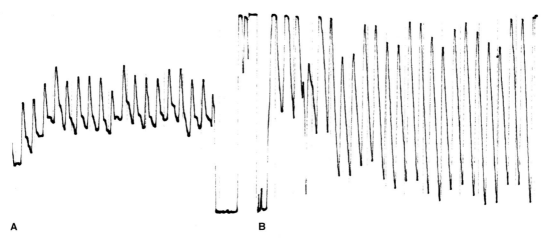

A   B

Figure 13–26. (A) Normal photoplethysmography pulse recordings during baseline resting state. **(B)** Normal photoplethysmography pulse recording during the hyperabduction maneuver.

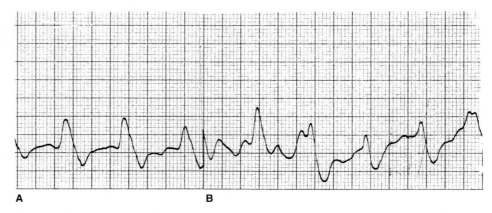

Figure 13–27. (A) Photoplethysmography pulse recordings during baseline resting state. **(B)** Abnormal photoplethysmography recording demonstrating reverse flow during the Adson maneuver.

tral analysis can confirm the vascularity with the swirling motion of the blood with color changes. Spectral analysis will demonstrate a low flow with a to-and-fro motion as the blood swirls in the dilated aneurysm (Fig. 13–30).

Pseudoaneurysm means false aneurysm. The dilated sac communicates with the true arterial lumen, and there is absence of the three layers of the arterial wall, hence the term "false aneurysm." These are usually the result of trauma and are sometimes seen following femoral

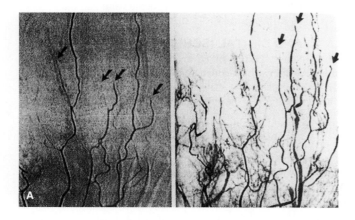

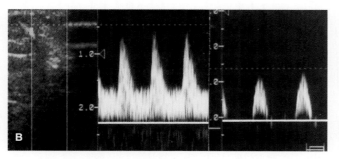

Figure 13–28. Raynaud's disease. **(A)** Angiogram shows absence of flow (arrows) followed by partial resolution after drug stimulation indicating vasospasm. **(B)** Waveforms before and after cold stimulation indicating vasospasm.

vascular reconstruction, percutaneous transluminal coronary angioplasty, cardiac catheterization, and intravenous injections by drug abusers.[1] They may be asymptomatic or present as a pulsating mass. Color flow Doppler readily demonstrates the pulsating mass adjacent to the native artery, and there is usually a neck or connective tract between the normal vessel and the aneurysm. Real-time imaging can identify the mass; however, it may not differentiate between a hematoma and an aneurysm. Doppler or color flow Doppler must be used to demonstrate the arterial flow and confirm the diagnosis. Spectral waveform analysis demonstrates a normal pulsatile triphasic waveform for the normal artery with a high-frequency/velocity shift in the neck that goes both forward and reverse because of the filling and emptying with the cardiac cycle. The aneurysmal sac will demonstrate a low-frequency shift with a to-and-fro pattern due to the swirling blood (Figs. 13–31, 32, 33).

A *dissecting aneurysm* usually develops secondary to a tear in the aorta; however, they may be seen extending to the abdominal aorta and are sometimes seen in the cerebral arteries. They are classically demonstrated on ultrasound by the intraluminal flap that separates the true and false lumen. Color flow Doppler will exhibit a change in color as the blood flow reverses into the false lumen. The waveform in the false lumen will be damped or absent (Figs. 13–34, 35).

A *mycotic aneurysm* is caused by an infectious process that involves the arterial wall. They often occur in multiple sites and are usually seen as a complication of bacterial endocarditis. In children, ultrasound or MRI may be used to identify and monitor treatment of the aneurysm because of the noninvasive nature and lack of radiation. The mycotic aneurysm exhibits the same ultrasound characteristics as the aneurysm (Figs. 13–36, 37).

Pseudoaneurysm Compression Techniques
Ultrasound-guided compression of the pseudoaneurysm is a safe and effective technique for inducing thrombosis and eliminating the aneurysm.[1] The procedure is to identify the

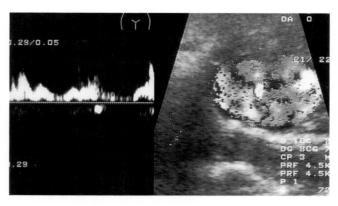

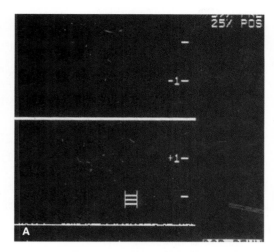

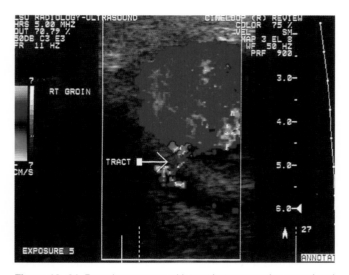

Figure 13–30. Aortic aneurysm. Spectral waveforms show a damped turbulent to and fro waveform. Color flow Doppler shows a swirling of colors consistent with aneurysm.

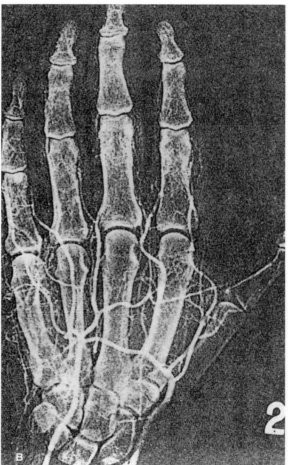

Figure 13–31. Pseudoaneurysm with tract between native vessel and aneurysm.

Figure 13–29. Raynaud's phenomenon. **(A)** Spectral analysis shows absence of digital flow. **(B)** Angiogram verifies digital occlusion.

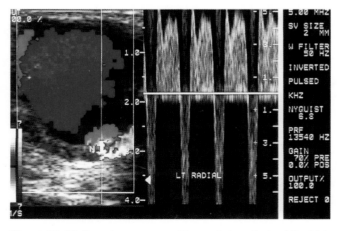

Figure 13–32. Pseudoaneurysm with spectral analysis of the high velocity jet with a forward and reverse flow in sync with the cardiac cycle.

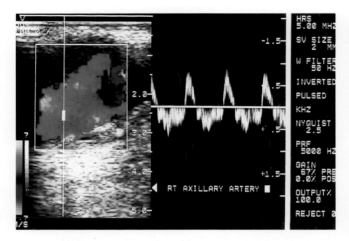

Figure 13–33. Pseudoaneurysm with spectral analysis of the to and fro pattern characteristic of an aneurysm.

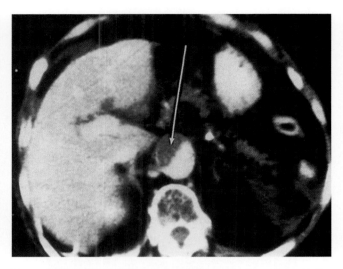

Figure 13–35. CT scan demonstrates the aortic dissection with the true lumen and false lumen (arrow).

pseudoaneurysm with color flow Doppler along with the tract or neck that connects the artery to the aneurysm. This is followed by manual compression of the pseudoaneurysm with sufficient pressure to obliterate the blood flow and holding for 15–20 minutes. The pseudoaneurysm is reassessed every 15–20 minutes with additional compression applied as required. The pedal pulses are checked throughout the compression to ensure the presence of distal blood flow (Figs. 13–38, 39).

Arterial Reconstruction and Grafts

There are a variety of surgical reconstruction procedures and grafts performed on the lower extremities. It is imperative that the sonographer know the type of surgery per-

formed and the exact graft schematic. Color flow Doppler is the method of choice for evaluating the arterial reconstruction and grafts. It has the capabilities of easily demonstrating patency, perigraft masses or fluid collections (hematomas or abscesses), hyperplasia, stenosis, and occlusion. An ABI complements the procedure by quantifying the flow and can monitor the improvement of flow or failure of the graft. Grafts of the lower extremities commonly involve the aorta, femoral, and popliteal arteries. They are usually identified by the arteries involved: aorto–femoral, femoral–femoral, femoral–popliteal, etc. Most grafts are attached using end to end or end to side anastomosis. The graft itself may be prosthetic (dacron or teflon) or autologous (saphe-

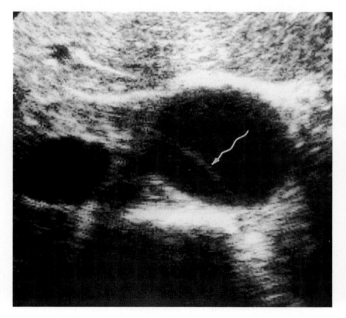

Figure 13–34. Dissecting aneurysm. Real-time image shows the thin membrane within the lumen (arrow).

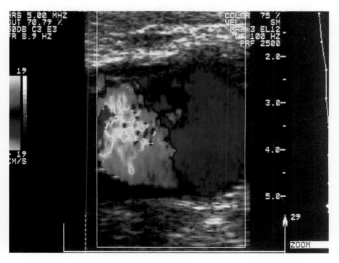

Figure 13–36. Mycotic aneurysm of the gluteal artery demonstrated by color flow Doppler.

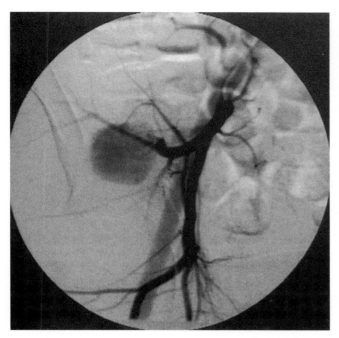

Figure 13–37. Mycotic aneurysm of the gluteal artery demonstrated by angiography.

nous vein). The saphenous vein graft is usually the standard to which other grafts are compared.[1]

Duplex and color flow Doppler provides assessment of patency and function. Some of the principal factors involved in graft failure are the low blood flow velocity, technical

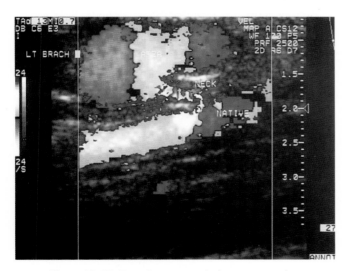

Figure 13–38. Pseudoaneurysm before compression.

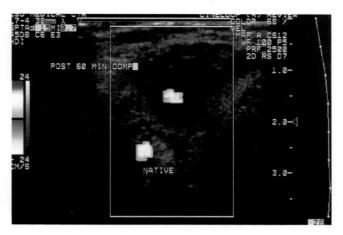

Figure 13–39. Pseudoaneurysm after compression.

errors at the anastomotic sites, or intrinsic graft problems. The measurement of graft flow velocity is a valuable tool. During the postoperative period, the normal blood flow is hyperemic, with antegrade flow throughout the cardiac cycle and relatively high-end diastolic velocities. The mature graft exhibits a triphasic pattern of peripheral arterial flow and because they are usually prosthetic conduits of fixed diameter, they have a constant velocity throughout the graft. Pseudoaneurysms may occur at the anastomosis site where narrowing or stenosis is more likely to occur. A decrease in peak systolic flow velocity to less than 45 cm/s in the graft indicates impending graft failure. No flow would indicate occlusion. Peak systolic velocities greater than 200 cm/s with spectral broadening and lumen reduction indicate severe stenosis[1] (Figs. 13–40 A, B).

Arteriovenous (AV) Fistula
An AV fistula is an abnormal communication between an artery and vein. This anomaly can be congenital or a result of trauma, infection, arterial aneurysm, or a malignancy.[10] It may resolve spontaneously or may cause hypertension or bleeding. Color flow Doppler demonstrates a mosaic pattern in the artery and vein at the point of injury and communication. The spectral waveform presents a high-velocity communication between the artery and the vein. There will be greatly increased velocities in the feeding artery because of the high-pressure gradient between the artery and the vein. There will be irregular amplitude caused by the turbulence with both venous and arterial sounds. There will also be turbulent venous flow with arterial pulsations in the draining vein[1] (Figs. 13–41 A, B).

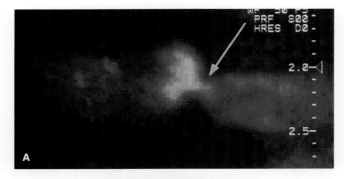

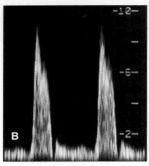

Figure 13–40. Graft stenosis. **(A)** Power angio shows the narrowed segment of the graft. **(B)** Spectral analysis show the increased peak systolic velocity.

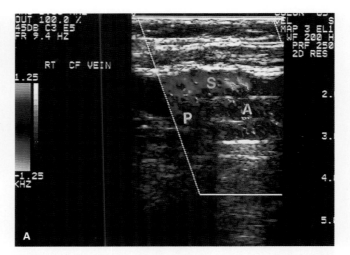

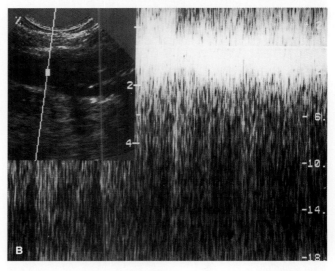

Figure 13–41. Arteriovenous fistula. **(A)** Color flow Doppler shows a mosaic color pattern in the superficial (S) and profunda (P) femoral veins with disturbed flow in the superficial femoral artery. **(B)** Spectral analysis shows a high-pitched turbulent waveform with arterial and venous signals mixed.

REFERENCES

1. Krebs CA, Giyanani VL, Eisenberg RL. *Ultrasound Atlas of Vascular Diseases.* Stamford, CT: Appleton & Lange; 1999.
2. Zwiebel WJ. *Introduction to Vascular Ultrasonography.* Philadelphia: WB Saunders; 2000.
3. Odwin CS, Dubinsky T, Fleischer AC. *Appleton & Lange's Review for the Ultrasonography Examinations.* Norwalk, CT: Appleton & Lange; 1993.
4. Jager KA, Phillips DJ, Martin RL. et al. Noninvasive mapping of lower limb arterial lesions. *Ultrasound Med Biol.* 1985; 11(3):515–521.
5. *ATL Ultramark9 Ultrasound System Reference Manual.* Bothell, WA: Advanced Technology Laboratories, Inc.; 1993.
6. Urdang L, Swallow HH. eds. *Mosby's Medical & Nursing Dictionary.* St. Louis: CV Mosby; 1983.
7. *Dorland's Illustrated Medical Dictionary.* 26th ed. Philadelphia: WB Saunders; 1981.
8. *Oncology Watch,* Nov. 14, 2000:8.
9. Williams PL, Warwick R, Dyson M, et al., eds. *Gray's Anatomy.* 37th ed. New York: Churchill Livingstone; 1989.
10. Hallet JW, Brewster DC, Darling RC. *Handbook of Patient Vascular Surgery.* 3rd ed. Boston: Little, Brown; 1995:6.
11. Powis RL, Schwartz RA. *Practical Doppler Ultrasound for the Clinician.* Baltimore: Williams & Wilkins; 1991:52.
12. Eisenberg RL, Dennis CA, May CR. *Radiographic Positioning.* 2nd ed. Boston: Little, Brown; 1995.
13. Tortora GJ, Grabowski SR. *Principles of Anatomy & Physiology.* 7th ed. New York: HarperCollins; 1993.
14. Schwartz SI, Shires GT, Spencer FC, Storer EH, eds. *Principles of Surgery.* 4th ed. New York: McGraw-Hill; 1984.
15. Gerlock AJ, Giyanani VL, Krebs CA. *Applications of Noninvasive Vascular Techniques.* Philadelphia: WB Saunders; 1988.
16. Cotran RS, Kumar V, Robbins SI. *Robbins Pathologic Basis of Disease.* 4th ed. Philadelphia: WB Saunders; 1989.

17. Cossman D, Ellison J, et al. Comparison of contrast arteriogram to arterial mapping with color flow duplex imaging in the lower extremities. *J Vasc Surg.* 1989; 10(5): 522–529.

18. Sanders RC, ed. *Clinical Sonography: A Practical Guide.* 2nd ed. Boston: Little, Brown; 1991.

19. Rutherford RB. *Vascular Surgery.* 2nd ed. Philadelphia: WB Saunders; 1984.

20. Taylor K, Burns P, Wells P: *Clinical Applications of Doppler Ultrasound.* New York: Raven Press; 1988.

21. Belanger A. *Vascular Anatomy & Physiology: An Introductory Text.* Pasadena, CA: Appleton Davies; 1986.

Questions

GENERAL INSTRUCTIONS: For each question, select the best answer. Select only one answer for each question, unless otherwise instructed.

1. What determines the Doppler shift frequency?

    (A) flow toward the transducer
    (B) flow away from the transducer
    (C) difference between the reflected and transmitted frequency
    (D) the velocity of the moving particles toward the transducer

2. The Doppler effect creates

    (A) change in frequency or Doppler shift when the reflector moves relative to the transducer
    (B) increase in frequency as the reflector moves away from the transducer
    (C) maximum frequency shift at 90°
    (D) requires angle correction for frequency measurements

3. Continuous wave Doppler has how many crystals in the transducer?

    (A) one
    (B) two
    (C) three
    (D) four

4. If flow is toward the transducer the frequency shift will be

    (A) lower
    (B) same
    (C) variable
    (D) higher

5. If the transmitted frequency is raised, the Doppler shift

    (A) increases
    (B) decreases
    (C) remains the same
    (D) will not be detected

6. Maximum Doppler shift frequency occurs at

    (A) 90°
    (B) 180°
    (C) 0°
    (D) 75°

7. What instrumentation is used for measurement of volume changes in the extremities to demonstrate blood flow?

    (A) continuous wave Doppler
    (B) Color flow Doppler
    (C) plethysmography
    (D) pulse volume recording

8. Which of the following is not true of the spectral analysis?

    (A) mathematical display of the frequency components in the Doppler signal
    (B) computer using the Fast Fourier Transform method
    (C) demonstrates the presence, direction, and characteristics of blood flow
    (D) Does not provide measurements of the blood flow

9. Name the components of the spectral analysis labeled on Fig. 13–42.

    (A) _____
    (B) _____
    (C) _____

10. Spectral broadening seen on the spectral analysis means

    (A) normal arterial waveform
    (B) increased bandwidth caused by disturbed flow
    (C) decreased bandwidth caused by disturbed flow
    (D) increased bandwidth caused by laminar flow

11. Which statement is *not* true about aliasing?

    (A) velocities exceed the Nyquist limit
    (B) wraparound of the waveform

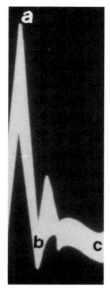

Figure 13–42. Spectral analysis waveform.

(C) higher velocities appear on the negative side of the baseline
(D) not controlled by the pulse repetition rate

12. Fig. 13–43 demonstrates

(A) spectral broadening
(B) aliasing
(C) turbulence
(D) monophasic waveform
(E) triphasic waveform

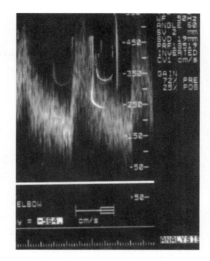

Figure 13–44. Spectral analysis waveform.

13. Fig. 13–44 demonstrates

(A) spectral broadening
(B) aliasing
(C) monophasic waveform
(D) triphasic waveform

14. Fig. 13–45 demonstrates

(A) dampened waveform
(B) aliasing of the waveform
(C) monophasic waveform
(D) triphasic waveform

15. Fig. 13–46 demonstrates

(A) spectral broadening
(B) aliasing
(C) turbulence

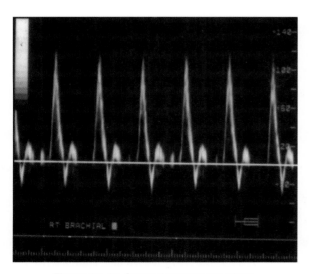

Figure 13–43. Spectral analysis waveform.

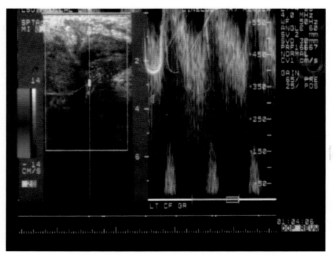

Figure 13–45. Spectral analysis waveform.

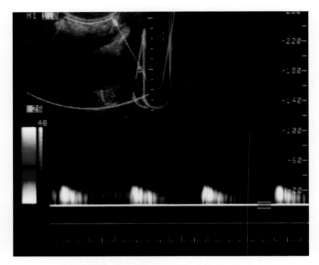

Figure 13–46. Spectral analysis waveform.

(D) monophasic waveform
(E) triphasic waveform

16. Fig. 13–47 demonstrates

(A) spectral broadening
(B) aliasing
(C) damping
(D) monophasic waveform
(E) triphasic waveform

17. Fig. 13–48 is

(A) Doppler equation
(B) Poiseuille's Law
(C) Reynolds number
(D) Bernoulli's equation

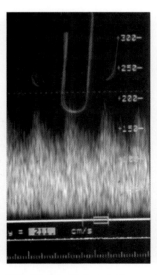

Figure 13–47. Spectral analysis waveform.

$$FS = \frac{2\ V\ Fo}{c\ +}\ \cos \theta$$

Figure 13–48. Physics equation.

18. A radiology procedure where a balloon catheter is placed in a vessel and dilated to eliminate stenotic lesions is called

(A) digital subtraction angiography
(B) magnetic resonance imaging
(C) positron emission tomography
(D) percutaneous transluminal angioplasty

19. What interventional procedure using a vascular catheter for introduction of a substance or device is used to control bleeding or stop the blood flow?

(A) transjugular intrahepatic portosystemic shunt
(B) embolization
(C) percutaneous angioplasty
(D) thrombolytic therapy

20. The physiology of circulation is called

(A) fluid dynamics
(B) circulatory system
(C) hemodynamics
(E) coronary circulation

21. Blood movement in concentric layers with the highest velocity in the center of the vessel that creates a parabolic flow profile is

(A) laminar flow
(B) disorganized flow
(C) boundary layer separation
(D) turbulent flow

22. What type of plethysmography identifies subcutaneous blood flow?

(A) air
(B) strain gauge
(C) impedance
(D) photoplethysmography

23. In the poststenotic flow zone, there may be frank swirling movements, which is called

(A) collateral flow
(B) vortices
(C) reversed flow
(D) laminar flow

24. Which statement is not true of the Reynolds number?

(A) defines the point where flow changes from laminar to disturbed

(B) is less than 2000 in the normal arterial circulation

(C) is not included in the basic principles of fluid dynamics

(D) predicts the stability of a fluid

25. Laminar flow tends to be disturbed if the Reynolds number exceeds what value?

(A) 500
(B) 700
(C) 1000
(D) 1500
(E) 2000

26. A turbulence in the blood flow distal to a narrowing of the vessel is

(A) poststenotic turbulence
(B) velocity jet
(C) laminar flow
(D) dampened flow

27. How is the velocity of blood flow related to the cross-sectional area of the blood vessel?

(A) inversely
(B) directly related
(C) not related
(D) variable

28. Blood pressure is

(A) volume of blood flowing through the vessel
(B) average pressure throughout the cardiac cycle
(C) pulse pressure in circulatory system
(D) pressure exerted by blood on the wall of a blood vessel

29. In a resting young adult the blood pressure is

(A) 100 mm Hg during systole and 50 mm Hg during diastole
(B) 120 mm Hg during systole and 40 mm Hg during diastole
(C) 150 mm Hg during systole and 70 mm Hg during diastole
(D) 120 mm Hg during systole and 70 mm Hg during diastole

30. The expansion and contraction of arteries after each systole of the left ventricle creates a pressure wave termed

(A) cycle
(B) waveform
(C) pulse
(D) mean

31. The resting pulse is

(A) between 50 and 100 pulses per minute
(B) over 100 pulses per minute

(C) under 50 beats per minute
(D) between 25 and 75 pulses per minute

32. Predisposing factors for arterial disease does not include

(A) smoking
(B) aging
(C) diabetes
(D) family history of arterial disease
(E) hypertension
(F) bradycardia

33. What is the most common symptom of lower extremity arterial disease?

(A) ulceration
(B) absence of pulses
(C) claudication
(D) cyanosis

34. Which of the following is not one of the classic five Ps for acute arterial ischemia?

(A) pain
(B) pallor
(C) pressure
(D) paresthesias
(E) paralysis
(F) pulselessness

35. The ankle brachial index is used in which examination?

(A) strain gauge plethysmography
(B) peripheral angiography
(C) peripheral venous evaluation
(D) segmental pressure arterial examination

36. If a patient falls into a claudication category on the segmental pressure examination, what additional testing is done?

(A) color flow Doppler
(B) peripheral angiography
(C) exercise with a treadmill or hyperemia testing
(D) impedance plethysmography

37. In performing the segmental arterial pressure examination, the pressure recording is obtained

(A) site where the cuff is inflated and deflated
(B) at the posterior tibial artery
(C) site below where the cuff is inflated and deflated
(D) site above where the cuff is inflated and deflated

38. In segmental arterial studies, the cuff at each site is inflated until the systolic pressure, sound or Doppler waveform

(A) appears
(B) disappears

(C) remains constant
(D) none of the above

39. What is used as the standard pressure for segmental arterial studies?

(A) posterior tibial artery systolic artery pressure
(B) common femoral artery systolic artery pressure
(C) brachial artery systolic artery pressure
(D) anterior tibial artery systolic artery pressure

40. The bilateral brachial pressures should be within

(A) 5 mm Hg
(B) 10 mm Hg
(C) 25 mm Hg
(D) 50 mm Hg

41. An ankle brachial index of 0.6–0.9 indicates

(A) normal value
(B) claudication
(C) severe occlusive disease
(D) occlusion

42. An ankle brachial index of 0.5 or less indicates

(A) normal value
(B) claudication
(C) severe occlusive disease
(D) occlusion

43. In performing a peripheral arterial disease and the vessels of the lower extremity are calcified with falsely elevated values on the segmental pressure recordings, what is required?

(A) color flow Doppler
(B) strain gauge plethysmography
(C) brachial pressures
(D) toe pressures

44. The normal toe pressure is what?

(A) equal to the brachial pressure
(B) equal to the ankle index pressure
(C) 60% of the brachial pressure
(D) 75% of the brachial pressure

45. Exercise normally does what to the blood flow?

(A) increases
(B) decreases
(C) remains unchanged
(D) creates a high variable

46. Composition of the arteries does not include

(A) intima
(B) media
(C) adventitia
(D) internal capsule

47. As sympathetic stimulation is increased, the smooth muscle of the artery contracts and narrows the vessel lumen. This is called

(A) vasodilatation
(B) vascular narrowing
(C) vasoconstriction
(D) vasospasm

48. Which artery is present only on right side of the upper extremity?

(A) brachiocephalic
(B) subclavian
(C) thyrocervical
(D) costocervical

49. Which arterial vessel is a direct continuation of the subclavian?

(A) vertebral
(B) common carotid
(C) axillary
(D) brachiocephalic

50. The terminal branches of the brachial artery are the

(A) axillary and subclavian
(B) palmar and digital
(C) radial and ulna
(D) radial and palmar

51. Which arterial vessel is a continuation of the external iliac and supplies the psoas major muscle, inferior epigastric, and deep circumflex?

(A) common femoral
(B) superficial femoral
(C) profunda femoral
(D) popliteal

52. Which vessel lies posterior to the medial aspect of the ankle?

(A) anterior tibial
(B) peroneal
(C) posterior tibial
(D) dorsalis pedis

53. Ischemia is secondary to

(A) excessive blood flow
(B) normal blood flow
(C) loss of blood flow
(D) none of the above

54. Embolism is

(A) sudden blocking of artery by clot or foreign material
(B) atherosclerotic plaque formation
(C) trauma to an artery with resulting occlusion
(D) dissection of an artery caused by trauma

55. What type of pain is present during exertion and disappears upon cessation of activity?

 (A) rest pain
 (B) claudication pain
 (C) trauma pain
 (D) normal exercise

56. The majority of arterial disease is caused by

 (A) genetic origin
 (B) atherosclerosis
 (C) cardiac disease
 (D) diabetes

57. Blood flow and pressures are not significantly diminished until at least what percentage of the cross-sectional area of the vessel is obliterated?

 (A) 25%
 (B) 50%
 (C) 75%
 (D) 95%

58. Other factors that influence a critical stenosis are

 (A) length of the stenosis
 (B) blood viscosity
 (C) peripheral resistance
 (D) A and C
 (E) all of the above

59. The most common site of atherosclerotic occlusion in the lower extremity is

 (A) common femoral artery bifurcation into superficial and deep femoral artery
 (B) profunda (deep) femoral artery
 (C) distal superficial femoral artery in the adductor canal
 (D) popliteal artery

60. Which artery in the lower extremity passes through the interosseous membrane and courses along the anterolateral aspect of the leg?

 (A) posterior tibial
 (B) anterior tibial
 (C) peroneal
 (D) dorsalis pedis

61. A stenosis or occlusion of the subclavian artery proximal to the vertebral artery is

 (A) subclavian steal
 (B) thoracic outlet syndrome
 (C) vertebral-basilar occlusive disease
 (D) vertebral artery stenosis

62. Subclavian steal is characterized by

 (A) turbulent erratic waveforms throughout the vertebrals
 (B) a monophasic waveform of the subclavian artery

 (C) a high-grade stenosis with increased velocities
 (D) reversal of blood flow within the vertebral artery

63. The hallmark clinical sign of subclavian steal is

 (A) pain in the upper extremity
 (B) numbness in the upper extremity
 (C) difference in BP of over 10 mmHg
 (D) absence of pulses

64. Intrinsic compression of the vessels by the clavicle, first rib, and the scalene muscles is characteristic of

 (A) subclavian steal
 (B) thoracic outlet syndrome
 (C) subclavian aneurysms
 (D) Raynaud's disease

65. Positioning maneuvers (military, hyperabduction, and Adson) are used during diagnostic testing for

 (A) Raynaud's disease
 (B) subclavian steal
 (C) thoracic outlet syndrome
 (D) Raynaud's phenomenon

66. A functional vasospastic disorder that affects the small arteries of the extremities is

 (A) Raynaud's disease or syndrome
 (B) Raynaud's phenomenon
 (C) thoracic outlet syndrome
 (D) subclavian steal

67. An obstructive arterial disease which has an underlying systemic or vascular abnormality is

 (A) Raynaud's disease
 (B) Raynaud's phenomenon
 (C) thoracic outlet syndrome
 (D) subclavian steal

68. Absence of the three layers of the arterial wall in an abnormal dilated vessel is

 (A) aneurysm
 (B) dissection
 (C) pseudoaneurysm
 (D) arteriovenous malformation

69. Which type of aneurysm is associated with an infectious process?

 (A) pseudoaneurysm
 (B) mycotic
 (C) dissecting
 (D) fusiform

70. Which type of aneurysm has two lumens?

 (A) pseudoaneurysm
 (B) mycotic
 (C) dissecting
 (D) saccular

71. In the evaluation of arterial reconstruction and grafts, what provides quantification of the flow of the entire extremity?

(A) color flow Doppler
(B) spectral waveform analysis
(C) ankle brachial index
(D) duplex scanning

72. A decrease in peak systolic flow velocity of less than 45 cm/s in the arterial graft indicates

(A) patency of the graft
(B) stenosis of the graft
(C) occlusion of the graft
(D) graft failure

73. A communication between the artery and the vein is

(A) pseudoaneurysm
(B) aneurysm
(C) AV fistula
(D) dissection

74. The resistive index is used to quantify

(A) arterial flow
(B) resistance
(C) turbulence
(D) volume of flow

75. Tachycardia means

(A) rapid heart rate
(B) slow heart rate
(C) normal heart rate
(D) irregular heart rate

76. Which of the following is not a noninvasive testing procedure?

(A) Doppler
(B) plethysmography
(C) segmental pressures
(D) angiography

77. The ankle brachial index is

(A) brachial systolic pressure divided by the ankle systolic pressure
(B) the ankle systolic pressure divided by the brachial systolic pressure
(C) brachial diastolic pressure divided by the ankle diastolic pressure
(D) ankle diastolic pressure divided by the brachial diastolic pressure

78. What is required before the performance of the vascular noninvasive examination?

(A) evaluation of blood pressure
(B) process screening

(C) patient history
(D) billing procedures

79. In performance of the segmental pressure examination of the lower extremities, how many cuffs are preferred?

(A) 2
(B) 3
(C) 4
(D) 5

80. What do most sonographic contrast agents use to increase reflectivity and improve the ultrasound image?

(A) iodine
(B) saline
(C) barium
(D) air bubbles

81. The two major pathways of the cardiovascular system are

(A) arterial and venous
(B) systemic and pulmonary circulation
(C) cerebrovascular and systemic circulation
(D) cerebrovascular, systemic, and pulmonary circulation

82. Which layer of the artery is the muscle layer?

(A) intima
(B) media
(C) adventitia
(D) tunica externa

83. What is the first branch of the subclavian?

(A) thyrocervical
(B) internal mammary
(C) costocervical trunk
(D) vertebral

Questions 84–85: Match the structures in Fig. 13–49 with the terms in Column B.

COLUMN A	COLUMN B
84. _____	(A) femoral artery
85. _____	(B) femoral vein

Questions 86–89: Match the structures in Fig. 13–50 with the terms in Column B.

COLUMN A	COLUMN B
86. _____	(A) profunda (deep) femoral vein and artery
87. _____	(B) femoral artery
88. _____	(C) greater saphenous vein
89. _____	(D) femoral vein

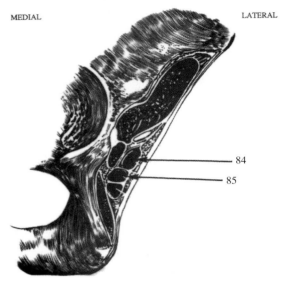

MEDIAL   LATERAL

——— 84
——— 85

Figure 13–49. Lateral surface of the right pelvic girdle. *(Reprinted with permission from Gray H, Clemente CD. Anatomy of the Human Body. Philadelphia: Lea & Febiger; 1985.)*

Questions 90–93: Match the structures in Fig. 13–51 with the terms in Column B.

COLUMN A	COLUMN B
90. _____	(A) lesser (small) saphenous
91. _____	(B) popliteal vein
92. _____	(C) greater saphenous
93. _____	(D) popliteal artery

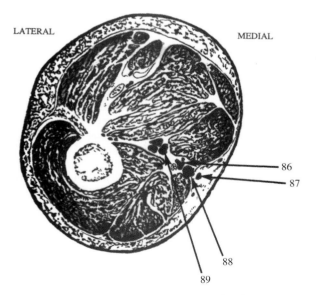

LATERAL   MEDIAL

——— 86
——— 87

88
89

Figure 13–50. Cross section proximal thigh. *(Reprinted with permission from Gray H, Clemente CD. Anatomy of the Human Body. Philadelphia: Lea & Febiger; 1985.)*

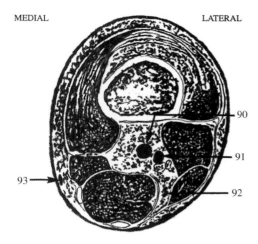

MEDIAL   LATERAL

——— 90
——— 91
93 ——→
——— 92

Figure 13–51. Cross section of the popliteal space. *(Reprinted with permission from Gray H, Clemente CD. Anatomy of the Human Body. Philadelphia: Lea & Febiger; 1985.)*

Questions 94–100: Match the structures in Fig. 13–52 with the terms in Column B.

COLUMN A	COLUMN B
94. _____	(A) internal iliac artery
95. _____	(B) popliteal artery
96. _____	(C) superficial femoral artery
97. _____	(D) profunda (deep) femoral
98. _____	(E) common femoral artery
99. _____	(F) distal aorta
100. _____	(G) external iliac artery

Questions 101–106: Match the structures in Fig. 13–53 with the terms in Column B.

COLUMN A	COLUMN B
101. _____	(A) peroneal artery
102. _____	(B) popliteal artery
103. _____	(C) plantar metatarsal arteries
104. _____	(D) digital arteries
105. _____	(E) anterior tibial artery
106. _____	(F) posterior tibial artery

Questions 107–110: Match the velocity waveforms in Fig. 13–54 with the terms in Column B.

COLUMN A	COLUMN B
107. _____	(A) 20–40% diameter reduction stenosis
108. _____	(B) 0% diameter reduction stenosis
109. _____	(C) 50–99% diameter reduction stenosis
110. _____	(D) 1–19% diameter reduction stenosis

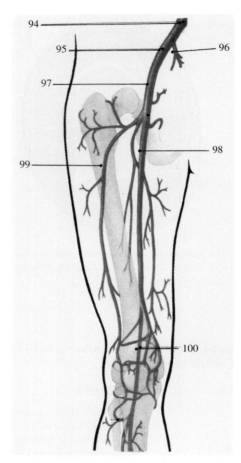

Figure 13–52. Arteries of the thigh. *(Reprinted with permission from Abbott Laboratories, North Carolina, IL. Medical illustration by Scott Thorn Barrows, AMI.)*

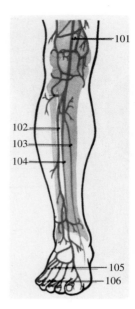

Figure 13–53. Arteries of the leg. *(Reprinted with permission from Abbott Laboratories, North Carolina, IL. Medical illustration by Scott Thorn Barrows, AMI.)*

111. Signs and symptoms of arterial disease of the lower extremity include

(A) intermittent claudication
(B) dependent rubor
(C) pallor on elevation
(D) impotence in males
(E) trophic skin changes
(F) all of the above
(G) A, B, D, and E

112. There are many known risk factors that play a part in the development of atherosclerosis of the extremities. These include

(A) family history
(B) cigarette smoking
(C) hypertension
(D) malignancies
(E) diabetes
(F) all of the above
(G) A, B, C, and E

113. The Doppler signal in Fig. 13–55 demonstrates

(A) triphasic flow
(B) marked spectral broadening
(C) normal velocity profile at 83 cm/s
(D) abnormal velocity profile at 83 cm/s
(E) A and C
(F) B and D

114. With a hemodynamically significant, short-segment stenosis, one would expect

(A) an increased peak-systolic velocity and an increased end-diastolic velocity
(B) a decreased peak-systolic velocity and a decreased end-diastolic velocity
(C) an increased peak-systolic velocity and a decreased end-diastolic velocity
(D) a decreased peak systolic velocity and an increased end-diastolic velocity

115. Information obtained from the pulsed-wave Doppler spectral display includes all the following except

(A) the source of origin of the Doppler signal
(B) pulsatility features of the waveform
(C) velocity or frequency shift of the blood flow
(D) direction of flow

116. Spectral broadening results in the loss of the clear spectral window below the peak-systolic velocity spectral waveform in systole. Which of the following statements is true?

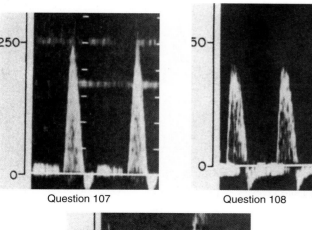

Question 107   Question 108

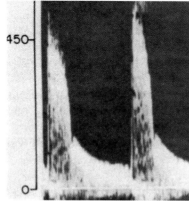

Question 109

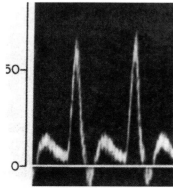

Question 110

Figure 13–54. Velocity waveforms. *(Reprinted from Bergan JJ, Yao JST: Arterial Surgery: New Diagnostic and Operative Techniques. Philadelphia: Grune & Stratton, 1988: 441.)*

    (A) A small sample volume placed centrally in the artery should decrease the size of the spectral window.
    (B) The spectral window filling occurs as flow disturbances produce vortices (swirling eddies) with varying flow direction.
    (C) Vortices (rotating flow) will show only forward flow and produce a narrow band of velocities demonstrating a clear spectral window.

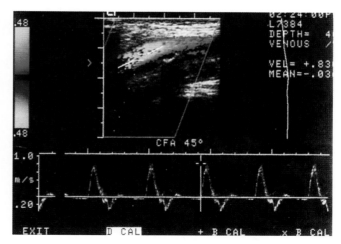

Figure 13–55. Doppler signal.

    (D) Loss of the spectral window occur only with stenotic lesions of 75% or greater.

117. Appreciable changes in pressure and flow do not occur until the diameter of an artery is reduced by 50% or greater. This degree of narrowing is called

    (A) critical stenosis
    (B) Reynolds number
    (C) Bernoulli's principle
    (D) Poiseuille's law

118. The principal control mechanisms affecting blood volume changes are

    (A) viscosity and blood vessel diameter
    (B) cardiac output and peripheral resistance
    (C) blood pressure gradients and inertial losses
    (D) energy losses and flow-reducing lesions

119. One advantage of using continuous wave Doppler is

    (A) the ability to differentiate overlying blood vessels
    (B) minimal spectral broadening
    (C) high velocities can be displayed without aliasing
    (D) control of the depth selection of the sample site

120. Factors affecting the Doppler shift frequency include

    (A) Doppler angle
    (B) transducer
    (C) velocity of the red blood cells
    (D) B and C
    (E) A, B, and C

121. As an arterial stenosis becomes hemodynamically significant, which statement is true about the hemodynamics of the stenosis?

    (A) flow volume increases, peak-systolic velocity decreases
    (B) flow volume decreases, peak-systolic velocity decreases

(C) flow volume decreases, peak-systolic velocity increases

(D) flow volume increases, peak-systolic velocity increases

122. The highest peak systolic velocity is found

(A) at the narrowest portion of the stenotic lesion
(B) just proximal to the stenotic lesion
(C) just distal to the stenotic lesion
(D) both proximal and distal to the stenotic lesion

123. The flow pattern throughout the stenotic lesion will be

(A) laminar
(B) mild scattering
(C) disturbed
(D) turbulence only on the outer edges

124. All other factors being constant, the artery with the smallest radius will have

(A) lower resistance to flow
(B) higher resistance to flow
(C) no change in the resistance
(D) variable resistance

125. Which of the following is not used to determine the severity of arterial stenoses?

(A) peak systolic velocity
(B) end diastolic velocity
(C) systolic velocity ratio
(D) volume flow

126. With a 50–99% diameter reduction in a peripheral artery, the waveform would

(A) be triphasic with no appreciable spectral broadening
(B) normal reverse components of waveform with mild spectral broadening
(C) loss of reverse component with a distal damped monophasic waveform
(D) proximal waveform will have diminished velocities and a monophasic waveform

127. In Fig. 13–56, color flow Doppler of the iliac artery shows

(A) normal iliac arterial graft
(B) iliac artery graft with stenosis
(C) iliac artery graft with occlusion
(D) iliac artery graft with pseudoaneurysm

128. In Fig. 13–57, spectral analysis of the distal iliac artery shows

(A) normal waveform
(B) site of stenosis
(C) proximal to a stenotic lesion
(D) distal to a stenotic lesion

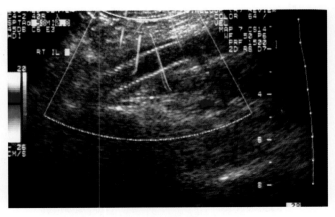

Figure 13–56. Color flow Doppler of the iliac artery.

129. In Fig. 13–58, segmental pressures and Doppler waveforms of the lower extremities show

(A) severe occlusive disease of the right lower extremity
(B) claudication disease of the left lower extremity
(C) bilateral severe occlusive disease
(D) bilateral mild claudication disease
(E) A and B

130. In Fig. 13–59, segmental pressures and Doppler waveforms of the lower extremities show

(A) normal segmental and pressure study
(B) bilateral claudication disease
(C) bilateral iliac artery occlusion
(D) occlusive disease on the right and claudication disease on the left

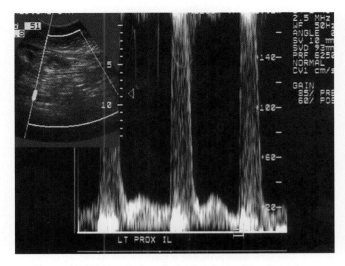

Figure 13–57. Spectral analysis waveform of the iliac artery.

BRACHIAL PRESSURE RIGHT 190

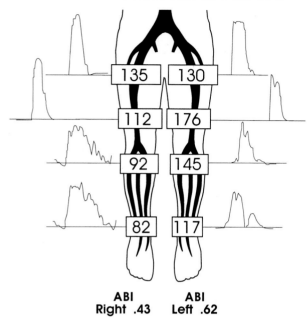

ABI
Right .43

ABI
Left .62

Figure 13–58. Arterial segmental pressure study.

131. Fig. 13–60 shows the maneuver position for arterial testing for

(A) thoracic outlet compression
(B) Raynaud's disease
(C) Raynaud's phenomenon
(D) subclavian steal

132. In Fig. 13–61, real-time image of the aorta shows

(A) normal aorta
(B) aortic dissection
(C) aneurysm with calcified wall
(D) pseudoaneurysm with classical tract

Questions 133–135: Match spectral analysis components in Fig. 13–62 with the terms in Column A.

COLUMN A	COLUMN B
133. zero baseline	_____
134. spectral window	_____
135. bandwidth	_____

Questions 136–145. Match the upper extremity arteries in Fig. 13–63 with the letters in Column B.

COLUMN A	COLUMN B
136. ulnar artery _____	(A)
137. axillary artery _____	(B)
138. brachial artery _____	(C)
139. radial artery _____	(D)
140. subclavian artery _____	(E)
141. vertebral artery _____	(F)
142. aortic arch _____	(G)
143. thyrocervical artery _____	(H)
144. common carotid artery _____	(I)
145. brachiocephalic artery _____	(J)

146. Fig. 13–64 is a diagram of what type of surgical graft?

(A) aortofemoral
(B) femoral–popliteal
(C) aorta
(D) femoral–femoral

147. In Fig. 13–65, the ankle brachial index seen is

(A) normal study
(B) claudication of the right and severe occlusive disease on the left
(C) normal on the right and claudication on the left
(D) bilateral severe occlusive disease

148. Blood flow information from a specific location is obtained by the

(A) velocity range
(B) Doppler angle
(C) field of view
(D) sample volume

149. The digital blood pressure is normally

(A) within 20–30 mm Hg of the brachial pressure
(B) the same as the brachial pressure
(C) within 10–20 mm Hg of the brachial pressure
(D) within 30–40 mm Hg of the brachial pressure

150. Normally, the flow velocity in an artery accelerates

(A) slowly
(B) rapidly
(C) moderately
(D) variable

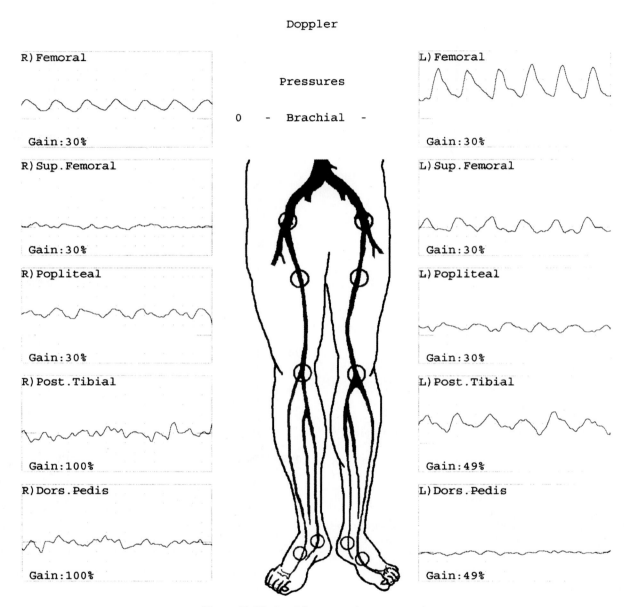

Figure 13–59. Arterial segmental pressure study.

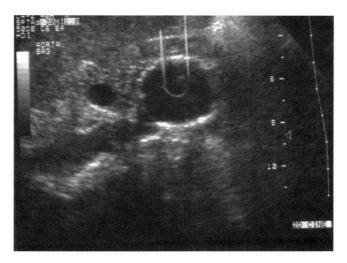

Figure 13–61. Real time longitudinal image of the aorta.

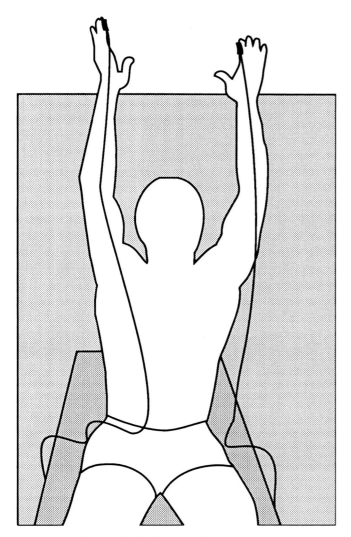

Figure 13–60. Arterial testing maneuver.

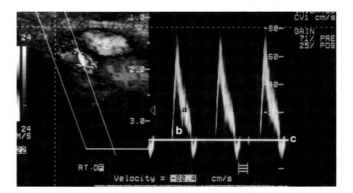

Figure 13–62. Spectral analysis waveform.

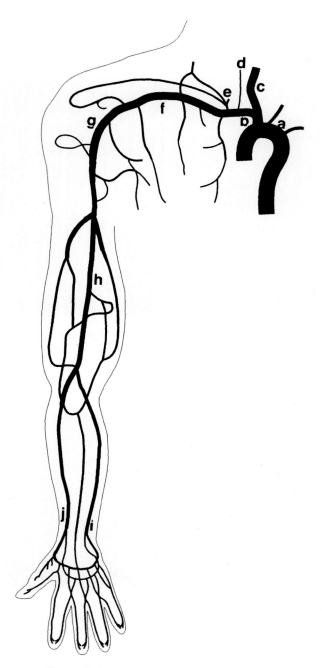

Figure 13–63. Upper extremity arterial anatomy.

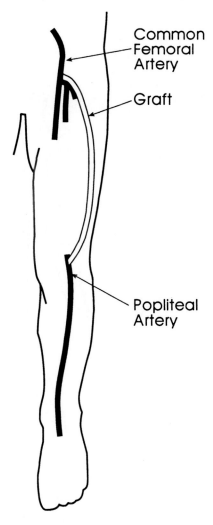

Figure 13–64. Surgical graft diagram.

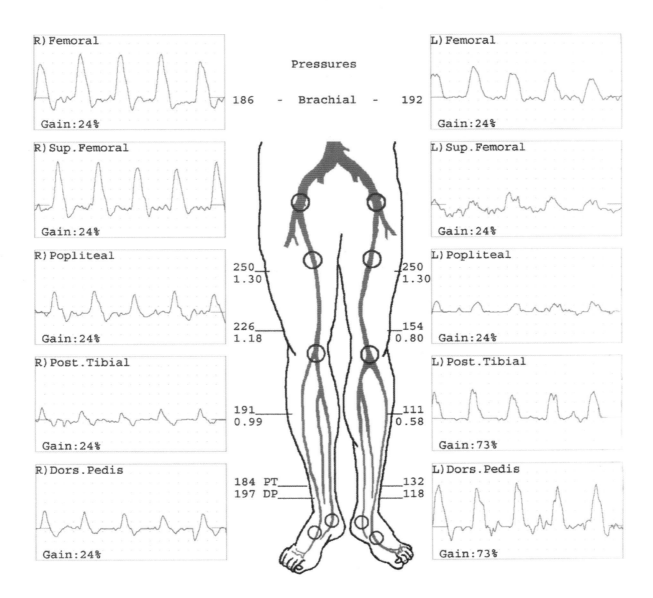

Figure 13–65. Arterial segmental pressure study.

Answers and Explanations

At the end of each explained answer there is a number combination in parentheses. The first number identifies the reference source; the second number or set of numbers indicates the page on which the relevant information can be found.

1. **(C)** The Doppler shift is the difference between the received and transmitted frequencies or the difference between the reflected and transmitted frequency and is defined in the Doppler equation. *(2:26; 1:5)*

2. **(A)** The Doppler effect is a change in frequency relative to motion. The frequency received is higher or lower than the transmitted frequency depending on whether the motion is toward or away from the transducer. *(2:26; 1:4)*

3. **(B)** Continuous wave Doppler has two inherent crystals in one transducer. One to receive and one to send continuously. *(1:14)*

4. **(D)** When we think of the Doppler principles we think of motion. For example, as a train moves closer to us the sound is louder, and as it is moves further away, the sound is lower. The sound frequency increases as it approaches the receiver and decreases as it gets farther from the receiver. *(1:4, 5)*

5. **(A)** If the Doppler frequency is higher, the Doppler shift frequency will be higher and, conversely, if the Doppler frequency is lowered, the Doppler shift frequency will be lower. This is defined by the Doppler equation, which states the Doppler frequency is proportional to both the reflector frequency and the ultrasound transmitted frequency. *(Study Guide; 2:35)*

6. **(C)** When the flow is toward the transducer at zero degrees the Doppler frequency shift is the greatest and reduced accordingly at other incident angles. A perpendicular or 90° angle of insonation results in no detected Doppler shift. Because zero degree is not feasible in most clinical applications; we avoid the 90° angle and maintain a 30–60° for clinical applications. *(2:26)*

7. **(C)** Plethysmography, Strain gauge plethysmography is one of the older noninvasive vascular techniques for measuring the outflow of venous blood to determine deep vein thrombosis. It has a specificity approximately 60–70% and a positive predictive value of only approximately 50%. Most laboratories now use color flow Doppler. Photoplethysmography is still in use in some laboratories for screening patients for reflux. It demonstrates the filling time of the veins and differentiates between superficial and deep venous incompetency. *(10:51; 2:353)*

8. **(D)** The spectral analysis displays the frequency distribution on a time scale. To process the Doppler signal and calculate all the frequency components the Fast Fourier Transform method is used. The spectral analysis determines the presence, direction, and characteristics of blood flow. The spectral analysis does provide the quantification and measurements of the blood flow. This cannot be achieved with color flow imaging alone. *(1:5; 2:33)*

9. a. peak systolic velocity
   b. flow reversal
   c. diastole *(1:6)*

10. **(B)** Spectral broadening means broadening or increase in the bandwidth with filling of the spectral window. This can range from mild to severe and is caused by disturbed flow. Disturbed flow produces increased frequencies and the formation of small eddies that increase the center stream and produce random motion of the blood cells. Spectral broadening is commonly seen with stenosis. *(1:6–7)*

11. **(D)** The Nyquist limit is controlled by the pulse repetition rate. Aliasing is seen with high velocities that exceed the Nyquist limit or ½ the pulse repetition rate. It is seen on the spectral analysis waveform display as a wraparound with the higher velocities appearing as a negative reading below the baseline. *(1:15; 2:35)*

12. **(E)** Triphasic waveform that is consistent with a high-resistance peripheral artery. It demonstrates a rapid systolic rise, prominent flow reversal, and forward flow in diastole. *(2:236)*

13. **(A)** Spectral broadening caused by stenosis of the vessel. There is an increase in the frequencies/velocities causing spreading of the bandwidth. Characteristic associated with disturbed flow and stenotic lesions.
(1:7)

14. **(B)** Aliasing (exceeding the Nyquist limit) is seen with mild spectral broadening and turbulence of the waveform secondary to a high-grade stenosis. *(1:15)*

15. **(D)** Damped monophasic waveform distal to a stenosis. This is because of the slow systolic acceleration and rounding of the systolic peak. The peak systolic velocity will be decreased and the diastolic velocity increased.
(2:64)

16. **(A)** The spectral waveform does not show aliasing or wraparound of the waveform. However, it does show spectral broadening with complete filling of the spectral window, turbulence, and increased diastolic flow.
(2:54)

17. **(A)** Doppler equation where: *(1:7; 2:26)*

FS = Doppler frequency shift (difference between original transmitted frequency and received frequency)
V = Velocity of the interface
Fo = Original transmitted frequency
Cos = Doppler angle (angle of incidence between the beam and the interface)
c = velocity of sound in the medium

18. **(D)** Percutaneous transluminal angioplasty (PTA) is the nonoperative dilatation of arterial stenoses using inflatable balloon-tip catheters. This procedure has been used to dilate or recanalize arteries or grafts in every anatomic region. It has less risks, shorter recovery time, and is less expensive than surgical revascularization.   *(10:69, 70)*

19. **(B)** Embolization is the introduction of a substance or device via a catheter into a vessel to occlude the vessel and eliminate blood flow.   *(7:431)*

20. **(C)** Hemodynamics is the study of the movement of blood and of the forces concerned. This term is commonly used in vascular ultrasound.   *(7:593)*

21. **(A)** Laminar flow is the normal flow pattern usually seen where blood flow is highest in the center and lowest near the walls creating a parabolic flow profile. Turbulent flow is where fast moving blood moves in diagonal directions secondary to sharp turns, tortuosity, or rough surfaces. Eddy currents are whorls or currents seen in rapid moving blood. Boundary layers are the blood adjacent to the arterial wall with slower flow.   *(Study Guide; 2:5, 54)*

22. **(D)** Photoplethysmograph (PPG) uses a light sensor that shines light into superficial skin layers, and a photoelectric detector measures the reflected light. PPG is a simple noninvasive test for assessing chronic venous insufficiency in postphlebitic patients.
(10:34)

23. **(B)** Vortice. The poststenotic zone is immediately past an arterial stenosis. The flow becomes disorganized with frank swirling movements, which are called vortices.   *(2:63)*

24. **(C)** The Reynolds number (RE) predicts the stability of a fluid and defines the point where flow changes from laminar to turbulent. If the RE exceeds 2000, laminar flow tends to be disturbed. This is a basic principle in fluid dynamics.   *(10:6; 2:6)*

25. **(E)** 2000   *(10:6; 2:6)*

26. **(A)** Poststenotic turbulence is commonly seen immediately distal to an arterial stenosis. In fact, this is usually one of the diagnostic criteria for identification of stenotic lesions. It is described as the flow stream distal to the stenotic lumen spreads out, the laminar flow pattern is lost, and flow becomes disorganized.   *(2:63)*

27. **(A)** Inversely. The volume flow is proportional to the fourth power of the radius so small changes in the radius can make large changes in the flow. The length of the vessel and the viscosity of blood do not change much in the cardiovascular system, so the changes in blood flow occur primarily as a result of changes in the radius of the vessel and the difference in the pressure energy level.   *(2:5)*

28. **(D)** Blood pressure is the pressure exerted on the wall of a blood vessel by the contained blood and the difference in the blood pressure within the vascular system provides the immediate driving force that keeps the blood moving. Pulse pressure is the difference between the systolic pressure and the diastolic pressure. The mean pressure is the average blood pressure throughout the cardiac cycle and blood flow is the volume of blood flowing through a vessel, organ, or circulatory system for a given period of time.   *(1:23)*

29. **(D)** 120/70 mm Hg. The systolic pressure is the peak blood pressure within a large artery approximately 120 mmHg. The diastolic pressure is the lowest pressure during the cardiac cycle, approximately 70 mmHg.   *(1:23)*

30. **(C)** The pulse is the pressure wave created by the expansion and contraction of the arteries during the cardiac cycle. The pulse pressure is the difference between the systolic pressure and diastolic pressure.   *(1:23)*

31. **(A)** Pulse rate or number of pulsations per minute varies and is normally 50 to 100 pulses per minute. *(7:1095)*

32. **(F)** The most significant risk factor is the unavoidable family history. Cigarette smoking, diabetes, aging, and hypertension all lead to the development of atherosclerosis. Bradycardia is slowness of the heart rate and pulse rate. *(10:5)*

33. **(C)** Pressure is not one of the symptoms of lower extremity arterial disease. Claudication is the most common symptom in lower extremity arterial disease. Other symptoms include coldness, cyanosis or color changes, or the absence of pulses. As the ischemia progresses to severe, symptoms will include rest pain, nonhealing ulcers, microemboli, or gangrene of the foot. *(10:24)*

34. **(C)** The classic five Ps for acute arterial ischemia are; pain, pallor, paresthesias, paralysis, and pulselessness. If a patient presents with these symptoms, the extremity is examined to assess the severity of the ischemia and to determine the urgency of further tests and treatment. *(10:24)*

35. **(D)** The ankle brachial index or ankle-brachial pressure is used for peripheral arterial examinations and segmental pressure examinations. Normally, the systolic ankle pressure should be equal to or greater than the systolic pressure. The ratio should be 1.0 or greater. *(10:38)*

36. **(C)** Patients with an ankle brachial index of 0.6–0.9, which falls in the claudication range require exercise testing. These patients with mild arterial disease usually have compensatory collateral flow. Collateral flow provides sufficient flow under resting conditions, but when the extremity is stressed or exercised, there will be claudication pain. Exercise testing normally increases the total limb blood flow; however, with significant arterial disease, ankle pressure will drop after exercise. The time it takes to return to the pre-exercise level is an indication of the severity of disease. *(1:269, 270; 17:38, 40)*

37. **(A)** The pressure is recorded at the site where the cuff is inflated and deflated, even though the Doppler probe is maintained in place at the posterior tibial artery. *(1:268, 269C; 10:37)*

38. **(B)** The cuff at each site is inflated until the systolic pressure, sound, or Doppler waveform disappears. The cuff is slowly released until the sound or Doppler waveform returns. The return of the Doppler sound is then recorded. *(1:269; 10:37)*

39. **(C)** The brachial artery systolic pressure is the standard for segmental arterial studies. The bilateral brachial pressures normally should be within 10 mm Hg of each other. The highest value of the two brachial systolic pressures is used. If the bilateral brachial pressures differ by more than 10 mm Hg, then an upper extremity arterial lesion is suspected. *(1:269)*

40. **(B)** As stated in the answer to question 39, the brachial systolic pressures should be within 10 mm Hg of each other. If there is a greater difference, an upper arterial lesion is suspected on the side with the lowest value. *(1:269)*

41. **(B)** Patients who have intermittent claudication have a pressure index in the range of 0.6–0.9 and are required to have exercise testing to evaluate the severity of disease. *(1:269)*

42. **(C)** An ankle index of 0.5 or less indicates severe arterial occlusive disease and exercise testing is not required. *(1:268; 10:38)*

43. **(D)** Diabetic patients who have calcified vessels may have systolic pressures at the ankle arteries that exceed 300 mm Hg. This exceeds the limit of the automated units to record the systolic pressure. Toes pressures are required using photoplethysmography and toe cuffs. *(1:270; 2:234)*

44. **(C)** The normal toe pressure is 60% of the brachial pressures. *(1:270)*

45. **(A)** Leg exercise increases blood flow. In the presence of significant arterial disease, the ankle pressure drops after exercise for two reasons; first, increased flow across the stenosis results in turbulence and a pressure drop; and second, blood flow is diverted into the higher resistance collaterals of the leg muscles. *(10:400; 1:269, 170)*

46. **(D)** The internal capsule is located in the brain. The composition of the arteries includes: the tunica intima (inner layer), the tunica media (middle layer), and the tunica adventitia (outer layer). *(1:21, 22)*

47. **(C)** Vasoconstriction is the decrease in the caliber of the vessels, especially constriction of arterioles, which leads to decreased blood flow to a part. *(7:1438)*

48. **(A)** The brachiocephalic or innominate arises on the right from the aortic arch and gives rise to the right common carotid artery and the right subclavian artery. On the left, there is no brachiocephalic, the left carotid artery arises from the aortic arch. *(9:734, 737)*

49. **(C)** The axillary artery is a direct continuation of the subclavian artery. The subclavian descends lateral to the lateral margin of the scalenus anterior to

the outer border of the first rib and then becomes the axillary artery. *(9:750)*

50. **(C)** Radial and ulnar artery. The brachial artery is a continuation of the axillary artery. It terminates about a centimeter distal to the elbow joining by dividing into the radial and ulnar arteries. *(9:658)*

51. **(A)** Common femoral artery is a continuation of the external iliac artery. It begins at the inguinal ligament midway between the anterior superior iliac spine and the symphysis pubis. It descends the thigh and becomes the popliteal artery as it passes through the adductor canal. *(9:781)*

52. **(C)** Posterior tibial artery lies posterior to the medial aspect of the tibia and ankle joint. This artery is the one most often used for segmental pressure examination. If the vessel has a low Doppler signal or there is no Doppler signal, alternative vessels are the anterior tibial and dorsalis pedis. *(9:788; 10:37)*

53. **(C)** Ischemia is defined as a deficiency of blood to a part because of the functional constriction or obstruction of a blood vessel. Hallett presents several clinical categories of chronic limb ischemia that are common in dealing with lower extremity arterial disease. *(7:681; 10:180)*

54. **(A)** Embolism is defined as a sudden blocking of an artery by clot or foreign material traveling through the blood stream. There are many origins of embolism, which include; air, coronary, infective, pulmonary, and tumors. *(7:431)*

55. **(B)** Claudication. This is a classical term used to describe peripheral arterial disease and the most common manifestation pf peripheral artery occlusive disease. It actually means to "limp." It is described as pain during exercise that ceases when the activity is stopped. *(10:157; 1:298)*

56. **(B)** Atherosclerosis is the cause of most arterial diseases today. It is defined by the World Health Organization as a combination of changes in the intima and media of the artery. These changes include focal accumulation of lipids, hemorrhage, fibrous tissue, and calcium deposits. *(10:4)*

57. **(C)** The blood flow and pressure are not significantly diminished until at least 75% of the cross-sectional area of the vessel is obliterated. This figure for cross-sectional area can be equated to a 50% reduction in lumen diameter. The formula for the area of a circle (area = $3.14 \times radius^2$) explains the relationship between the cross section and the vessel diameter. *(10:5)*

58. **(E)** Although the radius is the greatest influence on a critical stenosis other factors also influence the critical stenosis to a lesser extent. They include: length of stenosis, blood viscosity, and peripheral resistance. *(10:5)*

59. **(C)** The superficial femoral artery in the adductor canal is a common location of stenosis or occlusion in the lower extremity. This is one of two common anatomic sites. The other is the distal abdominal aorta and iliac arteries. *(10:157)*

60. **(B)** Anterior tibial artery. *(1:223)*

61. **(A)** Subclavian steal syndrome. Occurs more often in the left subclavian artery and is a common atherosclerotic lesion. It is usually discovered because the left brachial blood pressure is significantly lower than the right; however, other clinical symptoms may be present such as: claudication, dizziness, syncope, visual blurring, or ataxia. Subclavian steal is characterized by reversal of blood flow within the vertebral artery resulting from a hemodynamically significant stenosis or occlusion in the proximal subclavian or innominate artery. The steal is induced because of the decreased pressure in the vessel distal to the stenotic lesion, which leads to retrograde flow in the ipsilateal vertebral artery. This retrograde vertebral flow on the side of the lesion is taken from the contralateral vertebral artery, which is stealing it from the basilar artery. *(10:145; 1:114)*

62. **(D)** Reversal of flow in the affected vertebral artery is a classical sign of subclavian steal syndrome. It goes through several stages as the stenosis or occlusion progresses. Beginning with the deceleration of the antegrade flow during systole, followed by an alternating flow with reversal of flow in systole and reduced antegrade flow during diastole and culminating with a reversal of flow during the entire pulse. *(1:115)*

63. **(C)** A difference in bilateral blood pressure in the upper extremity of 10–20 mm Hg and a decreased peripheral pulse in the affected upper extremity is a hallmark sign of subclavian steal. *(1:116)*

64. **(B)** Thoracic outlet syndrome is defined as compression of the brachial plexus nerve trunks characterized by pain, paresthesia of fingers, vasomotor symptoms, and weakness of the small muscles of the hand. The subclavian artery leaves the chest by the thoracic outlet. It passes over the first rib, behind the clavicle, and between the anterior and middle scalene muscles. Because of the confines of the thoracic outlet the subclavian artery, the subclavian vein, and the brachial plexus are subject to compression. Noninvasive testing for this entity requires special maneuvers, which include: exaggerated military position, hyperabduction, and Adson maneuver. The rationale is to determine any obliteration of the blood flow, which relates to specific positions. *(7:1298; 2:249; 1:285)*

65. (C) Multimaneuvers are used for the evaluation of thoracic outlet syndrome. These positions are used to demonstrate an obliteration of blood flow relating to specific positions. During the maneuvers, the waveforms are recorded by Doppler or photoplethysmography to identify any change in blood flow. *(1:285)*

66. (A) Raynaud's disease is an innocuous vasospastic disorder; whereas, Raynaud's phenomenon is an underlying systemic or vascular abnormality with vascular occlusion. *(1:283)*

67. (B) Raynaud's phenomenon is associated with occlusive disease, whereas Raynaud's disease is associated with vasospasm. *(1:283)*

68. (C) Pseudoaneurysms (false aneurysms) do not have a true arterial wall and are usually the result of vascular injury caused by trauma or previous surgical reconstruction. The pseudoaneurysm lies outside the arterial wall; whereas, the true aneurysm is contiguous with the arterial wall. *(1:82)*

69. (B) Mycotic aneurysms are secondary to an infectious process that involves the arterial wall. *(1:197)*

70. (C) Arterial dissection usually develops secondary to a tear in the intimal layer, which allows blood to enter the wall of the vessel and the creation of two lumens. Characteristically, a moving flap is seen in the lumen of the vessel with real-time imaging. *(1:201–203)*

71. (C) Ankle brachial index quantitates the blood flow. The segmental pressures combined with the ABI provide an assessment of arterial disease in the entire extremity. It determines the level of disease and estimates the severity of the disease. This exam is often used for arterial screening of the lower extremities. Duplex and color flow Doppler provide anatomical detail and hemodynamics but cannot quantitate the flow. *(1:267; 2:208)*

72. (D) A decrease in peak systolic flow velocity to less than 45 cm/s would indicate impending graft failure. The normal graft has a hyperemic waveform (forward flow throughout the pulse cycle) and a systolic flow velocity of more than 45 cm/s. *(1:303)*

73. (C) Arteriovenous fistula is an abnormal communication between an artery and a vein. They may be the result of a congenital defect, created by surgical means as seen in the dialysis access graft (Brescia–Cimino), or caused by trauma as seen secondary to percutaneous biopsy procedures in the renal or liver transplant created trauma. *(7:506; 2:260)*

74. (B) The resistive index calculates and quantifies resistance to blood flow. A high-resistance waveform pattern has a high systolic peak and a low diastolic flow. The resistance can be calculated using the resistive index, systolic frequency (S), minus diastolic frequency (D), divided by the systolic frequency. *(18:27)*

75. (A) Tachycardia refers to a rapid heart beat and usually means a heart rate above 100 bpm. *(7:1307)*

76. (D) Angiography is an invasive procedures using computerized fluoroscopy for direct visualization of the arterial system after injection of a contrast medium. *(10:67)*

77. (B) The ankle/brachial index (ABI) is the measurement of the systolic blood pressure at the ankle divided by the brachial pressure. It is used to determine the presence and severity of arterial disease. *(1:27)*

78. (C) The patient history should always be obtained before the vascular examination. It provides valuable information as to the patients symptoms and related problems. It also ensures that a complete evaluation of the patient is performed. In some cases, the clinical history may be incorrect or the wrong examination is ordered. By talking to the patient and acquiring history and clinical information, we can make sure our information is correct and the correct exam is being performed. If it is not, we can take the necessary time to talk to the clinician to make sure our information is correct. *(10:17)*

79. (C) Segmental arterial pressures can be obtained using three or four cuffs. It is preferred to use four cuffs to differentiation between the common femoral artery and superficial femoral artery lesions. This is not possible with the three-cuff method. *(1:268)*

80. (D) Microbubbles of air are used for most sonographic contrast agents. The success of the more sophisticated contrast agents has been dependent on stabilization of these micro air bubbles because they are usually short lived in the peripheral circulation, and to transport them within the body by means of a carrier agent. *(2:87)*

81. (B) The cardiovascular system has two major pathways, the systemic circulation, and pulmonary circulation. The path of the blood from the left ventricle through the body is the systemic circulation and its passage from the right ventricle via the lungs to the left atrium is the pulmonary circulation. *(2:21; 9:683)*

82. (B) Tunica media is the fibromuscular middle layer that extends from the internal to external elastic lamina and is circumferential. It is the thickest layer of the arterial and aids in maintaining continuous circulation and appropriate blood pressure by controlling the diameter of the vessel lumen.

(2:22; 9:684)

83. **(D)** The vertebral artery is the first branch of the subclavian artery. It arises from the superoposterior aspect of the subclavian artery. *(1:105)*

84. **(A)** Femoral artery. *(Study Guide)*

85. **(B)** Femoral vein. *(Study Guide)*

86. **(D)** Femoral vein. *(Study Guide)*

87. **(B)** Femoral artery. *(Study Guide)*

88. **(C)** Greater saphenous vein. *(Study Guide)*

89. **(A)** Profunda (deep) femoral vein and artery.
(Study Guide)

90. **(D)** Popliteal artery. *(Study Guide)*

91. **(B)** Popliteal vein. *(Study Guide)*

92. **(A)** Lesser (small) saphenous vein.
(Study Guide)

93. **(C)** Greater saphenous vein. *(Study Guide)*

94. **(F)** Distal aorta artery. *(Study Guide)*

95. **(G)** External iliac artery. *(Study Guide)*

96. **(A)** Internal iliac artery. *(Study Guide)*

97. **(E)** Common femoral artery. *(Study Guide)*

98. **(C)** Superficial femoral artery. *(Study Guide)*

99. **(D)** Profunda (deep) femoral artery.
(Study Guide)

100. **(B)** Popliteal artery. *(Study Guide)*

101. **(B)** Popliteal artery. *(Study Guide)*

102. **(E)** Anterior tibial artery. *(Study Guide)*

103. **(F)** Posterior tibial artery. *(Study Guide)*

104. **(A)** Peroneal artery. *(Study Guide)*

105. **(C)** Plantar metatarsal arteries. *(Study Guide)*

106. **(D)** Digital arteries. *(Study Guide)*

107. **(A)** 20–49% diameter reduction stenosis.
(Study Guide)

108. **(D)** 1–19% diameter reduction stenosis.
(Study Guide)

109. **(C)** 50–99% diameter reduction stenosis.
(Study Guide)

110. **(B)** 0% diameter reduction stenosis.
(Study Guide)

111. **(F)** All of the above. Intermittent claudication is usually the first symptom of arterial disease. As the disease progresses to the point of rest pain, the trophic skin changes, dependent rubor, and pallor on elevation occur. If the level of disease is aortoiliac, it often renders the male impotent because the penile circulation branches from the internal iliac. *(19:5)*

112. **(F)** All of the above. Atherosclerosis is a disease process that is influenced by several risk factors: family history, smoking, hypertension, hyperlipidemia, diabetes mellitus, malignancies, and aging. *(10:5)*

113. **(C)** The Doppler signal shows normal triphasic flow with a peak systolic velocity of 83 cm/s, which is within the normal range of velocities. *(17:522–529)*

114. **(A)** A hemodynamically significant lesion is a 50% diameter reduction or greater. As the stenotic segment exceeds 50%, the peak-systolic velocities also increase. The ratio of systolic to diastolic velocities begins to fall. *(2:62, 63)*

115. **(A)** The source of origin of the Doppler signal is derived from the sample volume location on the 2-D image and not from the spectral display. Amplitude of the Doppler signal, pulsatility features of the waveform, velocity or frequency shift of the blood flow, and direction of flow are all obtained from the spectral display. *(2:33, 48)*

116. **(B)** A clear spectral window indicates laminar flow with little flow disturbances. A small sample volume placed in the central portion of the normal flow stream will produce a crisp, clear window. Flow disturbances, such as vortices and swirling eddies, will decrease the size of the spectral window and should demonstrate flow reversal as well. Spectral broadening can occur with moderate stenotic lesions as well as severe lesions. *(20:103–104)*

117. **(A)** Critical stenosis. The critical stenosis occurs with a diameter reduction of 50% or greater (area reduction of 75%) or greater. This is also called a hemodynamically significant lesion. *(20:23)*

118. **(B)** The two principal mechanisms that control blood volume are the cardiac output and the peripheral resistance. Cardiac output (mL/s) is the rate of blood flow per minute. Two factors that affect cardiac

output are heart rate and stroke volume. Peripheral resistance is controlled by the arterioles and arterial capillaries. These tiny vessels control the volume of blood flow.   *(20:157–159, 163–165)*

119. **(C)** The major advantage of continuous wave Doppler is that it can display high velocities without the phenomena of aliasing occurring. Unfortunately, it has no range resolution, and its sample size cannot be controlled.   *(21:108)*

120. **(E)** Doppler shift frequencies are affected by Doppler angle, transducer frequency, and the velocity of the red blood cells. As the Doppler angle decreases between the Doppler beam and the flow stream, there will be an increase in the frequency shift. If the transducer frequency decreases, the frequency shift will decrease. The velocity of the red blood cells will affect the Doppler shift. As the red blood cells move faster, the frequency shift will increase.   *(15:5–7)*

121. **(C)** As an arterial stenosis exceeds 60%, the peak systolic velocity will increase and the volume of the flow will decrease.   *(20:62)*

122. **(A)** The single most valuable Doppler finding is increased velocity in the stenotic zone for determining the severity of arterial stenosis.   *(2:55)*

123. **(C)** Disturbed flow is seen throughout the stenotic lesion and just distal to the stenosis in the post-stenotic zone. The maximal flow disturbance usually occurs within 1 cm beyond the stenosis.   *(2:63)*

124. **(B)** As the radius of an artery decreases, the resistance to flow will increase.   *(21:147–149)*

125. **(D)** Volume flow is not used in determining the severity of arterial stenosis. There are three stenotic zone velocity measurements commonly used to determine the severity of arterial stenoses: peak systolic velocity, end diastolic velocity, and the systolic velocity ratio (comparison of peak systole in stenoses to peak systole in the proximal normal segment.   *(2:55)*

126. **(C)** In a 50–99% diameter reduction of the artery, there will be a loss of reverse flow with forward flow throughout the cardiac cycle and distal to the stenosis the waveform will be damped and monophasic.   *(2:271)*

127. **(C)** Fig. 13–56. Iliac artery graft occlusion. The iliac graft is seen in a longitudinal plane with the characteristic corrugated appearance. Color Doppler identifies adjacent blood flow; however, there is absence of flow in the graft compatible with graft occlusion.   *(1:303, 307; 2:276)*

128. **(B)** Fig. 13–57. The proximal iliac artery demonstrates aliasing with velocity in excess of 200 cm/s and a loss of the reverse component which would indicate iliac artery stenosis. In the poststenotic zone there would be a damping monophasic waveform and with occlusion there would be no Doppler signal.   *(2:271)*

129. **(C)** Fig. 13–58. Bilateral severe occlusive arterial disease. Bilateral iliac artery stenosis with monophasic waveforms throughout the lower extremity and abnormal segmental pressures. The ABI is 0.4 on the right and 0.6 on the left indicating severe occlusive arterial disease. Normally, the waveforms would be triphasic, and there would be a pressure gradient of greater than 30 mm Hg between each cuff. The upper thigh pressure should be at lease 40 mmHG above the brachial pressure. Usually the cutoff for severe occlusive arterial disease is 0.5 or less; however, the waveforms indicate severe disease and exercise revealed a slow recovery time which would confirm the diagnosis.   *(1:268, 297)*

130. **(C)** Fig. 13–59. Bilateral iliac artery disease. Abnormal Doppler waveforms bilaterally with zero flow or severely damped monophasic flow. ABI could not be obtained because of absence of flow in the lower extremities.   *(13:12, 13)*

131. **(A)** Fig. 13–60. Position for thoracic outlet compression. It is the Adson maneuver using attached photo cells for photoplethysmographic recording of the waveform.   *(1:285–287)*

132. **(C)** Fig. 13–61. Shows an aneurysm with calcifications of the wall in the distal aorta. The focal dilatation is easily noted in comparison with the proximal portion as is the echogenic rim caused by wall calcification. A dissection of the aorta would have a moving membrane with two lumens.   *(1:199, 200)*

133. **(c)** Zero baseline   *(Study Guide;1:6; 13:3)*

134. **(b)** Spectral window   *(Study Guide;1:6; 13:3)*

135. **(a)** Bandwidth   *(Study Guide;1:6; 13:3)*

136. **(I)**   *(Study Guide;14:14, 15)*

137. **(G)**   *(Study Guide;14:14, 15)*

138. **(H)**   *(Study Guide;14:14, 15)*

139. **(J)**   *(Study Guide;14:14, 15)*

140. **(F)**   *(Study Guide;14:14, 15)*

141. **(D)**   *(Study Guide;14:14, 15)*

142. (A) *(Study Guide;14:14, 15)*

143. (E) *(Study Guide;14:14, 15)*

144. (C) *(Study Guide;14:14, 15)*

145. (B) *(Study Guide;14:14, 15)*

146. (B) Femoral–Popliteal (Fem–Pop) arterial graft.
(1:302, 303)

147. (C) ABI on the right is 1.03, which is normal. ABI on the left is 0.69, which is in the claudication range.
(1:268)

148. (D) Sample volume. The frequency spectrum shows the blood flow information from a specific location using the sample volume. The spectral analysis is the display of the frequency distribution within the signal, but the sample volume denotes the specific location. The Doppler angle governs the intensity of the reflected wave and the field of view governs the viewing area of the vessels.
(1:268)

149. (A) Digital blood pressure is normally within 20–30 mm Hg of the brachial pressure. This usually corresponds to a ratio of finger systolic pressure to brachial systolic pressure of greater than 80%.
(2:255)

150. (B) Very rapidly. Flow velocity in a normal artery accelerates very rapidly in systole. It produces an almost vertical deflection of the Doppler waveform at the beginning of systole.
(2:52)

REFERENCES

References appear on pages 590–591.

CHAPTER 14

NEUROSONOLOGY

Chandrowti Devi Persaud, Karen K. Rawls, Carol A. Krebs, and Charles S. Odwin

INTRODUCTION

Neurosonology had its beginning in the late 1960s and early 1970s. One of the first applications was the A-mode or amplitude mode to determine midline shifts. If, in fact, the midline was shifted, this was an indication of a tumor or pathology. As newer technology and gray-scale imaging emerged so did new applications. The A-mode midline shift examination was quickly replaced with computerized axial tomography. The realization that the open fontanelles in neonates offered a sonographic window to permit ultrasound scanning of the neonatal brain opened new technological advances. Gray-scale imaging became a mainstay in the neonatal department primarily to detect intracranial hemorrhage and monitor enlargement of the ventricles. Ultrasound was also being utilized in neurosurgery to localize lesions and pathology during the surgical procedure. The introduction of color flow Doppler added additional diagnostic capabilities for identifying vascular variances and anomalies in the neonate.[1] It was also a time when transcranial Doppler was introduced using the transtemporal window for examination of the adult patients. Neurosonology has been an ongoing expanding speciality for the last 30 years. It now requires the sonographer to have a well rounded knowledge encompassing anatomy, vascular hemodynamics, positioning, and instrumentation. Transcranial Doppler and vascular studies are included in the cerebrovascular section. This chapter deals primarily with neonatal neurology.

INSTRUMENTATION AND TECHNIQUE

Real-time gray-scale imaging using a 5 or 7.5 MHz frequency is most commonly used in the evaluation of the neonatal brain. Higher frequencies such as 10 MHz may be used for superficial structures. Duplex and color flow Doppler sonography are used to evaluate congenital vascular anomalies, cerebral perfusion, and vascular anatomy.[2]

The anterior fontanelle is used as an acoustic window in the first year of life. It starts to close at 9 months and is completely closed in 12 months.[2] Standard scanning planes and views for evaluations of the brain are coronal, sagittal, and axial.

Coronal. These scans are obtained through the frontal fontanelle (Fig. 14–1 A–F). The six standard scans are at the level of

- frontal horns (anterior to the foramen of Monro)
- foramen of Monro
- posterior aspect of the third ventricle through the thalami
- quadridgeminal cistern
- trigones of the lateral ventricles
- parietal and occipital cortex

Sagittal. These scans are obtained through the frontal fontanelle (Fig. 14–2 A,B). The three standard scans include:

- *Midsagittal plane,* which includes the following anatomical landmarks: cavum septi pellucidi, cavum vergae, corpus callosum, pericallosal artery, cingulate sulcus and gyrus, third ventricle, massa intermedia in the third ventricle (seen with hydrocephalus), quadridgeminal cistern, fourth ventricle, brain sten (pons and medulla), and the cisternal magna.[2]
- *Parasagittal* right and left planes which include the following anatomical landmarks: caudothalamic groove, caudate nucleus, thalamus, and anterior portions of the choroid plexus.
- *Parasagittal* slightly more lateral than the above on the right and left, which includes the following anatomical landmarks: the body, occipital and temporal horns of the lateral ventricles, and the glomus (largest) part of the choroid plexus. The frontal, parietal, temporal, and occipital lobes are seen surrounding the lateral ventricle.

Axial. These scans are obtained through the squamosal portion of either temporal bone. To obtain the desired images and anatomical landmarks, the transducer is angled superiorly. The ventricles are seen just above the choroid plexus. The lateral ventricular measurements are obtained in this position or the squamosal fontanelle.

MNEMONICS

Mnemonics are just one of many useful ways to formulate words that will help you remember. How fast you learn, and how much you retain after you learn, may be a big

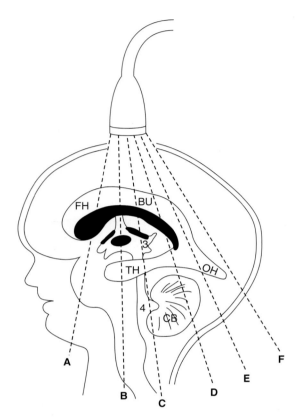

Figure 14–1. Schematic of the coronal planes.

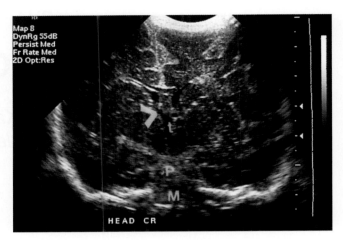

Figure 14–1B. Coronal sonogram represents plane B. Arrowhead = foramen of Monro, t = third ventricle, p = pons, m = medulla oblongata.

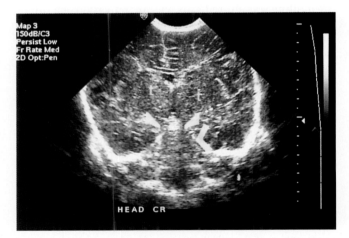

Figure 14–1C. Coronal sonogram represents plane C. t = thalamus, single arrowhead = tentorium, half-arrowheads = cerebral peduncles.

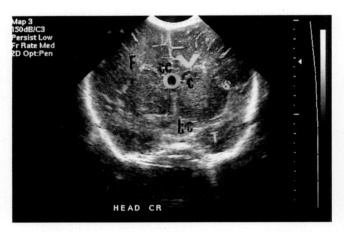

Figure 14–1A. Coronal sonogram represents plane A. Circle = cavum sept pellucidi, CC = corpus callosum, c = caudate nucleus, white arrowhead = lateral ventricle, F = frontal lobe, T = temporal lobe.

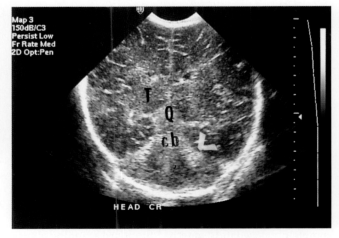

Figure 14–1D. Coronal sonogram represents plane D. T = thalamus, Q = quadridgeminal cistern, arrowhead = tentarium, cb = cerebellum.

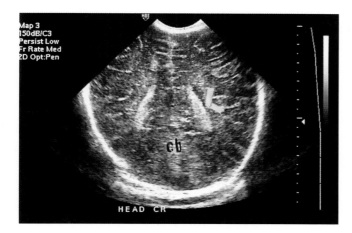

Figure 14–1E. Coronal sonogram represents plane E. Arrowhead = to chorid plexus, cb = cerebellum.

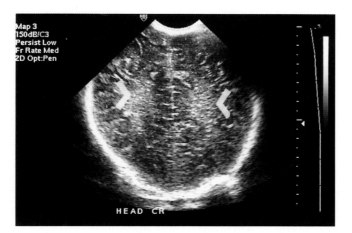

Figure 14–1F. Coronal sonogram represents plane F. Area between arrowheads = white matter of the occipital lobe and sulci.

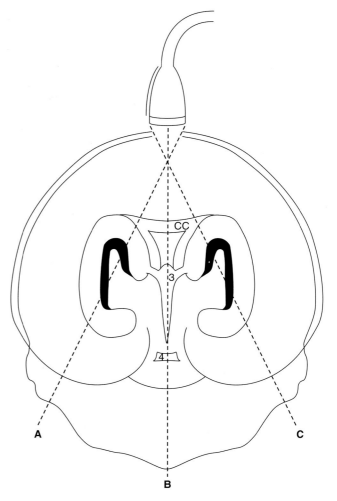

Figure 14–2. Schematic of the sagittal planes.

factor in taking examinations. The following are study groups. Formulate your own mnemonic device to help you remember them.

The mnemonic "SCALP" serves as a memory key for the five layers of the scalp listed below:

S	skin
C	connective tissue
A	aponeurosis epicranialis
L	loose connective tissue
P	pericranium

The mnemonic "PAD" serves as a memory key for the three layers of membranes called meninges, which cover the brain and spinal cord from inner to outer.
The three layers are as follows:

P	pia
A	arachnoid
D	dura

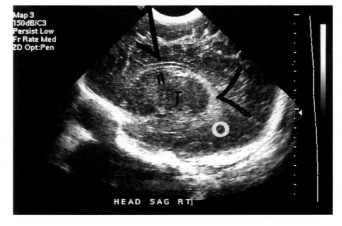

Figure 14–2A. Parasagittal sonogram represents plane A. Half-arrow = lateral ventricle, T = thalamus, n = caudate nucleus, arrowhead = choroid plexus, white circle = occipital lobe.

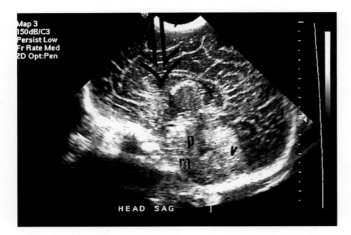

Figure 14–2B. Sagittal sonogram represents plane B. Large arrowhead = corpus callosum, V = cerebellar vermis, p = pons, m = medulla. Fourth ventricle is the small sonolucent area anterior to the cerebellar vermis.

A mnemonic for the 12 cranial nerves is "O,O,O Tell Ted And Frances About Going Vacationing After Halloween."

O	olfactory
O	optic
O	oculomotor
T	trochlear
T	trigeminal
A	abducens
F	facial
A	acoustic
G	glossopharyngeal
V	vagus
A	accessory
H	hypoglossal

A fontanelle is where several sutures meet and form a triangular space that encloses a membrane called a "soft spot." There are six fontanelles:

One posterior
Two mastoidal
Two sphenoidal

The mnemonic "MAPS" serves as a memory key for these fontanelles:

M	mastoidal
A	anterior
P	posterior
S	sphenoidal

The time of closure for the fontanelles vary. The posterior is the first to close at 2–3 months, with the anterior closing at 18 months, and the mastoid closing by 1 year.

The mnemonic "SAC" serves as a memory key for the three scanning planes used in neonatal cranial sonography.

S	sagittal scan taken along the axis of the sagittal suture (longitudinal in the skull)
A	axial scan taken from a lateral approach through the temporal bone.
C	coronal scan taken along the axis of the coronal suture (transverse in the skull)

TERMINOLOGY

The following definitions of the various anatomic structures associated with sonographic neurologic examinations will enhance your understanding of the anatomic diagrams in the subsequent text.

Arachnoid—The middle layer of meninges covering the brain and spinal cord.

Atrium (Trigone) of the Lateral Ventricles—This is where the anterior, occipital, and temporal horns join.

Brainstem—Part of the brain connected to the forebrain and the spinal cord. It consists of the midbrain, pons, and medulla oblongata.[1]

Caudate Nucleus—Consists of a head, body, and tail. It lies next to the lateral wall of the lateral ventricles.

Cavum Septi Pellucidi—A thin triangular hole filled with cerebrospinal fluid that lies between the anterior horns of the lateral ventricles. If located posteriorly, it is termed a cavum vergae. The cavum septi pellucidi has also been referred to as a fifth ventricle and the cavum vergae as a sixth ventricle.

Central Nervous System—The central nervous system consists of the cerebellum, cerebrum, spinal cord, pons (brain stem), and medulla.

Cerebellum—Portion of the brain that lies posterior to the pons and medulla oblongata below the tentorium.

Cerebral Hemispheres—These are paired brain matter separated from the midline by the falx cerebri.

Cerebrum—The largest part of the brain, which consists of two hemispheres.[1]

Choroid Plexus—Mass of special cells located in the atrium of the lateral ventricles. They regulate the intraventricular pressure by secreting or absorbing cerebrospinal fluid.[1]

Cistern—Enclosed space serving as a reservoir for cerebrospinal fluid.

Corpus Callosum—Large group of nerve fibers visible superior to the third ventricle that connects the left and right sides of the brain.[1]

Ependyma—The membrane lining the cerebral ventricles.[1]

Epidural—Lies outside the dura matter.

Falx Cerebri (interhemispheric fissure)—A fibrous structure separating the two cerebral hemispheres.

Germinal Matrix—Periventricular tissue including the caudate nucleus. Before 32 weeks gestation, it is fragile and bleeds easily.[1]

Gyri—Convolutions on the surface of the brain caused by infolding of the cortex.[1]

Massa Intermedia—Also called the interthalamic adhesion, this is the place of fusion between the third ventricle and the medial surface of the thalami.

Meninges—The brain coverings.[1]

Mesencephalon—Midbrain.

Parenchyma—Cortex tissue of the brain.[1]

Pia Mater—The innermost of the three membranes covering the brain and spinal cord.

Pineal Recess—Posterior recess on the third ventricle. There are two posterior recesses: the pineal and the suprapineal recess.

Prosencephalon—Forebrain.

Rhombencephalon—Hindbrain.

Subdural—Between the dura mater and the arachnoid.

Subependyma—Area immediately beneath the ependyma. In the caudate nucleus, it is the site of hemorrhage from the germinal matrix.

Subarachnoid—Between the arachnoid and the pia mater.

Sulcus—A groove or depression on the surfaceof the brain, separating the gyri.[1]

Suprapineal recess—One of the two posterior recesses on the third ventricle.

Sylvian Fissure—Lateral cerebri fissure.

Telea Choroidea—Point where the choroid attached to the floor of the lateral ventricles and located behind the foramen of Monro. Most common site of hemorrhage.

Tentorium—V shaped echogenic structure which separates the cerebrum and the cerebellum and is an extension of the falx cerebri.[1]

Thalamus—Two ovoid brain structures situated on either side of the third ventricle superior to the brainstem.[1]

Ventricle—A cavity within the brain containing cerebrospinal fluid.[1]

Vermis Cerebellum—Median part of the cerebellum which lies between the two hemispheres.

ANATOMY

It is essential to know the basic anatomy of the brain. The main parts of the brain are the cerebrum, cerebellum, and the brain stem.

Cerebrum

The cerebrum is divided into two cerebral hemispheres by the longitudinal fissure and connected by the corpus collosum. It is made up of six lobes. The lobes are named according to the skull bones they lie under.

Lobes of the brain and the main functions are:

- One frontal lobe—functions include personality, language, and judgement
- Two parietal lobes—functions include senses and muscle control
- Two temporal lobes—function is auditory
- One occipital lobe—function is vision

The cerebrum consists of an outer thin gray matter called cerebral cortex and inner white matter. On the surface, there are numerous ridges or convolutions gyri and sulci (grooves). Gyri appear hypoechoic and are marked off by sulci. Sulci appear echogenic. Prominent sulci are pericallosal sulcus, cingulate sulcus and the calcarine sulcus. Deep sulci are called fissures. Fissures appear echogenic and are the longitudinal, transverse, fissure of Rolando (central sulcus), and the Sylvian fissure (lateral sulcus).

Cerebellum

The cerebellum is divided by the vermis into two hemispheres and separated from the occipital lobe by the transverse fissure superiorly. It has an inner white matter and thin gray outer cortex. On the sonogram, it appears echogenic. Functions include muscle coordination and equilibrium.

Brain Stem

Superiorly the brain stem includes: diencephalon, midbrain, pons and the medulla oblongata inferiorly. It lies between the base of the cerebrum and the spinal cord. The diencephalon includes the thalamus and the hypothalamus. The midbrain includes the cerebral aqueduct, cerebral peduncle, and the corpora quadrigeminus. The brain stem functions mainly for automatic survival, controls the heartbeat and breathing, and acts as a relay station for sensory impulses and reflexes.

Basal Ganglia

The basal ganglia is the gray matter that lies deep within the cerebral hemispheres. It includes the caudate nucleus, putamen, and globus pallidus. The caudate nucleus is a common site for intracranial hemorrhage.

There are four ventricles. The first and second are called the right and left lateral ventricles. The lateral ventricles are the largest cerebrospinal filled cavities. Each lateral ventricle is arbitrarily divided into the frontal horn, body, occipital horn, and temporal horn. The third and fourth are below the first and second. Between the frontal horns of the lateral ventricle is the cavum septum pellucidum; between the bodies of the two lateral ventricles is the cavum vergae. The third ventricle is bridged by the massa intermedia. There are several foramens which include:

Foramen of Monro—Also termed intraventricular foramen, it divides the frontal horn anteriorly from the body of the ventricle posteriorly and connects the third ventricle with the lateral ventricle.

Aqueduct of Sylvius—Also called the cerebral aqueduct, it connects the third and fourth ventricle.

Foramen of Luschka—The opening in the roof of the fourth ventricle for circulation of the cerebrospinal fluid.

Foramen of Magendie—The opening in the roof of the fourth ventricle for circulation of the cerebrospinal fluid.

The following pages contain illustrations of anatomical structures. Study each illustration carefully, then close your examination book and try to form a photographic image of the illustration in your mind. Then draw and label the illustration on a separate sheet of paper without referring to the illustration. Although this process may sound difficult at first, it is a simple method of developing a photographic memory. As sonographers, we see hundreds of sonographic images each day and have probably used photographic memory without even realizing it. Go ahead and try this with the following illustrations (Figs. 14–3 to 14–30).

DISEASE AND PATHOLOGY

Intracranial Hemorrhage

The most common intracranial pathology in neonates and infants is intracranial hemorrhage. Clinical symptoms may include respiratory distress syndrome, hematocrit drop, prematurity (less than 32 weeks or 1850 grams) or problems during delivery. Most bleeds occur within 72 hours after birth. Later complications of hemorrhage include hydrocephalus and porencephalic cyst.[1]

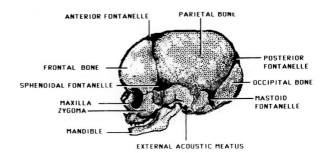

Figure 14–3. Diagram of a lateral view of the infantile skull.

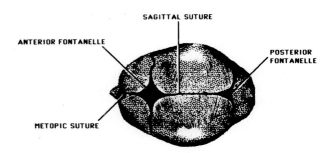

Figure 14–4. A diagram of a superior view of the infantile skull.

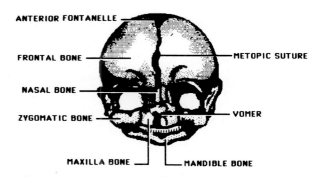

Figure 14–5. An anterior view of an infantile skull.

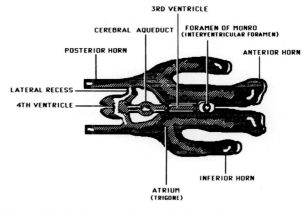

Figure 14–6. A diagram of the ventricular system, superior view.

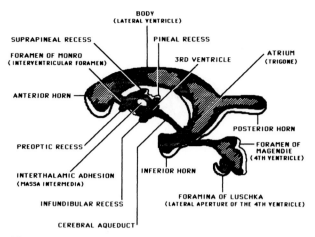

Figure 14–7. A diagram of the ventricular system, lateral view.

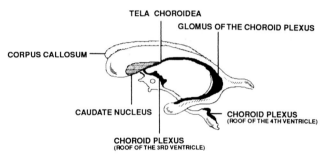

Figure 14–8. A diagram of the ventricular system and choroid plexus, lateral view.

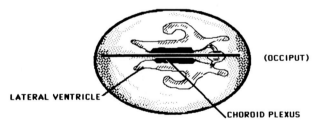

Figure 14–9. A diagram of an axial view at the level of the lateral ventricle.

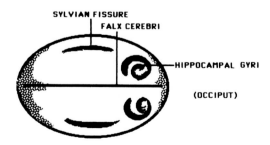

Figure 14–10. A diagram of an axial view at the level of the sylvian fissure.

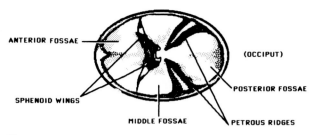

Figure 14–11. A diagram of an axial view at the base of the skull.

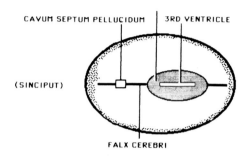

Figure 14–12. A diagram of an axial view at the level of the thalami.

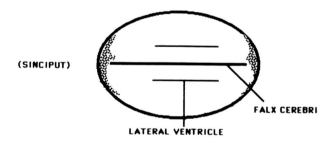

Figure 14–13. A diagram of an axial view at the level of the lateral ventricle.

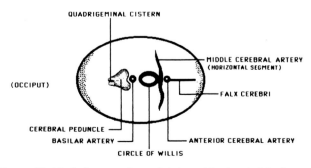

Figure 14–14. A diagram of an axial view at the level of the base of the skull.

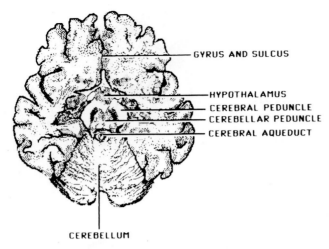

Figure 14–15. A diagram of a coronal section of the brain.

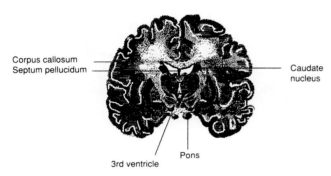

Figure 14–16. A diagram of a coronal section of the brain.

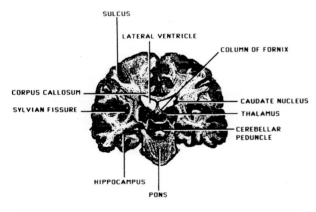

Figure 14–17. A diagram of a coronal section of the brain.

There are several types of hemorrhages according to the location. These include:

a. *SHE: subependymal* hemorrhage, which occurs in the caudate nucleus and can be seen inferior to the floor of the lateral ventricles[1] (Fig. 14–31).

b. *IVH: intraventricular* hemorrhage occurs within the ventricles and can completely fill the ventricles forming a cast[1] (Fig. 14–32).

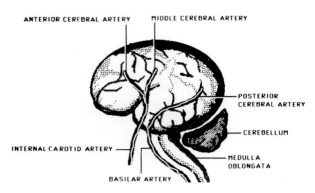

Figure 14–18. A diagram of the brain and arteries, sagittal section.

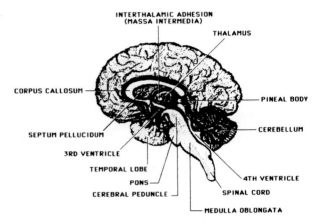

Figure 14–19. A diagram of the brain, sagittal section.

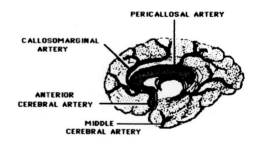

Figure 14–20. A diagram of the lateral aspect of the internal carotid artery divisions.

c. *IPA: intraparenchymal* hemorrhage occurs within the brain substance, usually near the caudate nucleus and lateral to the ventricles. Dilatation of the lateral ventricles is often associated with parenchymal hemorrhage[1] (Fig. 14–33).

d. *CPH: Choroid* and cerebella hemorrhage occur within the echogenic choroid and cerebellum. They may be difficult to distinguish; however, outline irregularity and increased echogenicity will suggest a hemorrhage.[1]

e. *GMH: germinal matrix hemorrhage* this is the site of many subependymal hemorrhages and is often associated with prematurity.

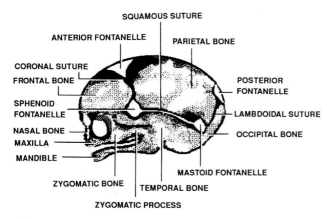

Figure 14–21. A diagram of a lateral view of the infantile skull.

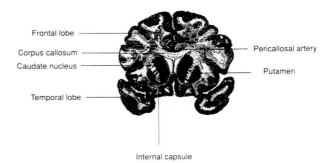

Figure 14–24. A diagram of a coronal section of the brain.

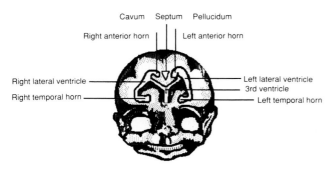

Figure 14–22. A diagram of an anterior view of the infantile skull with the ventricular system.

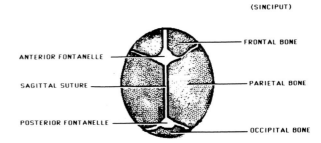

Figure 14–25. A superior view of an infantile skull.

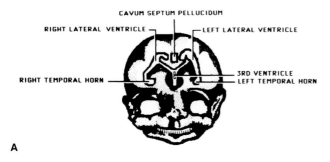

A

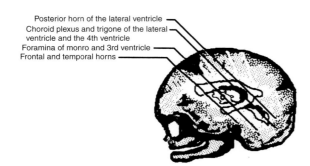

B

Figure 14–23. A diagram of **(A)** an anterior view and **(B)** a lateral view of the infantile skull with the ventricular system.

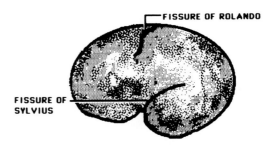

Figure 14–26. A lateral view of the brain.

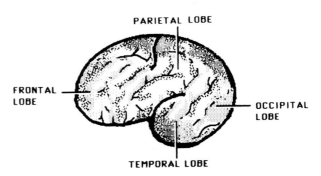

Figure 14–27. A lateral view of the brain.

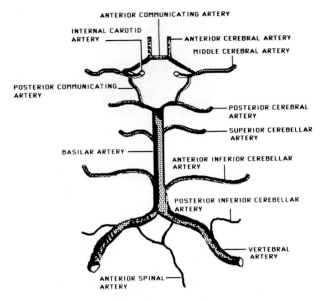

Figure 14–28. The circle of Willis.

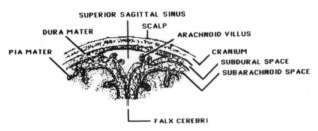

Figure 14–29. A diagram of a coronal section of the meninges and cortex.

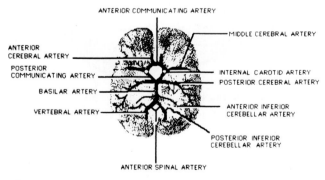

Figure 14–30. A diagram of the arteries at the base of the brain.

f. *SAH: subarachnoid hemorrhage* is located between the arachnoid and pia mater and may be difficult to see on ultrasound unless there is a large amount of blood present.

The sonographic appearance of intracranial hemorrhage changes with time. Early hemorrhages are echogenic and change to decreased echogenicity in a few weeks. The end result is often porencephalic cysts.[1]

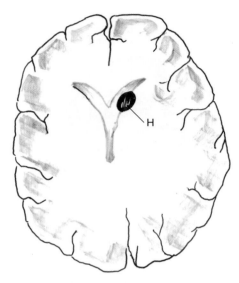

Figure 14–31. Subependymal hemorrhage (H).

Grading of Intracranial Hemorrhage[2]

Grade 1. This is a germinal matrix or subependymal hemorrhage. It is seen inferolaterally to the floor of the frontal horn or body of the lateral ventricle and medially to the head of the caudate nucleus.

Grade 2. This is an intraventricular hemorrhage presented with no dilatation and may coexist with germinal matrix hemorrhage.

Grade 3. This is an intraventricular hemorrhage with dilatation of the ventricle and may coexist with germinal matrix hemorrhage.

Grade 4. This is an intraparenchymal hemorrhage, which may coexist with germinal matrix and intraventricular hemorrhage with or without dilatation.

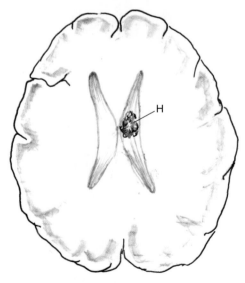

Figure 14–32. Intraventricular hemorrhage (H).

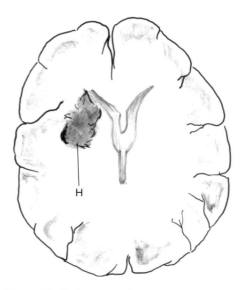

Figure 14–33. Intraparenchymal hemorrhage (H).

Porencephalic Cyst. This is a cyst arising from the ventricle that develops secondary to parenchymal hemorrhage[1] (Fig. 14–34).

Hydrocephalus. Ventricular dilatation is most often secondary to obstruction of the cerebrospinal flow pathways. This is typically associated with enlargement of the head, brain atrophy, and mental deterioration. It is first seen sonographically in the occipital horn, followed by the body and the anterior horn. It can be a minimal, moderate, or marked degree. The third and fourth ventricles are normally barely seen on the scan, so dilatation is easy to visualize.[1] Ultrasound monitors ventricular enlargement and if a shunt placement is required, it can assist in localization. In addition, ultrasound can provide follow up examinations for the shunt procedure to ensure patency[1] (Fig. 14–35).

Periventricular Leukomalacia. Periventricular leukomalacia (PVL) occurs in neonates who have had asphyxia.[1] It is a region of coagulation necrosis and rarified neutrophile areas that contain swollen axons or macrophages followed by a reaction of microglia cells and astrocytosis. Hemorrhage may accompany the infarction, and the areas of necrosis may liquify and cavitate.[3] Sonographically, this condition will present with lesions distinctly separate from the caudate nucleus and usually adjacent to the atrium of the lateral ventricles. There will be increased echoes at the external angle of the lateral ventricles, with extensions radiating anterior to the frontal horns. It may be asymmetrical or bilateral. The echo intensity decreases in 2–4 weeks, and cysts or cavities are seen later in the previously echogenic areas[4] (Fig. 14–36).

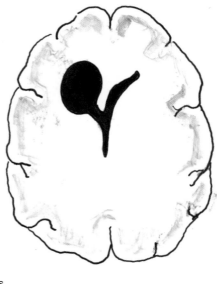

Stages

Echagenic Hemorrage

Resolution Changes of Hemorrhage

Mature Cystic Porencephalic Cysi

Figure 14–34. Porencephalic cyst.

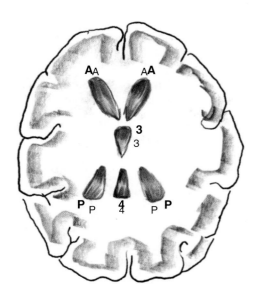

(obstruction with enlargement of the ventricles)
A = Anterior horn
P = Posterior horn
3 = Third ventricle
4 = Fourth ventricle

Figure 14–35. Hydrocephalus.

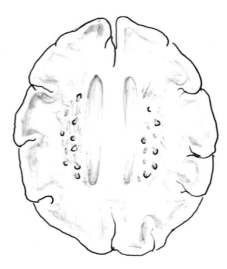

Figure 14–36. Periventricular leukomalacia.

Intracranial Infections

Encephalitis and Brain Edema. Encephalitis is inflammation of the brain. It is characterized sonographically with an overall increased echogenicity. Brain edema also shows increased echogenicity but has an additional finding; the ventricles become slitlike as a result of the brain swelling.[1]

Ventriculitis. Infection of the ventricles usually associated with encephalitis. It causes dilatation of the ventricles, and they may contain septa and debris. The brain becomes more echogenic, and often there are small cystic areas. The lining of the ventricles appears echogenic on ultrasound, and there may be holes in the borders of the ventricles.[1]

Brain Abscess. Abscesses vary in number and size. They may be lobulated and usually appear as a cystic type lesion with a nonhomogeneous echogenic material within. There is usually other signs of ventriculitis and encephalitis.[1]

Intracranial Calcifications. Calcifications in the brain may may be seen as a result of infections that occurred during pregnancy. For example, cytomegalovirus inclusion disease or toxoplasmosis. Sonographically, echogenic areas may be seen in the brain with associated shadowing[1] (Fig. 14–37).

Arachnoid Cyst. This is an uncommon benign cystic lesion that is lined in arachnoid tissue. These lesions have a normal cerebral hemisphere or vermis, but it is displaced and compressed anteriorly.[1] The exact etiology of this condition is unknown; however, it can be congenital, caused by previous trauma, infection, or infarction. Common locations of arachnoid cysts include middle cranial fossa anterior to the temporal lobe, the cerebral convexities, the posterior fossa, the suprasellar region, and the quadrigeminal plate cistern. Arachnoid cysts located in the midline may be associated with hydrocephalus. The arachnoid cyst is usually seen on ultrasound as an anechoic mass with well defined smooth margins. The ventricles may also be dilated[5] (Fig. 14–38).

Subdural Hemorrhage. This is a hemorrhage located between the dura mater and the arachnoid. Trauma can

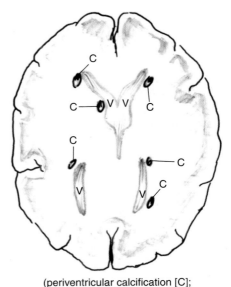

(periventricular calcification [C];
ventricles [V])

Figure 14–37. Cytomegalovirus.

cause a tearing of the dural folds or rupture of the medullary veins which cause a blood collection around the periphery of the brain. The cerebral surface will appear flattened with an echogenic space between the cranium and the cerebrum. On a coronal view, fluid can be seen within the inter-

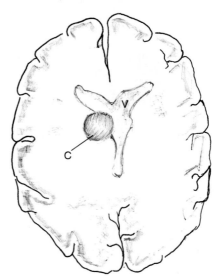

(cyst [C] medial and inferior to ventricle [V]
and superior to thalami)

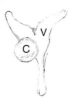

Figure 14–38. Arachnoid cyst.

hemispheric fissure, with blood collecting around the brain. The gyri are compressed and become more prominent and closer together.[1]

Agenesis of the Corpus Callosum.

The corpus callosum is the tract connecting the right and left cerebral hemispheres. This entity is defined as the absence of the corpus callosum. The corpus callosum may be hypoplastic, partially absent, or totally absent. Agenesis of the corpus callosum can be congenital or acquired. Acquired agenesis, for example, can occur as the result of intrauterine insult with anoxia or infarction in the distribution of the anterior cerebral artery. In the congenital type, the posterior portion of the corpus callosum is generally affected, whereas the anterior portion is affected in the acquired type.[5] The patients may be asymptomatic or have seizures, delayed development, hydrocephalus, or cerebral disconnection syndrome.

Real-time ultrasound shows a wide separation of the ventricular frontal horns with an asymmetrical appearance of the lateral ventricles. The third ventricle is high in position, which produces a "rabbit ear" appearance. The normal prominent corpus callosum is not seen on the midline sagittal scan.[5] CT, MRI, and ultrasound may be used to demonstrate this condition[5] (Fig. 14–39).

Holoprosencephaly.

This entity is defined as a congenital malformation with partial or complete failure of the primitive prosencephalon to form the cerebral hemispheres (telencephalon), and a thalmus and hypothalamus (diencephalon). This leads to a midline cleavage defect with failure to form the cerebral hemispheres and the thalamus. There is a common large ventricle with a horseshoe shape. There are three types of holoprosencephaly:

Alobar (severe form)—a single horseshoe-shaped ventricle with a thin cortical mantle. The thalami are fused, and the third ventricle is absent.[1] This type has severe abnormalities and is not compatible with life (Fig. 14–40).

Semilobar (moderate form)—Anterior horns of the ventricles are present. There is a single occipital horn with partial development of occipital and temporal horns. This form is usually associated with mental retardation.[1]

Lobar (mildest form)[1,5]—a less severe variant than the alobar with considerable cortex present.[1]

Risk factors include: maternal diabetes mellitus, toxoplasmosis, trisomies 13, 15, and 18, intrauterine rubella, and Meckel's syndrome. It can be associated with severe facial abnormalities, such as cleft palate, cleft lip, hypotelorism, trigonocephaly, cyclopia, ethmocephaly, and cebocephaly.

Real-time ultrasound demonstrates a large central ventricle draping over a bilobed fused thalamus in a horseshoe-shape appearance. The third ventricle is usually visible in some form with semilobar and lobar types and small or absence in the alobar type. The falx cerebri and interhemispheric fissure are present to a variable degree in the semilobar and lobar forms, and usually absent in the alobar forms. The corpus callosum is absent in the alobar form.

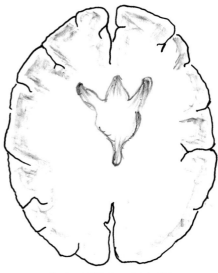

(enlarged 3rd ventricle [3] between lateral ventricles [V])

Figure 14–39. Agenesis of the corpus callosum.

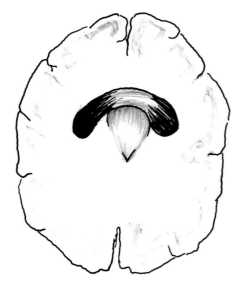

(single ventricle [V] & fused thalami [T])

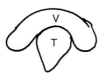

Figure 14–40. Alobar holoprosencephaly.

There is usually some residual brain tissue, depending on the type, with no differentiation of the frontal, temporal, and occipital horns.[5] CT, MRI, and ultrasound demonstrate holoprosencephaly; however, MRI is superior in showing the structural changes caused by holoprosencephaly.

Arnold–Chiari Malformation. This entity is characterized by inferior displacement of the cerebellum and the fourth ventricle into the upper cervical canal and is usually associated with cerebellar dysplasia.[5] There are four types:

Chiari 1 Malformation—Low-lying cerebellar tonsils below the foramen magnum. Cisterna magna is small or absent. There can be mild elongation and low position of the fourth ventricle. Complications include hydrocephalus and hydromyelia.

Chiari II Malformation—Inferior displacement of the medulla, fourth ventricle, inferior cerebellar tonsils, and vermis, and the presence of a myelocele or meningo-myelocele (Fig. 14–41).

Chiari III Malformation—Low occiput–high cervical cephalocele with a bony defect in the infraocciput, posterior rim of the foramen magnum, and posterior arch of the first cervical vertebra. Herniation of the cerebellum, brainstem, fourth ventricle, and upper cervical cord into the defect may occur.

Chiari IV Malformation—Severe cerebellar dysplasia associated with hypoplastic cerebellum, small brainstem, large posterior fossa, and CSF space not causing pressure effects.[5]

Patients may be asymptomatic, have headache, enlargement of the head from hydrocephalus, ataxia, incoordination, signs and symptoms of increased intracranial pressure, and a cervico–occipital soft tissue mass from encephalocele.[5]

Real-time ultrasound shows the cerebellum low in the posterior fossa. The third ventricle may be obscured by the massa intermedia, and the fourth ventricle may be small or absent. The posterior fossa may be small with the cisterna magna not visualized. Hydrocephalus may be present with the lateral ventricles dilated more than the frontal horns. A melocele or meningomyelocele may be seen at the cervico–occiptal junction.[5]

CT, MRI and ultrasound are used to demonstrate the anomaly. CT and MRI can more effectively demonstrate the bony defects in the occiput, foramen magnum, and C1 and C2 in addition to showing the myelocele or meningo-myelocele, fourth ventricle, and brain stem. [5]

Dandy–Walker Malformation or Syndrome. This process is characterized by a cyst in the infratentorial region with absence of the inferior cerebellar vermis and atresia of the foramina of Luschka and Magendie.[6] It is associated with hydrocephalus and presents on ultrasound with a large posterior fossa cyst that communicates with the fourth ventricle and enlargement of the posterior fossa. This condition has been associated with a higher incidence of other anomalies, such as agenesis of the corpus callosum, aqueductal stenosis, porencephalic cyst, encephalocele, holoprosencephaly, and lissencephaly.[6] There will be a small cerebellum and a large posterior fossa[5] (Fig. 14–42).

Hydranencephaly. This is a severe congenital malformation with a complete or almost complete absence of telencephalic structures. The cerebellum, basal portion of the temporal lobes, occipital lobes, and diencephalon are generally preserved. This anomaly is a result of severe intrauterine destructive process, although the exact etiology is uncertain. Neonates may be asymptomatic or have a large head with marked retardation. Transillumination of the skull is increased because of the thinness of the calvarium

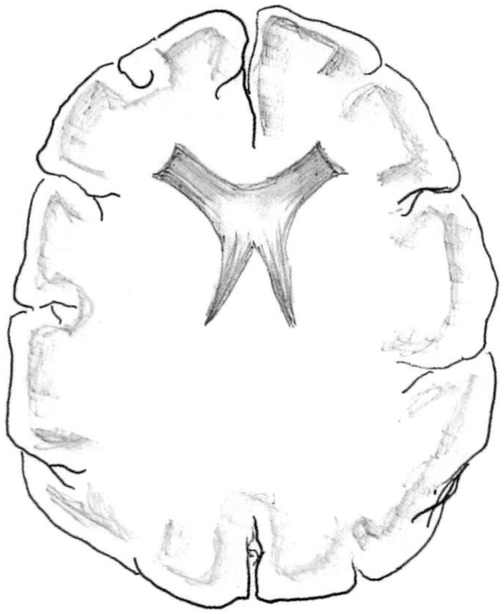

"Batwing" painted frontal horns

Figure 14–41. Arnold–Chiari II malformation.

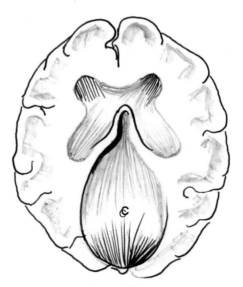

(posterior fossa cyst [C] communicating with the fourth ventricle)

Figure 14–42. Dandy–Walker cyst.

and increased intracranial fluid. Cerebral activity may be absent on an electroencephalogram.

Sonographically, this anomaly is seen as large bilateral cystic masses in the supratentorial region. Cerebral tissue may be present in the occipital and basal portions of the temporal lobes. The falx cerebri is usually attenuated and deviated[5] (Fig. 14–43).

Congenital Porencephaly. This anomaly is defined as the presence of cystic cavities within the brain matter. These cystic cavities may communicate with the ventricular system, the subarachnoid space, or both.[3]

Microcephaly. This condition is characterized by a decreased head size and reduction of brain mass. It features a typical disproportion in size between the skull and the face. The forehead slopes with a small brain, and the cerebral hemispheres are affected.[4]

Choroid Plexus Papilloma. That is a benign tumor that causes the choroid plexus to appear enlarged and echogenic. Hydrocephalus may develop because of obstruction of ventricular foramina.[1]

Corpus Callosum Lymphoma. The lymphoma presents as an echogenic mass within the corpus callosum. It has separated anterior horns that are pointed due to the maldevelopment of the corpus callosum.[1]

Cranioschisis. This condition is a splitting of the brain and caused by failure of the neural tube to close. The level

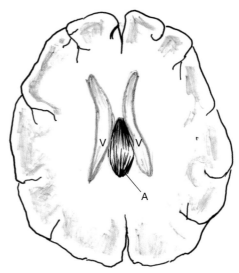

(midline vascular mass [A]
between dilated ventricles [V])

Figure 14–44. Vein of Galen aneurysm.

where the neural tube closes determines which anomalies will be present. Various anomalies include: anencephaly, encephalocele, and myelomeningocele.

Vein of Galen Aneurysm and Arteriovenous Malformation. The vein of Galen can become dilated or aneurysmal due to an increased flow from a deep cerebral arteriovenous malformation. The enlarged vein of Galen is seen posterior to the third ventricle and draining posteriorly into the dilated straight sinus and torcular herophili.[6] Sonographically, it appears as a cystic midline space with lateral ventricular dilatation.[2] This condition can be differentiated from other cystic anomalies with color flow Doppler or Doppler evaluation showing flow in the cystic space (Fig. 14–44).

REFERENCES

1. Sanders RC. *Clinical Sonography: A Practical Guide*, 2nd ed. Boston: Little, Brown; 1991.
2. Siege MJ. *Pediatric Sonography.* 2nd. ed. Philadelphia: Lippincott Raven; 1994.
3. Fleischer AC, Manning FA, Jeanty P, et al. *Sonography in Obstetrics & Gynecology Principles and Practice.* New York: McGraw-Hill; 2001.
4. Babcock DS. *Cranial Sonography of Infants. Syllabus: Categorical Course in Ultrasound.* 70th Scientific Assembly and Annual Meeting of The Radiological Society of North America, November 1984: 123–127.
5. Krebs CA, Giyanani VL, Eisenberg RL: *Ultrasound Atlas of Disease Processes.* Norwalk, CT: Appleton & Lange; 1993.
6. Aletebi FA, Fung KFK: Neurodevelopmental outcome after antenatal diagnosis of posterior fossa abnormalities. *Ultrasound Med.* 1999; 18:683–689.

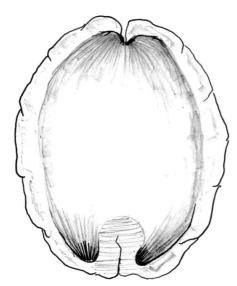

(fluid filled skull [F] with small portion of brain tissue [B])

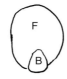

Figure 14–43. Hydranencephaly.

Questions

GENERAL INSTRUCTIONS: For each question, select the best answer. Select only one answer for each question unless otherwise instructed.

Questions 1–16: Identify the structures to which the lines point in Fig. 14–45, then place in Column A the letter corresponding to the appropriate item in Column B.

COLUMN A	COLUMN B
1. _____	(A) mastoidal fontanelle
2. _____	(B) sphenoid fontanelle
3. _____	(C) parietal bone
4. _____	(D) maxilla
5. _____	(E) orbit
6. _____	(F) occipital bone
7. _____	(G) coronal suture
8. _____	(H) frontal bone
9. _____	(I) zygomatic bone
10. _____	(J) nasal bone
11. _____	(K) temporal bone
12. _____	(L) mandible
13. _____	(M) anterior fontanelle
14. _____	(N) squamous suture
15. _____	(O) lambdoidal suture
16. _____	(P) zygomatic process

Questions 17–22: Identify the structures to which the lines point in Fig. 14–46, then place in Column A the letter corresponding to the appropriate item in Column B.

COLUMN A	COLUMN B
17. _____	(A) mastoidal fontanelle
18. _____	(B) coronal suture
19. _____	(C) sagittal suture
20. _____	(D) anterior fontanelle
21. _____	(E) parietal bone
22. _____	(F) posterior fontanelle

Questions 23–31: Identify the structures to which the line points in Fig. 14–47, then place in Column A the letter corresponding to the appropriate item in Column B.

COLUMN A	COLUMN B
23. _____	(A) dura mater
24. _____	(B) subdural space
25. _____	(C) pia mater
26. _____	(D) superior sagittal sinus
27. _____	(E) arachnoid villus
28. _____	(F) falx cerebri
29. _____	(G) subarachnoid space
30. _____	(H) scalp
31. _____	(I) cranium

Questions 32–37: Identify the structures to which the line points in Fig. 14–48, then place in Column A the letter corresponding to the appropriate item in Column B.

COLUMN A	COLUMN B
32. _____	(A) frontal lobe
33. _____	(B) sylvian fissure
34. _____	(C) fissure of Rolando
35. _____	(D) occipital lobe
36. _____	(E) parietal lobe
37. _____	(F) temporal lobe

Questions 38–50: Identify the structures to which the lines point in Fig. 14–49, then place in Column A the letter corresponding to the appropriate item in Column B.

COLUMN A	COLUMN B
38. _____	(A) corpus callosum
39. _____	(B) thalamus
40. _____	(C) cerebellum
41. _____	(D) pineal body
42. _____	(E) pons
43. _____	(F) spinal cord
44. _____	(G) cerebral peduncle
45. _____	(H) septum pellucidum
46. _____	(I) medulla oblongata
47. _____	(J) interthalamic adhesion
48. _____	(K) fourth ventricle
49. _____	(L) third ventricle
50. _____	(M) temporal lobe

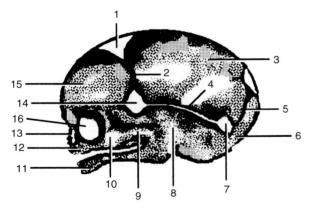

Figure 14–45. Lateral view of an infantile skull.

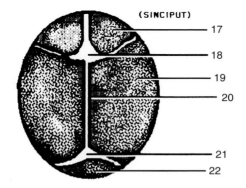

Figure 14–46. Superior view of an infantile skull.

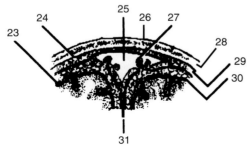

Figure 14–47. Diagram of a coronal section of the meninges and cortex.

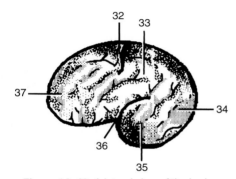

Figure 14–48. A lateral view of the brain.

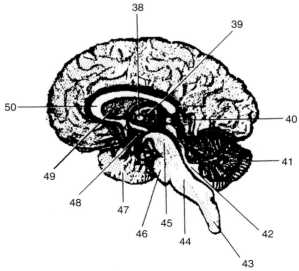

Figure 14–49. Diagram of a sagittal section of the brain.

Questions 51–59: Identify the structures to which the lines point in Fig. 14–50, then place in Column A the letter corresponding to the appropriate item in Column B.

COLUMN A	COLUMN B
51. _____	(A) third ventricle
52. _____	(B) anterior horn
53. _____	(C) inferior horn
54. _____	(D) foramen of Monro
55. _____	(E) lateral access
56. _____	(F) cerebral aqueduct
57. _____	(G) fourth ventricle
58. _____	(H) atrium
59. _____	(I) posterior horn

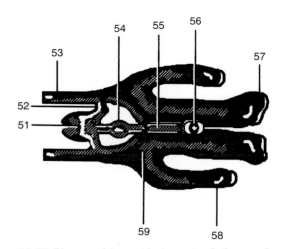

Figure 14–50. Diagram of the ventricular system in the superior view.

Questions 60–74: Identify the structures to which the lines point in Fig. 14–51, then place in Column A the letter corresponding to the appropriate item in Column B.

COLUMN A

60. _____
61. _____
62. _____
63. _____
64. _____
65. _____
66. _____
67. _____
68. _____
69. _____
70. _____
71. _____
72. _____
73. _____
74. _____

COLUMN B

(A) pineal recess
(B) body of lateral ventricle
(C) interventricular foramen
(D) posterior horn
(E) infundibular recess
(F) third ventricle
(G) preoptic recess
(H) frontal horn
(I) inferior horn
(J) collateral trigone
(K) suprapineal recess
(L) foramen of Magendie (fourth ventricle)
(M) cerebral aqueduct
(N) foramina of Luschka
(O) interthalamic adhesion

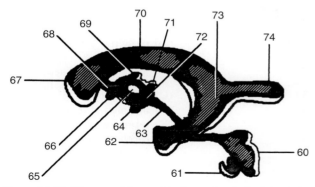

Figure 14–51. Diagram of the ventricular system in the lateral view.

Questions 75–80: Identify the structures to which the lines point in Fig. 14–52, then place in Column A the letter corresponding to the appropriate item in Column B.

COLUMN A

75. _____
76. _____
77. _____
78. _____
79. _____
80. _____

COLUMN B

(A) caudate nucleus
(B) choroid plexus of the third ventricle
(C) telea choroidea
(D) corpus colosum
(E) choroid plexus of the fourth ventricle
(F) glomus of the choroid plexus

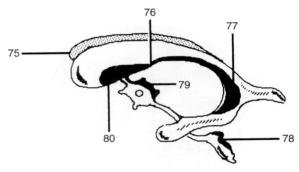

Figure 14–52. Diagram of the ventricular system in a neonate.

Questions 81–84: Identify the structures demonstrated in each scan plane where the lines project in Fig. 14–53, then place in Column A the letter corresponding to the appropriate item in Column B.

COLUMN A

81. _____
82. _____
83. _____
84. _____

COLUMN B

(A) foramina of Monro and third ventricle
(B) posterior horn of the lateral ventricle
(C) frontal and temporal horns
(D) choroid plexus and trigone of the lateral ventricle and the 4th ventricle

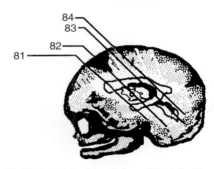

Figure 14–53. Diagram of a lateral view of the infantile skull with the ventricular system.

Questions 85–94: Match the structures where the lines point in Fig. 14–54 then place in Column A the letter corresponding to the appropriate item in Column B.

COLUMN A

85. _____
86. _____
87. _____
88. _____
89. _____
90. _____
91. _____
92. _____
93. _____
94. _____

COLUMN B

(A) lateral ventricle
(B) cerebellar peduncle
(C) pons
(D) corpus callosum
(E) caudate nucleus
(F) hippocampus
(G) sylvian fissure
(H) sulcus
(I) column of fornix
(J) thalamus

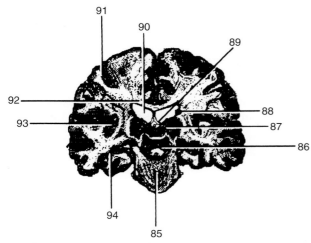

Figure 14–54. Diagram of a coronal section of the brain.

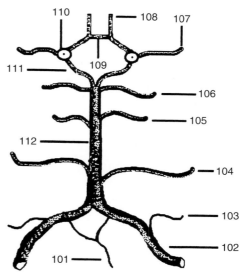

Figure 14–56. Circle of Willis.

Questions 95–100: Match the structures where the lines point in Fig. 14–55 then place in Column A the Letter corresponding to the appropriate item in Column B.

COLUMN A	COLUMN B
95. _____	(A) cerebral aqueduct
96. _____	(B) cerebellum peduncle
97. _____	(C) cerebellum
98. _____	(D) hypothalamus
99. _____	(E) gyrus and sulcus
100. _____	(F) cerebral peduncle

Questions 101–112: Identify the structures to which the lines point in Fig. 14–56, then place in Column A the letter corresponding to the appropriate item in Column B.

COLUMN A	COLUMN B
101. _____	(A) basilar artery
102. _____	(B) posterior cerebral artery
103. _____	(C) middle cerebral artery
104. _____	(D) internal carotid artery
105. _____	(E) anterior cerebral artery
106. _____	(F) anterior inferior cerebellar artery
107. _____	(G) vertebral artery
108. _____	(H) anterior communicating artery
109. _____	(I) posterior communicating artery
110. _____	(J) anterior spinal artery
111. _____	(K) posterior inferior cerebellar artery
112. _____	(L) superior cerebellar artery

Questions 113–120: Identify the structures to which the lines point in Fig. 14–57, then place in Column A the letter corresponding to the appropriate item in Column B.

COLUMN A	COLUMN B
113. _____	(A) internal carotid artery
114. _____	(B) posterior cerebral artery
115. _____	(C) vertebral artery
116. _____	(D) basilar artery
117. _____	(E) anterior cerebral artery
118. _____	(F) middle cerebral artery
119. _____	(G) cerebellum
120. _____	(H) medulla oblongata

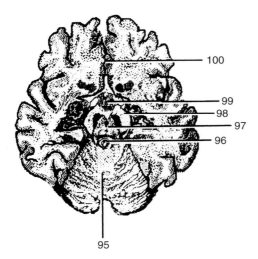

Figure 14–55. Diagram of a coronal section of the brain.

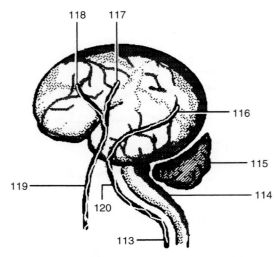

Figure 14–57. Diagram of the brain in the sagittal view.

Questions 121–124: Identify the structure to which the arrows point in Fig. 14–58, then place in Column A the letter corresponding to the appropriate item in Column B.

COLUMN A	COLUMN B
121. _____	(A) pericallosal artery
122. _____	(B) middle cerebral artery
123. _____	(C) callosomarginal artery
124. _____	(D) anterior cerebral artery

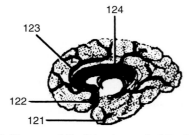

Figure 14–58. Diagram of the lateral aspect of the internal carotid artery and its branches.

125. The acoustic windows used most often in neonatal cranial sonography are

(A) anterior and posterior fontanelle
(B) anterior and sphenoidal fontanelle
(C) anterior and mastoidal fontanelle
(D) posterior and sphenoidal fontanelle

126. On sonography, cytomegalovirus in the neonate is associated with

(A) periventricular calcifications
(B) small cystic lesions
(C) encephalocele
(D) anencephaly

127. Another name for the sphenoid fontanelle is

(A) lambda
(B) the antrolateral fontanelle
(C) the posterolateral fontanelle
(D) bregma

128. The anterior fontanelle becomes progressively smaller and, in most cases, closes completely by the age

(A) 6 months
(B) 2–3 months
(C) 12 months
(D) 18 months

129. Another name for the mastoidal fontanelle is

(A) anterior fontanelle
(B) posterior fontanelle
(C) lambda
(D) posterolateral fontanelle

130. Which of the following statements about temporal and occipital horns are true?

(A) They both diverge laterally as they project from the body of the lateral ventricles.
(B) They both diverge medially as they project from the body of the lateral ventricles.
(C) The occipital horn is lateral, and the temporal horns are medial to the body of the lateral ventricles.
(D) The right temporal horn and the occipital horn are medial, and the left temporal horn is lateral.

131. The lateral ventricular ratio can be obtained by measuring the distance from the

(A) anterior wall to the posterior wall of the lateral ventricle
(B) midline to medial wall of the lateral ventricle and from the inner wall of the table of the skull
(C) medial wall to the lateral wall of the lateral ventricle
(D) midline to the lateral wall of the lateral ventricle and dividing this by the distance from the midline echo to the inner table of the skull

132. The axial scan is obtained by placing the transducer on the parietal bone just above the

(A) styloid process
(B) coronal suture
(C) glabella
(D) external auditory meatus

133. Which of the following statements regarding the germinal matrix is *not* true?

(A) it cannot be visualized as a distinct structure
(B) it lies just above the caudate nucleus
(C) it disappears between 32 weeks to term
(D) it is not a fetal structure

134. The normal location for the germinal matrix after 24 weeks gestation is

(A) above the caudate nucleus in the subependymal layer of the lateral ventricle
(B) within the choroid plexus
(C) inferior to the caudate nucleus
(D) within the choroid plexus in the trigone

135. The cisterna magna appears sonographically as

(A) echogenic space superior to the cerebellum
(B) echogenic space inferior to the cerebellum
(C) echo-free space superior to the cerebellum
(D) echo-free space inferior to the cerebellum

136. Vascular pulsations are sometimes seen in the sylvian fissure, which most likely represent the

(A) anterior cerebral arteries
(B) posterior cerebral arteries
(C) basilar artery
(D) middle cerebral arteries

137. Which of the following statements about the fissure and sulci is true?

(A) Fissure and sulci both appear echogenic.
(B) Fissure is echo-free and sulci echogenic.
(C) Sulci is echo-free and the fissure is echogenic.
(D) Fissure and sulci are both echo-free.

138. The cavum septum pellucidum is located

(A) lateral to the corpus callosum
(B) posterior to the third ventricle
(C) medial to the thalami
(D) between the frontal horns of the lateral ventricles

139. The third ventricle is located between the

(A) cavum septum pellucidum
(B) frontal horns of the lateral ventricles
(C) thalami
(D) corpus callosum

140. Increased echogenicity in the brain parenchyma is seen with

(A) subependymal hemorrhage
(B) intraventricular hemorrhage
(C) intraparenchymal hemorrhage
(D) choroid plexus hemorrhage

141. If dense echogenic material is seen in the ventricle it is called

(A) intraventricular hemorrhage
(B) intraparenchymal hemorrhage
(C) subarachnoid hemorrhage
(D) subependymal hemorrhage

142. After an intraparenchymal hemorrhage, the clot retracts and may result in a cystic area communicating with the ventricle. This is termed

(A) holoprosencephaly
(B) hydranencephaly
(C) hydrocephalus
(D) porencephaly

143. Which of the following is *not* a possible contributing factor to intracranial hemorrhage?

(A) maternal ingestion of aspirin during the final weeks of pregnancy
(B) extrauterine stress
(C) intrapartum hypoxia
(D) pleural effusion

144. A neonate is defined as

(A) child during the first 28 days after birth
(B) child from 29 days after birth to 1 year
(C) a fetus of 20 weeks of gestation to a child 28 days after birth
(D) conception to birth

145. The most common site for periventricular leukomalacia is

(A) white matter surrounding the ventricles
(B) gray matter surrounding the ventricles
(C) gray matter around the caudate nucleus
(D) white matter around the cerebellum

146. Disruption of organogenesis in brain development causes specific related brain defects. Such defects do *not* include

(A) diverticulation
(B) neural tube closure
(C) neuronal proliferation
(D) tuberous sclerosis

147. The term used to describe any hemorrhage within the cranial vault is

(A) subependymal hemorrhage
(B) germinal matrix hemorrhage
(C) intraventricular hemorrhage
(D) intracranial hemorrhage

Questions 148–151: Match the term in Column B with the types of hemorrhage in Column A.

COLUMN A

148. Cerebrospinal fluid—blood level in the ventricles
149. Echogenic foci in the region of the caudate nucleus
150. Echogenic area in the brain parenchyma
151. Enlarged irregular and highly echogenic choroid plexus

COLUMN B

(A) Intraparenchymal hemorrhage (IPH)
(B) Subependymal hemorrhage (SHE)
(C) Intraventricular hemorrhage (IVH)
(D) Choroid plexus hemorrhage (CPH)

152. Which type of intracranial hemorrhage is most common in premature infants?

(A) subdural hemorrhage
(B) intraventricular hemorrhage
(C) intraparenchymal hemorrhage
(D) subependymal germinal matrix hemorrhage

153. True coronal scans are performed at what angle with the orbitomeatal line?

(A) 60°
(B) 90°
(C) 150°
(D) They do not have an angle with the orbitomeatal line.

154. Which of the following does *not* designate the term "acoustic window" in cranial sonography?

(A) a procedure to bypass bone interface
(B) an opening through which ultrasound can travel with little or no obstruction
(C) an area in which ultrasound is obstructed
(D) an area in which ultrasound is not obstructed

155. Which of the following diseases is *not* a common cause of congenital infections of the nervous system?

(A) rubella
(B) toxoplasmosis
(C) gonorrhea
(D) syphilis
(E) cytomegalovirus

156. Which of the following are *not* sonographic findings of congenital infection of the nervous system?

(A) microcephaly with enlargement of the ventricles
(B) a prominent interhemispheric fissure and brain atrophy
(C) macrocephaly with enlargement of the ventricles
(D) calcification in the periventricular regions

157. According to the computed tomography grading system for intracranial hemorrhage, which of the following is a Grade I hemorrhage?

(A) subependymal hemorrhage with intraventricular hemorrhage and ventricular dilatation
(B) subependymal hemorrhage with intraventricular hemorrhage and no ventricular dilatation
(C) subependymal hemorrhage with intraventricular hemorrhage and intraparenchymal hemorrhage
(D) isolated subependymal hemorrhage

158. The foramen between the third and fourth ventricle is the

(A) cerebral aqueduct
(B) foramen of Monro
(C) foramen of Magendie
(D) foramen of Luschka

159. Which of the following is *not* true regarding hydranencephaly?

(A) Usually only the brain stem and portion of the occipital lobe remain.
(B) The falx is usually intact.
(C) The falx is usually not intact because the head is largely filled with fluid.
(D) There is a severe loss of cerebral tissue.

160. A Dandy–Walker cyst is usually associated with

(A) toxoplasmosis
(B) dysgenesis of the vermis of the cerebellum
(C) syphilis
(D) cytomegalovirus

161. The current treatment for hydrocephalus with increased intraventricular pressure is

(A) Javid's internal shunt
(B) ventriculoperitoneal (V-P) shunt
(C) radiation treatment
(D) ventriculoectomy

162. Which of the following is *not* a sign of hydrocephalus?

(A) skull bones halo sign on x-ray
(B) anterior fontanelle sinks
(C) bulging of the frontal bone of the skull
(D) rapid head growth
(E) decreasing size of ventricles

163. The most common cause of congenital hydrocephalus is

(A) aqueductal stenosis
(B) subarachnoid hemorrhage
(C) interventricular hemorrhage
(D) intracranial infection

164. Subperiosteal hematomas are also called

(A) cephalohematomas
(B) subependymal hemorrhages
(C) intraventricular hemorrhages
(D) choroid plexus hemorrhages

165. The cavum pellucidum begins to close at which week of gestation?

(A) 40 weeks
(B) 36 weeks
(C) 12 weeks
(D) 24 weeks

166. Which of the following best defines the Dandy–Walker syndrome?

(A) a cyst in the posterior fossa that does not communicate with the fourth ventricle
(B) a congenital cystic dilatation of the third ventricle
(C) congenital dilatation of the ventricular system
(D) a posterior fossa cyst that is continuous with the fourth ventricle

167. A differential diagnosis for hydranencephaly is

(A) severe hydrocephalus
(B) Dandy–Walker cyst
(C) arachnoid cyst
(D) intracranial teratoma

168. On cranial sonography, the middle cerebral artery is found in the

(A) region of the sylvian fissure and above the corpus callosum
(B) region of the sylvian fissure and in the circle of Willis
(C) genu of the corpus callosum and sylvian fissure
(D) genu of the corpus callosum and hippocampal sulcus

169. The most severe form of hemorrhage is

(A) germinal matrix hemorrhage
(B) intraventricular hemorrhage
(C) subependymal hemorrhage
(D) intraparenchymal hemorrhage

170. The forebrain is also called

(A) prosencephalon
(B) mesencephalon
(C) rhombencephalon
(D) myelencephalon

171. Which of the following vessels does *not* form the Circle of Willis?

(A) posterior cerebral arteries
(B) anterior cerebral arteries
(C) internal carotid arteries
(D) posterior and anterior communicating arteries
(E) external carotid arteries

172. Which of the following is true regarding noncommunicating hydrocephalus?

(A) It is also called nonobstructive hydrocephalus.
(B) The cerebrospinal fluid pathways within the brain are blocked.
(C) Cerebrospinal fluid is blocked within the ventricular system.
(D) none of the above

173. A Chiari II malformation is defined as

(A) a congenital abnormality of the brain with elongation of the pons and fourth ventricle and downward displacement of the medulla into the cervical canal
(B) congenital cystic dilatation of the fourth ventricle caused by atresia of the foramen of Magendie
(C) congenital formation of a holospheric cerebrum caused by a disorder of the diverticulation of the fetal brain
(D) none of the above

174. The main arteries supplying the brain are

(A) one vertebral and one carotid artery
(B) one basilar artery and carotid arteries
(C) two external carotid and two vertebral arteries
(D) two internal carotid and two vertebral arteries

175. The vertebral artery at the level of the pons is called the

(A) middle cerebral artery
(B) basilar artery
(C) internal carotid artery
(D) posterior cerebral artery

176. The greatest proportion of the cerebrospinal fluid is produced by

(A) choroid plexus
(B) caudate nucleus
(C) lateral ventricles
(D) movement of extracellular fluid from blood through the brain and ventricles

177. The sonographic findings of ventriculitis do not include

(A) echogenic ventricular walls
(B) septated ventricles
(C) normal-size ventricles with no debris within
(D) debris within the ventricles

178. How many cranial bones are there?

(A) 12
(B) 10
(C) 8
(D) 5

179. Blood between the arachnoid membrane and the pia mater is called

    (A) subarachnoid hematoma
    (B) subdural hematoma
    (C) epidural membrane
    (D) intraparenchymal hematoma

180. The amount of cerebrospinal fluid production in children is

    (A) 140 mL/week
    (B) 140 mL/day
    (C) 532–576 mL/day
    (D) 552–576 mL/week

181. The accumulation of blood between the dura mater and the inner table of the skull is called

    (A) subarachnoid hemorrhage
    (B) subdural hematoma
    (C) epidural hematoma
    (D) intraparenchymal hemorrhage

182. Another name for the temporal horn is the

    (A) anterior horn
    (B) posterior horn
    (C) inferior horn
    (D) lateral horn

183. The largest of all the horns is the

    (A) temporal horn
    (B) occipital horn
    (C) frontal horn
    (D) lateral horn

184. Which of the following are *not* midline structures?

    (A) third ventricle and fourth ventricle
    (B) cerebral hemispheres
    (C) cavum septum pellucidum
    (D) falx cerebri

185. The vein of Galen aneurysm is most likely to be located

    (A) anterior to the third ventricle
    (B) posterior to the foramen of Monro and superior to the third ventricle
    (C) posterior to the foramen of Monro and inferior to the third ventricle
    (D) posterior to the fourth ventricle

186. Which of the following is *not* a bacterial cause of intracranial infection?

    (A) haemophilus influenzae
    (B) herpes simplex
    (C) diplococcus pneumoniae
    (D) bacterial meningitis

187. The central fissure is also called

    (A) sylvian fissure
    (B) fissure of Rolando
    (C) lateral fissure
    (D) longitudinal fissure

188. The etiology of a porencephalic cyst is which of the following?

    (A) intracranial infection
    (B) infarction
    (C) intracranial hemorrhage
    (D) trauma

189. Numerous sulci can normally be identified on the premature brain, particularly in the sagittal scan. Identify the condition that would least be likely to obscure the normal sulcal pattern.

    (A) salmonella meningoencephalitis
    (B) subdural hematoma
    (C) intracranial infection
    (D) infarction

190. The germinal matrix is largest at which week of gestation?

    (A) 40 weeks (term)
    (B) 24–32 weeks
    (C) 32–40 weeks
    (D) 12–15 weeks

191. Which of the following is not an intracranial tumor?

    (A) dermoid tumor
    (B) choroid plexus papilloma
    (C) medulloblastoma
    (D) cyclopia

192. Periventricular leukomalacia is best described as

    (A) ischemic lesions of the neonatal brain characterized by necrosis of periventricular white matter
    (B) a disorder of premature newborns characterized by the increase in vascularity in the periventricular white matter
    (C) a disorder of premature newborns characterized by highly echogenic solid lesions in the parenchyma
    (D) an infection disorder with a decrease in definition of the parenchymal structures

193. Which of the following is not a common infection acquired in utero?

    (A) herpes simplex
    (B) leukomalacia
    (C) toxoplasmosis
    (D) cytomegalovirus

194. Which of the following results in the greatest number of neonatal deaths?

    (A) hypoxia
    (B) erythroblastosis
    (C) trauma at birth
    (D) premature placental separation

195. Which of the following is *not* a characteristic of lissencephaly

(A) decrease in the size of the sylvian fissure as the neonatal brain matures
(B) large ventricles
(C) less sonographic characteristics because of the inability to differentiate white from gray matter
(D) large sylvian fissures

196. If an infant has a ventriculoperitoneal (V-P) shunt and the fontanelles are bulging, the usual position to assist in drainage is the

(A) Trendelenburg position
(B) lithotomy position
(C) semi-Fowler's position
(D) Sims' position

197. The cerebellum is separated from the occipital lobe of the cerebrum by the

(A) interhemispheric fissure
(B) tentorium
(C) cerebellar vermis
(D) parieto-occipital sulcus

198. The central nervous system consists of the brain and spinal cord. The spinal cord is referred to as the distal continuation of the central nervous system. The terminal portion of the spinal cord is the

(A) filum terminale
(B) conus medullaris
(C) cauda equina
(D) pia mater

199. What region of the lateral ventricular system is the first to dilate in hydrocephalus?

(A) the third ventricle
(B) occipital horns
(C) frontal horns
(D) temporal horns

200. The correct placement for a ventriculoperitoneal (V-P) shunt catheter is

(A) frontal horns anterior to the foramen of Monro
(B) frontal horns posterior to the foramen of Monro
(C) trigone of the lateral ventricle
(D) the roof of the third ventricle

201. Which of the following is least associated with complete agenesis of the corpus callosum?

(A) absence of the septum pellucidum
(B) enlarged septum pellucidum
(C) wide separation of the lateral ventricle
(D) displacement of the third ventricle

202. Which of the following is *not* seen in septoptic dysplasia?

(A) septum pellucidum
(B) frontal horns
(C) thalamus
(D) occipital horns

203. When scanning neonates, excessive pressure should not be applied to the anterior fontanelle because it may

(A) cause increased heart rates
(B) cause slowing of the heart
(C) cause increased body temperatures
(D) cause irregularity of the heart rate

Match the definitions in Column B with the terms they define in Column A.

COLUMN A	COLUMN B
204. periventricular leukomalacia ___	(A) enclosed space located caudal to the cerebellum, between the cerebellum and the occipital bone, serving as a reservoir for cerebrospinal fluid
205. tentorium cerebelli ___	
206. sulci ___	(B) folds on the surface of the brain
207. choroid plexus ___	
208. cisterna magna ___	(C) special cells located in the ventricles that secrete cerebrospinal fluid
209. pia mater ___	
210. corpus callosum ___	(D) softening of the white matter surrounding the ventricles
211. cavum septum pellucidum ___	
212. insula ___	(E) congenital obstruction of the third and fourth ventricles resulting in ventricular dilation
213. gyri ___	
214. aqueduct stenosis ___	(F) group of nerve fibers above the third ventricle that connects the left and right sides of the brain
	(G) transverse division of dura mater forming a partition between the occipital lobe of the cerebral hemispheres and the cerebellum
	(H) a triangular area of cerebral cortex, lying deeply in the lateral cerebral fissure
	(I) grooves on the surface of the brain separating the gyri
	(J) cavity filled with cerebrospinal fluid that lies between the anterior horns of the lateral ventricle
	(K) the inner membrane covering the brain and spinal cord

Each of the following terms has an alternative name. Match the terms in Column A with the alternative term in Column B.

COLUMN A

215. interventricular foramen ___
216. atrium ___
217. subependymal hemorrhage ___
218. epiphysis cerebri ___
219. posterior horn ___
220. frontal horn ___
221. inferior horn ___
222. interthalamic adhesion ___

COLUMN B

(A) massa intermedia
(B) temporal horn
(C) anterior horn
(D) occipital horn
(E) pineal gland
(F) germinal matrix hemorrhage
(G) trigone
(H) foramen of Monro

223. When evaluating the intracerebral vessels of an infants brain, the optimal frequency range for a continuous-wave Doppler transducer is

(A) 1–3 MHz
(B) 4–5 MHz
(C) 1–10 MHz
(D) 5–10 MHz

224. When using a transcranial approach with the transducer placed 0.5–1 cm anterior to the ear and superior to the zygomatic process, the vessel that can be evaluated most accurately in the neonates brain is the

(A) middle cerebral artery
(B) anterior cerebral artery
(C) posterior cerebral artery
(D) posterior communicating artery

225. In a normal tracing of a cerebral vessel in a neonates brain, the maximum systolic velocity is equivalent to the

(A) peak height
(B) area under the curve
(C) slope
(D) minimum height

226. A Doppler tracing of an anterior cerebral artery in an infant with asphyxia can reveal

(A) low pulsatility and high diastolic forward flow
(B) low pulsatility and low diastolic forward flow
(C) high pulsatility and high diastolic forward flow
(D) high pulsatility and low diastolic forward flow

227. A Doppler tracing of an anterior cerebral artery in an infant with an intraventricular hemorrhage can reveal

(A) low pulsatility and low diastolic forward flow
(B) low pulsatility and high diastolic forward flow
(C) high pulsatility and high diastolic forward flow
(D) high pulsatility and low diastolic forward flow

228. The term craniosynostosis denotes

(A) premature fusion of the cranial sutures
(B) premature separation of the cranial sutures
(C) a bluish discoloration of the cranium
(D) a bluish discoloration of the scalp

229. Hypothermia denotes

(A) high memory
(B) low memory
(C) high temperature
(D) low temperature

230. When the parietal bones are relatively thin, lateral ventricular measurements can be obtained up to

(A) 5 years
(B) 6 months
(C) 2–3 years
(D) 6–12 months

231. In cranial sonography, a real-time linear array transducer is limited. Which of the following statements is *not* true of the linear array limitations?

(A) limited field of view
(B) inability to visualize the inner lateral table of both sides of the calvarium simultaneously
(C) able to examine only the central portion of the brain
(D) producing only a 90° pie-shaped image
(E) low signal-to-noise ratio and artifact

232. Which of the following sonography planes are most comparable with cranial computed tomography?

(A) axial
(B) coronal
(C) sagittal
(D) occipital

233. The choroid plexus is attached to the floor of the lateral ventricle. Its point of attachment is called

(A) telea choroidea
(B) interhemisphere fissure
(C) pineal body
(D) caudate nucleus

234. A structure often confused with the third ventricle in the fetus and neonate is the

(A) cavum septum pellucidum
(B) choroid plexus
(C) thalamus
(D) cavum vergae

235. Between 32 and 40 weeks, the incidence of germinal matrix hemorrhage drops. Approximately what percentage of germinal matrix hemorrhage occurs at 28 weeks of gestation?

(A) 25%
(B) 35%
(C) 40%
(D) 67%

236. The term isodense denotes the following

(A) same density
(B) same as sonolucent
(C) same as echogenic
(D) same as anechoic

237. Which of the following is associated with an intracranial hemorrhage?

(A) hyaline membrane disease
(B) sudden change in blood flow to the region of the germinal matrix
(C) increase in venous and arterial pressure
(D) expanded volume of plasma
(E) B and C
(F) all of the above

238. An infant is defined as a child

(A) from 29 days after birth to 1 year
(B) during the first 28 days after birth
(C) from 1–2 years after birth
(D) from 2–6 years after birth

239. Which of the following is not an imaginary line from the outer canthus to the external auditory meatus?

(A) orbitomeatal line
(B) canthomeatal line
(C) radiographic baseline
(D) Reid's baseline

240. Posterior fossa scans are performed at what angle with the orbitomeatal line?

(A) 150° from the orbitomeatal line and perpendicular to the clivus
(B) 150° from the canthomeatal line and parallel to the clivus
(C) 90° perpendicular to the orbitomeatal line and parallel to the clivus
(D) 120° perpendicular to the canthomeatal line and parallel to the clivus

241. If one sees echogenic material within the occipital horn, it would most likely be correct to assume that there is

(A) a choroid plexus in the occipital horn
(B) a choroid plexus in the lateral horn
(C) an intracranial hemorrhage because no choroid extends into this area
(D) an intracranial hemorrhage because the tail of the choroid extends into the occipital horn

242. Which of the following does *not* describe hydranencephaly?

(A) the head is largely filled with fluid
(B) the falx is usually intact
(C) the loss of cerebral tissue is severe
(D) the brainstem and a portion of the occipital lobe remain
(E) there is a presence of a single midline ventricle

243. The pericallosal artery is normally seen

(A) above the corpus callosum
(B) below the corpus callosum
(C) in the sylvian fissure
(D) between the hippocampal sulcus

244. Approximately how long after ventricular dilatation does the head circumference start to increase?

(A) 5–7 days
(B) 3–4 days
(C) 8 weeks
(D) 2 weeks

245. If hemorrhage is detected in a newborn on the first examination, studies should be performed

(A) every 3 days until 2 weeks of age
(B) every 3 days until 2 months of age
(C) every 5 days until 3 weeks of age
(D) every 7 days until 3 weeks of age

246. At which week of gestation is the choroid plexus prominent and may completely fill the lateral ventricle?

(A) last trimester
(B) first trimester
(C) mid trimester
(D) after birth

247. Hydranencephaly is defined as a

(A) holospheric cerebrum
(B) posterior fossa cyst
(C) congenital cystic dilatation of the fourth ventricle
(D) head largely filled with fluid and a severe loss of cerebral tissue

248. Which of the following does not describe holoprosencephaly?

(A) formation of a holospheric cerebrum
(B) disorder of diverticulation of the fetal brain
(C) cerebral hemispheres and lateral ventricles that develop as one vesicle
(D) large single midline ventricular cavity
(E) premature fusion of the cranial sutures either complete or partial

249. Which of the following statements about spinal and cranial nerves is true?

   (A) There are 12 pairs of cranial nerves and 12 pairs of spinal nerves
   (B) There are 12 pairs of cranial nerves and 10 pairs of spinal nerves
   (C) There are 15 pairs of cranial nerves and 15 pairs of spinal nerves
   (D) There are 20 pairs of cranial nerves and 20 pairs of spinal nerves

250. The spinal cord ends at about what vertebral level?

   (A) L2
   (B) L5
   (C) S2
   (D) S5

251. Which foramen connects the third ventricle to the fourth ventricle?

   (A) foramen of Monro
   (B) foramen of Luschka
   (C) foramen of Magendie
   (D) cerebral aqueduct

252. The two anterior recesses on the third ventricle are the

   (A) supraoptic and pineal recess
   (B) pineal and infundibular recess
   (C) infundibular and suprapineal recess
   (D) supraoptic and infundibular

253. Microcephaly is *not* associated with which of the following?

   (A) diverticulations
   (B) craniosynostosis
   (C) Meckel–Gruber's syndrome
   (D) chromosomal abnormalities
   (E) exposure to environmental teratogens

254. The two posterior recesses on the third ventricle are

   (A) preoptic and pineal recesses
   (B) pineal and infundibular recesses
   (C) infundibular and suprapineal recesses
   (D) pineal and suprapineal recesses

255. Another name for massa intermedia is

   (A) interthalamic adhesion
   (B) pineal recess
   (C) preoptic recess
   (D) infundibular recess

256. Which structure is *not* a partition of the dura mater?

   (A) falx cerebelli
   (B) falx cerebri
   (C) tentorium
   (D) cerebellum

257. Bleeding within the cerebral parenchyma is called

   (A) subdural hematoma
   (B) intraparenchymal hemorrhage

   (C) cerebellar hemorrhage
   (D) subarachnoid hematoma

258. Another name for the foramen of Monro is the

   (A) interventricular foramen
   (B) cerebral aqueduct
   (C) foramen of Luschka
   (D) foramen of Magendie

259. Which of the following is *not* part of the brain stem?

   (A) spinal cord
   (B) diencephalon
   (C) midbrain
   (D) pons

260. Midline facial anomalies are often associated with holoproencephaly. These malformations do not include which of the following?

   (A) cerebrocephaly
   (B) cleft palate
   (C) hypoplasia of the ethmoid bone
   (D) cyclopia
   (E) meningomyocele

261. The meninges covers the brain and spinal cord. Which of the following is *not* one of its layers?

   (A) dura mater
   (B) white matter
   (C) arachnoid membrane
   (D) pia mater

262. Which of the following is *not* an etiology of an arachnoid cyst?

   (A) abnormal mechanism of leptomeningeal formation
   (B) entrapment of subarachnoid space by adhesions
   (C) entrapment of cisternal space by adhesions
   (D) failure of development of the cerebral mantle

263. Which of the following does not occur as a result of a vein of Galen aneurysm?

   (A) cardiac failure
   (B) hydrocephalus
   (C) enlarged aorta
   (D) quadrigeminal cyst

264. Which of the following does *not* apply to an arachnoid cyst?

   (A) Arachnoid cysts lie between the pia mater and the subarachnoid space.
   (B) Arachnoid cysts do not communicate with the ventricles or the arachnoid space.
   (C) Arachnoid cysts contain cerebrospinal fluid.
   (D) Arachnoid cysts are usually found in the sylvian fissure, middle fossa, and interhemispheric fissure.
   (E) Arachnoid cysts are usually congenital and acquired.

265. Which of the following statements is true about the arachnoid granulations?

(A) Arachnoid granulations lie in the cingulate sulcus.
(B) Arachnoid granulations lie in the pericallosal artery where cerebrospinal fluid is reabsorbed by the blood.
(C) Arachnoid granulations lie in the sagittal sinus and reabsorb cerebrospinal fluid as it circulates.
(D) Arachnoid granulations lie in the ventricular system and reabsorb cerebrospinal fluid as it circulates.

266. Which of the following is *not* a characteristic of schinzencephaly?

(A) the corpus callosum is absent
(B) the septum pellucidum is absent
(C) the ventricle has an unusual shape
(D) the septum pellucidum is dilated

267. Eight out of 12 neonates with meningitis usually develop

(A) ventriculitis
(B) intracranial hemorrhage
(C) abscess
(D) encephalomalacia

268. Early scans of a preterm infant brain that has periventricular leukomalacia reveal

(A) increased echogenicity at the external angle of the lateral ventricles
(B) normal echogenicity surrounding the lateral ventricles
(C) cysts varying from a few small ones to multiple variably sized ones
(D) markedly decreased vascular pulsations

269. The main nutrient vessel of the subependymal germinal matrix tissue is the

(A) pericallosal artery
(B) callosal marginal artery
(C) posterior cerebral artery
(D) Heubner's artery

270. The most common infections acquired in utero are aoxoplasmosis, rubella, cytomegalovirus, and herpes simplex which is referred to as

(A) torch
(B) histogenesis
(C) cytogenesis
(D) organogenesis

271. Periventricular leukomalacia (PVL) is a result of infarction in the arterial boundary zones also known as

(A) cervical circulation
(B) watershed circulation regions

(C) ventriculofugal artery region
(D) ventriculopetal parenchymal artery region

272. There are four grades of intracranial hemorrhage. What grade of hemorrhage is demonstrated on the coronal and sagittal sonograms in Figs. 14–59 A and B?

(A) grade IV
(B) grade I
(C) grade III
(D) grade II

273. Which statement best explains the extent of the intracranial hemorrhage shown in Figs. 14–59 A and B?

(A) An intraparenchymal hemorrhage only is present.
(B) Parenchymal and germinal matrix hemorrhages are present.
(C) Germinal matrix, and intraventricular hemorrhages are present.
(D) Only intraventricular hemorrhage is present.

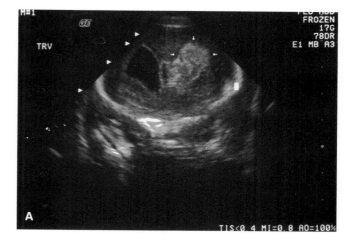

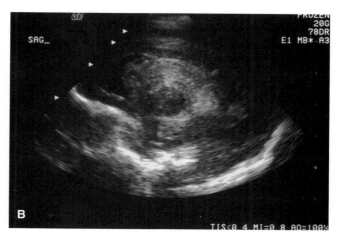

Figure 14–59. (A) Coronal sonogram. **(B)** Sagittal sonogram.

274. The sonogram shown in Fig. 14–60 was taken from a premature neonate. The sonographic findings demonstrate a

(A) lipoma
(B) bilateral germinal matrix hemorrhage
(C) unilateral germinal matrix hemorrhage
(D) none of the above

275. The abnormal sonographic findings shown in Fig. 14–61 show

(A) a Dandy–Walker cyst
(B) dilatation of the fourth ventricle because of obstruction at the foramen of Magendie
(C) atresia of the foramen of Magendie
(D) none of the above

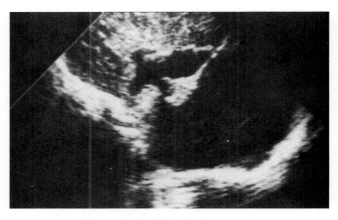

Figure 14–61. Midsagittal sonogram.

276. The arrows in Fig. 14–62 points to

(A) choroidal fissure
(B) sylvian fissure
(C) fissure of Rolando
(D) none of the above

277. The arrow in Fig. 14–63 points to

(A) cisternal magna
(B) vein of Galen
(C) vermi of the cerebellum
(D) none of the above

278. The sonograms shown in Fig. 14–64 A and B were taken from a 4-week-old premature neonate. The abnormal findings include

(A) arachnoid cyst
(B) enlarged ventricles and an area of porencephaly in the posterior horn of the right lateral ventricle
(C) enlarged ventricles with an area of porencephaly at the region of the body of the left lateral ventricle
(D) isolated porencephalic cyst

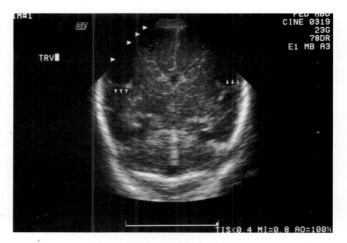

Figure 14–62. Coronal sonogram.

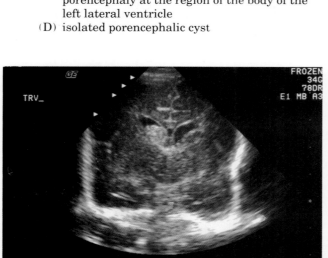

Figure 14–60. Coronal sonogram.

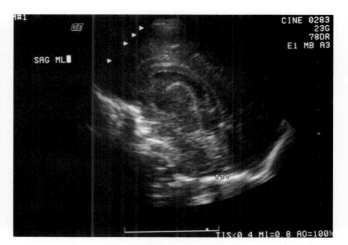

Figure 14–63. Sagittal sonogram.

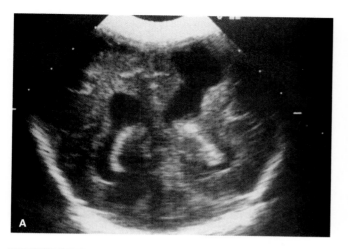

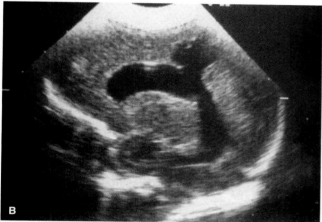

Figure 14–64. (A) Coronal sonogram. **(B)** Parasagittal sonogram.

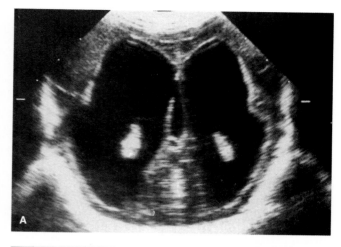

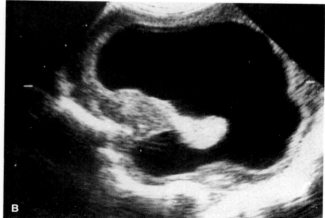

Figure 14–65. (A) Coronal sonogram. **(B)** Parasagittal sonogram.

279. The abnormal findings in Fig. 14–64 A,B are the result of

   (A) isolated germinal matrix hemorrhage
   (B) resolving intraparenchymal and intraventricular hemorrhages
   (C) subarachnoid hemorrhage
   (D) none of the above

280. The sonograms shown in Fig. 14–65 A,B were taken from a 1-month-old premature infant. The abnormal findings are

   (A) lobar holoprosencephaly
   (B) alobar holoprosencephaly
   (C) hydrocephalus
   (D) Dandy–Walker cyst

281. The bilateral echogenic structures seen in the sonolucent cavities in the coronal view in Fig. 14–65 A,B are

   (A) clots
   (B) choroid plexus
   (C) ethmoid and sphenoid bones
   (D) bilateral lipomas

282. The sonogram show in Fig. 14–66 is a midsagittal view of the head of a 1-month-old infant. Which statement best describes the abnormal findings?

   (A) an enlarged cavum septum pellucidum, enlarged third and fourth ventricles, a dilated foramen of Monro, dilated aqueduct of Sylvius
   (B) an enlarged lateral ventricle, an enlarged third ventricle, an enlarged fourth ventricle, a dilated foramen of Monro, and a dilated aqueduct of Sylvius
   (C) all abnormalities in (A) plus a posterior fossa cyst
   (D) a dilated cavum septum pellucidum only

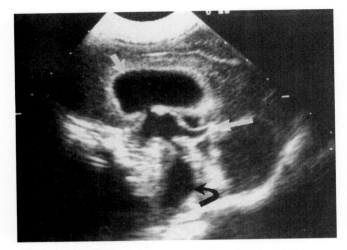

Figure 14–66. Midsagittal sonogram.

283. Identify the structure the long straight arrow points to in Fig. 14–66.

(A) foramen of Monro
(B) supraoptic recess
(C) infundibular recess
(D) pineal recess

284. Identify the enlarged structure the curved black arrow points to in Fig. 14–66.

(A) third ventricle
(B) fourth ventricle
(C) cerebrum
(D) quadrigeminal cistern

285. Identify the structure the short arrow points to in Fig. 14–66.

(A) one of the lateral ventricles
(B) cavum septi pellucidi
(C) cisterna magna
(D) a cyst in the interhemispheric fissure

286. The two sonolucent areas the arrows point to in Fig. 14–67 are

(A) bilateral porencephalic cyst in the temporal lobes
(B) forencephalic cyst in the frontal lobe
(C) temporal horns of the lateral ventricles
(D) frontal horns of the lateral ventricles

287. The sonographic findings in Fig. 14–68 A and B suggest

(A) subependymal hemorrhage
(B) resolving intraventricular hemorrhage and periventricular leukomalacia
(C) enlarged lateral ventricles
(D) parenchymal hemorrhage with enlarged ventricles

288. Fig. 14–69 is a midsagittal sonogram of the head of a 2-month-old premature infant. The slightly echogenic linear structure the arrow points to in the sonolucent cavity is

(A) septal vein
(B) anterior cerebral artery

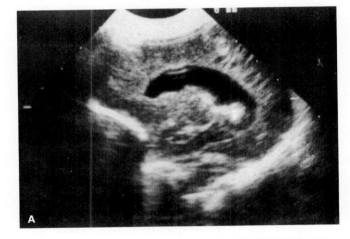

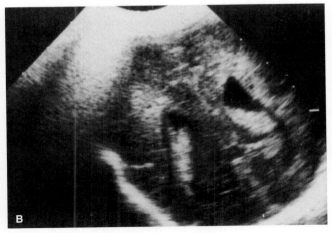

Figure 14–68. (A) Parasagittal sonogram. **(B)** Coronal sonogram.

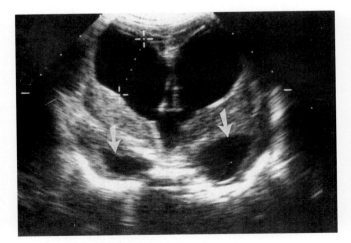

Figure 14–67. Coronal sonogram.

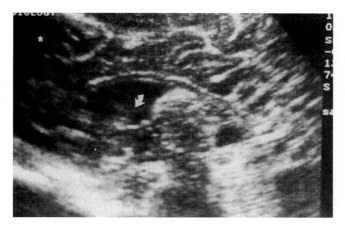

Figure 14–69. Midsagittal sonogram.

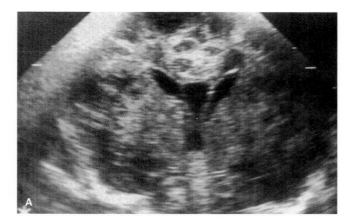

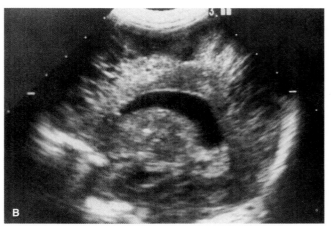

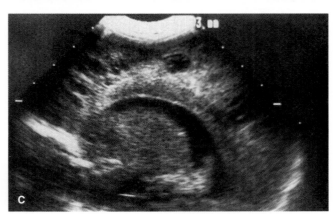

(C) corpus callosum
(D) pericallosal artery

289. Fig. 14–70 is a sagittal sonogram taken from a 2-week-premature neonate born at 31 weeks gestational age. The structure the arrow points to is

(A) clot in the third ventricle
(B) massa intermedia
(C) interthalamic adhesion
(D) pericallosal artery

290. The sonograms in Fig. 14–71 were taken from a 3-week-old neonate born at 31 weeks gestational age. Which statement is not true of the abnormal findings?

(A) encephalomalacia
(B) diffuse hemorrhagic infarction
(C) periventricular leukomalacia
(D) enlarged ventricles

Figure 14–71. (A) Coronal sonogram. **(B)** Parasagittal sonogram. **(C)** Parasagittal sonogram.

291. Fig. 14–72 is a magnified coronal sonogram from a full-term neonate with a history of persistent pulmonary hypertension. The incidental finding is

(A) arachnoid cysts
(B) multiple irregular-shaped cysts in the glomus part of the choroid plexus
(C) intraventricular hemorrhage
(D) porencephalic cysts

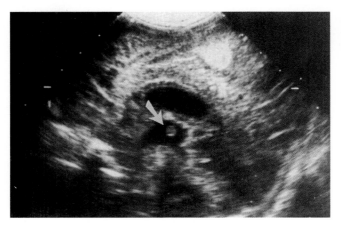

Figure 14–70. Sagittal sonogram.

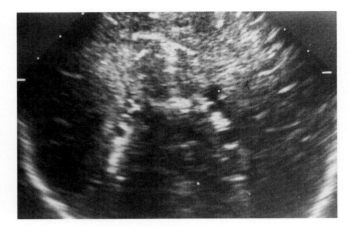

Figure 14–72. Coronal sonogram.

292. The bilateral sagittal cranial sonograms in Fig. 14–73 demonstrate

(A) porencephalic cysts that communicate with the ventricles
(B) periventricular leukomalacia

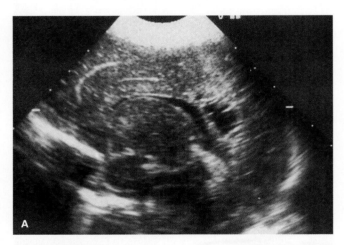

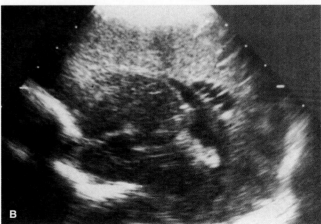

Figure 14–73. (A) Right parasagittal sonogram. **(B)** Left parasagittal sonogram.

(C) intraventricular hemorrhage
(D) B and C

293. At what level of the lateral ventricle is the coronal sonogram in Fig. 14–74 taken?

(A) occipital horns
(B) body
(C) frontal horns
(D) trigone region

294. Fig. 14–75 A–C were taken from a 2-day-old full-term neonate with abnormal chromosomes, kidneys, and upper and lower extremities. The abnormal intracranial findings include

(A) cysts within the lateral ventricles
(B) septated lateral ventricles
(C) bilateral germinal matrix cysts
(D) bilateral porencephalic cysts in the frontal lobe of the cerebrum.

295. The echogenic structure the straight arrow points to in Fig. 14–76 is the

(A) interhemispheric fissure
(B) sylvian fissure
(C) corpus callosum
(D) cingulate sulcus

296. The bilateral sonolucent structures the open arrows point to in Fig. 14–77 represent

(A) trigone region of the lateral ventricles
(B) bodies of the lateral ventricle
(C) frontal horns of the lateral ventricle
(D) porencephalic cysts

297. The straight black arrow in Fig. 14–78 points to

(A) calcarine sulcus
(B) circular sulcus
(C) tentorium
(D) cingulate sulcus

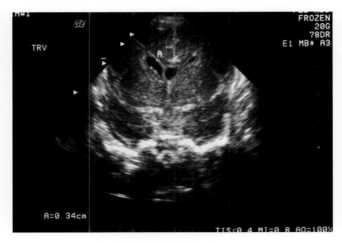

Figure 14–74. Coronal sonogram.

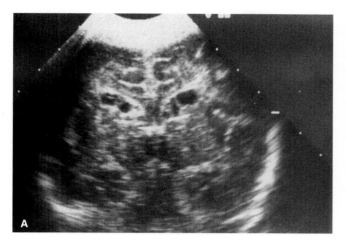

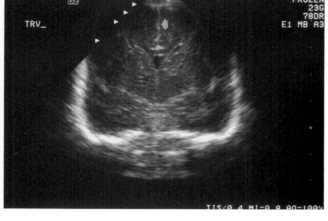

Figure 14–76. Coronal sonogram.

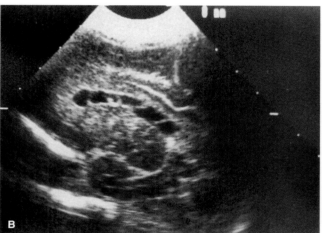

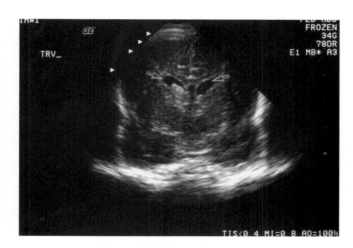

Figure 14–77. Coronal sonogram.

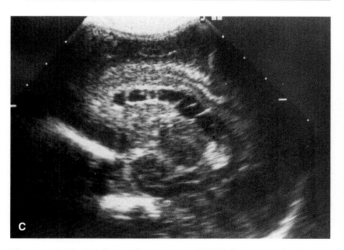

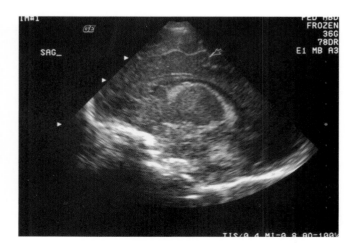

Figure 14–75. (A) Coronal sonogram. **(B)** Right parasagittal sonogram. **(C)** Left parasagittal sonogram.

Figure 14–78. Sagittal sonogram.

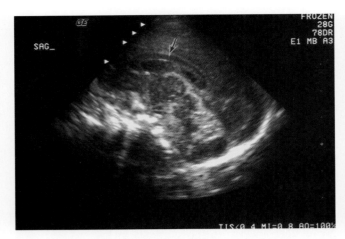

Figure 14–79. Midsagittal sonogram.

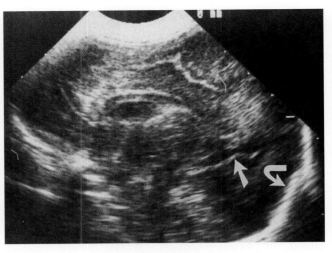

Figure 14–80. Sagittal sonogram.

298. The curved arrow in Fig. 14–79 points to

(A) corpus callosum
(B) interhemispheric fissure
(C) choroid plexus
(D) lateral ventricle

299. The straight arrow in Fig. 14–80 points to an echogenic line called the

(A) callosal sulcus
(B) central sulcus

(C) parieto-occipital sulcus
(D) cerebellar vermis

300. The highly echogenic structure that the curved arrow points to in Fig. 14–80 is the

(A) frontal bone
(B) temporal bone
(C) occipital lobe of the cerebrum
(D) occipital bone

Answers and Explanations

At the end of each explained answer there is a number combination in parentheses. The first number identifies the reference source; the second number or set of numbers indicates the page or pages on which the relevant information can be found.

Figure 14–45

1. **(M)** anterior fontanelle

2. **(G)** coronal suture

3. **(C)** parietal bone

4. **(N)** squamous suture

5. **(O)** lambdoidal suture

6. **(F)** occipital bone

7. **(A)** mastoidal fontanelle

8. **(K)** temporal bone

9. **(P)** zygomatic process

10. **(I)** zygomatic bone

11. **(L)** mandible

12. **(D)** maxilla

13. **(J)** nasal bone

14. **(B)** sphenoid fontanelle

15. **(H)** frontal bone

16. **(E)** orbit

Figure 14–46

17. **(B)** frontal bone

18. **(D)** anterior fontanelle

19. **(E)** parietal bone

20. **(C)** sagittal suture

21. **(F)** posterior fontanelle

22. **(A)** occipital bone

Figure 14–47

23. **(C)** pia mater

24. **(A)** dura mater

25. **(D)** superior sagittal sinus

26. **(H)** scalp

27. **(E)** arachnoid villus

28. **(I)** cranium

29. **(B)** subdural space

30. **(G)** subarachnoid space

31. **(F)** falx cerebri

Figure 14–48

32. **(C)** fissure of Rolando

33. **(E)** parietal lobe

34. **(D)** occipital lobe

35. **(F)** temporal lobe

36. **(B)** sylvian fissure

37. **(A)** frontal lobe

Figure 14–49

38. **(J)** interthalamic adhesion (massa intermedia)

39. **(B)** thalamus

40. **(D)** pineal body

41. **(C)** cerebellum

42. **(K)** fourth ventricle

43. **(F)** spinal cord

44. **(I)** medulla oblongata

45. **(G)** cerebral peduncle

46. **(E)** pons

47. **(M)** temporal lobe

48. **(L)** third ventricle

49. **(H)** septum pellucidum

50. **(A)** corpus callosum

Figure 14–50

51. **(G)** fourth ventricle

52. **(E)** lateral recess

53. **(I)** posterior horn

54. **(F)** cerebral aqueduct

55. **(A)** third ventricle

56. **(D)** foramen of Monro

57. **(B)** arterial horn

58. **(C)** inferior horn

59. **(H)** atrium

Figure 14–51

60. **(L)** foramen of Magendie

61. **(N)** foramina of Luschka

62. **(I)** inferior horn

63. **(M)** cerebral aqueduct

64. **(E)** infundibular recess

65. **(O)** interthalamic adhesion

66. **(G)** preoptic recess

67. **(H)** anterior horn

68. **(C)** foramen of Monro

69. **(K)** suprapineal recess

70. **(B)** body of lateral ventricle

71. **(A)** pineal recess

72. **(F)** third ventricle

73. **(J)** atrium

74. **(B)** posterior horn

Figure 14–52

75. **(D)** corpus callosum

76. **(C)** tela choroidea

77. **(F)** glomus of the choroid plexus

78. **(E)** choroid plexus of the fourth ventricle

79. **(B)** choroid plexus of the third ventricle

80. **(A)** caudate nucleus

Figure 14–53

81. **(C)** frontal and temporal horns

82. **(A)** foramina of Monro and third ventricle

83. **(D)** choroid plexus trigone

84. **(B)** posterior horn of lateral ventricle

Figure 14–54

85. **(C)** pons

86. **(B)** cerebral peduncle

87. **(J)** thalamus

88. **(E)** caudate nucleus

89. **(I)** column of fornix

90. **(A)** lateral ventricle

91. **(H)** sulcus

92. **(D)** corpus callosum

93. **(G)** sylvian fissure

94. **(F)** hippocampus

Figure 14–55

95. **(C)** cerebellum

96. **(A)** cerebral aqueduct

97. **(B)** cerebellum peduncle

98. **(F)** cerebral peduncle

99. **(D)** hypothalamus

100. **(E)** gyrus and sulcus

Figure 14–56

101. **(J)** anterior spinal artery

102. **(G)** vertebral artery

103. **(K)** posterior inferior cerebellar artery

104. **(F)** anterior inferior cerebellar artery

105. **(L)** superior cerebellar artery

106. **(B)** posterior cerebral artery

107. **(C)** middle cerebral artery

108. **(E)** anterior cerebral artery

109. **(H)** anterior communicating artery

110. **(D)** internal carotid artery

111. **(I)** posterior communicating artery

112. **(A)** basilar artery

Figure 14–57

113. **(C)** vertebral artery

114. **(H)** medulla oblongata

115. **(G)** cerebellum

116. **(B)** posterior cerebral artery

117. **(F)** middle cerebral artery

118. **(E)** anterior cerebral artery

119. **(A)** internal carotid artery

120. **(D)** basilar artery

Figure 14–58

121. **(B)** middle cerebral artery

122. **(D)** anterior cerebral artery

123. **(C)** callosomarginal artery

124. **(A)** pericallosal artery

125. **(A)** Although all of the fontanelles and sutures can be used as an acoustic window to bypass the bone interface, the anterior and posterior fontanelles are used most frequently because of easy access to the paraventricular structures.   *(1:24–25)*

126. **(A)** periventricular calcifications. Infection of the fetal brain includes toxoplasmosis, rubella, cytomegalovirus, and herpes simplex. (TORCH). These infections are acquired in utero; however, the diagnoses are usually made in the neonatal-infant period. All TORCH symptoms are characterized by periventricular calcifications.   *(27:197)*

127. **(B)** The anterolateral fontanelle. The sphenoidal fontanelles are positioned anatomically anterior and lateral.   *(5:345)*

128. **(D)** 18 months. The anterior fontanelle is the largest fontanelle and is the last to close.   *(5:346)*

129. **(D)** Posterolateral fontanelle. This is because the mastoidal fontanelles are positioned anatomically posterior and lateral.   *(5:345)*

130. **(A)** They both diverge laterally as they project from the body of the lateral ventricles. The temporal horns (inferior horns) of the lateral ventricles are curved downward and extend laterally from the body of the ventricles. The tip of their inferior end extends around the posterior aspect of the thalamus. The occipital horns (posterior horns) of the lateral ventricles extend laterally from the body of the lateral ventricle and into the occipital lobe.   *(2:183; 8:29–31)*

131. **(D)** The lateral ventricular width/hemispheric width ratio is obtained by measuring the distance from the middle of the falx cerebri (midline echo) to the lateral wall of the lateral ventricle and dividing this by the distance from the falx cerebri (midline echo) to the inner table of the skull. Both measurements are taken from the same image.   *(2:183; 27:64)*

132. **(D)** External auditory meatus. The transducer is placed on the parietal bone above the ear. The tube-like passage in the ear is called the external auditory meatus.   *(1:29)*

133. **(D)** It is a fetal structure. The germinal matrix cannot be depicted as a distinct structure by computed tomography or sonography. The germinal matrix is a structure of the fetus that begins early in gestation and regresses as pregnancy advances. By 32 weeks to term, it may be completely absent. The location of the germinal matrix is above the caudate nucleus in the subependymal region of the lateral ventricle.   *(2:183; 27:44)*

134. **(A)** Above the caudate nucleus in the subependymal layer of the lateral ventricle. The germinal matrix forms the entire subependymal layer of the lateral ventricles in early gestation. After 24 weeks of gestation, the germinal matrix is present only over the head of the caudate nucleus.   *(2:183; 27:45)*

135. (D) Echo-free space inferior to the cerebellum. The cisterna magna is anechoic (echo free) and normally can be relatively large. It is located inferior to the cerebellum and should not be confused with a cyst. *(2:183; 27:186)*

136. (D) Middle cerebral arteries. On real-time sonography, a dense echo representing the sylvian fissure can be seen near the lateral aspect of the brain on most coronal scans. The identification of symmetric pulsation in this fissure is the result of the middle cerebral arteries. *(1:95; 27:63)*

137. (A) The fissure and sulci both appear echogenic. The normal premature brain has numerous echogenic sulci. The echogenicity is caused by normal vascular structures. The fissures and cisterns also are echogenic. *(2:187; 27:121)*

138. (D) The cavum septum pellucidum is located between the frontal horns of the lateral ventricles. *(2:187; 27:42)*

139. (C) Thalami

140. (C) An intraparenchymal hemorrhage. Most intraparenchymal hemorrhages appear as increased echogenicity in the brain parenchyma and occur as a result of a subependymal hemorrhage. *(2:190; 27:126)*

141. (A) An intraventricular hemorrhage. These hemorrhages present as high-density echoes in the ventricles. They may present with clots or high-density cerebrospinal fluid blood levels. These findings are more evident with change of head position. *(27:123)*

142. (D) Porencephaly. About 2–3 months after the hemorrhage, necrosis and phagocytosis are completed and an anechoic area termed porencephaly can be depicted (fourth stage). *(2:190; 27:128)*

143. (D) Pleural effusion is not among the many possible causes of intracranial hemorrhage. There are many possible causes of intracranial hemorrhage: maternal ingestion of aspirin, infantile pneumothorax, hypoxia, extrauterine stress, hyaline membrane disease, acidosis, ischemia, hypertension, and hypercarbia. *(1:196; 7:100–107)*

144. (A) A child during the first 28 days after birth. *(9:2)*

145. (A) White matter surrounding the ventricles. This is the most common site for periventricular leukomalacia in premature infants. *(9:85–86)*

146. (D) Tuberous sclerosis. Developmental brain defects in organogenesis are classified in different groups such as neural tube closure, diverticulation, neuronal proliferation and neuronal migration, organization,

and myelination. Tuberous sclerosis is a disorder of histogenesis. *(27:91–93)*

147. (D) Intracranial hemorrhage. The term intraventricular hemorrhage was formerly used to refer to all types of cranial hemorrhage and caused some confusion in the terminology. The accepted term now is intracranial hemorrhage, which refers to any hemorrhage within the cranial vault. *(8:209; 27:117)*

148. (C) Intraventricular hemorrhages. This type of hemorrhage is presented as echogenic material within the ventricles. An echogenic clot or elevated levels of blood in the cerebrospinal fluid may be present with a gravitational effect. *(27:123)*

149. (B) Subependymal hemorrhage. This type of hemorrhage originates in the germinal matrix and for this reason is also called a germinal matrix hemorrhage. These hemorrhages present as highly echogenic foci in the region of the caudate nucleus. However, the most common site is the telea choroidea. *(27:121)*

150. (A) Intraparenchymal hemorrhage. This type of hemorrhage is present at first as a homogeneous, highly echogenic focus. However, as hemorrhagic resolution proceeds through its stages, a variety of heterogeneous sonographic appearances can be identified. *(27:128)*

151. (D) Choroid plexus hemorrhage. This type of hemorrhage can be difficult to diagnose because both the normal choroid plexus and a choroid plexus hemorrhage appear echogenic. However, a choroid plexus that is heterogeneous in texture, irregular in contour, and bulbous in the anterior region, with echogenic foci extending from the choroid plexus into the ventricle would strongly suggest hemorrhage. *(8:209; 27:126)*

152. (D) Subependymal germinal matrix hemorrhage is seen primarily in premature infants and is the most common in that age group. *(27:121)*

153. (B) 90°. Coronal scans should be performed at 90° from the orbitomeatal line (canthomeatal line), and the transducer should be angled to sweep from anterior to posterior. *(1:49)*

154. (C) The fontanelles are used as an acoustic window by allowing an opening through which ultrasound can travel with little or no obstruction to bypass bony interfaces. *(10:15)*

155. (C) The organisms associated most often with congenital infections of the nervous system are toxoplasmosis, rubella, cytomegalovirus, and herpes simplex (TORCH). Syphilis is associated but rare. Gonococcal infections are not among the organisms most often associated with congenital infections of the nervous system.   *(1:186; 27:197)*

156. **(C)** The sonographic findings include: periventricular calcifications, ventricular enlargement, and a small head (microcephalus).   *(1:185; 27:197–199)*

157. **(D)** An isolated subependymal hemorrhage. The grades are from Grade I to Grade IV. Grade I is an isolated subependymal germinal matrix hemorrhage.   *(8:210; 27:131)*

158. **(A)** Cerebral aqueduct. The foramen or passage between the third and fourth ventricles also is known as the aqueduct of Sylvius.   *(8:217)*

159. **(C)** Hydranencephaly is a congenital deformity characterized by severe loss of cerebral tissue. The falx, midbrain, basal ganglia, and cerebellum are intact.   *(8:191)*

160. **(B)** dysgenesis of the vermis of the cerebellum. Dandy-Walker cysts are associated with dysgenesis (defective development) of the cerebellar vermis.   *(8:191; 27:103)*

161. **(B)** A ventriculoperitoneal (V-P) shunt. The purpose of a V-P shunt is to decrease the intraventricular pressure caused by hydrocephalus by shunting the fluid from the ventricle into the peritoneal cavity.   *(8:242, 246)*

162. **(E)** A decrease in the size of the ventricles is not a sign of hydrocephalus. Hydrocephalus is dilatation of the ventricles caused by obstruction of cerebrospinal fluid. X-ray signs include skull bones halo sign and clinical signs include anterior fontanelle sinking, bulging of the frontal bone of the skull and rapid head growth.   *(9:221–312)*

163. **(A)** Aqueductal stenosis. This condition also can be associated with other abnormalities.   *(8:224)*

164. **(A)** Cephalohematomas. These are also called subperiosteal hematomas and refer to hemorrhages beneath the periosteum.   *(1:194)*

165. **(A)** 40 weeks. Between the septum pellucidum is a fluid-filled cavity called the cavum septum pellucidum. The dorsal extension of the cavum septum pellucidum is called the cavum vergae. The fornix is the anatomic landmark dividing this single structure into two names. The cavum vergae is the first to start closure at about 24 weeks of gestation. The cavum septum pellucidum begins to close at term (40 weeks).   *(8:218; 27:42)*

166. **(D)** Dandy-Walker syndrome is characterized by continuity of the fourth ventricle with a posterior fossa cyst and hydrocephalus.   *(8:191)*

167. **(A)** Severe hydrocephalus. The differential diagnoses for hydranencephaly are severe hydrocephalus, alobar holoprosencephaly, and massive subdural effusions.   *(8:191; 27:86)*

168. **(B)** Region of the sylvian fissure and in the circle of Willis. The middle cerebral artery is the continuation of the internal carotid artery.   *(7:87; 27:63)*

169. **(D)** Intraparenchymal hemorrhage. Extension of blood into the brain parenchyma is one of the most severe forms of hemorrhage.   *(7:101)*

170. **(A)** The prosencephalon. During embryologic development, the brain vesicles form the forebrain or prosencephalon, the midbrain or mesencephalon, and the hindbrain or rhombencephalon.   *(13:370)*

171. **(E)** External carotid arteries. The circle of Willis is formed by eight arteries: two posterior cerebral arteries (vertebral arteries), two anterior cerebral arteries, two internal carotid arteries, and one posterior and one anterior communicating arteries.   *(15:12)*

172. **(B)** The cerebrospinal fluid pathways within the brain are blocked. Hydrocephalus can be acquired or congenital. It is divided into noncommunicating or obstructive (blockage of cerebrospinal fluid within the brain) and communicating or nonobstructive (blockage of cerebrospinal fluid within the ventricular system).   *(16:1539)*

173. **(A)** A congenital abnormality of the brain with elongation of the pons and fourth ventricle and downward displacement of the medulla into the cervical canal. The elongation of the pons is characterized by displacement of the fourth ventricle.   *(27:95)*

174. **(D)** Two internal carotid and two vertebral arteries. These are the two main pairs of arteries that supply the brain with blood.   *(15:8)*

175. **(B)** Basilar artery. The pons is the anatomic level at which the vertebral artery changes its name to the basilar artery.   *(15:8)*

176. **(D)** Movement of extracellular fluid from blood. Only about 40% of cerebrospinal fluid is elaborated by the choroid plexus. The other 60% is produced by the movement of extracellular fluid from blood through the brain and ventricles.   *(27:155)*

177. **(C)** Normal sized ventricles with no debris within them. The sonographic findings of ventriculitis include echogenic ventricular walls, septated ventricles, debris within the ventricles, and ventricular dilatation.   *(20:83; 84, 91)*

178. (C) Eight. The skull is made up of one frontal bone, two parietal bones, two temporal bones, and one occipital, sphenoid, and ethmoid each.   *(39:190)*

179. (A) Subarachnoid hematoma. Below the arachnoid is the subarachnoid space, which is located between the arachnoid and pia mater.   *(18:31)*

180. (C) 532–576 mL/day. In an adult, the amount of cerebrospinal fluid produced daily is between 600 to 700 mL. In the child, it is less.   *(18:9; 27:156)*

181. (C) An epidural hematoma. The accumulation of blood between the dura mater and the inner table of the skull.   *(1:194)*

182. (C) The inferior horn (cornu).   *(18:29)*

183. (A) Temporal horn (cornu).   *(18:29)*

184. (B) Cerebral hemispheres. They are paired brain matter separated from the midline by the falx cerebri.   *(20:294)*

185. (B) Posterior to the foramen of Monro and superior to the third ventricle.   *(27:192)*

186. (B) Intracranial infections can be bacterial or viral.

Bacterial	Viral
Diplococcus pneumoniae	toxoplasmosis
Haemophilus influenzae	mumps
Bacterial meningitis	cytomegalovirus
Herpes simplex	*(1:184)*

187. (B) The central fissure is also called central sulcus or fissure of Rolando.   *(20:295)*

188. (C) The etiology of a porencephalic cyst is a subependymal hemorrhage that extends into the brain parenchyma, an infection, an infarction, or trauma.   *(1:153; 27:186)*

189. (B) Subdural hematoma. The gyri and sulci of the brain are more prominent with a subdural hematoma and are usually obscured in intracranial infections, infarctions, and intracranial hemorrhages.   *(27:209)*

190. (B) 24–32 weeks. The germinal matrix subsequently regresses in size and is absent at birth.   *(1:196)*

191. (D) cyctopia. This is a developmental anomaly, not a tumor.   *(1:226)*

192. (A) Ischemic lesions of the neonatal brain characterized by necrosis of periventricular white matter.   *(21:760)*

193. (B) Leukomalacia. The most common infections acquired in utero are toxoplasmosis, rubella, cytomegalovirus, and herpes simplex (TORCH).   *(27:197)*

194. (A) Hypoxia and ischemic injuries account for the greatest number of fetal deaths.   *(21:752)*

195. (A) Decrease in the size of the sylvian fissure as the neonatal brain matures. Lissencephaly is characterized sonographically by large sylvian fissures and ventricles.   *(27:111)*

196. (C) Semi-Fowler's position. This position assists in drainage and prevents pressure on the site.   *(28:89)*

197. (B) Tentorium.   *(39:338)*

198. (B) Conus Medullaris. The spinal cord is the distal continuation of the central nervous system. It terminates as the conus medullaris at the end of the second lumbar vertebrae.   *(44:125)*

199. (B) Occipital horns. A change in shape without a change in size occurs first in the frontal horns. However, the occipital horns enlarge first, and the frontal horns enlarge last.   *(27:158)*

200. (A) Frontal horns anterior to the foramen of Monro. The reason for this position is to avoid obstruction of the shunt tip by the choroid plexus. No choroid plexus extends into the frontal horns or the occipital horns of the lateral ventricle.   *(27:166)*

201. (B) Enlarged septum pellucidum. In complete agenesis of the corpus callosum, there is no septum pellucidum or corpus callosum. In addition, the third ventricle undergoes upward displacement.   *(27:105)*

202. (A) Septum pellucidum. In septo-optic dysplasia, schizencephaly, and agenesis of the corpus callosum, the septum pellucidum is absent.   *(27:108)*

203. (B) Cause slowing of the heart.   *(46:5)*

204. (D) Periventricular leukomalacia is softening of the white matter surrounding the ventricles. *(58:G8-G54)*

205. (G) Tentorium cerebelli is a transverse division of dura mater forming a partition between the occipital lobe of the cerebral hemispheres and the cerebellum.   *(58:G8-G54)*

206. (I) Sulci are grooves on the surface of the brain separating the gyri.   *(58:G8-G54)*

207. (C) The choroid plexus comprises special cells located in the ventricles that secrete cerebrospinal fluid.   *(58:G8-G54)*

208. **(A)** Cisterna magna is an enclosed space located caudal to the cerebellum, between the cerebellum and the occipital bone, serving as a reservoir for cerebrospinal fluid. *(58:G8-G54)*

209. **(K)** The pia mater is the inner membrane covering the brain and spinal cord. *(58:G8-G54)*

210. **(F)** The corpus callosum is a group of nerve fibers above the third ventricle that connects the left and right sides of the brain. *(58:G8-G54)*

211. **(J)** Cavum septum pellucidum is a cavity filled with cerebrospinal fluid that lies between the anterior horns of the lateral ventricle. *(58:G8-G54)*

212. **(H)** Insula is a triangular area of cerebral cortex, lying deeply in the later cerebral fissure. *(58:G8–G54)*

213. **(B)** Gyri are folds on the surface of the brain. *(58:G8–G54)*

214. **(E)** Aqueduct stenosis is a congenital obstruction of the third and fourth ventricles resulting in ventricular dilation. *(58:G8–G54)*

215. **(H)** Interventricular foramen — foramen of Monro *(18:30)*

216. **(G)** Atrium — trigone *(8:216)*

217. **(F)** subependymal hemorrhage — germinal matrix hemorrhage *(1:198)*

218. **(E)** epiphysis cerebri — pineal gland *(58:G42)*

219. **(D)** posterior horn — occipital horn *(18:30)*

220. **(C)** frontal horn — anterior horn *(18:30)*

221. **(B)** inferior horn — temporal horn *(18:30)*

222. **(A)** interthalamic adhesion — massa intermedia *(18:38)*

223. **(D)** 5–10 MHz. The continuous-wave Doppler transducer can either be flat or be a pencil probe with an ultrasonic frequency of 5–10 MHz. *(52:180)*

224. **(A)** Middle cerebral artery. This artery can be evaluated best through the cranial vault because the newborn skull has a single pliable bony layer without the dipole. *(54:499)*

225. **(A)** Peak height. *(55:678)*

226. **(A)** The fact that infants with asphyxia have low pulsatility and high diastolic flow probably repre-

sents a decrease in resistance of the cerebrovascular system in response to the asphyxia. *(57:599)*

227. **(D)** The fact that infants with an intraventricular hemorrhage have high pulsatility indexes and extremely low forward diastolic flow may represent an increase in resistance in response to the hemorrhage. *(57:599)*

228. **(A)** Premature fusion of the cranial sutures. The prefix cranio relates to the cranium or skull. The suffix synostosis pertains to closure of the sutures. *(27:83)*

229. **(D)** Low temperature. Hypothermia (lowered body temperature) is defined as the reduction of body temperature below 35°C or 95°F. The clinically dramatic consequences of keeping a neonate in a cold environment, such as an air-conditioned ultrasound room could result in shivering and lowered body temperature. *(26:643, 716)*

230. **(C)** 2–3 years. The parietal bones are relatively thin when compared with other cranial bones; therefore, measurements can be obtained up to 2–3 years after birth. *(2:180)*

231. **(D)** Linear-array real-time transducer produces a rectangular image. This type of transducer can be used to image the infant's brain. However, in visualizing the neonatal brain, it is limited because of the small size of the fontanelle compared to the size of the transducer. In addition, the rectangular image produced by linear-array real-time fails on many occasions to visualize the inner walls of both sides of the calvarium simultaneously. *(2:180–199)*

232. **(A)** Axial. The sagittal and coronal CT views are useful but subject to artifacts; therefore, the axial plane is most compatible with sonography. *(1:24)*

233. **(A)** Telea choroidea. The point at which the choroid attaches to the floor of the lateral ventricles is located behind the foramen of Monro. *(2:187; 27:121)*

234. **(D)** Cavum vergae. The cava septic pellucide and vergae lie between the frontal horns and bodies of the two lateral ventricles. The fornix divides the cavum septi pellucidi anteriorly and the cavum septum posteriorly. *(2:187; 27:42)*

235. **(D)** 67%. The incidence of germinal matrix hemorrhage varies with age. At 28 weeks, approximately two-thirds of fetuses have such hemorrhages. *(27:135)*

236. **(A)** Same density. The term isodense denotes "same density" as soft tissue. This term is used in computed tomography (CT). A hemorrhage, for example is presented as high density on CT and can become isodense after 5–10 days.   *(22; 27:117–119)*

237. **(F)** All of the above. All of the given choices are associated with intracranial hemorrhage.   *(7:100–107)*

238. **(A)** From 29 days after birth to 1 year.   *(9:2)*

239. **(D)** This imaginary line is called the orbitomeatal line, a radiographic baseline, or the canthomeatal line. The Reid's baseline is an imaginary line drawn from the infraorbital rim to the external auditory meatus.   *(12:86)*

240. **(A)** 150° from the orbitomeatal line and perpendicular to the clivus. The transducer should be positioned over the posterior fontanelle and should sweep anterior at 5 mm intervals.   *(1:51)*

241. **(C)** An intracranial hemorrhage because no choroid extends into this area. There is no choroid plexus in either the frontal or occipital horn.   *(27:44, 166)*

242. **(E)** A single midline ventricle is characteristic of holoproencephaly not hydranencephaly. The brainstem and a portion of the occipital lobe remain in hydranencephaly. It is a congenital deformity characterized by a fluid-filled head with massive disruption of the cerebral hemispheres. The falx cerebri, cerebellum, and basal ganglia are usually intact.   *(8:191; 27:84)*

243. **(A)** Above the corpus callosum. The pericallosal artery is the terminal branch of the anterior cerebral artery. It courses over the superior margin of the corpus callosum.   *(8:218)*

244. **(D)** Two weeks. Hydrocephalus occurs first, followed by an increased head circumference approximately 14 days later.   *(7:25)*

245. **(A)** Every 3 days until 2 weeks of age.   *(7:117)*

246. **(B)** The choroid plexus nearly fills the entire volume of the lateral ventricles in the first trimester.   *(27:74)*

247. **(D)** A head that is largely filled with fluid and a severe loss of cerebral tissue. This congenital deformity of the head is characterized by complete or almost complete absence of the cerebral hemispheres.   *(1:152; 8:191)*

248. **(E)** Holoprosencephaly is a developmental abnormality characterized by a single large midline ventricle and diverticulation of the forebrain. A premature fusion of the cranial sutures wither complete or partial is characteristic of craniosymostosis.   *(8:191–192)*

249. **(D)** There are 12 pairs of cranial nerves and 31 pairs of spinal nerves.   *(15:4)*

250. **(A)** L2. The spinal cord is shorter than the vertebral column and ends at about the second lumbar vertebra.   *(15:4)*

251. **(D)** The cerebral aqueduct. This is also called the aqueduct of Sylvius.   *(27:40)*

252. **(D)** The supraoptic recess also called the preoptic recess and the infundibular recess, which lies below the supraoptic recess.   *(8:38)*

253. **(A)** Diverticulations are not associated with microcephaly. Microcephaly is associated with Meckel–Gruber's syndrome, chromosomal abnormalities, rubella, toxoplasmosis, craniosynostosis, and exposure to environmental teratogens such as radiation.   *(27:84, 85)*

254. **(D)** The two posterior recesses on the third ventricle are the pineal recess and the suprapineal recess.   *(8:217)*

255. **(A)** Interthalamic adhesion. The place of fusion on the medial surfaces of the thalami on both sides of the third ventricle is called a massa intermedia or an interthalamic adhesion.   *(18:38)*

256. **(D)** The cerebellum is not a partition of the dura mater.   *(39:338)*

257. **(B)** An intraparenchymal hemorrhage. Any hemorrhage into the brain parenchyma is called intraparenchymal hemorrhage.   *(8:209–215)*

258. **(A)** Intraventricular foramen.   *(18:29)*

259. **(A)** Spinal cord. The brain stem consists of the diencephalon, the midbrain, the pons, and the medulla oblongata.   *(39:357)*

260. **(E)** Meningomyocele is not associated with holoproencephaly facial anomalies. The facial anomalies that can be associated with holoprosencephaly are cleft palate(fissure), cleft lip (fissure), cyclopia (single orbital fossa), cerebrocephaly (characterized by a defective nose and closed eyes), and ethmocephaly (characterized by a defect of the ethmoid bone.   *(1:174)*

261. **(B)** The brain is invested by three membranes termed PAD for pia, arachnoid, and dura mater.   *(18:1–4)*

262. **(D)** The causes of an arachnoid cyst are arachnoid lesions, entrapment of subarachnoid or cisternal space, and abnormal leptomeningeal formation.   *(1:153)*

263. **(D)** Quadrigeminal cyst is not caused by a vein of Galen aneurysm. However, it may be a differential diagnosis because of its location and cystic components. Doppler evaluation should exclude a differential diagnosis. *(27:192)*

264. **(A)** Arachnoid cysts lie between the arachnoid membrane and the dura mater and not between the pia mater and the subarachnoid space. Acquired arachnoid cysts are found in cisterns adjacent to the third ventricle, sella, and posterior fossa. *(27:87, 188, 189)*

265. **(C)** They lie in the sagittal sinus and reabsorb cerebrospinal fluid as it circulates. *(27:155, 156)*

266. **(D)** A dilated septum pellucidum is not a characteristic of schinzencephaly. It is characterized by agenesis of the corpus callosum and septum pellucidum in addition to unusually shaped frontal horns of the lateral ventricles. *(27:112)*

267. **(A)** Ventriculitis. These neonates initially develop meningitis, edema, and cerebritis. Eight of 12 neonates with meningitis develop ventriculitis. Late complications include subdural effusion, enlarged ventricles, and ventricular septations. *(27:199)*

268. **(A)** Increased echogenicity at the external angle of the lateral ventricles. Ischemic lesions may occur at the watershed boundary zones of the periventricular white matter and the centrum semiovale as periventricular leukomalacia. *(50:61)*

269. **(D)** Heubner's artery. This is the main nutrient vessel of the subependymal germinal tissue, which is destined to give rise to much of the glial cell population of the hemisphere. *(49:183)*

270. **(A)** TORCH is the acronym for the most common infections acquired in utero: toxoplasmosis, rubella, cytomegalovirus, and herpes simplex. *(27:197)*

271. **(B)** In the premature infant, the watershed zones are located in the periventricular white matter adjacent to the external margins of the lateral ventricles. The zones lie approximately 3–10 mm from the ventricular wall. *(27:28)*

272. **(A)** Grade IV hemorrhage *(27:133)*

273. **(C)** Germinal matrix and intraventricular hemorrhages. *(27:133)*

274. **(C)** Unilateral germinal matrix hemorrhage. *(27:125)*

275. **(A)** Dandy–Walker Cyst. *(34:73)*

276. **(B)** Sylvian fissure. *(36:821)*

277. **(A)** Cistern magna. *(36:821)*

278. **(C)** Enlarged ventricles with an area of porencephaly at the region of the body of the left lateral ventricle. *(27:128, 129)*

279. **(B)** Resolving intraparenchymal and intraventricular hemorrhages. The irregularity noted in the choroid plexus region is a sign of intraventricular hemorrhage. *(27:133)*

280. **(C)** Hydrocephalus. The abnormal finding is a severe form of posthemorrhagic hydrocephalus. *(40:111, 117)*

281. **(B)** Choroid plexus. *(20:37)*

282. **(B)** The abnormal findings in Fig. 14–66 revealed an enlarged lateral ventricle, an enlarged third ventricle, and enlarged fourth ventricle, a dilated foramen of Monro, and a dilated aqueduct of Sylvius. *(27:164)*

283. **(D)** Pineal recess. The recess is dilated. The recesses of the third ventricle are as follows: supraoptic, infundibular, pineal, and suprapineal. *(27:40, 41, 44)*

284. **(B)** Fourth ventricle. *(27:164)*

285. **(A)** One of the lateral ventricles. The ventricle is enlarged. *(41:129)*

286. **(C)** Temporal horns of the lateral ventricles. Both are enlarged. *(41:128)*

287. **(D)** A resolving intraventricular hemorrhage and periventricular leukomalacia. The lateral ventricles are enlarged, and small cystic areas are seen in the periventricular regions. *(40:120)*

288. **(A)** Septal vein. *(38:623)*

289. **(D)** Massa intermedia. The massa intermedia or interthalamic adhesion, is visualized best in the presence of ventricular dilatation. *(27:41; 40:89)*

290. **(C)** Periventricular leukomalacia. This neonate may have had a generalized cerebral edema that led to multiple areas of infarction termed encephalomalacia or porencephaly. *(27:213)*

291. **(B)** Multiple irregular-shaped cysts in the glomus part of the choroid plexus. A study done with fetuses that had simple choroid plexus cysts revealed a normal karyotype and no significant related abnormalities. Babies were delivered with no neurological abnormalities at the time of the neonatal examination. However, a study involving complex choroid plexus cysts revealed trisomy 18 and 21. *(43:78, 81)*

292. **(D)** (B and C.) The abnormality demonstrated is bilateral periventricular leukomalacia and intraventricular hemorrhage. *(40:12)*

293. **(C)** Frontal horns.   *(27:17)*

294. **(B)** Septated lateral ventricles. In these sonograms, multiple partitions are seen extending to the lateral walls of the ventricles. This particular case is congenital; however, septated ventricles usually occur in ventriculitis.   *(40:83)*

295. **(A)** Interhemispheric fissure. The structure is shown in the coronal view.   *(40:34, 36)*

296. **(C)** Frontal horns of the lateral ventricle. The horns are slightly dilated with a unilateral subependymal hemorrhage.   *(40:39)*

297. **(D)** Cingulate sulcus.   *(40:45)*

298. **(A)** Corpus callosum.   *(40:45)*

299. **(C)** Parieto–occipital sulcus.   *(40:45)*

300. **(D)** Occipital bone.   *(41:14)*

REFERENCES

1. Babcock DS, Han BK. *Cranial Ultrasonography of Infants.* Baltimore: Williams & Wilkins; 1981.
2. Winsberg F, Cooperberg PL. Real-time ultrasonography: clinics in diagnostic ultrasound. In: Rumack CM, Johnson ML, eds. *Real-Time Ultrasound Evaluation of the Neonatal Brain,* Vol. 10. New York: Churchill Livingstone; 1982.
3. King DL, William McK. *Diagnostic Ultrasound.* St. Louis: CV Mosby; 1974.
4. Ora BA, Eddy L, Hatch G, Solida B, et al. The anterior fontanelle as an acoustic window to the neonatal ventricular system. *J Clin Ultrasound.* 1980;8:65–67.
5. Williams PL, Warwick R. *Gray's Anatomy,* 36th ed. Philadelphia: WB Saunders; 1980.
6. Bartrum RJ, Crow HC. *Real-time Ultrasound: A Manual for Physicians and Technical Personnel.* Philadelphia: WB Saunders; 1983.
7. Sanders RC, Thomas LS. *Ultrasound Annual.* New York: Raven Press; 1982.
8. Howard WR, William JZ, Babcock DS, et al. *Seminars in Ultrasound,* Vol. 3, No. 3. New York: Grune & Stratton; 1982.
9. Fenichel GM. *Neonatal Neurology,* Vol. 2. New York: Churchill Livingstone; 1980.
10. Haller JO, Shkolnik A, Slovis T. *Clinics in Diagnostic Ultrasound, Vol. 8: Ultrasound Pediatrics.* New York: Churchill Livingstone; 1981.
11. Helen LB, Sandra KM. *The Developing Person: A Life Span Approach.* San Francisco: Harper & Row; 1980.
12. Mallet M. *A Handbook of Anatomy and Physiology for Student X-ray Technicians,* 4th ed. Chicago: American Society of Radiologic Technologists; 1962.
13. Hagen-Ansert S. *Textbook of Diagnostic Ultrasound,* 2nd ed. St. Louis: CV Mosby; 1983.
14. William M. *The American Heritage Dictionary of the English Language.* New York: American Heritage, 1971.
15. Goldberg S. *Clinical Neuroanatomy Made Ridiculously Simple.* Miami: Med Master; 1979.
16. Robbins S, Cortran R. *Pathologic Basis of Disease,* 2 ed. Philadelphia: WB Saunders; 1979.
17. Sutton D. *A Textbook of Radiology and Imaging,* Vol. 2, 3rd ed. New York: Churchill Livingstone; 1980.
18. Carpenter M. *Core Text of Neuroanatomy,* 2nd ed. Baltimore: Williams & Wilkins; 1978.
19. Farmer T. *Pediatric Neurology,* 3rd ed. Philadelphia: Harper & Row; 1983.
20. Hole J Jr. *Human Anatomy and Physiology,* 3rd ed. Dubuque, IA: Wm C Brown; 1984.
21. Gordon BA. *Neonatology, Pathophysiology and Management of the Newborn.* Philadelphia: JB Lippincott; 1975.
22. *Dorland's Illustrated Medical Dictionary,* 26 ed. Philadelphia: WB Saunders; 1981.
23. Schaffer AJ, Avery ME. *Diseases of the Newborn,* 4th ed. Philadelphia: WB Saunders; 1977.
24. Waechter EH, Blake FG. *Nursing Care of Children,* 9th ed. Philadelphia: JB Lippincott; 1976.
25. Hellman LM, Pritchard J, Wynn RM. *Obstetrics,* 14th ed. New York: Appleton-Century-Crofts; 1971.
26. Danforth DN. *Textbook of Obstetrics and Gynecology,* 2nd ed. New York: Harper & Row; 1971.
27. Rumack CM, Johnson MI. *Perinatal and Infant Brain Imaging: Role of Ultrasound and Computed Tomography.* Chicago: Year Book; 1984.
28. Thompson DE. *Pediatric Nursing: An Introductory Text,* 4th ed. Philadelphia: WB Saunders; 1981.
29. Marlow RD. *Textbook of Pediatric Nursing,* 5th ed. Philadelphia: WB Saunders; 1977.
30. Hafen QB, Karren JK. *Prehospital Emergency Care and Crisis Intervention,* 2nd ed. Englewood, CO: Morton; 1983.
31. Fleischer AC, James AE. *Real-time Sonography: Textbook with Accompanying Videotape.* Norwalk, CT: Appleton-Century-Crofts; 1985.
32. Rubin J. Intraoperative ultrasonography of the spine. *Am J Radiol.* 1983; 146:173–176.
33. Grant E, Kerner M, Schellinger D. Evaluation of porencephalic cyst from intraparenchymal hemorrhage in neonates: Sonographic correlation. *Am J Radiol.* 1982;138:467.
34. Grant E, Schellinger D, Richardson J. Real-time ultrasonography of the posterior fossa. *J Ultrasound Med.* 1983;2:73.
35. Taylor KWJ. Atlas of ultrasonography. In: Mannes E, Sivo J, eds: *The Neonatal Head,* Vol. 1, 2nd ed. New York: Churchill Livingstone; 1984.
36. Shuman W, Rogers J, Mack L. Real-time sonographic sector scanning of the neonatal cranium: technique and normal anatomy. *AJNR.* 1981; 2:349–356.
37. Babcock D, Ball W Jr. Postasphyxial encephalopathy in full-term infants: Ultrasound diagnosis. *Am J Radiol.* 1983;148:417–423.

38. Goldstein R, Filly R, et al. Septal veins: A normal finding on neonatal sonography. *Am J Radiol.* 1986; 161:623–624.

39. Hole JW Jr. *Human Anatomy and Physiology,* 3rd ed. Dubuque, IA: Wm C Brown; 1984.

40. Naidich TP, Quencer RM, eds. *Clinical Neurosonography: Ultrasound of the Central Nervous System.* New York: Springer-Verlag; 1986.

41. Levene M, Williams J, Fawer CL. *Ultrasound of the Infant Brain.* London: Spastics International Medical Publications, and Philadelphia: JB Lippincott; 1985.

42. *Dorland's Illustrated Medical Dictionary,* 26th ed. Philadelphia: WB Saunders; 1985.

43. Hertzberg S, Kay HH, Bowie JD. Fetal choroid plexus lesions. *J Ultrasound Med.* 1989;8.

44. Kapit W, Elson LM. *The Anatomy Coloring Book.* New York: Harper & Row; 1977.

45. Sanders RC. *Clinical Sonography: A Practical Guide.* Boston: Little, Brown; 1984.

46. Martin J. *Ultrasound Technology Series. Cranial Sonography in Infants: Technicare Ultrasound.* New Brunswick, NJ: Johnson & Johnson; 1983.

47. Pilu P, Louis P, Roberto R, et al. The fetal subarachnoid cisterns: an ultrasound study with report of a case of congenital communicating hydrocephalus. *J Ultrasound Med.* 1986; 5.

48. Bowerman RA, Zwischenberger JB, Andrews AF, et al. Cranial sonography of the infant treated with extracorporeal membrane oxygenation. *Am J Radiol.* 1985;145.

49. Wigglesworth JS, Pape KE. An integrated model for haemorrhage and ischaemic lesions in the newborn brain: Early human development. *Early Human Dev.* 1978;2(2):179–199.

50. Manger MN, Feldman RC, Brown WJ, et al. Intracranial ultrasound diagnosis of neonatal periventricular leukomalacia. *J. Ultrasound Med.* 1984;3:59–63.

51. Christtenen RA, Pinckney LE, Higgins S, et al. Sonographic diagnosis of lipoma of the corpus callosum. *J Ultrasound Med.* 1987;6:449–451.

52. Perlman JM. Neonatal cerebral blood flow velocity measurement. *Clin Perinatol.* 1985; 12:179–193.

53. Bada HS, Fitch CW. Uses of transcutaneous Doppler ultrasound technique in newborn infants. *Perinatol Neonatol.* 1983;7:27–35.

54. Raju TNK, Zikos E. Regional cerebral blood velocity in infants: a real time transcranial and fontanellar pulsed Doppler study. *J Ultrasound Med.* 1987; 6:497–507.

55. Gray PH, et al. Continuous wave Doppler ultrasound in evaluation of cerebral blood flow in neonates. *Arch Dis Child.* 1983; 58:677–681.

56. Grant EG, White EM, Schellinger D, et al. Cranial Doppler sonography of the infant. *Radiology.* 1987; 163:177–185.

57. Miles RD, Menice JA, Bashiru M, et al. Relationships of five Doppler measures with flow in vitro model and clinical findings in newborn infants. *J Ultrasound Med.* 1987; 6(10):597–599.

58. Tortora GJ, Anagnostakos NP. *Principles of Anatomy and Physiology,* 6th ed. New York: Harper & Row; 1990.

59. Olds SB, London ML, Ladewig PA. *Maternal-Newborn Nursing: A Family-Centered Approach,* 3th ed. Menlo Park, CA: Addison-Wesley; 1988.

60. Williams PL, Warwick R, Dyson M, et al., eds. *Grays Anatomy,* 37th ed. New York: Churchill Livingstone; 1989.